Encyclopedia
of
BIOETHICS

Encyclopedia of BIOETHICS

WARREN T. REICH, *Editor in Chief*

GEORGETOWN UNIVERSITY

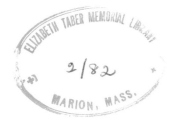

VOLUME 4

THE FREE PRESS
A Division of Macmillan Publishing Co., Inc.
NEW YORK

Collier Macmillan Publishers
LONDON

THE FREE PRESS
A Division of Macmillan Publishing Co., Inc.
866 Third Avenue, New York, N.Y. 10022

Collier Macmillan Canada, Ltd.

Library of Congress Catalog Card Number: 78–8821

Printed in the United States of America

printing number

3 4 5 6 7 8 9 10

Library of Congress Cataloging in Publication Data
Main entry under title:

Encyclopedia of bioethics.

Includes bibliographies and index.
1. Bioethics–Dictionaries. 2. Medical ethics–
Dictionaries. I. Reich, Warren T. [DNLM: 1. Bio-
ethics–Encyclopedias. QH302.5 E56]
QH332.E52   174′.2   78-8821
ISBN 0-02-926060-4

The *Encyclopedia of Bioethics* project was made possible by a grant
from the National Endowment for the Humanities. In funding the
project the Endowment matched gifts from non-federal sources
including The Joseph P. Kennedy, Jr. Foundation, the Raskob
Foundation, The Commonwealth Fund, The Loyola Foundation, Inc.,
and The David J. Greene Foundation, Inc. The views expressed in
this encyclopedia are not necessarily those of the Endowment or of
these foundations.

Contents

EDITORIAL ADVISORY BOARD   *vii*

PREFACE   *xi*

INTRODUCTION   *xv*

CONTRIBUTORS   *xxiii*

SPECIAL REVIEWERS   *xxxvii*

Encyclopedia of Bioethics

APPENDIX: Codes and Statements Related to Medical
Ethics   *1721*

ALPHABETICAL LIST OF ARTICLES   *1817*

SYSTEMATIC CLASSIFICATION OF ARTICLES   *1825*

ADDITIONAL RESOURCES IN BIOETHICS   *1839*

INDEX   *1845*

R

RACE DIFFERENCES IN INTELLIGENCE

See Genetic Aspects of Human Behavior, *articles on* race differences in intelligence *and* philosophical and ethical issues.

RACISM

I. RACISM AND MEDICINE   *James H. Jones*
II. RACISM AND MENTAL HEALTH
                        Aaron D. Gresson

I
RACISM AND MEDICINE

More than a century ago the eminent physician Dr. Oliver Wendell Holmes noted that "medicine, professedly founded on observation, is as sensitive to outside influence, political, religious, philosophical, imaginative, as is the barometer to the atmospheric density." In theory "it ought to go on its own straightforward inductive path," Dr. Holmes continued, but in practice there existed "a closer relation between the Medical Sciences and the conditions of Society and the general thought of the time, than would at first be expected" (Holmes, p. 177). Few examples of the interaction between society and medicine better illustrate the accuracy of this observation than the influence racial attitudes have exerted on the perception and response of white physicians to disease in Negroes in the history of medicine in the United States.

No less than other white Americans of the early nineteenth century, physicians were fascinated by the large number of ways in which black people appeared to be different. They were one of the first groups to study Negroes in a systematic manner, and, because they belonged to a profession that claimed to possess scientific knowledge about human beings, their views carried considerable weight. Physicians did not dissent as a group from white society's pervasive belief in the physical and mental inferiority of blacks as compared with whites. On the contrary, they did a great deal to bolster and elaborate racist attitudes. No difference between the races, real or imagined, went unnoticed, and topics such as the Negro's hair, facial features, posture and gait, odor, skin color, and cranium and brain size were discussed at great length.

There was a compelling reason for this preoccupation with establishing physical and mental distinctions between the races, one that transcended the disinterested pursuit of empirical facts. Most physicians who wrote about Negroes during the nineteenth century were Southerners who clung tenaciously to the existing social order; they justified slavery, and, after its abolition, insisted on second-class citizenship for blacks by arguing that blacks were incapable of assuming any higher station in life. Too many differences separated the races. And here "different" unquestionably meant "inferior." Thus, medical discourses on the peculiarities of Negroes offered, among other things, a pseudo-scientific rationale for keeping Negroes at the bottom of American society.

To support the view that black people were fundamentally different, vociferous advocates of Negro inferiority, such as Dr. Josiah Clark Nott of Mobile and Dr. Samuel A. Cartwright of New

Orleans, published numerous articles on diseases and physical properties that were allegedly peculiar to Negroes. Drs. Nott and Cartwright were merely the best known of a group of Southern physicians who helped inflame the controversy over slavery by writing about racial medicine. Among the diseases that were thought unique to Negroes were Cachexia Africana (dirt-eating) and Struma Africana (tuberculosis) (Haller, 1972, pp. 239–244). Influenced by such physicians, slave owners who wished to treat their bondsmen without benefit of professional help called upon Southern doctors to write medical manuals directed exclusively to the treatment of Negroes. Their request went unanswered. Instead, physicians continued to assert simply that blacks were medically inferior to whites without attempting to construct a plausible medical system based on racial differences. Their observations were perfect for polemics but useless for the care of sick Negroes.

Advocates of racial medicine argued that differences in natural immunity, degree of susceptibility, and relative severity of reactions to various diseases often separated the races. In many instances racial prejudice unquestionably influenced their views. Nowhere was this tendency more evident than when physicians debated the degree to which Negroes were susceptible to malaria and the relative virulence of the disease in blacks as compared with whites. In many instances Negroes did appear to be less susceptible to the disease and to have milder cases when they contracted it; there was no question of that, but the facility with which some physicians were willing to extrapolate from individual cases to an entire race suggests an attempt to explain a medical anomaly with a racial explanation that defended slavery. For, by arguing that blacks were relatively immune to malaria or suffered milder bouts with the disease, physicians in effect created a medical sanction for sending Negroes into the rice fields and canebrakes. In other words, they were helping to support the South's contention that the use of bondsmen to perform such unhealthy work was more humane than employing white laborers (Savitt, "Sickle Cell and Slavery," pp. 1–5).

For the most part, alleged differences between black and white patients did not produce separate remedies or treatments for the same disease. Bleeding, a standard treatment employed by physicians who practiced during the age of heroic medicine (other treatments included purging and vomiting), was routinely administered to blacks, despite the broadly held view that blacks could not tolerate the loss of blood as well as whites. There were, however, numerous instances in which physicians differentiated treatment on the basis of race.

The record of such cases tends to obscure the basic fact that for better or worse Negroes usually received the same treatment as their masters. Quite apart from the issue of humanitarian concern, the high cost of purchasing and maintaining slaves made the health of bondsmen a matter of solicitous concern to masters. If for no other reason than to protect their investments, it behooved masters to provide the best health care they could afford for their slaves. And because physicians declined to produce a comprehensive treatment manual devoted exclusively to Negroes, the only remaining course of action was to apply white medicine to black patients. For routine ailments masters treated their families and their slaves with the identical home remedies; when serious illnesses made it necessary to call in professional help, the same physicians treated whites and blacks. Indeed, a sizable portion of the income of many Southern physicians was derived from the care and treatment of Negro slaves (Postell, pp. 50–54, 66).

Physicians unquestionably saw the Civil War as a watershed in black health. Slavery, they argued, had provided an environmental hothouse in which the conditions necessary for the survival of an inferior and disease-prone race had been maximized through a system of total control. They argued that freedom would probably condemn the race to extinction, because the blacks lacked the knowledge and the self-control that were required for survival. Census data for the last three decades of the century appeared to support those fears. The Ninth Census (1870) showed that the black population had increased at a slower rate compared to the white population between 1860 and 1870, a disturbing development, as the opposite had usually prevailed during the antebellum period. While the Tenth Census (1880) reversed this trend and placed the percentage of black births ahead of whites, alarmists were quick to note that the apparent gains were reduced by a higher mortality rate among the blacks. Moreover, when the Eleventh Census (1890) again showed the birthrate among blacks to be lower than that of whites, predictions of the inevitable extinction of the Negro race abounded, notwithstanding the fact that many observers questioned the reliability of the censuses pertaining to Negroes. The specter of a vanishing race was given further credence when the nation's leading life insurance companies, led by Prudential, all but refused to write policies for Negroes (Haller, 1971, pp. 40–44).

Perhaps because of their Puritan heritage, Americans have always been intensely interested in (not to say preoccupied with) determining the degree of personal responsibility that individuals bear for the illnesses that beset them. The outcome of this determination has important consequences, for it defines how those who are well will regard those who are ill. People judged to have brought their illnesses upon themselves through personal faults can expect to receive less sympathy than people whose illnesses are thought to be totally gratuitous. Extending this principle from the individual to an entire race, white physicians of the late nineteenth and early twentieth centuries sought to explain the decline in black health in terms of self-destructive behavioral traits that were thought to be common in blacks. In addition to discussions of the Negro's weak constitution and inherent susceptibility to disease, physicians hammered away at the black man's distaste for honest labor, fondness for alcohol, proclivity to crime and sexual vices, disregard for personal hygiene, ignorance of the laws of good nutrition, and total indifference to his own health. A standard feature of the vast majority of medical articles on the health of Negroes was a sociomedical profile of a race whose members were rapidly becoming diseased, debilitated, and debauched and had only themselves to blame (McHatton, pp. 6–9).

By defining the problem in racial terms, many physicians absolved themselves of any responsibility for the Negro's deterioration. Few were willing to ponder the responsibility that might be assigned to a profession whose members worked strictly on a fee-for-service basis and whose services were often beyond the reach of the poor. Blaming the victim was much easier on the profession's collective ego and permitted physicians to project a certain self-righteousness in their pronouncements. A few physicians were downright mean and spoke of Negroes having earned their illnesses as just recompense for their wicked life-styles. And around the turn of the century, when race relations throughout the United States had reached their nadir, some physicians even suggested that disease held the ultimate solution to the race problem (Murrell, p. 307; McIntosh, p. 187).

But rank racial hatred among a relative handful of physicians was not nearly as important in determining the outlook for the health of black Americans at the turn of the century as the widespread sense of pessimism that existed among physicians of goodwill. Notions of constitutional inferiority, inherent susceptibility to disease, and behavioral traits deleterious to health formed a medical-sociological view of the problem that worked as much damage to Negro health as disease. Disease came to be seen as the rule rather than the exception in the race, a development that could not be reconciled with the tendency of Americans in general and physicians in particular to view disease as a form of social deviance. Physicians had come dangerously close to depicting the unhealthy Negro as the representative Negro, and as sickness replaced health as the normal condition of the race, the sense of horror and urgency with which society defines illness markedly diminished. The result was a powerful rationale for inactivity in the face of a health problem of epidemic proportions.

Health officials, in contrast to private physicians, looked at the same situation but reached a different conclusion. A large segment of the population was thought to be diseased and dying; urgent action was therefore required. It was fortunate that this realization on the part of health officials coincided with the rise of the great philanthropic foundations in the United States. The United States Public Health Service, assisted by state and local health officials, joined forces with the Rockefeller Foundation and resolved to apply the principles of the public health movement to the rural South. The programs they developed, such as the campaigns to eradicate hookworm and pellagra, were models of what could be accomplished to improve Negro health once support became available.

Because private medical care remained beyond the financial reach of many Negroes, state and local health officials were forced to provide low-cost or free treatment to those with communicable diseases. To counter cries of "state medicine," which these efforts raised from private physicians, public health officers argued that they could not protect the health of white people while black people were left untreated. Germs could not be segregated as easily as people (Allen, p. 194). And with each public health campaign that ensued, health officials demonstrated that the principles of scientific medicine worked equally well for both races. Certainly by the Second World War little doubt remained about what could be accomplished from a purely medical standpoint to improve the Negro's health if support and personnel were available.

By the 1920s and 1930s racial explanations of the health problems of blacks had clearly begun to disappear from the medical literature, a development which can be explained largely in terms of changes within the medical profession between World Wars I and II. Broad acceptance of the germ theory of disease put an end to racial explanations for most illnesses. Marginal medical schools were shut down. The closings not only eliminated centers of inferior training but vastly reduced the number of physicians who entered the profession each year. High admission standards in the remaining schools reduced the number further. And as a result of the introduction of similar curricula, the glaring disparities that marked the training and competence of earlier physicians were blunted, if not removed.

The introduction of state licensing boards also contributed to the creation of a homogeneous profession. Whereas the medical profession in the nineteenth century was so hopelessly divided into sects that physicians could not agree on the causes and cures for disease (let alone a common body of knowledge and training for admission into the profession), twentieth-century physicians quickly agreed that only those doctors who had been trained in the tradition of scientific medicine should practice medicine. State boards drove the quacks and the holdovers from sectarian medicine out of the profession, placing a virtual monopoly on health care in America in the hands of physicians with similar training and common ideas about the causes and cures of disease.

The physicians who emerged from this better-educated and more carefully self-regulated profession had reason to be confident. They commanded an esoteric body of knowledge that made it possible to monopolize services that society prized dearly, and their prestige rose in direct relation to their ability to diagnose accurately and treat effectively the public's illnesses. Success in these endeavors rested upon a veritable revolution in the practice of medicine after the First World War. Medical research and practice were divided into specialized fields; improved surgical techniques and safer anesthetics were developed, and numerous therapeutic drugs were discovered.

The rise of scientific medicine and the rationalization of the medical profession produced a new generation of physicians who rejected racial explanations for all but a few specific health problems. The argument that blacks suffered a higher death rate than whites because they were constitutionally inferior to whites simply could not be reconciled with the claim that medicine had become a scientific enterprise. Negroes were incontestably human, and the canons of science had to apply equally to them. Physicians had to be able to diagnose everyone correctly and treat everyone effectively. Racial inferiority and moral depravity as catchall explanations for health problems had become incongruent with the scientific laws upon which modern medicine was said to rest. No race could be beyond the pale of science.

Does that mean that racism disappeared from medicine with the rise of scientific medicine and the emergence of a rationalized profession? No. Segregation in medical institutions remained a problem until the civil rights movement produced federal legislation to end it. As late as the 1960s hospitals resembled schools; many either refused to admit blacks or isolated them in separate wards. Nor was it uncommon for white physicians to equip their offices and clinics with separate waiting rooms for black and white patients (Morais, pp. 1–5).

Moreover, racial discrimination unquestionably worked to hold down the number and quality of Negro physicians and nurses in the United States. Prior to the Second World War it was not unusual for medical and nursing schools (especially in the South) to refuse to admit Negroes or to admit them only at token levels. Consequently, the majority of black medical students was forced to attend Negro institutions with small claim to excellence (Davis, p. 443). Because white hospitals often refused to train black interns and nurses, the opportunity to shore up a meager education with first-rate clinical experience was also denied to many Negroes. Furthermore, discrimination pursued them into practice. The same hospitals usually withheld staff privileges from Negro physicians and refused to hire black nurses. Even in the North, where overt segregation often was not a problem, black physicians in many instances simply did not feel that they were welcome in white hospitals and declined to push the issue (Marquette, pp. 19–20). The sense of isolation from their white colleagues that treatment like this instilled in black physicians contributed to the establishment of separate professional organizations such as the National Medical Association.

Thanks to the civil rights legislation of the 1960s, racial discrimination has been all but eliminated as a barrier to the admission of blacks to medical schools in the United States. Moreover, black physicians can be seen on the staffs of the best medical schools and hospitals. Decades may pass, however, before the proportion of black physicians will begin to equal the proportion of Negroes in the general population, though affirmative action programs may be able to reduce the gap sooner. Much depends upon the success of desegregation programs in making quality education available to black youths so that they can qualify for admission to medical schools.

Unless the federal guidelines that have come into existence since the Second World War are rigorously enforced, the use of Negroes as subjects in potentially harmful human experiments will continue. Experiments such as the Tuskegee Study (a Public Health Service experiment involving hundreds of black men in Alabama that was conducted from 1932 to 1972 to learn the effects of untreated syphilis on the human body) show only too clearly the moral callousness with which some investigators have treated black people.

The problem of nontherapeutic human experimentation in most instances, however, relates to the social class of subjects, not their race. The poor and the ignorant of all races continue to supply a disproportionate share of the subjects used in experiments. Guidelines prohibiting abuses must be applied for the benefit of all.

The same argument speaks volumes about the distribution of health care in the United States. While it is true that blacks continue to suffer higher mortality rates than whites in the United States, the difference would no doubt shrink dramatically if blacks and whites of the same social class were compared. The poor of all races fail to receive the full benefits of modern medicine. The American medical profession has purged itself of unscientific explanations of disease; it has made enormous gains in desegregating its institutions; and it has abolished most, if not all, of the discriminatory policies that made it difficult for blacks to become well-trained physicians and nurses. The problem of creating an equitable system of health care for all Americans has yet to be solved.

In conclusion a few comments need to be made on this article's bearing on the professional ethics of physicians. At no point in time has the ethical code of physicians served to im-

munize them against the racial prejudices of American society. The aura of kindly and priestly healer that surrounds physicians has tended to blind the public to the fact that physicians are people before they become physicians, and they remain people after they become physicians. As people they tend to reflect the values and attitudes of their society. In the United States that society has consistently harbored deeply racist attitudes toward black people. Therefore, it should not come as a surprise that racism in medicine has run on parallel tracks with racism in society.

The vast majority of physicians never regarded the race question as an ethical issue for medicine. Race remained a social issue for them, and if racial attitudes impinged upon the patient–physician relationship, doctors were no more likely to be troubled by the results than they were to question how racism defined other contacts between the races.

Most of the progress that has been made on the racial front in medicine to date has been in response to pressures from outside the profession.

JAMES H. JONES

[For further discussion of topics mentioned in this article, see the entries: HUMAN EXPERIMENTATION, article on BASIC ISSUES; MEDICAL EDUCATION; and MEDICAL PROFESSION. Directly related is the other article in this entry, RACISM AND MENTAL HEALTH. For discussion of related ideas, see the entries: ORTHODOXY IN MEDICINE; and WOMEN AND BIOMEDICINE, article on WOMEN AS PATIENTS AND EXPERIMENTAL SUBJECTS.]

BIBLIOGRAPHY

ALLEN, L. C. "The Negro Health Problem." *American Journal of Public Health* 5 (1915): 194–203.

BYERS, J. WELLINGTON. "Diseases of the Southern Negro." *Medical and Surgical Reporter* 58 (1888): 734–737.

DAVIS, MICHAEL M. "Problems of Health Service for Negroes." *Journal of Negro Education* 6 (1937): 438–449.

DEUTSCH, ALBERT. "The First U.S. Census of the Insane (1840) and Its Use as Pro-Slavery Propaganda." *Bulletin of the History of Medicine* 15 (1944): 469–482.

ETHERIDGE, ELIZABETH W. *Butterfly Caste: A Social History of Pellagra in the South.* Westport, Conn.: Greenwood Publishing Co., 1972.

FARLEY, REYNOLDS. *Growth of the Black Population: A Study of Demographic Trends.* Chicago: Markham Publishing Co., 1970.

FREIDSON, ELIOT. *Profession of Medicine: A Study of the Sociology of Applied Knowledge.* New York: Dodd, Mead & Co., 1970. This work is indispensable for its insights into disease as social deviance and the rationalization of the American medical profession.

HALLER, JOHN S., JR. "The Negro and the Southern Physician: A Study of Medical and Racial Attitudes 1800–1860." *Medical History* 16 (1972): 238–253.

———. "The Physician versus the Negro." *Outcasts from Evolution: Scientific Attitudes of Racial Inferiority, 1859–1900.* Urbana: University of Illinois Press, 1971, pp. 40–68.

HOLMES, OLIVER WENDELL. *The Writings of Oliver Wendell Holmes.* 13 vols. Riverside ed. Vol. 9: *Medical Essays 1842–1882.* Boston: Houghton, Mifflin & Co., 1891.

MCHATTON, HENRY. "The Sexual Status of the Negro—Past and Present." *American Journal of Dermatology and Genito-Urinary Diseases* 10 (1906): 6–9.

MCINTOSH, JAMES. "The Future of the Negro Race." *Transactions of the South Carolina Medical Association,* 41st Annual Meeting, June 1891, pp. 183–188.

MARQUETTE, BLEECKER. "Helping the Negro Solve His Problem." *Nation's Health* 9, no. 1 (1927), pp. 19–21.

MORAIS, HERBERT MONTFORT. *The History of the Negro in Medicine.* International Library of Negro Life and History. New York: Publishers Co., 1967. Published under the auspices of the Association for the Study of Negro Life and History.

MURRELL, THOMAS W. "Syphilis in the Negro: Its Bearing on the Race Problem." *American Journal of Dermatology and Genito-Urinary Diseases* 10 (1906): 305–307.

POSTELL, WILLIAM DOSITE. *The Health of Slaves on Southern Plantations.* Social Science Series, no. 1. Baton Rouge: Louisiana State University Press, 1951.

SAVITT, TODD LEE. "Sickle Cell and Slavery: Were Blacks Medically Different from Whites?" Unpublished paper presented at the Southern Historical Association Meeting, November 1975, pp. 1–15.

———. "Sound Minds and Sound Bodies: The Diseases and Health Care of Blacks in Ante-Bellum Virginia." Ph.D. dissertation, Department of History, University of Virginia, 1975. To be published as *Medicine and Slavery: The Diseases and Health Care of Blacks in Ante-Bellum Virginia* by the University of Illinois Press.

STANTON, WILLIAM RAGAN. *The Leopard's Spots: Scientific Attitudes toward Race in America, 1815–1859.* Chicago: University of Chicago Press, 1960.

II
RACISM AND MENTAL HEALTH

People living under the oppression of racism have two major concerns: their physical survival and deliverance from the psychosocial stresses caused by oppression. Recent social changes have suppressed some of the more critical threats to physical well-being and have enabled many oppressed persons to direct more attention to psychosocial concerns, including better mental health. Generally, however, racism in mental health services has hindered this search for better mental health.

Racism in mental health practice is an international, multiracial phenomenon. The following discussion will focus mainly on some of the racist features of mental health practice that have interfered with the provision of quality mental health services to blacks, although the issues raised are applicable to other minority groups.

Scope and context of the problem

Historically, the mental health of Afro-Americans has been of minimal concern to society. The dominant concerns have been the *control* of blacks' physical existence and *confinement* of their sociopolitical activities to the black ghetto. Recent social and political events have mandated certain changes in this regard, including more serious attention to black mental hygiene (Grier and Cobbs; Thomas and Sillen). However, many feel that an already established history of oppression in mental health practice, coupled with widespread racist feelings, renders this a difficult change to accomplish (Deutsch). Moreover, many feel it virtually impossible to distinguish racism in mental health practice from other forms of oppression stemming from forces such as sexism and poverty. This difficulty of differentiation may actually have a salutary effect with respect to bioethics; namely, it can encourage the search for social change policies and strategies of implementation that do not alleviate the unjust treatment of one oppressed minority through the creation of conditions that are unjust to another oppressed minority (de la Noë; Benedict, R.).

An exact understanding of the subtleties of racism in mental health practice remains important for avoiding honest misunderstandings between mental health-care providers and their patients (Bernard). Insight into these subtleties can be gained by noting the primarily racist dynamics in current mental health practice as seen through a consideration of the dominant theory of black personality, and the theory's bearing on several race-related trends in mental health care.

Some racist underpinnings of mental health care: the case of theory

Mental health theory draws its guiding principles of illness and intervention from both general and abnormal psychology. Generally these principles have been seen as universal and applicable to all humans. Prior to the advent of transcultural psychiatry, that approach to theory-building and intervention presented no major concerns (Wittkower and Fried). This was true despite earlier suggestions by cultural anthropologists that Euro-American theories of mental illness and health did not necessarily hold for other societies (Mead). But parochialism worsened as ethnocentric prejudices led to the identification of one particular pattern of behavioral adaptation as superior to all others, with complete disregard for the adaptiveness of different behavioral patterns (modal personality) within different sociocultural settings. Such ethnic bias forced the popular question: "What is *normal* behavior?" (Benedict and Jacks; Gaylin) and led to a polarization of mental health theorists. In an attempt to resolve the debate, some theorists asserted that mental illness could be operationally defined in terms of *failure to adjust* to dominant conceptions of proper behavior (Ausubel). Symptoms of this "failure" included, among others, transgenerational poverty, "chronic unemployment," "sexual promiscuity," and illegal and violent behavior (Parsons). Such characteristics of identification have been very influential in mental health theory. They have largely become the dominant conceptual framework by which less acute illness is identified and treated.

Blacks, along with others, have been very much affected by ideological maneuvers of that sort. For blacks such theorizing is racist. First, it is declared that oppression damages the psyche and that blacks reflect such damage (called the "mark of oppression") because they have been oppressed. This view of black modal personality is seen as "liberal" because (1) environment, not heredity, is blamed for it and (2) such behavioral tendencies are justified and, perhaps, necessary for the oppressed person. Then, mental illness is operationally defined in terms of some of those very behavioral tendencies previously conceded as adaptive for the oppressed person. Consequently, *normal* behavior (under oppression) becomes *abnormal* behavior because it is not the same as the behavior of non-oppressed persons, who represent the normal insofar as mental health is concerned. Such a sequence of defining leads to the ludicrous proposition (held as true by many) that all blacks are, at least partially, mentally ill (Maas; Thomas and Sillen). Thus, for all practical purposes, the dominant theory of black personality is essentially a theory of pathology: group mental illness. This kind of theorizing not only lends "scientific" support to traditional stereotypes of black personality, it also provides the legitimization for a return to the traditional forms of relating with blacks: control and containment (Mason). The influence of this theory of black personality is evident in current discussions of

the means of controlling urban racial protest and violence. Such theory-building seems as racist as the biosocial theories of racial inferiority developed in America during the era of slavery (Montagu; Szasz).

Some see the numerous versions of the pathology theory of black personality as racism per se (Fanon; Thomas and Sillen). Others consider it racist because of its apparent facilitation of certain racist trends in mental health care. For example, one trend that has been viewed as race-related is the disproportionate extent to which black mental health patients are given somatic therapy (drugs and electroshock) as opposed to psychotherapy (Maas; Thomas and Sillen). Presumably, severity of illness is the main criterion for this therapeutic trend. However, in these cases severity of illness has often been defined in terms of black negativism—violence and hostility—toward hospital staff and therapists. It is noteworthy that this mode of determining acuteness is conceptually linked to the part of the dominant theory of black personality that says all blacks have tremendous amounts of "repressed" rage toward the white man (Grier and Cobbs). It is perhaps valid to suggest that many white mental health personnel, like the traditional slave lords, are in continuous fear of black revolt and are therefore more readily disposed to employ more punitive methods of control and containment with black mental health patients. In such cases, it would seem that notions such as "repression" and "black aggression" have been uncritically integrated into mental health practice.

Concepts such as the above often stymie scientific advancement and contribute to "therapeutic lag": They misrepresent client behavior and motives, desensitize the therapist to a wide range of potentially important information about the client as a unique individual, and undermine the development of a more humanistic, broad-based mental health perspective and practice.

Those concepts have sometimes become so entrenched in the dominant perspective of the mental health establishment that its claim of "scientific neutrality" is seriously questioned. For example, its ideological involvement can be seen in the use of projective tests in identifying supposedly mentally ill blacks. The items used in personality tests such as the Minnesota Multiphasic Personality Inventory (MMPI) are designed to identify a person's degree of mental health by measuring the degree to which his or her attained rating deviates from a normative standard (statistically treated scores of a sample of presumably normal men and women). The MMPI, considered by many as the best test of its kind, is a cause of considerable concern. Blacks have consistently scored farther from the norm than whites and would, according to the rationale of the test, seem more psychopathological than their white counterparts (Baughman). This empirical finding seems to substantiate the pathology theory of black modal personality. There is a serious problem, however: The MMPI was standardized by *using normal groups of white men and women—no blacks were included.* The hint of racism is easily suggested inasmuch as the test has separate norms for *males* and *females* because of observed modal differences in *their* personalities, and yet modal differences are not unlike nor as great as those existing between blacks and whites.

Relevant to the prima facie racism in this continued abuse of projective tests is the extremely slow pace at which social epidemiological models of mental illness have penetrated mental health theory (Bernard; Wittkower and Fried). Nor has the culture and personality research been more influential in this regard. Well over a half century has come and gone since cultural anthropologists, working with the Rorschach test, first documented its tendency to identify as neurotic and psychotic persons who were not only happy, well-adjusted, and well-integrated members of their respective cultures but were also often gifted (Mead). And prior to the claim that such mental health practices were racist, they had already been viewed as instances of "ethnocentric prejudice" (Benedict and Jacks).

Availability and efficacy of mental health services for blacks

The presence of racism in mental health theory has led many to question to what degree traditional mental health intervention will significantly alleviate black emotional difficulties. The availability and the success of present services for blacks represent additional bases for questioning the ultimate outcome of such therapeutic intervention.

Racism and its long-term effects have profoundly influenced service availability. Racism has been such a pervasive part of American history that its impact sometimes even dominates therapeutic encounters where both patient and therapist are black (Grier and Cobbs). This observation serves to suggest the added pressures

and tensions extant between white therapist and black patient and partially explains the documented centrality of race issues in therapy even when they seem irrelevant (Milner). The presence of racial tension in therapy has produced some important consequences. First, white therapists often avoid individual therapy even when time and money seem unimportant factors. Second, white therapists tend to adopt a patterned response to black patients regardless of the presenting problems or mitigating circumstances. This patterned response has been described as defensive, overly accommodating, permissive, and pessimistic regarding the possibility of therapeutic success (Bernard; Maas).

Where encounters such as the above have occurred, many white therapists have sought to explain the client's negativism with a plethora of concepts such as "regression," "transference reaction," "primitivism," and so on. None of those notions is sensitive to the historical and political realities characterizing the everyday lives of blacks. Herein is one practical consequence of the racism earlier attributed to mental health theory: Therapists are unlikely to deal directly with their own incompetence and racial ambivalence, but rather seek to use their theories and concepts of personality as a means of (1) containing the patient by encouraging him simply to talk, take pills, and receive shock treatment (Brooks; Shannon) or (2) explaining his negativism when these procedures are seen as ineffective.

Blacks are not typically quick to seek help (Maas). Some progressive and comprehensive mental health programs have recognized and accepted the necessity of carrying services to the homes, schools, and communities in which blacks live. Most mental health practitioners have, however, resisted this trend. Some critics of therapy view their resistance as a mere matter of preference and tradition. Others view it as yet another instance of "polite racism," based on an aversion for personal contact with blacks and the poor. The latter view has been more convincing in those instances where avoidance of interaction with the black community has also been accompanied by an unwillingness (1) to encourage younger, more liberal mental health workers in their community orientation (Bernard) and (2) to allocate the resources needed to increase the ranks of black mental health workers who might be better prepared and more willing to carry their services to the community (Brooks).

Ethics and mental health practice: a postscript

Racism is present in and affects theories of psychopathology, modes of identifying the mentally ill, preferred styles of intervention, routine therapist–patient interaction, and resistance to the implications of transcultural psychiatry for the American setting (Wittkower and Fried). Further, many millions of happy, emotionally healthy blacks are potentially stigmatized and stereotyped by the pathology perspective of black personality (Shannon; Brooks). Such mislabeling not only is detrimental to therapy but has even more ominous ramifications for the whole issue of control and containment.

Some therapists have begun to seek alternative theoretical and interventional paradigms (Petro and French; Shannon). These new therapeutic approaches are partially sensitive to the ethical underpinnings of the dominant psychotherapeutic styles, and recognize their potentially nondemocratic thrust (Breggin; Lederer).

Bioethics has also reflected a growing sensitivity to the interrelationships among environmental conditions, sociopolitical dynamics, and oppressive biomedical policy and practice (Williams). However, many feel that the confusion and racist ambivalence characterizing current mental health practice are likely to endure unless bioethical analysis and sensitivity are intensified and result in action-oriented policy statements.

AARON D. GRESSON

[*Directly related are the entries* MENTAL HEALTH; MENTAL HEALTH SERVICES; *and* MENTAL ILLNESS. *Other relevant material may be found under* GENETIC ASPECTS OF HUMAN BEHAVIOR, *article on* RACE DIFFERENCES IN INTELLIGENCE; *and* INFORMED CONSENT IN MENTAL HEALTH. *See also:* HEALTH AND DISEASE; *and* MEDICINE, ANTHROPOLOGY OF. *Compare:* WOMEN AND BIOMEDICINE, *article on* WOMEN AS PATIENTS AND EXPERIMENTAL SUBJECTS.]

BIBLIOGRAPHY

AUSUBEL, DAVID P. "Personality Disorder is Disease." *American Psychologist* 16 (1961): 69–74.

BAUGHMAN, EMMETT EARL. *Black Americans: A Psychological Analysis.* Foreword by M. Brewster Smith. New York: Academic Press, 1971.

BENEDICT, PAUL K., and JACKS, IRVING. "Mental Illness in Primitive Societies." *Psychiatry* 17 (1954): 377–389.

BENEDICT, RUTH. "Postwar Race Prejudice." *An Anthropologist at Work: Writings of Ruth Benedict.* Compiled by Margaret Mead. Boston: Houghton Mifflin Co., 1959, pp. 361–368.

BERNARD, VIOLA W. "Composite Remedies for Psychosocial Problems." *Psychiatric Care of the Underprivileged.* Edited by Guido Belsasso. International Psychiatry Clinics, vol. 8, no. 2. Boston: Little, Brown & Co., 1971, pp. 61–85.

BREGGIN, PETER ROGER. "Psychotherapy as Applied Ethics." *Psychiatry* 34 (1971): 59–74.

BROOKS, CAROL. "New Mental Health Perspectives in the Black Community." *Social Casework* 55 (1974): 489–496.

DE LA NOË, FRANÇOIS. "Freedom as the Bond of Union." *Proceedings of the First International Congress on Humanism and Ethical Culture: Amsterdam, August 21–26, 1952, at the Municipal University.* Utrecht: Humanistisch Verbond, 1953, pp. 121–126.

DEUTSCH, ALBERT. *The Mentally Ill in America: A History of Their Care and Treatment from Colonial Times.* 2d rev. ed. New York: Columbia University Press, 1949.

FANON, FRANTZ. *The Wretched of the Earth.* Translated by Constance Farrington. Preface by Jean-Paul Sartre. New York: Grove Press, 1963.

GAYLIN, WILLARD. "In Matters Mental or Emotional, What's Normal?" *New York Times Magazine,* 1 April 1973, pp. 14, 54, 56–57.

GRIER, WILLIAM H., and COBBS, PRICE M. *Black Rage.* Foreword by Fred K. Harris. New York: Basic Books, 1968.

LEDERER, WOLFGANG. "Some Moral Dilemmas Encountered in Psychotherapy." *Psychiatry* 34 (1971): 75–85.

MAAS, JEANNETTE P. "Incidence and Treatment Variations between Negroes and Caucasians in Mental Illness." *White Racism and Black Americans.* Edited by David G. Bromley and Charles F. Longino, Jr. Foreword by Shirley Chisholm. Cambridge, Mass.: Schenkman Publishing Co., 1972, chap. 29, pp. 550–557.

MASON, B. J. "Brain Surgery to Control Behavior: Is It a New Threat to Blacks?" *Current,* no. 149 (1973), pp. 28–34.

MEAD, MARGARET. "Creativity in Cross-Cultural Perspective." *Creativity and Its Cultivation: Addresses Presented at the Interdisciplinary Symposia on Creativity, Michigan State University.* Edited by Harold H. Anderson. New York: Harper & Row, 1959, chap. 14, 222–235.

MILNER, ESTHER. "Some Hypotheses Concerning the Influence of Segregation on Negro Personality Development." *Psychiatry* 16 (1953): 291–294.

MONTAGU, ASHLEY. *The Biosocial Nature of Man.* New York: Grove Press, 1956. Reprint. Westport, Conn.: Greenwood Press, 1973.

PARSONS, TALCOTT. "Definition of Health and Illness in the Light of American Values and Social Structure." *Patients, Physicians, and Illness: A Sourcebook in Behavioral Science and Health.* Edited by E. Gartley Jaco. New York: Free Press, 1972, chap. 7, pp. 97–117.

PETRO, OLIVE, and FRENCH, BETTY. "The Black Client's View of Himself." *Social Casework* 53 (1972): 466–474.

SHANNON, BARBARA E. "The Impact of Racism on Personality Development." *Social Casework* 54 (1973): 519–525.

SZASZ, THOMAS S. "The Sane Slave: A Historical Note on the Use of Medical Diagnosis as Justificatory Rhetoric." *American Journal of Psychotherapy* 25 (1971): 228–239.

THOMAS, ALEXANDER, and SILLEN, SAMUEL. *Racism and Psychiatry.* New York: Brunner/Mazel, 1972.

WILLIAMS, PRESTON H., ed. *Ethical Issues in Biology and Medicine: Proceedings of a Symposium on the Identity and Dignity of Man.* Sponsored by Boston University, School of Theology and the American Association for the Advancement of Science. Cambridge, Mass.: Schenkman Publishing Co., 1973.

WITTKOWER, E. D., and FRIED, J. "Some Problems of Transcultural Psychiatry." *International Journal of Social Psychiatry* 3 (1958): 245–252.

RAPE

See WOMEN AND BIOMEDICINE, *article on* WOMEN AS PATIENTS AND EXPERIMENTAL SUBJECTS.

RATIONING OF MEDICAL TREATMENT

The economist understands "rationing" as a policy of allocating goods when supply and demand are out of balance at established price levels, and it includes such techniques as pricing and queuing. Although the term "allocation" is more common in ethical and medical literature, "rationing" and "allocation" will be used interchangeably in this discussion of the distribution of scarce medical resources.

The rationing of medical treatment is only partially a medical problem. Certainly medical personnel will be involved in rationing decisions, because only they can determine which persons can respond to specific treatments. But often they make rationing decisions with little accountability to the public. The prevalence and effects of such medical discretion become visible to the public only in dramatic cases where the decision to provide one patient with kidney dialysis (a process whereby the functions of a failing kidney can be taken over by a machine, which filters waste products such as urea from the patient's blood) or a major organ transplant condemns another patient to death. Beecher's discussion (pp. 275–281) of a few historical examples of rationing new substances and techniques (e.g., anesthesia, insulin, and penicillin) indicates that "in many cases no very extensive, thought-out policies were involved" (pp. 275–281). Individual decisions often have serious social effects before any public policy is formulated.

An increased interest in public accountability of physicians extends to the rationing of medical treatment. Because of this broad public concern with justice and utility, ethicists together with lawyers, physicians, and others should try to identify the moral issues to be considered in establishing or modifying a system of rationing. Although one may not be able to design a perfect system, the ethicist may be able to identify unjust and unjustified systems.

How might the ethicist proceed? One way is to examine existing societal practices for their underlying principles, which can then be used to determine how medical treatment should be rationed. For example, practices such as the military draft may embody principles that are acceptable to the public, philosophically defensible, and relevant to other social practices, including the allocation of medical resources. This approach has the advantages of concreteness and immediate applicability to policy. Another approach is to start with moral principles—their content, form, and validation—and then apply them to determine the justifiability of social practices. Thus one might trace the implications of the principles of fairness and utility for several practices, including systems of rationing medical resources. The first approach is more inductive, the second more deductive.

Whichever approach is used, the ethicist as well as the lawyer will look for analogies. Analogical reasoning is required by the principle of universalizability, viz., similar cases must be treated in a similar way. Although some lawyers and ethicists (Abram and Wadlington, pp. 615–620) interested in systems of rationing have examined the principles underlying social responses to abortion, euthanasia, and artificial insemination, most (Childress; Katz; Ramsey; Rescher; Sanders and Dukeminier; "Scarce Medical Resources") have found the closest analogy in dramatic cases of killing survivors to eat their flesh or jettisoning fellow passengers after shipwrecks in order to save some lives when not all can survive. Nevertheless, there are several dissimilarities: those involved in shipwrecks are deciding for themselves as well as for others, and often they must kill rather than merely let die. But according to Ramsey (p. 254), there is no difference between these cases as far as the selection process is concerned.

Furthermore, the shipwreck cases concern life and death decisions. There are good reasons for focusing the discussion of rationing on *lifesaving* resources whose deprivation results in death. For an ethical framework may yield different conclusions about rationing resources important for health broadly understood and resources absolutely indispensable for life. Who shall live when not all can live? That question is explicit in the rationing of scarce *lifesaving* medical resources such as kidney transplants. It is implicit in discussions of medical priorities that may be "incorrigible to moral reasoning" (Ramsey, p. 240; cf. p. 268). Examples of the latter include choosing among various social needs, of which medical care is only one, and between preventive and rescue medicine.

Selection procedures

A system for rationing scarce lifesaving medical resources hinges on two questions: (1) What should be the criteria of selection? (2) Who should make the decisions? The first question is fundamental, for the second varies with the criteria that must be applied. For example, while a lay committee may help formulate and apply criteria of social worth, it has no function in a system that uses the standard of "first come, first treated." Two different sets of criteria appear to be necessary. Sometimes called rules of exclusion and rules of final selection ("Scarce Medical Resources"), one set establishes the pool from which the final selections are made according to another set of criteria (although, of course, the two may overlap).

Rules of exclusion. Although they are not entirely free of controversy, rules of exclusion are generally more acceptable than rules of final selection because they usually involve minimum standards (e.g., age and medical acceptability) that are more objective and more easily applied. They may, of course, incorporate arbitrary distinctions and unfounded judgments. The numerous actual and possible criteria of exclusion can be arranged in three basic categories: the constituency factor, the progress-of-science factor, and the prospect-of-success factor (Rescher, pp. 176–177). The constituency factor includes considerations such as clientele boundaries (for example, veterans' hospitals), geographic boundaries, minimum and maximum age groups, and ability to pay. Doubts of a moral nature can be raised about all of these, especially the last one. In an experimental stage, the progress of science may dictate that only patients without other complicating diseases and within a certain age range be included. At any stage, a scarce medical resource should only be distributed to those patients who have some reasonable prospect of benefiting from it.

Some specific criteria, such as the ability to pay, are morally dubious, and the constituency factor may be inappropriate in a life and death situation (analogous to emergency room care). Furthermore, age may be merely an objective but arbitrary standard, or it may be important in relation to medical acceptability or social worth. Indeed, the most widely endorsed criteria fall under "medical acceptability," which will, of course, vary in the experimental and established stages of any medical treatment. While medical discretion is less objectionable in the experimental stage, "medical acceptability" should never serve as a cloak for judgments of social worth. If such judgments are to be made at all, they should be conscious, deliberate, and subject to public scrutiny rather than concealed in medical jargon.

It has been argued that judgments about medical acceptability should be made as though the supply were unlimited. By making scarcity irrelevant in this first stage, physicians would exclude only those who could not possibly benefit from the treatment ("Scarce Medical Resources," pp. 654, 656).

Psychosocial factors are closely related to medical acceptability but are even more susceptible to corruption by judgments of social worth. For chronic dialysis and heart transplants, some commentators report that "only mentally deficient or actively psychotic patients would likely be rejected on nonmedical grounds" (Christopherson and Lunde). Nevertheless, some physicians view "cooperativeness" as absolutely indispensable in dialysis. Although psychological factors are important, they may not be as critical for kidney transplantation as for dialysis; for instance, the incidence of suicide among patients on dialysis is "more than 100 times the normal population" (Abram, Moore, and Westervelt). Although the medical profession alone can determine the criteria of medical suitability, including psychosocial considerations, society can and should demand accountability by asking whether a particular psychological or environmental criterion or some other factor such as age is really medically significant. Again, the best approach to determining the pool for final selection is to forget that the resource is limited and to exclude only those patients whose medical and psychological condition would certainly prevent successful treatment.

Several more or less objective but possibly arbitrary classifications have been proposed for the first step of determining the pool (and occasionally for final selection): age, number of dependents, sex, etc. Some of these classifications, such as age, may be relevent to judgments of medical suitability for some treatments, while other classifications, such as the number of dependents, may be relevant only to judgments of social value. Whatever their final adequacy, such objective classificatory schemes may be preferable to ad hoc judgments of social worth. Thus, Paul Freund (p. xiii) would permit "a mechanical selection on the basis of age" rather than judgments of social value, which would require a total assessment of a person's worth in comparison with other persons.

Rules for final selection. The rules for final selection are even more controversial. Although the major alternatives are social worth criteria or some form of chance (randomization, lottery, or "first come, first treated"), several specific criteria have been proposed for this stage, and some of them overlap the criteria for the first stage. Rescher, for example, lists two biomedical and three social factors that should be considered in final selection. The biomedical factor includes the relative likelihood of success of treatment and life expectancy, while the social factor includes family role, potential future contributions, and past services. The consideration of potential future contributions is based on utility, while the consideration of services rendered is based on equity or justice or on utility (Rescher, pp. 177–183).

If "family *role*" involves numbers of dependents rather than quality of relationships (e.g., the value of a particular father for his family may be negative rather than positive), it is objective and easily determined, although its relevance to final selection may be questioned. If it concerns quality of relationships, it is closer to other social considerations that involve more or less total and comparative evaluations of persons. Since the major arguments deal with the legitimacy of such comparisons in life and death situations, it is not necessary to separate justice and utility, although the latter is even more problematic since it depends on calculating future societal needs and a person's probable contribution to satisfying those needs. For the sake of brevity, this article will consider only the utilitarian factor.

A major point in arguments for utilitarian selection is that medical institutions and personnel are trustees of society and its interests. Rescher writes:

In "choosing to save" one life rather than another, "the society," through the mediation of the particular medical institution in question—which should certainly look upon itself as a trustee for the social interest—is clearly warranted in considering the likely pattern of future *services to be rendered* by the patient (adequate recovery assumed), considering his age, talent, training, and past record of performance. In its allocations . . . society "invests" a scarce resource in one person as against another and is thus entitled to look to the probable prospective "return" on its investment [Rescher, p. 178; cf. Shatin, p. 99].

As trustees of society, medical institutions and personnel are clearly accountable to that society, but whether accountability calls for utilitarian selection depends on how the society understands itself and its members. Trusteeship does not necessarily require such an allocation system, for society may have a stake in protecting the patient-physician relationship from utilitarian calculations (including the language of investment and return).

Another argument for utilitarian selection is that the use of chance mechanisms or "first come, first treated" is "literally irresponsible, a rejection of the burden. Its refusal to be rational is a deliberate dehumanization, reducing us to the level of *things* and blind chance" (Fletcher). For Fletcher the development of "criteria for selection" is "the number one task of medical ethics." However, rational persons may indeed responsibly choose to use some form of chance because it preserves several of their values better than any other approach to rationing scarce lifesaving medical resources.

Among their reasons may be the absence of acceptable social worth criteria in a pluralistic society. The defenders of utilitarian selection reply that "the fact that the standard is difficult to apply is certainly no reason for not attempting to apply it" (Rescher, p. 178). But the critics point out that the standard itself is unclear. Because of the plurality of standards of social worth, different communities often make different judgments. In the absence of clearly articulated standards, the anonymous lay committee that chose patients for dialysis in the Swedish Hospital in Seattle used such arbitrary standards as Scout leadership and church participation. "The Pacific Northwest is no place for a Henry David Thoreau with bad kidneys," as Sanders and Dukeminier (p. 378) remarked. Conceding that our rationing is already determined by an unacknowledged scale of values, Leo Shatin (pp. 96–101) urges that we use attitude and opinion surveys in order to develop a scale of social values consistent with the explicit and implicit convictions of the society.

Even if the standards are articulated, defended, and applied fairly, a basic objection remains: "The more nearly total is the estimate to be made of an individual, and the more nearly the consequence determines life and death, the more unfit the judgment becomes for human reckoning" (Freund, p. xiii). We do not know enough to make total assessments of persons, particularly when such assessments determine life and death.

Many critics of utilitarian selection also offer other reasons for randomization, lottery, or "first come, first treated" (Childress; "Scarce Medical Resources"; Ramsey; cf. Rescher). First, such methods of allocation enable us to preserve some of our most important values, including equality of opportunity, while solely comparative assessments violate personal dignity, which cannot be reduced to one's social functions. Second, trust between patient and physician can best be established, maintained, and strengthened when patients are not subject to such comparative assessments and are not treated merely as means to some social end. Third, from a psychological standpoint, rejected candidates for scarce lifesaving medical resources and their families can better cope with their rejection if it is based on chance rather than on judgments of social worth. Fourth, we could imagine a hypothetical situation (inspired by John Rawls's interpretation of justice as fairness) in which several persons must choose a system for rationing scarce lifesaving medical resources to themselves and their children. If we suppose that those devising the system are (1) self-interested and (2) ignorant of their talents and abilities (in order to ensure a *fair* setting in which no one's interests are favored), it would be rational for them to choose some form of chance rather than social worth criteria (Childress). Fifth, a committee would not be necessary for the final stage, unless unusual circumstances demanded an inquiry into the warrants for an exception. Sixth, the use of chance in final selection would probably result in increased resources, since wealthy and powerful citizens would try to minimize their chances of being excluded. Finally, Paul Ramsey (p. 259) uses a theological analogy: "In allocating sparse medical resources among equally needy persons, an extension of God's indiscriminate care into human affairs requires random selection and forbids godlike judgments that one man is worth more than another."

These different systems of allocation often rest on different models of the cases that the system will handle. Should the system be designed for the "hard" or the "easy" cases? And which side should bear the burden of proof? How heavy should the burden be for those who would argue for exceptions? For example, according to societal values and philosophically defensible principles, it may be clear that a system should prefer the research scientist who is a person of high moral character and the father of five children over the convicted mass murderer. If this "easy" case is taken as the model, the system is likely to stress social worth and put the burden of proof on exceptional procedures such as the use of chance when there are no substantial differences between the applicants. Thus, although Rescher (p. 183) includes retrospective and prospective social worth in his allocation system, he suggests that "if there are no really major disparities within this group . . . then the final selection is made by *random* selection."

If, on the other hand, "hard" cases are the model for the system, random choice, a lottery, or "first come, first treated" may be preferred. For example, if there is no focused community and if one must choose between physicians, lawyers, teachers, laborers, businessmen, etc.— each of whom is apparently dispensable from a functional standpoint and is roughly comparable in past contributions and moral virtue— how can one choose? By what criteria? By what certitude of society's needs and this candidate's indispensability? If these unfocused settings and "hard" cases are taken as normal, social worth judgments seem inappropriate and even impossible.

A pluralistic community may well become focused as a result of a disaster. In a focused community judgments about social worth are limited to the specific qualities and skills that are essential for the survival of that community; they are not total and do not concern the person as a whole. Ramsey (pp. 257–258) gives three examples: the decision to allocate penicillin to men "wounded in brothels" rather than those wounded in battle among U.S. Armed Forces in North Africa in 1943 on the grounds that the former could more easily be made fit for combat. Second, the preservation of as many of the crew as are necessary for handling a lifeboat after a shipwreck. Third, triage in disaster medicine: priority should be given to victims who can be restored so that they can help others. Here is a specific and minimal common good of survival, essential for any other goods. "Triage decisions are all a function of the narrowly defined, exceptional purposes to which a community of men may have been reduced. In these terms, comparative social worthiness can be measured" (ibid., p. 258).

The paradigm of triage suggests a way of legitimating exceptions within a system that uses chance or objective standards such as age in the final selection. For example, a system could impose the following burden of proof on those who advocate an exception for patient X: only if X's contribution is indispensable to attaining (or preventing) a certain state of affairs, and only if society values (or fears) that result so much that it would deny Y a second transplant or would remove Z from dialysis in order to save X (cf. "Scarce Medical Resources," p. 664).

Recent practice in the United States

Dialysis has been subjected to the most careful and extensive examinations from moral, sociological, and other standpoints. Because of the attention it has received, it can serve as a paradigm for other scarce resources, although the federal government has covered most of the patient costs since 1972 through the Social Security Act. Several studies of the actual procedures and criteria for selecting recipients of dialysis treatment have shown that the likelihood of success in medical and social terms (including job rehabilitation) is the most important criterion. "Such factors as the congeniality of the patient as an individual, economic burdens of dependents if the patient wasn't selected, 'demonstrated social worth,' 'future social contribution' . . . were considered of minor importance by the majority of centers, although from one-fifth to one-third rated them important" (Katz and Procter, p. 24; cf. Abram and Wadlington). Forty-two percent of the dialysis centers (reporting in a 1967–1968 survey) evaluated "future social contribution" as distinct from job rehabilitation. One of the most remarkable statistics was the predominance of male patients: excluding the Veterans Administration hospitals, the patients were sixty-six percent male and thirty-four percent female (Katz and Procter, p. 27). These percentages are out of line with the normal incidence of renal failure among males and females and thus suggest another sort of social worth evaluation.

Another study ("Scarce Medical Resources," pp. 659–660) identified a number of hospitals that avoided social comparisons among patients mainly by using "first come, first treated" (although the Los Angeles County–USC Medical Center used a lottery). Furthermore, practically all institutions used one form of the "first come, first treated" rule, for they did not drop patients from dialysis or refuse a second or third transplant merely because a superior patient in terms of social worth appeared. Whether they hold that the expectations established by granting a person dialysis constitute a promise, a commitment, or even a contract, no dialysis centers—to my knowledge—drop inferior patients when better ones arrive. A waiting list is considered acceptable, and it is certainly a limit to a strict calculation of consequences. A more difficult question is whether changes in the patient's physical or psychological condition (including cooperativeness) should justify termination of dialysis treatment or refusal of another needed transplant.

No system of rationing scarce lifesaving medical resources will realize all society's values, but it is necessary to have a system in particular hospitals even if there is no standard system for the country as a whole. Reasons can be given for rejecting some systems as arbitrary, unfair, unjust, and impractical. If ethicists, lawyers, and others can identify the moral and social consequences of choosing one system over another, their contribution will help solve the difficult problems of rationing lifesaving medical treatment.

JAMES F. CHILDRESS

[Directly related is the entry JUSTICE. *This article will find application in the entries* HEART TRANSPLANTATION; KIDNEY DIALYSIS AND TRANSPLANTATION; LIFE-SUPPORT SYSTEMS; *and* ORGAN TRANSPLANTATION, *article on* ETHICAL PRINCIPLES. *For the macroallocational problem, see* HEALTH CARE, *articles on* RIGHT TO HEALTH CARE *and* THEORIES OF JUSTICE AND HEALTH CARE. *See also:* DECISION MAKING, MEDICAL; ETHICS, *article on* RULES AND PRINCIPLES; *and* SUICIDE.]

BIBLIOGRAPHY

ABRAM, HARRY S.; MOORE, GORDON L.; and WESTERVELT, FREDERIC B. "Suicidal Behavior in Chronic Dialysis Patients." *American Journal of Psychiatry* 127 (1971): 1199–1204.

ABRAM, HARRY S., and WADLINGTON, WALTER. "Selection of Patients for Artificial and Transplanted Organs." *Annals of Internal Medicine* 69 (1968): 615–620.

BEECHER, HENRY K. "Scarce Resources and Medical Advancement." *Daedalus* 98 (Spring 1969): 275–313.

CHILDRESS, JAMES F. "Who Shall Live When Not All Can Live?" *Soundings* 53 (1970): 339–355. Reprint:

Readings on Ethical and Social Issues in Biomedicine. Edited by Richard W. Wertz. Englewood Cliffs, N.J.: Prentice-Hall, 1973, pp. 143–153.

CHRISTOPHERSON, LOIS K., and LUNDE, DONALD T. "Selection of Cardiac Transplant Recipients and Their Subsequent Psychosocial Adjustment." *Seminars in Psychiatry* 3 (1971): 36–45.

"Due Process in the Allocation of Scarce Lifesaving Medical Resources." *Yale Law Journal* 84 (1975): 1734–1739.

FLETCHER, JOSEPH F. *The Greatest Good of the Greatest Number: A New Frontier in the Morality of Medical Care.* Sanger Lecture, no. 7. Richmond: Medical College of Virginia, Virginia Commonwealth University, n.d.

FOX, RENÉE C., and SWAZEY, JUDITH P. *The Courage to Fail: A Social View of Organ Transplants and Dialysis.* Chicago: University of Chicago Press, 1974.

FREUND, PAUL. "Introduction." *Daedalus* 98 (Spring 1969): viii–xiv. This issue of *Daedalus* concerns "Ethical Aspects of Experimentation with Human Subjects."

KATZ, AL. "Process Design for Selection of Hemodialysis and Organ Transplant Recipients." *Buffalo Law Review* 22 (1973): 373–418.

KATZ, ALBERT H., and PROCTER, DONALD M. "Social-Psychological Characteristics of Patients Receiving Hemodialysis Treatment for Chronic Renal Failure." Contract no. PH-108-66-95. Xeroxed. Rockville, Md.: Kidney Disease Control Program, U.S. Department of Health, Education and Welfare, July 1969. No longer available.

O'DONNELL, THOMAS J. "The Morality of Triage." *Georgetown Medical Bulletin* 14 (1960): 68–71.

RAMSEY, PAUL. *The Patient as Person: Explorations in Medical Ethics.* New Haven and London: Yale University Press, 1970.

RAWLS, JOHN. *A Theory of Justice.* Cambridge: Harvard University Press, 1971.

RESCHER, NICHOLAS. "The Allocation of Exotic Medical Lifesaving Therapy." *Ethics* 79 (1969): 173–186.

SANDERS, DAVID, and DUKEMINIER, JESSE, JR. "Medical Advance and Legal Lag: Hemodialysis and Kidney Transplantation." *UCLA Law Review* 15 (1968): 357–413. Part of a symposium on Reflections on the New Biology.

"Scarce Medical Resources." *Columbia Law Review* 69 (1969): 620–692.

SHATIN, LEO. "Medical Care and the Social Worth of a Man." *American Journal of Orthopsychiatry* 36 (1966): 96–101.

THIELICKE, HELMUT. "The Doctor as Judge of Who Shall Live and Who Shall Die." *Who Shall Live?* Edited by Kenneth Vaux. Philadelphia: Fortress Press, 1970, pp. 146–186.

WESTERVELT, FREDERIC B. "A Reply to Childress: The Selection Process as Viewed from Within." *Soundings* 53 (1970): 356–362. Reprint. *Readings on Ethical and Social Issues in Biomedicine.* Edited by Richard W. Wertz. Englewood Cliffs, N.J.: Prentice-Hall, 1973, pp. 154–158.

RECOMBINANT DNA RESEARCH

See RESEARCH, BIOMEDICAL; RESEARCH POLICY, BIOMEDICAL.

REDUCTIONISM

I. PHILOSOPHICAL ANALYSIS   *Ned Block*
II. ETHICAL IMPLICATIONS OF PSYCHOPHYSICAL
    REDUCTIONISM   *Ruth Macklin*

I

PHILOSOPHICAL ANALYSIS

"Reductionism" is used to designate a variety of doctrines so disparate that it is hard to find anything common to them all, other than being hated in common by one group of thinkers and adored by another. Some of those doctrines are that all events are determined by past events in accordance with laws of nature (determinism); that the mental processes underlying creativity and consciousness can be decomposed into simple, mechanical "information" processes, like the elementary operations of a digital computer (mechanism); and that the sciences of man can be "value free." But the core doctrine, the one that links the others together, insofar as they are linked at all, is the doctrine that mental phenomena, such as thinking, wanting, itching, and, more generally, all phenomena of living organisms are nothing but physical and chemical phenomena. That doctrine will be the concern of this article.

Philosophers have construed such reductionist claims as claims about the reduction of one branch of science to another. Thus reductionism with respect to mentality is analyzed as the claim that psychology is reducible to physiology or to physics and chemistry. A widely accepted analysis of reducibility is in terms of two conditions: definability and derivability (Nagel; Hempel, 1966). Using reduction of biology to physics and chemistry as an example, the definability condition is that each term of each true biological theory is definable in terms of some true physicochemical theory. These definitions are not intended to capture the *meanings* of the defined terms; rather, what is intended is the provision of necessary and sufficient conditions for the application of the biological term in physicochemical terms. The derivability condition is that the laws of each true biological theory are derivable from the laws of some true physicochemical theory, plus the definitions specified in the definability condition (and statements of boundary conditions—though this point will be ignored in what follows).

Oppenheim and Putnam divided all nature into the following reductive "levels": (1) elementary particles, (2) atoms, (3) molecules,

(4) cells, (5) multicellular living things, (6) social groups (Oppenheim and Putnam; Wimsatt, "Reductionism"). The entities of each level are decomposable (without remainder) into entities of any given lower level. The authors hypothesize that the branch of science whose domain is a given level reduces to the next lowest branch, and that since reduction is transitive (if A reduces to B and B to C, then A reduces to C), all branches are reducible to elementary particle physics. They adduce the following considerations in favor of this hypothesis: (1) successes at reduction in the history of science; (2) evolution: items at each level—below 6—evolved out of items at the next lowest level; (3) ontogenesis: each individual of level *n* developed out of lower level parts; and (4) synthesis: individuals of level *n* can often be synthesized out of items at lower levels. The argument based on the last three points assumes that if something could develop or is causally produced out of a set of parts, then its features can be explained in terms of features of and relations among the parts.

On the present account of reduction, to say that psychology is reducible to physics and chemistry is to say that for each true psychological theory there is some true theory of physics and chemistry such that each term of the former is definable in terms of the latter, and the laws of the former are derivable from the latter—plus definitions. But it is not obvious that we can meaningfully talk in this way about unknown true theories of psychology, physics, and chemistry (Hempel, 1969). We can distinguish among branches of science *now* by reference to their distinctive concepts or vocabulary. But we have no idea what the distinctive concepts of future theories might be. Otherwise we would more or less have those theories. Further, branches of science have a way of coalescing and splitting, and borderlines often shift. Phenomena that at one point seem to be in the domain of one branch of science can often be seen later to be in the domain of another. Thus current reductionist claims may be absurd from the standpoint of future science.

The present account of reduction is highly idealized; actual reductions depart from it in various ways. Testosterone might be characterized biologically as the hormone produced by the testes which has such and such effects. But, given the definition of "testosterone" in terms of its physicochemical structure, it is clear that testosterone could be produced synthetically, thus falsifying the biological characterization.

More significantly, the deeper understanding a more basic theory provides almost always shows the "laws" of the more superficial theory to be false, strictly speaking. Thus insofar as the laws of classical thermodynamics of gases (e.g., the entropy of a closed system always increases) can be reduced to the laws describing the molecules out of which the gases are composed, it is found that the original laws are only *approximately* true (e.g., the entropy of a closed system sometimes decreases).

Reduction and identity

Part of the intuitive idea behind full-blown reductionism is that everything—objects, events, states, processes, etc.—is physical. The classical analysis of reduction in terms of definability and derivability seems to miss this important idea. After all, even if all biological laws are derivable from physics, must all biological objects, events, states, etc. then be (identical to) physical objects, events, states, etc.? Does reductionism in the classical sense require entity reduction? In Quine's terminology, does ideological reduction require ontological reduction?

Suppose that a theory contains the "law" that sufficiently great temperature decreases in water cause freezings, and another theory contains the "law" that sufficiently great mean molecular kinetic energy decreases in conglomerates of H_2O molecules cause formations of molecular lattice structures. Suppose the first theory is reducible to the second. Is each freezing *identical* to a lattice formation? Is each temperature decrease *identical* to a molecular kinetic energy decrease? Or are these entities merely correlated? That is, if something simultaneously decreases in temperature and mean molecular energy, are there *two* decreases, or just one? Kim (1966) has pointed out that correlations and identities would serve equally well for the purposes of deriving the reduced laws from the reducing laws; he argues (mainly with respect to the case of reduction of the mental to the physical) that all *science* can establish are the correlations. He says any observation that would confirm or refute such identities would also confirm (or refute) such correlations; thus, he concludes that identity is just a speculative and metaphysical interpretation of correlation (Kim, 1966; Brandt and Kim). But if Kim's argument were right, it would apply equally well to *objects* as to events. If a postulate correlating temperature decreases with freezings will suffice for reduction, so will a postulate correlating (rather than identifying) parcels of water with parcels of H_2O. Just as no "observation" can distinguish between the claim that freezings *are* lattice formations and the claim that freezings *are correlated with* lattice formations, no "observation" can distinguish between the claim that water *is* H_2O and the claim that occurrences of samples of water and H_2O *are correlated*. But it is mad to suppose water and H_2O are correlated but not identical. Why is it that whenever there is water in the bathtub (sink, glass) there is H_2O there too? Is this correlation just a brute fact? Of course, to say that water and H_2O are identical is not scientifically to explain the correlation, but to say this, is satisfactorily to *answer the question* why they are correlated (Bromberger); indeed, one of the major methodological purposes of supposing x and y to be identical is to *rule out* scientific explanations of the correlation of x and y.

Suppose two groups of historians of the distant future discover a strange correlation between facts about Mark Twain and facts about Samuel Clemens. They were born, married, and died on the same dates, made various trips to the same places at the same times, and so forth. Why this correlation? "Aha" exclaims one of the historians, "Mark Twain *is* Samuel Clemens." Since he is right, no scientific explanation of the correlation is necessary or possible. On the other hand, in cases where such identity claims are not true, substantive explanations of correlations are in order. Consider the correlation of electrical and thermal conductivity. This correlation is explainable in terms of the fact that the mechanisms of transmission of heat and electricity are the same.

Another methodological purpose of identity (as opposed to correlation) is to transmit explanatory power. If Mark Twain was known to be injured on May 1, and Samuel Clemens was known to be hospitalized on May 2, the identity but not the correlation of states of Mark Twain and states of Samuel Clemens allows us to explain the latter in terms of the former. Likewise, if it is known how a molecular kinetic energy decrease caused a molecular lattice formation, then the identity of the molecular lattice formation with the freezing allows us to understand how a molecular kinetic energy decrease caused a freezing. Without such an identity, we would have a causal explanation of something correlated with a freezing, and not an explanation of the freezing itself (Block, 1971; Causey, 1972; Wimsatt, "Reductive Explanation").

The upshot is that normally reducibility in the definability–derivability sense (ideological reducibility) does ensure ontological reducibility. The application of this point to the mind–body problem is that, if psychology is reducible to physics in the derivability–definability sense, unless there is some relevant difference between the psychology–physiology reduction and other reductions, mental events are identical to physical events.

Behaviorism and functionalism

One popular quasi-reductionist view that does not quite fit either of the two models so far discussed is behaviorism—the view that mentality is reducible to dispositions to behave in certain ways in certain circumstances. Behavioristically inclined philosophers have tended to suppose that behaviorism is true in virtue of the meanings of mental terminology, that is, that mental terms can be analyzed in terms of dispositions to behave (Ryle). Thus, for example, "wanting goal G" might be analyzed partly in terms of a disposition to do action A if A leads to G. However, there are many actions that lead to G which one might not be disposed to do even if one wants G—for example, one might not *know* an action leads to G. Thus the analysis of "wanting G" should be corrected so as to involve reference to the disposition to do A if one *believes* A will lead to G. Desire cannot be characterized in terms of dispositions to behave without appeal to beliefs. Every attempt to analyze mental terms in terms of behavioral dispositions alone has failed, and the pattern in the failures convinces most students of the subject that what one is disposed to do is a function of one's whole mental organization. Many philosophers who find something attractive about behaviorism in spite of its obvious flaws have thus been led to a doctrine known as "functionalism," the view that mental states can be characterized in terms of their total causal role, i.e., their causal relations to sensory inputs, behavioral outputs, and other mental states as well.

Is reductionism true?

Fodor and Putnam developed an argument against reductionism in psychology, which applies to some other branches of science as well (Fodor, 1965, 1974; Putnam, 1964; Block and Fodor). The idea behind the Fodor–Putnam argument is that entities at one level can have realizations at lower levels which differ so much from one another that there is no lower-level property that is coextensive with the original (upper-level) property. So the "definability" condition on reductions could not be met. For example, you cannot define a mental property in terms of a neural configuration of the brain if creatures without brains can have that very mental property. More generally, we know that a given type of information processing can be accomplished by machines that are physically quite different, e.g., a device made of cardboard working on mechanical principles, and an electrical device. So, if machines can have psychological properties, it seems unlikely that there will be physical properties coextensive with those psychological properties. (For an opposed view, see Kalke.) Of course, it is possible that we are the only creatures that shall exist or shall have existed in the universe and that we shall die out. If so, there would be a physical property that *happened* to be coextensive with any given mental property (for example, the property of being in the physical state that realized the first pain, or the physical state that realized the second pain, etc.) But as Davidson has pointed out, even if we were to find a complex physical predicate that happened to apply just in case "pain" applies, nothing but a brute enumeration that we could not make could rationally convince us we had found it (Davidson).

Physicalism and functionalism

If the argument against reductionism sketched above is right, there is no physiological or physical state that must be common to all creatures in pain. It follows that pain can't *be* a physiological or physical (type of) state; if physicalism is the doctrine that pain is a physical (type of) state, physicalism is false. The possibility remains that pain might be a more abstract state, say a functional state of the sort mentioned above—a state characterized in terms of its causal relations to inputs and other mental states.

Many philosophers have pointed out that, if functionalism is true, physicalism is false (Fodor, 1965; Putnam, 1967; Block and Fodor). The ground is the by now familiar argument that there is every reason to doubt there will be any interesting physical similarities among the disparate physical systems that can realize a given set of causal relations of the sort functionalists have in mind. Oddly, some philosophers have used functionalism to argue *for* physicalism (Armstrong; Lewis, 1966, 1972). This view requires that human pain is one brain state and Martian pain is another. In order to avoid contradiction (one thing identical to two different things) this view must confine itself to

talking about restricted universals like *human pain* and *Martian pain*, and give up saying what it is *in virtue of which* Martians and humans can both be in *pain*.

While functionalism seems an improvement over reductionist theses such as physicalism and behaviorism, it shares some of their difficulties (Block, 1978; Block and Fodor, pp. 172–173 and 179–181). The major difficulty is provided by the "absent qualia argument": Two states might be functionally identical, yet one has while the other lacks qualitative content. Imagine an artificial body that contains thousands of tiny men who know your functional description and use it to duplicate your functional organization, making the body do just what you would do in any input situation. If such a device is conceivable, it would presumably have no pain, even if it is in the functional state that functionalists want to identify with pain.

Weaker versions of reductionism

Thus far, we have encountered three major reductionist doctrines: (1) ideological reduction: e.g., the laws and terms of psychology are respectively definable in and derivable from physics; (2) ontological reduction, e.g., *each* pain is a physical event or state of a given type; and (3) physicalism, e.g., *pain* is a type of physical state. What distinguishes (2) from (3) is that (2) says each concrete, particular pain-event is a physical event (or state) while (3) amounts to much the same thing as the claim that the property of being in pain is a physical property. While (3) is about a universal, (2) is about particulars. Why is this distinction important? The last two sections have pointed out that, because human psychology is realizable by a sufficiently disparate variety of physical systems, there will be no physical property in common to all systems in pain. If this is right, (1), (2), and (3) are all false. But it remains possible that a weakened version of (2) is true: Perhaps each particular pain event is a physical event of some type or other. This can be true even if pains in different organisms (or in one organism at different times) are physical events of different types.

Thus (1), (2), and (3) all require that there be a physical property in common to all organisms in pain, while the weakened version of (2) does not require this. Another materialist doctrine that does not require the common physical property is: Each organism that has mental states is decomposable without remainder into physical objects. Materialists may have been reductionists because of failure to see that one can be a materialist in either of the weak senses just mentioned without being committed to any of the strong reductionist doctrines mentioned in the previous paragraph.

Reducibility and methodology

Reducibility in the classical sense has less to do with methodology of science than one might suppose. Even if psychology is not reducible to physics, it is still of importance to psychological thinking to study the physiological mechanisms that make psychological processes possible. For example, psychologists should not postulate information-processing capacities that physiological mechanisms are unlikely to be capable of realizing. Further, even if psychology is not totally reducible to physics, it may be reducible in large part. Finally, there will always be mental phenomena that require physical explanation. Just as evolutionary biology must appeal to physics for a partial explanation of mutations (cosmic rays hitting genes), so psychology will need to appeal to physiology to explain mental disturbances due to strokes and brain tumors. Thus, whether or not psychology is reducible to physics, psychology will certainly fail to be "complete."

If psychology is reducible to physics, however, it does not follow that psychologists should trade in their tape recorders and stopwatches for electron microscopes. A given rigid, round peg may not fit in a given rigid, square hole; this fact may be in principle deducible from elementary particle physics (plus characterizations in elementary particle physics of the peg and hole), but it would be foolish to suppose that the possibility of such a derivation shows we needn't bother finding explanations in terms of "upper-level" properties like rigidity and shape. First, the deduction is possible only in principle, not in practice. Second, formulating even the rough outlines of such a derivation depends on *already having* the explanation in terms of shape and rigidity. Finally, it is not clear whether the elementary particle account adds anything to the explanation in terms of shape and rigidity (Putnam, 1973, goes further, denying the elementary particle account is explanatory at all). Moreover, it could turn out that reductionism is true, but the only way to discover certain physical laws would be by doing one of the special sciences. For example, there could be laws of physics that come into play only in very complex biological

systems, e.g., brains of certain size. Chomsky has speculated that such a phenomenon could explain the sudden emergence of language in the phylogenetic scale. The laws of physics discoverable outside of neurophysiology might not predict (even in principle) what goes on inside the human brain. But this does not entail that neurophysiology fails to be reducible to physics. For it could be that (if all neurophysiological terms are definable in terms of physics) the missing laws could be imported into physics by translation of neurophysiological laws into the vocabulary of physics. In spite of their neurophysiological origin, the new laws, being universally true counterfactual supporting statements in the vocabulary of physics, would be laws of physics. So reductionism is compatible with the position that in some cases physicists should adopt the method of the special sciences, rather than vice versa.

NED BLOCK

[*For further discussion of topics mentioned in this article, see the entries:* BEHAVIORISM, *article on* PHILOSOPHICAL ANALYSIS; *and* MIND–BODY PROBLEM. *Directly related is the other article in this entry,* ETHICAL IMPLICATIONS OF PSYCHOPHYSICAL REDUCTIONISM. *Other relevant material may be found under* FREE WILL AND DETERMINISM; *and* PAIN AND SUFFERING, *articles on* PSYCHOBIOLOGICAL PRINCIPLES *and* PHILOSOPHICAL PERSPECTIVES.]

BIBLIOGRAPHY

ARMSTRONG, D. M. *A Materialist Theory of the Mind.* International Library of Philosophy and Scientific Method. Edited by Ted Honderich. London: Routledge & Kegan Paul; New York: Humanities Press, 1968.

BECKNER, MORTON. "Reduction, Hierarchies and Organicism." *Studies in the Philosophy of Biology: Reduction and Related Problems.* Edited by Francisco José Ayala and Theodosius Dobzhansky. Berkeley: University of California Press, 1974, pp. 163–177.

BLOCK, NED JOEL. "Correlationism." "Physicalism and Theoretical Identity." Ph.D. dissertation, Harvard University, 1971, chap. 3, pp. 1–96.

———. "Troubles with Functionalism." *Perception and Cognition: Issues in the Foundations of Psychology.* Minnesota Studies in the Philosophy of Science, vol. 9. Edited by C. Wade Savage. Minneapolis: University of Minnesota Press, 1978.

———, and FODOR, J. A. "What Psychological States Are Not." *Philosophical Review* 81 (1972): 159–181.

BRANDT, RICHARD, and KIM, JAEGWON. "The Logic of the Identity Theory." *Journal of Philosophy* 64 (1967): 515–537.

BROMBERGER, SYLVAIN. "Why-Questions." *Mind and Cosmos: Essays in Contemporary Science and Philosophy.* University of Pittsburgh Series in the Philosophy of Science, vol. 3. Edited by Robert G. Colodny. Pittsburgh: 1966, pp. 86–111.

CAUSEY, ROBERT L. "Attribute-Identities in Microreductions." *Journal of Philosophy* 69 (1972): 407–422.

———. "Polanyi on Structure and Reduction." *Synthese* 20 (1969): 230–237.

DAVIDSON, DONALD. "Mental Events." *Experience and Theory*. Edited by Lawrence Foster and Joe William Swanson. Amherst: University of Massachusetts Press, 1970, pp. 79–102.

FODOR, JERRY A. "Computation and Reduction." *Perception and Cognition: Issues in the Foundations of Psychology*. Minnesota Studies in the Philosophy of Science, vol. 9. Edited by C. Wade Savage. Minneapolis: University of Minnesota Press, 1978.

———. "Explanations in Psychology." *Philosophy in America*. Edited by Max Black. Muirhead Library of Philosophy. Edited by H. D. Lewis. Ithaca, N.Y.: Cornell University Press; London: George Allen & Unwin, 1965, pp. 161–179.

———. "Special Sciences (Or: The Disunity of Science as a Working Hypothesis)." *Synthese* 28 (1974): 97–115.

GRENE, MARJORIE, ed. *Interpretations of Life and Mind: Essays around the Problem of Reduction*. New York: Humanities Press; London: Routledge & Kegan Paul, 1971.

HEMPEL, CARL GUSTAV. *Philosophy of Natural Science*. Prentice-Hall Foundations of Philosophy Series. Edited by Elizabeth Beardsley and Monroe Beardsley. Englewood Cliffs, N.J.: Prentice-Hall, 1966.

———. "Reduction: Ontological and Linguistic Facets." *Philosophy, Science, and Method: Essays in Honor of Ernest Nagel*. Edited by Sidney Morgenbesser, Patrick Suppes, and Morton White. New York: St. Martin's Press, 1969, pp. 179–199.

HULL, DAVID L. "Reduction in Genetics—Biology or Philosophy?" *Philosophy of Science* 39 (1972): 491–499.

KALKE, WILLIAM. "What Is Wrong with Fodor and Putnam's Functionalism?" *Nous* 3 (1969): 83–93.

KEMENY, JOHN G., and OPPENHEIM, PAUL. "On Reduction." *Philosophical Studies* 7 (1956): 6–19.

KIM, JAEGWON. "On the Psycho-Physical Identity Theory." *American Philosophical Quarterly* 3 (1966): 227–235.

———. "Phenomenal Properties, Psychophysical Laws, and the Identity Theory." *Monist* 56 (1972): 177–192.

LEWIS, DAVID K. "An Argument for the Identity Theory." *Journal of Philosophy* 63 (1966): 17–25.

———. "Book Reviews: *Art, Mind, and Religion*." *Journal of Philosophy* 66 (1969): 22–27, in particular, sec. 3, pp. 23–25, a review of "Psychological Predicates" by Hilary Putnam.

———. "Psychophysical and Theoretical Identifications." *Australasian Journal of Philosophy* 50 (1972): 249–258.

NAGEL, ERNEST. *The Structure of Science: Problems in the Logic of Scientific Explanation*. New York: Harcourt, Brace & World, 1961.

OPPENHEIM, PAUL, and PUTNAM, HILARY. "Unity of Science as a Working Hypothesis." *Concepts, Theories and the Mind–Body Problem*. Minnesota Studies in the Philosophy of Science, vol. 2. Edited by Herbert Feigl, Michael Scriven, and Grover Maxwell. Minneapolis: University of Minnesota Press, 1958, pp. 3–36.

POLANYI, MICHAEL. "Life's Irreducible Structure." *Science* 160 (1968): 1308–1312.

PUTNAM, HILARY. "Brains and Behavior." *Analytical Philosophy, Second Series*. Edited by R. J. Butler. New York: Barnes & Noble; Oxford: Basil Blackwell & Mott, 1965, pp. 1–19.

———. "Psychological Predicates." *Art, Mind, and Religion*. Proceedings of the Sixth Oberlin Colloquium in Philosophy, Oberlin College, 1965. Edited by W. H. Capitan and D. D. Merrill. Pittsburgh: University of Pittsburgh Press, 1967, pp. 37–48.

———. "Reductionism and the Nature of Psychology." *Cognition* 2 (1973): 131–146. See also Andrew Lugg. "Discussion: Putnam on Reductionism." *Cognition* 3 (1974–1975): 289–293; Hilary Putnam. "Reply to Lugg." *Cognition* 3 (1974–1975): 295–298.

———. "Robots: Machines or Artificially Created Life?" *Journal of Philosophy* 61 (1964): 668–691.

RYLE, GILBERT. *The Concept of Mind*. New York: Barnes & Noble; London: Hutchinson & Co., 1949.

SCHAFFNER, KENNETH F. "Approaches to Reduction." *Philosophy of Science* 34 (1967): 137–147.

SKLAR, L. "Types of Inter-Theoretic Reduction." *British Journal for the Philosophy of Science* 18 (1967): 109–124.

WIMSATT, WILLIAM C. "Reductionism, Levels of Organization, and the Mind–Body Problem." *Consciousness and the Brain: A Scientific and Philosophical Inquiry*. Edited by Gordon Globus, Grover Maxwell, and Irwin Savodnik. New York: Plenum Press, 1976, chap. 8, pp. 205–267.

———. "Reductive Explanation: A Functional Account." *PSA 1974: Proceedings of the 1974 Biennial Meeting Philosophy of Science Association*. Edited by Robert S. Cohen, C. A. Hooker, Alex C. Michalos, and J. W. Van Evra. Boston Studies in the Philosophy of Science, vol. 32. Synthese Library, no. 101. Dordrecht, Netherlands: D. Reidel Publishing Co., 1976, pp. 671–710.

II
ETHICAL IMPLICATIONS OF PSYCHOPHYSICAL REDUCTIONISM

In any inquiry into the implications of a theoretical or methodological viewpoint, it is important to distinguish between what follows from the position itself and what might be the consequences of people's beliefs about the position. Nowhere is this distinction more easily overlooked than in the case of psychophysical reductionism. It is often thought that a reductionist view of human beings would, if true, have widespread implications for ethics generally and for bioethics in particular. But the implications of reductionism for bioethics depend, in large part, on just which reductionist theory is under consideration and what its alternatives are taken to be.

The general difficulty often thought to exist with respect to any reductionist account of persons, regardless of its specific details, is this: If human thought, feeling, and action can be analyzed or explicated wholly in terms of biochemical, electrophysiological, or other physical states or processes, then there is no place for value concepts such as human dignity, rationality, responsibility, and a host of other notions central to our view of persons as capable of moral behavior. If humans are nothing but "machines," even of a very complex or sophisticated sort, how can we meaningfully consider ourselves *responsible* for our actions in a way that makes praise and blame, reward and punishment, appropriate? Such questions can be answered by showing that the difficulties laid at the door of reductionism are properly to be located either within *materialism* (physicalism) or *determinism*. Since it is often the case that, when applied to persons, reductionism entails both materialism and determinism, it is easy to see how the issues may get confused.

Motivations for holding a reductionist view

It is no doubt true that the primary motivation underlying reductionist accounts of persons has been to demonstrate that human beings, like everything else amenable to scientific inquiry, can in principle be fully understood by the methodology of science. The unity of science would seem to require that human beings not be construed as unique entities, composed of material and nonmaterial stuff, making them unlike any other known subject of scientific study. If the methods of science are to be applied to humans as well as to other animate creatures and to inanimate matter, this demands an account of persons such that their behavior and properties can meet the requirements of public observability. Moreover, theories arising from such scientific inquiry must be testable as well as systematically interconnected with well-established theories in other domains (e.g., biology, chemistry, and physics). Making such interconnections requires that human thought, feeling, and behavior be explainable in terms of lawlike propositions; hence the connection between reductionism and determinism. These same considerations stemming from the unity of science would seem to demand a basic commitment, with regard to the nature of persons, similar to that made by physicists, namely, that the universe is composed of matter and its transformations.

Reductionism and determinism

Confusion about the implications of reductionism for bioethics is likely to stem from what is thought to be the necessary denial of the doctrine of free will. It seems natural to assume that a reductionist conception of persons necessarily entails a thoroughgoing determinism. If the problems posed for ethics by reductionist theories of persons are no different from the problems engendered by psychological determinism, then reductionism would seem to have no special implications for bioethics—at least, none that are not already posed by a form of determinism that is incompatible with positing human freedom.

We must make two further assumptions before concluding that a materialist reduction raises problems for bioethics. First, it must be shown why a physicalistic account of persons must be fully deterministic. It is sometimes argued that, since modern physics is itself not fully deterministic (by reference to the Heisenberg principle of indeterminacy in quantum theory), there is reason to think that neural events in humans might also include an irreducible element of randomness. But to show that indeterminism rather than determinism is the case at the neurophysiological level does not yet address the issue of whether we can ascribe free will to persons. Indeterminism seems no more helpful in support of a free will hypothesis than does determinism itself. The second assumption we need to make is that determinism is incompatible with human freedom. If, as the compatibilists or "soft" determinists have argued, the truth of determinism is not inconsistent with postulating genuine freedom, then even a determinist reductionism poses no special problems for bioethics.

But let us assume the worst, for the moment: that determinism is true, that it is a feature of reductionist theories, and that it is incompatible with ascribing free will to persons. What follows for bioethics? For one thing, the distinction between criminal acts and acts that are the product of a deranged mind would presumably be lost. If we could no longer distinguish between human acts as freely chosen or determined, then we would lose the ethical basis for treating criminals differently from the so-called criminally insane. An example of a thoroughgoing determinist's own account of the consequences of accepting his behaviorist view is B. F. Skinner's (1971) explicit disavowal of the concepts of freedom and dignity. Here it is evident that the determinist feature of Skinner's theory, rather than its reductionist aspect, is responsible for his rejecting the meaningfulness of ethical concepts. While Skinner's account can properly be termed reductionistic, it consists of a *behaviorist* reduction rather than a *materialist* reduction (1959). Skinner is as concerned to eliminate mental events as are materialists, but he replaces all talk of mental or "inner" states or processes by a language referring solely to observable behavioral events.

Along with the notion of human freedom, another concept that many believe would have to be abandoned if determinism were true is that of rationality. Judgments to the effect that persons or their actions are rational or irrational contain an element of appraisal. Rational behavior is that which is appropriate to the circumstances; irrational behavior *ought* to be other than it is, since irrational acts are self-destructive or pointless or both. If determinism precludes the ability to appraise actions in this way, or if it eliminates the possibility of giving a rational justification for actions (as distinguishable from causal explanation), then there would seem to be significant consequences for bioethics. As determinists we could no longer deliberate over whether or not a patient's wish to die is a "rational" one. Debates about whether or not there is a class of "rational suicides" would have to be curtailed. We would be left with explanations of human behavior—however powerful they may be—but would be forced to abandon the notions of appraisal and justification.

These alleged consequences of the truth of psychological determinism are themselves debatable. Some have argued that determinism does not entail all of the unhappy results just sketched. The point is, however, that if such implications do exist, they stem not from the reductionist aspects of such theories, but rather from the determinist features. If a nondeterminist reductionist account is even conceivable, then the dire consequences for bioethics that stem from determinism simply would not obtain.

Reductionism as a denial of Cartesian dualism

It now appears that the implications of reductionism for bioethics can meaningfully only be assessed by examining specific alternative theories. To fix ideas, it would be helpful to look at one prominent antireductionist theory: Cartesian dualism (Descartes). This theory has been important historically, and is explicitly antireductionist since it holds that persons are composed of two essentially different substances: (1) mind (or soul), and (2) matter. According to this view, human bodies are governed by deterministic laws (the human body is

a machine), but human minds are not so governed. Instead, minds are characterized by their rational nature (ability to reason) and by the possession of free will.

If the alternative to a reductionist account of persons is some form of Cartesian dualism, then there do seem to be significant implications for bioethics. Since freedom and rationality are held to be unique attributes of the human mind or soul and cannot properly be viewed as qualities of bodies, any attempt to reduce mental events, states or properties to bodily events, states or properties will have crucial consequences for ethics. Similar consequences would follow for those religious conceptions of human life that rest on belief in the existence of a human soul distinct from the body. Views maintaining that the uniqueness of human beings lies in their possession of a rational soul implanted by God and having the attribute of freedom would be inconsistent with a materialistic reductionism. Still further implications for this religious conception would exist if it is held that the soul is separable from the body at death and is immortal. A great many choices and actions on the part of religious persons are likely to rest on their belief in life after death and on the relationship between deeds committed in their mortal life and what happens to them in an afterlife. As an example, consider the belief held by Jehovah's Witnesses that accepting blood transfusions is a sin. Members of this sect refuse even lifesaving transfusions rather than be "cut off" from a chance at immortality.

Pragmatic consequences

Whatever conclusions are reached in an analysis of theoretical issues pertaining to reductionism, there are some significant considerations that may arise in practice. The discussion so far has focused on what follows from reductionist theories themselves; but there may be practical consequences for bioethics that might arise if people came to *believe* that reductionism were true.

It might be thought that the solution to the problem of when a fetus can be considered human, or a person, would result from the truth of reductionism. That this is not the case can easily be seen. Leaving aside the particular theistic view pinpointing the time at which the soul enters the body (the Cartesian alternative to reductionism), every proposal for deciding this issue is irrelevant to the truth or falsity of reductionism. Even granting that the genetic make-up of the unique individual is determined at the moment of conception, writers on the subject have identified the beginning of personhood with everything from "quickening" or viability of the fetus to the time at which the infant becomes a social being relating to other persons. So reductionism seems irrelevant to conceptual and moral decisions in bioethics pertaining to the onset of personhood and to abortion.

Similarly, it might be thought that the truth of reductionism has some bearing on issues in bioethics at the other end of the human life span: determination of time of death, or what may be done to a corpse after death (autopsy, taking organs for transplantation). But here again, decisions that bear on fixing the time of death need to employ a criterion that can be used in practice by physicians. Whether the criterion is brain death, cessation of all vital functions, or some other, determination of the time at which death occurs involves a pragmatic decision. Even if the antireductionist position of Cartesian dualism were true, it would make no difference in the domain of medical practice since there could be no operational criteria for determining when the soul had left the body. Further, in this connection, it should be noted that the sorts of religious proscriptions against tampering with the dead body that one finds in Orthodox Judaism are irrelevant to the truth or justification of any reductionist theory.

A rather different set of implications for bioethics might arise from people's beliefs about reductionism in the following way. If it were widely held that a reductionist account of human beings is true, this might affect the funding of various forms of research. For example, those who allocate funds might decide to put more money into neurophysiological or biochemical research, if based on the reducing theories, or into behavioral research, if behaviorist reductions are believed true, while eliminating or severely curtailing funds for research into motivational or psychodynamic aspects of personality theory. This would be a theoretical error, as well as a practical mistake. Even if some form of reductionism were true, research at the level of the "reduced" theory is necessary in order to carry out the reduction in the first place, as well as to construct bridging laws between phenomena at both levels of analysis as new findings are obtained. Whether a reductionist doctrine is of the ideological or ontological variety, terms or laws denoting states or events

at the level of the reduced theory as well as the reducing theory are necessary, both for theoretical advances and for heuristic purposes.

A final possible implication concerns modes of therapeutic intervention. Of the wide range of therapies currently in use for behavioral or affective disorders, some employ the rational or deliberative processes, while others bypass them. For example, psychoanalytic approaches in particular, and "talk" therapies generally, invoke the patient's or client's conscious thoughts and feelings in the therapeutic encounter as well as in the aspects of therapy the patient or client is asked to work on at home. On the other hand, the techniques of behavior modification, the use of psychotropic drugs, electrode implantation in the brain, and, in the extreme, psychosurgery are interventions aimed at curing or ameliorating behavioral or emotional disorders. If some form of psychophysical reductionism were true, would this set up a presumption in favor of using therapies that bypass rather than employ the rational reflective or deliberative processes in humans? Even if talk therapies "work," would it not be more appropriate to choose modes of intervention that are likely to be much more effective and efficient?

These last two questions are stated in a form that appears to conflate the issues it was earlier urged should be kept separate: what people's responses are, in fact, likely to be, and what the reaction to reductionism ought to be. The answer to either question is neither clear nor simple. On the one hand, the appropriateness of some modes of intervention rather than others is closely linked to their respective efficiency and effectiveness. On the other hand, there are deep-seated commitments to promoting and using the rational processes—commitments it would be hard to dismiss or show to be misconceived even if reductionism were true. But the question of whether efficiency and effectiveness are the chief values to use in choosing among therapeutic interventions seems, once again, to be irrelevant to the truth or falsity of reductionism. Even if mental events, states, or processes can be *explained* wholly by being reduced to physical or behavioral events, states, or processes, there may be other values to be gained by retaining modes of therapy that emphasize self-awareness and the search for better communication and interaction with other persons.

RUTH MACKLIN

[*Directly related is the previous article in this entry,* PHILOSOPHICAL ANALYSIS, *as well as the entries* BEHAVIORISM; FREE WILL AND DETERMINISM; *and* MIND–BODY PROBLEM. *Other relevant material may be found under* ABORTION, *article on* CONTEMPORARY DEBATE IN PHILOSOPHICAL AND RELIGIOUS ETHICS; CADAVERS, *article on* GENERAL ETHICAL CONCERNS; DEATH, DEFINITION AND DETERMINATION OF; INSTITUTIONALIZATION; PERSON; *and* SUICIDE.]

BIBLIOGRAPHY

[See the bibliography appended to the preceding article for a more complete selected list of works dealing with reductionism. Additionally, the following works are cited in this article.]

DESCARTES, RENÉ. *Meditations on First Philosophy* (1641). Translated by Laurence J. Lafleur. 2d rev. ed. The Library of Liberal Arts. Indianapolis: Bobbs-Merrill Co., 1960.

SKINNER, B. F. "Are Theories of Learning Necessary?" *Cumulative Record.* The Century Psychology Series. New York: Appleton-Century-Crofts, 1959, pp. 39–69. Original appearance. *Psychological Review* 57 (1950): 193–216.

———. *Beyond Freedom and Dignity.* New York: Alfred A. Knopf, 1971. Especially "Freedom," chap. 2, pp. 26–43; "Dignity," chap. 3, pp. 44–59; and "What Is Man?" chap. 9, pp. 184–215.

REFUSAL OF TREATMENT

See RIGHT TO REFUSE MEDICAL CARE.

RELATIVISM

See ETHICS, *article on* RELATIVISM.

RELIGION AND MEDICINE

See entries on the major religions: BUDDHISM; CONFUCIANISM; EASTERN ORTHODOX CHRISTIANITY; HINDUISM; ISLAM; JUDAISM; PROTESTANTISM; ROMAN CATHOLICISM; TAOISM. *See also* RELIGIOUS DIRECTIVES IN MEDICAL ETHICS; ETHICS, *article on* THEOLOGICAL ETHICS; MENTAL HEALTH, *article on* RELIGION AND MENTAL HEALTH; MIRACLE AND FAITH HEALING; HEALTH AND DISEASE, *article on* RELIGIOUS CONCEPTS; PAIN AND SUFFERING, *article on* RELIGIOUS PERSPECTIVES; PASTORAL MINISTRY.

RELIGIOUS DIRECTIVES IN MEDICAL ETHICS

I. JEWISH CODES AND GUIDELINES
Isaac N. Trainin and Fred Rosner
II. ROMAN CATHOLIC DIRECTIVES *Bernard Häring*
III. PROTESTANT STATEMENTS *Thomas Sieger Derr*

I
JEWISH CODES AND GUIDELINES

Codes of Jewish law

The eternal guide to Jewish conduct and practice is the Torah with the absolute divine truths enshrined therein. In its narrow sense, the Torah means the Pentateuch or Five Books of Moses. In its broader sense, the Torah includes all of Jewish religious and moral law and lore. The term "biblical law," as used by the rabbis, refers to commandments and ordinances that derive from the Pentateuch. Amplification of biblical law, including observances, ordinances, and even new enactments instituted by classic rabbinical authority, is called "rabbinic law."

Talmud is the comprehensive term for the compilation of traditional interpretations and applications of the Torah. The Torah is called the written law, and the Talmud is the oral law. The Talmud consists of Mishnah and Gemara. The former, compiled in the second century by R. Judah the Patriarch, is a manual of interpretative and traditional Jewish legal teachings, which reduces to writing the legal matter of the oral law. Much more voluminous than the Mishnah is the Gemara, which provides analysis, discussion, dissection, and commentary of the Mishnaic nucleus. There are six divisions or Orders in the Talmud comprising sixty-three tractates or treatises.

The earliest attempts to arrange topically the massive material of Jewish law include the *She'iltot* of R. Ahai Gaon (eighth century) and the *Halakhot Gedolot* of R. Simon Kaira (ninth century). An important eleventh-century codifier of Jewish law is R. Isaac of Fez, known as Alfasi. His code closely follows the Talmud but omits all the argumentation and discussion leading up to the legal conclusions.

The greatest single code of Jewish law ever produced is the monumental work of Moses Maimonides (1135–1204) called the *Mishneh Torah.* It is a fourteen-book systematic compilation of all biblical and talmudic law, presented with brilliant clarity and orderliness.

In the thirteenth century several codes appeared, including the *Sefer Mitzvot Gadol, Sefer Mitzvot Katan, Mordekhai, Beit Habehirah,* and the codes of R. Moses ben Nachman (Nachmanides), R. Solomon ben Adret ("Rashba"), and R. Asher ben Yehiel ("Asheri" or "Rosh"). The latter's son, Jacob (fourteenth century), wrote the next landmark code, called the *Tur,* which displaced many of the earlier codes. No major codes were written for the next two hundred years.

In the sixteenth century R. Joseph Karo wrote his famous code of Jewish law called the *Shulhan Arukh*, based heavily on the earlier codes of Alfasi, Maimonides, and Asheri. Karo's code was augmented by the glosses of R. Moses Isserles, followed by numerous commentators and decisors, and became the accepted standard work, which, together with Maimonides's *Mishneh Torah*, it remains to this day. Over the past four centuries, questions not specifically dealt with in the *Shulhan Arukh* or other codes are answered in Responsa. The Respondent analyzes the legal literature bearing on the subject of the query, cites the rulings of previous authorities, and arrives at a decision for the specific case at hand. This type of "case law" becomes legal precedent for future rulings.

Jewish guidelines in medical ethics

Although no separate codes of Jewish medical ethics exist, the classical codes of Jewish law including the *Mishneh Torah* and the *Shulhan Arukh* contain sections dealing with medicine and the treatment of patients. Such codes are, in nature and scope, roughly comparable to the corpus of canon law. The Responsa literature also contains numerous questions and answers specifically dealing with medical ethics and practice. Several recent books (see bibliography) specifically address the issues of medical ethics from the Jewish viewpoint. These publications, however, are not binding upon individuals or hospitals, since Judaism has no central authority like the Vatican, and therefore, by definition, none of these "contemporary codes of Jewish medical ethics" can be compared to the Ethical and Religious Directives for Catholic Health Facilities. Since Jewish hospitals, unlike their Catholic counterparts, are usually administered as secular institutions, those contemporary codes would in effect serve mainly as guidelines and be regarded as binding only by those individuals and hospitals that conscientiously submit to certain traditions of Jewish religious law. One exception is the strictly orthodox Shaare Zedek hospital in Jerusalem, where such rules of Jewish medical ethics are enforced as a matter of hospital policy.

An attempt to provide some authoritative guidance on Jewish teachings related to medical theory and practice is the compendium *Medical Ethics* published by the Committee on Religious Affairs of the Federation of Jewish Philanthropies of New York (Tendler). This compendium provides a concise summary of the rulings of traditional Jewish law on the religious and moral issues encountered in the practice of medicine. It is intended as guidance to the boards of directors and hospital administrators who establish hospital policy, the individual physician, and to all concerned with health care.

Although many theologians and physicians joined to produce the compendium, the conclusions and the rulings represent but generalities. It is quite impossible, in a work of such limited scope, to provide specific answers to the many complex questions that arise in medical practice.

Authority of directives

The principles of Jewish medical ethics, described in the compendium and other books on the subject, are based on the Torah and are founded on the concept of the supreme sanctity of human life including the dignity of man as a creation in the image of God. They are based on the religious precept to mitigate suffering and sickness. The needs of the sick and their families for spiritual guidance must therefore be met and their sensitivities respected.

Jewish ethical insights are most frequently phrased in legal terms. This reflects the essential quality of traditional Judaism—that religious obligations are seen as regulated by precise norms rather than imprecise sentiments or principles. This fact also accounts for the differences of opinions within the traditional community. As in all legal systems there are those who are strict constructionists and others who are more liberal. Since Judaism does not have a central authority that makes decisions for all Jews, individual members of the community choose to follow the authorities they deem to be most reliable.

The viewpoints expressed in *Medical Ethics: A Compendium* represent a significant statement within the Jewish community, including many issues on which there is a consensus. However, there are others on which some interpreters of Jewish law might differ with some opinions expressed in the compendium.

It is important to recognize the interface of medical ethics and religion. Judaism does not intrude into the physician's medical prerogatives, provided the considerations in question are purely medical in character. However, modern medicine has moved into new areas in which great moral issues are involved. Organ transplantation, hemodialysis, genetic engineering, abortion, contraception, euthanasia, and drug addiction raise serious moral issues. In those areas Judaism offers a message and an opinion. The validity of this opinion is confirmed by thousands of years of empirical evidence, accumulated while maintaining the moral structure of our society. Only through the full cooperation of both the physician and the rabbi can there be established for Jews a moral code of conduct that will enable medical science to make its great contribution without violating the fundamental integrity and worth of the individual.

Judaism, the founding monotheistic religion, embodies within its philosophy and legislation a system of ethics, a definition of moral values. It emphatically insists that the norms of ethical conduct may be governed neither by the accepted notions of public opinion nor by the whims of the individual conscience. Moral values are not matters of subjective choice or personal preference. Right and wrong, good and evil are absolute values that transcend the capricious variations of time, place, and environment as well as human intuition or expediency.

Jewish law has the advantage of being heir to a rich millennial tradition of intimate partnership between Judaism and medicine. Many of the principal architects of Jewish law, and some of the most outstanding authorities of the Talmud, codes, commentaries, and other rabbinical writings, were themselves medical practitioners; Maimonides is an outstanding example. The literary depositories of Jewish law, from the Bible and Talmud to the medieval and modern rabbinical literature, are replete with discussions on religious and moral problems raised in the practice of medicine. The conclusions reached frequently reflect practical experience in medicine no less than respect for the medical profession and infinite regard for human life and health inculcated by Jewish teachings.

Jewish health service

The healing of the sick is a Jewish religious precept. Any person who has the power to save life and does not exercise it, but stands idly by, violates the biblical command: "Thou shalt not stand upon thy neighbor's blood." The religious and moral obligations of the physician necessitate that he perform his duties without regard for the financial, social, or religious status of his patient.

The task of the healer is to help his Jewish patients regain their spiritual strength and confidence, as well as their physical well-being. Anything that strengthens the will to live facilitates the patient's recovery. Consequently, during this trying period of illness the religious needs of the patient may assume particular importance. The provision of kosher food, Sabbath and Holy Day observance, and general regard for the religious scruples of the patient can be of inestimable help in the healing process.

The early purpose of Jewish hospitals in the United States was the treatment of Jewish patients who, it was believed, needed a medical environment that was Jewish. After approximately 1920, when Jewish patients needed the Jewish medical environment less and less as they began to lose their foreignness, the Jewish hospitals tended to find, as a rationale, the necessity of providing opportunities for Jewish physicians who were victims of severe discrimination in hospital staff appointments elsewhere. When medical discrimination declined after about 1950, the Jewish hospitals, many of which by then had only ten to twenty-five percent Jewish patients, tended to be rationalized once again, this time as a Jewish service to the community at large.

Jewish hospitals and health services in the United States are supported by Jewish federations. In addition to general hospitals, such federations maintain nursing homes and homes for the aged and infirm. They finance home care programs carried out by doctors, nurses, therapists, and social workers, and health programs conducted in Jewish community centers. Their help extends to family welfare agencies with counseling, homemaker and housekeeping services, and mental health programs such as "halfway houses" to ease the adjustment of the mentally ill from institution to home life, vocational rehabilitation centers, neighborhood health centers, child care centers, and summer camps.

To assist hospital administrators in treating Jewish patients, Agudath Israel of America, an orthodox Jewish organization that sponsors diversified programs for Jews, has published *The Jewish Patients' Bill of Rights*. Patterned after an American Hospital Association Patient's Bill of Rights, the Agudath Israel publication lists what a Jewish patient can expect from a hospital administration but is not legally binding.

The *Bill of Rights* includes such things as being served kosher food, deferred advance payment until the close of the Sabbath or a festival, observance of Jewish rituals, refusal of outpatient appointments scheduled for the Sabbath or festivals, and the right to consult with spiritual advisers before deciding whether to undergo medical procedures that might pose religious questions.

ISAAC N. TRAININ AND
FRED ROSNER

[*Directly related are the entries* JUDAISM; ABORTION, *article on* JEWISH PERSPECTIVES; CADAVERS, *article on* JEWISH PERSPECTIVES; CONTRACEPTION; EUGENICS AND RELIGIOUS LAW, *article on* JEWISH RELIGIOUS LAWS; ORGAN TRANSPLANTATION, *article on* ETHICAL PRINCIPLES; POPULATION ETHICS: RELIGIOUS TRADITIONS, *article on* JEWISH PERSPECTIVES; REPRODUCTIVE TECHNOLOGIES, *article on* ETHICAL ISSUES; SEXUAL ETHICS; *and* STERILIZATION, *article on* ETHICAL ASPECTS. *See also:* ETHICS, *article on* THEOLOGICAL ETHICS; HEALTH AND DISEASE, *article on* RELIGIOUS CONCEPTS; MEDICAL ETHICS EDUCATION; MIRACLE AND FAITH HEALING, *article on* CONCEPTUAL AND HISTORICAL PERSPECTIVES; *and* PAIN AND SUFFERING, *article on* RELIGIOUS PERSPECTIVES. *See* APPENDIX, SECTION I, DAILY PRAYER OF A PHYSICIAN ("PRAYER OF MOSES MAIMONIDES"), *and* OATH OF ASAPH; *and* SECTION III, A PATIENT'S BILL OF RIGHTS.]

BIBLIOGRAPHY

FELDMAN, DAVID MICHAEL. *Birth Control in Jewish Law: Marital Relations, Contraception, and Abortion as Set Forth in the Classic Texts of Jewish Law.* New York: New York University Press, 1968.

JAKOBOVITS, IMMANUEL. *Jewish Medical Ethics: A Comparative and Historical Study of the Jewish Religious Attitude to Medicine and Its Practice.* New York: Bloch Publishing Co., 1968. New ed. 1975.

The Jewish Patients' Bill of Rights. New York: Agudath Israel of America, n.d. Pamphlet.

ROSNER, FRED. *Modern Medicine and Jewish Law.* Studies in Torah Judaism, no. 13. Edited by Leon D. Stitskin. New York: Yeshiva University, Department of Special Publications, 1972. Reprint. New York: Bloch Publishing Co.

TENDLER, M. D., ed. *Medical Ethics: A Compendium of Jewish Moral, Ethical & Religious Principles in Medical Practice.* 5th ed. New York: Federation of Jewish Philanthropies, Committee on Religious Affairs, 1975.

II
ROMAN CATHOLIC DIRECTIVES

In Roman Catholic perspective, Jesus Christ has entrusted to his disciples the mission to continue his own healing ministry throughout the ages. Therefore, it is important for the self-understanding of the Church to cooperate with the healing profession while striving for a genuine identity in its own healing ministry and deciphering the "signs of the times." Religious and ethical directives promulgated by the hierarchy strive to give expression to the Church's self-understanding of its mission and to read the "signs of the times" by providing direction for Catholic health-care institutions in their efforts to carry on Christ's healing mission. Such directives play a decisive role in determining the nature and extent of Catholic institutional participation in the overall health-care delivery system. In situations where the Catholic hospital is the only health-care facility in an area, such directives often determine the nature of medical service that will be available to the entire community. The directives often are also a powerful force in molding the personal convictions and influencing the private practice of individual Catholic doctors. At times the specific nature of the directives and the manner in which they are proposed as binding for Catholic health-care institutions can result in conflict between freedom of conscience and fidelity to official Church teaching. For these reasons the importance of such directives and their impact on the health-care ministry of the Church cannot be overestimated.

Catholic teaching recognizes the fact that ethical guidelines for medical practice need to reflect the expertise, knowledge, and experience of the men and women of the healing profession. Pope and bishops, therefore, who share the official teaching office in the Church are expected in formulating directives to engage in a constructive dialogue with the medical community. Such dialogue will help the directives to bring home the light of the Gospel to support a profound understanding of human dignity and sound medical practice.

An ethical code can be offered with quite diverse intentions and goals: (1) It can be a prophetic vision opening new horizons for the future and promoting mature discernment; (2) it can state the common convictions of well-informed Catholic doctors, moralists, and patients and offer criteria for action in areas where equally sincere people have a difference of opinion; (3) it can offer guidelines for further reflection and dialogue between doctor and patient without trying to impose uniform decisions in concrete cases; (4) it can state in a binding form what has to be considered morally wrong by all and under all circumstances, or (5) it can be proposed as a pragmatic policy or as a "fence around the law."

Ethical and religious codes in the United States and Canada

In most countries there exists no code of ethics for the medical profession in Catholic health facilities proposed by local hierarchies. One of the reasons might be that prior to the Second Vatican Council, in most countries, episcopal conferences were not yet organized, while associations of Catholic doctors did exist; bishops could be confident that the associations were the best means to maintain a Christian vision of medical practice.

The Ethical and Religious Directives for Catholic Hospitals of the Catholic Hospital Association of the United States and Canada was first published in 1949. While prior to that time many of the American and Canadian dioceses had medical-moral codes for local use, the Directives were intended to update these diocesan codes and make them more complete. A need was soon felt for a briefer version of the Directives, and in 1954 the Code of Medical Ethics for Catholic Hospitals was published. This soon became the official code in many dioceses in the United States and Canada. The Moral Code of the Catholic Hospital Association of Canada, largely based on the earlier Directives, was approved by the Canadian hierarchy in October 1954. A revised version of the Directives was issued in 1955 (Kelly).

In the post–Vatican II era, new and complex questions raised by advances in medical technology, new developments in moral theology, a new openness to pluralism and ecumenism, and the rapidly changing role of the Catholic hospital accentuated the need for a revision of the 1955 Directives. On 9 April 1970 the Canadian bishops promulgated their revised version in the form of the Medico-Moral Guide. In November 1971 the U.S. bishops approved as the national code, subject to the approval of the bishops for use in their dioceses, their revised version in the form of the Ethical and Religious Directives for Catholic Health Care Facilities (Dedek, pp. 201–214). Although the two documents contain similar specific directives, their preambles reflect profoundly different understandings of the role of directives in reaching medical-moral decisions.

The Medico-Moral Guide of the Canadian bishops recognizes a distinction between the level of guidelines and that of the concrete decision. It emphasizes the uniqueness of concrete decision making, especially in complex situations. The preamble states it well: "The Guidelines should serve to enlighten the judgment of conscience. They cannot replace it." The emphasis is on respect for the conscience of both the doctor and the patient. The bishops call for the establishment of Medico-Moral Committees on which doctors and theologians should be represented and the advice of specialists carefully considered. The norms are worded in a way that reflects the present consensus but allows and encourages freedom and personal responsibility in matters of legitimate dissent.

The Ethical and Religious Directives for Catholic Health Facilities issued by the U.S. bishops reflect a quite different understanding of the relation of the Directives to the concrete medical-moral decision. As their preamble states:

These Directives prohibit those procedures which, according to present knowledge, are recognized as clearly wrong. The basic moral absolutes which underlie these Directives are not subject to change, although particular applications might be modified as scientific investigation and theological development open up new problems or cast new light on old ones.

It further states that "any attempt to use a Catholic health facility for procedures contrary to these norms would indeed compromise the board and administration in its responsibility to seek and protect the total good of its patients, under the guidance of the Church."

Consultation among theologians, physicians, and other medical and scientific personnel is encouraged, but "the moral evaluation of new scientific developments and legitimately debated questions must be finally submitted to the teaching authority of the Church in the person of the local bishop."

The tenor of this preamble presents the specific directives as apodictic law, which is to be implemented without exception. There is no recognition of the role of conscience in decision making nor any acknowledgment of the existing ethical pluralism on many of these issues both within and outside the Church. Even the mildest forms of probabilism are excluded, and the role ascribed to the local bishop as controller even regarding "legitimately debated questions" seems to be in sharp contradiction to the spirit of the Second Vatican Council. That Council's document, *The Constitution on the Church in the Modern World,* says:

Laymen should also know that it is generally the function of their well-formed conscience to see that the divine law is inscribed in the life of the earthly city. Let the laymen not imagine that their pastors are always such experts, that to every problem which arises, however complicated, they can readily give him a concrete solution, or even that such is their mission [art. 43].

The next paragraph of the same Constitution stresses the unavoidable diversity of opinions and convictions among sincere and committed Christians and that this can contribute to the ongoing search for better knowledge of truth.

The Directives not only ignore the problem of legitimate pluralism but even seem to exclude the traditional approach of probabilism. It is noteworthy that they eliminated the more open-minded text of the Directives of 1955, which said, "In questions legitimately debated by theologians, liberty is left to physicians to follow the opinions which seem to them in conformity with the principles of sound medicine" (Catholic Hospital Association of Canada, 1955, no. 3, p. 1).

The Medico-Moral Guidelines of the Canadian bishops and the Ethical and Religious Directives of the U.S. hierarchy thus represent two fundamentally different approaches to the relationship between ecclesiastical norms and concrete medical-moral decisions.

For some, the U.S. Directives provide the kind of certain and authoritative answers that are needed to safeguard the Church's strong witness to respect for life and moral values. Others are equally convinced that such directives reflect an excessively biological and legalistic approach to morality and allow little room for promoting genuine dialogue and discernment, for honoring sincere conviction, and for uniting people of differing opinions, at least on the essential issues.

The U.S. Directives: specific issues

The reactions to the U.S. Directives were quite diverse—and the differences among Roman Catholics and others are traceable both to the underlying rationale of the Directives and to the diversity of opinion that exists on the specific prohibitions. In the first category, the preamble states that the absolutes underlying the Directives are not subject to change; however, the wording and tone of the Directives do not help one to discern between "underlying absolutes" and concrete application. The following issues addressed by the Directives reflect the areas of greatest concern and most serious impact for Catholic involvement in the health-care field.

1. All contraception is declared to be always wrong (#19). The Canadian bishops, after quoting the 1968 papal encyclical *Humanae Vitae*, in which contraception had been declared immoral, refer to their own nuanced pastoral statement in which they help people resolve conflict situations with peace of mind (Dedek, p. 204). At least a dozen major episcopates have promulgated similarly nuanced statements. On the other hand, the Directives of the U.S. bishops seem not to tolerate any application in Catholic health facilities of differing teachings and convictions on this question.

2. The condemnation of all forms of direct sterilization is equally absolute (#20). In the interpretation of what is to be considered "direct sterilization" the Directives are much narrower than the legitimate diversity that exists in Catholic theology and in episcopal pronouncements throughout the world. While the preamble calls for a holistic vision of therapy, this very approach is excluded regarding sterilization. The Directives allow only therapeutic sterilization where diseased organs are concerned, but not where such a sterilization might be necessary for the mental and bodily health of the whole person and for the health of a marriage. There is no allowance of a psychosomatic medicine, at least in this respect. A strict interpretation of the Directives, enforceable by the local bishop, would, for instance, prohibit a doctor in a Catholic health facility from performing a sterilization as a part of a total therapy in the case of pregnancy psychosis, repulsion by the husband, extreme danger for the mental health of a spouse, and the breakdown of a marriage when there is no diseased reproductive organ or other diseased organ directly influenced by the reproductive organ (#20).

3. "Masturbation as a means of obtaining seminal specimens" is among those things that are recognized as "clearly wrong" (#21). Were probabilism not excluded, a case could easily be made that the label "masturbation" should not be applied to a massage undertaken in order to obtain seminal specimens. The prestigious *Lexikon für Theologie und Kirche*, published under the auspices of the German bishops, speaks strongly in favor of the licitness of this procedure (Vodipivec, p. 296).

4. Artificial insemination with the sperm of the husband is radically excluded, while assisted insemination is allowed. On this point, too, a case for differing probable opinions could easily be made (Lobo, pp. 149–152).

5. No difference is allowed between the moral evaluation of procedures that impede implantation and those that expel a fetus from the uterus (#12) (Häring, "New Dimensions"). Most typical is the treatment of the termination of an ectopic pregnancy (#16). Although there is, generally speaking, not the slightest hope that the embryo in an ectopic pregnancy will reach the phase of viability, according to the Directives it cannot be removed, except in the case in which the "affected part" ("e.g. cervix, ovary, Fallopian tube") is so dangerously damaged "as to warrant its removal." This approach implies the foreseeable destruction of fertility, while a removal of the embryo, done prior to this dangerous development, could save the integrity of the body and the fertility. This intellectual maneuver manifests how narrowly the concept of "direct" and "indirect" is understood. Only very few doctors, Catholic or others, will consider this sound medicine. The malice of abortion is to deprive the fetus of its right to life. But what, then, if the embryo has in any event no chance whatsoever? Must the doctor then wait until an organ of the mother is so dangerously affected that the embryo can be removed together with the organ in order to qualify the action as "indirect" action?

6. It is in the case of ectopic pregnancy that the underlying presuppositions of the Directives we have already discussed can be seen: The normative value is based on the physical structure of the act, and not on its total personal meaning for the individual involved. Persons and their health can be sacrificed for the sacredness of the physical structure of an act. It is a radical option in favor of a biochemical understanding of medicine and against an anthropological, psychosomatic, and holistic understanding of health and therapy. It is true that the Directives (#6) state: "Ordinarily the proportionate good that justifies a medical or surgical procedure should be the total good of the patient himself." But, wherever sexual aspects or the concept of responsible transmission of life appears, the prohibitions exclude what "ordinarily" should be expected.

Conclusion

The diversity of approach to Church directives and widespread pluralism on many medical-moral issues have been the source of much of the current tension in the Catholic health-care community. A special Commission on Ethical and Religious Directives for Catholic Hospitals sponsored by the Catholic Theological Society of America has offered an excellent analysis of the situation with positive recommendations for "a prompt revision of the 1971 Directives" (Dedek, p. 199).

In January 1972 the Health Affairs Committee of the U.S. Catholic Conference appointed an Advisory Committee on Ethical and Religious Directives composed of medical experts, theologians, hospital administrators, nurses, chaplains, and legal counsel to work at the task of clarifying, updating, and revising the present Directives. Although no sudden or simple resolution of the current dilemma is envisioned, a willingness to search and struggle together offers hope for a more effective articulation of the Gospel values as they relate to the health-care field.

BERNARD HÄRING

[*Directly related are the* APPENDIX, SECTION I, ETHICAL AND RELIGIOUS DIRECTIVES FOR CATHOLIC HEALTH FACILITIES; *and the entry* ROMAN CATHOLICISM. *Other relevant material may be found under* ABORTION, *article on* ROMAN CATHOLIC PERSPECTIVES; CONTRACEPTION; EUGENICS AND RELIGIOUS LAW, *article on* CHRISTIAN RELIGIOUS LAWS; ORGAN TRANSPLANTATION, *article on* ETHICAL PRINCIPLES; POPULATION ETHICS: RELIGIOUS TRADITIONS, *article on* ROMAN CATHOLIC PERSPECTIVES; REPRODUCTIVE TECHNOLOGIES, *article on* ETHICAL ISSUES; SEXUAL ETHICS; *and* STERILIZATION, *article on* ETHICAL ASPECTS. *See also:* ACTING AND REFRAINING; CARE; DEATH AND DYING: EUTHANASIA AND SUSTAINING LIFE, *article on* ETHICAL VIEWS; DOUBLE EFFECT; MEDICAL ETHICS EDUCATION; MIRACLE AND FAITH HEALING, *article on* CONCEPTUAL AND HISTORICAL PERSPECTIVES; NATURAL LAW; PAIN AND SUFFERING, *article on* RELIGIOUS PERSPECTIVES; *and* PASTORAL MINISTRY.]

BIBLIOGRAPHY

Catholic Hospital Association. *Code of Medical Ethics for Catholic Hospitals.* St. Louis: 1954.
———. *Ethical and Religious Directives for Catholic Hospitals.* St. Louis: 1949. 2d rev. ed. 1955.
Catholic Hospital Association of Canada. *Moral Code.* Ottawa: 1955.
———. *Survey of Medico-Moral Committees Established in Catholic Hospitals across Canada.* Ottawa: 1972.
Catholic Theological Society of America. "Catholic Hospital Ethics: Report of the Commission on Ethical and Religious Directives for Catholic Hospitals (1971)." *Linacre Quarterly* 39 (1972): 246–268. *Hospital Progress* 54, no. 2 (1973), pp. 44–56.
CRONIN, DANIEL A. "Toward Realistic Relationships Between Bishops and Hospitals." *Hospital Progress* 56, no. 10 (1975), pp. 64–67.
CURRAN, CHARLES E. *New Perspectives in Moral Theology.* Notre Dame, Ind.: Fides Publishers, 1974.

DEDEK, JOHN F. *Contemporary Medical Ethics.* New York: Sheed & Ward, 1975.

HÄRING, BERNARD. *Ethics of Manipulation: Issues in Medicine, Behavior Control, and Genetics.* Crossroad Book. New York: Seabury Press, 1976.

———. *Medical Ethics.* Rev. ed. Notre Dame, Ind.: Fides Publishers, 1975.

———. "New Dimensions of Responsible Parenthood." *Theological Studies* 37 (1976): 120–132.

KEEFE, DONALD J. "A Review and Critique of the CTSA Report." *Hospital Progress* 54, no. 2 (1973), pp. 57–69.

KELLY, GERALD. "Review of Existing Codes: An Analysis of Their Background, Differences and Significance." *Hospital Progress* 37, no. 3 (1956), pp. 53, 80.

KOSNIK, ANTHONY R. "Developing a Health Facility Medical-Moral Committee." *Hospital Progress* 55, no. 8 (1974), pp. 40–44.

LOBO, GEORGE V. *Current Problems in Medical Ethics: A Comprehensive Guide to Ethical Problems in Medical Practice.* Allahabad, India: St. Paul Society, 1974.

McCORMICK, RICHARD A. "Not What Catholic Hospitals Ordered." *America* 125 (1971): 510–513.

MAIDA, ADAM J. *Ownership, Control and Sponsorship of Catholic Institutions.* Harrisburg: Pennsylvania Catholic Conference, 1975.

"Pastoral Constitution on the Church in the Modern World (Gaudium et Spes)." *The Documents of Vatican II.* Edited by Walter M. Abbott and Joseph Gallagher. New York: Geoffrey Chapman, America Press, 1966, pp. 199–308.

PELLEGRINO, EDMUND D. "The Catholic Hospital: Options for Survival." *Hospital Progress* 56, no. 2 (1975), pp. 42–52.

Policy Manual for Committee to Advise on Requests for Obstetrical/Gynaecological Sterilization Procedures. Rev. ed. London, Ont.: St. Joseph's Hospital, 1974.

VODIPEVEC, MIRAN. "Samenuntersuchung." *Lexicon für Theologie und Kirche.* 10 vols. and supps. Edited by Josef Höfer and Karl Rahner. Freiburg: Verlag Herder, 1964, vol. 9, col. 296.

YOUNG, GLADYS SHIRLEY. "Family Life Services in Catholic Hospitals in Ontario." D.H.A. Thesis, School of Hygiene, University of Toronto, 1975.

III
PROTESTANT STATEMENTS

Authority of bioethical statements

Protestant churches do not issue codes of ethics in medical practice, in the sense of promulgated *rules* meant to cover most foreseeable problems in at least a general way. Even where there are occasional rules, as among some of the minor sectarian groups with a special focus on one or more medical issues, they are addressed to particular questions and are not systematized into complete codes.

There are, however, many *statements* on specific topics in bioethics, which emanate from various levels of church organization. They may come, for example, from a church agency such as a board of social responsibility and may or may not find approval in the denominational governing assemblies. These latter bodies, representing a wider constituency, may appoint special task forces or call special study conferences, whose findings will typically be issued as a report "commended" to church members for "study and reflection." Sometimes such a report, or its recommendations, will be accepted by vote of the denominational assembly; other resolutions may also be voted by the assembly.

It will be evident that the weight of such statements varies with their source and with the degree of unanimity behind the statement. Agreement is often impossible, in which case a report will note the differences of opinion in the study group. The complexity of many issues in bioethics is often reflected in a report's tone of modesty and uncertainty. Its impact may be further reduced by poor dissemination in the nonhierarchical structures typical of most Protestant churches. It is probably fair to say that most laymen, except for the minority who read denominational magazines, do not hear of these statements unless their minister informs them from the pulpit.

In addition to these practical difficulties, the authority of statements is limited by the Protestant tradition of private judgment. "God alone is Lord of the conscience." The principle of ecclesiastical direction in ethical matters would be difficult for Protestants to accept in any case: The Reformation doctrine of the "calling," by which all professions are equally holy as places where God is to be served, creates a bias against anything that looks like clerical directives to other professions such as medicine. The statements are not binding on doctors, nurses, or social workers, not even in church-sponsored hospitals. Small wonder, then, that the authority of bioethical directives from Protestant church groups rests in the first instance not on their ecclesiastical provenance but on their intrinsic merit.

That said, it remains true that these statements have their effectiveness and their uses. Lacking magisterial authority, they are nevertheless guides to the conscience and may function effectively in forming opinions, particularly in fields like bioethics, where the complexity of the issues inhibits the formation of hard and fast positions. By the fact of their standing as church documents they at least compel attention and invite scrutiny in areas where guidance is appreciated. They may find their way into sermons or church educational literature or serve as resource material for study groups. Where the task force that produced a statement is of recognized expertise, and where its work bears the marks of serious wrestling with the ethical questions in the context of a faith commitment, the results tend to commend themselves to a Protestant laity taught to find moral guidance not so much in rules as in an enlightened mind transformed by faith.

Bioethical statements may also be used by church agencies who quote them as bases for representations or remonstrances before public bodies, such as legislatures or government administrative departments. Sometimes a change in law is requested, although there are different Protestant views on the relation of law to morality. In a pluralistic society few would want to impose on others an opinion derived specifically from confessional sources; and there is some feeling that the law ought to stay out of most bioethical issues, which are judged to be matters of private moral conduct. On the other hand, many Protestants want the church to witness in public forums to its convictions, lest it abdicate all responsibility for influencing the moral climate of society. Some would go farther and urge also that, as law should lead and educate public opinion, it should find workable ways to express values like respect for life, even if such values are considered "religious" in origin.

Health-care delivery

Because they regard medicine as a gift of God, many Protestant church groups are critical of the health-care system for failing to reach large segments of the world's population. Poor distribution of health services becomes a case of injustice. Many modern statements, echoing the declaration of the World Health Organization, speak of medical care as a fundamental human "right" and define its desirable extent as "the highest attainable standard of health." Where private resources have proved inadequate to the task—as, it is charged, in the United States—then a publicly sponsored national health service is called for, extending broadly to mental health, dentistry, outpatient care, and other areas not covered by existing insurance schemes. The principle of equal access for all to this "right" means that ability to pay must not become a barrier, whatever method of financing is used. Yet there are drawbacks to national plans, and statements are likely to express the hope that elements of voluntary choice and local flexibility may be preserved.

Although statements characteristically call for an increased use of paraprofessionals to meet the demands posed by such an extension of medical services, it is clear that social resources would still be severely strained. Accordingly many groups, including the Christian Medical Commission of the World Council of Churches (which is mainly but not entirely Protestant), have begun to question the focus of traditional care. The emphasis on curative medicine is said to be wasteful, leading to the centralization of practice in expensive hospitals. Better to stress preventive or "primary" care—nutrition, sanitation, examinations, and so on—and dispense these services through modest and widely dispersed community centers. When health maintenance gets more attention than crisis care, the demands of distributive justice will be better met.

Medical practice and research

One principal subject of statements in bioethics from the "mainstream" Protestant churches has been contraception and family planning, though even here the tradition has a short history. Theologically reasoned defenses of contraception, as *church* pronouncements, date from the Anglican communion's Lambeth Conference of 1958, though of course the position is older (Fagley). In general the current Protestant view is that procreation, though a blessing and one of the purposes of marriage, is not the sole purpose. Sexuality also serves the communion of the couple; and birth control helps to keep these two purposes in harmony. All medically acceptable means of contraception are approved, though there has been some reluctance in the recent past concerning sterilization (cf. Church of England, 1962, pp. 8–11); and the way in which some methods blur the line between prevention of conception and abortion has not gone unnoticed (*Déclaration du Conseil*). It is also generally argued in Protestant church documents that contraception should be universally available, together with an effective education program, partly at least to cut down on the number of abortions. And finally, in the light of recent awareness of the seriousness of the world population problem, many Protestant statements speak of family limitation not simply as a right but as a duty.

Protestant church declarations on abortion vary considerably and are undergoing steady evolution. There is general agreement on rejecting two extreme views—on the one hand that abortion is always to be condemned, or on the other hand that it may be used as simply another method of birth control. In between there are many differences. As recently as 1961 the National Council of Churches, in the United States, could claim as the general Protestant position the view that abortion should be condemned except to save the mother's life or health. Most, though not all, statements still insist on assigning a high value to the fetus from the moment of conception. It is nascent *human* life and deserves to be protected. To say anything less is to court disrespect for all life. Even those statements, fewer in number, which indicate that the value of the fetus increases as it develops still tend to consider abortion at any stage a regrettable extinction of life. The 1969 statement of the American Methodist Board of Christian Social Concern, which regarded the early fetus as "not a person, but rather tissue with . . . potentiality," is an exception to this generalization. Yet, significantly, it was not supported at the highest level of church authority: The denomination's 1972 General Conference statements speak of "the sanctity of unborn life" and regard abortion as at best an unfortunate necessity ("Birth and Death"; United Methodist Church, "Responsible Parenthood," p. 42).

The burden of proof is clearly upon those who would claim that certain circumstances justify violating the fetus. Protestant statements argue that there are such exceptional circumstances but differ considerably on their extent. Justification would come, in the first instance, from showing that the developing life conflicted with another life with a prior claim: the mother's, or perhaps also her existing family's. All agree that danger to the mother's life or bodily health is an indication for abortion, but some—an increasing number—would expand the category of "health" so that it would include also mental stress, and even unfavorable social circumstances likely to produce such stress. Some would make the prospect of a deformed or handicapped child a further indication for abortion, while others would consider such a reason only if it would damage the mother's mental health.

On the value of abortion laws, Protestant church statements vary with the differences noted above on the relation of law to morality. Some would maintain legal guidelines under which abortion would be sanctioned, the limits thus standing as the law's witness to the value of becoming life. Others, noting especially that

the presence of laws leads to dangerous illegal abortions, would leave the decision to the woman and her doctor and, where appropriate, include consultation with her husband or guardian. Abortion would thus be "on request" of the woman, although not, the statements reiterate, as a matter of simple convenience but only after careful consideration of the moral gravity of the procedure. And in order that abortion not be undertaken only because no alternatives are available, there is general agreement on the need for supportive family services.

The third area where there is a significant number of Protestant church statements is euthanasia or, more broadly, death and dying. There seems to be general agreement now on the right of a terminally ill patient to refuse treatment and avoid the prolongation of his dying, and thus in effect to exercise some choice in the manner and timing of death. Even if the patient is unable to express his wishes, some argue, those who are responsible for him may choose to discontinue extraordinary measures keeping him alive, so that his disease may take its inevitable course more quickly. These are all cases of passive or indirect euthanasia. A defense of active euthanasia, direct killing as opposed to "letting die," is conspicuous by its absence in Protestant church statements; and a recent and thorough Anglican study argues against it at considerable length (Church of England, 1975).

Other issues beyond these three tend to be too sporadically addressed to generalize. Some, like artificial insemination, have a history of occasional interest. Others, like genetic control or embryo transplants, are new concerns that have yet to generate a significant body of Protestant church opinion. Judging by the reasoning of earlier bioethical statements, new procedures will be welcomed insofar as they contribute to human health. But they will also be watched warily lest they infringe on the well-being of the individual for the sake of an alleged good for the species or, erring in the opposite direction, treat the individual without reference to the larger context of family and society in which he or she lives.

THOMAS SIEGER DERR

[*Directly related are the entries* PROTESTANTISM; ABORTION, *article on* PROTESTANT PERSPECTIVES; CONTRACEPTION; EUGENICS AND RELIGIOUS LAW, *article on* CHRISTIAN RELIGIOUS LAWS; POPULATION ETHICS: RELIGIOUS TRADITIONS, *article on* PROTESTANT PERSPECTIVES; REPRODUCTIVE TECHNOLOGIES, *article on* ETHICAL ISSUES; SEX-

UAL ETHICS; *and* STERILIZATION, *article on* ETH-ICAL ASPECTS. *For further discussion of topics mentioned in this article, see the entries:* HEALTH CARE, *articles on* RIGHT TO HEALTH-CARE SERVICES *and* THEORIES OF JUSTICE AND HEALTH CARE; LAW AND MORALITY; *and* REPRODUCTIVE TECHNOLOGIES, *article on* ARTIFICIAL INSEMINATION. *See also:* CARE; DEATH AND DYING: EUTHANASIA AND SUSTAINING LIFE, *article on* ETHICAL VIEWS; ETHICS, *article on* THEOLOGICAL ETHICS; HEALTH AND DISEASE, *article on* RELIGIOUS CONCEPTS; MEDICAL ETHICS EDUCATION; MENTAL HEALTH, *article on* RELIGION AND MENTAL HEALTH; MIRACLE AND FAITH HEALING, *article on* CONCEPTUAL AND HISTORICAL PERSPECTIVES; PAIN AND SUFFERING, *article on* RELIGIOUS PERSPECTIVES; *and* PASTORAL MINISTRY.]

BIBLIOGRAPHY

[The following items are merely a representative selection of statements, or summaries and discussions of statements, from a variety of Protestant traditions on a broad range of bioethical issues.]

"Abortion." *Church and Society* 61, no. 1 (1970), pp. 8–11. Statement adopted by the 1970 General Assembly of the Presbyterian Church in the United States.

American Friends Service Committee. *Who Shall Live? Man's Control over Birth and Death.* New York: Hill & Wang, 1970. Discussion of Quaker views on contraception, abortion, euthanasia, and genetic control. Appendix summarizes and quotes abortion statements of Baptists, Anglicans, Unitarians, and Presbyterians.

"The Artificial Prolongation of Life." *Church and Society* 65, no. 1 (1974), pp. 65–66. Statement adopted by the 186th General Assembly (1974) of the United Presbyterian Church.

"Birth and Death." *Book of Discipline of the United Methodist Church.* Edited by Emory Stevens Bucke. Nashville, Tenn.: United Methodist Publishing House, 1972, p. 86.

Christian Medical Commission, World Council of Churches. "Position Paper on Health Care and Justice." *Contact*, no. 16, August 1973, pp. 1–6.

Church of England. *Artificial Insemination by Donor: Two Contributions to a Christian Judgment.* London: Church Information Office, 1959. Report of a Church of England study group, reaffirming an earlier study critical of artificial insemination by donor.

———, National Assembly, Board for Social Responsibility. *Abortion: An Ethical Discussion.* London: Church Information Office, 1965, 1973. Report of a Church of England study group, with new preface.

———, National Assembly, Board for Social Responsibility. *On Dying Well: An Anglican Contribution to the Debate on Euthanasia.* London: Church Information Office, 1975. Supersedes an earlier Anglican study, *Decisions about Life and Death.*

———, National Assembly, Board for Social Responsibility. *Sterilization: An Ethical Inquiry.* London: Church Information Office, 1962. Report of a Church of England study group.

———, National Assembly, Board for Social Responsibility. *Vasectomy: A Guide to Personal Decisions.*

London: Church Information Office, 1973. A joint study sponsored by the Church of England and the British Methodist Church.

CLEMENTS, LESLIE C., and PICHAL, ROSE MARIE, eds. *Report on the Consultation, "Pastoral Care of Those Confronted with Abortion," October 6–11, 1974.* Geneva: Office of Family Ministries, and Portfolio on Social Services, World Council of Churches, 1975.

Conseil de la Fédération protestante de France. *La Sexualité: Pour une réflexion chrétienne.* Paris: Le Centurion, 1975.

CREIGHTON, PHYLLIS, ed. *Abortion: An Issue for Conscience.* Toronto: Anglican Church of Canada, 1974. A study done by a "Task Force on Human Life" appointed at the request of the General Synod.

Déclaration du Conseil de la Fédération protestante de France sur l'éducation sexuelle, la régulation des naissances et l'avortement. Paris: Bureau d'information protestant, 1973.

"Erklärung des Rates der Evangelischen Kirche in Deutschland zu den Rechtsfragen des Schwangerschaftsabbruchs." *Zeitschrift für evangelische Ethik* 16 (1972): 244–246.

Erklärung des Rates der Evangelischen Kirche in Deutschland zum Urteil des Bundesverfassungsgerichts in der Frage des Schwangerschaftsabbruch. Hannover: Evangelische Kirche in Deutschland, 1975.

FAGLEY, RICHARD M. "Protestant Thought on Population Problems." *Engage/Social Action* 2, no. 5 (1974), pp. 51–61. Summarizes recent church statements.

"Freedom of Choice Concerning Abortion." *Social Action* 38, September 1971, pp. 9–12. Statement adopted by the 8th General Synod of the United Church of Christ, June 1971.

"Genetics and the Quality of Life: Report of a Consultation: Church and Society/Christian Medical Commission: Zurich, June 1973." *Study Encounter* 10, no. 1 (1974), pp. 1–26. Entire issue. Reprint. *Genetics and the Quality of Life.* Edited by Charles Birch and Paul Abrecht. New York: Pergamon Press, 1975, pp. 200–223.

KUNST, HERMANN; WILKENS, ERWIN; WRAGE, KARL HORST; FORSTER, KARL; MIKAT, PAUL; and WÖSTE, WILHELM. *Das Gesetz des Staates und die sittliche Ordnung.* Gütersloh: Gütersloher Verlagshaus Gerd Mohn; Trier: Paulinus-Verlag, 1970. Report of a joint Roman Catholic–Protestant study group, published with a foreword by the reigning bishops. Includes the relation of law to ethics, divorce, pornography, and abortion.

"National Health Care." *Engage/Social Action* 3, no. 9 (1975), pp. 35–38. Statement of the 1975 General Synod of the United Church of Christ.

"Organ Transplants." *Church and Society* 61, no. 1 (1970), pp. 71–77. Statement on transplants and death, adopted by the 1970 General Assembly of the Presbyterian Church in the United States.

"The Rights and Responsibilities of Christians Regarding Human Death." *Engage/Social Action* 4, no. 4 (1976), p. 37. Statement of the 1973 General Synod of the United Church of Christ.

"Sexuality and the Human Community." *Church and Society* 61, no. 1 (1970), pp. 5–7. Statements on contraception and abortion adopted by the 1970 General Assembly of the United Presbyterian Church.

"Toward a National Public Policy for the Organization and Delivery of Health Services." *Church and Society*

61, no. 6 (1971), pp. 55–64. Statement adopted by the 1971 General Assembly of the United Presbyterian Church.

United Church Board for Homeland Ministries. *National Health Care: The Time Is Now.* Study packet prepared at the request of the 1973 General Synod of the United Church of Christ.

United Methodist Church, Program Council, "Health Care." *The Book of Resolutions of the United Methodist Church.* Nashville, Tenn.: United Methodist Publishing House, 1972, pp. 37–41.

————, Program Council. "Responsible Parenthood." *The Book of Resolutions of the United Methodist Church.* Nashville, Tenn.: United Methodist Publishing House, 1972, pp. 41–43.

Wort des Rates der Evangelischen Kirche in Deutschland anlässlich des Inkrafttretens der neuen strafrectlichen Bestimmungen zum Schwangerschaftsabbruch. Hannover: Evangelische Kirche in Deutschland, 1976.

Zumbro Valley Medical Society, Medicine and Religion Committee. *Religious Aspects of Medical Care: A Handbook of Religious Practices of All Faiths.* St. Louis: Catholic Hospital Association, 1975. Sketchy, but gives useful glimpses of church positions on medical ethics among smaller sectarian groups as well as major denominations.

RENAL DIALYSIS

See KIDNEY DIALYSIS AND TRANSPLANTATION.

REPRODUCTIVE TECHNOLOGIES

*The articles in this entry, unlike the articles in some of the other composite entries, were planned as an interdependent unit. Thus, each of the first five articles—*SEX SELECTION, ARTIFICIAL INSEMINATION, SPERM AND ZYGOTE BANKING, IN VITRO FERTILIZATION, *and* ASEXUAL HUMAN REPRODUCTION—*presents a state-of-the-field survey and introduces the ethical issues and positions involved in the development or use of that particular reproductive process. The sixth article,* ETHICAL ISSUES, *then serves as an all-encompassing statement and discusses in detail those ethical principles that can be applied to all of the first five articles. The seventh article,* LEGAL ASPECTS, *summarizes the legal issues involved in the use and control of these five kinds of reproductive technologies.*

I. SEX SELECTION   *Gale Largey*

II. ARTIFICIAL INSEMINATION   *Mark S. Frankel*

III. SPERM AND ZYGOTE BANKING   *Mark S. Frankel*

IV. IN VITRO FERTILIZATION   *Luigi Mastroianni, Jr.*

V. ASEXUAL HUMAN REPRODUCTION
                         Robert L. Sinsheimer

VI. ETHICAL ISSUES   *Richard A. McCormick*

VII. LEGAL ASPECTS   *John A. Robertson*

I
SEX SELECTION

Sex selection—variously discussed within the literature as sex control, sex determination, sex predetermination, and sex preselection—refers to means whereby the sex of an offspring can be chosen. Although a simple and an effective means of sex selection has not been developed, research scientists generally agree that it will inevitably be available.

Justification of sex selection

The impetus and justification for sex selection research and development are related to two basic aims of medical science: (1) the control of diseases—in this case, sex-linked and sex-influenced ones such as hemophilia and Parkinsonism (for others, see Montagu, pp. 77–78); and, (2) the promotion of human happiness. In this regard, it is assumed that the parents would be happier because an offspring would be of the preferred sex and the offspring would be happier because they would not experience being of an "unwanted" sex.

A secondary justification is expressed in terms of an assumed need to reduce the birthrate. It is contended that the availability of sex selection would reduce the total number of births because parents would not have to bear additional children in order to have one or more of a particular sex (Markle and Nam, pp. 73–83; McDonald, pp. 137–146).

Finally, sex selection research is said to be justified as contributing to the accumulation of knowledge about reproduction. It is maintained that in the absence of any evident negative consequences of such research, it is justifiable to further sex selection knowledge.

Critics of the foregoing justifications counter-argue the following: (1) there are few serious sex-linked diseases that are not already treatable; (2) it is inappropriate to utilize scarce medical resources in research and development of a nonessential innovation, i.e., one for which the purpose is primarily to fulfill a parental whim; (3) an adequate social and psychological impact assessment has not been conducted—especially with regard to its potential sexist application and imbalancing of the sex ratio; and, (4) utilization of such an innovation would further undermine the privacy of decisions regarding reproduction because a medical practitioner would probably be involved (Gribnau, p. 1229; Lappé and Steinfels, pp. 3–7).

Sex selection research and development

The effort to select the sex of offspring traces back to the Egyptian culture (1350 B.C.); and, over the centuries, numerous theories and much folklore have evolved among nearly all cultures. For example, the Hebrew Talmud suggested that placing the marriage bed in a north–south direction favored the conception of boys. In many of the Slavic countries, if a couple preferred a boy, the wife was advised to pinch her husband's right testicle during intercourse. German folklore held that if the father wanted a boy he was to take an ax to bed with him.

It was not, however, until recently that biological knowledge reached a point whereby a scientifically effective means of sex selection has become increasingly feasible. Research and development has led to several different proposed methods of sex selection, among which a critical ethical distinction may be drawn between those that would apply prior to conception and those that would apply after conception.

Preconception methods. Proposed preconception methods are premised upon the established biological fact that the sex of an offspring is determined by the type of sperm that fertilizes the egg. In the typical human male ejaculate there are an estimated 300 million sperm. Some of them are andro-(Y-bearing) sperm, while others are gyno-(X-bearing) sperm. If one of the former fertilizes an egg, the genetic basis for a male offspring is provided; whereas if a gynosperm impregnates an egg, the basis for a female is provided. Thus, the aim of preconception research is simply to provide a means whereby one could control which type of sperm fertilized the egg.

The development of a preconception means of sex selection has followed several lines of investigation. Geneticists have presumed that sex determination depends not simply on the presence of an X or Y chromosome, but specifically on a gene or genes present in the particular chromosome. It has been tentatively concluded that the presence of the H-Y antigen, located on the Y chromosome, is necessary for male development. But at this point geneticists have not discovered a means for manipulating the antigen for the purpose of sex selection.

A second line of inquiry relates to spermatogenesis. The objective of this research is to ascertain factors (e.g., biochemical conditions, body temperature, and stress) that may influence the production of andro- and gynosperm. In this regard, scientists hope to determine: (1)

if the supposition is accurate that human males generally produce disproportionately more andro- than gynosperm; (2) why there are individual differences among a group of males; and (3) why a given individual male may differ in his production over a given time span. Research discoveries relating to biochemical, genetic, and sociopsychological factors that are involved in spermatogenesis would greatly advance the prospect for an effective means of sex selection.

Another approach to sex selection focuses upon conditions affecting the movement of the sperm within the reproductive tract. It has been assumed that while the androsperm are generally more motile (though shorter-lived) than the gynosperm, specific biochemical conditions nonetheless affect that motility. For example, it has been noted that an acidic environment is more favorable to the motility and survival of gynosperm, whereas an alkaline environment is more favorable for androsperm. In this regard, it is interesting that the conditions of ovulation and orgasm increase alkalinity within the reproductive tract. In addition, studies indicate that androsperm deposited near the womb or cervix have greater chances than if deposited within the vagina because the secretions of the latter tend to be more acidic than those of the former.

Thus, on the basis of the foregoing findings and assumptions, a sex selection means is already regarded by many as available. In fact, procedures based upon the foregoing findings and widely publicized in the popular press are now being utilized by prospective parents. It has been reported that under clinical conditions a group of forty-eight parents were about eighty-five percent successful in procreating a child of the preferred sex (Rorvik and Shettles). Replication of the results is, however, conspicuously absent in the literature.

A fourth proposed approach to sex selection is premised upon the supposition that androsperm are smaller and less dense than gynosperm (Shettles, p. 123). It is speculated, therefore, that a diaphragm could be inserted within the female reproductive tract and that it would filter out the gynosperm, sequentially allowing only the androsperm to reach the egg. However, the validity of this theory has not been verified.

A quite different method of sex selection would require a special treatment of male semen followed by artificial insemination. Through any or a combination of four treatments—centrifugation, electrophoresis, agglutination, or albumin isolation—a medical practitioner would separate the andro/gynosperm, then artificially inseminate the female with the preferred sperm.

The centrifugation method of separation is based on the notion that the gynosperm are heavier than the androsperm and that the two can therefore be separated at high speeds. Utilizing this technique, animal breeders have found that by artificially inseminating with the more readily sedimented portion of a semen portion, impregnation probability decreased, but when it did occur the proportion of males increased (Lindahl, p. 784).

The second technique, electrophoresis, is based upon the finding that for some unknown reason when sperm are subjected to an electric current, the androsperm tend to group around the cathode, while the gynosperm, around the anode. Animal experiments involving fertilization with sperm that had been subjected to electrophoresis achieved about seventy percent success in the prediction of the sex of the offspring (Sevinç, pp. 7–9). The technique has not, however, been attempted with humans.

The agglutination technique is premised upon the finding that gynosperm have a greater density than androsperm, and that they will therefore sediment more rapidly in a gravitational field. In artificial insemination experiments with rabbits it has been reported that sperm from the bottom of a sedimentation column, which presumably had the highest density, yielded only twenty-five percent males (Branham, p. 479). It should, however, be noted that the results of subsequent experiments have failed to confirm the initial claims.

Finally, there is some evidence that sperm may be separated because the androsperm are more motile than the gynosperm. In this regard, the devised technique involves placing sperm diluted in Tyrode's solution on top of a bovine serum albumin, then isolating out the highly motile sperm contained in the albumin. There has been one report that sperm fractions derived through this technique contain up to eighty-five percent androsperm of which about ninety-four percent are motile (Ericsson, Langevin, and Nishino, p. 421). But, here again, subsequent studies have not confirmed that report.

Postconception methods. Proposed postconception sex selection methods are based upon advances in microsurgery and the technology of determining the sex of an embryo/fetus prior to birth. One such method involves the removal of the blastocyst from the mother, determination of its sex, followed by reimplantation of the blastocyst in the uterus if it is of the desired sex. This procedure has been attempted in rabbits. While only twenty percent of the reimplantations developed, all of them were of the predicted sex (Gardner and Edwards, p. 348). The foregoing procedure would be greatly advanced if the blastocysts could be created outside the mother; however, even then it would have limited application because of the expensive and complicated microsurgical techniques it requires.

A more likely postconception method is contingent upon advances in prenatal diagnostic techniques whereby the sex of a fetus *in utero* may be determined. Currently, through amniocentesis (perforation of the uterus to permit drainage of a portion of amniotic fluid for antenatal diagnosis of the fetus) the sex of the fetus may be determined as early as the twelfth week of the pregnancy (Nelson and Emergy, pp. 23–24; Hudson, pp. 523–528). As further medical developments assure earlier predetermination of sex and easier means of abortion, use of this sex selection method becomes more probable—particularly in cases where there is a risk of sex-linked diseases.

In sum, research and development aimed toward finding a simple and effective means of sex selection has been quite diverse. And it is probable that not one but several different techniques of sex selection will be developed within the foreseeable future. Some require the direct involvement of a medical practitioner, others do not. Some require treatment of the father, some treatment of the mother, and still others treatment of both parents. Some apply prior to conception, others after conception. Some are medically complicated and expensive, others less so. And finally, some of the methods have a high degree of medical effectiveness but are not apt to be widely used, while others have a lower degree of effectiveness but are more likely to be used. It should be recognized, too, that at this stage of development the adverse effects (e.g., teratogenic) of the respective techniques is undetermined.

Any discussion of the social and psychological impact of sex selection must therefore cautiously recognize the diversity of the proposed means.

Social impact

The social impact of sex selection is contingent upon what methods become available, the extent to which government regulates the use of the respective methods, the extent to which they are effectively used by couples, and the sex preferences of these couples.

Progress in the development of sex selection is largely dependent upon research support given to it by both government and private sources—particularly the pharmaceutical industry. Research and development by the government is influenced by public opinion and concern about sex-linked diseases. Research and development by private enterprise is based primarily upon the prospective market, that is, how many couples would be willing to pay how much in order to fulfill their sex preferences.

In considering the societal context of the development and diffusion of sex selection methods, it is useful to compare it with similar birth control methods—keeping in mind that the latter have greater importance to the public than sex selection. Governmental regulations would probably parallel those governing birth control methods. The rhythm–douching method would be difficult to regulate because it would be essentially self-administered. A method requiring a drug, abortion, or artificial insemination would probably be more closely regulated. In this regard, consumer protection tests and regulations will undoubtedly contribute to the time lag between its development and diffusion.

If widespread diffusion occurs, perhaps the most significant governmental concern will involve assessing the social impact of sex selection. Leaders may have to deal with such questions as: At what point is an imbalanced sex ratio societally dysfunctional? If, for example, the use of sex selection increases the number of male births by, say, ten percent, should its use be regulated? To what extent are the norms and ethics of society premised upon a relatively balanced number of males and females? If a lack of females resulted in an increase in male homosexuality or polyandry, would there be sufficient ethical grounds to urge the curtailment of the use of sex selection? And, if so, how much of an increase?

On the other hand, if sex selection is shown to be an effective means for curtailing sex-linked defects, the question may arise: To what extent should society require its use? What sex-linked defects, if any, should society be empowered to curtail through the enactment of laws governing the right to reproduce children of a particular sex?

Before proceeding on the assumption of a significant social impact which might require diffi-

cult ethical and policy decisions, let us deal with another question: If a simple and effective means of sex selection becomes available, will couples use it?

The answer is complicated at this point because of the hypothetical nature of the methods and also because it is not known how effective the pharmaceutical industry can be in creating a market for such an innovation. There are, however, various reasons why couples may not use sex selection. They include: (1) an indifference with regard to the sex of their children, (2) a belief that sex selection is unnecessarily tampering with nature, (3) religious values, (4) a belief that it constitutes sexist behavior, (5) a willingness to risk chance since there is an almost fifty–fifty chance of having a child of the preferred sex, (6) the probability that most of the methods increase the length of time needed for most females to become pregnant once they desire to become so, (7) objections to the nature of particular methods, (8) cost of the methods, and (9) disagreements between spouses over whether they should use a method and, if they do, what specific method and sex they prefer.

Nonetheless, assuming that the aforementioned objections are minimized and a significant number of couples do effectively utilize sex selection, the further question arises: What are the social and psychological risks and benefits?

The foremost concern of social scientists is that extensive use of sex selection might lead to an imbalanced sex ratio in ethnic groups and societies that have traditionally shown a very strong preference for males (Stinner and Mader, pp. 181–188). Furthermore, if the imbalance were serious, it would necessitate changes in sexual, marital, familial, political, and other norms. For example, the institution of monogamy is suited for a balanced sex ratio, but polygamy for one that is imbalanced.

It is fortunate, though, that the likelihood of such a serious imbalance may be lessening due to a declining preference for males in many societies. For example, in India, the strong son-preference is apparently lessening with the modernization of the society (Repetto, pp. 70–76; Lahiri, p. 323). In the People's Republic of China, a concerted governmental campaign was initiated in 1975 explicitly to lessen the son-preference. In the United States, as well as in many other societies, it may be assumed that the women's movement may lessen the male preference by advancing the status of women.

It should be noted, too, that some groups may sustain a strong son-preference but at the same time be resistant to the adoption of sex selection methods (Largey, 1973, p. 318).

A second sociological concern is that, since many couples prefer a male for the first child, the first-child personality traits will become accentuated in the male population, whereas the later-child traits will find emphasis among females. In this respect, a limited study has indicated that only nine of fifty-eight young suburban American couples jointly agreed that they preferred a male for the first child and that they would be willing to use a means of sex selection to fulfill their first-child sex preference (Largey, 1972). The extent to which the finding may be generalized is clearly limited; nonetheless, it does suggest the need to be cautious in assuming spouse agreement regarding the preferred sex of the first child and the willingness of couples to utilize a sex selection technique to actualize a preference. It should be recognized that many couples would chance the sex of their first child and only use sex selection, if at all, for a second or third child. Of course, the question still remains: What percentage increase of first-born males, if any, would constitute a social condition inconsistent with the good of society? And at what point, if any, should society be permitted to regulate parental rights to reproduce children of a particular sex?

The third concern is that tension and conflict may emerge if some groups, such as women's groups, exert pressures against the research, development, and sale of sex selection methods due to the sexist implications. Such pressures will raise several ethical issues, e.g., the legitimacy of interfering with research dealing with sex-linked diseases and the legitimacy of an individual couple's engaging in reproductive behavior that they know will contribute to social problems and especially sexism.

Finally, there are questions to be dealt with at the intersocietal level. It is plausible that sex selection would not adversely affect American society but may generate social problems in India. If so, what rules should govern its diffusion?

On the other side, the potential benefits of sex selection are twofold: (1) it might facilitate familial adjustments; and (2) it might contribute to decreasing the birth rate. Regarding the first, it is speculated that if couples were able to select the sex of their offspring they would be more content, their children's sexual devel-opment would be less problematic, and familial relationships would improve (Pohlman, pp. 274–280). This potential benefit must, however, be weighed against potential problems—disagreements between the spouses over the sex preferred and cases in which the method does not work effectively.

Regarding a reduced birthrate, it is speculated that with the availability of sex selection couples would no longer have to bear additional children in order to have one or the other of a particular sex. While a seemingly obvious benefit—especially as the desired family size decreases and with it the opportunity to fulfill sex preferences by chance—it should be noted that recent empirical studies have indicated that expressed son-preferences in both developing countries and the United States did not affect actual fertility levels (Repetto, pp. 70–76; Cutright, Belt, and Scanzoni, pp. 242–248). Furthermore, some couples might have additional children if they were able to select the sex (Serow and Evans, p. 319).

In sum, the social impact of sex selection and the ethical questions associated with it depend to a large extent upon the nature of the methods that are made available, the willingness of couples to utilize those available, the strength of sex preferences, the understanding of what constitutes sexism, and the kinds of societal regulations that are promoted to control the use of sex selection.

GALE LARGEY

[*Directly related are the subsequent articles in this entry,* ETHICAL ISSUES *and* LEGAL ASPECTS. *Other relevant material may be found under* EUGENICS; GENETIC DIAGNOSIS AND COUNSELING; *and* PRENATAL DIAGNOSIS. *For discussion of related ideas, see the entries:* ABORTION; CONTRACEPTION; FUTURE GENERATIONS, OBLIGATIONS TO; HUMAN EXPERIMENTATION; *and* POPULATION POLICY PROPOSALS, *article on* DIFFERENTIAL GROWTH RATE AND POPULATION POLICIES: ETHICAL ANALYSIS.]

BIBLIOGRAPHY

BHATTACHARYA, B. C.; BANGHAM, A. D.; CRO, R. J.; KEYNES, R. D.; and ROWSON, L. E. A. "An Attempt to Predetermine the Sex of Calves by Artificial Insemination with Spermatozoa Separated by Sedimentation." *Nature* 211 (1966): 863.

BRANHAM, J. M. "Separation of Rabbit Semen into Two Populations of Spermatozoa by Centrifugation." *Journal of Reproduction and Fertility* 22 (1970): 469–482.

CUTRIGHT, PHILLIPS; BELT, STEPHEN; and SCANZONI, JOHN. "Gender Preferences, Sex Predetermination, and Family Size in the United States." *Social Biology* 21 (1974): 242–248.

ERICSSON, R. J.; LANGEVIN, C. N.; and NISHINO, M. "Isolation of Fractions Rich in Human Y Sperm." *Nature* 246 (1973): 421–424.

ETZIONI, AMITAI. "Sex Control, Science, and Society." *Science* 161 (1968): 1107–1112.

GARDNER, R. L., and EDWARDS, R. G. "Control of the Sex Ratio of Full Term in the Rabbit by Transferring Sexed Blastocysts." *Nature* 218 (1968): 346–348.

GRIBNAU, F. W. J. "Selecting the Sex of One's Children." *Lancet* 1 (1974): 1228–1229. Letter to the editor.

HUDSON, ELIZABETH A. "The Cytological Difference between Amniotic Fluids of Male and Female Fetuses." *British Journal of Obstetrics and Gynaecology* 82 (1975): 523–528.

JONES, R. J. "Sex Predetermination and the Sex Ratio at Birth." *Social Biology* 20 (1973): 203–211.

LAHIRI, SUBRATA. "Preference for Sons and Ideal Family in Urban India." *Indian Journal of Social Work* 34 (1974): 323–336.

LAPPÉ, MARC, and STEINFELS, PETER. "Choosing the Sex of Our Children: A Dream Come True or . . .?" *Hastings Center Report* 4, no. 1 (1974), pp. 3–7.

LARGEY, GALE. "Sex Control and Society: A Critical Assessment of Sociological Speculations." *Social Problems* 20 (1973): 310–318.

———. "Sex Control, Sex Preferences, and the Future of the Family." *Social Biology* 19 (1972): 379–392.

LINDAHL, PER ERIC. "Separation of Bull Spermatozoa Carrying X and Y Chromosomes by Counter-streaming Centrifugation." *Nature* 181 (1958): 784.

McDONALD, JOHN. "Sex Predetermination: Demographic Effects." *Mathematical Biosciences* 17 (1973): 137–146.

MARKLE, GERALD E., and NAM, CHARLES B. "Sex Predetermination: Its Impact on Fertility." *Social Biology* 18 (1971): 73–83.

MONTAGU, M. F. ASHLEY. *The Natural Superiority of Women*. New York: Macmillan, 1968, pp. 77–78.

NELSON, M. M., and EMERGY, A. E. H. "Amniotic Fluid Cells: Prenatal Sex Prediction and Culture." *British Medical Journal* 1 (1970): 523–526.

PARKS, GERALD S. "Y-Linked Genes and Male-Sex Determination." *New England Journal of Medicine* 293 (1975): 1095.

POHLMAN, EDWARD. "Some Effects of Being Able to Control Sex of Offspring." *Eugenics Quarterly* 14 (1968): 274–281.

REPETTO, ROBERT. "Son Preference and Fertility Behavior in Developing Countries." *Studies in Family Planning* 3 (1972): 70–76.

RHINE, SAMUEL A.; CAIN, JEFFREY L.; CLEARY, ROBERT E.; PALMER, CATHERINE G.; and THOMPSON, JOSEPH F. "Prenatal Sex Detection with Endocervical Smears: Successful Results Utilizing Y-body Fluorescence." *American Journal of Obstetrics and Gynecology* 122 (1975): 155–160.

RORVIK, DAVID M., with SHETTLES, LANDRUM BREWER. *Your Baby's Sex: Now You Can Choose*. New York: Dodd, Mead & Co., 1970.

"Selecting the Sex of One's Children." *Lancet* 1 (1974): 203–204. Editorial.

SEROW, W. J., and EVANS, V. J. "Demographic Effects of Prenatal Sex Selection." *Population Index* 36 (1970): 319.

SEVINÇ, AFIF. "Experiments on Sex Control by Electrophoretic Separation of Spermatozoa in the Rabbit." *Journal of Reproduction and Fertility* 16 (1968): 7–14.

SHETTLES, LANDRUM BREWER. "Conception and Birth Sex Ratios." *Obstetrics and Gynecology* 18 (1961): 122–130.

STINNER, WILLIAM F., and MADER, PAUL DOUGLAS. "Son Preference among Filipino Muslims: A Causal Analysis." *Social Biology* 22 (1975): 181–188.

WALTER, STEPHEN D. "Sex Predetermination and Epidemiology." *Social Science and Medicine* 9 (1975): 105–110.

WESTOFF, CHARLES F., and RINDFUSS, RONALD R. "Sex Preselection in the United States: Some Implications." *Science* 184 (1974): 633–636.

II
ARTIFICIAL INSEMINATION

Artificial insemination (AI) is a relatively simple medical procedure which provides an alternative to childlessness. However, by altering the natural processes of procreation and providing human beings with the potential for exercising control over the generation and quality of human life, AI also raises complex ethical, legal, and social issues.

To perform AI, semen is introduced by means of a syringe into the female vagina, cervical canal, or uterus in order to induce pregnancy. The procedure has a high probability of success, depending on such variables as the quality of the semen specimen and the timing of the insemination (Guttmacher). There is no evidence of any increased mortality or abnormality rate in the progeny. AI is of two basic types: homologous, when the semen is obtained from the husband (AIH); and heterologous, when the semen is acquired from a donor (AID). Reasons for using AIH include physical or psychological difficulties which preclude cervical insemination through intercourse and some cases of oligospermia (deficient sperm count), whereby a number of ejaculates are pooled so that the spermatozoa can be separated from the semen and subsequently inseminated in concentrated form. AID is medically indicated in instances of the man's sterility, possible hereditary disease, rhesus incompatibility, or in most cases of oligospermia. Applying these criteria, an estimated total of ten thousand conceptions through AI occur annually in the United States (Sagall).

Some of the more formidable ethical questions AI raises concern its relationship to marriage and the consequences it has for the meaning of parenthood. One ethical perspective (Ramsey) argues that the bond between marriage and procreation is inseparable; that man is not merely a reproductive mechanism. Since AI divides the sexual unity between husband and wife, it violates the covenant of marriage

(AID is especially considered to be a gross unfaithfulness toward one's spouse). Furthermore, AI is an assault on the concept of parenthood by transferring procreation to the laboratory; it dehumanizes parenthood by separating the biological potential from the human potential. Another view, however, suggests that faithfulness in marriage is more than a legal requirement or a sexual monopoly. Rather, it is a personal covenant nourished by love, with the love and care that the child receives being crucial factors. For many childless couples, therefore, AI may be a truly human and loving act (Fletcher). The ethical friction, then, between these two contrasting views is whether the use of AI, especially AID, to induce pregnancy within the marital relationship is intrinsically immoral and dehumanizing; or rather, is it a special and human way of expressing marital love and of accepting the moral responsibilities of parenthood when physical problems preclude natural procreation?

If husband and wife consent to the procedure, AIH presents no real legal difficulties. However, a common legal problem that arises when a donor's semen is used is whether a child so conceived is legitimate. The problem occurs because the child conceived by AID is not the true biologic offspring of both the husband and wife. Unfortunately, inconsistent rulings in the few judicial cases on the subject preclude a definitive resolution of this legal issue. While some American states (e.g., Georgia, Kansas, New York, Oklahoma) have enacted statutes that confer legitimacy on a child conceived by AID, in the majority of states a child so conceived may well be declared illegitimate by the courts. Yet to subject an AID child who is conceived as a result of careful planning and husband–wife consent to the social stigma of an illegitimate child who is unwanted and unplanned would appear to be unjust.

The selection of donors for AID raises a number of ethical and social questions. Since the donor has no control over the use of his semen, responsibility for how the semen is used now rests with the physician. However, the nature and limits of his responsibility remain undefined. For example, what criteria should a physician use in selecting a "suitable" donor? Are there minimal medical and genetic tests that should be conducted? Although there is a danger of transmitting infectious or genetic diseases through AI, present methods of donor selection and testing vary widely. Such differences mean that prospective recipients and the community have no minimum standards of practice upon which to rely. The absence of procedures designed to test the biologic and genetic adequacy of the donated semen suggests the taking of highly unethical risks from which the inseminated female, her husband, and their progeny might suffer.

To protect the rights and welfare of all parties involved in AID, a consent agreement between the recipient and the physician should be executed. The emotional effects of donor insemination, its ambiguous legal status, and the possibility of transmitting infectious and genetic diseases are compelling reasons for obtaining informed consent. But what information should such agreements include? Are recipients entitled to know the donor's health status and semen quality? Should they be given a genetic profile of the donor? The ethical and legal responsibilities of the physician performing AI to inform his patients remain unclear at the present time.

AI may also be used to influence the genetic quality of the human species by making available genetic material from carefully selected donors (Muller). There are certainly humane reasons for using AID to prevent the birth of a potentially defective child (negative eugenics). But is there similar justification for a technological breeding program designed to "improve" the human race (positive eugenics)? Questions such as what human qualities should be considered "desirable" and by whom those choices should be made raise profound ethical and social issues. A disproportionate use of certain donors would also result in the eventual reduction of genetic variability in the population. The genetic diversity of the human species has long been recognized as necessary for ensuring the adaptability to future environments, so essential to survival in the face of constant evolutionary change. It may be morally and biologically unwise, therefore, to tamper with human genes without greater knowledge regarding the conditions of future environments.

MARK S. FRANKEL

[*Directly related are the subsequent articles in this entry,* ETHICAL ISSUES *and* LEGAL ASPECTS. *For further discussion of topics mentioned in this article, see the entries:* EUGENICS; GENE THERAPY; *and* GENETIC DIAGNOSIS AND COUNSELING. *Other relevant material may be found under* CONFIDENTIALITY; FUTURE GENERATIONS, OBLIGATIONS TO; LIFE; SEXUAL ETHICS; *and* LAW AND MORALITY.

See APPENDIX, SECTION I, PRINCIPLES OF MEDICAL ETHICS, *and* ETHICAL AND RELIGIOUS DIRECTIVES FOR CATHOLIC HEALTH FACILITIES.]

BIBLIOGRAPHY

FLETCHER, JOSEPH F. "Artificial Insemination: Our Right to Overcome Childlessness." *Morals and Medicine.* Princeton: Princeton University Press, 1954, pp. 100–140.

GUTTMACHER, ALAN F. "Artificial Insemination." *Annals of the New York Academy of Sciences* 97 (1962): 623–631.

MULLER, HERMAN J. "Human Evolution by Voluntary Choice of Germ Plasm." *Science* 134 (1961): 643–649.

RAMSEY, PAUL. "Parenthood and the Future of Man by Artificial Donor Insemination, Etcetera, Etcetera." *Fabricated Man.* New Haven: Yale University Press, 1970, pp. 104–160.

SAGALL, ELLIOT L. "Artificial Insemination: I. Legality Considerations." *Medical Counterpoint*, October 1972, pp. 55–60.

WOLSTENHOLME, G. E. W., and FITZSIMONS, DAVID W., eds. *Law and Ethics of AID and Embryo Transfer.* Ciba Foundation Symposium, n.s., no. 17, Amsterdam: Associated Scientific Publishers, 1973.

III
SPERM AND ZYGOTE BANKING

Sperm, ovum, and zygote banking promises humans greater control over their reproductive processes and evolution. Sperm banking—the freezing and preservation of sperm at low temperatures—has developed to the point where facilities are now available in a number of American cities (Frankel). With minor variations, the most accepted cryopreservation (low-temperature preservation) technique is the immersion of sperm in liquid nitrogen at $-196.5°C$. Although the fertilizing capacity of frozen sperm is approximately two-thirds of that of fresh sperm, more than five hundred normal births have resulted from its clinical use (Sherman). Sperm banking has a long history of use in livestock breeding and is also used to preserve the "seeds" of endangered animal species. In humans, it is used as a way of overcoming infertility; as "fertility insurance" for men who wish to undergo vasectomy (irreversible surgical procedure that prevents the passage of sperm into the male ejaculate) while hoping to retain their fertility for future use; and in research into human genetic diseases and reproductive processes. In the future it may permit couples to predetermine the sex of their children or be used to further eugenic goals.

No human ovum banking—the cryopreservation of an unfertilized egg—is at present being done. For practical reasons, there is greater incentive to proceed with the freezing of fertilized eggs (zygotes). Animal research has shown that the freezing process is complicated by a tough membrane which surrounds the ovum, and the more fully developed fertilized egg is better able to survive the freezing and thawing process. Yet, once these technical difficulties are resolved, human ovum banking will be possible and the ethical and social questions it raises will be similar to those of sperm banking.

In zygote banking—the cryopreservation of fertilized eggs—oocytes (eggs) are first removed from the female ovary by laparoscopy, a minor surgical operation that involves the insertion of a needlelike instrument into the egg sac. The eggs are then fertilized by sperm in vitro (outside the female body) and can be frozen to temperatures ranging from $-196°C$ with liquid nitrogen to $-269°C$ with liquid helium (Edwards; Whittingham, Leibo, and Mazur). While this procedure has uses similar to those of sperm banking, undoubtedly its most controversial application in humans would be the implantation of a frozen zygote into the female uterus (not necessarily that of the original egg donor) for routine gestation and birth. Work with frozen zygotes has thus far been entirely with animals, with some successes reported with mice and rabbits.

Ethical and social issues associated with sperm and zygote banking emerge in several dimensions. Both techniques must still be considered experimental, with their degree of safety still unknown. The total number of pregnancies from the use of frozen sperm stored longer than six months is very small, which means that the genetic and biological consequences of long-term cryopreservation are uncertain. Furthermore, there are now no procedures for determining the genetic and biologic "fitness" of a zygote prior to implantation. Yet, there is evidence that demonstrates that irreversible damage can occur during the freezing process. And although experiments indicate that animal zygotes are highly resistant to induced damage, it is uncertain whether conducting diagnostic tests on human zygotes would itself cause unsuspected anomalies. The prominent issue of medical safety, then, relates to potential progeny. Under what circumstances should it be morally permissible to use frozen sperm or zygotes for the purpose of generating new life? What ethical responsibilities are there to any child whose conception and future development are subject to these manipulative procedures? Should children damaged by such procedures be entitled to compensation for their suffering? Since there is at present no way of predetermining the dangers to the human embryo from these techniques, there are those who argue that they should never be tried on humans (Kass; Ramsey). For them, these procedures are an unethical form of experimentation. Others, however, contend that such an argument, if applied to all research, would stifle medical progress. Moreover, they insist that the benefits to be gained far outweigh the risks and that animal experimentation has provided sufficient evidence to allow for the use of these procedures on humans (Edwards; Sherman).

The availability of sperm and zygote banking for therapeutic and contraceptive purposes raises several ethical issues regarding informed consent. Because both are clearly experimental techniques, prospective users should be informed that their use will not necessarily result in pregnancy. This is especially important, since many infertile couples will be anxious to consent to any procedure that offers them the slightest hope of conception. It is too easy to exploit, even unintentionally, the desperation of such a couple, and it would be cruel and unethical to engender false expectations. Similarly, men may use sperm banking to block out their anxiety over the irreversibility of vasectomy, assuming that their fertility will be assured at some later date. No assurances can be made, however, and it would be unethical to allow such men to undergo vasectomy in the belief that their sperm will maintain its fertilizing capacity after freezing. There is also the question of how much information about the uses of extra sperm, eggs, or zygotes should be provided to prospective donors. Consent forms now used by American sperm banks fail to make clear the possible research uses, e.g., in vitro fertilization with donor sperm (Frankel). Persons seeking to store their sperm or eggs should be informed of the possible research that may be performed and its consequences.

The use of sperm and zygote banking to ameliorate infertility and to promote various eugenic goals will require a considerable supply of sperm and eggs. Since sperm specimens from different donors vary in their capacity to endure the process of freezing, storage, and thawing, a good deal of trial and error will be involved in order to identify the "best" sperm. In order to attract these highly sought-after specimens, it may be necessary to compensate donors. Compensation is already common practice among American sperm banks (ibid.) and raises several questions about the impact on contemporary social values. If sperm and eggs are treated in practice as market place commodities, what will be the consequences for the donation of such vital organs as eyes or kidneys? To what extent will the buying and selling price of frozen sperm or zygotes determine the quality of the product and its consequences for the recipient? Will this lead to a bank's promise of "eugenically desirable" sperm or zygotes to the highest bidder? And will individual donors view compensation as a sign that they no longer need be concerned with the consequences of their act? The search for the "best" sperm or eggs will eventually lead to those donors whose sperm or eggs exhibit the greatest fertilizing capacity after freezing. Such donors will thus be the genetic parents of a greater proportion of progeny than would be expected from their normal history of fertility. Unless such frequently used donors are examined thoroughly for possible genetic disease traits, harmful recessive genes could inadvertently proliferate throughout the population. The matter of genetic testing is complicated, however, by the fact that the majority of diseases cannot now be detected. How, then, can society maximize the safety and well-being of prospective users and their progeny? And what are the responsibilities of the physician who requests the sperm or zygote for clinical use? Should he be held morally and legally responsible for the procurement practices adopted by the banks? At this time, the nature of the responsibility between the physician and the bank remains undefined.

The right of ownership over donated eggs, sperm, or zygotes also remains ambiguous. Does the donor relinquish ownership upon donating egg or sperm? Do they then become the property of the bank? What is the status of the sperm or eggs after the donor's death? Are the spouse or heirs entitled to assume ownership? Should the physician/scientist be given certain "rights of research" over stored sperm or zygotes? Under what circumstances should it be morally and legally permissible to perpetuate in vitro a human zygote? If the zygote should then mature into a viable fetus, whether by accident or by intent, who should have responsibility for its care? And what interests does society have in the ultimate use or disposal of human sperm or zygotes?

Sperm and zygote banking also have eugenic

applications. A couple in which both partners are carriers of complementary recessive genes could prevent the birth of a potentially afflicted child by substituting their sperm or eggs with those of a donor known to be free of such genes or by simply requesting a "defective-free zygote." Promoters of such negative eugenics contend that every child should have the "right" to be born with a sound physical and mental constitution (Glass). A program of positive eugenics could also be implemented, whereby "superior" human beings could be bred by mating eggs and sperm from donors possessing certain desirable features. Frozen sperm and eggs would permit a high degree of selectivity among donors to assure such preferred matching (ibid.). These techniques might also be used to predetermine the sex of children, either to avoid sex-linked diseases or to satisfy parental preferences. The availability of such programs, however, raises some troublesome questions. Will they promote an unhealthy preoccupation with "good genes," perhaps to the psychological or physical detriment of those who now suffer from such disability? Should highly valued medical resources be used to satisfy a couple's desire for a boy or girl? And what of the ethical propriety of discarding zygotes when they do not measure up to preferred genetic standards, or of fetal abortion should the offspring be of the "wrong" sex? At issue in such eugenic programs is not only the biologic and genetic quality of the human species, but the quality of its social and cultural values as well.

MARK S. FRANKEL

[*Directly related are the subsequent articles in this entry*, ETHICAL ISSUES *and* LEGAL ASPECTS. *For further discussion of topics mentioned in this article, see the entries*: EUGENICS, *article on* ETHICAL ISSUES; FETAL RESEARCH; *and* RESEARCH, BIOMEDICAL. *See also*: ABORTION, *article on* CONTEMPORARY DEBATE IN PHILOSOPHICAL AND RELIGIOUS ETHICS; CONTRACEPTION; HUMAN EXPERIMENTATION, *article on* BASIC ISSUES; SEXUAL ETHICS; *and* STERILIZATION.]

BIBLIOGRAPHY

EDWARDS, R. G. "Fertilization of Human Eggs in Vitro: Morals, Ethics and the Law." *Quarterly Review of Biology* 49 (1974): 3–26.

FRANKEL, MARK S. "Role of Semen Cryobanking in *American Medical Association* 220 (1972): 1346–1350. (1974): 619–621.

GLASS, BENTLEY. "Science: Endless Horizons or Golden Age?" *Science* 171 (1971): 23–29.

KASS, LEON R. "Babies by Means of In Vitro Fertilization: Unethical Experiments on the Unborn?" *New England Journal of Medicine* 285 (1971): 1174–1179.

RAMSEY, PAUL. "Shall We 'Reproduce'? I. The Medical Ethics of In Vitro Fertilization." *Journal of the American Medical Association* 220(1972):1346–1350.

SHERMAN, J. K. "Synopsis of the Use of Frozen Human Semen since 1964: State of the Art of Human Semen Banking." *Fertility and Sterility* 24 (1973): 397–412.

WHITTINGHAM, D. G.; LEIBO, S. P.; and MAZUR P. "Survival of Mouse Embryos Frozen to −196° and −269° C." *Science* 178 (1972): 411–414. Reprint. *Selected Readings: Genetic Engineering and Bioethics.* 2d ed. Edited by Robert A. Paoletti. New York: MSS Information Corp., 1974, pp. 100–107.

IV
IN VITRO FERTILIZATION

Fertilization (the union of egg with sperm) is obviously a prerequisite of procreation. In an effort to explore the biological, biophysical, and biochemical events in the fertilization process, techniques to achieve fertilization in vitro (within a glass) have been developed for egg and sperm of several laboratory animals. Laboratory fertilization of human eggs has also been achieved. Such human studies, not unexpectedly, have raised ethical questions. The purpose of this article is to review the techniques that have been developed for human in vitro fertilization, to evaluate the technical problems associated with these techniques, and to consider the experimental and therapeutic purposes of such procedures and their ethical implications.

Technical procedures

Human ovum recovery. Work with human ova must at present be viewed as experimental. With few exceptions, ovum recovery is carried out in volunteers during the course of a medically indicated abdominal operation (laparotomy) or laparoscopy. Laparoscopy, a technique for visualizing the abdominal contents, involves placing a telescope through a small incision in the umbilicus. It is used extensively in evaluating female infertility and for tubal sterilization.

During laparotomy or laparoscopy a small number of ova are aspirated by needle puncture. They are then placed in a nourishing liquid culture medium. Removal of ova does not significantly increase the risk of the procedure to the patient. There is no evidence that removal of oocytes (eggs prior to maturation) causes damage to the ovary. The normal female has 400,000 to 500,000 oocytes at birth, so there is no danger of depleting the supply of eggs.

If the operative procedure is performed not

for purposes of maintaining or improving the patient's health but solely to recover oocytes for culture, fertilization, and transfer, the issues are compounded. One would then be obliged to consider a more complex risk-benefit ratio. In the initial phases of experimentation the questions asked by the experimenter would include the risk to the mother (in the procedure itself), and the benefits to her (a successful pregnancy), as well as the risk to the fetus (possibility of deformity).

In some centers patient volunteers are pretreated with pituitary hormones in order to obtain properly conditioned ova for fertilization. The use of pituitary hormones allows standardization of the menstrual cycle and simultaneous maturation of several ova containing follicles. These hormones have been used extensively for the induction of ovulation in infertile patients, and this treatment has been responsible for occasional production of ovarian cysts and multiple births. Treatment with gonadotropins (hormones formed in the pituitary gland and acting on the sex organ) imposes an additional risk, that of the hormonal treatment itself, although thus far no complications have been reported when it has been used for ovum recovery.

Ovum culture and insemination. On recovery, oocytes are cultured in vitro under controlled conditions. Semen is obtained by masturbation. Spermatozoa are separated from the semen by centrifugation, and washed; measured amounts are placed in culture chambers containing the oocytes. In several mammalian species, spermatozoa must be conditioned through exposure to the female reproductive tract before they acquire the ability to fertilize. This conditioning process, referred to as capacitation, does not appear to be as complicated or as prolonged in the human as in some of the lower mammals. It is apparently completed in vitro, possibly through exposure to the fluid recovered from the follicle (follicular fluid) along with the egg. Conditions of culture are critical if development is to proceed normally, and a proper balance of nutrients and carefully monitored temperature and oxygenation are important. The percentage of human ova that proceed through the blastocyst stage, the point at which they would ordinarily implant in the uterine wall, is small. Embryonal development to that stage has, however, been documented in the human.

Transfer of the fertilized ovum. If a cultured embryo is to be transferred to the uterine cavity for implantation, placement must be timed to coincide with development of the endometrium (uterine lining). At present there is no way to be sure that in vitro conditions are sufficiently well controlled for development not to occur faster or slower than would occur in vivo (in the living body). Normally the endometrium is progressively modified following ovulation. The endocrinologic events that occur following removal of an oocyte from its follicle (artificial ovulation) are still not completely understood. Discrepancy between the stage of development of the embryo and the level of maturation of the endometrium would predictably result in a high rate of implantation failure. Although successful cases have been widely reported, transfer to the uterus with continued development to viability has not as yet been documented in the scientific literature.

Experimental and therapeutic purpose of human in vitro fertilization

Most investigators share the opinion that at this time in vitro fertilization of the human ovum is of importance solely for biologic experimentation. The potential use of the technique with ovum transfer is a separate and more demanding issue. Opinion on the appropriateness of this use is divided. Since fertilization, on the one hand, and transfer of the product, on the other, involve risks of a different order of magnitude, the experimental and therapeutic purposes of each are best considered separately.

In vitro fertilization and culture. Since fertilization occurs in the fallopian tube (the conduit between the ovary and the uterus), the process is inaccessible and can be observed and evaluated best in vitro. Although animal models are useful in establishing important basic knowledge, one cannot confidently make inferences from the laboratory animal to Homo sapiens. There are substantial differences in fertilization even among closely related laboratory species. Understanding of *human* fertilization could result in development of systems for evaluation of human infertility or for more efficient methods of conception control. Examples of how in vitro fertilization could be used are considered below.

1. The effectiveness of antifertility agents could be tested in vitro. In this way medications could be initially evaluated without subjecting a patient to the effects of an untried drug.

2. The in vitro system could be used to evaluate the fertilizability of ova of patients with infertility and to assess the structural and bio-

chemical normality of the conceptus in patients who have had repeated spontaneous abortion.

3. The effect of noxious agents, or teratogens, on the human conceptus (product of conception) could be evaluated in vitro. Such a screening system is much needed.

4. In vitro fertilization is being used for genetic studies in order to understand the mechanisms behind the production of such conditions as Down's syndrome (mongolism). Knowledge gained from such experimentation could lead to the development of methods to predict or prevent such unfortunate consequences of defective reproduction.

5. The recently fertilized ovum is a totipotential cell and in vitro culture systems could be used to advance our understanding of normal and abnormal cell growth and differentiation.

Laboratory procedures for human in vitro fertilization and ovum culture involve no significant risk to the donors of ova and spermatozoa. The pivotal issue relates to the status of the in vitro created embryo itself. Does the embryo constitute new human life, and if so is the experimenter responsible for its inevitable demise? The purposes for which the experiments are designed clearly involve cessation of culture with observations on the embryo from the one-cell stage through the blastocyst at six to seven days. Predictably technology will eventually allow more advanced development.

Embryo transfer.· Following in vitro fertilization and culture, the ovum may be transferred to a recipient uterus for implantation. The obvious practical application of this technology, once developed, is to obviate the necessity of the fallopian tube. In patients with absent or severely damaged tubes one might someday remove an ovum from the ovary, fertilize it, culture the product, and return it to the uterus. The incidence of tubal disease has increased recently as a result of the rising prevalence of gonorrhea, which may severely damage the fallopian tubes.

Ovum donor treatment—removing an ovum from a female donor, fertilizing with a husband's spermatozoa, and returning it to his wife, whose eggs are defective (genetically abnormal or damaged by disease) or absent—has also been suggested. The male counterpart of this procedure is artificial insemination using a donor's specimen. In the latter the wife has normal gametes and the husband has absent or defective spermatozoa. An extension of this approach is the transfer of the in vitro produced embryo to the uterus of a surrogate mother. This would allow an ovum donor with a diseased or absent uterus, or one who is unable or unwilling to proceed through pregnancy, to procreate without actually bearing a child.

It has been suggested that systems of in vitro fertilization, culture, and transfer could be used for "genetic engineering." Substitution of one gene for another is not at this point feasible. Cloning, i.e., removal of the nucleus from an egg and substituting the nucleus of a body cell, has been cited as a possibility. Theoretically this system would provide the egg with the complete genetic composition of the donor from whose cell the nucleus had been removed, and thus one would produce a genetically identical offspring. Cloning has not been accomplished in mammalian eggs. It has, however, been carried out in the amphibian. In practical terms these procedures will require thousands of attempts using various approaches and can be developed only in the experimental laboratory mammal.

The risk of returning an in vitro fertilized embryo to the uterus must be scrutinized with great care. Animal evidence that the offspring are normal does not guarantee that the procedures would work equally well in the human. Statistically valid proof in animals that present techniques predictably produce normal offspring has not as yet been presented. Indeed, successful experiments have not been carried out in the monkey, and results in other laboratory species are far from conclusive.

Those who favor human embryo transfer concede that it is impossible to guarantee that genetic normality of in vitro handled material but suggest that it is equally true that each normally produced conceptus has no guarantee of future health. Nature's way of handling at least some genetic abnormalities is through spontaneous abortion. Under normal conditions fetal wastage is in excess of fifty percent, i.e., more than fifty percent of human conceptuses are destined to abort, many before the skipped menstrual period. Genetic screening in mid-trimester pregnancy allows evaluation of the chromosomal integrity of the fetus. These techniques uncover only the most obvious genetic disease. If the fetus were shown to be abnormal a decision would have to be made as to whether the defective fetus should be aborted. It is true that the mammalian ovum is particularly hardy and can be manipulated vigorously in the laboratory and yet continue through normal development. For example, cells from donor mouse embryos can be placed into the embryo of the recipient with subsequent normal development of the product. Such experiments do not, however, support the safety of actual in vitro fertilization and cleavage.

Those who have taken the position that transfer experiments are now, and will continue to be, unacceptable espouse the view that there is no way to evaluate the risk of damage to a child so generated from experiments in the laboratory animal. The possibility of misuse of such techniques for "genetic engineering" has been raised. It is suggested that, although controlled reproduction is not now within the realm of possibility, at some point in the future these techniques may become feasible unless experimentation in this area is curtailed. The premise here is that appropriate societal safeguards may not be possible and, even if generally agreed upon now, may not be observed in the future.

While some scientists express confidence that present technology will soon allow successful clinical application of ovum transfer, others, on reasonable ground, believe that such predictions have little validity. In any case, it is reasonable, and in the view of some essential, to consider the ethical decisions that face society in anticipation of such biotechnical advances. Meanwhile, optimistic predictions of future success victimize patients with tubal infertility who are led to believe that a solution to their infertility problem is close at hand. Clinicians treating infertility know that often their patients are willing and enthusiastic subjects. Investigators in the area of in vitro fertilization should be aware of the impact of overly optimistic statements concerning the possibility of the use of these techniques. Those treating infertile patients should temper their enthusiasm for new and untried approaches with an extreme degree of caution.

LUIGI MASTROIANNI, JR.

[Directly related are the subsequent articles in this entry, ETHICAL ISSUES and LEGAL ASPECTS. For further discussion of topics mentioned in this article, see the entries: EUGENICS; FETAL RESEARCH; and HUMAN EXPERIMENTATION. For discussion of related ideas, see the entries: ABORTION; FETAL–MATERNAL RELATIONSHIP; GENETIC SCREENING; and SEXUAL ETHICS.]

BIBLIOGRAPHY

"Asexual Reproduction and Genetic Engineering: A Constitutional Assessment of the Technology of Cloning." *Southern California Law Review* 47 (1973–1974): 476–584.

DE KRETZER, D.; DENNIS, P; HUDSON, B.; LEETON, J; LOPATA, A.; OUTCH, K.; TALBOT, J.; and WOOD, C. "Transfer of a Human Zygote." *Lancet* 2 (1973): 728–729.

DZIUK, PHILIP. "Embryo Transfer: An Experimental Tool with Practical Applications." *BioScience* 25 (1975): 102–106.

EDWARDS, R. G., and STEPTOE, P. C. "Physiologic Aspects of Human Embryo Transfer." *Progress in Infertility*, 2d ed. Edited by S. J. Behrman and R. W. Kistner. Boston: Little, Brown & Co., 1975, pp. 377–409.

"Genetic Engineering: Reprise." *Journal of the American Medical Association* 220 (1972): 1356–1357.

KASS, LEON R. "Babies by Means of In Vitro Fertilization: Unethical Experiments on the Unborn?" *New England Journal of Medicine* 285 (1971): 1171–1179.

———. "Making Babies—The New Biology and the 'Old' Morality." *Public Interest*, no. 26 (1972), pp. 18–56.

MASTROIANNI, LUIGI, JR. "Fertilization and the Tubal Environment." *Hospital Practice* 7, no. 3 (1972), pp. 113–119.

RAMSEY, PAUL. "Shall We 'Reproduce'? I. The Medical Ethics of In Vitro Fertilization." *Journal of the American Medical Association* 220 (1972): 1346–1350.

———. "Shall We 'Reproduce'? II. Rejoinders and Future Forecast." *Journal of the American Medical Association* 220 (1972): 1480–1485.

SCHUMACHER, GERHARD F. B.; BRACKETT, B. G.; FLETCHER, JOSEPH; MARIK, J. J.; MASTROIANNI, LUIGI, JR.; SHETTLES, L. B.; TEJADA, R.; and TYLER, EDWARD T. "In Vitro Fertilization of Human Ova and Blastocyst Transfer: An Invitational Symposium." *Journal of Reproduction Medicine* 11 (1973): 192–204.

SEITZ, H. M., JR.; BRACKETT, B. G.; and MASTROIANNI, LUIGI, JR. "Fertilization." *Human Reproduction: Conception and Contraception*. Edited by E. S. E. Hafez and T. N. Evans. Hagerstown, Md.: Medical Department, Harper & Row, 1973, pp. 119–131.

WOLSTENHOLME, G. E. W., and FITZSIMONS, DAVID W., eds. *Law and Ethics of AID and Embryo Transfer*. Ciba Foundation Symposium, n.s., no. 17, Amsterdam: Associated Scientific Publishers, 1973.

V

ASEXUAL HUMAN REPRODUCTION

Nonsexual (also called asexual) reproduction is a common mode in simpler life forms. Single-celled organisms most frequently reproduce by direct binary fission (although sexual modes may be elicited by specific environmental conditions). Fungi and simple multicelled organisms such as coelenterates (e.g., jellyfish) can reproduce by budding, releasing a single cell or a detached cluster of cells capable of regenerating the organism.

Nonsexual reproduction provides (most often) faithful genetic perpetuation. The progeny of a single cell or a single organism reproducing asexually is a *clone;* all of the individuals of a clone are genetically identical.

Reproduction in more complex forms is most commonly achieved by sexual means, involving the participation of highly specialized germ cells, sperm and eggs. The fertilized egg cell has the unique capability to develop into the mature organism.

By introduction of the element of chance into the determination of the set of genetic characters (the genotype) of each descendant, sexual reproduction provides increased genetic variety and thus, most often, affords evolutionary advantage.

However, the *potential* exists for the asexual reproduction of higher organisms and has long been recognized in plants. Ordinarily sexual plant forms have been propagated by grafting, from cuttings, and, in the laboratory, even from single cells of a mature organism after appropriate culture. The differentiation of plant cells (the specialization of individual cells for a particular function) appears, in at least some instances, to be plastic and reversible, permitting such reformation of the entire organism.

Until recently, similar propagation by asexual reproduction has not been possible in more complex animals. It has not been possible to reverse the developmental process which gives rise (from the fertilized egg) to the specialized cells of the adult; such differentiated cells, when isolated, could not be induced to repeat the ordinary embryonic process.

The development of the technique of nuclear transplantation has created a new potential for the asexual reproduction and cloning of higher animal forms. This potential is based upon the concept that each nucleus present in every cell of the adult organism is believed to contain the entire genetic complement of that organism. The developmental program gives rise to the diverse types of differentiated cells by control of the *expression* of the various genetic factors in each cell type.

Thus, for instance, the nucleus within an adult intestinal cell is genetically identical to that of the fertilized egg which gave rise to that adult (although it is in a very different functional state). Further, when the nucleus of a differentiated cell is extracted and mechanically inserted into an enucleated egg cell of the same species the program of expression of the transplanted nucleus is reset to that of the fertilized egg, i.e., it will direct the egg cell to begin the developmental process characteristic of that species.

The product of this development beginning with the transplanted nucleus will be an individual genetically identical to that adult from which the nucleus was taken. Since many nuclei could be obtained from the cells of one adult and each transplanted into an appropriate egg cell, a large number of genetically identical organisms could thereby be produced by this cloning process.

(Such individuals could conceivably differ in their cytoplasmic inheritance. The mitochondria —small, bacteria-size organelles found in the extranuclear cytoplasm of all cells of higher organisms—possess their own genetic material, distinct from that found in the nucleus. The mitochondrial genes give rise to what is known as cytoplasmic inheritance, which obeys different rules from those governing ordinary nuclear inheritance. However, the genetic content of a mitochondrion is less than .001 percent of that of the nucleus; also, the potential diversity of mitochondrial genes among the members of a species is unknown. Hence variability of cytoplasmic inheritance among the members of a nuclear transplant clone is not likely to be of much significance.)

Nuclear transplantation has been successfully accomplished in insects and in amphibia with a modest percentage of success. In these instances the fertilized egg develops in an external medium.

Attempts at asexual reproduction of mammals by nuclear transplantation have so far been unsuccessful. However, as far as is known, the difficulties are technical rather than intrinsic. The mechanical introduction of the nuclear transplant into the much smaller volume of a mammalian egg (a mouse egg has 1/3500 the volume of a frog egg) is likely to be far more disruptive than in the amphibian. Attempts to introduce the nucleus by cellular fusion have so far been unsatisfactory, possibly because of the need either to strip the egg of its normal protective layers or to perforate those layers.

If a successful nuclear transplant into a mammalian egg can be achieved, the necessary subsequent steps for cloning are already in hand, at least in certain species. Mouse eggs, for instance, can be fertilized in vitro, cultured in the test tube to the blastocyst stage (a small cluster of embryonic cells), implanted into the uterus of a hormonally prepared female mouse, and brought to full term with an appreciable percentage of success. The extension of such techniques to man would not seem likely to pose major technical difficulty.

The potential applications of cloning to agriculture, if and when technically feasible, are evident and would not seem to involve significant ethical issues. The potential application of cloning to man, however, involves very basic questions of ethical principle and social policy.

We are, in fact, already familiar with accidental clones: identical twins. The physical and psychological similarities of identical twins have often been remarked. Indeed, comparisons of correlations within sets of identical twins with those within sets of fraternal twins are one of the most powerful means to ascertain the relative contributions of genetic and environmental factors to individual characteristics.

Cloning of human beings has been proposed as a means to perpetuate and to increase the proportion in the human population of particular genotypes, selected for certain qualities exemplified in the life of the prototype, e.g., intellectual or artistic or athletic ability, physical beauty, sturdiness of health, lack of genetic disease, longevity, docility, submissiveness, etc. It is implicit in such proposals that genetic factors are the predominant components that contribute to such qualities (and indeed the twin studies are cited as evidence).

The validity of this assumption (as to the relative importance of genetic and environmental factors) is inherently constrained to the range of environmental variation over which it has been (and could be) tested in each particular instance. In particular the correlations within twin sets can be demonstrated only within the range of environments available within the given epoch of their lives (and in practice, the range available is even more constrained).

Further, the relation between genotype and realized social role is obscure and potentially subject to profound temporal modification. As a specific instance, even if largely genetic, the qualities that make an individual the greatest physicist or painter of his day may or may not be those needed to advance the science or the art in a subsequent era.

The central ethical issue involved in human cloning concerns the generation of human beings for some specific social purpose. Cloning implies the germinal subordination of the individual to the demands of society, in the sense that one's genes become the product not of chance, but of social decision, based upon historically accepted values and individual precedents.

The social issues involved in human cloning concern the criteria for the choice of genotypes to be cloned and the politics of that decision-making process. Different choices could lead to very diverse social orders ranging from a specialized, insect-like society to a homogeneous society, with a much reduced diversity of genetic potential.

If introduced on a small experimental scale (as is likely), human cloning would create extraordinary issues for both the clonees and their sponsors. It is uncertain how the clonees would react to their special and preselected status. It is uncertain how the rest of society, and particularly their "normal" cohorts, would react to them. The sponsors of the clonees would both wish to monitor the progress of the experiment and bear a special responsibility to its subjects. The entire society, which sets at least minimal standards for the preservation of individual human dignity, would have a stake in the project.

If adopted on a large scale, human cloning would inevitably result in major and irreversible social change, including marked reduction in human genetic and (possibly) social diversity. The consequences of such a transition with respect to the prospects for human conflict or for intellectual, artistic, or social progress are difficult to foresee. Cloning could come to be the accepted, cultured, superior mode of human reproduction and the present unpredictable genetic lottery regarded as barbaric. Or cloning could be seen as a repression of potential human individuality and thus a denial of our most basic humanity.

The ethical and social quandaries associated with cloning are but facets of the quandaries associated with the broader prospect of intervention into the human biological inheritance. What responsibilities do we have to our descendants with respect to their genetic endowment? Cloning would specify such endowment precisely; specific genotypes would be the consequence of deliberate decisions, based upon observed lives. Is human wisdom adequate for such a project? At present our ability to forecast the efficacy of cloning is grievously limited by our ignorance of the extent of specific human genetic predestination. The same ignorance thereby shrouds sharp definition of the attendant ethical and social issues.

ROBERT L. SINSHEIMER

[*Directly related are* GENE THERAPY, *article on* CELL FUSION AND HYBRIDIZATION; *and the subsequent articles in this entry,* ETHICAL ISSUES *and* LEGAL ASPECTS. *See also:* GENETIC CONSTITUTION

AND ENVIRONMENTAL CONDITIONING; *and* GENE THERAPY, *article on* ETHICAL ISSUES.]

BIBLIOGRAPHY

BURHOE, RALPH WENDELL, ed. *Science and Human Values in the 21st Century.* Philadelphia: Westminster Press, 1971.

EDWARDS, R. G., and FOWLER, RUTH E. "Human Embryos in the Laboratory." *Scientific American* 223, no. 6 (1970), pp. 44–54.

GRAHAM, CHRISTOPHER F. "Genetic Manipulation of Mouse Embryos." *Advances in the Biosciences.* Vol. 8: *Workshop on Mechanisms and Prospects of Genetic Exchange.* Edited by Gerhard Raspé. New York: Pergamon Press, 1972, pp. 263–273.

GURDON, J. B. "Transplanted Nuclei and Cell Differentiation." *Scientific American* 219, no. 6 (1968), pp. 24–35.

HARRIS, HENRY. *Cell Fusion.* Cambridge: Harvard University Press, 1970.

HILTON, BRUCE; CALLAHAN, D.; HARRIS, M.; CONDLIFFE, P.; and BERKLEY, B., eds. *Ethical Issues in Human Genetics.* New York: Plenum Press, 1973.

KASS, LEON R. "Making Babies—The New Biology and the 'Old.'" *Public Interest,* no. 26 (Winter 1972), pp. 18–56.

MUKHERJEE, ANIL B., and COHEN, MAIMON M. "Development of Normal Mice by In Vitro Fertilization." *Nature* 228 (1970): 472–473.

RAMSEY, PAUL. *Fabricated Man.* New Haven: Yale University Press, 1970.

SONNEBORN, TRACY MORTON, ed. *The Control of Human Heredity and Evolution.* New York: Macmillan Co., 1965.

STEWARD, F. C. "The Control of Growth in Plant Cells." *Scientific American* 209, no. 4 (1963), pp. 104–113.

———. "The Croonian Lecture, 1969. From Cultured Cells to Whole Plants: The Induction and Control of Their Growth and Morphogenesis." *Proceedings of the Royal Society of London* ser. B, 175 (1970): 1–30.

VANDENBERG, STEVEN G., ed. *Progress in Human Behavior Genetics.* Invitational Conference on Human Behavior Genetics. Baltimore: Johns Hopkins Press, 1968.

WOLSTENHOLME, GORDON ETHELBERT WARD, ed. *Man and His Future: A Ciba Foundation Volume.* Boston: Little, Brown & Co., 1963.

VI
ETHICAL ISSUES

Introduction

The term "reproductive technologies" must be properly limited before its ethical dimensions are set forth. This article will not deal with abortion, contraception, delivery (including Caesarean sections, induced labor), amniocentesis, therapeutic interventions for mother or child (e.g., ectopic pregnancies), and genetic screening, even though they may all legitimately qualify as reproductive technologies in the broader sense.

The meaning of "reproductive technologies." The term "reproductive technologies" will be limited here to all procedures that replace, in part or totally, the natural (by sexual intercourse) process of conception and of *in utero* gestation. Practically this would include (1) artificial insemination (homologous, when the insemination is from the husband's semen [AIH] and heterologous when the insemination is from a donor [AID]), (2) in vitro fertilization (with sperm of husband or donor, with ovum of wife or donor) with subsequent implantation (in wife or host womb) or without it (artificial placenta), and (3) cloning. Other technologies such as sperm banking, ovum banking, and zygote banking are generally ancillary and instrumental to those procedures. The ancillary procedures may raise specific ethical and policy problems rooted in effectiveness, danger, confidentiality, selection criteria, etc. On the other hand they may raise very few problems. For instance, few would have any problem with totally artificial gestation (artificial placenta) if it were the only way of possibly saving an otherwise doomed fetus, that is, if the artificial placenta were therapeutic in purpose. However, the main ethical issues cluster around the three technologies noted.

Several things should be remarked about the use of these three technologies. First, they progressively increase in the replacement of so-called natural processes. Just as artificial insemination replaces sexual intercourse, so in vitro fertilization does that and more. It replaces tubal fertilization and natural implantation, and could conceivably replace natural gestation. Second, many of the arguments used to justify or condemn one type of intervention reappear where another type is involved. However, even though there is an overlapping in the application of principles, there is sufficient difference in the procedures to make it necessary to discuss each individually.

Motive for intervening. The reproductive interventions in question, or at least most of them, may be motivated by a variety of considerations:

1. They could be *individual* or *personal* in purpose, even though such purposes have social dimensions (marriage, parenthood). Thus AID could be and is employed to overcome the husband's infertility secondary to oligospermia and azoospermia, or when fertilization by husband is undesirable because of hereditary disease. Similarly, in vitro fertilization followed by artificial implantation could be used where the wife suffers from tubal blockage. Or again, embryonic transfer to a surrogate womb might be attempted where the wife is a habitual and intractable spontaneous aborter. Finally, under personal

motivation would be included embryonic transfer to a host womb in situations where the only reason is convenience or dislike of pregnancy.

2. Reproductive interventions could be *eugenic* in purpose (planned breeding). Such eugenics are either positive or negative. Positive eugenics is "preferential breeding of so-called superior individuals in order to improve the genetic stock of the human race" (Hirschhorn, p. 63). The best known of such eugenicists is Herman J. Muller who proposed sperm banks from preferred donors to assure the continuance of desirable traits in the race. Negative eugenics is defined as "the discouragement or the legal prohibition of reproduction by individuals carrying genes leading to disease or disability" (ibid.). This purpose can be implemented in a variety of ways (e.g., genetic counseling, sterilization, and in its most intense form, abortion). These means have their own ethical aspects and problems.

The reproductive technologies discussed in this article would fall into the category of either personal interventions or interventions of positive eugenics. In other words, they are not by and large examples of negative eugenics.

The ethical discussion of such interventions could occur, then, at two distinguishable levels: the level of the personal and the level of positive eugenics. The types of ethical problems raised differ depending on the level of discussion. Furthermore, there are ethical assumptions hidden in the very level one chooses as the appropriate one to discuss the interventions. Thus one who derives the moral character of AID exclusively from the level of positive eugenics assumes that there is no objection to be made in terms of its possible violation of marital fidelity, the notion of parenthood, etc.

Interventions for positive eugenics

The ethical problems associated with any regime of positive eugenics, and therefore one that would use the reproductive technologies mentioned above, are enormous. In showing why both scientists and nonscientists have a powerful aversion to positive eugenics, R. A. Beatty has put the problems as clearly as possible:

First, wherever it has been attempted on a large scale it has been in the hands of evil men. Secondly, there is no proper measure of indefinable qualities such as nobility or courage; and if we cannot measure a character, we cannot select for it. Thirdly, even if selection were effective, the results would not necessarily be something to look forward to with pleasure. The controllers of positive eugenics would probably be leaders of religious or political power

groups. Desirable human qualities—those tending to perpetuate the power group—would no doubt include submissiveness to the power group and readiness to act rashly on its behalf. Undesirable qualities would probably include gentleness and the questioning of the power group's authority. With relief, one must conclude that mankind is simply not ready for positive eugenics [Beatty, p. 60].

Similar objections to reproductive technologies as the tools of positive eugenics have come from others. Bentley Glass refers to "frightful dilemmas" (Glass, p. 119). For example, how does one judge a "good" genotype when what is the optimum in one set of circumstances may be inferior in another? In selecting for certain characteristics, one sacrifices other desirable traits and compromises overall adaptability. Who does the judging, and with what criteria? Is technical intelligence even with reduced emotional and moral development to be preferred to a less developed IQ in a person of profoundly human qualities (compassion, generosity, love)? Similar questions and objectives are registered by the community of ethicists (Häring, p. 170).

A further problem with approaching reproductive technologies as tools of positive eugenics is that positive eugenics is simply unworkable. Hirschhorn notes that "neither positive nor negative eugenics can ever significantly improve the gene pool of the population and simultaneously allow for adequate evolutionary improvement of the race" (Hirschhorn, p. 67). Similarly, Peter Medawar argues that a regimen of selective inbreeding is not scientifically acceptable. The reason for this is that the end product of selective inbreeding (the supercattle, supermice, etc.) were expected to fulfill two functions. "The first function was to be end-product itself, to be the usable, eatable, or marketable goal of the breeding procedure. The second function was to be the parents of the next generation of super animals" (Medawar, p. 75). In order to fulfill the second function, the end product had to be homozygous or one that would breed true with regard to the desirable qualities that conditioned the selection process. Medawar argues that most geneticists think this view mistaken. On that basis he asserts that "it is *populations* that evolve, not the lineages and pedigrees of old-fashioned evolutionary 'family trees,' and the end-product of an evolutionary episode is not a new genetic formula enjoyed by a group of similar individuals, but a new spectrum of genotypes, a new pattern of genetic inequality, definable only in terms of the population as a whole" (ibid., p. 90). Medawar concludes that the newer genetic conception (that it is *populations* that breed true, not its individual members) means that "the goal of positive genetics, in its older form, cannot be achieved, and I feel that eugenic policy must be confined . . . to *piecemeal genetic engineering* [emphasis in original]" (ibid.). By that phrase Medawar means negative eugenics in the individual setting.

Because positive eugenics is scientifically problematic and because the ethical problems inseparable from it (were it workable) are enormous, the ethical discussion of reproductive technologies has generally taken a more modest path—the assessment of technologies as they relate to marriage, parenthood, sexual love, or the good of the child.

Interventions for personal purposes

In the following sections ethical appraisals of specific reproductive interventions will be offered and analyzed. Before proceeding to that, however, it will be useful to note some general orientations to reproductive interventions.

Many in the scientific community, e.g., Joshua Lederberg, R. G. Edwards, R. Francoeur, along with such ethicists as Joseph Fletcher and William Hamilton, contend that the principal reproductive interventions already mentioned can be fully justified. Those writers share some definite presuppositions (to be examined at length later), three of which seem to be central to their arguments. First, they incline toward a consequentialistic or teleological normative position. That is, they hold that an act or practice is right and just if, on balance, it does more good than harm and helps to minimize human suffering. Second, they incline to the view that sharply distinguishes between sexual love and the generation of human life, seeing in them quite disparate activities. As Fletcher puts it, we have succeeded in separating completely "babymaking from lovemaking" (Fletcher, 1971, p. 781). Third, they regard parenthood as a relationship essentially and primarily defined by acts of nurturing, not by acts of begetting.

Some members of the scientific community, e.g., Leon Kass, and the majority of religious ethicists initially approach the issues of reproductive interventions with a great deal more caution, principally because they share a different set of presuppositions. First, they are not pure teleologists in their moral thinking. That is, they argue that factors other than consequences need to be taken into account in offering a valid ethical evaluation of any human act, although many such writers do believe that a proportionately

good enough end can justify the deliberate, direct intent to effect some kinds of disvalues or evils. Second, they maintain that a meaningful and reciprocal relationship between sexual love and the generation of human life exists and that it is no mere evolutionary accident that human beings come into existence through an act that is also capable of expressing love between a man and woman. Third, while recognizing that acts of nurturing life are distinct from acts of generating life and that acts of nurturing are included within the meaning of parenthood, they also affirm that acts of generating life are parental in nature and carry with them responsibilities for nurturing the life generated.

In the following discussions of specific reproductive interventions and in the analysis of the arguments employed, the presuppositions of the two groups will become more manifest and will be subjected to critical scrutiny.

Artificial insemination

Since artificial insemination among humans, though known and performed in the nineteenth century, did not become common until the twentieth century, the ethical discussion of the procedure is heavily located in this period.

Artificial insemination by donor. In this section attention will center on the arguments offered by those who belong to the second group of authors previously mentioned. Their presuppositions will become evident in the exposition of their arguments.

Roman Catholic appraisals. Within the Catholic community, there never was and still is not much wavering on AID, although occasionally individual authors manifest doubts or even endorse it as ethically acceptable. It was and still generally is seen as morally wrong, and for several reasons, not all of equal weight. First, and above all, it violates the marriage covenant wherein exclusive, nontransferable, inalienable rights to each other's bodies and generative acts are exchanged by spouses. Even the more personalistic approaches to marriage subsequent to the Second Vatican Council have not substantially altered that appraisal. Second, as Pius XII worded it, "So it must be, out of consideration for the child. By virtue of this same bond, nature imposes on whoever gives life to a small creature the task of its preservation and education. Between the marriage partners, however, and child which is the fruit of the active element of a third person—even though the husband consents—there is no bond of origin, no moral or juridical bond of conjugal procreation" (Pius XII, 1950,

p. 252). Third, once conceded the right, even by their own husbands, to be inseminated artificially by the seed of another man, wives might too easily conclude that it would be preferable to receive the seed in the natural way (sexual intercourse). Thus, adulteries would be multiplied to the detriment of marriage. Fourth, the human stud-farming mentality toward marriage would be fostered. (These last two considerations are but supportive teleological arguments, that is, arguments built on possible and probable consequences.)

One of Catholicism's leading theologians, Karl Rahner, has put the matter as follows:

Now this personal love which is consummated sexually has within it an essential inner relation to the child, for the child is an embodiment of the abiding unity of the marriage partners which is expressed in marital union. Genetic manipulation [Rahner means AID here], however, does two things: it fundamentally separates the marital union from the procreation of a new person as this permanent embodiment of the unity of married love; and it transfers procreation, isolated and torn from its human matrix, to an area outside man's sphere of intimacy. It is this sphere of intimacy which is the proper context for sexual union, which itself implies the fundamental readiness of the marriage-partners to let their unity take the form of a child [Rahner, p. 246].

Rahner adds other confirmatory arguments. For example, the donor remains anonymous, thus refusing his responsibility as father and infringing the rights of the child so conceived. Furthermore, AID commonly practiced would lead to two new races, the technologically bred supergroup and the ordinary, unselected group, and this at the very time we are attempting to dismantle all other forms of discrimination.

Jewish appraisals. Most rabbinic opinion sees AID as an abomination. With arguments very similar to those used in Catholic literature, Jakobovits summarizes the rabbinic attitudes: "By reducing human generation to stud-farming methods, AID severs the link between the procreation of children and marriage, indispensable to the maintenance of the family as the most basic and sacred unit of human society. It would enable women to satisfy their craving for children without the necessity to have homes and husbands" (Jakobovits, pp. 248–249). Other reasons are also offered for regarding AID as prohibited: possibility of incest, lack of genealogy, problems of inheritance.

However, while that is the dominant rabbinic view, it is not universal. Dr. Soloman B. Freehof writes: "My own opinion would be that the possibility of the child marrying one of his own kin is far fetched, but that since according to Jewish law the wife has committed no sin and the child is 'kosher,' then the process of artificial insemination should be permitted" (quoted in Friedman, p. 104). Rabbinic opinion continues to be divided on whether AID should be regarded as adultery and the child illegitimate.

Protestant appraisals. The ethical analysis in the Protestant community reveals several diverging points of view. Joseph Fletcher argues that AID is not a violation of the marriage bond because (1) marriage is not a physical monopoly, and mutual consent by husband and wife protects AID against the accusation of broken faith, and (2) the donor's relationship to the wife is completely impersonal (Fletcher, 1954, p. 139).

Contrarily, Helmut Thielicke argues that the psychophysical totality of the marriage is threatened by the presence of the AID child, which is a factual incarnation of the division of the one-flesh unity of husband and wife. He states: "The problem is presented by the fact that here a third person enters into the exclusive psychophysical relationship of the marriage, even though it is only his sperm that 'represents' him" (Thielicke, p. 259). Similarly, Paul Ramsey utterly rejects AID on the theological grounds that it separates what may not be separated: "To put radically asunder what God joined together in parenthood when He made love procreative, to procreate from beyond the sphere of love . . . or to posit acts of sexual love beyond the sphere of responsible procreation (by definition, marriage) means a refusal of the image of God's creation in our own" (Ramsey, 1970, p. 39). Thus, the spheres of responsible procreation and personal love must be held together if our conduct would reflect the creative love of God.

While accepting the substance of Ramsey's argument and giving a qualified "no" to AID, others add further practical objections. For example, in light of the demographic and ecological facts of our time, adoption serves the common good better than AID. Furthermore, when done for eugenic reasons, AID creates the enormous problem of deciding what qualities we should breed for and who decides this (Smith). Still others note that both AID and adoption involve sacrifice and risks. However, adoption and AID enjoy a markedly different status and acceptance in the community. For adoption there is a "more complete supportive network helping the parents to adjust emotionally to their sterility and evaluate themselves as parents" (Richards, p. 323). This, plus the radical asymmetry of the parents' relationship to the AID child and the psychological difficulties involved in that asymmetry, means AID is the riskier of the two options and ought to be rejected as such.

Artificial insemination by husband. When AIH is under discussion, the matter is remarkably different.

Developments within Roman Catholicism. Within Catholicism AIH was for years defended by some as at least probably permissible, if semen was obtained in a licit (nonmasturbatory) way. The reasons adduced against AID were not there, and the method seemed a defensible way of overcoming the sterility problems of the couple. In 1949 Pius XII intervened and said AIH "must be absolutely eliminated." In support of his rejection he noted:

We must never forget this: it is only the procreation of a new life according to the will and plan of the Creator which brings with it—to an astonishing degree of perfection—the realization of the desired ends. This is, at the same time, in harmony with the dignity of the marriage partners, with their bodily and spiritual nature, and with the normal and happy development of the child [Pius XII, 1949].

In 1951 Pius XII returned to the subject in more detail. He stated:

To reduce the cohabitation of married persons and the conjugal act to a mere organic function for the transmission of the germ of life would be to convert the domestic hearth, sanctuary of the family, into nothing more than a biological laboratory. . . . The conjugal act in its natural structure is a personal action, a simultaneous natural self-giving which, in the words of Holy Scripture, effects the union "in one flesh." This is more than the mere union of two germs, which can be brought about artificially, that is, without the natural action of the spouses. The conjugal act as it is planned and willed by nature, implies a personal cooperation, the right to which the parties have mutually conferred on each other in contracting marriage [Pius XII, 1951, p. 850].

The argument, then, of Pius XII, was that even AIH is immoral, because the child so born is not the fruit of an act *of itself* the expression of personal love. The hidden assumption in this argument would seem to be that the child must always be conceived of an act *of itself* a personal expression of love if marriage is not to be converted into a biological laboratory. That is the import of the phrase "willed by nature." Recent Catholic theologians have suggested that this is only generally true. That is, if procreation were

commonly and routinely to occur via AIH, a long step would have been taken toward biologizing and mechanizing marriage, thus undermining it. However, if AIH is not a substitute for sexual intercourse, but in relatively rare cases its complement, the reasoning would not seem to support the absolute prohibition. This has led a number of theologians to maintain the probable moral licitness of AIH, at least in some instances of infertility, e.g., Häring, Curran, Lobo.

Protestant and Jewish approaches. A tolerant attitude is certainly dominant in the Protestant and Jewish communities. The very ethicists who most clearly and sometimes severely condemn AID, e.g., Ramsey, Thielicke, Smith, and Jakobovits, have little problem with AIH as a morally legitimate intervention to overcome infertility. For at least many ethicists the self-stimulation that produces the semen is not seen as problematic, either because it is not an invariably necessary procedure or because it does not (as finally procreative in purpose) fall within the class of prohibited masturbatory acts. Furthermore, there is no foreign (donor) intrusion into the marital covenant or the psychophysical totality that is marriage.

Analysis of the arguments. It is clear, then, that the ethical aspects of artificial insemination have been approached from the dominant perspective of the meaning of marriage, parenthood, and the family. Furthermore, the majority opinion of ethicists has been that AID, by the introduction of donor semen, separates procreation from marriage, or the procreative sphere from the sphere of marital love, in a way that is either violative of the marriage covenant or likely to be destructive of it and the family.

Here it is opportune to examine in more detail the views of those writers, previously referred to, who operate with a different set of presuppositions. Obviously, they would not agree with this approach to the question. Some argue that sexual intimacy and procreation are and should be distinct human acts each governed by "totally distinct ethics" (Francoeur, p. 109). Still others would argue that "the demand of love in relation to parenthood is fulfilled in ensuring that all children born into this world, *by whatever means* [emphasis added], be reared in a family" (Hamilton, p. 743). This position rests on the conviction that parenthood is, in its deepest sense, not principally a matter of biological begetting but a more broadly human function—a man and a wife accepting responsibility for caring for and rearing a child.

A possible counterstatement to that approach would be one that argues that in Christian conviction the same sexual love that generates ought to become *in principle* the parental love that nurtures (McCormick, 1969). Parents do not love their children simply because the children are there and need love. They ought to love them because they have loved each other and because the children are the visible fruit and extension of that love. That is, it has been said—sometimes clumsily to be sure—that conjugal love is by its very nature "ordained for the procreation and education of children, and finds in them its ultimate crown" (Vatican Council). Just as education is, in a sense, a continuation of procreation, so there ought to be a basic identity and continuity in the love that procreates and the love that nurtures. Therefore to separate the acts that nurture from the act that generates, and then to associate parental love only with the former, is to undermine the very foundation of the love that nurtures. To limit the notion and love of parenthood to "caring for and rearing a child" is therefore a radical attack on several basic humano-Christian values (the meaning of human sexuality, the meaning of marriage and parenthood).

This argument must be properly understood; otherwise it could be used to show that adoption is an attack on some basic humano-Christian values. The argument is that we ought not to separate *in principle* the acts that generate from the acts that nurture, that the notion of parenthood ought *in princple* to include both. Obviously conceptions occur *in fact* where marriage is impossible or inadvisable, and adoption offers the best resolution of the situation. Just as obviously, marriages *in fact* break up and remarriage occurs. In these situations it is clear that the child can be (and ought to be) loved, cared for, and protected within a family context wherever possible. The argument insists only that these are surrogate arrangements and that we ought to try to avoid them in principle insofar as possible.

The Hamilton approach holds that parenthood is not a biological but a human function. It identifies the human function with accepting responsibility for rearing a child. Summarily, caring for and rearing a child is human, procreating him is biological. But since parenthood and parental love are obviously human, procreation as such does not pertain to them.

Here, it might be argued, we are face to face once again with an all too familiar and destructive dualism, where persons love and care in many ways, but not in their sexual intercourse. Ultimately such an attitude is rooted in a principle that depreciates the body and disallows its participation in the specifically human. This is the area and these the concepts and arguments that have by and large surrounded discussion of AID. It is important because it sets the stage for some of the ethical arguments that will be used in assessing in vitro fertilization and cloning.

There has been little discussion of AID where the husband is fertile but the wife sterile. That would involve an anonymous (preferably) ovum, and perhaps uterus, donor to provide the husband his self-fulfillment as a father. It is not properly AID as it has been discussed but represents a reproductive intervention that raises some of the problems associated with AID. Thus on the very principles espoused where artificial insemination is concerned, those against AID would be a fortiori opposed to such procedures. For they involve an even greater intrusion into or threat to the marital covenant and family. In this light sperm banks and ovum banks whose *sole purpose* is some form of AID would share in the moral acceptance or rejection attributed to the AID procedure itself. (It is possible, of course, that such storage could serve other therapeutic purposes, for example, research on infertility problems.)

Ultimate factors in decision making. At this point it is important to make a methodological point about the arguments and analyses used in the discussion of artificial insemination, because such a methodological consideration will be operative in the assessment of other reproductive interventions.

The point to be underlined is the relationship of an ultimate moral judgment to the reasons used to express it. Some theologians involved in the discussion of reproductive interventions insist that there is a "moral instinct of faith" (Rahner). The "instinct" under discussion can be called by any number of names; but the point is that there is a component to moral judgment that cannot be adequately subject to analytic reflection. But it is this component that is chiefly responsible for one's ultimate judgments in concrete moral questions. In that sense the ultimate judgments are not simply the sum of the rational considerations and analyses one is capable of objectifying. For that reason Rahner states explicitly that "all the 'reasons' which are intended to form the basis for rejecting genetic manipulation," such as AID, "are to be understood, at the very outset, as only so many references to the moral faith-instinct (and as so many appeals to it, to have the courage to take a clear decision). For in my view the moral faith-instinct is aware of its right and obligation to reject genetic manipulation, even without going through (or being able to go through) an adequate process of reflection" (Rahner, p. 243).

Something very similar to this is used by the scientist Peter Medawar. What is the line between a humanizing use of technology and a dehumanizing one? The answer we give in practice "is founded not upon abstract moralizing but upon a certain natural sense of the fitness of things, a feeling that is shared by most kind and reasonable people even if we cannot define it in philosophically defensible or legally accountable terms" (Medawar, p. 84).

This nondiscursive element in ethical discourse is important. One of the central assertions of those who regard AID (and a fortiori more drastic reproductive interventions) as morally wrong is that procreation of a human being ought not occur outside the covenanted relationship of marriage. While various warrants (some biblical, some teleological) can be gathered to support that assertion, it remains true that it cannot be proved by rational arguments or analytic reasoning in a totally satisfactory way. This will be viewed as a fatal weakness only if one fails to realize that in all moral judgments concerned with basic human values there is a prethematic and instinctive component that cannot be totally recovered in analytic discourse. For our knowledge of those values or goods is not first of all discursive.

In that sense the arguments pro and con AID, in vitro fertilization, etc., important as they are, are always more or less imperfect, more or less incomplete, more or less persuasive. They only externalize, rationalize, and communicate a spontaneous sense of the rightness or wrongness of things. To think otherwise would almost invariably convert moral judgments in this area into technological judgments. It is in this sense that the "natural sense of the fitness of things" (Medawar) or "moral instinct of faith" (Rahner) underlies and animates the positions and arguments on reproductive interventions.

In vitro fertilization

R. G. Edwards notes that there are three areas of medicine that could benefit greatly from the studies surrounding in vitro fertilization: (1) Some forms of infertility (blockage of the oviduct) could possibly be cured; (2) knowledge useful for contraceptive technology could be gained; and (3) knowledge and methods could be obtained leading to the alleviation of genetic disorders and even other deformities (Edwards, p. 27).

The simplest instance of in vitro fertilization is extraction of the wife's oocytes by laparoscopy, fertilization with husband's sperm followed by laboratory culture to the blastocyst stage, then embryo transfer (implantation) into the wife's uterus. The procedure would be aimed at overcoming sterility due to obstruction of the fallopian tubes. This is the "simplest" instance because it does not raise the further issues of donor sperm, host wombs, and totally artificial gestation.

The ethical issues involved in such a procedure are multiple, even if only this simplest form is in question. They involve considerations of justice, the beginning of human life, and the value of life, in addition to the questions of parenthood and sex. First, there is question of embryo wastage. Only one or two of the eggs taken from the mother would be transferred back into her. The remaining embryos would be discarded (ibid., p. 28). Those who are convinced that human personhood begins with fertilization would reject in vitro fertilization on that ground alone, for it would involve the deliberate destruction of human life to achieve a pregnancy.

However, other ethicists argue that there is a genuine doubt about whether we are dealing with a human person at this stage of development. The existence of such a doubt leads to a variety of conclusions. Some say that the very probability of human personhood constitutes "an absolute veto against this kind of experimentation" (Häring, p. 198). Others, while remaining basically negative, argue that given such a positive doubt, "the reasons in favor of experimenting might carry more weight, considered rationally, than the uncertain rights of a human being whose very existence is in doubt," (Rahner, p. 236). Finally, there are some who would undoubtedly agree with Joseph Fletcher that the product of in vitro fertilization is but human tissue, "fallopian and uterine material" (Fletcher, 1974, p. 88).

Edwards's response to these serious ethical concerns seems unconvincing. He notes that in discarding embryos experimenters are doing nothing more than women who use intrauterine contraceptive devices. However, rather than an argument supporting embryo wastage, this could be viewed as an objection against intrauterine devices—to the extent that they achieve contraceptive effectiveness by expelling embryos. The same response could be made to his assertion that, "in a society which sanctions the abortion of a fully-formed fetus, the discarding of such a minute, undifferentiated embryo should be acceptable to most people" (Edwards, p. 28). Such an argument says nothing of the moral rightness or wrongness of abortion, but only of a particular society's toleration or sanctioning of it. As a form of ethical argument, it is equivalent to saying that a society that tolerates obliteration bombing of cities should not object to a little selective torture of enemy prisoners. While that may be true in terms of ethical consistency, it says nothing about the moral rightness or wrongness of either procedure.

The second serious ethical problem with in vitro fertilization is its experimental character. It has been argued that, given the unknown hazards associated with laboratory culture and embryonic transfer, and the inability to overcome such unknown hazards, in vitro fertilization with subsequent implantation constitutes potentially hazardous experimentation with a human subject without his consent (Ramsey, 1972; Kass, 1971). That is, risks are chosen for the future human being without his consent. More concisely, the experimental phase of this technology can only be shown to be risk-free by exposing a certain number of subjects to unethical experiments. Therefore we can never get to know how to perform such procedures in an ethical way. The argument does not rest on ascription of personal status to the embryo who is eventually discarded during development of the technology (though, as noted above, some ethicists would see a serious problem here too). Rather, it points to the possible harm to be inflicted on living children who come to be born after in vitro fertilization and laboratory culture. There is at present no way of finding out whether the viable progeny of these procedures will be deprived or retarded. Nor would a willingness to practice abortion on the deformed solve the problem, since many such deformities cannot and will not be identifiable by amniocentesis.

Others contend that this argument is not altogether persuasive, for procreation by natural processes produces a certain percentage of deformed, crippled, or retarded children. Thus the natural process of sexual intercourse also imposes serious hazards on future children without their consent and is no less "experimental" in this sense than laboratory fertilization with embryo transfer. Thus the problem is to bring the dangers associated with in vitro fertilization procedures to an acceptable level. No one has insisted that "natural" procreation be completely safe for the fetus before it is undertaken. Even in the most severe cases (women with phenylketonuria, whose offspring are virtually certain of receiving damage during gestation), it is argued that we do not constrain such couples from procreating except by moral suasion. "If we accept the morality of couples making this childbearing decision, can we deny the needs of a couple childless because of the woman's blocked oviducts?" (Lappé, p. 105.)

A double possible response could be made to this argument. First, we have no way of knowing the comparative risk ratios of the two methods of reproduction, since discovering the percentage of risk of in vitro procedures would expose a certain, perhaps very large, number of human subjects to serious risk without their consent. Second, when it is known that husband and wife are carriers of the same severe recessive, genetic disease the course of moral responsibility demands that they not run the hazards of procreation. Therefore, when faced with the possible deformities from in vitro technology, the proper response is not to point to similar deformities in natural processes as justification for creating them by technology, but to use that technology to diminish them in the natural processes.

At some point, then, this discussion opens on the morality of risk-taking even within so-called natural procreative processes. What is the responsible course for couples who are carriers for the same deleterious recessive disease (e.g., phenylketonuria) when there is a one-in-four chance that the child will be afflicted? Many, if not all, philosophers and theologians who have discussed the problem hold that running such a risk is morally irresponsible, and indeed that partners with such recessive defects ought not as a general rule to marry. As Medawar puts it, "if anyone thinks or has ever thought that religion, wealth, or color are matters that may properly be taken into account when deciding whether or not a certain marriage is a suitable one, then let him not dare to suggest that the genetic welfare of human beings should not be given equal weight" (Medawar, p. 93). The problem remains, however, of where to draw the line where risk-taking is involved. Some would argue that a one-in-four chance of a seriously afflicted child is a tolerable risk. Others would disagree.

Here, however, several points must be made to

structure the ethical discussion. First, even though abstention from childbearing may be the only responsible decision in these cases, it is another matter altogether whether this abstention should be compelled by law. Second, there is a line to be drawn where inherited defects are involved. Some diseases are relatively minor and manageable; others are enormously crippling and catastrophic for the child. Finally, in a highly technological and comfort-oriented society, the fear of having a defective child can easily become pathological. That is particularly possible in a society unwilling (unable?) to adjust itself to the needs of its most disadvantaged citizens.

The third set of arguments against in vitro fertilization concerns what it is likely to lead to, especially through the mentality it could easily foster. For instance, if in vitro fertilization is successfully (with safety and normality) introduced to treat sterility *within a marriage*, will there not be extensions beyond the marriage if either husband's sperm or wife's ovum is defective? And this raises all the ethical and theological problems associated with AID. Furthermore, the standard use of in vitro fertilization for infertility involves viewing infertility as a disease. But the accuracy of that description has been challenged not only because sterility is not a disease in the ordinary sense, but above all because viewing it as a disease tends to undermine, in thought and practice, the bond between childbearing and the marriage covenant (Kass, 1972). Those who have no problem with AID would see little force in this type of argument, or would see it overridden by the value of providing the couple with their own child. But that is where the issue is.

If these arguments are overcome, there remain other issues of ethical relevance. For instance, would children conceived by in vitro fertilization suffer any identity or status problems? Would they experience a possibly harmful pressure to research their mental, physical, and emotional development? If the technology were widely used, would that distort the priorities of the health-care system in a way that would do harm by neglect in other more urgent areas?

In vitro fertilization can also be undertaken with donor sperm, to be followed by embryonic transfer to the wife of the sterile husband, or to a host womb. Or it could occur with the sperm of the husband and an egg of another woman to be implanted in the wife (adopted embryo). Where donor sperm or ovum is used, not only is there

the issue of unknown hazards imposed without consent, but once again the relation of procreation to marriage becomes the focus of concern. The issue is intensified when a host or surrogate womb (not the wife's) is used for the pregnancy, for not only does one of the agents of fertilization come from outside the marriage, but the entire period of pregnancy and delivery is outside the marriage.

Such a rather exotic arrangement raises further formidable problems. What if the surrogate "mother" were to become disenchanted with the pregnancy and desire an abortion? What if the genetic parents desired such an abortion and tried to force the surrogate mother to undergo one? What if the genetic husband and wife are determined to have a healthy child and refuse to accept the deformed or retarded child that is born of the surrogate mother? There are additional ethical problems with the social identity of the child. Who is truly the child's mother? Who has rights and responsibilities with regard to such a child? A society, it can be argued, that already has enormous problems with marital stability would be unwise in the extreme to add freely to those problems.

Cloning

The reproductive technology known as cloning represents the most intense intervention of all. It not only removes insemination and fertilization from the marriage relationship, but it also removes one of the partners from the entire process. Its purported advantages are eugenic in character (removal of deleterious genetic material from the gene pool, and programming the genotype in such a way as to maximize certain desirable traits—e.g., intelligence, creativity, artistic ability).

There are those who judge such procedures as desirable and moral in terms of their consequences and advantages (Fletcher, 1971, 1974). If such manipulative reproduction would heighten the intelligence (or artistic, or creativity) quotient of the race, or provide solutions to some particularly difficult and intractable human problems, it is good. To the objection or at least suspicion that there might be something inhuman in laboratory reproduction of human beings, it is asserted that "man is a maker and a selector and a designer, and the more rationally contrived and deliberate anything is, the more human it is" (Fletcher, 1971, pp. 779–781). On this basis it is concluded that "laboratory reproduction is radically human compared to conception by ordinary heterosexual intercourse. It is willed, chosen, purposed and controlled, and surely these are among the traits that distinguish *Homo sapiens* from others in the animal genus" (ibid., p. 781).

Whether such value judgments are the only ones capable of supporting the ethical character of cloning may be debatable. However, they do suggest that there comes a point in the moral discourse surrounding reproductive technologies when one must step aside from the casuistry of individual interventions and view the future possibilities and directions in aggregate and in the light of overall convictions about what the "human" is. When that is done, some of the following questions arise. Will such reproductive interventions, even if they provide certain short-term remedies or advantages, actually improve the overall quality of human life? If so, how is the improvement to be specified? What is the notion of the human that functions in the description of an "improvement"? And who decides this? If the development and application of such technology are likely to be humanly destructive, why will they be such? And if the more advanced forms of reproductive technology threaten some profoundly cherished human values and institutions (parenthood, marriage, the family), and are therefore something to be avoided, or at least stringently controlled, how are these values threatened, and where was the first wrong step or threatening one taken? Those are the questions that will be asked for decades as technology becomes increasingly sophisticated.

Conclusion

In summary, then, the ethical character of reproductive interventions is to be determined by considerations clustering around benefits and such human values as sexuality and parenthood. Those most strongly in favor of encouraging such interventions point to the benefits (overcoming sterility, healthy child, eugenic improvement). Here they manifest their underlying teleological or consequentialist approach in making moral judgments. In addition, they offer an interpretation of the values of human sexuality and parenthood that (1) treats the procreative dimension of sexuality primarily as a mere biological function and (2) defines parenthood principally in terms of acts of nurturing life, not generating life. Those who oppose such interventions believe that the benefits to be secured are short-term at best and fear that the interventions will, over the long run, prove detrimental to such basic human values as parenthood, marriage,

the family, and the inviolability of the child. For them, too, human procreativity is not merely a biological function, and parenthood includes acts of begetting as well as acts of nurturing.

If the questions surrounding these values are not asked, not asked seriously, not asked publicly, not asked continually, and in advance of the use of reproductive technologies, the danger is that we will identify the humanly and morally good with the technologically possible. That is why so much is at stake in reproductive interventions—not only in the conclusions that are drawn, but in the criteria and form of moral reasoning involved.

There is not only an ethics of reproductive technology; there is an ethics of public policy or regulation of reproductive technology. The human values at stake are so great that the question arises: Should there be regulation of the technological application of research in human reproduction, and what kind of regulation? The answers given will depend to some extent on the ethical assessments of the procedures. For instance, if in vitro fertilization is judged to be unethical, some sort of regulation might be judged to be fitting.

In a situation where there is no ethical consensus, regulation becomes problematic. However, very many would be likely to agree that the issue of human embryo manipulation is so important that at least procedural cautions or regulations, self-imposed if possible, are appropriate. The following policies deserve serious consideration (cf. Kass, 1971, 1972; Lappé):

1. a profession-wide, self-imposed moratorium on experiments leading directly to human egg implantation, at least until such time as the safety of such procedures is assured and consensus can be reached about this;
2. exhaustive studies involving implants with higher primates to assess risk and normality of offspring so produced;
3. establishment of international professional bodies to evaluate research in mammalian and human reproduction.

RICHARD A. MCCORMICK

[*Directly related are the other articles in this entry, and the entry* EUGENICS, *article on* ETHICAL ISSUES. *See also:* ABORTION; CONTRACEPTION; GENE THERAPY, *article on* ETHICAL ISSUES; GENETIC DIAGNOSIS AND COUNSELING; HUMAN EXPERIMENTATION; SEXUAL ETHICS; *and* STERILIZATION, *article on* ETHICAL ASPECTS.]

BIBLIOGRAPHY

BEATTY, R. A. "The Future of Reproduction." *Selected Readings: Genetic Engineering and Bioethics.* Edited by Robert A. Paoletti. New York: MSS Information Corp., 1972, pp. 51–61.

EDWARDS, R. C. "Reproduction: Chance and Choice." *Genetic Engineering.* Edited by David Paterson. London: British Broadcasting Corp., 1969, pp. 25–32.

FLETCHER, JOSEPH FRANCIS. "Ethical Aspects of Genetic Controls: Designed Genetic Changes in Man." *New England Journal of Medicine* 285 (1971): 776–783.

———. *The Ethics of Genetic Control: Ending Reproductive Roulette.* Garden City, N.Y.: Anchor Books, 1974.

———. *Morals and Medicine: The Moral Problems of the Patient's Right to Know the Truth, Contraception, Artificial Insemination, Sterilization, Euthanasia.* Foreword by Karl Menninger. Princeton: Princeton University Press, 1954.

FRANCOEUR, ROBERT T. *Utopian Motherhood: New Trends in Human Reproduction.* Garden City, N.Y.: Doubleday & Co., 1970.

FRIEDMAN, BENJAMIN. "Symposium on Artificial Insemination: The Religious Viewpoints: Jewish." *Syracuse Law Review* 7 (1955): 104–106.

GLASS, BENTLEY. "The Human Multitude: How Many Is Enough?" *Genetic and Reproductive Engineering.* Edited by Darrel S. English. New York: MSS Information Corp., 1974, pp. 110–122.

HAMILTON, MICHAEL. "New Life for Old: Genetic Decisions." *Christian Century* 86 (1969): 741–744.

HÄRING, BERNARD. *Ethics of Manipulation: Issues in Medicine, Behavior Control, and Genetics.* Crossroad Book. New York: Seabury Press, 1975.

HIRSCHHORN, KURT. "On Re-doing Man." *Selected Readings: Genetic Engineering and Bioethics.* Edited by Robert A. Paoletti. New York: MSS Information Corp., 1972, pp. 62–71.

JAKOBOVITS, IMMANUEL. *Jewish Medical Ethics: A Comparative and Historical Study of the Jewish Religious Attitude to Medicine and Its Practice.* New York: Philosophical Library, 1959.

KASS, LEON R. "Babies by Means of In Vitro Fertilization: Unethical Experiments on the Unborn?" *New England Journal of Medicine* 285 (1971): 1174–1179.

———. "Making Babies—The New Biology and the 'Old' Morality." *Public Interest,* no. 26 (1972), pp. 18–56.

LAPPÉ, MARC. "Risk-taking for the Unborn." *Hastings Center Report* 2, no. 1 (1972), pp. 1–3.

McCORMICK, RICHARD A. "Current Theology: Notes on Moral Theology: January–June, 1969 (Genetic Engineering)." *Theological Studies* 30 (1969): 680–692.

———. "Genetic Medicine: Notes on the Moral Literature." *Theological Studies* 33 (1972): 531–552.

MEDAWAR, PETER BRIAN. *The Hope of Progress: A Scientist Looks at Problems in Philosophy, Literature, and Science.* Garden City, N.Y.: Anchor Press/Doubleday, 1973.

PIUS XII. "Iis quae interfuerunt Conventui Unionis Catholicae Italicae inter Obstetrices, Romae habito." *Acta Apostolicae Sedis* 43 (1951): 835–854. Translated as "Apostolate of the Midwife: An Address by His Holiness to the Italian Catholic Union of Midwives, October 29, 1951." *Catholic Mind* 50 (1952): 49–64.

———. "Participantibus conventus internationalis quarti medicorum Catholi corunt." *Acta Apostolicae Sedis* 41 (1949): 557–561. Translated as "To Catholic Doctors: An Address by His Holiness to the Fourth International Convention of Catholic Doctors, Castelgandolfo, September 29, 1949." *Catholic Mind* 48 (1950): 250–253.

RAHNER, KARL. "The Problem of Genetic Manipulation." *Theological Investigations.* Vol. 9: *Writings of 1965–67(1).* Translated by Graham Harrison. New York: Herder & Herder, 1972, chap. 14, pp. 225–252. Translation of "Zum Problem der Genitischen Manipulation." *Schriften zur Theologie.* Einsiedeln: Benziger Verlag, 1967, vol. 8, pp. 286–321.

RAMSEY, PAUL. *Fabricated Man: The Ethics of Genetic Control.* New Haven: Yale University Press, 1970.

———. "Shall We 'Reproduce'? I. The Medical Ethics of In Vitro Fertilization." *Journal of the American Medical Association* 220 (1972): 1346–1350.

———. "Shall We 'Reproduce'? II. Rejoinders and Future Forecast." *Journal of the American Medical Association* 220 (1972): 1480–1485.

RICHARDS, RICHARD P. "Ethical and Theological Aspects." *Soundings* 54 (1971): 315–324.

SMITH, HARMON L. *Ethics and the New Medicine.* Nashville, Tenn.: Abingdon Press, 1970.

THIELICKE, HELMUT. *The Ethics of Sex.* Translated by John W. Doberstein. New York: Harper & Row, 1964.

Vatican Council. 2d, 1962–1965. "Pastoral Constitution on the Church in the Modern World." *The Documents of Vatican II.* Edited by Walter M. Abbott. An Angelus Book. New York: Guild Press, America Press, Association Press, 1966, pp. 199–308, especially pt. 2, chap. 1, sec. 48, p. 250. *Gaudium et Spes.*

VII
LEGAL ASPECTS

This article surveys legal issues in the use of novel means of controlling the reproductive process. Few such techniques have moved beyond the experimental or merely theoretical stage of development, with artificial insemination alone at present available. The main legal problems posed are questions of access and state regulation, quality control, and the legal effect of resulting relationships. With a few exceptions the law is as undeveloped as the technology, creating confusion, ambiguity, or uncertainty, which in the absence of further judicial or legislative action could impede the development and diffusion of techniques for fulfilling individual procreative choices.

Access and state regulation

A key issue underlying the entire topic is whether the state may constitutionally prohibit the development of reproductive techniques, such as research on embryo transfer and cloning, or their application in particular circum-

REPRODUCTIVE TECHNOLOGIES: Legal Aspects   *1465*

stances. Although it is typical of this particular area that the question has not yet been directly resolved by the courts, the U.S. Supreme Court in a series of recent cases involving contraception, abortion, and marriage has recognized a doctrine of procreative privacy granting the individual wide autonomy in reproductive decisions, subject to regulation only upon the showing of a compelling state interest. Given autonomy in deciding whether to use contraception, to choose a mate, to be sterilized, or to abort, individuals appear to be also free to make reproductive decisions involving unconventional means such as artificial insemination, in vitro fertilization with embryo transfer, and the like, at least where conventional means of reproduction are unavailable. Thus, the application of adultery or fornication laws to heterologous (donor) artificial insemination would probably be held unconstitutional. The issue might never arise, however, because the trend both in the United States and in other countries is to permit infertile couples to select AID (artificial insemination by donor) as a solution to their problems.

Since few would argue that use of these devices does not fall into the sphere of reproductive choice, the main question here is likely to be whether there are any state interests that would justify limitation of individual autonomy over reproductive choices. Suggested reasons for limitation include the risk of zygote, fetal, or offspring deformity; sex ratio imbalances; denial of unique genotype to offspring; changes in concept of person; and abuse by the government. The weight of these concerns varies, and perhaps will change over time. Some of them may not be proper governmental concerns at all, and others are merely speculative. All are subject to the principle that fundamental rights may be restricted only if there are no alternative means of achieving a compelling state interest.

Costs to others. Prohibitions on research or use of embryo transfer, implantation, or cloning techniques, because they are likely to produce zygote or fetal abnormalities requiring abortion, may not be constitutionally valid if *Roe* v. *Wade* (the 1973 U.S. Supreme Court decision on abortion) is interpreted to mean that previable stages of fetal development have no intrinsic worth. While prevention of offspring deformities has a different status, the question is whether prenatal monitoring and lawful abortion would

prevent such births as effectively as a ban on the use of those techniques. Similarly, methods of sex selection could not automatically be banned because of expected societal sex ratio imbalances without a showing that less restrictive alternatives, such as tax incentives or subsidies, would not prevent the harm. Even cloning could not be banned to protect the well-being of clones, unless it could be shown that genetic, as opposed to environmental, factors had a dominant effect on personality or that knowledge of being a clone created psychosocial disabilities, and keeping one's origin a secret was impossible.

By the same token, there will be few situations in which the state's interest in requiring a person to use a particular reproductive technique would override a contrary personal choice. Laws requiring artificial insemination of infertile couples where a male factor is present, laws mandating abortion, and similar positive state intrusions into reproductive choices are probably as unconstitutional as state prohibitions on use of those techniques. Even if constitutional in a particular jurisdiction, such a policy would conflict in nearly all cases with a principle granting individuals maximum autonomy in reproductive choices.

Harm to integrity and concept of person. Although a person's use of a reproductive technology will seldom produce the tangible costs to others that justify regulation, technological control of the procreative process may impair our notions of the integrity or concept of the person as a unique, randomly assorted genotype, not fabricated or programmed to meet the needs or plans of others. The root issue in determining the limits of individual reproductive freedom will be the extent to which this idea or value achieves societal and constitutional recognition. Three reasons suggest that such considerations will not achieve legally recognized status, though they may well influence private behavior. First, several reproductive techniques that allow the individual to assert considerable control over the randomness of reproduction are widely used: selection of marriage partners, genetic screening, contraception, abortion, heterologous and homologous artificial insemination, and birth induction techniques. The new techniques such as in vitro fertilization, zygote transplants, egg and sperm banking, and the like, while extending control in significant ways, are not logically so discontinuous that prohibiting them, while allowing the former, can be justified. Second, the notion of integrity of the person as based on a randomly assigned genotype involves very basic philosophical considerations that are almost religious in nature. Elevating a particular notion of what is uniquely human into law, at the expense of the reproductive freedom of those who think otherwise, may amount to the establishment of a religion, contrary to the First Amendment. Third, if the reproductive choices of some are offensive to others, it is socially efficient to give those offended an entitlement to prevent the transaction only if the offense is very great or very pervasive. If not, it may well be that the cost to Y of allowing X to reproduce freely is less than the cost to X and others similarly situated of a converse entitlement. That is, society may well conclude that not having a child at all is much worse for X than Y's being offended at the techniques that X must use to reproduce.

Special problems of access. Although the state may not prohibit the access of married adults to reproductive technologies in most circumstances, it may be able to deny minors and perhaps unmarried persons the same access, though the latter is open to question on equal protection and due process grounds. AID, for example, may enable single women to bear a child in situations where sexual preference or social situation bars sexual intercourse. A state-funded clinic or hospital doing AID probably could not deny insemination services to a single woman without showing a substantial reason for the discrimination. Regulations that set minimum standards of quality but do not substantially impair access, such as restricting artificial insemination or zygote transfer to licensed physicians and clinics, or that regulate donor selection and storage procedures in sperm cryobanks are clearly desirable and would be constitutional if reasonably related to protecting the health or safety of users. However, the government is not required to fund research in this area or directly to make these techniques available as long as no unjustified discrimination among techniques for resolving fertility problems occurs. Finally, the state could constitutionally regulate the number of offspring to be fathered by single donors as long as individual procreative choices were not unduly impaired and the regulation were rationally related to a health or welfare goal. If the sperm and ova cryobanking industry grows, government regulation consistent with free access would appear desirable.

In sum, the right of procreative privacy will permit an individual a wide range of reproductive interventions to solve problems of infertility or sex-linked disease, or otherwise control reproductive outcomes, and few will be the circumstances justifying state limitations on development or use of those techniques.

Quality control: liabilities and obligations in use of reproductive interventions

The use of novel reproductive technologies is likely to give rise to questions of liability under traditional tort, contract, and criminal law as injuries and unexpected or unlawful outcomes occur.

Consent. One question concerns the extent of disclosure required to make a person's consent to use of these procedures legally valid. Developing case law of informed consent, as well as statutory enactments with regard to AID, suggest that a physician or other person (sperm bank) will have a legal obligation to disclose details of a procedure, particularly its likely risks and benefits, and the risks and benefits of alternative procedures, to a user, and will be liable in damages if they do not, though the precise content of disclosures will vary with the jurisdiction. A signed, written consent form detailing all information relevant to a person deciding whether to utilize a particular technique should minimize these problems. At the extreme, use of AID, harvesting of ova, etc., without consent could constitute a civil battery and possibly be subject to criminal liability.

Injury to a participant. A second area of liability is injury to one of the participants in performing the reproductive intervention. The instruments used in AID could lead to infection, or disease could be transmitted from the donor. Laparoscopy for removing eggs has a risk of complications as well as infection. Zygote transplantation may also injure the recipient, and a surrogate mother could be injured in carrying the child to term. Finally, the resulting child could also be injured because of the technical manipulations that must occur, or because of a "defective" sperm or egg cell. While no such cases have yet reached the courts, existing principles of tort law give some idea of the likely outcome. The physician or other intervenor could be liable to the parents, or to the donor, or to the offspring on a theory of (1) strict liability, (2) negligence, or (3) contract.

Strict liability would impose liability without any determination of fault or negligence, simply because of an unfortunate result. While it is possible that courts would impose strict liability because of the delicate nature of the procedure, its effect would be to raise the price of these services (because of the higher cost of insurance) or deter many physicians from employing them. A more likely possibility is the use of a negligence standard, with physicians and other intervenors being liable to the injured party if it can be shown that their actions fell below the required standard of care and this deviation caused the resulting injury. The standard of care would most likely be set by the practice of other professionals in the circumstances, though if this appears insufficient to protect consumers, a court could impose a more objective standard. Finally, reproductive interventions will be provided in accordance with implied or express terms of contractual arrangements between the parties, which also could lead to liability, as when the result guaranteed by a physician did not occur, or a particular technique or donor type was not used as agreed.

Whether the rule is strict liability or negligence, difficult problems of damage may arise when the "parents" or offspring seek damages for the birth of a deformed or otherwise impaired child. The damage could occur because of physical manipulation of egg, sperm, or zygote; because of introduction of infection or disease; or because of the occurrence of an insufficient examination or monitoring of the donor of an egg, of sperm, or of a surrogate womb to assure the absence of genetic defects. If liability were established in tort (e.g., if the physician failed to examine the donor of sperm or egg) or contract (if the physician guaranteed or warranted a healthy offspring), the parents probably would get damages for their medical expenses, pain and suffering, and, if the child were deformed, the additional costs of raising and caring for it. But the deformed offspring could not recover, because its claim appears to be that it should not have been born at all, and courts have generally agreed that claims of "wrongful life" will not be compensated. However, these cases could be distinguished, because here the child's claim is that it should have been born healthy and unimpaired, rather than not have been born at all, and because liability will give further incentives to physicians to use care in doing these procedures. It is unlikely that the offspring could sue the parents here, unless the offspring were intentionally injured.

Other liability problems. Several other instances of liability should be noted. A donor of egg or sperm could be liable to parents and/or child for neglecting to disclose illness or genetic defects that led to injury, though liability for such results, to preserve donor anonymity, may be better placed on the physician or clinic. This seems particularly warranted where cryobanking (freezing) techniques give the physician ample time to karyotype (view the chromosomal characteristics of) and test donor specimens. A donor may also seek to hold the physician/clinic or even the parent liable, if the donor status was disclosed to his or her spouse, the public, or the resulting offspring, resulting in embarrassment or psychological injury. Purchasers of sperm cryobank services would also have claims against the bank for improper handling, spoilage, insufficient disclosure, or use without consent, subject to particular contractual arrangements. Persons providing insemination and similar services would also be liable to the couple and offspring for breach of confidentiality or privacy if they unjustifiably disclosed to others the couple's use of AID. Finally, while one may speculate that a surrogate mother might seek to hold the biological or social parents liable for injuries suffered during the surrogate motherhood, assumption of the risk doctrines and specific contract between the parties will control the outcome. Similarly, biological or social parents might hold the surrogate liable for actions during the pregnancy that violated the contract or imposed a high risk of birth defects or abortion on the fetus.

In summary, use of a wide range of reproductive interventions will raise many traditional and novel questions of liability, confronting the law with the choice of imposing the costs on one or another of the several involved parties. In making this choice, the law will probably try to maximize the social interest in individual procreative autonomy by minimizing the possibility of untoward outcomes, balanced against fairness and the need to encourage development of knowledge.

Legal effect of reproductive interventions on resulting relationships

The third major area of legal concern is family law problems involving the legal status, relationship, rights, and duties of the various parties toward each other after a successful reproductive intervention. The main problems concern the legal status and rights of the offspring of AID, embryo transfer, or surrogate mother-hood vis-à-vis the egg or sperm donor, the surrogate mother, and the social parents; the effect of such a birth on relations between a married couple; and the effect of the birth on donor and surrogate mother vis-à-vis the offspring and the social parents. These questions generally do not arise with homologous insemination, with sex selection techniques, or with in vitro fertilization with husband sperm and implantation in the uterus of the egg donor, because they maintain the unity of genetic, biological, and social parenthood. Where a technique separates genetic and biological from social parentage, as in the paradigm case of AID, certainty of result and stability of family relations require clear legal answers, which have not always been forthcoming.

Legal status of the child. An important issue is the legal status of the child born as a result of an egg or sperm provided by a donor outside the marriage. While there is some precedent that the offspring of AID is illegitimate because the husband was not the biological father, there is a legislative and judicial trend in many jurisdictions to recognize the child as legitimate for all purposes. However, since clarification has occurred in only a few states, the legal status of AID offspring in the majority of jurisdictions remains unclear—a situation that appears to serve no useful social purpose and may possibly deter wider use of AID. In that case, the husband, depending on the legitimation procedure of the state, may legitimate the child by adoption, formal acknowledgement, or open acceptance. Legal status, however, may never become a problem, for the obstetrician delivering the child, who often will not know its origin, will name the husband as the father on the birth certificate, and a question of legitimacy is unlikely ever to arise.

While the cases and statutes address only AID, there would appear to be no logical basis to treat heterologous egg donation differently. On the other hand, the legal status of the offspring of a surrogate mother or artificial womb has not yet been considered, perhaps because the technique is still highly speculative. In that situation, if the goal of public policy is to facilitate realization by persons of their reproductive choice, then courts and legislatures should recognize the offspring as the legitimate child of the genetic parents (if a married couple), though a formal adoption procedure after the

birth would accomplish the same end. While one could argue that the heterologous donor of sperm or egg is the parent of the resulting child, with parental obligations and rights, such a result would advance none of the social interests at stake and is unlikely to be reached by the courts. Until detailed legislative codes specifying legal relationships are enacted, providers and consumers of these services should be aware of the resulting status ambiguity in many jurisdictions and plan accordingly, e.g., in drawing up wills.

Effect on marital relationship. A second area of concern is the effect of resort to a novel reproductive technique on the rights, duties, and relationship of a married couple. Conception by AID without spousal consent or ratification could constitute grounds for divorce, depending on the jurisdiction, though it is unlikely that anonymous donorship or banking of sperm or egg by a spouse would be similarly treated. Removal of an egg from one partner, and AID with reimplantation, or donorship of an egg from another with AID and implantation would probably be treated similarly. An important question in this area concerns the rights and duties of a husband whose wife has conceived a child by AID. In the leading case of *People* v. *Sorenson*, it was held that the father was obligated to provide support to the offspring if he consented to the AID. Other cases indicate that the husband would have support obligations if he later acquiesced in and accepted the child, even without a formal adoption. Cases have also indicated that the social father has rights concerning adoption, custody, and visitation of the offspring of AID, at least where he consented to it, despite his not being the biological father. Again, the law, if the goal of policy is to maximize individual autonomy in the procreative process, should minimize the disruptive effect on marital relations of consensual AID.

Donor or surrogate relationship. A third area of concern is the relationship between the donor of egg/sperm or surrogate mother, and the offspring. Questions here are whether the biological/genetic parent is legally a parent for purposes of support, consent to adoption, right of visitation and custody; and whether the offspring has a right to know or learn the donor's identity and be supported by or inherit property through him. These questions have not yet been faced by courts or legislatures. A sound solution would be to deny the donor or surrogate any parental rights, duties, or obligations vis-à-vis the offspring, with the sole possible exception of a duty to the offspring not to injure it in donation or surrogate motherhood. Even here, protection of the offspring may best be accomplished by holding the physician or clinic responsible for such outcomes, with no right of recovery, except by the physician or clinic, against the donor. This policy would give certainty and stability to relationships and encourage the donorship essential to a wider use of these techniques. It would then follow that the offspring would not be an heir or child of the donor for estate or support purposes, and possibly would have no right to learn who the donor was, even if he learned he was artificially conceived.

Legal status of fetus. A final highly speculative issue concerns the legal status and relationship of a zygote or fetus that is conceived in vitro and raised in an artificial or surrogate womb. The problem will be less acute if development of the zygote or fetus is aborted prior to viability. Current Anglo-American law recognizes personhood only upon a live birth, making it unnecessary (as long as public policy continues to grant the nonviable fetus little legal protection) to determine relationships prior to that time. A resulting birth, however, would raise the question of whether the genetic parents (who may be anonymous donors) or the biological parent (a surrogate mother or physician/scientist in charge of the laboratory) should be assigned the responsibility of social parentage, or whether the child shall be without a social parent until adoption occurs. Solutions here include prohibition of surrogate or artificial procreation unless a commitment for social parentage has been made, prohibition of artificial fetal development beyond a few weeks, or assigning of parental responsibility to genetic or biological parent. Again, the solution will depend on social goals and the interests that one wants to advance.

Conclusion

In summary, although some uncertainty in the legal status of relationships resulting from novel reproductive choices now exists, the uncertainty appears not to be so great as to disrupt family relations or to deter infertile couples from using these techniques. Given the long existence of AID, the absence of detailed legislative codes probably reflects societal unwillingness fully to accept individual control of the reproductive process. Until general societal attitudes shift to permit individuals greater control of their reproduction, the legal clarification necessary to facilitate the full range of reproductive interventions will be lacking.

JOHN A. ROBERTSON

[*Directly related are the other articles in this entry, and the entry* GENETICS AND THE LAW. *For further discussion of topics mentioned in this article, see the entries:* CONFIDENTIALITY; GENETIC SCREENING; INFORMED CONSENT IN THE THERAPEUTIC RELATIONSHIP; PRENATAL DIAGNOSIS; *and* PRIVACY. *Other relevant material may be found under* ABORTION, *article on* LEGAL ASPECTS; CONTRACEPTION; GENE THERAPY, *article on* ETHICAL ISSUES; MEDICAL MALPRACTICE; *and* STERILIZATION, *article on* LEGAL ASPECTS.]

BIBLIOGRAPHY

In re Adoption of Anonymous. 345 N.Y.S. 2d 430. 74 Misc. 2d 99 (Surr. Ct. King's County, 1973).

Anonymous v. Anonymous. 246 N.Y.S. 2d 835, 41 Misc. 2d 886 (Sup. Ct., Suffolk County, 1964).

Ark. Stat. Ann. sec. 61-141(c) (1971).

ATALLAH, LILLIAN [Pseudonym]. "Report from a Test-Tube Baby." *New York Times Magazine,* 18 April 1976, pp. 16–17, 48–52.

BEHRMAN, SAMUEL J. "Artificial Insemination." *Progress in Infertility.* Edited by Samuel J. Behrman and Robert W. Kistner. Boston: Little, Brown & Co., 1975, pp. 779–789.

Cal. Civil Code sec. 7005 (West) (1975).

Canterbury v. Spence. 464 F. 2d 772 (D.C. Cir. 1972).

CAPRON, ALEXANDER MORGAN. "Informed Decision-making in Genetic Counseling: A Dissent to the 'Wrongful Life' Debate." *Indiana Law Journal* 48 (1973): 581–604.

Coleman v. Garrison. 281 A. 2d 616 (Del. 1971).

Doornbos v. Doornbos. 23 U.S. L.W. 2308 (Super. Ct. Cook County, Ill., 13 Dec. 1954).

EDWARDS, ROBERT G., and SHARPE, DAVID J. "Social Values and Research in Human Embryology." *Nature* 231 (1971): 87–91.

Eisenstadt v. Baird. 405 U.S. 438. 31 L. Ed. 2d 349. 92 S. Ct. 1029 (1972).

FIUMARA, N. J. "Transmission of Gonorrhoea by Artificial Insemination." *British Journal of Venereal Disease* 48 (1972): 308–309.

FRANKEL, MARK S. *The Public Policy Dimensions of Artificial Insemination and Human-Semen Cryobanking.* Program of Policy Studies in Science and Technology, The George Washington University, Monograph no. 18. Washington: 1973.

Ga. Code Ann. sec. 74–101.1(b) (1973).

Gleitman v. Cosgrove. 277 A. 2d 689 (N.J. 1967).

GOSS, DONALD A. "Current Status of Artificial Insemination with Donor Semen." *American Journal of Obstetrics and Gynecology* 122 (1975): 246–252.

Griswold v. Connecticut. 381 U.S. 479. 14 L. Ed. 2d 510. 85 S. Ct. 1678 (1965).

Gursky v. Gursky. 242 N.Y.S. 2d 406. 39 Misc. 2d 1083 (Sup. Ct. King's County, 1963).

Helling v. Carey. 519 P. 2d 981. 83 Wash. 2d 514 (1974).

HORNE, HERBERT W., JR. "Artificial Insemination, Donor: An Issue of Ethical and Moral Values." *New England Journal of Medicine* 293 (1975): 873–874. Editorial.

Kan. Stat. Ann. sec. 23–128 (1968).

Karp v. Cooley. 493 F. 2d 408 (5th Cir. 1974).

KINDREGAN, HARRY D. "State Power over Human Fertility and Individual Liberty." *Hastings Law Journal* 23 (1972): 1401–1426.

KRAUSE, HARRY D. *Illegitimacy: Law and Social Policy.* Indianapolis: Bobbs-Merrill Co., 1971.

L. v. L. [1949] 1 All E. R. 141 (P. Div'l Ct. 1948).

Loving v. Virginia, 388 U.S. 1. 18 L. Ed. 2d 1010. 87 S. Ct. 1817 (1967).

MacLennan v. MacLennan. [1958] Sess. Cas. 105. [1958] Scots. L.T.R. 12.

MOTULSKY, ARNO G. "Brave New World?" *Science* 185 (1974): 653–663.

N.Y. Domestic Relations Law sec. 73 (McKinney 1974).

OAKLEY, MARY ANN B. "Test Tube Babies: Proposals for Legal Regulation of New Methods of Human Conception and Prenatal Development." *Family Law Quarterly* 8 (1974): 385–400.

Okl. Stat. Ann. tit. 10, sec. 551 (West 1967).

Orford v. Orford. 49 Ont. L. R. 15. 58 D.L.R. 251 (1921).

People ex rel. Albajian v. Dennet. 184 N.Y.S. 2d 178. 15 Misc. 2d 260 (Sup. Ct. N.Y. County, 1958).

People v. Sorenson. 437 P. 2d 495 (Cal. 1968).

RAMSEY, PAUL. "Shall We 'Reproduce'? I. The Medical Ethics of In Vitro Fertilization." *Journal of the American Medical Association* 220 (1972): 1346–1350.

———. "Shall We 'Reproduce'? II. Rejoinders and Future Forecast." *Journal of the American Medical Association* 220 (1972): 1480–1485.

Roe v. Wade. 410 U.S. 113. 35 L. Ed. 2d 147. 93 S. Ct. 705 (1973).

Skinner v. Oklahoma. 316 U.S. 535. 86 L. Ed. 1655. 62 S. Ct. 316 (1942).

Slater v. Slater. [1953] 1 All E.R. 246 (C. A. 1952).

SMITH, GEORGE P., II. "Through a Test Tube Darkly: Artificial Insemination and the Law." *Michigan Law Review* 67 (1968): 127–150.

STRICKLER, RONALD C.; KELLER, DAVID W.; and WARREN, JAMES C. "Artificial Insemination with Fresh Donor Semen." *New England Journal of Medicine* 293 (1975): 848–853.

Strnad v. Strnad. 78 N.Y.S. 2d 390. 190 Misc. 786 (Sup. Ct. N.Y. County, 1948).

Symposium on Legal and Other Aspects of Artificial Insemination by Donor (A. I. D.) and Embryo Transfer, London, 1972. *Law and Ethics of A.I.D. and Embryo Transfer.* CIBA Foundation Symposium, n.s. no. 17. New York: Elsevier, 1973.

Troppi v. Scarf. 187 N.W. 2d 511. 31 Mich. App. 240 (1971).

RESEARCH, BEHAVIORAL

Ethical issues in behavioral and social science research have increasingly become matters of public debate, governmental regulation, and active concern within the research community itself. In part, this development can be viewed as fallout from the growing awareness of the implications and occasional abuses of biomedical experimentation. In part, the recent concern with the ethics of behavioral research represents a direct response to activities within the field itself, traceable to the increase in the sheer amount of behavioral research and to its occasionally controversial nature. Controversies have typically focused not so much on the research itself as on the use of some of the tools or products of behavioral research in public life, such as the use of intelligence or achievement tests in educational and occupational selection, of behavior modification techniques in social control, or of opinion polling in the political process.

Two broad categories of ethical issues confronted by behavioral research can be distinguished: those relating to the processes of behavioral research and those relating to its products. Questions about the *processes* of research refer to the experiences of the specific individuals (or groups or communities) who participate as subjects—how they are recruited, how they are treated in the course of their participation, and what short-run and long-run consequences their participation has for them. Considerations of long-run consequences of participation—particularly when they involve consequences for a group or community—merge into questions about the *products* of research. These refer to the kinds of knowledge that the research generates and the uses to which the knowledge is put. The central issue here revolves around the fear that behavioral research may provide tools for controlling and manipulating human behavior and, particularly, that the tools may be used by some segments of society at the expense of others.

Types of behavioral research

In reviewing ethical issues relating to the processes of behavioral research, I shall refer to three principal types of research procedure, all designed to derive data from direct observations of and interactions with individual human subjects, but differing in the way the data are obtained: (1) experimental manipulation, (2) questioning of respondents, and (3) behavioral observation. The three procedures represent different research traditions, but they are often combined in the same investigation.

Experimental manipulation. The most common examples of the first tradition are controlled laboratory experiments, particularly popular among psychologists. By varying the definition of the situation, the experimental instructions, or the subject's activities or experiences in the situation, the experimenter creates different psychological or social conditions and observes their effects on the subject's behavior. Studies in this genre that have raised ethical concerns included experiments designed to create different degrees of psychological stress, and the well-known obedience experiments in which subjects were induced to deliver apparently painful and dangerous shocks to another subject, when in fact that other "subject" was the experimenter's accomplice and received no shocks at all (Milgram). Experiments on the effects of drugs, psychosurgery, or manipulation of physiological states on behavior fall in the same category, but this entry will deal with them only tangentially. Experimental manipulation also occurs in field experiments in which the experimenter—unbeknown to the subjects—introduces manipulations in a natural setting. For example, ethical questions have been raised about studies of helping behavior in which the experimenter stages certain emergencies in a public situation and observes the responses of passersby under varying conditions. In another type of field experiment, alternative experimental treatments (or an experimental and a control treatment) are deliberately introduced in an ongoing organization or group of organizations, and their effects on various behavioral, attitudinal, or organizational dimensions are compared. Such experiments may compare different decision-making patterns in business organizations, for example, or different teaching styles in educational institutions. An extension of this type of research is the large-scale social experiment, such as the New Jersey–Pennsylvania Income Maintenance Experiment, designed to evaluate new social policies by studying their effects on sample communities (Rivlin and Timpane). Each community is selected to participate in one or another version of the program being tested or to serve as a control group. Finally, we can include in the category of experimental manipulation laboratory simulations in which subjects are asked to play such real-life roles as those of national decision makers, business executives, or—as in a study that has aroused considerable ethical controversy (Zimbardo et al.)—prison guards and inmates. Such simulation studies are generally not controlled experiments, although they may be, but they do involve the deliberate staging of a set of events and experiences in order to study their effects on the subjects' behavior.

Questioning of respondents. The second type of research procedure involves the questioning of respondents about their personal characteristics, life histories, experiences, interpersonal relations, attitudes, beliefs, values, fantasies, past behaviors, or behavioral intentions. The Census, insofar as it is used as a research tool in collecting population statistics and exploring national trends, falls in this category. The most common procedure within this broad research tradition is the sample survey, which is used in opinion polling, market research, and a wide variety of theoretical and applied studies to assess the attitudes, expectations, or practices of a population through interviews with a representative sample of that population. Personal interviews are also used with special populations—for example, to study the job satisfaction of workers in a plant, the adjustment of immigrants, the inner conflicts of neurotic patients, or the political views of legislators. Finally, the category includes the use of written questionnaires, attitude scales, and tests of aptitude, achievement, or personality in research on a variety of populations for a variety of purposes. Ethical questions, focusing on consent and the invasion of privacy, have been raised, for example, by the distribution of such questionnaires in public schools, particularly when they have dealt with such controversial issues as sex, religion, and parent–child relations.

Behavioral observation. The third type of research procedure obtains data through direct observation of ongoing behavior. One subvariety is structured observation, in which the investigator assigns special tasks to subjects or arranges special interaction situations—such as group discussions or mother–child interactions—in a laboratory setting and then watches the subjects' performance. Typically, observations are recorded (or subsequently coded) in terms of a systematic set of behavioral categories. Another approach is naturalistic observation of public events, ranging from the play behavior of children, through the interactions of strangers on trains, to the reactions of crowds at football games or political demonstrations. The most common observational procedure is participant observation, which has been used extensively, most often by anthropologists and sociologists, in the study of small societies, communities, organizations, total institutions, and social movements. Ethical problems in participant observation are particularly pronounced when the investigator disguises his role as observer (Erikson). An example of such a procedure is provided by Humphreys's study of male homosexual activities in public restrooms, which was heavily criticized by Warwick (1973; reprinted in Humphreys) and others.

Consent and deception

In behavioral as in biomedical research, a sine qua non of ethical practice is the subjects' voluntary informed consent to participation. Consent represents a right in itself, constituting a central feature of the right to privacy and to respect for one's personal dignity. At the same time, it is a guarantor of other rights: The principle of consent enables prospective subjects to determine and protect their own interests—to decide what risks in terms of long-term damage or short-term stress they are willing to take in return for the anticipated personal and societal benefits. The various risks entailed by research participation are greatly exacerbated by the absence of consent. Conversely, many ethical problems are substantially reduced, if not eliminated, when there is a genuine opportunity for voluntary and informed consent.

The conditions for genuinely voluntary and informed consent, however, are often lacking in behavioral, as well as biomedical, research. Limits on obtaining such consent are imposed by certain systemic factors, mostly having to do with power differentials between those who sponsor and carry out research and those who serve as its subjects. Typically, subjects are in positions of relative disadvantage both within the larger social system and within the research situation itself (Kelman, 1972).

In behavioral as in biomedical research, there is a tendency to recruit subjects disproportionately from particular groups within the social system—groups that are dependent or powerless by virtue of their age, their physical and mental condition, their minority status, their economic and political position, their educational level, their social deviance, or their condition of captivity within various institutions. In behavioral and social research, the disproportionate use of these groups is due not only (as in biomedical research) to their greater availability, but also to two customary definitions of research problems, which have converged on disadvantaged groups: On the one hand, research is often carried out within the framework of sponsoring agencies concerned with the control of social deviance and the management of social dependency; on the other hand, there is a strong tradition of "social problems" research concerned with improving the conditions of disadvantaged groups and individuals.

Given the subjects' power deficiency within the social system, the truly *voluntary* nature of their consent becomes problematic. They may not feel free to withhold consent, and they are particularly vulnerable to various subtle forms of pressure or coercion, including the pressures generated by positive inducements, which a desperately deprived population cannot resist. Such vulnerability helps to explain why, in biomedical research, ethically questionable procedures are more likely to be employed with disadvantaged and powerless subjects. For example, Barber et al. (pp. 54–57) found that studies characterized by a relatively high ratio of risks to expected benefits (either to the subjects or to science) were more likely to utilize ward or clinic patients than private patients. The dramatic cases of abuse of subject rights in biomedical research that have come to light in recent years have involved studies of cancer using aged ward patients, syphilis using poor blacks, birth control using welfare recipients, and the effects of LSD using military personnel. Investigators have found it easier, with such populations, to sidestep the requirements of voluntary consent.

The subjects' power deficiency within the research situation derives from the structure of that situation as being defined and owned by the investigator. The investigator's expertise and the trappings of the situation enhance his apparent legitimacy, and subjects generally feel neither competent nor entitled to question his procedures. Under such circumstances, the truly *informed* nature of their consent becomes problematic. Being unaware of the dimensions of the situation, subjects typically do not know what information to seek when deciding on participation, nor do they feel free to challenge the investigator's explanations. Their decisions are thus heavily dependent on what the investigator chooses to communicate to them.

The principle of informed consent is severely compromised when the investigator deliberately misrepresents the situation and deceives the subjects about the purpose or other features of the research. When investigators provide false or incomplete information to subjects, it is generally for one or both of the following reasons: because full disclosure might affect subjects' decision to participate, or because it might alter the reactions the investigator wishes to observe. In biomedical research the second consideration enters into drug studies in which subjects are not informed that they are or might be receiving placebos; more typically, however, where deception is used, it is because investigators anticipate that subjects would refuse to participate if all the facts were disclosed to them. By contrast, when deception is used in behavioral research, it is largely for the second reason—although the two reasons may blend together. It is generally assumed that many of the phenomena that behavioral scientists hope to observe would be destroyed if subjects knew the true object of the observations. Indeed, Campbell has argued persuasively that the most valid and nontrivial findings in behavioral science come from research in which subjects are unaware that they are being observed at all (Campbell). There is now increasing epistemological controversy about the range of behaviors that are actually affected by awareness and about the success of deception in assuring the spontaneity of subject reactions. Insofar as the common assumptions are correct, however, deception for behavioral scientists is often integral to the nature of their research, rather than just a means of assuring subjects' cooperation.

The use of deception to avoid refusals to participate is a clear violation of the principle of informed consent, since the investigator is deliberately falsifying or withholding information that he knows to be material to the subjects' decision. On the other hand, the use of deception to assure spontaneous subject reactions, unaltered by awareness of the investigator's purpose, can be more readily justified within a utilitarian framework. Still, it presents serious ethical problems even for utilitarians. The problems are most severe when deception is used in a study that entails risks of long-term damage or short-term stress.

By deceiving the subjects about the nature of the research, the investigator deprives them of the opportunity to decide whether they want to expose themselves to those risks. The *effect* of the deception—regardless of its purpose—is to deny subjects information that might well be material to their decision to participate. Even when the research does not entail potential harm or discomfort, however, the use of deception is ethically objectionable (Kelman, 1968; Warwick, 1973, 1975). It deprives the subjects of the respect to which they are entitled as fellow human beings and violates the trust that is basic to all human relationships. Most directly, it may undermine the basis of trust between social scientists and the public and thus help to "pollute" the research environment. Beyond that, it may contribute to the climate of distrust within the society at large and to the generalized expectation that statements and events are never to be taken at face value. Moreover, the use of deception may have a deleterious effect on social values, reinforcing an attitude of cynicism and further legitimizing the already widespread practices of misinformation and manipulation.

Thus, the use of deception poses a difficult dilemma for behavioral researchers. Some have called for a complete moratorium on deception, even if it meant abandoning some lines of research (Warwick, 1975). Many consider that position too extreme, though they agree that the frequency of deception in research must be reduced, the extent and form of deception limited, and adequate protection built in to circumscribe its practice and consequences. They defend continued use of deception under such controlled conditions, not only because they consider it essential to valid research but also because they are convinced—from experience and a limited amount of empirical evidence—that subjects do not consider the information withheld material to their decision to participate, that participation in such research does not cause long-term damage, and that any short-term discomfort or resentment is dissipated through appropriate debriefing procedures. Paradoxically, some of the same investigators also argue that in some of the field studies in which subjects are unaware that they are being observed it is often better not to debrief them, because revealing the deception might increase rather than relieve their discomfort.

Clearly the issues are not settled. Thus, as long as the use of deception is condoned under certain carefully delimited circumstances, it is incumbent upon investigators, review committees, and the research community to weigh the following kinds of questions with respect to each piece of research or general line of research in which deception is being considered: (1) Has the availability of alternative procedures that would meet the same objective without using deception been fully explored? (2) Can certain compromises be introduced to mitigate deception, such as obtaining subjects' prior consent to participate in experiments, some of which might involve deception, or obtaining proxy consent from spokespersons of the subject population? (3) Does the value of the research warrant this ethical shortcut? Specifically, how likely is it that the proposed methods will in fact achieve the desired purpose? (4) Are the risks entailed by participation in the study—in terms of lasting damage, temporary stress, invasion of privacy, and effects on social values—really minimal? (5) Is there a sound basis for the assumption that the information withheld or falsified would be immaterial to subjects' decision to participate? Have peers of the subjects been consulted and do they share this assumption? (6) Finally, are debriefing procedures adequate to correcting misinformation, alleviating stress, and restoring trust once the observations have been completed?

Risks entailed by research processes

As in biomedical research, a common approach to ethical evaluation of procedures used in behavioral research is to assess risks relative to potential benefits. Benefits are largely in the form of contributions to scientific knowledge and to the general social welfare or public enlightenment generated by such knowledge. Participation in the research may also provide benefits to the individual subject in the form of financial remuneration, opportunity to make a contribution, enjoyable experiences, new insights, help with personal (psychological or social) problems, improvements in the conditions of the subject's group or community, and specific services integral to the research program, such as child care, innovative educational experiences, or income supplementation. Risks can be grouped in three broad categories: long-term damage, short-term stress or discomfort, and invasion of privacy.

Long-term damage. The only areas of behavioral research that present significant risks of physical damage are those linked to biomedicine—such as psychosurgery, psychopharmacology, or psychophysiology. In principle, there is the possibility that strictly psychological or social interventions may create anxiety in a subject to the extent of inducing self-directed violence, or hostility to the extent of inducing violence against others. In practice, there is little or no evidence that this has been a serious problem.

By contrast, the risk of long-term psychological damage must be very seriously considered. It is conceivable that the stresses, anxieties, self-discoveries, or experiences of rejection that might be created in an experiment, a depth interview, or a self-analytic group discussion might induce psychotic reactions in vulnerable individuals. There is little evidence that this has in fact happened in a research context, but experience in other settings makes it imperative to use vigilance whenever such stressful procedures are used in research. There is clearly a need for careful screening of subjects, for continual monitoring of subjects' reactions, and for the ready availability of help and support when needed.

More subtle kinds of potentially harmful psychological effects may occur when an experiment provides a subject with experiences or induces him to take actions that reveal unacceptable weaknesses in him and thus lower his self-esteem or self-confidence. Similarly, an experiment may create anxieties in the subject about himself or the world that he cannot entirely shake. Kelman describes several examples of such research, including experiments in which college-age subjects were led to believe, wrongly, that they had homosexual tendencies; even though they were subsequently debriefed, such an experience may create lingering self-doubts about sexual identity in that age group (1968).

It is precisely this type of potential long-term damage that has been central to the critiques of Milgram's obedience research mentioned above. For example, it has been argued that—aside from the intense temporary stress experienced by all subjects in the experiment—the obedient subjects were entrapped into committing acts they considered unworthy by an individual they had reason to trust; this may have led, for at least some subjects, to changes in their self-images or their future ability to trust adult authorities (Baumrind). Even though subjects were reassured at the end of the experiment that they had actually not been administering shocks and that their reactions had not been atypical, they were left with the knowledge that they had been willing to obey authority to the point of harming another human being. The question arises whether the subjects have made a disturbing discovery about themselves and society with potentially damaging long-term effects. In response to that possibility, Milgram arranged follow-up interviews with a selected sample of his subjects, conducted by a psychiatrist a year after completion of the experiment. The psychiatrist concluded that there was no evidence of traumatic reactions or lasting damage in the subjects (Katz, p. 400). It may well be, as Milgram argues, that the same psychological mechanisms that enable subjects to carry out the experimenter's demands in the first place also enable them to justify their actions retrospectively and to integrate them with their self-images. Nevertheless, despite the apparent absence of clinical damage, such experiences may leave some subjects with lowered self-esteem or heightened cynicism. The experimenter has a moral obligation to ensure that subjects do not leave the experiment with a net decline in their psychological well-being. At the very least, this principle implies that psychologically risky experiments should include careful debriefing and follow-up procedures that will help subjects work through their experiences and build constructively upon them. Beyond that, it raises the serious question whether such experiments should be carried out at all, given the risks they entail. From a utilitarian perspective, the answer would depend on one's assessment of the social benefits derived from the experiments. Thus, some writers have ethically justified the Milgram experiments on the ground that the insights they produce may enhance human welfare and freedom (Crawford); others consider them unjustified, in part, because they challenge their validity and hence their significance (Baumrind; Orne and Holland).

In addition to the psychological damages discussed so far, participation in behavioral research may occasionally expose subjects to the risk of material or social damages in the sense of a net loss in certain goods or services. Thus, in certain field experiments, members of the control group not only may be deprived of benefits extended to the experimental group, but may actually be worse off than they would have been had the experiment not been carried out at all. The problem is exacerbated when deception makes informed consent impossible. For example, Rosenthal and Jacobson randomly selected an experimental group of children in an elementary school and informed their teachers—ostensibly on the basis of a special test—that those children could be expected to show unusual intellectual gains. The research, in an important demonstration of the effects of self-fulfilling prophecies, found that the experimental-group children actually made significantly greater gains in IQ by the end of the school year than did the undesignated control-group children. There is evidence that the teachers perceived the experimental-group children more favorably, and it can be presumed that they interacted with those children in a qualitatively different way,

which facilitated their intellectual development (Rosenthal and Jacobson). By the same token, the control-group children were arbitrarily denied opportunities that they might have had in the absence of the experiment to impress their teachers favorably and thus to receive the type of attention that might have facilitated their development.

Large-scale social experiments may create disadvantages not only for the control group but also for nonparticipants, if their impact on a larger social system is to increase competition for a desired commodity. Thus, Brown describes a saturation experiment in selected cities that provides housing allowances to all families that meet certain criteria. This experiment is likely to affect the housing market throughout the community, placing the individuals who do not meet the criteria for inclusion in the experiment at a competitive disadvantage and leaving them worse off than they would have been in the absence of the experiment (Brown). The same can be said, of course, of various social programs that may have harmful consequences for some members of the community (Schultze). Acceptance of social experiments, however, is generally not subject to the formal and informal political processes that are designed ideally to assure "a rough balance of equity" (ibid., p. 125) in the development of social programs. On the other hand, as Schultze points out, comparable safeguards could be introduced in social experimentation, e.g., by requiring the consent of local governing bodies. Special problems may also arise in certain social experiments by virtue of their novelty (Brown), or of their random (and thus arbitrary) assignment of individuals or groups to different treatments. Members of the experimental group, although receiving the intended benefits of the social experiment, may also find themselves worse off as a result of their participation. In particular, there are certain material or psychological risks associated with termination of the experiment that are difficult to foresee at the time the participant's initial consent is sought.

Finally, potential long-term damage also includes the possibility of "diffuse injury," which affects not an identifiable individual or even a class of individuals, but the entire body politic. The concern here is that the processes of behavioral research may contribute to the weakening of certain social values. For example, some critics have argued that polling, particularly when it focuses on the intentions of the voters over the course of an election campaign, distorts the political process; defenders have countered that it is merely an extension of normal procedures, which, in fact, contributes to the democratic process by sensitizing politicians to the concerns of the public. To take another example, critics of field experiments on helping behavior, mentioned above, have argued that the proliferation of such experiments may help to rationalize nonintervention by bystanders in crisis situations; defenders have countered that findings of such research may, in fact, encourage helping behavior by sensitizing the public to the prevalence and causes of nonintervention.

Short-term stress or discomfort. While there is considerable disagreement about the amount and nature of long-term damage risked by participation in behavioral research, it is generally agreed that the subjects often experience a certain amount of short-term stress or discomfort. Since these effects are temporary and reversible, they are ethically less troublesome. Nevertheless, imposition of such costs on the subjects can only be justified by the potential benefits of the research to the subjects themselves and to the larger society. It is also essential to assure, through appropriate debriefing procedures, that the effects of the experience have indeed been overcome.

In considering short-term risks, it may be useful to think of the generic issue involved as that of imposition or intrusion. Even in the absence of stress or discomfort, participation in research takes up subjects' time. This in and of itself represents a cost to the subject—particularly if the task lacks inherent interest—that can only be justified by commensurate benefits. The greater the amount of time demanded, the clearer the justification must be. In this view, short-term stress or discomfort adds to the degree of imposition represented by a particular piece of research. As with time, the greater the amount of stress, the clearer must be the justification (in terms of personal and societal benefits) for imposing the experience on subjects. By the same token, the more stressful and time-consuming participation in the study is likely to be for the subjects, the more essential it is to assure their voluntary and informed consent.

There is another issue that sometimes accompanies short-term stress or discomfort, which is far more difficult to enter into cost–benefit calculations: Participants in some studies may be subjected to experiences that are degrading and deprive them of their dignity. Thus, much

of the negative reaction to the Milgram obedience experiments and the Zimbardo prison simulation was based not so much on the risk of long-term damage or even short-term stress entailed by these studies as on the fact that subjects were induced to engage in behavior that they and others considered unworthy. Other degrading experiences would be ones in which research participants lose control over their reactions, are made to appear foolish, or are subjected to insults. More generally, being lied to in and of itself represents a form of degradation in that it deprives people of the respect to which they are entitled. The last example underlines the point that degrading experiences need not necessarily be accompanied by acute stress, although they often are. The issue goes beyond calculable short-term or long-term risks for the subject to the larger ethical question of decent treatment of fellow human beings. Thus, in evaluating studies that expose subjects to potentially degrading experiences, we must consider the joint risks of short-term stress to the subject and of diffuse injury to the social values governing human relationships.

Invasion of privacy. The risks represented by invasion of privacy can probably be subsumed under the categories of long-term damage and short-term stress. However, since invasion of privacy is an issue so central to behavioral and social research, it merits treatment under a separate category. If we conceive of privacy as "the freedom of the individual to pick and choose for himself the time and circumstances under which, and most importantly, the extent to which, his attitudes, beliefs, behavior and opinions are to be shared with or withheld from others" (Ruebhausen and Brim, p. 1189), we can see why behavioral research—with its heavy emphasis on precisely such personal facts and feelings—inevitably runs the risk of violating the right to privacy. Such violations occur to the extent that subjects are unable to determine what information about themselves they will disclose and how that information will be disseminated.

A major reason for concern about privacy is that public exposure of people's views or actions may have damaging consequences for them. The ethical problem is exacerbated by the semi-coercive context in which such research is sometimes carried out. Concern about consequences dwells not only on the risk of specific penalties but also on the possibility that public exposure may lead to disapproval and embarrassment. All such risks can be virtually eliminated if investigators eschew even the most subtle and indirect forms of coercion in eliciting information from subjects, and if they rigidly adhere to guarantees of confidentiality.

Maintaining the confidentiality of an individual's data is a practicable goal. The most effective procedure, now in fairly common use, is to destroy identifying information so that it becomes impossible to associate the names of subjects with their data. What is far more difficult is to maintain the anonymity of a group and thus to protect its members from possibly damaging or embarrassing consequences. The problem becomes even more complex when the research involves large population groups, particularly when its prime focus is on comparison between such groups. For example, concerns have been expressed about research yielding unfavorable comparisons between ethnic minorities and the majority population on various psychological or social dimensions. Although the findings of such research or their interpretation are often of questionable validity, they may be damaging to minority group members by reinforcing negative stereotypes and supporting social policies that are irrelevant or detrimental to their interests. A closely related issue, best described as invasion of cultural privacy, arises when members of a society feel that a foreign investigator who has come to study them presents them to the outside world as objects of curiosity, ridicule, or derogation. To minimize negative consequences of group exposure, investigators must inform subjects or their spokespersons of such possible consequences when their agreement to participate is solicited and must take special care (where possible, after consultation with group representatives) that findings about the group are reported accurately, fairly, and respectfully.

Invasion of privacy refers not only to the consequences of unwanted wider publicity but also to individuals' loss of control over their self-presentation in the immediate situation. Thus, whenever people are observed without their knowledge, their privacy is invaded in the sense that they are deprived of the opportunity to decide how to present themselves to the observer. The degree of intrusiveness varies over different situations. Unacknowledged observations in a public situation are not especially problematic, since people expect to be observed by others, even if not specifically by social scientists. At the other extreme are participant observation studies in which observers gain access to their subjects through misrepresentation. Examples are provided by the Humphreys study, cited earlier, or even more clearly by studies in which the investigator joins an organization under false pretenses. Subjects in these situations are induced to say or do things in the presence of an outsider that they may wish to reserve for fellow group members. They are thus denied the opportunity to decide what to reveal or not reveal to a nonmember. Observations obtained under false pretenses can be justified more readily if the situation to which the investigator gains access is one that is in principle subject to public scrutiny. Thus, Rosenhan and his collaborators gained secret admission to psychiatric hospitals to observe, from the patient's vantage point, the process of psychiatric diagnosis and the hospital experience (Rosenhan). There is no question that the investigators' deception deprived the hospital staff of the opportunity to control their self-presentations. Yet it can be argued that the staff's actions vis-à-vis their patients are not protected by the right to privacy and that the observations made in the Rosenhan study served the larger public interest.

Even in a public situation, unacknowledged observations become more problematic when the investigator deliberately introduces experimental manipulations in the natural setting. The invasion of privacy is relatively mild when "the experimental treatment falls within the range of the respondent's ordinary experience, merely being an experimental rearrangement of normal-level communications" (Campbell, p. 371). It becomes severe when the experimenter stages a dramatic event that represents a disturbing imposition and a source of conflict to the subjects. Unlike the subjects in such field experiments, those in laboratory experiments generally know that they are being observed and thus maintain greater control over their self-presentation. Their control is reduced, however, when they are deceived about the purposes of the experiment.

In research using questioning procedures, the loss of control over self-presentation may also become an issue. The issue arises when respondents are presented with indirect questions, so that they are unaware of the dimension that is being assessed, or with questions that they would prefer not to answer, but feel under pressure to entertain.

Issues involving loss of control are more difficult to resolve than those involving the consequences of publicity, because they are integrally linked to the nature of the research procedures themselves—procedures such as unobtrusive measurement or deceptive experimentation. Thus the question often is not how to avoid coercion and assure confidentiality, but whether to do the research at all. In most cases the intrusiveness of the procedures is mild, and there is general consensus that their use is justified. Certain procedures, however—involving various forms of misrepresentation—have been the subject of considerable debate within the research community. The consensus now would justify their use, if at all, only under special circumstances and with appropriate safeguards and correctives (American Psychological Association).

There is, finally, a third reason for concern about invasion of privacy, and it raises issues that may be even more difficult to resolve than those involving the long-term or immediate effects of exposure. This concern is based on the feeling that one's private (physical or psychological) space has been violated—that the boundary between self and environment has been overstepped. The preservation of such a private space would seem essential to a person's sense of an autonomous self. Observations and questions in certain areas may be experienced, by their very nature, as intrusions into private space. The specific areas defining that space vary across cultures, across individuals within a given culture, and across time for the same individual. A blanket prohibition of research that might conceivably touch on such areas—which would include, among others, the topics of sex, personal health, death, religion, ethnicity, politics, money, and parent–child relations—would destroy or trivialize social research. What is needed instead is careful planning of research that potentially violates private space; sensitivity to messages from subjects that their boundaries have been overstepped; and mechanisms to protect subjects against pressures to reveal more than they are ready to reveal and against negative reactions to intrusive inquiries.

Risks entailed by research products

In discussing possible damaging consequences of research participation for the group, society, or population segment to which the subjects belong—particularly the invasion of cultural privacy and the publication of unfavorable group comparisons—we have already touched on the risks entailed by the products of behavioral and social research. The ethical issues here pertain not to the process of the research and the implications of a subject's participation in it, but to the types of knowledge generated by the research. What are the dangers that the research products might have detrimental consequences for the society or for certain segments of it? These issues are discussed more fully elsewhere (Kelman, 1972, and associated references) and can only be alluded to here.

The central ethical issue raised by the products of social research is that they often consist of knowledge capable of helping to control and manipulate human behavior. Who is likely to use that knowledge, over whom, and to what ends? Perhaps the most troubling issue is the possible *differential* control of some segments of the population over others—particularly the danger that the more powerful groups will use the knowledge to the detriment of the powerless. An example of such a possibility that has aroused considerable controversy is the use of behavior modification in institutional contexts, such as prisons. Although the method is designed to give clients better control over their environments, its use in such contexts may well have the effect of giving the institution unwarranted control over its inmates. Perhaps the clearest illustration of the use of social research by the powerful for the direct manipulation of the powerless is provided by counterinsurgency activities. Ethical issues surrounding such research shook the international research community in the 1960s, with Project Camelot serving as the focal point of the debate (Horowitz).

Apart from the question of direct application of research findings to the control and manipulation of disadvantaged populations, there is the broader question about research traditions that are largely formed by the perspective of social control. For example, much of the research on social deviance focuses on the carriers of the deviance—that is, the psychological and social characteristics of deviant individuals and groups—rather than the systemic processes that may give rise to deviant behavior. The products of such research lend themselves more readily to controlling deviant behavior and changing the deviants than to changing institutionalized patterns of discrimination and oppression. Research on the characteristics of deviant populations is perfectly legitimate, but ethical problems arise when this research tradition becomes the dominant perspective for analyzing deviance as a societal phenomenon and for formulating policy.

A related problem arises from the products of research on ethnic group differences. Since the definition of the problems and the choice of methods for such research typically reflect the perspective of the majority population, it is not surprising that the findings often reveal psychological, social, or cultural "deficiencies" in minority groups. Such findings may then be used to justify discriminatory practices or to support policies designed to correct the group's deficiencies rather than to remove structural inequalities. Research on group characteristics must be recognized as a highly precarious basis for policy formation, unless it is balanced by an analysis of the structural relations between the groups and the institutional context in which they operate.

Risks entailed by research products, which usually involve the possibility of harm to a group, need to be considered more fully than they have been in the evaluation of behavioral (as well as biomedical) research, though we must also remain alert to the possibility that ethical controls in this domain can easily turn into political constraints. The most effective way of minimizing the risks is to make sure that all segments of the population have an opportunity to bring their perspectives to bear on the formulation of research problems and the interpretation and utilization of findings. In the long run, this requires broadening the base of the research enterprise through diversification or democratization of the community of research producers and users.

Mechanisms of protection and accountability

Behavioral as well as biomedical research in the United States is now subject to various external controls, including government regulation and institutional review committees, designed to ensure the protection of human subjects. Despite understandable misgivings, many investigators not only have accepted such controls as a fact of life but consider them necessary and just. It is increasingly recognized that treating the rights of subjects as an internal matter, to be handled entirely within the research community, is tantamount to having a conflict of interests adjudicated by one of the interested parties. This analysis makes it clear that there must be some public involvement in the protection of subject rights. Ideally, the involvement should include representatives of the very populations from which subjects are drawn, since they are in the best position to view the issues from the subjects' perspectives and to reflect the subjects' interests. Thus, institutional review committees would include not only the investigator's peers, who are able to bring to the evaluation an understanding of the background and requirements of the proposed research, but also the peers of the subjects.

The development of external controls has been accompanied by developments within the research community itself. Indeed, such internal mechanisms are essential if ethical practice is to be a fully integrated part of the research enterprise rather than an adjustment to outside pressures. The American Psychological Association has had an ethics committee since 1940 and a code of ethics since 1953. Until recently the code was largely concerned with ethical issues in professional practice and covered research ethics only sketchily. In 1972, however, a series of new principles, developed by an Ad hoc Committee on Ethical Standards in Psychological Research through a careful and extensive process of deliberation and consultation, were incorporated in the code. The committee's statement provides a thoughtful and balanced discussion of risks entailed in the process of research but touches only briefly on the risks entailed by the products of research. The American Anthropological Association began a thorough exploration of ethical issues in the wake of the debate over Project Camelot and has since developed a code and a committee. Its Principles of Professional Responsibility, adopted in 1971, focus on research in foreign cultures and address, among others, the issues of secrecy and research sponsorship. The American Sociological Association has also developed a Code of Ethics in recent years, administered since 1971 by a standing ethics committee. At the international level, developments have been extremely slow so far. A series of "advisory principles" for ethical conduct of cross-cultural research, developed by a group of U.S. investigators in consultation with many scholars from around the world (Tapp et al.), has served as a starting point for deliberations over a possible international code within the International Association for Cross-Cultural Psychology. The established ethical codes are all supported by enforcement procedures, with expulsion from the professional association serving as the ultimate sanction. Their main purposes, however, are to raise researchers' consciousness of ethical issues, to establish norms and standards within the research community, to provide explicit guidelines, and to serve as training instruments.

In addition to developing mechanisms of protection and accountability, the research community can engage in research relevant to questions of ethical research practice. Studies have been done and proposed on the effectiveness of debriefing procedures, the long-term effects of research participation, and the reactions of subjects to research in which they have participated or to hypothetical research situations. Findings of such research can be useful inputs into evaluations of research proposals and deliberations about ethical issues, but ethical questions generally cannot be settled by empirical data.

Finally, a major task—to which behavioral scientists are increasingly addressing themselves —is the development of alternative research procedures that do not involve deception; that minimize intrusiveness, imposition, and other costs to the subject; and that maximize subjects' benefits. The general direction in which such methodological innovation would move can be characterized as *participatory research*, in which subjects' positive motivations to contribute to the research enterprise as active collaborators with the investigator are elicited. Certain forms of role playing or simulation, elite interviews, and action research exemplify this approach. These methodological innovations must go hand in hand with a reexamination of the epistemological assumptions that have dominated the field. Such a process of reexamination, which is already under way, is likely to contribute not only to ethical practice but also to enrichment of the research enterprise.

HERBERT C. KELMAN

[*Directly related are the entries* BEHAVIOR CONTROL; HUMAN EXPERIMENTATION; INFORMED CONSENT IN HUMAN RESEARCH; PRIVACY; *and* RISK. *This article will find application in the entries* ELECTRICAL STIMULATION OF THE BRAIN; GENETIC ASPECTS OF HUMAN BEHAVIOR; HYPNOSIS; PSYCHOPHARMACOLOGY; PSYCHOSURGERY; RACISM, *article on* RACISM AND MENTAL HEALTH; *and* SEX THERAPY AND SEX RESEARCH. *For problems of experimenting on special populations, see:* ADOLESCENTS; AGING AND THE AGED, *article on* HEALTH CARE AND RESEARCH IN THE AGED; ANIMAL EXPERIMENTATION; CHILDREN AND BIOMEDICINE; MENTALLY HANDICAPPED; PRISONERS, *article on* PRISONER EXPERIMENTATION; *and* WOMEN AND BIOMEDICINE, *article on* WOMEN AS PATIENTS AND EXPERIMENTAL SUBJECTS. *See also:* BEHAVIORISM; COMMUNICATION, BIOMEDICAL; CONFIDENTIALITY; RIGHTS; *and* TRUTH-TELLING. *For discussion of related ideas, see the entries* RESEARCH, BIOMEDICAL; RESEARCH POLICY, BIOMEDICAL; *and* THERAPEUTIC RELATIONSHIP. *See* APPENDIX, SECTION II: DIRECTIVES FOR HUMAN EXPERIMENTATION; *and* SECTION IV, AMERICAN PSYCHOLOGICAL ASSOCIATION.]

BIBLIOGRAPHY

American Psychological Association, Ad hoc Committee on Ethical Standards in Psychological Research. *Ethical Principles in the Conduct of Research with Human Participants.* Washington: 1973.

BARBER, BERNARD; LALLY, JOHN J.; MAKARUSHKA, JULIA LOUGHLIN; and SULLIVAN, DANIEL. *Research on Human Subjects: Problems of Social Control in Medical Experimentation.* New York: Russell Sage Foundation, 1973.

BAUMRIND, DIANA. "Some Thoughts on Ethics of Research: After Reading Milgram's 'Behavioral Study of Obedience.'" *American Psychologist* 19 (1964): 421–423.

BROWN, PETER G. "Informed Consent in Social Experimentation: Some Cautionary Notes." Rivlin, *Ethical and Legal Issues*, chap. 3, pp. 79–104.

CAMPBELL, DONALD T. "Prospective: Artifact and Control." *Artifact in Behavioral Research.* Edited by Robert Rosenthal and Ralph L. Rosnow. New York: Academic Press, 1969, chap. 8, pp. 351–382.

CRAWFORD, THOMAS J. "In Defense of Obedience Research: An Extension of the Kelman Ethic." *The Social Psychology of Psychological Research.* Edited by Arthur G. Miller. New York: Free Press, 1972, pp. 179–186.

ERIKSON, KAI T. "A Comment on Disguised Observation in Sociology." *Social Problems* 14 (1967): 366–373.

HOROWITZ, IRVING L., ed. *The Rise and Fall of Project Camelot: Studies in the Relationship between Social Science and Practical Politics.* Cambridge: MIT Press, 1967.

HUMPHREYS, LAUD. *Tearoom Trade: Impersonal Sex in Public Places.* Enl. ed. Chicago: Aldine Publishing Co., 1975.

KATZ, JAY. *Experimentation with Human Beings: The Authority of the Investigator, Subject, Professions, and State in the Human Experimentation Process.* New York: Russell Sage Foundation, 1972.

KELMAN, HERBERT C. "The Human Use of Human Subjects." *A Time to Speak: On Human Values and Social Research.* San Francisco: Jossey-Bass, 1968, chap. 8, pp. 202–225.

———. "The Rights of the Subject in Social Research: An Analysis in Terms of Relative Power and Legitimacy." *American Psychologist* 27 (1972): 989–1016.

MILGRAM, STANLEY. *Obedience to Authority: An Experimental View.* New York: Harper & Row, 1974.

ORNE, MARTIN T., and HOLLAND, CHARLES C. "On the Ecological Validity of Laboratory Deceptions." *International Journal of Psychiatry* 6 (1968): 282–293.

RIVLIN, ALICE M., and TIMPANE, P. MICHAEL, eds. *Ethical and Legal Issues of Social Experimentation.* Washington: Brookings Institution, 1975.

ROSENHAN, DAVID L. "On Being Sane in Insane Places." *Science* 179 (1973): 250–258.

ROSENTHAL, ROBERT, and JACOBSON, LENORE. *Pygmalion in the Classroom: Teacher Expectation and Pupils' Intellectual Development.* New York: Holt, Rinehart & Winston, 1968.

RUEBHAUSEN, OSCAR M., and BRIM, ORVILLE G., JR. "Privacy and Behavioral Research." *Columbia Law Review* 65 (1965): 1184–1211.

SCHULTZE, CHARLES L. "Social Programs and Social Experiments." Rivlin, *Ethical and Legal Issues*, chap. 5, pp. 115–125.

TAPP, JUNE LOUIN; KELMAN, HERBERT C.; TRIANDIS, HARRY C.; WRIGHTSMAN, LAWRENCE S.; and COELHO,

George V. "Continuing Concerns in Cross-Cultural Ethics: A Report." *International Journal of Psychology* 9 (1974): 231–249.

Warwick, Donald P. "Social Scientists Ought to Stop Lying." *Psychology Today*, February 1975, pp. 38–40, 105–106.

————. "Tearoom Trade: Means and Ends in Social Research." *Hastings Center Studies* 1, no. 1 (1973), pp. 27–38.

Zimbardo, Philip G.; Haney, Craig; Banks, Curtis W.; and Jaffe, David. "The Psychology of Imprisonment: Privation, Power, and Pathology." *Doing unto Others: Joining, Molding, Conforming, Helping, Loving.* Edited by Zick Rubin. The Patterns of Social Behavior series. Englewood Cliffs, N.J.: Prentice-Hall, 1974, pp. 61–73.

RESEARCH, BIOMEDICAL

The present entry does not deal explicitly with the concrete ethical issues arising in the context of biomedical research. Rather, it discusses the foundations and goals of such research, with an emphasis on the canons of scientific research professions, the responsibility of the scientific community for experimental medicine, the decisions on research priorities, the right to profit from scientific research, and the question of auto-experimentation. The entry alludes to, but does not detail, the philosophical and sociological perspectives on the issues involved, and offers an explanation of the entire biomedical research endeavor as background material for understanding properly the specific issues discussed in the entries Animal Experimentation; Communication, Biomedical; Human Experimentation; Informed Consent in Human Research; Medical Ethics under National Socialism; Research Policy, Biomedical; Risk; *and* Science: Ethical Implications.

Biomedical research is a construction that is used so commonly that it may be difficult to imagine that, just twenty years ago, it did not exist. Research means, according to *Webster's Third New International Dictionary*, "Studious inquiry or examination; especially: critical and exhaustive investigation or experimentation having for its aim the discovery of new facts and their correct interpretation, the revision of accepted conclusions, theories, or laws in the light of newly discovered facts, or the practical applications of such new or revised conclusions, theories or laws." While the word "biomedical" suggests a simple amalgam of biology and medicine, at least one dictionary definition indicates a broader conceptualization: "Of, relating to, or involving biological, medical, and physical sci-

ence." Biomedical research, as used here, means research having as its ultimate aim the advancement of the goals of medicine. In order to understand more fully the scope of biomedical research, one must first consider modern concepts of the domain and orientation of medicine. It will be seen that the philosophy of science and the methodology of research have become firmly established in the practice of medicine. Succeeding sections of this article will deal with the concerns of biomedical research in relation to various conceptions of medicine; the problems deriving from blending the conflicting traditions of research and medical practice; and some of the tensions associated with recent developments in the social control of biomedical research.

The domain of medicine

Henry Sigerist, in the introduction to his monumental work on the history of medicine, states: "The scope of medicine is so broad that it includes, under any circumstances, infinitely more than the physician's actions. The task of medicine may be outlined under the following four headings: 1. Promotion of health; 2. Prevention of illness; 3. Restoration of health; and 4. Rehabilitation" (Sigerist, p. 7).

In the traditional medical model, the focus is on the last two functions and their extensions. A person who feels ill initiates contact with a physician with the hope—and increasingly in the twentieth century, the expectation—that he or she will be treated and consequently rendered healthy. The physician first makes a diagnosis, naming the disease that is causing the patient to feel ill. Based upon the diagnosis the physician can perform the other functions expected of him or her (Feinstein, p. 385): The physician can provide (1) a prognosis, predicting what will become of the patient, and (2) therapy designed to cure the disease; to delay the progress of or compensate for its disabling manifestations; or to relieve symptoms (make the patient feel better). Finally, the physician is expected to care for the patient, with all that the word "care" implies.

The principal focus of the medical profession and of biomedical research is on disease. In the modern concept of a disease, it is a distinct entity the presence of which is verifiable objectively; it has a cause, and if we can identify the cause the physician can either cure or prevent it or the means for its cure or prevention inevitably will be developed by the biomedical researcher. This view of disease presupposes that it is something distinct from the person who contracts it and that if rid of it the person will be normal (healthy).

The doctrine that each disease is a distinct entity the presence of which is verifiable objectively was established firmly in the closing years of the eighteenth century by a group of Parisian physicians whose intellectual leader was Xavier Bichat (Shryock, 1948, pp. 129 ff.). Their philosophical perspective was largely that of the French *idéologues* who accepted the philosophical empiricism of Locke; their concentration was on the careful observation of phenomena and their correlations and an avoidance of speculation and theory. Under their influence, two major traditions of medical science—each of which had yielded a classification of disease— were fused: (1) careful and systematic observation of the living sick person (clinical observation) and (2) systematic dissection of the dead person (necropsy), which yielded a body of knowledge known as morbid anatomy (forerunner of pathology, the study of diseases).

Morbid anatomy became the dominant science of clinical medicine, because at the time it was the only science of the human body that could provide objective evidence of concrete abnormalities. Most diseases were named by what abnormality was found at necropsy. Thus, if a disease produced inflammation of the liver, it was named hepatitis (*hepar* = liver; *itis* = inflammation). During the late eighteenth and most of the nineteenth century, most maneuvers now recognized as the modern physical examination were developed. The ultimate test of a diagnostic maneuver was that it could predict what would be found at necropsy, and the ultimate test of a physician was that he or she could predict what would be found at necropsy (Feinstein, pp. 106–108).

Through the remainder of the nineteenth and into the twentieth century, other natural sciences were applied with increasing success to the description of normal and abnormal structure and function, to the identification of the causes of diseases, and to the mechanisms through which they produce malfunction and disability. With time, names began to be assigned to diseases according to their causative agents, e.g., streptococcal sore throat (named for the bacteria that cause it); or by the physiological (high blood pressure) or biochemical (phenylketonuria) aberrations through which they might be identified.

While the scientific disciplines used to identify and explain disease have evolved, the necessity of objective verification remained constant. Lack of objective verification may cast doubt on the legitimacy of a discipline, on a proposed disease entity, or on the credibility of a patient. Thus, the specialty of dynamic psychiatry was admitted very slowly and grudgingly into the traditional medical profession. Early acceptance of organic psychiatry into departments of neurology was based on the fact that anatomical abnormalities, if any, were found in the brain and that some mental illnesses were caused by infection (e.g., syphilis), vitamin deficiency, or hormonal imbalances (Shryock, 1948, pp. 290 ff.). Full acceptance of dynamic psychiatry was delayed until the mid-twentieth century, when it was demonstrated that some severe behavioral disorders responded favorably to either surgery (frontal lobotomy), electroconvulsive therapy, or drugs (tranquilizers).

The modern examination of a patient by a physician evolved in the same philosophical tradition. A patient must receive an "adequate" examination consisting first of a complete "history" including a systematic quest for complaints that the patient may have neglected to mention and for diseases that may either be familial or related to environment or habits. This is followed by a physical examination in which the physician will look at or into, feel, and listen to virtually every part of the body, generally with the aid of various instruments. Measurement is emphasized, e.g., the rate of the pulse, the size of the liver, the loudness of the heart sounds. Next, the examination is continued in various laboratories; blood and urine samples are collected for microscopic examination and chemical and physical testing. Electrocardiograms and X-rays of the chest are routine.

After the initial examination the physician formulates an "impression" (equivalent to hypothesis) as to what might be wrong. Evidence of the possible presence of various diseases is pursued with further diagnostic testing. When all the necessary data are available, the physician makes a diagnosis (equivalent to a theory). At this point the other functions of the physician begin.

If there is objective evidence of disease, a diagnosis is made; if not, a problem is presented to both physician and patient. Until recently a dichotomy was made between organic and functional illness. The former classification was assigned to patients having validated diseases, while the latter was a suspect set. Patients with functional illness were informed that there was nothing wrong, i.e., stop complaining, or else it was delicately suggested that they might see a psychiatrist—a suggestion that until recently was usually resisted and frequently rejected (Cassell, p. 27). The sick role was described vividly by a sociologist (T. Parsons) as one in which an individual might be excused from usual obligations only on the conditions that (1) the role was legitimized by a physician and (2) the sick person was obligated to cooperate with the physician's healing efforts. The paradigmatic experience was that of the requirement of a note from a doctor to permit return to school or work after an alleged illness. Consider the plight of the person with a functional illness.

Since the Second World War several things have happened to change the composition of medicine. Three have had a profound impact on the orientation of biomedical research. First, the concept of disease has begun to expand. Disease, always recognized as a type of abnormality, gradually came to be equated with any deviance from accepted norms (Freidson, pp. 205 ff.). But now increasingly the deviations derived their objective verification through the devices of the social and behavioral as well as the natural sciences. The identification of some sorts of children with learning disabilities as diseased or sick led to the development of therapies that often enhance their abilities; however, it reversed the model presented earlier. In some cases they are diagnosed by school authorities and sent home with a note *to* the doctor. Illegitimate classification of a group may be associated with the social stigmatization of being sick without any possibility of therapy (Makarushka). As we label as diseases such things as alcohol abuse and drug abuse, inappropriate aggression, and deviant sexual behavior, we begin to blur the distinctions between sin, crime, and disease (V. Parsons). A deviant may now be offered the choice between the criminal role and the sick role. The physician, accustomed to playing legitimizer, may now be called upon to function as illegitimizer (Freidson, pp. 239 ff.).

And yet, through naming these deviations diseases, thereby including them in the purview of biomedical research, application of the natural sciences has begun to yield correlations that may result in explanatory theories. Consistent biochemical changes have been found in association with various behaviors; they are curiously similar for hunger, lust, and aggression. These findings present new and increasingly formida-

ble problems. For example, explanation of all behavior in biological terms would lead to the disappearance from our culture of such concepts as free will or individual responsibility and their replacement by biological determinism (Connell).

Second, as a consequence of the success of the struggle against infectious diseases—until the early twentieth century the perennial greatest killers of people—a new constellation of diseases has emerged to dominate the lists of causes of death. These include the familiar triad of heart disease, cancer, and stroke. Treatment of these diseases is most effective if begun before they become manifest as illness. For example, high blood pressure, by producing relentless destruction of arteries over a period of many years, eventually produces heart attacks, strokes, and kidney failure, which, in turn, cause disability and death. Treatment of high blood pressure, begun before the patient feels ill, will retard greatly the rate of development of disabling and lethal complications. Similar statements may be made for some of the other major chronic diseases such as abnormalities of fat metabolism. The physician, who is accustomed to dealing with patients who feel ill, is increasingly called upon to work with people who, although they may have diseases, feel well (Cassell).

Third, as a consequence of these and other factors, strong forces have developed within and without the medical profession to change its primary orientation toward the maintenance of health rather than the treatment of disease. There has been an increasing emphasis on the approaches of public health and preventive medicine, and both of these disciplines have influenced the practice of medicine. The World Health Organization provides the following definition in its constitution: "Health is a state of complete physical, mental and social well-being and not merely the absence of disease or infirmity" (WHO, p. 459). Unlike disease, the presence of health is not objectively verifiable. Thus, the researcher has difficulty focusing on health as a definitive objective.

Public health, which is concerned with maintaining the health of populations, had its origins in the development of sanitation techniques for purposes of preventing contagious diseases. A story of one of its early successes demonstrates the characteristic nature of its approaches and emphasizes that it is not always necessary to know the final cause of a disease in order to prevent it (Burton and Smith, p. 29). During an epidemic of cholera in London in 1854, John Snow observed that most fatally infected people seemed to have used the water pump at Broad Street. He persuaded the city authorities to remove the handle from the pump; almost immediately thereafter the epidemic disappeared.

In the twentieth century the domain of public health has been extended to manipulations of the environment generally so as to maintain physical, mental, and social health. Among its concerns are improvement of working conditions (to prevent occupational diseases), urban planning (to reduce mental illness, drug abuse), clean air and water, highway safety, and so on.

Preventive medicine, which is concerned with doing something to or for an individual person in order to prevent future disease, also had its origins in the combat against infectious diseases (ibid., pp. 16 ff.). One of its notable early triumphs was the finding in the eighteenth century that persons could be protected from severe cases of smallpox by deliberately infecting them with material from persons with mild cases; subsequently, it was found that even more satisfactory protection could be afforded by deliberate infection with a closely related and much milder disease, cowpox (*vaccinia*). The latter finding was based on Edward Jenner's observation that milkmaids who contracted cowpox retained a permanent immunity to smallpox.

In the late nineteenth and early twentieth centuries, vaccines were developed that produced lasting protection against many of the major infectious diseases. Further, it was discovered that many severe diseases were due to nutritional deficiencies that could be prevented by appropriate diets, and the probability of acquiring some other diseases, e.g., emphysema and venereal diseases, could be minimized through modification of personal habits. The approaches of preventive medicine have been extended into preventive therapy with a current emphasis on early detection of such diseases as high blood pressure and glaucoma so that they might be treated before disabling or lethal complications ensue.

The shifting orientation toward health has had a significant impact on the social structure of the medical profession (ibid., pp. 67–108). Medical practice increasingly is referred to as part of the "health-care delivery system." Recent manifestations of this shifting orientation include the health maintenance organization (where ill and well alike are examined and/or treated), multiphasic screening procedures, and outreach operations.

Biomedical research in relation to medicine

A revolution in medical education was launched in 1910 by Abraham Flexner, who proposed in his report to the Carnegie Foundation that American medical schools should be reconstructed to emulate the highly successful European (particularly German) university-based model. He suggested that all medical schools should have full-time faculties, that the teachers of medicine should be actively engaged in research, and that medical students should be educated in what he called the laboratory sciences (Flexner). By the late 1930s all American medical schools conformed to the Flexnerian model.

The disciplines that came to be known as the biomedical sciences are those that Flexner identified as the laboratory sciences. In general, they have comprised most of the first two years of the medical school curriculum; they are commonly referred to as the basic sciences to distinguish them from the primary focus of the second two years, the clinical studies. There is a general tendency to refer to research in these disciplines as biomedical research, whether or not it conforms to the definition used here.

The sciences include anatomy (the study of bodily structure), physiology (the study of bodily function), biochemistry, pathology, pharmacology (the study of drugs), and microbiology (the study of microorganisms, many of which can cause disease). With the addition of statistics, behavioral sciences, immunology, and genetics, this model remains generally intact. In the twentieth century, biochemistry, "efforts to explain biological phenomena in terms of the specific properties of chemical substances present in living organisms," emerged as the natural science having the greatest power to provide an explanatory theory for the nature of health and disease as well as the development of remedies (Fruton). The approaches of biochemistry now dominate most research and explanatory theory in the aforementioned sciences.

If we accept the expanded definition of medicine developed in the preceding section, it becomes apparent that biomedical research includes parts of almost all the natural, behavioral, and social sciences as well as many aspects of engineering. For example, while it is absurd to say that sociology is a biomedical science, it is clear that its research approaches are being applied to the development of explanatory theory for health and diseases and, further, that social research may suggest approaches to the improvement of public health and to the development of improved medical facilities (Kreider and Mamlin).

Although the researcher is more attracted to the study of disease than of health, this does not mean that he or she eschews the study of normal processes. The concept of a normal process presents no problem to the researcher; rather, it is the totality of the concept of health that defies scientific validation. The researcher knows that an understanding of disease—deviation from normal—is contingent upon a thorough understanding of the normal. As stated earlier, a disease is conceived as a distinct entity that has a cause; if we can identify the cause, the physician can either cure or prevent it, or the means for its cure or prevention inevitably will be developed by the biomedical researcher. The last part of this statement may be recognized as an article of faith that forms the basis for the mainstream of modern biomedical research (Thomas).

The foundations for this article of faith were established by the proof of the germ theory of disease and the consequent successes of immunization and chemotherapy (Shryock, 1948, pp. 224 ff.). In 1876 Robert Koch first demonstrated beyond doubt that a specific disease (anthrax) was caused by specific bacteria. He developed a set of tests (Koch's postulates), which must be satisfied if an organism is to be accepted as the cause of a disease. Within a short period of time, the bacteria that caused many diseases were identified. Aside from firmly fixing the concept of "one disease, one cause" in the tradition of biomedical research, this event had three other important practical consequences.

First, it was possible to isolate these bacteria and grow large numbers of them in pure culture. These cultured bacteria could be treated in various ways so as to render them less virulent. The less virulent bacteria could be administered to normal persons causing little or no illness but conferring a lasting immunity to the disease (immunization). Subsequently, very similar techniques have been applied to the isolation of viruses and the development of immunizations (vaccines) to them.

Second, it was found that some dyes selectively stained certain cells—either bacteria or the cells of animal tissues—but not others. Presumably, their affinity for specific cells was based upon their chemical properties. It occurred to Paul Ehrlich that some poisonous chemicals might be developed that would have an affinity for bacteria but not normal cells. Such chemicals

would be "magic bullets" in that they would kill the cause of the disease without killing the cells of the diseased. Among the chemotherapeutic agents (chemical therapies) found by this approach are sulfa drugs (derivatives of the original analine dyes with which Ehrlich worked) and antibiotics.

Third, it was possible to inject these bacteria into animals and to produce in them the same diseases they caused in humans (animal models). Thus it became possible to perform increasingly sophisticated studies on the nature of disease. Further, it became possible to test the new vaccines and chemotherapeutic agents to see if they truly effected prevention or cure without seriously damaging the animal.

Lewis Thomas has categorized the therapeutic activities of physicians as the "high technology," "halfway technology," and "nontechnology" of medicine. High technology is based upon fundamental understandings of the causes of disease. When we learn the specific cause of a disease we should expect to develop a cure (e.g., an antibiotic) or a prevention (e.g., a vaccine). Meanwhile, not knowing the causes of most diseases we struggle to develop halfway technology. That is a technology designed to make up for disease —to compensate for its incapacitating effects or to relieve its symptoms—or to postpone death. Current examples of halfway technology include artificial kidneys for patients with kidney failure, coronary bypass surgery for patients with angina pectoris, drug treatment of psychotic disorders, and so on. The best of halfway technology is based upon sound understanding of the fundamental mechanisms of disease, e.g., what is wrong anatomically, physiologically, biochemically, and so on, but not on a knowledge of the final causes of disease. Finally, the nontechnology of medicine includes those things physicians do that are usually subsumed under the rubric "caring for." It includes the large part of any good doctor's time that is occupied by providing reassurance, comfort, and so on.

As Thomas sees it, we currently understand the major crippling diseases of the twentieth century at about the same level that we knew infectious diseases in the mid-nineteenth. He views disease as essentially an unnatural state and predicts its ultimate eradication. This is not to say that we will achieve immortality; he sees death as the culmination of the normal aging process rather than as necessarily a complication of disease.

Not all agree with this philosophy. René Dubos, for example, agrees that we will identify the causes of some diseases and eradicate them (pp. 346 ff.). However, he believes that most of the current major diseases have multiple causes; in general, they reflect a failure on the part of human beings to adapt to the social and other stresses presented by an ever-changing environment. Because the environment and social structure are constantly changing, humans never will become perfectly adapted. Thus, each time period and each type of civilization will have its peculiar burden of diseases created by unavoidable failures of adaptation. He sees the struggle against diseases as never ending and the concept of perfect health as a utopian creation of the mind. Those who accept the Dubos view are more inclined to emphasize the approaches of public health than what one might call the mainstream of biomedical research.

The expression "biomedical research" ordinarily calls to mind research on human subjects. Yet the vast majority of biomedical research activity is conducted on animals or their tissues, cells, or even parts of cells (Comroe and Dripps). Some is done on plants, and some utilizes nothing derived from living sources, e.g., developmental engineering designed to improve devices such as cardiac pacemakers. Because a need for prior animal experimentation is emphasized in such documents as the Nuremberg Code and the Declaration of Helsinki, it is often thought that its purpose is to try something out on animals to see if it is sufficiently safe to be tried in humans. However, much of biomedical research is devoted to the development of animal models of human disease (McCance; Lindsey and Capen). The purposes of developing animal models are essentially those established in the development of the germ theory. The models provide efficient systems for the studies of mechanisms of disease, providing the basis for the development of more effective halfway technologies. Additionally, the availability of animal models greatly facilitates searches for causes, cures, and preventions.

Conflicts between medical practice and research

There are important conflicts between the traditions and motivations of physicians and researchers. As much as we have attempted to fuse science with medicine, much of the practice of medicine is not scientifically based. Much of what the physician does in practice is dictated by authority (Green). For centuries the authority was Hippocrates (fifth century B.C.) as updated by Galen (second century A.D.); no physician dared challenge the teachings of Galen until the Renaissance was well established. Subsequently, while some authority (or the statements of some authorities) has been established through the scientific method, the vast majority of physicians' activities—particularly the caring functions—have no scientific validation. Further, the average physician, who has not participated in what scientific validation there is, must accept the statements of the new authorities with faith that the science upon which they are based is sound.

The researcher, by contrast, challenges authority. If there is one overriding ethic in research it is to learn and to tell the truth (Visscher, pp. 7–11). Authority, as established in the Hippocratic Corpus, instructs the physician to use treatment to help the sick according to *his* ability or judgment but never to injure or wrong them. Put another way, to help, or at least to do no harm. Truth is dispensed to the patient as cautiously and judiciously as any powerful remedy with a clear weighing of the potential adverse consequences. For thousands of years, the physician has known that a sick person who is convinced that he or she will feel better as a consequence of taking some remedy almost always will (Bok; Shapiro). Thus, while administering remedies, some of which were fantastic and nearly all of which were inert, the ancient physician uttered some mystical or magical incantation. The post-Renaissance physician was admonished by authorities to label a prescription with something in Latin that had no meaning to the patient (and often no meaning at all), e.g., tincture of Condurango; the modern physician finds that labeling a drug with a long chemical name has similar effects. At times, the modern physician knowingly prescribes an inert substance called a placebo (from the Latin: I shall please), usually to produce relief of symptoms.

Similarly, it is in the tradition of the physician not to tell the patient the truth about diagnosis or prognosis unless the physician is reasonably certain that on balance the consequences of so doing will produce more benefit than harm (Blumgart).

There are several other important conflicts. Physicians, by virtue of both the immediacy of contact with patients and the expectations of patients, are impelled to do something. Scientists, who can select their problems, are impelled to learn something. Physicians, whose "problems" select them, are constrained by their oath to conduct their practices with utmost confidentiality, and by modern medical ethics to shun advertising. Scientists, whatever their primary motivations, can achieve their rewards only through publication.

The conflicting motivations of the physician and the researcher produce the most dramatic tensions when both functions are being performed simultaneously by the same individual (Katz). Some authors have argued that these conflicts are essentially irreconcilable and—in the interests of protecting the patient who might also be asked to play the role of subject—that the roles of physician and researcher should always be played by different individuals (Fried, pp. 160 ff.; Beecher, pp. 289–292). Others argue that the roles should not be separated because in the final analysis the best assurance that the welfare of research subjects will be protected derives from the motivations, or "conscience," of the physician.

Another controversial issue that derives from recognition of these conflicts is the role of self-experimentation in assuring the validity of research on human subjects. Point five of the Nuremberg Code requires that: "No experiment should be conducted where there is an a priori reason to believe that death or disabling injury will occur; except, perhaps, in those experiments where the experimental physicians also serve as subjects." This point was based on the premise that no person so rational as a scientist would ever deliberately take such risks unless the importance of the knowledge to be gained were extremely high. However, a survey of the history of self-experimentation reveals that, although some self-experimenters are firmly and properly placed in the heroic tradition of medicine (e.g., members of Walter Reed's Yellow Fever Commission), many have taken extreme risks for relatively unimportant goals and, further, their results were often invalid owing to lack of proper controls (Ivy). Since the trials at Nuremberg, there has been a growing recognition that the occasionally overpowering motivations of investigators may lead them to erroneous or, at least, quite different value judgments from those of lay subjects. The 1975 Declaration of Helsinki makes no mention of self-experimentation, and the National Institutes of Health Code for Self-experimentation (Beecher, pp. 304–305) requires the same standards of "group consideration" of proposed research, whether it is to be done on oneself or on normal volunteers. In general, however, an expression of willingness on the part of investigators to participate as subjects in their own proposed research lends credibility to their suggestion that the benefits to be expected merit the taking of the risks (Beecher, p. 233; Cowan).

Efforts to distinguish research from practice are often confounded by the fact that most physicians state that much of the practice of medicine consists of experimentation (Green; Moore). As noted earlier, much diagnostic activity involves observation followed by experimentation. Therapy also relies heavily upon application of the experimental method in the sense that experimentation means to try something out to see if it works. For example, the physician will ordinarily first select a drug likely to produce the desired result with the least possible risk of adverse reactions. Ordinarily, the initial dose of the drug is low; it is gradually increased to a level that produces optimal therapeutic results with minimal side effects. If unacceptable side effects are produced before optimal benefit can be achieved it is customary to change to another medication and repeat the same process. While such activity is experimentation, the experimenter is proceeding with the motivations of the physician. It is not likely that the welfare of the patient will be assigned a priority subsidiary to the ends of research.

The U.S. National Commission for the Protection of Human Subjects of Biomedical and Behavioral Research (hereinafter referred to as the Commission) began in 1976 to develop definitions of research and practice that take these distinctions into account (preliminary draft: 24 February 1976):

[R]esearch . . . refers to a class of activities designed to develop or contribute to generalizable knowledge. . . . By contrast, the practice of medicine . . . refers to a class of activities designed solely to enhance the well-being of an individual. . . . Uncertainty is inherent in therapeutic practice because of the variability of physiological and behavioral human response. This kind of uncertainty is, itself, routine and accepted [National Commission, pp. 1, 2].

A third class of activities, therapeutic innovation (Moore), is identified by the Commission as a "deviation from common practice in drug administration or in surgical, medical, or behavioral therapy [which is] tried in the course of rendering treatment" (National Commission, p. 2). Therapeutic innovation in this sense also includes innovations in diagnostic or prophylactic techniques or procedures. Much recent commentary in the lay media as well as in professional literature inappropriately tends to equate these departures from customary practice with research. The prevailing view that such innovations should be conducted in accord with the standards of research to the extent that adherence to such standards does not subjugate the goals of practice is reflected in the preliminary draft of the report of the Commission.

The tensions between the motivations and value systems of the researcher and physician are exemplified well in the widely used, peculiarly twentieth-century device known as the randomized clinical trial (RCT). The problems associated with the RCT have been discussed extensively (Fried). While the RCT was designed primarily to test new drugs (Hill), subsequently it has been applied to the study of the validity of old drugs, of surgical interventions, and even of social innovations such as multiphasic screening. The RCT has the following elements:

1. The significance of its results is established through statistical analysis. Frequently, in order to generate sufficiently large numbers for statistical analysis in a reasonably short period of time it is necessary to involve several medical centers in the study; thus, the design of the protocol and the evaluation of the results may be conducted in a center remote from that in which any particular patient-subject is being studied.

2. It is a controlled study. That is to say, the new therapy is administered to part of the subject population while another part—as similar as possible in all important respects—receives either another therapy or no therapy. The purpose of having simultaneous controls is to avoid the fallacy of *post hoc ergo propter hoc* reasoning.

Controlled experimentation and statistical analysis are not twentieth-century innovations. The credibility of the former was established firmly in the eighteenth century when James Lind applied it to demonstrate clearly that scurvy could be treated successfully by feeding afflicted persons citrus fruits (Green). The power of statistical analysis to resolve otherwise irreconcilable conflicts over the relative merits of a particular form of therapy was established in the nineteenth century. One of its first triumphs was to demonstrate quite clearly that blood-letting—in the early part of that century the most popular form of therapy for all fevers—was much more dangerous than no therapy at all (Shryock, 1948, pp. 135 ff.).

In the twentieth century additional features were introduced to the RCT. First, the suggestibility of patients, known and used to advantage by physicians for centuries, was acknowledged as a cause of some apparent drug-induced results. This is overcome by "blinding" the subjects, i.e., not letting them know which therapy they are receiving. When the therapy is designed to produce relief of symptoms, the control group often receives a placebo.

Subsequently, it was acknowledged that the biases of investigators might also influence results. Their proclivities to assign patients to what they consider the most promising treatment group are overcome by random selection of treatment and control groups. Similarly, biases in the interpretation of results are eliminated through use of the "double-blind" technique. That is, neither the investigator nor the subject knows until the conclusion of the study who is in which treatment (or control) group.

One can easily see how—in the negotiations for informed consent for participation in an RCT—nearly all the traditions and motivations of the physician must be suspended. Similarly, the effects on expectations and wishes of many patients may be devastating. There are those who argue that the entire process is so technological and dehumanizing that its use should be sharply curtailed (Fried). On the other hand, there are scientists (Hill) and physicians (Chalmers, Block, and Lee) who hold that the power of the RCT to develop sound information on the relative merits of therapies is so great that it would be unethical to introduce a new therapy without this sort of validation.

Socialization of biomedical research

The history of the socialization of biomedical research has been traced in detail in relation to the social, economic, and political forces that helped to shape it (Shryock, 1947). Research originated as a very private enterprise; the popular image of one man working alone was once quite correct. By the late nineteenth century, as biomedical research became increasingly successful in generating explanatory theory for diseases and means for their prevention or cure, it began to attract the attention of financial patrons. Early patronage was provided largely from private sources; philanthropists financed the creation of research institutes in universities and drug companies established research and development departments. Governmental support began slowly in the nineteenth century, accelerated greatly during the Second World War, and, in recognition of its success in developing remedies for war-induced injuries and infections then applicable to treating the diseases of civilians, continued to expand during the next two decades. By the 1970s biomedical research had become, for practical purposes, a public utility (Cooper).

Researchers, according to their tradition, wish to pursue knowledge, if not merely for its own sake at least in relation to problems they consider important. The public demands relevance (ibid.). The public tends to define health as its primary objective, while most biomedical researchers would prefer to concentrate on disease (Seldin). If health is the objective, biomedical research is forced to compete for funds with public health, ecology, urban planning, highway safety, and so on.

Medical care is expensive, and its expense is due in large part to halfway technologies. There are those who argue that we should stop developing new technologies in favor of learning how to distribute efficiently what we have now. Others propose that we might choose not to develop a new, expensive technology unless it can be distributed equitably among all persons (Outka). On the other hand, if we concentrate on learning the causes of disease we can expect to develop specific cures and preventions that tend not only to be inexpensive but also to render obsolete the very expensive halfway technologies and nontechnologies (Thomas). For example, during the polio epidemics of the summer months of the early 1950s, the wards of most city hospitals were crowded with iron lungs, and the efforts of the staff were largely devoted to care of polio victims. By the late 1950s, after distribution of the polio vaccine, iron lungs had all but disappeared, and the efforts of the staff were diverted to other problems.

Increasingly, the public tries to ensure the achievement of its research objectives through priority funding of "mission-oriented" or "targeted research" (Comroe and Dripps). The researcher, perplexed by this, argues that one cannot commission discoveries; these are nearly always accidents. One cannot legislate that a scientist such as Wilhelm Roentgen, while exploring a fundamental problem in physics, will accidentally discover the X-ray. Rather, one can through legislation create environments in which young prospective scientists will learn how to do research and how to deal with discoveries, i.e., their validation and their application to the solution of problems.

Comroe and Dripps identified the ten most important advances in the treatment of cardio-vascular and pulmonary diseases—which currently account for more than half the deaths in the United States—and analyzed the sorts of research upon which they were based. Research was defined as "clinically oriented" (analogous to "mission-oriented"), even if performed entirely on animals, tissues, cells, or fragments of cells, if the author mentioned even briefly an interest in a medical problem. By these criteria, forty-one percent of key articles leading to the development of the ten most important advances were not clinically oriented. Thus, they conclude, if the public chooses to fund only clinically oriented research, it will sacrifice such advances as the development of antibiotics, polio vaccine, and so on.

While priorities for research funding in the United States are established by the public through its representatives in Congress, responsibility for determining which specific projects will be funded is delegated to agencies such as the National Science Foundation and the National Institutes of Health. These agencies, in turn, call upon biomedical researchers to serve on review groups, called study sections, which evaluate the scientific merit of each research proposal. Those with highest scientific merit are recommended for funding. The deliberations of study sections were conducted in strictest confidence until the mid-1970s, when it was determined that research proposals as well as detailed accounts of the deliberations of study sections are available for public scrutiny under the Freedom of Information Act (Morgan, Keyes, and Sherman). Scientists protest that this decision will actually harm the interests of the public it was meant to serve. Scientists do not deem a truth worth considering until the work has been completed and accepted for publication after rigorous review by the editorial board of a journal. Premature release of the activities of scientists may create false impressions that breakthroughs in the treatment of various diseases are closer than they really are. This, in turn, may create false hopes and expectations among the public. Additionally, opening the process of peer review is likely to diminish the necessary candor on the part of members of study sections, thus undermining their effectiveness in assuring preferential funding of high-quality research. Opening the review process may also threaten the interests and traditions of scientists. For example, since much of the reward system in research is based upon being recognized as the first to report an important new finding, researchers tend to resist any move that might increase the possibilities of plagiarism.

The activities of biomedical researchers may, at times, jeopardize the interests and welfare of other human beings. In recognition of this fact, university hospitals began in the 1950s to establish committees designed to review proposed research on human subjects with a view toward safeguarding their rights and welfare (Cowan). Subsequently, federal regulation was developed requiring all institutions that received federal funds for research on human subjects to establish such committees, to which was assigned the general name of institutional review boards (IRBs). At first IRBs comprised almost exclusively biomedical researchers and physicians. With time, membership on IRBs expanded to include lawyers, clergy, representatives of the community of research subjects, and other lay persons. Various observers have pointed out that the system of protection of subjects' rights and welfare is imperfect. The federal government has responded by requiring increasingly complex review procedures. Researchers, who never were quite comfortable about having their activities reviewed and criticized by nonresearchers but who complied more or less willingly, have begun to protest the ever-increasing requirements for both complex protective procedures and formal documentation of compliance (Visscher). Among other things, they suggest that the entire IRB system might collapse under the sheer weight of the bureaucracy involved (Cowan) or that the energies of those responsible for safeguarding the rights and welfare of subjects might be dangerously diverted from the important to the trivial (Ingelfinger). Meanwhile, others argue that IRBs—still dominated by professionals and investigators—do not truly reflect the wishes and values of the lay public (Veatch); accordingly, they propose new procedures, such as a review mechanism composed exclusively of lay persons.

Although most public attention has focused on the rights and welfare of human research subjects, researchers have recognized that some of their activities might present risk to other humans. When an area of research seems to present a particularly serious threat, researchers have called moratoria to provide suitable time to study a problem to learn if and how they might proceed safely. Such a moratorium was called on recombinant DNA research when it became apparent that the research presented grave dangers to the public. For example, it could lead to

the development of new strains of bacteria and viruses that might be highly dangerous and that there is no way to combat (Cohen). After extensive study and discussion by scientists, lawyers, ethicists, journalists, and others, the moratorium was terminated, allowing the research to go forward only in limited areas and only with strict precautions.

Another mechanism developed by researchers for social control of their activities recognizes that all of their social rewards are contingent upon publication. Thus, editors of scientific journals are now held accountable for reviewing submitted papers not only for scientific merit but also for whether the work was performed in accord with established ethical standards. When a manuscript is identified that seems to have violated some ethical standard, the editor should either refuse to publish it (DeBakey) or publish it along with an editorial in which the questions of ethical impropriety are raised (Levine).

Summary

Biomedical research is defined as research having as its ultimate aim the advancement of the goals of medicine. The domain of medicine is defined most narrowly in the traditional medical model, which focuses the attention of the physician on a patient who either feels ill or has a disease, the presence of which is subject to objective verification. The broadest view of the domain of medicine holds that the primary concern of the profession is the maintenance of health, a state of complete physical, mental, and social well-being, not merely the absence of disease. Thus, biomedical research may be seen—according to the traditional medical model—primarily as the application of the natural sciences; in relation to the broader view of the domain of medicine, biomedical research is extended to include some aspects of virtually all natural, behavioral, and social sciences.

Since early in the nineteenth century there has been a systematic effort to blend the scientific method into the practice of medicine. And yet there are important conflicts between the traditions, assumptions, and motivations of physicians and researchers. As a consequence of these conflicts serious problems may be presented to patients, subjects, physicians, and investigators. These problems are exemplified well in the peculiarly twentieth-century device known as the randomized clinical trial.

Research began as a lonely pursuit, and medicine has been called one of the last major remnants of the cottage industry tradition. In the late twentieth century biomedical research and the practice of medicine have become essentially public utilities. This change in the perception of the two enterprises is associated with major controversies over their priorities, goals, and values. Some examples are provided of current controversies within the biomedical research and medical practice enterprises and between spokespersons for biomedical research and the public.

ROBERT J. LEVINE

[*For further discussion of topics mentioned in this article, see the entries:* CARE; CONFIDENTIALITY; ENVIRONMENTAL ETHICS, *article on* ENVIRONMENTAL HEALTH AND HUMAN DISEASE; HEALTH CARE, *article on* HEALTH-CARE SYSTEM; LIFE-SUPPORT SYSTEMS; MASS HEALTH SCREENING; MEDICAL EDUCATION; PUBLIC HEALTH; TECHNOLOGY; THERAPEUTIC RELATIONSHIP; *and* TRUTH-TELLING. *Directly related are the entries* ANIMAL EXPERIMENTATION; COMMUNICATION, BIOMEDICAL; HUMAN EXPERIMENTATION; INFORMED CONSENT IN HUMAN RESEARCH; MEDICAL ETHICS UNDER NATIONAL SOCIALISM; RESEARCH POLICY, BIOMEDICAL; RISK; *and* SCIENCE: ETHICAL IMPLICATIONS. *This article will find application in the entries* CADAVERS; CRYONICS; DRUG INDUSTRY AND MEDICINE; GENE THERAPY; HEART TRANSPLANTATION; ORGAN TRANSPLANTATION, *article on* MEDICAL PERSPECTIVE; *and* REPRODUCTIVE TECHNOLOGIES. *For problems of conducting biomedical research on special populations, see:* ADOLESCENTS; AGING AND THE AGED, *article on* HEALTH CARE AND RESEARCH IN THE AGED; CHILDREN AND BIOMEDICINE; FETAL RESEARCH; INFANTS, *article on* MEDICAL ASPECTS AND ETHICAL DILEMMAS; MENTALLY HANDICAPPED; PRISONERS, *article on* PRISONER EXPERIMENTATION; *and* WOMEN AND BIOMEDICINE, *article on* WOMEN AS PATIENTS AND EXPERIMENTAL SUBJECTS. *See* APPENDIX, SECTION II: DIRECTIVES FOR HUMAN EXPERIMENTATION; *and* SECTION III, DECLARATION ON THE RIGHTS OF MENTALLY RETARDED PERSONS, *and* PEDIATRIC BILL OF RIGHTS.]

BIBLIOGRAPHY

BEECHER, HENRY K. *Research and the Individual: Human Studies.* Boston: Little, Brown & Co., 1970.

BLUMGART, HERRMAN L. "The Medical Framework for Viewing the Problem of Human Experimentation." *Experimentation with Human Subjects.* Edited by Paul A. Freund. New York: George Braziller, 1970, pp. 39–65.

BOK, SISSELA. "The Ethics of Giving Placebos." *Scientific American* 231, no. 5 (1974), pp. 17–23.

BURTON, LLOYD EDWARD, and SMITH, HUGH HOLLINGSWORTH. *Public Health and Community Medicine for the Allied Medical Professions.* 2d ed. Baltimore: Williams & Wilkins Co., 1975.

CASSELL, ERIC J. "Illness and Disease." *Hastings Center Report* 6, no. 2 (1976), pp. 27–37.

CHALMERS, THOMAS C.; BLOCK, JEROME B.; and LEE, STEPHANIE. "Controlled Studies in Clinical Cancer Research." *New England Journal of Medicine* 287 (1972): 75–78.

COHEN, STANLEY N. "Recombinant DNA: Fact and Fiction." *Science* 195 (1977): 654–657.

COMROE, JULIUS H., JR., and DRIPPS, ROBERT D. "Scientific Basis for the Support of Biomedical Science." *Science* 192 (1976): 105–111.

CONNELL, ALASTAIR. "The Nature of Responsibility." *Ethical Responsibility in Medicine.* Edited by Vincent Edmunds and C. Gordon Scorer. Edinburgh: E. & S. Livingstone, 1967, pp. 1–22.

COOPER, THEODORE. "Socialization of Medical Research." *Clinical Research* 20 (1972): 299–304.

COWAN, DALE H. "Human Experimentation: The Review Process in Practice." *Case Western Reserve Law Review* 25 (1975): 533–564.

DeBAKEY, LOIS. "Ethically Questionable Data: Publish or Reject?" *Clinical Research* 22 (1974): 113–121.

DUBOS, RENÉ. *Man Adapting.* New Haven: Yale University Press, 1965.

FEINSTEIN, ALVAN R. *Clinical Judgment.* Baltimore: Williams & Wilkins Co., 1967.

FLEXNER, ABRAHAM. *Medical Education: A Comparative Study.* New York: Macmillan Co., 1925.

FREIDSON, ELIOT. *Profession of Medicine: A Study of the Sociology of Applied Knowledge.* New York: Dodd, Mead & Co., 1970.

FRIED, CHARLES. *Medical Experimentation: Personal Integrity and Social Policy.* New York: American Elsevier Co., 1974.

FRUTON, JOSEPH S. "The Emergence of Biochemistry." *Science* 192 (1976): 327–334.

GREEN, F. H. K. "The Clinical Evaluation of Remedies." *Lancet* 2 (1954): 1085–1091.

HILL, AUSTIN BRADFORD. "Medical Ethics and Controlled Trials." *British Medical Journal* 1 (1963): 1043–1049.

INGELFINGER, FRANZ J. "The Unethical in Medical Ethics." *Annals of Internal Medicine* 83 (1975): 264–269.

IVY, A. C. "The History and Ethics of the Use of Human Subjects in Medical Experiments." *Science* 108 (1948): 1–5.

KATZ, JAY. "The Regulation of Human Research—Reflections and Proposals." *Clinical Research* 21 (1973): 785–791.

KREIDER, SIDNEY D., and MAMLIN, JOSEPH J. "Health Care Research in the Public General Hospital: A Symposium Summary." *Clinical Research* 20 (1972): 305–309.

LEVINE, ROBERT J. "Ethical Considerations in the Publication of the Results of Research Involving Human Subjects." *Clinical Research* 21 (1973): 763–767.

LINDSEY, J. RUSSELL, and CAPEN, CHARLES C., cochairmen. "Symposium: Animal Models for Biomedical Research: VI. Metabolic Disease." *Federation Proceedings* 35 (1976): 1192–1236. Part of a series of symposia sponsored by the Institute of Laboratory Animal Resources and the American College of Laboratory Animal Medicine.

McCANCE, R. A. "The Practice of Experimental Medicine." *Proceedings of the Royal Society of Medicine* 44 (1951): 189–194. President's address.

MAKARUSHKA, JULIA LOUGHLIN. "The Requirement for Informed Consent in Research on Human Subjects: The Problem of the Uncontrolled Consequences of Health-Related Research." *Clinical Research* 24 (1976): 64–67.

MOORE, FRANCIS D. "Therapeutic Innovation: Ethical Boundaries in the Initial Clinical Trials of New Drugs and Surgical Procedures." *Experimentation with Human Subjects.* Edited by Paul A. Freund. New York: George Braziller, 1970, pp. 358–378.

MORGAN, THOMAS E.; KEYES, JOSEPH A.; and SHERMAN, JOHN F. "Confidentiality of Research Grant Protocols." *Clinical Research* 24 (1976): 5–12.

National Commission for the Protection of Human Subjects of Biomedical and Behavioral Research. "The Boundaries between Biomedical and Behavioral Research and Accepted and Routine Practice." Draft. Xerographically reproduced typescript. 24 February 1976. 4 pp. Belmont Manifesto. Appeared as the second entry under Tab. 4 in the tentative agenda for the 16th meeting of the National Commission, held on 12–13 March 1976. Draft was prepared at the 15th meeting of the National Commission, held on 13–16 February 1976 at the Belmont Conference Center, Elkridge, Maryland.

OUTKA, GENE. "Social Justice and Equal Access to Health Care." *Perspectives in Biology and Medicine* 18 (1975): 185–203.

PARSONS, TALCOTT. *The Social System.* Glencoe, Ill.: Free Press, 1951.

PARSONS, VICTOR. "Social Aberrations—Sin, Crime or Disease?" *Ethical Responsibility in Medicine.* Edited by Vincent Edmunds and C. Gordon Scorer. Edinburgh: E. & S. Livingstone, 1967, pp. 117–135.

SELDIN, DONALD W. "The Intimate Coupling of Biomedical Science and Physician Education." *Clinical Research* 23 (1975): 280–286.

SHAPIRO, ARTHUR K. "A Contribution to the History of the Placebo Effect." *Behavioral Science* 5 (1960): 109–135.

SHRYOCK, RICHARD HARRISON. *American Medical Research Past and Present.* New York Academy of Medicine, Committee on Medicine and the Changing Order, Monograph Studies. New York: Commonwealth Fund, 1947.

————. *The Development of Modern Medicine: An Interpretation of the Social and Scientific Factors Involved.* Rev. ed. New York: Alfred A. Knopf, 1948.

SIGERIST, HENRY E. *A History of Medicine.* Vol. 1: *Primitive and Archaic Medicine.* Department of the History of Medicine, Yale University, Publication no. 27. New York: Oxford University Press, 1951.

THOMAS, LEWIS. "Commentary: The Future Impact of Science and Technology on Medicine." *Bioscience* 24 (1974): 99–105.

VEATCH, ROBERT M. "Human Experimentation Committees: Professional or Representative?" *Hastings Center Report* 5, no. 5 (1975), pp. 31–40.

VISSCHER, MAURICE B. *Ethical Constraints and Imperatives in Medical Research.* American Lecture Series, no. 983. A monograph in the Bannerstone Division of American Lectures in Behavioral Science and Law. Springfield, Ill.: Charles C. Thomas, 1975.

World Health Organization. *The First Ten Years of the World Health Organization.* Geneva: 1958.

RESEARCH POLICY, BIOMEDICAL

Value implications

"Research policy" suggests a paradox that lies at the core of public support of scientific research. In its fundamental sense, "research" suggests a systematic investigation of some phenomenon or phenomena by means of the empirical method. "Policy," on the other hand, suggests a course or plan—usually governmental—designed to influence future decisions and activities.

"Research policy" immediately raises two questions: (1) How much, if at all, should the conduct of biomedical research be supported by public resources? (2) How much should the conduct of research, including the setting of its goals, be subject to public control?

In the United States the question concerning the amount of resources to be invested in research has been answered through the complex rough-and-tumble of the political processes of authorization, appropriation, and allocation. Consequently, the question is answered anew by each succeeding Congress and by each new administration.

In England and Europe, including the Scandinavian countries, the public support of research is a function of some relatively stable aspect of the overall economy of the nation. In England, for example, a fixed percentage of the total budget for health is set aside for biomedical research support. Similar systems prevail throughout most of the countries that subsidize research.

The question of whether the goals of research should be set by the political process remains unclear. Generally speaking, investigators in the United Kingdom and Western Europe have been free of external direction. In the United States the issue has been debated in every decade. Scientists have long contended that research achievement, particularly in basic science, has been and continues to be possible only if investigators are given freedom to follow their own insights and the logic of the discipline in which they are laboring. For the most part, the political forces that generate support for biomedical research have respected the freedom of investigators working in areas of fundamental or basic research.

However, in the realm of "applied" science, goals external to scientific purposes have been identified and imposed on the work of biomedical investigators. The degree to which it is appropriate and wise to direct, target, or constrain biomedical research has been and continues to be the central and most difficult public policy question raised in relation to biomedical research.

A complaint frequently voiced by scientists is that society often tends to co-opt their services to such a degree that the freedom of inquiry is endangered. In recent years the opposite complaint has been raised by environmentalists and other critics, who contend that the needs of science may exert such influence on public policy that society itself may be co-opted in the service of science. For example, it has been charged that the rights of human subjects of research have been transgressed by investigators supported by public funds who are seeking new research knowledge. Most recently it has been alleged that public safety has been breached by investigators who wish to conduct research using recombinant DNA techniques to produce new combinations of genetic material.

The tension between the goals and values of public policy and the needs of scientists to follow the logic of the life-science disciplines appears to be inevitable. This tension has produced a complex partnership between public officials and the scientific community. It has also produced a series of public debates and compromises around which much of the history of the development of public biomedical research policy revolves. Some of the highlights of that historical development in the United States are presented below.

History of the development of U.S. biomedical research policy

Early years. Almost from the beginning of its history, the U.S. government recognized, at least in a limited way, its obligation to provide health care for some segments of the society. Under President John Adams in 1798, Congress authorized the establishment of the Marine Hospital Service for sick and disabled seamen as a division of the Treasury Department. The decision to provide public support for health research did not develop for almost another century, with the establishment in 1887 of the one-room bacteriological laboratory for the investigation of cholera and other infectious diseases at the Marine Hospital, Staten Island, N.Y., under the direction of Dr. Joseph J. Kinyoun.

In the years that followed, public research policy was expressed in terms of the need to prevent, diagnose, and treat infectious categorical

diseases such as yellow fever, cholera, and smallpox. Each succeeding Congress expanded the mission of the Marine Hospital Service and assigned new research responsibilities to its laboratory (designated the Hygienic Laboratory in 1891). The Marine Hospital Service was renamed the "Public Health and Marine Hospital Service" in 1902, and in 1912 became part of the more comprehensive "Public Health Service" (PHS).

It was soon seen that if biomedical research were to produce effective techniques for combating disease, it must consider not only the health needs of the public, but the state of the art in related scientific disciplines. Consequently, the Fifty-seventh Congress created an Advisory Board to the Biologics Control Division, which became the National Advisory Health Council in 1930. Its creation marked the formal beginning of the participation of nongovernmental scientific experts in the formulation of national biomedical research policy. From that time forward policymakers within the government and experts from the scientific community would work together, though not always in harmony, to develop a public research policy intended to respect the freedom of scientific disciplines while striving to meet the utilitarian goals of a public that assigned an ever expanding public health role to the government.

In 1918 the Chamberlain–Kahn Act provided for the study of venereal diseases. The PHS (by then under direction of a Surgeon General) used this new authority to make grants-in-aid of research to twenty-five institutions. That action established a precedent for the federal government to seek assistance of scientists employed by nonfederal institutions in implementing public policy. The venereal diseases research program marked the beginning of a federal policy which assumes that public goals can be achieved through investigator-initiated research supported by tax dollars under nonspecific authority.

The 1920s witnessed a strongly contested debate concerning the appropriate mission of the PHS. On one hand Senator Joseph Ransdell, backed by Surgeon General Lewis R. Thompson, contended that research supported by the federal government should "take in all the ills that flesh is heir to." On the other hand, Senator Matthew M. Neely supported legislation that would have required the bulk of federal biomedical research dollars to be marshaled in a concentrated effort to overcome cancer. In enacting the Ransdell view into law in 1930, the Congress reorganized and expanded the Hygienic Laboratory and redesignated it the National Institute of Health (NIH). The Neely bill was unsuccessful in 1930, but the concept of a targeted research effort concentrated on a single disease category remained alive in Congress and in the public mind. The contest between proponents of federally supported research (guided principally by the opportunities perceived by the scientific community) and proponents of "categorical" or "targeted" research (guided by goals set by political process) has been repeated again and again in the development of public health research policy.

In 1937 Senator Hugh Bone and Congressman Warren G. Magnuson successfully sponsored companion bills in each House of Congress establishing a national institute to launch a major targeted research attack on cancer, the disease most feared by Americans. The Bone–Magnuson Act (P.L. 75–244) authorized the National Cancer Institute to conduct and foster research and studies relating to the cause, prevention, and methods of diagnosis and treatment of cancer. This act became the prototype of future targeted health research legislation. It identified a specific research category or target; required an advisory council composed of members from outside the government to review and approve all extramural research projects (thus extending the partnership between government and the scientific community); included authority for training investigators; added a small but significant international dimension to U.S. research efforts; and called for coordination of federal and state health agencies.

The war years. The Second World War brought profound changes to health research. The Committee for Medical Research was created by President Franklin D. Roosevelt to mount a research program aimed at reducing the effects of war-related disease and injury. In conjunction with the National Research Council of the National Academy of Sciences, the committee mobilized the community of biomedical scientists in an extraordinary outpouring of creative energy. Spectacular results have been attributed to the work coordinated by the committee, including development of wide use of penicillin, sulfanilamides, gamma globulin, adrenal steroids, and cortisone, as well as development of many other drugs and techniques, which led to the saving of thousands of lives. The momentum generated by research efforts during the war years

led to continued expansion of research efforts for two decades.

In 1944 the Congress enacted P.L. 78–410, landmark legislation known as the Public Health Service Act. It consolidated all of the authorities under which the PHS operated and divided the PHS into the Office of the Surgeon General, the Bureau of Medical Services, the Bureau of State Services, and the National Institute of Health. It included authority for clinical research within PHS medical facilities. The act gave the Surgeon General broad (noncategorical) powers to conduct and support research in the fundamental problems of diseases and disabilities and made the National Cancer Institute a division of the NIH.

The Public Health Service Act included research and research training authority without "time" or "dollar" limits. That meant, in effect, that there was no authorization ceiling or dollar limit imposed a priori on the appropriations process whereby Congress funded the PHS. Funding levels for biomedical research depended exclusively on appropriations bills reported to the House and the Senate. Thus the chairmen of two Congressional health appropriations subcommittees had, for many years, complete control over the levels of biomedical research funding. No parallel for this extraordinary funding process can be found in any other country that supports biomedical research.

Postwar developments. In 1946 the NIH was successful in securing the transfer of fifty projects from the wartime Office of Scientific Research and Development. Consequently the NIH research budget shot from $180,000 in fiscal 1945 to $850,000 in fiscal 1946 and to $8,000,-000 in fiscal 1947. The sudden growth of the NIH budget helped to avert the possibility that the newly created National Science Foundation might take over federal support of biomedical research. An upward spiral of research budgets continued for twenty years.

In 1946 the National Institute of Mental Health was created, and in 1948 the Congress authorized creation of the National Heart Institute and changed the name of the National "Institute" of Health to the National "Institutes" of Health. These changes brought categorical research programs directly under the broad, general (noncategorical) authority of the Public Health Service Act. It was almost as if the Congress were saying: "The scientist is to conduct health-related research at government expense in whatever way the state of the art, scientific opportunity, and his or her own creative bent indicates; however, whenever possible, special emphasis is to be given to research relating to the categorical missions of the research institutes." The directors of the categorical institutes have, for the most part, interpreted the Public Health Service Act and its amendments as requiring the conduct and support of both basic and applied research.

The distinctions between basic research and applied research and technology, and between fundamental and categorical or targeted research, are by no means clear. These terms have no commonly accepted univocal meaning. Nevertheless, they do connote very different emphases, which are reflected in the policy swing between support of biomedical research relying on the interests of the investigator for its direction and support of research planned to fulfill goals dictated by public policy.

In the quarter-century from 1950 to 1975, the number of research institutes within the NIH grew from two to eleven. These included not only additional institutes related to categorical diseases or to organs subject to disease, but also the Institute for General Medical Sciences (dedicated to basic research), the Institute for Environmental Health Sciences, the Institute for Child Health and Human Development, and the Institute on Aging. Thus growth in categorical disease research was balanced by increases in support for noncategorical biomedical research.

Period of growth.   Federal support for health research has grown from $27 million in 1947 to upwards of $3 billion in 1976. This dramatic expansion is attributable in no small degree to the efforts of Mrs. Mary B. Lasker and the health lobby which she orchestrated. Between 1955 and 1968, under the directorship of Dr. James A. Shannon and with the support of Senator Lister Hill and Representative John Fogarty, chairmen of the appropriations subcommittees, the NIH enjoyed steady growth and consolidation of its programs. Those thirteen years witnessed a remarkable harmony between federal policies and the health research community. In the context of expanding budgets, both public policy and biomedical research goals appeared to reach a happy balance.

Peer review.   In 1958 the NIH brought about a reorganization of the Division of Research Grants, which developed and perfected the peer review system for selecting the most meritorious grant applications. This review of research projects by peers of the researcher has often been called the "lynchpin" of federal support of scientific research. Not only does it seek to maintain fairness and justice in the apportionment of federal dollars, it gives assurance of high-quality research and seeks a middle ground between public goals and the demands of science. This system has been adapted and utilized by most of the federal agencies that conduct or support research and technology and by Sweden, England, France, and other countries. Despite occasional criticism, the system has operated virtually without scandal for many years.

Policy for protection of human subjects. Since its inception in 1953, the Clinical Center of the NIH has ranked as one of the largest and best research hospitals in the world. It houses laboratory facilities for clinical support of research on resident patients and outpatients who agree to participate in its research programs. In 1953 a Clinical Center policy was published requiring that research subjects give informed consent prior to their participation in research. This document was the first written U.S. policy for the protection of human subjects of biomedical research.

In 1960 the National Institutes of Health awarded a grant to Boston University to recommend a policy for the protection of human subjects of research. In 1966, guided by the report of the Boston study and by experience with the Clinical Center policy, the Surgeon General issued a Public Policy for the Protection of all Human Subjects who participate in research conducted or supported by PHS funds. This policy was revised several times and was reissued in expanded form as the Department of Health, Education, and Welfare (DHEW) policy in 1971.

In 1974 the Congress created the National Commission for the Protection of Human Subjects of Biomedical and Behavioral Research to serve as an advisory body to the Secretary of Health, Education, and Welfare in policy matters pertaining to ethical, social, and legal aspects of biomedical and behavioral research.

The federal policy for the protection of human subjects is built on the doctrines of informed consent and a favorable risk-benefit ratio. It requires that all research carried out in institutions that receive federal support from DHEW must be scrutinized by Institutional Review Boards.

Current developments

Erosion of harmonious partnership. In the late 1960s the steady growth of the national biomedical research effort and the harmonious partnership of federal and nonfederal agents in the promotion of that effort eroded quickly. At the time, the United States was divided over the conduct of a costly, controversial war; President Johnson called for additional domestic spending to fuel the domestic service programs of his "war on poverty."

In 1968 Senator Lister Hill of Alabama led the Senate in raising the appropriations of the NIH, but in 1969 Congress cut $20 million from the NIH budget, the largest cut in its history. Coupled with rising inflation, this was a major reversal and marked the beginning of relatively level budgets for biomedical research. Only the cancer research budget has continued to grow at a steady rate.

The debate over targeted research. In 1971, upon receipt of the report of a panel of experts that called for a carefully planned, targeted approach to the conquest of cancer, Senator Edward Kennedy introduced legislation for creation of a separate cancer agency to wage a war on cancer. Much of the rhetoric surrounding this bill likened the proposed cancer initiative to the "moon shot," which had, as a result of a ten-year crash program, placed a man on the moon. Not to be outdone by his Democratic rival, President Nixon proposed, and Congress enacted in 1971, a supplemental appropriations act which included $100 million for cancer research. Meanwhile a fierce debate that produced deep divisions within the scientific community occurred over the Kennedy bill. Proponents argued that the "state of the art" in cancer research called for a massive targeted research effort. Opponents contended that the Kennedy bill was simply "throwing money" at a disease, and that a separate cancer agency would "tear the fabric" of biomedical research, which depended—in the main—on investigator-initiated discoveries rather than on targeted planning that could be programmed by Congress.

However, the House of Representatives, under the leadership of Congressman Paul Rogers, was reluctant to separate the Cancer Institute from the NIH. When a compromise between Senate and House versions of the National Cancer Act of 1971 was finally reached, views of both camps were included in the act. The Cancer Institute was to be a "separate agency within the National Institutes of Health." What this meant in practice was that the Director of the Cancer Institute, while continuing to report to the Director of the NIH, was authorized to bring budgetary concerns directly to the President. A three-member President's Cancer Panel was to oversee the administration of the cancer program, and the Cancer Council would be replaced by a new, larger Cancer Advisory Board appointed by the President. Furthermore, the Cancer Institute was to mount a major control and demonstration program intended to bring the latest research findings quickly to the mainstream of health-care delivery.

Once again the pendulum had swung away from investigator-initiated research and was now swinging in the direction of research targeted and directed by public policy. This tactic brought a monetary bonanza to cancer research. The budget of the Cancer Institute climbed from $233 million in 1971 to $691 million in 1975, while budgets of most of the other research institutes remained relatively level and in some cases declined.

The targeted or categorical approach to research has been in fashion since 1971. In 1972 the Congress enacted, with time and dollar limits, the National Sickle Cell Anemia Control Act, the National Cooley's Anemia Control Act, and the National Heart, Blood Vessel, Lung and Blood Act. In 1972 the Congress also created a Multiple Sclerosis Commission, which, in more recent years, has been joined by a Huntington's Chorea Commission, a Diabetes Commission, an Arthritis Commission, and an Epilepsy Commission. Each of these efforts represents an attempt to draw public attention and increased dollar support to a given categorical research field; on the other hand, each has created additional administrative burdens, which increase the cost of research.

Ethical and policy dimensions: an overview

Public policies for the governance of biomedical research are expressed primarily through the acts and attitudes of the Congress. In its authorizations and appropriations the U.S. Congress plays a more active role than does the British Parliament, the German Bundesrat, or other lawmaking bodies in countries that support research with public funds. At times U.S. congressional support has been inappropriate and misguided. On the whole, it has been generous toward research and enlightened in its understanding of the need to balance research disciplines and public needs.

In the 1970s, in response to voices raised on many sides, Congress has tended to place tighter controls on those who wish to conduct research. The Department of Health, Education, and Welfare, responding to advice from the congressionally created Commission for the Protection of Human Subjects, has limited the kind of research that may be conducted on the human fetus. Special provisions for research involving prisoners, the mentally disabled, children, and candidates for psychosurgery have also been promulgated.

Constraints have been placed on the shipment of etiologic and radioactive materials that are essential to the conduct of research. The Freedom of Information Act has been invoked to open the contents of research grant applications and contract proposals to the public—a matter which has produced several court cases, many congressional hearings, and much evidence for the Congress to sift. The Federal Advisory Committee Act has challenged and changed the functioning of the peer review system and may produce further changes, which could affect the quality of review of grant applications and contract proposals. The Privacy Act has imposed complex administrative burdens with the intention to protect the privacy of identifiable individuals whose records are under the control of research agencies. The Federal Reports Act has regulated the methods used by investigators to seek information. The Medical Devices Act and the Toxic Substances Control Act have placed further curbs on the conduct of research. A broad public debate has arisen relating to the technique of recombining genetic material from one species into another. Congress, state legislatures, and city governments have all participated in the debate over a process that promises rich benefits, but contains potential hazards for humankind or other species. Regulation of techniques for recombining genetic material appears to be inevitable.

The National Environmental Protection Act requires publication of an environmental (including economic) impact statement before any major program that might change the environment may be undertaken. It has slowed the development of recombinant DNA molecule research and may be expected to be applied to all forms of research that contain potential hazards for individuals, communities, or the public at large.

Biomedical research in the United States has flourished, as nowhere else, under a generally enlightened public policy of partnership between government officials and the scientific community, with the public represented at every stage. The tension between public goals and disciplinary demands of science has, for the most part, been resolved in constructive and ingenious ways. The pendulum has swung first in one direction then in the other in a constantly self-correcting process. At present the emphasis has shifted toward increased public direction and control of biomedical research.

For the future, scientists must anticipate with greater sensitivity public needs or fears, learn better to explain their work, and share responsibility in a fashion wider than has been customary. The public, for its part, must come to understand the delicacy of the scientific enterprise, which depends in the last analysis on the creativity of a tiny minority of gifted and trained individuals who must have reasonable freedom to pursue their insights.

The value of biomedical research to society has been, and continues to be over any brief time span, difficult to assess. Over a longer period, the pursuit of research findings not only affects the health and life-styles of individuals but also shapes institutions and constitutes a considerable influence in the economic history of the developed nations. It provides aesthetic achievements comparable to those of music, art, and drama, and brings advances in medical care that confer significant benefits on many. On the other hand, biomedical research policy requires careful attention to societal priorities, the rights of individuals, the allocation of power and benefits, and the impact of biomedical technologies on contemporary society.

CHARLES R. MCCARTHY

[*Directly related are the entries* HEALTH POLICY, *article on* EVOLUTION OF HEALTH POLICY; *and* HUMAN EXPERIMENTATION, *article on* SOCIAL AND PROFESSIONAL CONTROL. *Other relevant material may be found under* RESEARCH, BEHAVIORAL; RESEARCH, BIOMEDICAL; *and* SCIENCE: ETHICAL IMPLICATIONS. *See* APPENDIX, SECTION II, U.S. GUIDELINES ON HUMAN EXPERIMENTATION.]

BIBLIOGRAPHY

EHRENREICH, BARBARA, and EHRENREICH, JOHN. *The American Health Empire: Power, Profits and Politics.* Health-PAC Book. New York: Random House, 1970. A report from the Health Policy Advisory Center.
Federation of American Societies for Experimental Biology, American Biology Council. "Contributions of the Biological Sciences to Human Welfare." *Fed-*

eration Proceedings 31, no. 6, pt. 2 (1972), pp. TF13—TF139.

FREDRICKSON, DONALD S. "The Public Governance of Science." Columbia University Bicentennial Lecture, 1976. To be published in *Man and Medicine* 3 (1978).

GREENBERG, DANIEL S. *The Politics of Pure Science.* New York: New American Library, 1967.

McCARTHY, ESTELLE, and McCARTHY, CHARLES. *The Power Picture.* New York: Friendship Press, 1973.

National Institutes of Health, Office of the Director. *The Training Programs of the Institutes of the National Institutes of Health, Fiscal Year 1974.* 2 vols. Bethesda, Md.: 1972.

PRIMACK, JOEL, and HIPPEL, FRANK VON. *Advice and Dissent: Scientists in the Political Arena.* New York: Basic Books, 1974.

REDMAN, ERIC. *The Dance of Legislation.* New York: Simon & Schuster, 1973.

SHANNON, JAMES AUGUSTINE, ed. *Science and the Evolution of Public Policy.* New York: Rockefeller University Press, 1973.

STRICKLAND, STEPHEN P. *Politics, Science, and Dread Disease: A Short History of United States Medical Research Policy.* Cambridge: Harvard University Press, Commonwealth Fund Book, 1972.

United States, National Institutes of Health, *The National Institutes of Health Almanac.* DHEW Publication no. (NIH) 76-5. Bethesda, Md.: 1976.

———, Public Health Service. *The Public Health Service To-Day.* DHEW Publication no. (OS) 76-50048. Washington: Government Printing Office, 1976.

ZUCKERMAN, SOLLY. *Scientists and War: The Impact of Science on Military and Civil Affairs.* New York: Harper & Row, 1967.

RESEARCH WITH HUMAN SUBJECTS

See HUMAN EXPERIMENTATION.

RESUSCITATION

See DEATH AND DYING: EUTHANASIA AND SUSTAINING LIFE; LIFE-SUPPORT SYSTEMS.

RETARDATION or RETARDED

See MENTALLY HANDICAPPED.

RIGHT TO CONFIDENTIALITY

See CONFIDENTIALITY; PATIENTS' RIGHTS MOVEMENT; PRIVACY. *See also* RIGHTS.

RIGHT TO DIE

See DEATH AND DYING: EUTHANASIA AND SUSTAINING LIFE; RIGHT TO REFUSE MEDICAL CARE. *See also* RIGHTS.

RIGHT TO FERTILITY CONTROL

See ABORTION; CONTRACEPTION; STERILIZATION; PRENATAL DIAGNOSIS; POPULATION POLICY PROPOSALS. *See also* RIGHTS.

RIGHT TO FOOD

See FOOD POLICY. *See also* RIGHTS.

RIGHT TO HEALTH or RIGHT TO HEALTH CARE

See HEALTH CARE, *articles on* RIGHT TO HEALTH-CARE SERVICES *and* THEORIES OF JUSTICE AND HEALTH CARE; INSTITUTIONALIZATION; PRISONERS, *article on* MEDICAL CARE OF PRISONERS; AGING AND THE AGED, *article on* HEALTH CARE AND RESEARCH IN THE AGED. *For discussion of questions dealing with the rights to mental health, genetic health, environmental health, etc., see the entries dealing with those topics. See also* RIGHTS.

RIGHT TO INFORMATION

See INFORMED CONSENT IN HUMAN RESEARCH; INFORMED CONSENT IN MENTAL HEALTH; INFORMED CONSENT IN THE THERAPEUTIC RELATIONSHIP; CONFIDENTIALITY; TRUTH-TELLING. *See also* RIGHTS.

RIGHT TO LIFE

See LIFE; PERSON; ABORTION; DEATH AND DYING: EUTHANASIA AND SUSTAINING LIFE. *See also* RIGHTS.

RIGHT TO PRIVACY

See PRIVACY; CONFIDENTIALITY. *See also* RIGHTS.

RIGHT TO REFUSE MEDICAL CARE

Interventions by persons providing health care proceed, as a general matter, only upon the permission of the patient. The restatement of what is usually called the doctrine of informed consent in terms of a right to refuse medical care has several significant consequences. First, the rights formulation makes apparent that, although "consent" may connote *agreement*, the heart of the doctrine is the necessity of a *decision* by the patient—which may be negative or affirmative —on whether to go forward with the intervention. Informed consent is intended to serve many other purposes as well, including the promotion of more rational decision making and of careful reflection about the procedures by the professionals carrying them out (Katz and Capron, pp. 82–90). Nonetheless, the fundamental objective of the doctrine is to preserve an individual's right to accept or decline proposed diagnosis, prevention, or therapy as he or she chooses.

Second, a rights-based analysis compels one to consider the duties created by the patient's exercise of the right, which will vary with the persons owing them. A physician, for example, is under a duty to adhere to his or her patient's decision about which medical alternative will be employed or, if the patient's choice is unacceptable to the physician, to secure someone else to care for the patient. In the absence of compelling reasons to the contrary, the state, usually acting through the judiciary, must honor a patient's refusal of treatment by declining to compel an unwanted intervention and by penalizing unauthorized overriding of the patient's wishes. The bases in law of the right to refuse treatment thus extend beyond tort law (battery and negligence), which underlies the doctrine of informed consent, to include criminal law and contract law. In contrast to the duties of physicians and state officials, a patient's family has no legal duty to assent to his or her decision but also no legal authority to overrule it. Nonetheless, since the right to refuse treatment arises from ethical as well as legal principles, family members could be said to have a moral duty to respect the patient's decision and indeed to support the patient in the face of the contrary wishes of others.

Third, describing the relative interests of the participants in health care in terms of a right to refuse treatment is one manifestation of the rights-consciousness of the modern age. The libertarian and humanistic principles on which the right is grounded have played central roles on the political stage for the past three centuries, but it is only recently that those principles have been enunciated in the sphere of medical care. The result has been to borrow from rules intended to restrict the coercive power of governments. Article 5, Point 1, of the 1951 European Convention on Human Rights, for example, states: "Everyone has the right to liberty and security of person." It has been argued that this codifies the patient's right to bodily integrity against interference by physicians (van Till, p. 32).

Finally, speaking about the right reminds one of the wavering commitment of both medicine and law to the principle of self-determination. If informed-consent strictures were really taken seriously by professionals there would probably be no occasion to turn to the stiffer and more absolute vocabulary of rights.

Importance of the right

The important role to be played by the right of refusal can be seen in both teleological and deontological terms, that is, in terms of consequences and of inherent moral duties. As a matter of the objectives being sought by modern medicine, the view is increasingly widely held that medical care sometimes produces more harm than good, particularly for terminal patients. It can be physically detrimental, dehumanizing for those who give and receive it, and wasteful of scarce resources. A right of patients to refuse such care would act as a brake on the phenomenon of unwanted treatment. It bears emphasis, however, that the right in question is distinct from a right not to be subjected to excessive medical intervention. Though both may serve similar objectives, the latter has reference to an external standard of excessiveness while the former is a right of choice, referring solely to a patient's subjective evaluation of reasonableness. As a matter of process or of the duties owed by people to one another, the asserted right to refuse treatment reflects a more broadly based desire to return to individuals control over their own lives (Ramsey, pp. 1–11). Health practitioners supporting vigorous use of biomedical technology have been rather taken aback to find themselves addressed in language reminiscent of the post-eighteenth-century movements for political liberation from tyranny. But the fervor should not be surprising, as it corresponds to a heightened concern with personal autonomy in the face of an increasingly routinized and impersonal world.

Despite the vigor with which the right is asserted, it may be qualified by countervailing interests. Particularly when a refusal of treatment seems likely to lead to a patient's death, serious ethical and legal doubts arise for commentators and decision makers alike. Yet it is precisely in cases of life-preserving treatment that the right has been most strongly advocated, and with good reason: it would be rather hollow to recognize a so-called right to decline medical care and then to disallow its exercise when a patient feels so strongly about the choices at issue that he or she is willing to risk death.

Conflicting claims or interests

As with all rights, articulation of a right to refuse care necessitates an examination of competing claims or interests. In addition to (1) the interests of the individual, at least six important interests weigh in the balance on the collective side: (2) protecting people from their own imprudence, (3) maintaining a healthy population to support society, (4) avoiding harm to third parties, (5) minimizing health-care and other costs, (6) safeguarding public morality and decency, and (7) reinforcing the principle that life is sacred.

1. Individual interests—autonomy and dignity. The concept of personal autonomy has particular importance in the context of medical care. In all circumstances, autonomy suggests that one has the liberty to follow one's will. But that notion of personal freedom has further consequences when the exercise of self-determination concerns one's body, as is true for medical decisions. Autonomy then implies protection of personal integrity as well. Without extending the concept as far as the autonomous Kantian will—making its own laws free from influences of pleasure or pain—it can be seen that freedom from physical or psychological interference is a necessary aspect of genuine self-determination in medical care.

Not all commentators would denominate personal autonomy the central personal interest underlying the right to accept or refuse treatment. In recent constitutional jurisprudence in the United States the concept of privacy has been pressed into service as the basis for declaring invalid statutes that circumscribe too tightly decisions about procreation. Although the courts have declined to recognize an absolute right in individuals to do completely as they please with their bodies, a broad right to make medical decisions has been acknowledged even when the exercise of the right can harm other living or potential people, impinge on other public interests, or expose the patient to an increased risk of death (In re *Yetter*, pp. 623–624).

Similarly, both humanistic and theistic commentators find in human beings' capability for conscious choice a dignity or moral selfhood that must be respected (Fletcher, pp. 9–14). The extraordinary fashion in which medicine can now combat illness has lent added impetus to the notion that human dignity is determined by the quality of life and not its mere existence.

Whether the core concept is denominated privacy, selfhood, dignity, or personal autonomy is less important than understanding its general contours, which encompass social and official respect for free choice concerning personal behavior and security from unwanted interferences in one's physical and psychological integrity. In a just society, the protection of that interest is not only a matter of individual concern but should also enter the scales on the collective side as well.

2. Precluding self-harm. Paternalism has made itself felt in health matters as elsewhere in society. Legislation that licenses health practitioners and regulates food and drugs, even to the point of prohibition, provides a relevant example. Such laws are meant to protect consumers, but do so by preventing individuals from selecting their own risks. The paternalism involved, however, falls short of that which would have to be asserted to counter a patient's refusal of treatment. Unlike coerced treatment, protective regulations are defended because individual consumers are usually ignorant of the hazards created by an industry or profession and are impotent to eliminate them. Moreover, compelled treatment is an active intervention in a person's body, not a mere limitation on the direct harm he or she can do to himself or herself (Cantor, pp. 247–248).

In ethical rather than legal terms, however, society may be justified in reminding an individual of the generally accepted expectation that people will attempt to maintain good health. A person who is ill is accorded the many special privileges that go with the sick role but is expected to reciprocate by devoting himself or herself to the task of regaining health by seeking out and cooperating with technically competent assistance (Parsons, pp. 436–437). On its face, a refusal of indicated treatment means that the individual has violated societal norms. For protection of the errant individual, society can thus be seen as having legitimate reasons to countermand some choices.

3. Benefiting society. Beyond harm to himself or herself, a person's refusal of treatment can also impinge on other interests that society desires to have protected. An organized society has an interest in its own preservation, which is in turn dependent on the existence of a healthy and productive population. It is unlikely, however, that such a large number of people would decline helpful treatment as seriously to undermine a society's ability to survive. Refusals of health care by a large number of people would indicate that strongly held values were being threatened by the proferred care, and to compel such care would be a massive assault on the very values of personal liberty and security, which societies are organized to protect. Carried to its logical extension, assigning high value to the promotion and preservation of the collectivity would justify forcing people to undergo experimental procedures if such might yield information of value to science and society. Yet the whole weight of ethical codes and commentary, as well as governmental regulations, is against coerced participation in human research (Katz). This provides further evidence that as regards medical care the common welfare is subordinate to individuals' perception of their own welfare (Pius XII, pp. 785–789). Nonetheless, the public interest in avoiding the spread of a dangerous, contagious disease may outweigh the individual's refusal of such medical steps as quarantine or vaccination (*Jacobson* v. *Massachusetts*).

4. Protecting others. A related societal interest is protecting identifiable third parties from the economic and psychological harm that occurs when a refusal of treatment leads to serious injury or death. It is difficult to construct a persuasive argument for such an interest when the persons being protected by society are adults, although they may be saddened or even economically inconvenienced by patients' actions. Similarly, while some courts have given deference to the judgment and feelings of the physicians whose treatment recommendations are rejected by their patients, the harm to the physician's dignity or professional self-image seems very small when compared to the harm to the patient who is forced to undergo a treatment he or she has rejected. Furthermore, it misconceives medical ethics and professional training to say that physicians or other health-care personnel violate their professional duties when they fail to treat to the fullest. The supremacy of physicians' consciences over patients' choices finds no real support in the law, and physicians' legitimate interest in avoiding later liability can be met when necessary by prior approval (Byrn, pp. 29–33).

Society's interest in protecting third parties is strongest when the people affected are the patient's minor dependents. The results of refusing treatment have been compared to the neglect or abuse of children, for which parents are subject to punishment (*Application of President*, p. 1015). Yet this rationale seems doubtful on several grounds. First, if the patient acts with the concurrence of the spouse it seems farfetched to say the family is being abandoned. Moreover, the future well-being of the children may be provided for through "material provision and family and spiritual bonds," as a court decided in refusing to order a blood transfusion for the thirty-four-year-old father of two children (In re *Osborne*, p. 375).

Even more important, society typically does not intervene in family decisions outside the context of compulsory education, and even there broad discretion is preserved. Parents every day inflict untold emotional harm and even economic deprivation on their children without call-

ing down the forces of the state as *parens patriae*. Little attempt is made to second-guess parental choices about how to spend time and money; about where and how to live; about marriage, separation, or divorce; and about engaging in activities that risk life or health (such as smoking cigarettes, driving or riding in motor vehicles, and consuming unhealthy foods). Many of these are trivial matters to parents, although they may have dire consequences to children's well-being. They are free from interference as a matter of principle in most Western societies, but also because they would be difficult to monitor and regulate (Cantor, pp. 251–254). It would be ironic if a choice about medical treatment, which is of great importance to a patient, were to be constrained by collective intervention merely because it is more visible and is subject to control through medical personnel.

5. Minimizing costs. More controversial is the interest, which some have asserted, in the avoidance of health-care and other costs that may be deemed "unnecessary." Declining efficacious treatment often worsens a patient's condition and may even lead to permanent disability and the need for further care for the patient and for his or her dependents. Yet it is not self-evident that the refusal of treatment should consequently be regarded as illegitimate. First, much of the burden resulting from such a refusal is not monetizable and will never be borne by the collectivity; moreover, society may not even absorb all of the measurable costs, since the injured person may draw on his or her own resources or private insurance. Second, even when the patient wishes to rely on collectively financed health and disability insurance, it is unfair to condition the funds on the patient's not refusing treatment unless a similar limitation is placed on the use of the insurance fund for the adverse consequences of other voluntarily assumed risks. It has been held that a patient's rejection of corrective surgery, especially when religiously motivated, is not a valid basis for excluding the refuser from disability benefits (*Montgomery* v. *Board*, p. 185).

6. Safeguarding public feelings. The remaining societal interests implicated by a refusal of treatment are somewhat more amorphous. The state may assert an interest in protecting public morality from being endangered by a refusal of treatment. By public morality is meant a concern for the moral sensibility of people in a society who must live with or be aware of the acts of others that offend them although the actors cause no direct, palpable harm to anyone other than themselves. Suicide by a person without dependents provides a relevant example—no one is injured but the person who commits it, and yet it has long been condemned by religious teaching and until recently even prohibited by public law. The prohibition rests on practical reasons (which reiterate, in effect, many of the societal interests already surveyed here, such as the harm to society's productive capacity) but also on the moral or aesthetic revulsion felt by many people for an act that goes contrary to social mores and the instinct of self-preservation. Nevertheless, the legislation of morality is much more controversial at present than in the past century, because its efficacy is doubted, its enforcement is problematic, and—like the kindred doctrine of paternalism—its achievement costs so dearly in harm to other values, such as personal privacy, bodily integrity, and self-determination (Cantor, pp. 245–246).

7. Upholding life's sacredness. All societies have many laws and moral rules that testify to the great importance placed on the preservation of human life. At stake are both real and symbolic interests. The sanctity of human life is not only a basic value in the ethical systems of Judeo-Christian cultures, but the protection of people from life-endangering conduct provides a central rationale for the existence of social institutions capable of exercising coercive force. Yet, as a factual matter, the usual assumption—that people wish to have the state use its power to protect their lives—is obviously inapplicable to the person who declines lifesaving treatment. In such a case, the threat to life and health comes not from a third person but from a disease or injury that the person chooses not to combat in the recommended fashion, and he or she can be protected only if society overrides the interest in self-determination and bodily integrity.

In support of official intervention to override a refusal of treatment, an analogy is often made to the laws on suicide. The comparison of treatment refusal with suicide seems apt if the latter is defined in the objective fashion advocated by Durkheim as "all cases of death resulting directly or indirectly from a positive or negative act of the victim himself, which he knows will produce this result" (Durkheim, p. 44). Yet this definition does not comport with the law—nor with prevailing ethical theories—as to the conduct and intent that are necessary for a death to be a suicide.

Viewed as a physical matter, the cause of death in suicide is something done by the patient that cuts off life, while declining potentially life-sustaining treatment merely permits an existing illness or injury to bring about death. But focusing on causation might erroneously suggest that a relevant distinction can be drawn between "natural death" and other kinds, or between different categories of treatment; the right to refuse treatment does not depend upon death's coming from "natural causes" or upon the treatment's being "extraordinary" or the like. The comparison of suicide and refusal of treatment must thus go beyond the physical to the moral and legal as well.

The distinction between positive acts and acts of omission provides one of the most controversial and perplexing topics in bioethics. In particular, the existence of any morally relevant distinction is denied by those who advocate the permissibility of voluntary, active euthanasia premised upon the assumed licitness of passive euthanasia (Rachels). For the present discussion, it is enough to observe that omission is equivalent to action only when a person is under a duty to act. If there is no duty for patients to accept medical procedures, then a refusal of such procedures, even when it eventuates in death, cannot be equated either morally or legally with an affirmative act causing death.

Suicide and treatment refusal are also not comparable when one considers what is being chosen in each case. The law distinguishes between acting with knowledge of possible or even probable consequences and acting with the specific intent to take human life, notwithstanding Durkheim's contrary position. The objective of suicide is, by definition, death, although in many instances the act results from an emotionally disturbed person's desire for comfort and assistance, and attempted suicide is today treated as a mental health rather than a criminal matter (Brooks, pp. 702–712). Treatment refusal, on the other hand, is the rejection of a proffered medical intervention but not the choice of death, though the patient's choice may increase the risk of death. Treatment may be refused when it employs procedures that are a religious anathema or are personally unacceptable; when it will not restore the patient to his or her desired level of functioning, or otherwise does not justify its costs with sufficient benefits; or when the patient wishes relief from the pain and indignities it produces or prolongs. Judicial opinions, such as *Application of President of Georgetown College* and *John F. Kennedy Memorial Hospital* v. *Heston*, that have compelled treatment based on the analogy to preventing suicide have had to dismiss the criminal law's traditional requirement of specific intent and to misstate the patient's asserted claim as a right to choose to die.

Suicide is a real as well as a symbolic affront to the sanctity of life (and to public sensibilities) since it not only takes a life but signifies that life is worthless (Williams, pp. 254–273). But to decline treatment a person need not reject life, any more than when he or she engages in other behavior that is valued on its own merits although dangerous. Thus, since treatment refusals are at most choices *involving* death rather than choices *of* death, the reasoning that supports state intervention to prevent suicide does not extend to declinations of potentially lifesaving medical procedures. Reciprocally, the acceptance of a right to refuse health care does not imply acceptance of a right of suicide.

Permitting people to refuse lifesaving treatment may not in itself defile the sanctity of life, some argue, but it drives in a wedge that opens the way to active, involuntary euthansia. The point is often illuminated by pointing to the horrors of Nazi Germany that followed upon apparently benign initial steps. Yet the feeling of certainty said to derive from insisting upon utmost efforts to preserve human life is merely the result of moral and legal line-drawing. If the rationale for the right to refuse treatment is clearly articulated and accepted in social mores, society is not left to career madly down a slippery slope to inevitable euthanasia without any morally persuasive distinctions to grab hold of (Maguire, pp. 131–140).

The balancing of public and private duties

The suggestion that one can "weigh" the interests of the individual against those of society so as to determine the validity of a refusal of medical care is at best metaphorical. In sheer numbers alone, the collective claims and interests overwhelm the individual ones, and the facts of a particular case or the views of the decision maker obviously can endow several of the collective concerns with overwhelming weight. Yet many of the claims and interests asserted on behalf of society against the right to refuse treatment appear on analysis to be inapplicable or of dubious merit, and none is persuasive enough to override the right completely. It remains to be seen whether in actual practice the social interests may together be sufficient in particular cases to outweigh, or at least to qualify, the individual's interest in autonomy.

It is important to remember that the determination of social interests and their balancing against individual interests is a matter for public institutions. Refusals of treatment arise most commonly in private settings, such as the physician–patient relationship, which do not directly involve state authority, as a judicial hearing would. When only private interests are at stake, the protection of law and tradition is all on the patient's side. And even when societal interests are presented, in the context of medical care they have with increasing frequency given way to individual interests, as illustrated by the recent ethical commentary, legislative reform, and judicial decisions on abortion, which involve the more troublesome issue of a patient's right to insist upon, rather than to forbid, a particular medical procedure.

The right in practice

Aside from public health measures such as vaccination, the largest exception in actual practice to the requirement of consent, and the reciprocal right to refuse, is in the involuntary hospitalization and treatment of persons believed to be mentally ill. (Hospitalization is itself regarded as a form of treatment, to be supplemented by drugs, surgery, or psychotherapy as required.) While some mental patients are also adjudged incompetent, which places the matter on an entirely different footing, the majority are deprived of their freedom because they are believed to be a threat to the safety of themselves or others, although this may actually mean no more than that their behavior makes them annoying. Regrettably, the experience with involuntary mental patients starkly demonstrates the dangers inherent in overriding the right to refuse treatment (Kittrie, pp. 340–371). Study after study has shown that many mental hospitals do not provide such patients with adequate care and all too often become warehouses for society's unwanted and forgotten. Those deplorable findings have given force to the argument that patients held involuntarily in hospitals have at the very least a right to receive treatment; since the rationale for the state's incarcerating them is that though they have committed no crime their mental condition makes them dangerous, the state is obliged to help them overcome the condition that leads to their confinement. This justifiable emphasis on the obligation to provide adequate care does not negate each patient's continuing right to decline specific procedures. While society's interest in protecting the patient and others from actual injury may justify a brief period of involuntary hospitalization and treatment, continued forced treatment and detention against the wishes of the patient violates the right to refuse medical procedures when the patient has not been found incompetent to exercise choice concerning medical care (Brooks, pp. 877–924).

Although fewer in number, the most difficult cases are those in which a patient's refusal of treatment risks imminent death. Physicians and nurses who wish to press ahead even when further treatment holds little prospect of restoring adequate human functioning for an appreciable period of time are, of course, reflecting a widely held belief in the sanctity of life as well as deeply ingrained professional norms and personal unwillingness to give up a battle while any chance of even a temporary victory over death and disease remains. This situation can amount to duress, depriving the patient of voluntary choice unless the refusal of further treatment creates an obligation in the health-care personnel to give alternative, palliative care including necessary dosages of painkillers.

If a patient does not share, or at least acquiesce in, the determination of the health personnel to proceed, the latter may call upon agents of the state, such as legislators, prosecutors, or most commonly judges, for support. U.S. courts have uniformly declined to order surgery or other major interventions over the objections of competent patients, "even when the best medical opinion deems it essential to save [the patient's] life" (*Palm Springs General Hospital* v. *Martinez*). Apparently more troublesome for the courts are the religiously motivated refusals of minor treatment that promise a full recovery of health, such as the unwillingness of Jehovah's Witnesses to accept blood transfusions. When presented with emergency requests to approve such involuntary lifesaving intervention, some courts have acceded on the rationale of preserving the status quo pending full argument of the case, particularly when doubt existed about the patient's real wishes or about his or her ability to reach a competent decision, given the exigency of the situation (*Application of President*, p. 1005). Nevertheless, although the irreversibility of a mistake understandably inclines judges to order temporary treatment, there is actually no way to maintain the status quo, at least not in those cases in which the patient objects to the treatment itself, such as an amputation or a blood transfusion. Moreover, the special protection given to the free exercise of religion has been found to give further weight to the patient's choice (In re *Estate of Brooks*, p. 441).

Thus it is not surprising that, when the desire of a competent patient to refuse treatment is clear, the only interest consistently held to outweigh the patient's right is direct harm to identifiable third persons, usually minor children who would be left without parental nurture and support. Even on this factor the authorities are divided, and the trend in the law appears to favor upholding a patient's wishes to the extent that they can be accomplished without posing an immediate physical danger to another life, such as that of a baby in the process of being born to a woman who forbids blood transfusions for herself (Byrn, p. 34).

The conundrum of treatment refusal and competency

Most instances of refusal of treatment remain within the private realm of physician, patient, and family members and do not become a visible part of public decision making so as to implicate directly the range of social interests discussed here. Although it is not possible to know the number of cases in which treatment is given without the necessary consent (and thus at the risk of liability for an unauthorized invasion of the person), physicians seek explicitly to override their patients' refusals only when they regard such decisions as very irrational or in conflict with official rules. The judgment of irrationality, for which the treatment personnel are seeking social concurrence when they move into the public arena, may stem from the conclusion that the patient is mentally unbalanced or holds beliefs that fall outside acceptable limits.

Although a court could compel treatment of a protesting competent adult, the initial determination typically sought in cases of treatment refusal is that the patient is incompetent. Particularly when the alleged incompetence is rooted in the condition for which treatment has been recommended or in the patient's refusal of treatment, the allegation deserves skeptical review in each case. Since the oddity or normality of people's conduct is a prime basis for ordinary judgments about their sanity, it is understandable that a patient's refusal to undergo a procedure recommended by qualified health personnel raises doubts about whether the patient is competent. Yet if this line of thinking is not held in check, it will obliterate any right to refuse medical care. Given the factual difficulties involved in determining incompetence and its far-reaching consequences, decision makers should be reluctant to declare it regarding treatment refusal. In one case, for example, the judge upheld a sixty-year-old mental hospital patient's firm refusal to undergo a biopsy and corrective surgery for suspected carcinoma of the breast, even though the grounds for her decision were not entirely reasonable and she had become increasingly delusional since the time of her original refusal (In re *Yetter*, pp. 622–624). This case, like *Estate of Brooks*, illustrates that formerly competent patients who have expressed their wishes regarding treatment need not be classed with children and other patients who were never competent.

Besides skepticism about physical incompetency, reappraisal of the legal incompetence of minors is warranted. The developing autonomy of young people may best be respected by honoring their unwillingness to undergo major interventions—as, for example, a teenage kidney patient who wishes to cease dialysis—although their guardians' concurrence is needed to authorize treatment (Veatch, pp. 149–152).

Incompetent patients

A person's incompetence does not, of course, alter the interests of society regarding him or her, though it may give the societal interests new content (the inability to be self-protective, for example, elevates the importance of official paternalism) and may diminish those interests of the individual that depend for their force on an ability to exercise self-choice.

Even when incompetence has been declared, a patient's opposition to treatment is still entitled to some deference. On a scale, as the harm of nontreatment increases and the patient's rationality decreases, disregarding his or her wishes is more acceptable, though it is never easy to subject an aware albeit incompetent patient to an intervention that he or she actively rejects.

When a patient's physical condition forecloses communication, it may still be proper for treatment to be withheld based upon the decision of a physician, hospital ethics committee, guardian *ad litem*, judge, or some combination of these. But only those cases in which the decision is predicated on what are perceived as the patient's actual wishes—and perhaps cases of familial guardianship—bear any relationship to the right to refuse treatment. In the other cases, regardless of the terms used, the decision not to treat represents what is thought by the decision maker to be most socially desirable or most in line with what a "reasonable patient" would do under the circumstances. For example, in the *Quinlan* decision, the New Jersey Supreme Court held that the fact that an unconscious patient is incapable of exercising his or her right to refuse treatment should not be allowed to extinguish this important right, which the court found to have constitutional roots (In re *Quinlan*). Yet, even when the guardians who order treatment ended are family members, such decisions are properly discussed as examples of involuntary passive euthanasia, not as part of the right to refuse, so long as the basis for the guardians' authority is the conclusion that anyone in the patient's position would wish to cease treatment because it can only prolong dying and not restore "cognitive and sapient life," as the *Quinlan* court declared.

Since the right to refuse treatment is a right to exercise choice about one's own person, it can reasonably be argued that it has no application when direct self-choice does not exist. The importance of the right, however, has led legislators and judges to find means to permit people to decide, while still competent, the manner in which they wish to be treated if they become incompetent (In re *Estate of Brooks*). It has been objected that any decision reached prior to the actual time of treatment will be too hypothetical: The healthy person giving directions is not faced with the actual details of treatment, the prospects of recovery, or the imminence of death. Nevertheless, it seems possible for a person to specify, at least in general terms, the limits of treatment he or she desires to receive according to the amount of pain and deterioration involved and the degree of recovery of physical and mental functions that are expectable as a result of various medical options. Advance resolution of the matter not only preserves the right to refuse undesired treatment but may also allay concern about the heavy financial and emotional burden that extended care of an incompetent terminal patient could place on one's family. Discussions with family members and physicians are very important, but greater protection is provided by the further step of drafting a careful, written statement, beginning perhaps with one of the model "Living Wills" that are now available (Bok, pp. 368–369). To be an extension of the right to refuse treatment, such documents need to be precise about the circumstances under which actions will or will not be taken, about the persons who are empowered to authorize or refuse treatment for the incompetent, and about the means for interpreting the documents and resolving disputes as to their meaning.

Although they depart from the conventional legal rule that the authority of the agent ceases with the incompetence of the principal, directions on terminal care are coming to have legal status, through legislation and judicial acceptance. Some states now provide that a power of attorney survives incompetency, and others allow an individual to designate a Committee of the Person to carry out directions in case of incompetence (Maguire, pp. 169–171). California has gone a step farther; in 1976 it adopted a Natural Death Act which specifies a Directive to Physicians that patients may execute to require the termination of lifesaving medical care. Unfortunately the statute, which applies only when death is imminent despite medical intervention, is so narrowly drafted that it may undermine patients' assertions of their wishes in the vast majority of cases. To err on the side of life and patient dignity, such documents must be regarded as subject to repudiation by patients even after they become incompetent—to avoid the prospect of physicians relying on prior written directions to terminate care while a patient pleads to have it continued.

A second circumstance in which it may make sense to speak of a right to refuse treatment for incompetents arises when the person declining treatment is a member of the incompetent's family with guardianship responsibility, as for example the parents of a young child. If the family is, as some believe, the relevant unit in modern society for making decisions about medical care, then there is no need to speak of "incompetence" so long as capable family members are available to decide about treatment for a patient who is incapable of deciding. In this view, affirmative evidence (such as a conflict of interest, gross irrationality, or a failure to consider the patient's welfare) would be required to justify the state in ruling the family incompetent and replacing it with another surrogate (Capron, pp. 424–429). This view is not generally accepted in actual practice, however, and decisions by a next-of-kin guardian to cease treatment are typically reviewed for reasonableness by medical professionals who, in order to avoid subsequent liability, may then seek governmental sanction for the decision to cease treatment (Veatch, pp. 125–131).

ALEXANDER MORGAN CAPRON

[*Directly related are the entries* DEATH AND DYING: EUTHANASIA AND SUSTAINING LIFE, *article on* ETHICAL VIEWS; HEALTH AS AN OBLIGATION; INFORMED CONSENT IN THE THERAPEUTIC RELATIONSHIP; PATERNALISM; PATIENTS' RIGHTS MOVEMENT; PRIVACY; *and* RIGHTS. *Other relevant material may be found under* ACTING AND REFRAINING; BEHAVIOR CONTROL, *article on* FREE-DOM AND BEHAVIOR CONTROL; DECISION MAKING, MEDICAL; LAW AND MORALITY; LIFE; *and* SUICIDE.]

BIBLIOGRAPHY

BOK, SISSELA. "Personal Directions for Care at the End of Life." *New England Journal of Medicine* 295 (1976): 367–369. Argues lucidly in favor of patients using instructions, written in advance, to retain control of terminal care; provides carefully drafted new model directions.

BROOKS, ALEXANDER D. *Law, Psychiatry and the Mental Health System.* Boston: Little, Brown & Co., 1974. Comprehensive collection of legal and other materials on the relationships between the mental health professions and society.

BYRN, ROBERT M. "Compulsory Lifesaving Treatment for the Competent Adult." *Fordham Law Review* 44 (1975): 1–36. A critical review of American cases, concluding that the right to refuse treatment is not equivalent to a right to die.

CANTOR, NORMAN L. "A Patient's Decision to Decline Life-Saving Medical Treatment: Bodily Integrity versus the Preservation of Life." *Rutgers Law Review* 26 (1973): 228–264. Excellent analysis of American case law on the refusal of medical care; argues strongly in favor of competent patients' having an unqualified right to refuse care.

CAPRON, ALEXANDER MORGAN. "Informed Consent in Catastrophic Disease Research and Treatment." *University of Pennsylvania Law Review* 123 (1974): 340–438. Develops a theory of informed consent and explores its implications for medical practice and research in light of recent court decisions.

DURKHEIM, ÉMILE. *Suicide: A Study in Sociology.* Translated by John A. Spaulding and George Simpson. New York: Free Press, 1951. The classic, pioneering study.

FLETCHER, JOSEPH FRANCIS. *Morals and Medicine: The Moral Problems of the Patient's Right to Know the Truth, Contraception, Artificial Insemination, Sterilization, Euthanasia.* Foreword by Karl Menninger. Princeton: Princeton University Press, 1954. Paperback ed. Boston: Beacon Press, 1960. A Protestant theologian's careful and influential examination of problems of conscience that face physicians in informing their patients and treating them.

KATZ, JAY, ed. *Experimentation with Human Beings: The Authority of the Investigator, Subject, Professions, and State in the Human Experimentation Process.* New York: Russell Sage Foundation, 1972. Provides a comprehensive and analytically arranged selection of historical materials and current literature on human experimentation, including many complete case studies.

———, and CAPRON, ALEXANDER MORGAN. *Catastrophic Diseases: Who Decides What?* New York: Russell Sage Foundation, 1975. An analysis of the roles of patients, physician-investigators, public officials, and others in decision making about new treatments of major illness, such as hemodialysis and organ transplantation.

KITTRIE, NICHOLAS. *The Right to Be Different: Deviance and Enforced Therapy.* Baltimore: Johns Hopkins Press, 1971. Criticizes the extension of state authority that has occurred in many fields under the guise of therapy.

MAGUIRE, DANIEL C. *Death by Choice.* Garden City, N.Y.: Doubleday, 1974. Lucid defense of the "human right to die humanly," and a powerful critique of present laws and much of the ethical literature on the subject.

PARSONS, TALCOTT. *The Social System.* Glencoe, Ill.: Free Press, 1951. Basic sociological description of modern society, including the medical profession and its clientele.

PIUS XII. "Iis qui interfuerunt Conventi primo internationali de Histopathologia Systematis nervorum, 13 September 1952" [Address to the First International Congress on the Histopathology of the Central Nervous System]. *Acta Apostolicae Sedis* 44 (1952): 779–789. Sets forth the moral limits of permissible experimental treatment, which is justified by three interests —medical science, the individual, and the community.

RACHELS, JAMES. "Active and Passive Euthanasia." *New England Journal of Medicine* 292 (1975): 78–80. Succinct and forceful argument against the view of organized medicine that active euthanasia is always forbidden.

RAMSEY, PAUL. *The Patient as Person: Explorations in Medical Ethics.* The Lyman Beecher Lectures at Yale University, 1969. New Haven: Yale University Press, 1970. Primarily addresses organ transplantation but elaborates generally on the ethics of medical practice.

VAN TILL, H. A. H. "Diagnosis of Death in Comatose Patients under Resuscitation Treatment: A Critical Review of the Harvard Report." *American Journal of Law and Medicine* 2, no. 1 (1976), pp. 1–40. Considers the impact of irreversible coma on the decision to terminate resuscitative treatment as well as on the definition of death.

VEATCH, ROBERT M. *Death, Dying, and the Biological Revolution: Our Last Quest for Responsibility.* New Haven: Yale University Press, 1976. Fits ethical theories into the social, legal, and medical contexts of caring for grievously ill patients.

WILLIAMS, GLANVILLE L. *The Sanctity of Life and the Criminal Law.* James S. Carpentier series, 1956. New York: Alfred A. Knopf, 1957. Scholarly dissection of, and important recommendations about, the law as it touches on matters of life and death in medical practice.

COURT DECISIONS

Application of President of Georgetown College. 331 F. 2d 1000 (D.C. Cir. 1964). Certiorari denied. 377 U.S. 978. 12 L. Ed. 2d 746. 84 S. Ct. 1883 (1964).

In re Estate of Brooks. 32 Ill. 2d 361. 205 N.E. 2d 435 (1965).

In re Osborne. 294 A.2d 372 (D.C. Cir. 1972).

In re Quinlan. 70 N.J. 10. 355 A. 2d 647 (1976).

In re Yetter. 62 Pa. D. & C. 2d 619 (Northampton County Court of Common Pleas 1973).

Jacobson v. Massachusetts. 197 U.S. 11. 25 S. Ct. 358 (1905).

John F. Kennedy Memorial Hospital v. Heston. 58 N.J. 576. 279 A.2d 670 (1971).

Montgomery v. Board of Retirement of the Kern County Employees' Retirement Association. 33 Cal. App. 3d 447. 109 Cal. Rptr. 181 (Ct. App. 1973).

Palm Springs General Hospital v. Martinez. Civil No. 71–12687 (Fla., Dade County Cir. Ct. 1971).

RIGHT TO REPRODUCE

See CONTRACEPTION; STERILIZATION; ABORTION; PRENATAL DIAGNOSIS; POPULATION ETHICS: ELEMENTS OF THE FIELD; POPULATION ETHICS: RELIGIOUS TRADITIONS; POPULATION POLICY PROPOSALS. *See also* RIGHTS.

RIGHTS

I. SYSTEMATIC ANALYSIS   *Joel Feinberg*
II. RIGHTS IN BIOETHICS   *Ruth Macklin*

I
SYSTEMATIC ANALYSIS

Positive rights and moral rights

Some of our most cherished rights are conferred and protected by constitutions, statutes, and other rules of law, but there are many familiar examples of rights that do not have their source in legal rules and may not even be recognized by juridical law. Some of the latter are rights conferred by the rules of nonpolitical institutions such as private clubs or libraries, or even by rule-structured games such as chess or baseball. Others, like the old lady's right to the young man's seat on the subway train, may derive from unwritten conventions, tradition, or mere custom. Those rights conferred by institutions, both legal and nonlegal, may be grouped with the conventional rights, and classified generically as *positive rights*. In essential contrast to them are a heterogenous collection of entitlements that can be denominated generically *moral rights*. Moral rights are rights that exist prior to and independently of any social conventions or legal or institutional rules. Although it seems clear that there are rights in the generically moral category, philosophers have often found such rights to be conceptually puzzling and have differed widely in their accounts of them.

Some writers think of moral rights not as actual rights of any kind, but rather as rationally prescribed legislative goals. A moral right so conceived is what ought to be made a positive (legal or conventional) right and would be a positive right in a more just legal system or moral code. Thus Maurice Cranston, speaking of the "human rights" declared by the United Nations, writes: "The intention of the sponsors of that Declaration was to specify something that everybody *ought* to have. In other words, they were moral rights" (Cranston, p. 10). This account of human rights, however, cannot be reconciled with some familiar uses of the language of moral rights. It cannot explain what is meant, for example, by talk of persons *exercising* their moral rights before those rights were legally recognized, as in the case of demonstrators arrested for illegal picketing. And the view that a moral right is simply what ought to be a *legal* right cannot without emendation explain what it could be to have a moral right to rebel against a tyrannical government. Since the right to rebel against established authority *could not* be a legal right conferred by the government in power, it could not very well be an ideally legal right. Finally, the account of moral rights as mere political ideals or "goals of legislative aspiration" cannot make sense out of many homely examples of moral rights that we all take for granted. One might very well acknowledge, for example, a parent's right to be spoken to civilly by his children and a student's right to be graded without prejudice by his teachers while denying that those undoubted rights ought to be legal rights at all. Such moral rights, then, cannot plausibly be construed as mere ideally legal or properly legal rights. We think of them, instead, as rights that can be exercised, stood upon, waived, or infringed, quite apart from what the law might say about the matter.

Rights as claims

The common character of all rights consists in their being rationally demonstrable claims. To have a claim to something is to be in a position, morally or legally, to demand that thing as properly one's own or one's due. The basis of a claim is always some evidence or some reasons that can be put forward relevantly and cogently in its support. Thus the numbered token given to a restaurant customer by the hat check girl in exchange for his coat and hat later supports, indeed establishes, his claim to that hat and coat, and under the rules of the practice of garment-checking puts him in a position to make claim to a certain coat and hat as his due. Normally the evidentiary support given to his claim by the receipt is so conclusive that it establishes his claim as *valid*, and hence not *merely* a claim, but a right to the coat and hat in question. In exceptional circumstances, however, the genuine claim to a given coat established by his receipt may not be valid. The cloakroom attendant may have made two tokens with the same number and given them to two different customers quite by mistake. Both customers may then have a claim to the same coat and neither claim will be conclusive until reinforced by other reasons (one's name printed in indelible ink on the lining, a sales receipt from the store of purchase, etc.). In a similar fashion receipts, canceled checks, IOUs, deeds, and titles support claims to the possession of property, and in the conclusive cases establish claims as valid, which is to say, as rights. But not all claims are supported by reasons of this kind. Sometimes, one can support one's claim against another by citing previous promises or agreements or by invoking legal rules. In other cases one makes claim to a title itself, by demonstrating that one has satisfied the conditions specified by some rule for the ownership of title, as when an inventor applies for his patent rights. Especially in the case of moral rights, the kinds of reasons that may support claims, and in conclusive cases establish them as rights, are diverse indeed.

When the evidence or reasons offered in support of another's claim are sufficiently cogent, they have a coercive effect upon our judgments, so that we feel impelled to acknowledge that the claims they support are genuine rights. Because the supporting considerations seem to have the character of binding reasons, we feel that it would not only be morally perverse to withhold recognition of the rights; it would be contrary to reason itself. In such cases, we feel that we have no more choice in making the judgment that the other person does indeed have a right than we do when we report the findings of our senses. That is why, in those cases, we fall so naturally into objective modes of speech and report that the person has the right as a kind of finding and not merely as a recommendation or a "legislative" decision to confer some benefit on him. In virtue of the reasons he can put forward to "coerce" our judgment, we acknowledge his right as something he already possesses quite independently of, and prior to, our recognition of it. The claimant in that case has a kind of "moral power" over us which we feel constrained to respect, and that gives him a certain dignity in our eyes. In that respect, a right-holder's making claim to what is rightfully his is significantly different from mere petitioning, begging, praying, or pleading; and receiving one's rights stands in sharp contrast to receiving a gift or a favor, or benefiting from another's mercy, charity, or noblesse oblige.

Moral and legal rights

It is essential to the notion of a claim that it be addressed to someone or other. Generally speaking, a right is a valid claim that a person can make in either or both of two directions. On the one hand, some of an individual's rights are claims he can make against individuals—either against specific private persons for assistance, repayment of debts, compensation for losses, performance of contract, and the like—or claims against all other individuals, "the world at large," to noninterference in his private affairs. On the other hand, an individual citizen can also make claims against the state not only for specific services and promised repayments, and noninterference in his private affairs (claims analogous to those he has against other citizens) but also claims to the legal enforcement of the valid claims he has against other private individuals and organizations. All enforcement claims against the state, of course, are associated with prior claims against private parties that the state is bound to enforce, but not all claims against individuals are backed up by enforcement claims against the state. One's right not to be spoken to rudely, for example, is not legally enforcible.

Many or most of our rights, however, give rise to double claims, both against other individuals and against the state to force performance from others of what is our due, or to protect us by threat of punishment from the unwanted interference of other individuals. My legal right not to be punched in the nose has that double character: It is a claim against all other citizens to their noninterference and a claim against the state to its protection. So indeed do some of my claims against the state itself, for example, my claim against the Internal Revenue Service to a refund of a tax overpayment, and against the courts for its enforcement. All such double-barrelled claims are *legal rights*.

Reason-backed claims against other individuals, or against the state (e.g., not to be victimized by the passage into law of invidious legislation) that are *not* at the same time legally valid claims against the state for enforcement are often called *moral rights merely*. A moral right is a claim backed by valid reasons other than, or in addition to, legal rules and addressed to the conscience of the claimee or to public opinion. When such claims are also enforcible by law, they are at once *both moral and legal rights*. Finally, when legally enforcible claims are arbitrary and supported by no respectable reasons (e.g., a slaveowner's right to beat and starve his slave), they are *legal rights merely*.

Rights and duties

The word "right," in both legal and moral discourse, is not without its ambiguities. In at least one of its various senses, that in which to have a right is to be at liberty, it has no necessary relation to duties whatever. (The "natural rights" that Thomas Hobbes thought all persons would possess even in a "state of nature" were rights only in this sense.) According to legal usage, to say that Doe is at liberty to do or have X is to say that Doe has no duty to refrain from or relinquish X (Hohfeld). But it may be that no one else has any duties in respect to X either, in which case Doe has no claim against anyone to noninterference with, or protection of, his "right" (liberty). On the other hand, what legal writers call a "claim-right," or a "right in the strict sense," is a rather more valuable possession. (The "natural rights" said by John Locke and the American founding fathers to belong to all persons were rights in this stronger sense.) To say that Doe has a claim-right to do or have X is to say that (1) Doe is at liberty to do or have X, and (2) his liberty is the ground of other people's duties to grant him X or not to interfere with him in respect to X. Thus, if Doe has a claim-right against Roe to be repaid a ten-dollar loan, then because of that right, Roe has a duty to Doe to repay the ten dollars, a duty from which Doe, and only Doe, can release him. Claim-rights are said to be negative when logically correlated with other people's duties to omit (e.g., Roe's duty not to punch Doe in the nose); positive when logically correlated with other people's duties to act (e.g., Roe's duty to repay his debt to Doe); *in rem* when logically correlated with the duties of other people generally (e.g., everyone's duty to stay off Doe's land without his consent to enter); and *in personam* when logically correlated with the duties of specific, namable individuals (e.g., debtors, promisors, parents, spouses).

The distinctions between positive and negative and between *in rem* and *in personam* cut across one another, generating four possible categories of rights according to the location and character of the corresponding duty: positive *in personam* rights, negative *in personam* rights, positive *in rem* rights, and negative *in rem* rights. Most legal rights are either positive *in personam* (for example, a creditor's right to be repaid a certain sum by his debtor) or negative *in rem* (for example, a person's right not to be improperly interfered with, molested, or assaulted by anyone). The familiarity of these examples has tempted some legal commentators to suppose that the other two classes are in fact empty or nearly empty, and that all *in rem* rights are negative, and nearly all *in personam* rights are positive. But in the twentieth century the idea that there can be positive *in rem* rights has steadily gained ground. The right to be rescued from serious danger, for example, can be thought of as a right to the positive assistance—not literally of "the whole world" but of anyone who happens to be in a position to help—just as the analogous negative *in rem* right to the exclusive possession of one's land is a right to the passive noninterference of anyone at all who happens to be in a position to trespass. Negative *in personam* rights in the law, on the other hand, are quite exceptional. Salmond writes that they are "usually the product of some agreement by which some particular individual has deprived himself of a liberty which is common to all other persons" (Salmond, p. 286), and gives as an example the sale by one merchant to another of the "goodwill" of his business, which is an agreement *not* to enter into competition with him for a certain period of time. That would be for the first party to give up a liberty shared in common by all businessmen and to confer thereby on the second a "right of exemption from competition," which is both *in personam* (directed at one specific party) and negative (requiring that party's omission).

In both law and morals, however, there are apparent examples of duties not linked to other people's rights and rights not linked to other people's duties, so it would seem that the doctrine of the correlativity of rights and duties does not hold universally. Examples of duties without other people's rights are perhaps less controversial than examples of rights without other people's duties. The law imposes duties on motorists to stop at red lights even when no other automobiles or pedestrians are in sight. That legal duty cannot plausibly be interpreted then as a duty to other motorists, or to legislators long since dead, or to the traffic signal itself. It is simply a duty without a correlative right. Similarly my moral duty to be charitable is not correlated with the right of any particular worthy recipient to my help. My duty is to be charitable to some worthy cause or other. When I discharge it by contributing to some persons I do not thereby violate the rights of the others. It has been suggested that these and similar examples derive their force from the fact that the word "duty" has gradually evolved a sense in which it is applied to any conduct thought to be morally required quite apart from whether there is a beneficiary to whom that conduct is "due" (Feinberg, 1973, p. 63).

Rights without correlative duties

The existence of rights without correlative duties is a more controversial matter. One of the most widely discussed examples is that of the "human rights" to acquire, or to have the opportunity to acquire, the goods that are necessary to the fulfillment of the most basic human needs and without which a person cannot live a minimally decent life. Those goods are said to include adequate nutrition, decent working conditions, health care, education, rest, and leisure (UNESCO, 1949). But clearly there are times and places in which such goods are in such short supply that it is quite impossible to provision everyone. In a famine every person may indeed still possess a human right to be fed, but in the case of many starving individuals there may be no other individuals who can plausibly be said to have the duty to feed them. The very humanity of the deprived persons continues to be the basis of a claim to be given food in a sense analogous to that in which the cloakroom check supports the claim to receive one's hat and coat from the hat-check girl. But in the latter case, when a fire has destroyed the restaurant and killed its owner and the cloakroom attendant, the claim to one's coat may survive, but there is no coat and there may be no person with the duty of returning it or its equivalent. The claim to one's coat established by the numbered token remains a valid claim, for there is nothing deficient about *it*, just as the claim to enough food to survive remains a valid claim even in a famine, since the humanity of its claimant is unimpaired and undiminished. But where there is no other person with a duty to fulfill the claim, its validity does the claimant no good.

Nevertheless, there is a real point in insisting that the deprived claimant has a genuine right to the fulfillment of his basic needs even in hopeless conditions of scarcity, for that mode of expression emphasizes that the reason why no other person has a duty to help him has nothing to do with his qualification for the help. He has not failed in any way; rather circumstances have failed him. It would be misleading, therefore, to say that he has a "mere claim," however strong, but one that is not in the final analysis a valid claim or right. The deprived claimant in conditions of scarcity remains in a position morally to make a claim, even when there is no one in the corresponding position to do anything about it, but should circumstances change so that the corresponding position finds an occupant, then that person instantly assumes a duty to help. Another consequence of the view that all persons have human rights even to goods in short supply is that it provides a basis for ascribing duties to governments and responsible agencies to work for the alleviation of the shortages, so that the valid claims of other human beings in the future will not go unanswered.

JOEL FEINBERG

[*Directly related are the following article,* RIGHTS IN BIOETHICS, *and the entries* BEHAVIOR CONTROL, *article on* FREEDOM AND BEHAVIOR CONTROL; DEATH AND DYING: EUTHANASIA AND SUSTAINING LIFE, *article on* ETHICAL VIEWS; HEALTH CARE, *article on* RIGHT TO HEALTH-CARE SERVICES; JUSTICE; LAW AND MORALITY; PATIENTS' RIGHTS MOVEMENT; PRIVACY; RATIONING OF MEDICAL TREATMENT; RIGHT TO REFUSE MEDICAL CARE; *and* TRUTH-TELLING, *article on* ETHICAL ASPECTS. *Other relevant material may be found under* CIVIL DISOBEDIENCE IN HEALTH SERVICES; CONFIDENTIALITY; FOOD POLICY; FUTURE GENERATIONS, OBLIGATIONS TO; INFORMED CONSENT IN HUMAN RESEARCH; INFORMED CONSENT IN MENTAL HEALTH; *and* INFORMED CONSENT IN THE THERAPEUTIC RELATIONSHIP.]

BIBLIOGRAPHY

BENN, STANLEY I. "Rights." *Encyclopedia of Philosophy.* 8 vols. New York: Macmillan Co., 1967, vol. 7, pp. 195–199.

———, and PETERS, RICHARD S. *Social Principles and the Democratic State.* London: Allen & Unwin, 1959, 1967, chap. 4, pp. 88–104.

BRAYBROOKE, DAVID. "The Firm but Untidy Correlativity of Rights and Obligations." *Canadian Journal of Philosophy* 1 (1972): 351–363.

CRANSTON, MAURICE WILLIAMS. *What Are Human Rights?* Preface by Reinhold Niebuhr. New York: Basic Books, 1963; London: Bodley Head, 1973.

FAWCETT, JAMES EDMUND SANDFORD. "The International Protection of Human Rights." *Political Theory and the Rights of Man.* Edited by David Daiches Raphael. Bloomington: Indiana University Press, 1967, chap. 10, pp. 119–133.

FEINBERG, JOEL. "The Nature and Value of Rights." *Journal of Value Inquiry* 4 (1970): 243–260.

———. *Social Philosophy.* Prentice-Hall Foundation of Philosophy Series. Englewood Cliffs, N.J.: Prentice-Hall, 1973, chaps. 4–6, pp. 55–97.

HOBBES, THOMAS. *Leviathan.* Edited with an introduction by C. B. Macpherson. Baltimore: Penguin Books, 1968.

HOHFELD, WESLEY NEWCOMB. *Fundamental Legal Conceptions: As Applied in Judicial Reasoning.* Edited by Walter Wheeler Cook. Foreword by Arthur L. Corbin. New Haven: Yale University Press, 1919, 1946.

LOCKE, JOHN. *The Second Treatise of Government (An Essay Concerning the True Original, Extent and End of Civil Government) and A Letter Concerning Toleration.* Edited with a revised introduction by J. W. Gough. Oxford: Basil Blackwell, 1966.

LYONS, DAVID. "The Correlativity of Rights and Duties." *Nous* 4 (1970): 45–57.

MARSHALL, GEOFFREY. "Rights, Options, and Entitlements." *Oxford Essays in Jurisprudence: A Collaborative Work.* 2d ser. Edited by A. W. P. Simpson. Oxford: Clarendon Press, 1973, chap. 9, pp. 228–241.

McCLOSKEY, H. J. "Rights." *Philosophical Quarterly* 15 (1965): 115–127.

RICHARDS, B. A. "Inalienable Rights: Recent Criticism and Old Doctrine." *Philosophy and Phenomenological Research* 29 (1969): 391–404.

SALMOND, JOHN WILLIAM. *Jurisprudence.* 11th ed. Edited by Glanville Williams. London: Sweet & Maxwell, 1957, chaps. 10–11, pp. 259–299.

UNESCO, ed. *Human Rights: Comments and Interpretations: A Symposium.* Introduction by Jacques Maritain. New York: Columbia University Press; London: Allen Wingate, 1949. Reprint. Westport, Conn.: Greenwood Press, 1973.

II
RIGHTS IN BIOETHICS

Rights as claims

Rights in bioethics are not essentially different from the kinds embodied in the generic concept of moral and legal rights. Consider, for instance, the claim that there exists a right on the part of everyone to adequate health care—a bioethical example of a problem in distributive justice. Or take the claims in support of a woman's right to terminate her pregnancy—a right construed by the U.S. Supreme Court as an instance of the constitutionally guaranteed right to privacy. This article will follow the categories set out in the preceding article, with the aim of showing how rights in bioethics are examples of the broader notion of rights.

As the previous article states, "The common character of all rights consists in their being rationally demonstrable claims. . . . The basis of a claim is always some evidence or some reasons that can be put forward relevantly and cogently in its support." That characteristic holds for both moral and legal rights, but the most problematic cases of rights in bioethics lie largely in the area of *moral rights merely*, rather than in the sphere of legal rights. While conflicts of rights may occur in both law and morality, there are some features of moral rights that pose special problems. When there is disagreement about the existence or nature of rights in particular cases, it is generally easier to put forward relevant and cogent reasons or evidence in support of the claim that something is a legal right than it is to justify claims about moral rights. For example, the patient may be said to have a right to confidentiality in the doctor–patient relationship. Aside from legal requirements concerning confidentiality, disagreements remain about where the moral presumptions ought to lie. If a patient confides to his psychiatrist that he intends to commit suicide, and the psychiatrist has good grounds to believe that the patient will carry out his stated intention, is the doctor justified in breaching confidentiality, thereby overriding the patient's right? Psychiatrists have claimed that there exists "a right to prevent an act of suicide" (Williams); but against this alleged right, a more commonly claimed right has long been argued for by others: a person's "right to suicide" or, put more generally, the right of everyone to determine the time and manner of his own demise (Motto).

It is only within the past three centuries that the emergence and general spread of the notion of rights has taken place. The embodiment of human rights in significant documents like the Declaration of Independence, the Declaration of the Rights of Man and of Citizens, and the Universal Declaration of Human Rights of the United Nations conferred the status of *positive rights* on claims that either had not been made earlier or remained as mere ideals. Within the field of bioethics, claims asserting a variety of rights began to multiply in the last several decades. That movement emerged partly out of the concerns expressed after the Second World War regarding atrocities perpetrated by the Nazis in the name of biological and medical research on human subjects. Those concerns were translated into the requirements for informed consent in medical experimentation in the Nuremberg Code, which mandated that subjects of experimentation must grant their fully voluntary and informed consent to any request from a researcher to participate in a medical experiment. The requirement of informed consent relies on what have long been regarded as fundamental human rights of self-determination and of freedom from bodily assault by others. As articulated by Justice Benjamin Cardozo: "Every human being of adult years and sound mind has a right to determine what shall be done with his own body; and a surgeon who performs an operation without his patient's consent commits an assault, for which he is liable in damages" (*Schloendorff* v. *New York Hospital*).

Additional rights on the part of patients generally, as well as special populations, have been increasingly asserted in the field of bioethics: the rights of children, the mentally ill, the elderly, prisoners, the mentally retarded. In such claims asserting the rights of special populations, there is an appeal to their basic human attributes—qualities that impose duties on others to act or forbear from acting in ways that violate what are held to be the fundamental rights of persons as expressed in statutes, declarations, or generally agreed-upon moral principles.

Problems in assessing rights claims in bioethics

The issues that face decision makers in the biomedical arena (whether the decisions involved are those of an individual physician or of health policymakers) often come down to assessing claims about rights in bioethics. Problems in assessing rights claims fall into four basic categories: (1) conflicts of rights; (2) the status of entities to which rights are attributed; (3) the correlativity between rights and duties; and (4) the impossibility of satisfying the rights of everyone under certain conditions.

1. Conflicts of rights. Problems arise in both the moral and legal domains when two or more legitimate rights come into conflict. A prominent example is that of involuntary commitment to mental institutions. The right of an innocent person to preserve his or her liberty is pitted against society's right to protection when the person to be involuntarily confined is judged by psychiatrists to be "dangerous to others" but has committed no criminal act. Another instance of a conflict of rights occurs in cases where a person rejects a particular medical treatment on religious grounds. Members of the Jehovah's Witness sect refuse to accept blood transfusions, based on the constitutional (First Amendment) right to freedom of religion, but they do accept other medical treatments. Witnesses have granted consent for open-heart surgery while refusing to consent to the blood transfusions often deemed medically necessary in such operations. On the other side, it has been claimed that "it is also the physician's inherent, albeit uncodified, right not to have constraints applied to a therapeutic program, which he regards as necessary for the patient's welfare or survival" (Schechter, p. 73). In both examples, debate continues to rage over which rights ought to take precedence when conflicts occur. Regardless of the evidence or reasons put forward relevantly and cogently in support of such claims, decisions concerning the priority of one person's rights over those of another are bound to be controversial where the rights in conflict appear to be legitimate.

2. Bearers of rights. The second class of problems concerning the evaluation of rights claims arises out of the need to determine what properties it is essential to have in order to qualify as a bearer of rights. Disagreements arise concerning the status of entities to which rights are attributed: Is the fetus a creature to whom rights can properly be ascribed? Are nonexistent entities, such as future generations of people, those to which rights can correctly be attributed? In the latter example, there are various acts or bioethical policies that are held to rest on the ascription of rights to future generations. Some claims address environmental considerations, as in assertions that future generations have a right to clean air and water; at other times, it is the right of future generations to genetic health that is invoked in arguments for positive or negative eugenics programs.

In the former example, if the question of whether or not the fetus is the proper sort of entity to qualify as a bearer of rights is answered in the affirmative, then the problem reverts to the first category—that of conflicts of rights. The alleged rights of the fetus become subsumed under the more general "right to life" (Kass), so an immediate conflict emerges between the presumed right on the part of the fetus and the rights of the mother—usually phrased in the abortion context as "the right to control one's own body" (Brody; Thomson). To resolve such conflicts, a judgment must be made about which rights weigh more heavily, or under what precise conditions the rights of the mother take precedence over the rights of the fetus. The abortion case serves as a good example of the resolution of a problem about rights in bioethics *by law,* although antiabortionists continue to maintain that the fetus has a right to life on *moral* grounds in spite of the fact that the courts have declared that the "right of privacy . . . is broad enough to encompass a woman's decision whether or not to terminate her pregnancy" (*Roe* v. *Wade*).

3. Rights and correlative duties.   The third category of problems pertaining to rights in bioethics arises out of the correlativity between rights and duties. If it is asserted that everyone in society has a right to adequate health care, then the question arises whether there is a correlative duty on the part of some person, group, or agency to provide health-care services. Even if it is cogently argued that it is meaningless or unrealistic to claim that a right to health care exists in the absence of a corresponding duty to provide it, many questions remain about the most *just* way of allocating health-care services, as well as what the limits of such services ought to be. The Universal Declaration of Human Rights of the United Nations proclaims for each person the right to an adequate standard of living and well-being of oneself and one's family, including food, clothing, housing, and medical care and the necessary social services. It is obvious that the rights of an enormous number of people are

being violated if those rights claims represent a correct list of what people can properly demand as their due.

4. Limits in satisfying rights.   In addition to posing problems about the correlativity of rights and duties in bioethics, the last example points directly to the fourth class of problems in assessing rights claims in bioethics. This category includes the one discussed at the end of the preceding article: the difficulty posed by the impossibility of satisfying valid rights claims when goods or services are in short supply. Whatever particular right might be claimed in such cases, the problem of allocating scarce medical resources will sometimes result in failure to satisfy the legitimate claims of some people. The things in short supply may be blood, organs for transplantation, available facilities in a hospital intensive care unit, or medical services generally, as in rural or remote areas. Since such allocation decisions in bioethics are properly viewed as problems in distributive justice, the determination of whose rights ought to be recognized or which rights have priority becomes a function of the particular theory of distributive justice that is used for allocating medical goods or services.

A related difficulty occurs when rights claims are impossible to fulfill because of barriers other than scarcity of resources. The problem is exemplified in a question posed by a leading biologist: "Is it not equally a right of every person to be born physically and mentally sound, capable of developing fully into a mature individual?" (Glass, p. 252). A plausible response to such a query might be that, when the conditions necessary for satisfying a particular rights claim are technologically or scientifically impossible to fulfill, the claim that a desirable state of affairs is a *right* of persons must be withdrawn.

Positive rights

Because of the continuing proliferation of rights claims in the field of bioethics, it is useful to examine rights referred to in the previous article as *positive rights*. This category includes rights conferred by institutions, both legal and nonlegal, as well as rights derived from conventions, tradition, or custom. Whether they are of recent origin or have long been recognized, positive rights in bioethics may still fall prey to some of the problems noted in the preceding section, such as the difficulty posed by rights that come into conflict. The following discussion is not meant to be exhaustive but is intended to cover the most prominent examples of rights invoked in bioethics.

Legally established rights. While it is sometimes the case that rights are conferred by legislative statutes, the majority of legally established rights in bioethics have originated in court cases at the state or federal level. One of the most notable of these is the U.S. Supreme Court decision on abortion in 1973 (*Roe* v. *Wade*). As noted earlier, the Court argued that a woman's decision whether or not to terminate her pregnancy properly falls under the constitutionally guaranteed right of privacy. When proabortionists argue on moral (as opposed to strictly legal) grounds, they invoke a woman's "right to decide what happens in and to her body." But the general right of privacy is broader in scope than the special "right to control one's own body" invoked in connection with abortion. For example, in a case where it was argued that a patient has the right to refuse life-prolonging medical treatment, the "right to die" has been presented to the courts as part of the right of privacy.

The last example serves to underscore the point that rights in bioethics are instances of larger moral and legal rights recognized in society. Use of the phrase "the right to die" is a good example of how confusing the language of rights can become. What may be referred to in the moral language of rights as "the right to die" must, in the legal domain, be subsumed under a different category since no constitutional right to die exists. Further confusion stems from the fact that legally the right to die has been based on the right to be left alone and so ought properly to be called "the right to be let die." A range of court cases establishing legal precedents in the United States involves patient refusals of medical treatment on religious grounds. Most commonly invoked where Jehovah's Witnesses refused blood transfusions, the "right to die" was originally viewed in such cases as being an instance of the First Amendment right that proclaims religious freedom for all.

More recently, however, the courts have broadened the basis for allowing patient refusal of medical treatment to include written statements by competent patients, which become effective after the patient lapses into an incompetent state. So it is not only life-preserving treatments (such as blood transfusions) where the competent patient is viewed as having the right to refuse treatment; it is also in cases of life-prolonging therapy that the patient's "right to die" has

been recognized. The Natural Death Act, passed by the California Legislature in 1976, is an instance of a legislative enactment of that positive right. As in the case of abortion, disagreement persists in the moral arena despite the fact that the right to die has been ensured by law. A range of ethical problems surrounds the exercise of rights on behalf of a person who is comatose or otherwise incompetent to make decisions about treatment refusal at the time such choices must be made.

Even greater controversy exists over whether or not the right to die as claimed in cases of terminal illness properly extends into the domain of suicide (Murphy). The sorts of cases in which "death with dignity" is an issue are usually quite different from situations in which suicide attempts are made. Until quite recently suicide was illegal according to most state laws. While the legal situation has changed, doubts remain on the part of many people about the morality of suicide. Staunch defenders of individual liberty maintain that attempts on the part of individual physicians, hospitals, or agents of the law to prevent a person from taking his own life are in violation of the fundamental human right of self-determination or liberty.

This last value consideration leads to another example of judicially established rights: the right to treatment. The recognition that involuntary confinement in a mental institution or other hospital on grounds that a person is judged "dangerous to self or others" constitutes an infringement of individual liberty eventually led to a number of landmark decisions (*Rouse* v. *Cameron*; *Wyatt* v. *Stickney*; *Donaldson* v. *O'Connor*). These court cases are often cited as establishing the "right to treatment" for those confined in institutions. In rendering its opinion in *Wyatt* v. *Stickney*, the court listed many subsidiary rights that must be met. They included a right to the least restrictive conditions necessary for treatment, the right to be free from isolation, a right not to be subjected to experimental research without consent, a right to a comfortable bed and privacy, the right to adequate meals, the right to an individualized treatment plan with a projected timetable for meeting specific goals, among numerous others. But however long such a list of rights may be, there are those who invoke rights of individual liberty with equal force in voicing their objections to involuntary hospitalization no matter what grounds are cited for commitment and regardless of what treatments are offered. A leading spokesman for this position has asserted that "calling involuntary mental hospitalization a 'medical right' is like calling involuntary servitude in antebellum Georgia a 'right to work' " (Szasz, p. 167).

Rights established in declarations, codes, and bills. There is a middle ground between *legally* established rights and those referred to in the preceding article as "moral rights merely." It consists of rights claims made by official organizations, such as the American Hospital Association, the World Health Organization, or the United Nations; it also includes statements that assert the rights of special populations, such as children, the handicapped, or the mentally retarded. Those declarations and bills lack the force of law, but they may establish a strong moral presumption in favor of society's recognizing the rights asserted in them. It is appropriate to consider such claims as affirming positive rights, since they exist in the form of published documents put forward either by the governing body of an organization or institution, or else by vote of the members of a group in adopting a constitution or set of principles.

The principles stated in the Constitution of the World Health Organization include a definition of the concept of health with the following claim about rights: "The enjoyment of the highest attainable standard of health is one of the fundamental rights of every human being without distinction of race, religion, political belief, economic or social condition." The WHO Constitution also includes a statement about the responsibility of governments for the health of their people—a responsibility that would seem to embody a *duty* of governments correlated with the *right* of every human being to the highest attainable standard of health.

The American Hospital Association has proclaimed two sets of patients' rights. The first, called A Patient's Bill of Rights, lists twelve specific rights. Some of them are put in the most general form, such as the first right affirmed in the Bill: The patient has the right to considerate and respectful care. Others are highly specialized rights, such as the patient's right to obtain information as to any relationship of his hospital to other health-care and educational institutions insofar as his care is concerned. What remains unclear about the Patient's Bill of Rights, as well as similar documents, is the recourse a patient has if his rights according to such declarations are violated. Unlike the situation with legally estab-

lished rights, there is usually no clearly stated procedure or publicly known method by which a patient can bring grievances against the hospital or its staff. The second statement of patients' rights by the American Hospital Association is entitled The Right of the Patient to Refuse Treatment. This document explicitly states that the patient's right to refuse medical or surgical procedures is often governed by state laws or court decisions, so the hospital must, in such cases, comply with existing statutes and obtain legal advice on an ongoing basis. That is a case where the rights embodied in a bill or declaration intersect with legally established rights.

A similar instance of positive rights that fall somewhere in the middle ground between "moral rights merely" and rights that enjoy full legal status appears in a decision rendered by the Board of Regents of the University of the State of New York. Acting under their responsibility for licensing the medical profession, the Regents handed down a verdict in a case involving the use of patients as subjects of medical research. The decision affirmed a right of patients and at the same time ascribed a duty to physicians in the form of denying them a right:

A patient has the right to know he is being asked to volunteer and to refuse to participate in an experiment for any reason, intelligent or otherwise, well-informed or prejudiced. A physician has no right to withhold from a prospective volunteer any fact which he knows may influence the decision [Langer].

An example of a declaration of rights aimed at a special population is the Declaration of General and Special Rights of the Mentally Handicapped, which was adopted by the International League of Societies for the Mentally Handicapped in 1968 and in modified form by the General Assembly of the United Nations in 1971. The main precept of this and related documents is that mentally retarded persons are held to have all the fundamental rights of anyone else of their age and nationality. Among these are the right to education and training appropriate to developmental status, the right to guardianship or other form of protective advocacy, and the right to marry and to procreate. Here is another case of a conflict of rights, constituting a direct clash between the laws of some states that prohibit retarded persons from marrying or that allow for involuntary sterilization, on the one hand, and a contrary right proclaimed but not legally mandated in the Declaration of General and Special Rights of the Mentally Handicapped.

Conclusion

In addition to the many rights in bioethics discussed in this article, there are numerous others that have been claimed on behalf of persons generally, as well as particular groups. Among them are the right to be well born, the right to genetic health, the right to a sound environment, the right to a balanced population, the right to know the truth about one's medical condition and prognosis. It is evident that some of these alleged rights are difficult if not impossible to fulfill, since it is not within the power of any single individual or even a government to take all the necessary steps to satisfy such rights. But as with any moral ideal, rights claims in bioethics serve an important function in setting forth the human needs and conditions requisite for attaining a just society.

RUTH MACKLIN

[*This article builds upon the previous article,* SYS-TEMATIC ANALYSIS. *For further discussion of topics mentioned in this article, see the entries:* ABORTION, *article on* LEGAL ASPECTS; DEATH AND DYING: EUTHANASIA AND SUSTAINING LIFE, *article on* ETHICAL VIEWS; FUTURE GENERATIONS, OBLIGATIONS TO; INFORMED CONSENT IN MENTAL HEALTH; RATIONING OF MEDICAL TREATMENT; *and* RIGHT TO REFUSE MEDICAL CARE. *Also directly related are the entries* CONFIDENTIALITY; HEALTH CARE, *article on* RIGHT TO HEALTH-CARE SERVICES; INFORMED CONSENT IN HUMAN RESEARCH; INFORMED CONSENT IN THE THERAPEUTIC RELATIONSHIP; STERILIZATION, *article on* LEGAL ASPECTS; *and* TRUTH-TELLING, *article on* ETHICAL ASPECTS. *Other relevant material may be found under* EUGENICS; FOOD POLICY; JUSTICE; *and* PRIVACY. *See* APPENDIX, SECTION II, NUREMBERG CODE; *and* SECTION III, A PATIENT'S BILL OF RIGHTS, *and* DECLARATION ON THE RIGHTS OF MENTALLY RETARDED PERSONS.]

BIBLIOGRAPHY

BRODY, BARUCH. "Abortion and the Law." *Journal of Philosophy* 68 (1971): 357–369.
Donaldson v. O'Connor. 493 F.2d 507 (5th Cir. 1974).
GLASS, BENTLEY. "Human Heredity and Ethical Problems." *Perspectives in Biology and Medicine* 15 (1972): 237–253.
KASS, LEON R. "Implications of Prenatal Diagnosis for the Human Right to Life." *Ethical Issues in Human Genetics: Genetic Counseling and the Use of Genetic Knowledge.* Edited by Bruce Hilton, Daniel Callahan, Maureen Harris, Peter Condliffe, and Burton Berkley. Fogarty International Proceedings, no. 13. New York: Plenum Press, 1973, pp. 185–199.
LANGER, ELINOR. "Human Experimentation: New York Verdict Affirms Patient's Rights." *Science* 151 (1966): 663–666.
MOTTO, JEROME A. "The Right to Suicide: A Psychiatrist's View." *Life-Threatening Behavior* 2 (1972): 183–188.
MURPHY, GEORGE E. "Suicide and the Right to Die." *American Journal of Psychiatry* 130 (1973): 472–473.
REDLICH, FRITZ, and MOLLICA, RICHARD F. "Overview: Ethical Issues in Contemporary Psychiatry." *American Journal of Psychiatry* 133 (1976): 125–136.
Roe v. Wade. 410 U.S. 113. 35 L. Ed. 2d 147. 93 S. Ct. 705 (1973).
Rouse v. Cameron. 373 F.2d 451 (D.C. Cir. 1966).
SCHECHTER, DAVID CHARLES. "Problems Relevant to Major Surgical Operations in Jehovah's Witnesses." *American Journal of Surgery* 116 (1968): 73–80.
Schloendorff v. New York Hospital. 211 N.Y. 125. 105 E. 92 (1914).
SZASZ, THOMAS. "Involuntary Mental Hospitalization." *Biomedical Ethics and the Law.* Edited by James M. Humber and Robert F. Almeder. New York: Plenum Press, 1976, pp. 151–171.
THOMSON, JUDITH JARVIS. "A Defense of Abortion." *Philosophy and Public Affairs* 1 (1971): 47–66.
WILLIAMS, GLANVILLE. "Euthanasia." *Medico-Legal Journal* 41 (1973): 14–34. See especially sections on suicide, pp. 26–29.
Wyatt v. Stickney. 344 F. Supp. 373 (M.D. Ala. 1972).

RIGHTS OF PATIENTS

See PATIENTS' RIGHTS MOVEMENT; TRUTH-TELLING; PRIVACY; CONFIDENTIALITY; INFORMED CONSENT IN THE THERAPEUTIC RELATIONSHIP. *See also* RIGHTS.

RIGHTS OF THE INSTITUTIONALIZED

See INSTITUTIONALIZATION; PATIENTS' RIGHTS MOVEMENT; HOSPITALS. *See also* RIGHTS.

RIGHTS OF THE MENTALLY ILL AND THE RETARDED

See MENTALLY HANDICAPPED; INFORMED CONSENT IN MENTAL HEALTH. *See also* RIGHTS.

RIGHTS OF WOMEN

See WOMEN AND BIOMEDICINE. *See also* RIGHTS.

RISK

Life is inherently risk-filled, if we understand "risk" as a chance of injury or loss. In ordinary discourse "risk" may refer to the *amount* of possible loss or to the *probability* of that loss. In all our acts we run risks and impose them on others. Frequently we are unaware of the risks for ourselves and others; often, however, we consciously and deliberately assume or impose risks. Some of those risks are justifiable, others are not. This entry will discuss some moral issues in assuming and imposing risks in biomedical activities, including public policies.

Few, if any, important factors in risk assumption and imposition in the biomedical area are unique. Although the physician–patient relationship, the investigator–subject relationship, and policymaking in biomedicine raise significant ethical questions, the similarities to other human activities are striking. Indeed, biomedical ethics is the application of general moral principles to a particular set of roles, relations, and acts whether the issue is truth-telling, distributive justice, assuming and imposing risks, or some other issue.

One important set of distinctions concerns the parties who bear the risks and gain the benefits of particular acts, policies, and technologies: (1) The risks and benefits may fall on the same party, e.g., in therapy; (2) party A bears the risks, while party B gains the benefits, e.g., in nontherapeutic experimentation; (3) both parties may bear the risks, while only one party gains the benefits, e.g., a nuclear-powered artificial heart; (4) both parties may gain benefits, while only one party bears the risks, e.g., persons in the vicinity of a nuclear energy plant may bear significantly greater risks than other persons who also benefit from that plant.

It is also necessary to distinguish between "voluntary" and "involuntary" risks and benefits. Some may voluntarily assume risks because they desire the benefits, either for themselves or for others. But risks are sometimes imposed on individuals against their will; such risks may be involuntary because the individuals involved do not want to take the risks for the benefits in question. Of course, one may inquire about the quality of a person's consent to or acquiescence in risks by probing the degree of voluntariness and the informational basis of the decision. Apparently we are willing to tolerate more risk in voluntary activities over which we have some control than in involuntary activities (Starr, p. 41).

Risk taking

Some studies of why people take chances—particularly the studies by Goffman—illuminate risk-taking conduct. Goffman contends that modern society has conspired to create "safe and momentless living" and that individuals try to offset this situation by significant risk-filled action that allows them to express themselves or to display their character. Although Goffman draws on dramatic forms of risk taking such as gambling or bullfighting, his analysis also encompasses more ordinary activities. Individuals also engage in various forms of risk avoidance and denial of risk to create security. They may try to cope by making realistic efforts to minimize risks, e.g., through physical care, or engage in defensive behavior, e.g., rituals based on superstition, that does not alter what happens but affects the emotional states associated with it (Goffman, pp. 174–181).

Several issues emerge from voluntary risk taking in accord with one's own risk-benefit analysis or life plan. According to an ancient myth Thetis could choose for her son, Achilles, either a short, heroic, and exciting life or a long, tranquil, and obscure one. While she chose the certainty of the former, nonmythic persons most often choose among life plans that have different degrees of risk of injury, death, etc. One of the most penetrating and helpful analyses of risk posits that "a person's life plan establishes the magnitudes of risk which he will accept for his various ends at various times in his life" (Fried, p. 177). Each person's life plan includes what Fried calls a "risk budget." Although Fried concentrates on budgeting risks of death in relation to goals and purposes in different periods of life as well as to the life plan as a whole, one's life plan implies budgets of other sorts of risks as well as budgets of time, energy, and money. Despite the fact that some people may have incoherent projects or may live unreflectively, most appear to have several significant goals in their life plans that they are not willing to sacrifice in order to prolong life or avoid risks of death. Indeed, one's style of life is determined largely by matters for which one will take serious risks. The willingness to risk death for particular ends such as success, friendship, and religious convictions shows the value of those ends (ibid., p. 167).

Paternalism

In general, liberal moral and political theories insist that individuals be allowed to bear whatever risks they voluntarily choose as long as those risks do not pose threats of harm for others. For instance, a person without dependents should be allowed to refuse a particular treatment even if his decision should greatly increase the likelihood of death. Because the liberal tradition tends to view each person's life plan, including its risk budget, as inviolable, it generally rejects paternalistic interventions, i.e., restricting a person's liberty for that person's own welfare or safety when there are no risks to others. Nevertheless, even John Stuart Mill, in *On Liberty*, allowed one exception to his condemnation of paternalistic interferences in the affairs of persons who are in the maturity of their faculties: No person should be allowed to sell himself into slavery, for it is "not freedom to be allowed to alienate his freedom." Gerald Dworkin argues that rational persons would consent to paternalistic interferences in decisions "which are far-reaching, potentially dangerous and irreversible," and would agree to an "enforced waiting period" before being permitted to act on decisions that are usually made under extreme pressures, e.g., dueling or committing suicide (Dworkin, p. 112). But he also contends that rational persons would require authorities to carry the burden of proof for paternalistic interference, to demonstrate the nature and magnitude of risks, and to choose the alternative that would least restrict liberty while reducing the risks.

In actual practice, it is not enough merely to distinguish individual and social decisions to assume risks, for often individuals determine their risks within options that are already limited in significant ways by social, usually governmental, decisions (*Perspectives*, pp. 148 ff.). For example, while individuals may make their own decisions concerning smoking cigarettes, the government regulates some of the public advertising and requires manufacturers to place a warning label on each package of cigarettes. Such policies do not restrict an individual's freedom to assume the risks of smoking; they rather provide information about the risks involved. In a second set of cases, individual risk taking is already limited by prior governmental action. "This category of decisions exemplifies compromise between a person's freedom of choice and governmental coercion to limit that freedom in the name of greater benefit and/or safety" (ibid., p. 148). Examples are building codes that set minimum design and construction standards and Food and Drug Administration regulations that require proof of a drug's efficacy and safety. In these cases the intention is not only to provide more information so that risk taking can be genuinely informed, but also to set a maximum level of risk. Thus, the individual's range of risks is limited. In a third set of cases, a social decision preempts the individual's choice of risks—for example, when the government tries to diminish the risk to health from air pollution by establishing and enforcing certain standards for industries and automobiles. Since individuals cannot easily avoid exposure to polluted air, and since the good of clean air is not divisible, clean air must be treated as a public good.

Dworkin distinguishes "pure" paternalism, which restricts X's liberty in order to reduce X's risk taking, from "impure" paternalism, which restricts X's freedom in order to reduce Y's risk taking when Y could easily avoid those risks (Dworkin, p. 111). Prohibiting individuals from using cigarettes is "pure" paternalism, while prohibiting the manufacture and sale of cigarettes is "impure" paternalism. Some commentators contend that we should attack the sources of some avoidable risks since individual choices are not really "voluntary" because of their "social preconditions" or "collective and structural aspects"—e.g., cigarette smoking in the context of widespread advertising (Beauchamp). Such a contention may wrongly assume that "voluntary" is equivalent to "unmotivated" or "uninfluenced." Some policies presuppose that risk taking can be "voluntary"; their intent is to ensure that private risk taking is "informed." They attempt to inform individuals about risks, particularly the probability and magnitude of harm in the distant future. Only if one is reasonably informed can one be said to choose freely certain risks.

Often apparently paternalistic policies are justified on the grounds that they are not merely paternalistic, since the risk takers in question also impose certain risks or burdens on others or society. If, as some argue, health is largely the responsibility of individuals, and if individuals willfully take certain risks by commission or omission, how should a society that has limited medical resources respond to their medical needs? If its educational programs fail to reduce the risk taking, should it increase the taxes of those who take risks so that it can increase its medical resources? Should it deny risk takers' claims for scarce medical resources when others who did not take those risks also need those resources? Numerous unanswered ethical and political questions emerge from the related issues of risk, paternalism, and allocation of scarce resources.

Ethical issues in risk imposition

Ordinary moral consciousness and most moral theories recognize a prima facie duty not to injure or harm others. Furthermore, they usually hold that this duty of nonmaleficence has priority over and is more stringent than the duty of beneficence. That is, it is easier to justify and excuse failures to fulfill the duty of beneficence than the duty of nonmaleficence, the latter encompassing risk imposition as well as intentional injury or harm. The Hippocratic Oath includes both promotion of good and avoidance of harm: "I will apply dietetic measures for the benefit of the sick, according to my ability and judgment; I will keep them from harm and injustice." The form that is commonly used is of obscure origin but accurately reflects the medical ethos: *primum non nocere* (first of all, do no harm) (Jonsen).

While tort law is more concerned with the imposition of risks than with intentional infliction of injury, the line between the two is not always clear. For instance, the line between negligence (defined as "conduct which falls below a standard established by the law for the protection of others against unreasonable risk of harm") and intent to injure becomes harder to draw as the probability of an injury to another becomes greater; substantial certainty of harm is often viewed as indistinguishable from an intent to harm (Prosser, pp. 145–146).

In cases of risk imposition, law and morality recognize a standard of "due care." This standard of due care, which invokes the notion of a "reasonable man," is met when the goals sought are sufficiently weighty and important to justify the risks (both degree and amount) imposed on others. Grave risks require very important goals for their justification, and emergencies (e.g., danger of an epidemic) may justify risks that ordinary utility calculations will not.

While a justifiable course of action requires a balance of probable benefit over costs, including risks, such weighing is not sufficient for justification. For example, courses of action A and B have favorable risk-benefit ratios in a particular situation, but they are not equally justifiable since A's ratio is more favorable. Thus, an additional standard is involved: which course of action has the best risk-benefit ratio.

Some moral and legal discussions view risk imposition as only a matter of balancing probable benefits and risks in relation to alternative courses of action. Such discussions are unsatisfactory if they do not consider other factors, such as special moral relations (e.g., between physician and patient), that give rise to obligations and that also specify "due care." Other moral and legal interpretations hold that balancing risks and benefits is not sufficient and stress the rights of parties, the principle of fairness, and so forth. Charles Fried's penetrating analysis of risk imposition posits a "risk pool," an interpersonal correlate to the "risk budget" and an implication of fairness or the Kantian principle of right, which affords a person "the fullest freedom to impose risk of death upon others compatible with an equal right on the part of others to impose risks of death upon him according to universal laws" (Fried, p. 185). The notion of a "risk pool" is that "all persons by virtue of their interactions contribute, as it were, to a common pool of risks which they impose upon each other, and on which they may draw when pursuing ends of the appropriate degree of seriousness" (ibid., p. 189).

Issues of rights and fairness emerge with special urgency when one party gains most of the benefits and another party bears most of the risks. As previous examples suggest, this distributional question appears not only in nontherapeutic experimentation but also in decisions about allocating resources. Some technologies impose substantial risks on one party for the sake of another; for example, the debate about the totally implantable nuclear-powered artificial heart focused in part on the risk of radiation for the families and associates of recipients (U.S. DHEW, pp. 111–113). The distribution of risks and benefits is especially complicated when "future generations" are involved. Since it is unfair for living persons to deplete the resources of, and impose other serious risks on, future generations, we may have to renounce some benefits that would otherwise be obtainable. Nevertheless, there is little agreement about the basis, extent, and implications of an obligation to future generations.

While physicians have a duty of personal care toward their patients, this duty does not imply that physicians must care for each patient as though there were no other patients under their care. In some cases, very extensive and intensive care would statistically reduce the risk of later complications, relapses, etc. For example, if patients recovering from certain operations were kept in hospitals for longer periods, their risks might decrease appreciably. But since no hospital or physician can limit care to one patient, it must allocate time, energy, space, treatment, and so forth. Medical practice thus reflects some rough criteria of acceptable degrees of risk for certain conditions. Although the society and the medical profession have not made explicit decisions in most instances, it is possible to ascertain the standard of "due care" in medical practice.

Physicians must make other judgments about risk imposition where risks and benefits fall on the same party. For example, "every medical and surgical procedure, even the most established, carries some uncertainty about its efficacy and safety" (Fox and Swazey, p. 142). Since the evaluation of risks and benefits will vary according to life plans and risk budgets, it is only fair for patients to be able to consent to or refuse particular therapies or procedures.

Risk-benefit analysis

Since risk can be construed as one sort of cost, many of the issues raised by risk-benefit analysis appear in more general cost-benefit analyses. The case can be made that patients, physicians, researchers, and policymakers—particularly the last—all use some form of cost-benefit analysis. Most often it is a rough and partly intuitive analysis in which the metaphorical character of "weighting," "balancing," and "calculating" is evident. Decision analysts insist that a more formal and systematic approach to cost-benefit analysis is both possible and productive. Indeed, they ask, what alternative do we have (Raiffa, p. 272)?

It is not possible in this article to cover the great variety of approaches and methods that fall under, or are related to, the general rubric of cost-benefit analysis. Some advantages and difficulties may be associated with one particular method but not with another. Nevertheless, what is common to the methods is important: "an effort to make comparisons systematically in quantitative terms, using a logical sequence of steps that can be retraced and verified by others" (Goldman, p. 31).

Proponents identify several advantages of cost-benefit analysis (Raiffa, pp. 268–272). It forces the decision maker to seek information from various sources, to be rigorous, to articulate his thought process indicating the factors that he considers and how he weights them, and to analyze organic wholes, not merely parts. It facilitates communication by encouraging expert testimony in clear, quantitative form and permits participants to ascertain the areas of agreement and disagreement so that they can more easily resolve their differences. Even if the method does not provide conclusive answers about what ought to be done, it may indicate which options should be rejected because they are ineffective or because their costs, including their risks, outweigh the benefits.

Critics do not always distinguish principled and practical objections to cost-benefit or risk-benefit analyses. Nevertheless, some flaws may be inherent in the method, while others may simply result from the inadequacies of particular techniques that can, in principle, be corrected. Still other objections may focus on abuses of analysis or may merely be rejections of particular conclusions that are drawn from some analyses. Indeed, it is only fair to emphasize that many of the difficulties of cost-benefit analysis confront any decision maker regardless of his theoretical perspective. For instance, every decision maker has to consider the effects of an act or policy. Yet it may be difficult to determine the connection between exposure to radiation and some disease because of the lapse of time between exposure and negative symptoms, or because the symptoms are relatively common, or because a later generation experiences the symptoms while the present generation gains the benefits (*Perspectives*, p. 15).

Most criticisms of cost-benefit analysis focus on the restatement of important factors in quantitative form. It is difficult and perhaps impossible, the critics say, to restate some factors in decision making in numbers, to assign any meaningful statistical weight to them. One danger is that "intangibles" that are relevant to the decision will be overlooked because they cannot be included in the formal, systematic, quantitative analysis. Furthermore, any attempt to restate decision factors in quantitative form involves the values of the analyst who may or may not give reasons for them. As one defender of analysis writes: "Human judgment is used in designing the analysis, in deciding what alternatives to consider, what factors are relevant, what the interrelations between these factors are, and what numerical values to choose, and in interpreting the results of the analysis" (Goldman, p. 8). These value judgments may be overlooked, because the analysis appears to be scientific and value-free.

While it is impossible to separate facts and values, description and evaluation, in the determination and weighting of factors in decision making, some interpreters apparently think of the determination of *probability* of risk and benefit as value-free. Certainly it is more value-free than the determination and weighting of decision factors, but

. . . the values of those performing the analysis dictate the manner in which uncertainty as to potential adverse consequences will be resolved. To some, the absence of evidence that there will be injury connotes the belief that injury will not in fact result; to others, the absence of proof that injury will not result connotes the belief that injury may result. A basic question, therefore, is whether uncertainty will be resolved optimistically or pessimistically, and the manner in which the resolution is accomplished reflects the value judgments of those who perform the analysis [Green, p. 799].

Description and evaluation are not separated even in the determination of probability of risk because of "opposing dispositions or outlooks toward the future" such as confidence and hope or fear and anxiety (Gustafson, p. 153).

Whether we should concentrate more on the risks or the benefits depends in part on value assumptions. Some scientists insist that we pay too much attention to the possible hazards of biomedical research, e.g., recombinant DNA molecule research, and new technologies, e.g., totally implantable, nuclear-powered hearts, and not enough to their benefits. Other interpreters, however, contend that the benefits in the biomedical area tend to be more immediate and obvious, while the risks are more difficult to identify and assess. They hold that the society should err on the side of underweighting benefit and overweighting risk (Green, p. 807). They could argue that such an approach will result in better policies in an uncertain world. A moral conviction may also undergird their argument: The duty of noninjury has priority over the duty of doing good, i.e., of producing benefits. Or they may hold that there is a difference between what happens and what one (even a society) does. From a utilitarian perspective, one is equally responsible for what happens and for what one does. But personal and social integrity may require that some benefits be passed up or at least postponed in order to avoid imposing certain risks on others (Williams).

It is not clear that scientific views about risks and benefits should be taken as decisive in formulating public policies, although they are, of course, indispensable. Because description and evaluation are joined, even those scientific views

rest on value judgments that have no special claim to authority in the political process. The issue is, "Who decides?" While scientists may have special perspectives and skills to help society identify and enumerate benefits and risks, "it is by no means clear that they are particularly qualified to participate in the actual balancing of benefits and risks in the making of the decision" (Green, pp. 799–800). The "balancing" is appropriately left to the political process, which may, of course, determine that such matters should be handled by a more expert group within statutory mandates and limits, e.g., some regulatory agencies such as the Food and Drug Administration or the Environmental Protection Agency in the United States.

JAMES F. CHILDRESS

[For further discussion of topics mentioned in this article, see the entries: DECISION MAKING, MEDICAL; and PATERNALISM. For discussion of related ideas, see the entries: FUTURE GENERATIONS, OBLIGATIONS TO; JUSTICE; RIGHTS; and TECHNOLOGY, article on TECHNOLOGY ASSESSMENT. Other relevant material may be found under FREE WILL AND DETERMINISM; INFORMED CONSENT IN THE THERAPEUTIC RELATIONSHIP; RATIONING OF MEDICAL TREATMENT; RESEARCH POLICY, BIOMEDICAL; RIGHT TO REFUSE MEDICAL CARE; and SOCIALITY.]

BIBLIOGRAPHY

BEAUCHAMP, DAN E. "Public Health as Social Justice." *Inquiry* 13 (1976): 3–14.

CALABRESI, GUIDO. *The Costs of Accidents: A Legal and Economic Analysis.* New Haven: Yale University Press, 1970.

DARBY, WILLIAM J. "Acceptable Risk and Practical Safety: Philosophy in the Decision-Making Process." *Journal of the American Medical Association* 224 (1973): 1165–1168.

DWORKIN, GERALD. "Paternalism." *Morality and the Law.* Edited by Richard Wasserstrom. Belmont, Calif.: Wadsworth Publishing Co., 1971, pp. 107–126.

FOX, RENÉE C., and SWAZEY, JUDITH P. *The Courage to Fail: A Social View of Organ Transplants and Dialysis.* Chicago: University of Chicago Press, 1974.

FRIED, CHARLES. *An Anatomy of Values: Problems of Personal and Social Choice.* Cambridge: Harvard University Press, 1970.

GOFFMAN, ERVING. *Interaction Ritual: Essays on Face-to-Face Behavior.* Garden City, N.Y.: Doubleday & Co., Anchor Books, 1967.

GOLDMAN, THOMAS A., ed. *Cost-Effectiveness Analysis: New Approaches in Decision-Making.* Washington Operations Research Council. New York: Frederick A. Praeger, 1967.

GREEN, HAROLD P. "The Risk–Benefit Calculus in Safety Determinations." *George Washington Law Review* 43 (1975): 791–807.

GUSTAFSON, JAMES M. "Basic Ethical Issues in the Bio-Medical Fields." *Soundings* 53 (1970): 151–180.

JONSEN, ALBERT R. "Do No Harm: Axiom of Medical Ethics." *Philosophical Medical Ethics: Its Nature and Significance.* Proceedings of the Third Trans-Disciplinary Symposium on Philosophy and Medicine, Farmington, Conn., 11–13 December 1975. Edited by Stuart F. Spicker and H. Tristram Engelhardt, Jr. Philosophy and Medicine, vol. 3. Edited by H. Tristram Engelhardt, Jr. and Stuart F. Spicker. Boston: D. Reidel Publishing Co., 1977, pp. 27–41.

LOWRANCE, WILLIAM W. *Of Acceptable Risk: Science and the Determination of Safety.* Los Altos, Calif.: William Kaufmann, 1976.

MILL, JOHN STUART. *On Liberty.* Edited by Currin V. Shields. Library of Liberal Arts, no. 61. Indianapolis: Bobbs-Merrill; New York: Liberal Arts Press, 1956.

OKRENT, DAVID, ed. *Risk–Benefit Methodology and Application: Some Papers Presented at the Engineering Foundation Workshop, September 22–26, 1975, Asilomar, California.* UCLA-ENG-7598. Los Angeles: University of California, School of Engineering and Applied Science, Energy and Kinetics Department, 1975.

Perspectives on Benefit–Risk Decision Making. Report of a Colloquium Conducted by the Committee on Public Engineering Policy, 26–27 April 1971. Washington: National Academy of Engineering, 1972.

PREST, A. R., and TURVEY, R. "Cost–Benefit Analysis: A Survey." *Economic Journal* 75 (1965): 683–735.

PROSSER, WILLIAM L. *Handbook of the Law of Torts.* 4th ed. Hornbook Series. St. Paul, Minn.: West Publishing Co., 1971.

RAIFFA, HOWARD. *Decision Analysis: Introductory Lectures on Choices under Uncertainty.* Series in Behavioral Science: Quantitative Methods. Reading, Mass.: Addison-Wesley, 1968.

SCHELLING, THOMAS C. "The Life You Save May Be Your Own." *Problems in Public Expenditure Analysis.* Papers presented at a conference of experts held 15–16 September 1966. Edited by Samuel B. Chase, Jr. Washington: Brookings Institution, 1968, pp. 127–176.

STARR, CHAUNCEY. "Social Benefit versus Technological Risk." *Science* 165 (1969): 1232–1238.

United States; Department of Health, Education, and Welfare; National Heart and Lung Institute; Artificial Heart Assessment Panel. *The Totally Implantable Artificial Heart—Economic, Ethical, Legal, Medical, Psychiatric, Social Implications.* DHEW Publications no. (NIH) 74–191. Bethesda, Md.: National Institutes of Health, 1973.

WILLIAMS, BERNARD. "A Critique of Utilitarianism." *Utilitarianism For and Against* by J. J. C. Smart and Bernard Williams. Cambridge: Cambridge University Press, 1973, pp. 77–155.

RISKS AND BENEFITS

See RISK; TECHNOLOGY, *article on* TECHNOLOGY ASSESSMENT.

ROMAN CATHOLICISM

By the 1950s medical ethics flourished in the Roman Catholic tradition as a well-developed and firmly established discipline. Many books on medical ethics existed then in all the major European languages (e.g., Bonnar; Healy; Kelly; Kenny; Niedermeyer, 1935; O'Donnell, 1956, 1976; Paquin; Payen; Pujiula; Scremin). In addition there were periodicals exclusively devoted to medical morality in many of the same countries, such as *Arzt und Christ, Cahiers Laënnec, Catholic Medical Quarterly, Linacre Quarterly,* and *Saint-Luc Medicale.* The existence of a well-developed discipline of medical ethics in Roman Catholicism distinguishes this tradition from most others. This article will focus on the monolithic discipline of medical ethics that existed in Roman Catholicism in the 1950s. Specifically, the following aspects will be discussed: (1) the general context, (2) the historical development, (3) the specific characteristics, (4) the moral principles, and (5) the particular questions considered. A final section (6) will summarize the very significant developments that have occurred since the 1950s.

The general context

The Christian tradition, rooted in both the Old and the New Testaments and exemplified in the story of the Good Samaritan, has always encouraged the care for the sick. Sickness, in the Christian perspective, has a number of dimensions. God as the author and giver of life is also recognized as the healer. Sickness and death have been associated with the power of sin in the world, but sickness is also a sign of human weakness and fragility; human beings can and should try to heal and overcome sickness if possible, but ultimately all will die. In the suffering connected with sickness the Christian tradition sees not only an evil to overcome if possible but also a mysterious sharing in the suffering, death, and resurrection of Jesus.

Corresponding to the multiple understandings of sickness were the different aspects of the care of the sick fostered by the Church. The spiritual care of the sick ultimately developed into the sacrament of anointing, one of the seven sacraments in the Roman Catholic Church. Recently, the Church has recognized a false emphasis in restricting that sacrament to the moment of death (it had been generally known as the sacrament of extreme unction before the Second Vatican Council in the early 1960s) and has renewed the emphasis on the sacrament as the anointing of the sick. The sacrament celebrates the presence of Jesus in the community as the healer of sickness but also as the Lord who through his death and resurrection has transformed sin, sickness, suffering, and death itself. Prayers for healing exist both in the sacrament and in the Christian life in general, but the believer knows that healing will not always come. The relationship between sickness and sin is seen in demonic possession and the rite of exorcism. However, the Church, while acknowledging the possibility both of miraculous cures by God and of possession by the devil, has generally been quite cautious in those two areas. Obviously in both cases the dangers of illusion and deception are most prevalent. Also in this connection the Church has been aware of the danger of magic and superstition in connection with healing. In other cultures healing was often associated with such superstitious practices, but they were continually condemned in the Christian tradition.

The Christian tradition in general and the Catholic tradition in particular have emphasized that God usually works mediately through secondary causes and not immediately without the help of human causes. Acceptance of this principle of mediation characterizes much of Roman Catholic theology and ethical thought. In the area of healing, human means of curing illness have been encouraged, for in that way the doctor is cooperating in God's work, although ultimately sickness and death will triumph. To relieve suffering and strive for healing are viewed as working with God and in no way an offense to divine providence, since the creature is called to responsibly take care of one's life and health. Thus the Christian tradition encouraged medicine as well as prayer and fought against superstition and magic as opposed to both faith and reason.

The Christian church has fostered and sponsored the establishment of hospitals to care for the sick and the dying. Catholic institutional involvement in hospitals and the care for the sick has continued to be a very vital aspect of the mission of the Catholic Church. Communities of religious men and women within the Church have dedicated themselves to the apostolate of caring for the sick and the dying. In the first millennium of Christianity it was not uncommon for clerics also to be medical doctors. However, abuses crept in, especially by clerics' devoting all their time to medicine so that prohibitions against the practice of medicine by clerics were introduced at the Fourth Lateran Council in 1215. The present Code of Canon Law (Canon 139§2) continues to forbid clerics or priests to practice medicine or surgery with-

out special permission, but such permission has customarily been given where there is necessity —e.g., in missionary countries—or some other good reason. Religious women and men who are not clerics have been encouraged to serve as doctors and nurses. Similarly, the Church has held in high regard vocations in the health-care field for all its members.

In addition, the Catholic tradition has affirmed that in theory there can be no contradiction between faith and reason and has cultivated human reason and the arts. In the Middle Ages universities sprang up under the auspices of the Church, and the natural sciences were encouraged in those institutions. Likewise, until the fifteenth century many of the leading theologians and thinkers of the Church were also experts in some aspects of biology and the physical sciences—e.g., Augustine, Hugh of St. Victor, Albert the Great, and Roger Bacon. Obviously, there have been some tensions between medicine and the Roman Catholic Church, as exemplified in the problem of obtaining cadavers for medical research, but on the whole the Roman Catholic tradition has fostered and encouraged the practice of medicine.

Historical development

Many factors contributed to the growth of what ultimately became the discipline of medical ethics. Catholic theology stressed the importance of works, for faith alone was not enough. The penitential practices of the Roman Catholic Church emphasized the need to know if certain actions were sinful or not. Casuistry focused discussion on the morality of particular acts. The discipline of canon law with its complete legislation on marriage, including such questions as sterility and impotence, called for a knowledge of biology and medicine. Concern for baptism, especially in the womb, occasioned a great interest in embryology.

The historical development of medical ethics in the Roman Catholic tradition is closely connected with moral theology in general. Unfortunately the definitive history of Catholic moral theology has not been written; but there are some rather generic overviews (e.g., Häring, 1961–1966, vol. 1, pp. 3–31).

Early development. The first 600 years after Christ are generally referred to as the Patristic Age, because the principal writers were the Fathers of the Church. Specific moral teachings were developed and proposed in a pastoral rather than a systematic or academic perspective. Many subjects of interest to the later development of medical ethics were first discussed at that time. Clement of Alexandria, for example, often called the founder of the first school of Christian theology, invoked the procreative rule to condemn contraception (Noonan, pp. 56–138). From the earliest times abortion was condemned, but influential figures like Jerome and Augustine accepted a theory of delayed ensoulment according to which the human soul came into the body some time after conception.

The most creative development in the period from the seventh to the twelfth century concerns the *Libri Poenitentiales (Penitential Books)*, which came into existence with the new format of the sacrament of penance, involving the confession of sins to a priest, who then gave absolution without a long period of penance. These penitential books consisted of an arrangement of sins by subject matter together with the prescribed penance the priest should give for every wrong act. In the penitentials one finds those actions which the Church considered wrong and sinful. In the midst of many other wrong acts, such as stealing, lying, cheating, and adultery, one also finds abortion, contraception, and other matters connected with marriage and what was later called medical ethics.

The twelfth century set the stage for the development of modern canon law in the Roman Catholic Church. Popes, various universal councils, particular councils, and local bishops had issued laws and legislation for the Church. About 1140 Gratian, traditionally identified as an Italian Camaldolese monk, collected and put in order many of the various laws and norms that had come into existence. His work, known as the *Decretum* or *Decree* of Gratian, was later accepted as the basis for church law. In 1234 Pope Gregory IX published an official collection of laws known as the *Decretals*, which among other things speak about medical inspection to prove the existence of impotency and the nullity of the marriage (*De Probationibus*). In 1331 Pope John XXII formed the church judges into a college of judges, which was called the Roman Rota. In his decretal *Ratio iuris exigit*, he mentioned medical skills and knowledge that help the work of the tribunal. Thus from the early stages in the development of canon law the role and importance of biological and medical science, especially in the area of marriage, are recognized.

The thirteenth century. The thirteenth century also witnessed the growth and development of scholastic theology, which achieved its high point in Thomas Aquinas, whose philosophical and theological approach was later accepted as normative. Thomas Aquinas (d. 1274) proposed a highly systematic theology in his famous *Summa Theologiae*. In the second part of this work Thomas treats the questions connected with the moral life of the Christian in the context of a threefold understanding—the human being related to God as ultimate end, the human being as an image of God insofar as one is capable of self-determination, and the humanity of Christ as our way to God. The natural law theory proposed by Aquinas has become the characteristic approach of Roman Catholic moral theology.

The fourteenth to the eighteenth century. For many theoretical and practical reasons, in the centuries after Aquinas moral theology developed as a distinct discipline in itself and generally became separated from systematic theology. Its concerns became more and more practical with a heavy emphasis on casuistry, closely connected with both canon law and the penitential practice of the Church. In the third tome of his four-volume *Summa* the Archbishop of Florence, St. Antoninus (d. 1459), considers the functions and obligations of different states in life—married people, virgins and widows, temporal rulers, soldiers, lawyers, doctors, merchants, judges, craft workers, etc. The discussion of the functions and obligations of doctors extends for five large pages and mentions the following: competence; diligence; care for the patient; the obligation to tell the dying patient, which is obligatory when the patient is not prepared for death but is counseled even if the patient is prepared for death; the possibility of accepting and caring for dying patients and receiving a fee from them; the proper fee or salary for the doctor (the doctor is bound to care for the sick when they cannot pay); the obligation not to prescribe remedies, such as fornication, that are against the moral law; and the question of abortion. Antoninus became a most important source, frequently cited by later theologians, e.g., Sylvester Prieras (d. 1523).

Beginning in 1621 Paolo Zacchia, a Roman doctor, published a multivolume work entitled *Quaestiones medico-legales*, which might be called the first work on medical ethics. Here Zacchia treated many diverse subjects—age, birth, pregnancy, death, mental illness, poison, impotence, sterility, plagues, contagious diseases, virginity, rape, fasting, mutilation of parts of the body, and conjugal relations.

Zacchia's work was well known and often referred to by moral theologians and canon lawyers and was recognized as a standard reference until the nineteenth century.

After Zacchia there were a few other works devoted to what might be called pastoral medicine or medical ethics. For example, Michiel Boudewyns, a doctor in medicine and philosophy, published in Antwerp in 1666 *Ventilabrum medico-theologicum* containing the questions and cases most often faced by doctors. The author describes his own work as necessary for theologians, confessors, and especially doctors. In the seventeenth and eighteenth centuries monographs also appeared on particular subjects. Theophilus Raynaudus in 1637 in his *De ortu infantium* writes about the morality of caesarean sections in the various circumstances that might arise in birth. P. Florentinius in 1658 published *Disputatio de ministrando baptismo* in which he talked about the sacrament of baptism and the products of conception which were doubtfully human. F. E. Cangiamila (d. 1763) in his *Sacra embryologia* discusses questions connected with embryology such as the animation of the fetus and intrauterine baptism.

However, despite these significant developments in the seventeenth and eighteenth centuries, one still cannot speak of a well-developed and distinct discipline of pastoral medicine or medical ethics in Roman Catholic theology. In the same two centuries Catholic moral theology in general was characterized by the growth of the manuals known as the *Institutiones theologiae moralis*. During that period acrimonious debate arose between laxists and rigorists, a debate which came to a solution in the sane middle course adopted in the work of St. Alphonsus Liguori (d. 1789), who expounded a position of moderate probabilism. The work of Alphonsus was approved by subsequent popes. Alphonsus's approach to moral theology thus became the examplar in format, content, and method for much of Catholic moral theology until the mid-1900s. His discussion of moral theology under the general division of the ten commandments and the sacraments incorporated medical knowledge especially in his considerations of marriage, baptism, care for the sick and dying, and abortion.

The nineteenth and twentieth centuries: pastoral medicine and medical ethics. In the nineteenth century the discipline called pastoral medicine fully bloomed and took its part as a separate discipline in the Roman Catholic tradition. Obviously, the newer developments in biological and medical science and the need for theologians and confessors to be aware of that knowledge encouraged the growth of pastoral medicine. The term comes from the most important works of this type, which often bore titles with the words "pastoral medicine," in them. Probably the most influential of many such works was written in 1877 by a German physician, Carl Capellmann, and later translated into Latin and many modern languages. In his introduction Capellmann describes his purpose as providing the priest with the medical knowledge needed to carry out his ministry and communicating to doctors the moral principles necessary to ensure that they act in accord with Christian morals. The chief areas covered by Capellmann are the fifth commandment, including questions of abortion, medical operations, and the use of medicine; the sixth commandment, including masturbation, pollution, marriage; the commandments of the Church, such as fasting and abstinence; the sacraments, particularly baptism, holy communion, extreme unction; and impotence in marriage; plus other topics of lesser importance. Other significant books of the same type were published by Debreyne, Eschbach, and Antonelli. A number of others were also published in various modern languages at the end of the nineteenth and the beginning of the twentieth century so at that time one could recognize the existence of a developed discipline called pastoral medicine.

The trend continued and grew in the twentieth century. These problems were still considered in general treatises on moral theology, but books on pastoral medicine, medical deontology, and medical ethics flourished in all modern European languages. In Germany, Albert Niedermeyer published a multivolume work on pastoral medicine, which included a complete and updated treatment of the topics covered in the older works as well as material dealing with psychiatry and psychotherapy. In the United States many books were written on medical ethics, often textbooks for use in Roman Catholic medical or nursing schools. Also the existence of Catholic hospitals following Catholic ethical codes stimulated the need for books and articles on these subjects.

As the twentieth century progressed, more and more monographs appeared on subjects in medical ethics. Areas of medical ethics became favorite topics for doctoral dissertations in the area of Roman Catholic moral theology. Also the journals existing in different languages published articles on the subject. Thus by the 1950s there was a large body of literature and a distinct field in Roman Catholic theology generally known as medical ethics, although occasionally the more popular nineteenth-century term "pastoral medicine" was still used.

Specific characteristics

Roman Catholic medical ethics as it existed in the 1950s, like all Roman Catholic moral theology at that time, was distinguished by three specific characteristics: natural law methodology, authoritative church teaching, and the Church's understanding of conscience.

Natural law methodology. Natural law is a complex term that has a number of aspects. From the more theological perspective, natural law theory recognizes that reason and human nature constitute a source of ethical wisdom and knowledge for the Christian. Catholic theology historically has recognized both faith and reason, scripture and the natural law. The twentieth-century textbooks in medical ethics acknowledge that their teaching was primarily based on natural law and not on the scriptures.

The philosophical aspect of the question of natural law concerns the precise meanings of human reason, human nature, and natural law itself. Here the Roman Catholic textbooks in medical ethics, like all the Roman Catholic ethical considerations in the first part of the twentieth century, appealed to the teaching of Thomas Aquinas and often summarized that teaching in the beginning of their discussions. According to Thomistic theory, the eternal law is the plan of divine wisdom insofar as it directs all activity and all change toward a final end. The eternal law is ultimately grounded in the very being of God.

The natural law is the participation of the rational creature in the eternal law. God directs all creatures to their end in accord with their own natures. There are laws by which the physical universe is governed, such as the law of gravity. However, human beings are governed according to their rational nature. The human being is an image of God precisely insofar as he or she is endowed with reason, free will, and the power of self-determination. Through reason the rational creature directs one's own activity toward one's proper end and thus is not merely passively directed by God to the end. Right reason is able to recognize the threefold natural inclinations within human nature—the inclina-

tions we share with all substances, the inclinations we share with animals, and the inclinations we have as rational beings. Thus the natural law is understood as human reason directing the individual to one's own end in accord with one's nature.

The natural law in the best of the Catholic tradition was recognized as an unwritten or unformulated law—the very law of one's being as a rational creature. However, on the basis of the ontological structures of rational human nature, reason is able to arrive at universally valid principles or prescriptions of the natural law. The first principles of the natural law are known intuitively by human reason: Good is to be done, evil is to be avoided, act according to right reason. Human reason on the basis of the first principles can then deduce the secondary principles of the natural law, such as adultery is wrong and stealing is forbidden.

Roman Catholic medical ethicists in the 1950s claimed that the secondary principles, since they are based on human nature, are universally obliging. There could be a growth in our knowledge of the implications of the principles and even in a clearer formulation of the principles, but there can be no substantial change in the statement of the principles.

According to one respected medical moral text (Kelly, pp. 19–20), what is true of the secondary principles is also true of some of the particular applications. There can be no question of notable change in what is said about direct abortion, direct attacks on fetal life, contraception, contraceptive sterilization, immoral fertility tests, and so forth. In these points the application of the general principle is so immediate and logical that a change in the morality of the procedure is inconceivable. Some of the condemnations are nothing more than restatements of the general principles. Changes, however, are not only possible but desirable in applications that are justified on the principle of sufficient reason. Certain drastic measures such as castration in the treatment of carcinoma or lobotomy in treating mental illnesses can be justified on the basis of proportionate reason in the present, but it is hoped that less drastic remedies will be found in the future.

Authoritative church teaching. A second distinctive characteristic of Roman Catholic medical ethics involves the authoritative teaching office of the Church. Acceptance of the gospel message calls for faith and works. The Roman Catholic Church recognizes a special God-given teaching office and function belonging to the pope and the bishops as well as to councils of the Church.

Early councils in the Church as well as letters of popes and other bishops spoke about specific moral questions such as abortion and marriage. Mention has already been made of authoritative collections of canon law beginning in the twelfth century. The papal teaching office—especially the Congregation of the Holy Office, which deals with faith and morals—made significant interventions in moral matters in the seventeenth and eighteenth centuries. The existence of papal encyclicals addressed to all the bishops and faithful of the world and speaking on specific areas of faith or morals became really prominent only in the nineteenth century.

The growth and development of medical ethics in the nineteenth and twentieth centuries corresponded with the greater emphasis on the papal teaching office in the Roman Catholic Church. Between 1884 and 1902, for example, the Holy Office responded to a number of inquiries about abortion and eliminated some of the exceptions that had not been expressly condemned. The Holy Office declared that one could not safely perform a craniotomy or directly kill the fetus to save the life of the mother, nor could one extract an ectopic pregnancy (Bouscaren, pp. 3–24). Encyclicals on marriage by Pope Pius XI, *Casti Connubii* in 1930, and by Pope Paul VI, *Humanae Vitae* in 1968, strongly reiterated the condemnation of artificial contraception.

Perhaps the most significant development in the matter of authoritative church teachings was the number of allocutions and addresses given by Pope Pius XII, very often dealing with questions of medical ethics. This corpus of papal teaching shows a wide-ranging interest in the problems of medical ethics as well as a penetrating knowledge of medicine and its problems. To various medical groups Pope Pius XII spoke on such subjects as the duties of the medical profession, blood donors, artificial insemination, contraception, sterilization, abortion, the moral limits of medical research in experimentation, genetics, painless childbirth, transplants, death, and the means necessary to preserve life. Obviously, the interest and concern of Pope Pius XII also sparked the growth and development of the discipline of medical ethics.

It is important to recognize the various grades or degrees of the hierarchical magisterium or teaching authority in the Roman Catholic Church. In the nineteenth century the distinction became formalized between the infallible church teaching to which one owed the assent of faith and the authoritative or authentic, noninfallible teaching to which the faithful owed the religious assent of intellect and will. It was generally acknowledged in the 1950s that teaching in the area of medical ethics ordinarily does not fall under the category of infallible teaching, which in reality is very limited. Gradations were also recognized in the various forms of the ordinary noninfallible papal teaching office. However, Pius XII, in the encyclical *Humani Generis*, 1950, declared that whenever the pope goes out of his way to speak on a controverted subject it is no longer a matter for free debate among theologians. In the light of such an understanding in the 1950s, any Roman pronouncement or decree both theoretically and practically ended debate about a specific question. It must be pointed out that the pope usually would not intervene when Catholic theologians were divided on a particular point and also that the papal teaching office recognized the need for theological input and advice.

The role of conscience. A third specific characteristic of Roman Catholic moral theology and medical ethics is the understanding of conscience. In traditional Catholic thought, conscience is the subjective norm of morality, whereas law, basically the eternal law with all its parts, is the objective norm of morality. Conscience is a dictate of practical reason declaring that a particular action is right or wrong.

A true conscience is had when the judgment of conscience conforms to the objective moral norm, i.e., human nature or the natural law; otherwise the conscience is erroneous. An erroneous conscience can be vincibly or invincibly erroneous, depending on whether or not one is morally responsible for the lack of conformity with the objective moral norm. The individual must always follow one's conscience, but there is guilt in following a vincibly erroneous conscience.

A certain conscience is a moral judgment made without fear of error based on evidence or motives that are sound. A doubtful conscience exists when the intellect suspends judgment because of insufficient evidence. A certain conscience must always be obeyed and is also a necessary requirement for moral action. A doubtful conscience must become certain in practice before one can act.

The controversy about probabilism in the

seventeenth and eighteenth centuries involved the question of how one goes from a doubtful conscience in theory to a certain conscience in practice. The theory of moderate probabilism, which was ultimately accepted, appeals to the basic understanding that the human will is free, and moral obligation can be known only through reason. According to this theory, if moral necessity is not certainly proposed by reason, the freedom of the will remains. In practice, one can follow a truly probable opinion in favor of freedom from the law or obligation even though the opinion in favor of the obligation may be more probable. However, there are some instances, such as danger to the life of another, in which probabilism cannot be used. The practical question was often asked whether or not a particular opinion is probable. Probability was determined by the intrinsic force of the argument but in practice was often reduced to the fact that a number of theologians or recognized authorities held a particular position. It was generally assumed, certainly until the 1950s, that a noninfallible teaching of the papal magisterium, either directly from the pope or through a Roman congregation such as the Holy Office, did not allow for dissent in theory or in practice.

Moral principles

Since the method of natural law talked about establishing the principles of natural law and then applying these principles to particular cases, it is evident that Roman Catholic medical ethics did speak about a number of important principles. In fact, the textbooks in the 1950s often began their discussion with a very brief summary of the more important principles governing medical ethics, somewhat along the following lines. Recall that these principles were generally accepted by all Catholic medical ethicists; only in the 1960s did the monolithic Catholic medical ethics begin to change.

The right to life. Human beings are made by God, who is the author of life and has dominion over all life. A right enables the person who possesses it to achieve one's end. The right to life is a natural right since it flows from the natural law itself. The right to life is inalienable, that is, it may not be renounced. The human being as creature does not have absolute power or full dominion over one's own life or body, for the individual is a steward or administrator over one's life. The right to life is inviolable; otherwise it would not truly be a right.

However, the Roman Catholic ethical tradi-

tion recognized that there are cases where the life of another may be taken; for example, killing another as a necessary way of defending one's life. Just war was acknowledged as a moral possibility. The possibility of capital punishment was generally accepted in the Catholic tradition. Accidental killing was also recognized as a possibility. The most precise formulation of the principle was that the direct killing of an innocent person on one's own authority is always wrong.

Right of use or stewardship. Much in the area of medical ethics follows from the moral principle that the individual possesses the right of use, limited by natural finality, of the faculties and powers of one's human nature. Since the individual is a user and not a proprietor, one does not have unlimited power to destroy or mutilate one's body or its functions (Pope Pius XII discussed this principle in his Address to the First International Congress on the Histopathology of the Nervous System, 14 September 1952). The principle of stewardship is the basis for the care one should have over one's own body as well as the justification in general for surgery and other procedures.

Principle of totality. One of the principles governing mutilation of the body was called by Pope Pius XII the principle of totality. Thomas Aquinas pointed out that a member of the body existed for the good of the whole body and could be disposed of according as it would benefit the whole. A diseased member may be removed if this is for the good of the whole. In the 1952 address mentioned above, Pius XII described the principle of totality, which maintains that the good of the whole is the determining factor in regard to the part, and one can dispose of the part in the interest of the whole.

The popes and Roman Catholic moralists were very aware of the abuses of totalitarian governments in sacrificing individuals for the good of the state, so they carefully spelled out the meaning and limits of the principle of totality. The part must have its entire finality and meaning in terms of the whole individual. Since the individual person does not exist totally for the good of the state, the individual cannot be totally subordinated to the state. The obvious example where the principle of totality applies is to the individual organs and functions of the total bodily organism. However, in 1958 Pope Pius XII, in his Address to the International College of Neuro-Psychopharmacology, commented that to the subordination of the particular organ to the organism and its own finality one must add the subordination of the organism to the spiritual finality of the person. Each single organ is subordinated not only to the good of the body but to the good of the person. The principle of totality was applied to many medical procedures, operations, and treatments that may often suppress or sacrifice a part for the good of the whole.

Principles regarding sexuality and procreation. In traditional Roman Catholic thought, the faculties and powers of human beings must be used according to the purpose for which they were evidently made by God and intended by nature; for example, the finality of speech is perverted if used to communicate to another as one's own judgment what is directly contrary to one's thought. The sexual function and organs have a twofold purpose—procreation and the love union of husband and wife. (An older terminology referred to procreation as the primary purpose of marriage and sexuality.) The human being thus can never go against the God-intended procreative purpose of human sexuality. Any use of human sexual powers is immoral when it impedes the very purpose for which God created these powers. As a result contraception and contraceptive sterilization are wrong. The individual person may not positively interfere to thwart the sexual act or faculty of its God-given finality. Note how, according to this reasoning, the sexual organs and functions differ from other organs. The sexual organs exist not only for the good of the individual but also for the good of the species. Since the whole meaning and finality of human sexuality are not restricted to the individual, the species-oriented dimension of human sexuality can never directly be subordinated to the good of the individual. Hence, the principle of totality could not be used to sacrifice the species aspect of the sexual organs and functions, for the good of the individual (Healy, pp. 11, 156–161, 171–184).

The principle of double effect. Catholic moral theology has recognized the existence of conflict situations. What is the morality of actions that have two or more effects including a bad effect? The principle of double effect was employed by all medicomoral textbooks to solve these dilemmas. According to Kenny (pp. 5, 6), who merely records the traditional criteria, one can perform an act with two effects, one good and one bad, if the following conditions are present: 1. The act must be good in itself or at least morally indifferent. 2. The good effect must follow as immediately from the cause as the evil effect. 3.

The intention of the individual must be good. 4. There must be a proportionately grave cause for doing the action. This principle was used at times to justify the possibility of indirect killing, indirect abortion, indirect sterilization, and indirect cooperation.

Cooperation and scandal. Especially in terms of the work of doctors and nurses questions arose about cooperation and scandal. Cooperation was generally defined as participation in the wrong or sinful act of another. Formal cooperation, described as intending the evil act, is always wrong. Immediate material cooperation, defined as participation in actually performing the wrong act and sometimes also called formal cooperation, is likewise always wrong. Mediate material cooperation, which presupposes there is no intention to do evil and involves doing an act that is good or indifferent, may be permitted if there is a sufficient reason for so doing. In such a case the individual person neither intends nor does an immoral act. The morality of mediate material cooperation according to O'Donnell (1953, p. 47), is to be judged in light of the principle of the double effect, with special attention to the proportion between the cooperation (proximate or remote, how necessary or unnecessary, to the wrong act of the other) and the gravity of the offense in connection with which another will make use of one's cooperation.

On the basis of these principles a casuistry was developed concerning mediate material cooperation. A doctor, for example, can never do an immoral operation, since that involves at least immediate material cooperation. A nurse's cooperation in such an operation is usually seen as only mediate material cooperation and might be justified—especially if it were not that proximate—by a number of reasons such as the possibility of losing one's position, which would make it impossible for the nurse to accomplish a measure of good in the hospital.

Scandal is a sinful or seemingly sinful word, action, or omission that tends to incite or tempt another to sin. Direct scandal in which the sin of the other is intended is always wrong. Indirect scandal, in which the sin of the other is not intended but only permitted, may be allowed under two conditions: if the act giving scandal is in itself not morally wrong and if there is a sufficient reason for doing such an act. Much of the classic Roman Catholic literature of the 1950s employed these principles governing cooperation and scandal in their discussion of matters in medical ethics.

Specific questions

Obligations of physicians and rights of patients. The textbooks of medical ethics in the 1950s considered many of the questions originally posed by Antoninus of Florence more than 500 years ago—professional competence, the obligation to attend patients, selection of remedies, correction of errors, fees, and newer additions such as ghost surgery and fee splitting. Special emphasis was often given to a number of important questions such as the obligations of secrecy and truthfulness, especially informing the patient about death.

The professional secret is a committed secret binding in justice, wherein the contract of secrecy is not explicitly put into words but is implied by reason of the professional position (e.g., doctor, lawyer) of the one who receives the secret knowledge. Professional secrecy obliges the doctor to keep the secret of the patient as long as the patient retains the right to the secret. A professional secret may be divulged when common necessity calls for it; for example, the law can ask doctors to report all gunshot wounds to the proper authorities. The professional secret may be divulged, but need not be when the patient has become an unjust aggressor and is threatening harm to an innocent third party under the cover of professional secrecy.

All human beings are obliged to tell the truth, but there are some special applications to the doctor–patient relationship, especially in terms of informing the patient about his or her condition. Patients in general have a right to know about the nature of their illness. However, the physician must also take into account the medical, psychological, spiritual, and material interest of the patient. Healy (p. 43) suggests some practical ways in which the doctor might avoid directly answering the question posed by the patient without lying if there are certain reasons why the patient should not be told at that particular time. Very important is the obligation to inform the patient about impending death. Directive eight of the Ethical and Religious Directives for Catholic Health Facilities offers a principle common in Roman Catholic medical ethics literature:

Everyone has the right and duty to prepare for the solemn moment of death. Unless it is clear, therefore, that a dying patient is already prepared for

death as regards both spiritual and temporal affairs, it is the physician's duty to inform him of his critical condition or to have some other responsible person impart this information [Dedek, p. 209].

Sexuality and the transmission of life. The finality of the sexual organs and faculties and the limited stewardship that individuals have over them constitute the basis for the condemnation of contraception and contraceptive or direct sterilization. Human beings cannot positively interfere in the sexual act or the sexual faculty to deprive them of their God-given procreative purpose.

However, Roman Catholic teaching has accepted the basic principle of responsible parenthood: While always open to the gift of life, couples should have the number of children they can properly care for and educate as good Christians and human beings. Acceptance of responsible parenthood gradually appeared in formal Roman Catholic teaching. Pope Pius XII in his 1951 Address to Midwives recognized that there were medical, eugenic, economic, and social indications justifying the limitation of the number of children. The *Pastoral Constitution on the Church in the Modern World* of the Second Vatican Council (n. 50) likewise endorses the concept of responsible parenthood. However, contraception and contraceptive sterilization are —in this same teaching—always wrong. Rhythm or the use of the infertile periods is permitted because there is no positive interference with the God-given purpose of the sexual faculty or act. There are various forms of the use of the infertile period. The form most recently advanced is the so-called natural family planning or Billings method, which has been acknowledged by some to be a highly effective means of family limitation.

The Catholic tradition as found in the medical moral textbooks in the 1950s has not emphasized procreation to such an extent that it gives no importance to all other purposes of sexuality. Catholic teaching has opposed masturbation as a means of obtaining semen for fertility tests, even though procreation would thereby be facilitated. Pope Pius XII in May 1956, in an address to the Second World Conference of Fertility and Sterility, explicitly condemned masturbation as a means of obtaining semen for semen analysis because it is an unnatural act. The pope was merely giving the long-standing teaching of Catholic moralists based on the understanding that the purpose and finality of the sexual act justified it only in the context of marriage, and the act must be both procreative and expressive of the love union (Kelly, p. 219).

On three different occasions Pope Pius XII spoke about and condemned artificial insemination, but again the condemnation was in keeping with the Catholic understanding of the nature and finality of the sexual act. AID (artificial insemination from a donor) was condemned because the child must be the fruit of the bodily gift of the parents. AIH (artificial insemination from the husband) is wrong because it goes against the nature of the sexual act. Emphasis was also given to the technological and mechanistic aspects of artificial insemination as opposed to the personal love union of husband and wife in the sexual act (Kenny, pp. 90–96).

The beginning of life and birth.   Catholic theology acknowledges a possible theoretical doubt about when human life begins, but in practice all must act as if human life is present from the first moment of conception. Since the fetus in the womb is defenseless, Catholic theology all the more feels the need to speak out in its defense. Direct abortion is always wrong. Indirect abortion is permitted for sufficient reasons. The two most often proposed examples of indirect abortion are the removal of the cancerous uterus when the woman is pregnant and the removal of the fallopian tube or the cervix containing an ectopic pregnancy. Caesarean sections were also still discussed in the textbooks of medical ethics. Premature delivery of a viable fetus is morally acceptable if there is a proportionate reason justifying the danger to the fetus involved in such a procedure. Inducement of labor follows the same general principle.

Care for health, surgery, and other procedures. The basic obligation to care for health comes from the stewardship we rational creatures exercise over our lives and bodies. The patient has a right to use all moral means possible to overcome pain even though in some way all will know the meaning of suffering in human existence. However, the Catholic tradition recognizes the right of the person freely to accept pain as a form of participation in the redemptive suffering and death of Jesus. The danger of habit-forming drugs is often discussed in this context of using drugs to relieve pain.

Surgery and other procedures to suppress bodily organs and functions other than the sexual organs and functions are permitted by the principle of totality, provided they are for the proportionate good of the individual. Alleviative surgery (to alleviate pain) and preventive and corrective surgery are permitted if the good of the person proportionately justifies the harm done. Cosmetic surgery can also be justified, but if the operation involves any danger it is much harder to justify.

Organ transplants raised a problem, especially when the organ was taken from another living donor. Here the one person is mutilated not for his or her own good but for the good of another. Pope Pius XII in his Address to Oculists and Cornea Donors, 14 May 1956, pointed out that the principle of totality cannot justify such transplants, because the mutilation is not for the good of the individual who is harmed. Some Roman Catholic moralists, therefore, considered organ transplants among the living as immoral operations, but others justified them on the basis of the principle of fraternal charity. However, even those allowing such transplants cautioned that the donors cannot gravely endanger their lives or seriously impair their functional integrity even for the sake of helping the neighbor (O'Donnell, 1976, pp. 106 ff.).

Death and dying.   On the basis of the teaching that the individual does not exercise full dominion but only stewardship over life, Roman Catholic moral teaching consistently opposed suicide and euthanasia. In addition to natural law arguments, references were frequently made to scriptural arguments and to the evil consequences that would flow from euthanasia. However, painkillers could be given to the dying person even though an indirect effect of these drugs might be the hastening of the death of the patient.

Clearly distinct from euthanasia is the teaching that one does not have to use extraordinary means to preserve human life. The teaching arose in the context of the positive obligation to care for health. Positive obligations do not hold in the face of moral impossibility. By the sixteenth century there was much discussion in the moral literature about the means necessary to preserve life, and the discussion was developed in the seventeenth century by Cardinal de Lugo in his discussion of ordinary and extraordinary means (Cronin, pp. 47–87). The principle is long established that, generally speaking, an individual has no obligation to use extraordinary means to preserve life. A well-accepted contemporary description views extraordinary means as all medicines, treatments, and operations that cannot be obtained or used without excessive expense, pain, or other inconvenience, or if used would not offer a reasonable hope of benefit (Kelly, pp. 129). From such an ethical perspective there is no difference between not using an artificial respirator to sustain life for a few hours or even days or shutting off the respirator already in use.

Even before recent discussions about changing the understanding of the moment of death, Roman Catholic medical ethics discussed that question. The traditional theological definition of death as the separation of the soul from the body lacks precision. Exactly when death occurs is beyond the competency of the Church or theology and belongs to the competency of medical science. Such a position was taken by Pope Pius XII in his address to an International Congress of Anesthesiologists on 24 November 1957.

Other questions.   Under the heading of the spiritual care of the patient, questions concerning informing the patient about death and especially the celebration of the sacraments of baptism and anointing of the sick (extreme unction) were considered. On the question of medical experimentation the textbooks generally followed the teaching of Pope Pius XII in his Address to the Eighth Congress of the World Medical Association, 30 September 1954, in distinguishing between experimentation for the good of the individual and experimentation in the strict sense for the good of others. For the good of the individual, experimentation is allowed provided no certainly effective remedy is available, if the dubious treatment most likely to help the patient is chosen, and if the consent of the patient is at least reasonably presumed. Experimentation for the good of others (experimentation in the strict sense as opposed to therapy) may be permitted for the proportionate good of others and of science if the subject freely consents, if no experiment that directly inflicts grave injury or death is used, and if all reasonable precautions are taken to avoid even the indirect causing of grave injury or death. Later, theologians and ethicists would probe these criteria more deeply and apply them to the cases of children, prisoners, and others whose ability to consent was in some way or other diminished or lacking.

Current trends

Significant developments have occurred in Roman Catholic moral theology since the 1950s and have greatly changed the monolithic discipline of medical ethics described above. It was only in 1963 that articles began appearing in serious scholarly journals disagreeing with the hierarchical teaching that condemns artificial contraception. New developments that often crystallized in the discussion over artificial contraception affected especially two of the distinctive characteristics of Catholic moral theology and medical ethics: natural law and the teaching authority of the Church.

A number of criticisms were directed against the concept of natural law as proposed in the manuals of theology and of medical ethics. A more historically conscious approach is called for, one that gives more emphasis to growth, development, and change and likewise emphasizes the individual, the particular, and the contingent more than is done in the older natural law theory. In this context a more inductive and not such a totally deductive methodology is called for. Newer approaches put more emphasis on the personal and less on the (merely) "natural" and call for a greater stress on the subject. Morality, according to some, cannot be based only on the finality and purpose of the faculty seen in itself apart from the total person. Above all, many contemporary Roman Catholic moral theologians disagree with the physicalism of the older approach according to which the moral aspect of the human act is identified with the physical aspect of the act. The distinction is often proposed between physical or premoral evil on the one hand and moral evil on the other. Physical or premoral evil can be justified for a proportionate reason.

Methodological difficulties with natural law led to the adoption of newer and different methodological approaches to moral theology and thus to medical ethics. Various trends in philosophical and theological thought—such as pragmatism, phenomenology, linguistic analysis, and transcendental Thomism—are currently being used by Roman Catholic ethicists. No longer can one speak of a monolithic natural law theory in Roman Catholic moral theology or medical ethics. There exists even now a pluralism of methodological approaches, but most of them are only in the incipient stages and need to be systematically developed and explored. On the other hand, there are some Roman Catholic ethicists still using the natural law approach as it has been handed down in the manuals of medical ethics.

Recent developments have also affected the understanding of the authoritative teaching of the church in moral matters. Reaction to the encyclical *Humanae Vitae* in 1968 condemning artificial contraception brought to the fore the possibility of dissent within the Roman Catholic Church. Appeal was made to the official documents of the Church themselves and to the historical tradition to justify the possibility of dissent from specific moral teachings of the hierarchical magisterium. The *Constitution on the Church* of the Second Vatican Council (n. 25) called for Catholics to give a religious submission of intellect and will to the authoritative teaching of the Roman Pontiff even when he is not speaking infallibly, but according to many theologians (e.g., Komonchak; Curran et al.), the proper understanding of this teaching allows for the possibility of dissent.

Other contemporary developments in Roman Catholic theology also lead to the possibility of dissent. Contemporary ecclesiology (the theology of the Church) has emphasized in all matters the concepts of collegiality and shared responsibility in the Church. In particular, the teaching office of the Church is not totally identified with the God-given hierarchical teaching office, hence some tension can and will exist. Newer methodological approaches stress that on specific moral questions the church can never have the degree of certitude that excludes the possibility of error. On the other hand, there are theologians who strongly argue against recent developments, which are condemned as forms of subjectivism, relativism, or utilitarianism. In practice these theologians do not allow dissent (Dubay).

The newer developments have been applied to many of the particular questions in medical ethics. The understanding of morality as based on the finality and purpose of the sexual faculty and act has been challenged by a good number of Roman Catholic moral theologians who now accept contraception, sterilization, and masturbation for seminal analysis, AIH, and for some even AID where there are sufficient or proportionate reasons. In addition, many theologians reject the principle of double effect as it has been proposed in the textbooks, especially because of the condition that emphasizes the physical causality of the act by requiring that the good effect must be equally immediate as the evil effect. To a much lesser extent there has even been some dissent on the question of when human life begins and how it affects the question of abortion. A few theologians (Maguire) argue for the possibility of active euthanasia in

some circumstances. However, on all these questions the official position of the hierarchical teaching office has not changed, and some theologians also vigorously defend these teachings. Now books on medical ethics that incorporate some of these new developments are beginning to appear (Häring, 1973; Dedek; Curran), but at the same time newer editions of older books (O'Donnell, 1976; McFadden) have been published in which the teaching of the hierarchical magisterium and the methodology proposed in the textbooks of the 1950s have been upheld.

CHARLES E. CURRAN

[For further discussion of topics mentioned in this article, see the entries: ABORTION, article on ROMAN CATHOLIC PERSPECTIVES; CONTRACEPTION; DEATH AND DYING: EUTHANASIA AND SUSTAINING LIFE; DOUBLE EFFECT; POPULATION ETHICS: RELIGIOUS TRADITIONS, article on ROMAN CATHOLIC PERSPECTIVES; RELIGIOUS DIRECTIVES IN MEDICAL ETHICS, article on ROMAN CATHOLIC DIRECTIVES; REPRODUCTIVE TECHNOLOGIES, article on ETHICAL ISSUES; SEXUAL ETHICS; and STERILIZATION, article on ETHICAL ASPECTS. Other relevant material may be found under HEALTH AND DISEASE, article on RELIGIOUS CONCEPTS; MEDICAL ETHICS, HISTORY OF, section on EUROPE AND THE AMERICAS, articles on MEDIEVAL EUROPE: FOURTH TO SIXTEENTH CENTURY, NORTH AMERICA: SEVENTEENTH TO NINETEENTH CENTURY, and NORTH AMERICA IN THE TWENTIETH CENTURY; PAIN AND SUFFERING, article on RELIGIOUS PERSPECTIVES. See also: HOSPITALS; NURSING; and OBLIGATION AND SUPEREROGATION. See APPENDIX, SECTION I, ETHICAL AND RELIGIOUS DIRECTIVES FOR CATHOLIC HEALTH FACILITIES.]

BIBLIOGRAPHY

[For important church documents in chronological order from the earliest times, see Denzinger, below. Official church documents since 1908 have been promulgated in *Acta Apostolicae Sedis*. English translations of important papal declarations can be found in *The Pope Speaks*, which began publication in 1954. Textbooks in medical ethics often give references to the major addresses of Pope Pius XII on these subjects, e.g., Kenny, 2d ed., p. 272.]

ANTONELLI, GIUSEPPE. *Medicina pastoralis in usum confessariorum et curiarum ecclesiaticarum.* 3 vols. Rome: F. Pustet, 1906.

ANTONINUS [ARCHBISHOP OF FLORENCE]. *Summae summarum* [Summa theologica]. 4 vols. in 2. Lyons: Apud Vincentius de Portonariis, 1542.

BONNAR, ALPHONSUS. *The Catholic Doctor.* 2d ed. London: Burns, Oates & Washbourne; New York: Kenedy & Sons, 1939.

BOUDEWYNS, MICHIEL. *Ventilabrum medico-theologicum quo omnes casus, tum medicos, cum aegros, aliosque concernentes eventilantur.* Antwerp: Apud Cornelium Woons, 1666.

BOUSCAREN, TIMOTHY LINCOLN. *Ethics of Ectopic Operations.* 2d ed. Milwaukee: Bruce Publishing Co., 1944.

CANGIAMILA, FRANCESCO EMMANUELE. *Sacra embryologia, sive, de officio sacerdotum, medicorum, et aliorum circa aeternam parvulorum in utero existentium salutem libri quatuor.* Munich and Ingoldstadt: J. F. X. Grätz, 1764.

CAPELLMANN, CARL FRANZ. *Medicina pastoralis.* 4th ed. Aachen: Rudolph Barth, 1879. Translated by William Dassel as *Pastoral Medicine.* New York: F. Pustet, 1879.

CRONIN, DANIEL A. *The Moral Law in Regard to the Ordinary and Extraordinary Means of Conserving Life.* Rome: Pontificia Universitas Gregoriana, 1958.

CURRAN, CHARLES E. *New Perspectives in Moral Theology.* Notre Dame, Ind.: Fides Publishers, 1974.

———; HUNT, ROBERT E.; HUNT, JOHN F.; and CONNELLY, TERRENCE R. *Dissent in and for the Church: Theologians and "Humanae vitae."* New York: Sheed & Ward, 1969.

DEBREYNE, PIERRE J. C. *La Théologie morale et les sciences médicales.* 6th ed. Edited by Ange E. A. Ferrand. Paris: Poussielgue frères, 1884.

DEDEK, JOHN F. *Contemporary Medical Ethics.* New York: Sheed & Ward, 1975.

DENZINGER, HEINRICH J. D., and SCHÖNMETZER, ADOLFUS. *Enchiridion symbolorum, definitionum et declarationum de rebus fidei et morum.* 32d ed. Barcelona: Herder, 1963.

DUBAY, THOMAS. "Current Theology: The State of Moral Theology: A Critical Appraisal." *Theological Studies* 35 (1974): 482–506.

ESCHBACH, ALPHONS. *Disputationes physiologico-theologicae de humanae generationis oeconomia, de embryologia sacra, de abortu medicali et de embryotomia, de colenda castitate.* Paris: Vict. Palmé, 1884.

FIORENTINI, GIROLAMO [FLORENTINIUS]. *Disputatio de ministrando baptismo humanis foetibus abortiuorum.* Lyons: Apud Claudium Chancey, 1658.

FLOOD, PETER, ed. *New Problems in Medical Ethics.* 4 vols. Translation, by Malachy Gerard Carroll, of *Cahiers Laënnec.* Westminster, Md.: Newman Press, 1953, 1954, 1956, 1960.

———, ed. *New Problems in Medical Ethics.* Nos. 1–4. Translation, by Malachy Gerard Carroll, of *Cahiers Laënnec.* Cork: Mercier Press, 1962, 1963. A series with content overlapping the Newman Press edition, but arranged differently. In part published under the imprint of Divine Word Publications: Techny, Ill.

HÄRING, BERNARD [BERNHARD]. *The Law of Christ: Moral Theology for Priests and Laity.* 3 vols. Translated by Edwin G. Kaiser. Westminster, Md.: Newman Press, 1961–1966.

———. *Medical Ethics.* Edited by Gabrielle L. Jean. Notre Dame, Ind.: Fides Publishers, 1973.

HEALY, EDWIN F. *Medical Ethics.* Chicago: Loyola University Press, 1956.

KELLY, GERALD A. *Medico-Moral Problems.* St. Louis: Catholic Hospital Association, 1958.

KENNY, JOHN P. *Principles of Medical Ethics.* Westminster, Md.: Newman Press, 1952. 2d ed. 1962.

KOMONCHAK, JOSEPH A. "Ordinary Papal Magisterium and Religious Assent." *Contraception: Authority and Dissent.* Edited by Charles E. Curran. New York: Herder & Herder, 1969, pp. 101–126.

LIGUORI, ALFONSO MARIA DE'. *Theologia moralis.* 4 vols. Edited by Leonardi Gaude. Opera moralia Sancti Alphonsi Mariae de Ligorio, vols. 1–4. Rome: Vatican, 1905–1912.

McFADDEN, CHARLES J. *The Dignity of Life: Moral Values in a Changing Society.* Huntington, Ind.: Our Sunday Visitor, 1976. First published as *Medical Ethics for Nurses.* Philadelphia: F. A. Davis Co., 1946. 2d ed. *Medical Ethics.* 1949.

MAGUIRE, DANIEL C. *Death by Choice.* Garden City, N.Y.: Doubleday, 1974.

MAZZOLINI, SILVESTRO [PRIERAS, SYLVESTER]. *Summa sylvestrina* [Summa summarum]. 2 vols. Venice: H. & N. Polum, 1601.

NIEDERMEYER, ALBERT. *Handbuch der Speziellen Pastoral Medizin.* 6 vols. Vienna: Herder, 1948–1952.

———. *Pastoralmedizinische Propädeutik, Einführung in die geistigen Grundlagen der Pastoral-Medizin und Pastoral-Hygiene.* Salzburg: A. Pustet, 1935.

NOONAN, JOHN THOMAS, JR. *Contraception: A History of Its Treatment by the Catholic Theologians and Canonists.* Cambridge: Harvard University Press, Belknap Press, 1965.

O'DONNELL, THOMAS JOSEPH. *Medicine and Christian Morality.* New York: Alba House, 1976.

———. *Morals in Medicine.* Westminster, Md.: Newman Press, 1956.

PAQUIN, JULES. *Morale et médecine.* Montreal: L'Immaculée conception, 1955.

PAYEN, GEORGES. *Déontologie medicale d'après le droit naturel: Devoirs d'état et droits de tout médecin* (1922). New ed. Zi-ka-wei [near Shanghai]: T'ou-se-we, Imprimerie de la mission catholique, 1935. 1st ed. Paris: Baillière. Originally written in Chinese for students of Aurora University, Shanghai.

PUJIULA, JAIME. *De medicina pastorali: Recentiores quaestiones quaedam exponuntur.* 2d ed. Turin: Marietti, 1953.

RAYNAUD, THÉOPHILE [THEOPHILUS RAYNAUDUS]. *De ortu infantium contra naturam per sectionem caesaream, tractatio qua reliqui item conscientiae nodi ad matrem alvo gerentem.* Lyons: G. Boissat, 1637.

SÁNCHEZ, TOMÁS. *De sancto matrimonii sacramento.* 3 vols. Venice: 1606.

SCREMIN, LUIGI. *Dizionario de morale professionale per i medici.* 5th ed. Rome: Editrice Studium, 1953.

SURBLED, GEORGES. *La Morale dans ses rapports avec la médecine et l'hygiène.* 4 vols. Paris: Victor Retaux, 1892–1898.

THOMAS AQUINAS. *Summa theologiae.* 4 vols. Turin: Marietti, 1950–1952.

ZACCHIA, PAOLO. *Quaestiones medico-legales.* 3 vols. Lyons: Anisson & Joannis Posuel, 1701.

ROME

See MEDICAL ETHICS, HISTORY OF, *section on* EUROPE AND THE AMERICAS, *article on* ANCIENT GREECE AND ROME.

S

SANCTITY OF LIFE

See LIFE.

SAUDI ARABIA

See MEDICAL ETHICS, HISTORY OF, *section on*
NEAR AND MIDDLE EAST AND AFRICA, *articles on*
CONTEMPORARY ARAB WORLD *and* CONTEMPO-
RARY MUSLIM PERSPECTIVE. *See also* ISLAM.

SCIENCE AND RELIGION

See PURPOSE IN THE UNIVERSE; EVOLUTION.

SCIENCE: ETHICAL IMPLICATIONS

The question of the implications of science for
ethics means widely different things to different
people. It can be as limited and personal as the
responsibilities of scientists for their work, as
broad as the effect of science and technology on
human values in their historical development, or
as technical as whether a science of ethics is
possible. We shall take the central problem
(within which the other problems find a place)
to be an assessment of the different kinds of
influence the development of science has had
and can have on morality and ethical theory.
"Science" as used here includes not only results
of the sciences, natural and social, but also
scientific method, outlook, and temper, as well
as technological applications. To these may be
added occasional direct study of moral phenomena, particularly in psychology and social
science. Inquiry here is not directed particularly
to causal analysis; there is certainly a complex

interaction of social practice, moral beliefs, ethical theories, and science, in which each has
some effects on all the rest.

The following account will deal in order with
(1) some historical instances of the influence
of science on ethics, (2) theoretical conflicts
about the relation of science and ethics, (3) the
twentieth-century impact of technology, (4)
some central problems in contemporary morality
that need the aid of science, (5) theoretical
shifts in moral philosophy under the impact of
a scientific outlook, (6) the effects of scientific
advance on formulation of moral problems, and
(7) moral responsibilities of scientists and technologists.

Historical instances of the influence of science

The clearest modern influence of science on
ethics is seen in the great scientific revolutions,
or the emergence of new fields of science.

The seventeenth-century rise of physical
science gave intellectual shape to a growing
individualism, and its Newtonian model (individual particles going their own inertial way, forming larger configurations through mutual pressures according to universal law) was exploited
by some philosophers for the understanding of
man. Sense experiences, including pleasure and
pain, explain the formation of human desires,
and conflict of desires in turn begets patterns of
harmony through institutions to maintain survival and order necessary for achievement of desires. Moral beliefs lie in these patterns. In
Hobbes, a psychology based on self-interest
was taken for granted; in Hume and Adam
Smith a natural human feeling of sympathy

gave a different cast to the same overall model. Other variants, especially in French and German philosophy, had all obligation emanate from individual will and contractual relations. The tentative, experimental, and cumulative method of science, with its expectation of continual revision as against claims to dogmatic truth, became the intellectual foundation for freedom of thought and expression as an ethical demand in modern liberalism.

The Darwinian revolution was the next great scientific influence on ethics. It established the evolutionary continuity of man with the rest of nature, bringing all human works and forms of life within the study of change and development. It dislodged the earlier views of morality as dependent on an unchanging human nature by showing that basic human drives and impulses were products of natural selection in the struggle for existence. While Darwin's own moral theory rested on the Hume–Smith concept of sympathy, which he saw as a selective consequence of cooperation in the higher animals, the dominant evolutionary views of morality took ideological shape from T. H. Huxley's picture of nature "red in tooth and claw." Huxley contrasted ethics with and defended it against the aggressive struggle of nature, as the gardener constantly battling against the encroaching jungle. Herbert Spencer transferred the struggle for existence and survival of the fittest into the social domain, justifying the predatory business ethics with this "Social Darwinism" (Hofstadter).

Under the influence of evolutionary and developmental ideas, innumerable attempts were made to establish moral patterns. Some saw growth of more cohesive social groups, from kin and village to a coming universalism; others generalized struggle into an ethics of power and group domination. Some extrapolated curves of increased adjustment to environment, or increased rationality. Prince Kropotkin saw cooperation as primary in biological and social phenomena rather than struggle; human history exhibits increasing mutual aid and moral sympathy, temporarily thwarted by power and political interference. Perhaps most comprehensive in the social and psychological sciences—both destined for wide twentieth-century influence—were Marx and Freud. One sets morality into a social evolutionary framework, the other into the full development of the individual.

Marx saw morality as part of the social superstructure reflecting the economic organization.

Dominant morality reflects dominant class interests, while rising classes grow their morality in the struggle. Eventually, with the full flowering of productive capacities, an all-human morality can develop. Men's struggles, becoming conscious, give mankind a direct role in fashioning their future rather than simply reflecting historical drifts (Engels). Freud treated morality as expressing the superego, representing internalized parental rules under early childhood emotional sanctions. By showing the deep unconscious roots of morality in the building of a self, his psychology appeared to question the genuinely rational character of moral decision. Both Freud and Marx present a determinist view, but Marx is hopeful of mankind's collectively achieving a freedom through knowledge. Freud, especially as his later speculations about a death instinct gave a biological basis for nonrational aggression, proved more pessimistic, though in a given individual growing insight into his own motivations extended his freedom.

In the first part of the twentieth century, anthropology revealed the great variety of moral beliefs; later, turning from isolated items to systematic cultural patterns, it emphasized understanding morality in fuller sociocultural context: for example, Eskimo abandonment of aged parents did not signify absence of filial affection but reflected the hard conditions of Eskimo survival, refracted in consoling myths. This is comparable to recent models of a "lifeboat ethics"; just as a lifeboat already loaded will be swamped if it takes on everyone calling for help, so advanced technological societies (assuming world scarcity of food) should limit assistance to rapidly developing countries, thereby abandoning less progressive ones to starvation. The theory of moral relativism generalized from anthropological work was often taken to mean that any moral beliefs established in a culture were beyond outside criticism. But sometimes more systematic analysis of culture allowed for underlying constant moral categories or underlying universal social bases for morality. It also became clear that the primary motivation of anthropological doctrines of moral relativism had been a plea for tolerance as against ethnocentric dogmatism.

Theoretical conflicts of science and ethics

By the early twentieth century the impact of science on ethics was sufficient to make that question itself a subject of reflection by scientists and philosophers. Three general positions were advanced during more than half a century of debate.

The first assumed that science was now in a position to give us a scientific ethics. Sometimes it was directly biological in spirit; sometimes, adding from psychological and social science, it took several directions. For example, the scientist might furnish a ground plan for the human being, a set of instincts or demands to be satisfied, or needs whose frustration would cripple human functioning whatever the ends to which persons or cultures devoted themselves. While earlier lists jumped directly from instincts, drives, and needs to social institutions—for example, from an aggressive instinct to a moral acceptance of war or from a hoarding instinct to inevitability of private property—later (especially post-Freudian) psychologies sought to determine virtues and attitudes that would be productive of a balanced or happy life. Surprisingly, these post-Darwinian theories did not make as much use of historical-evolutionary development as the nineteenth century had. (Spencer had a keen sense of human development in which basic shifts from early military to later industrial life brought changes in attitudes toward the morality of war and the congruence of egoism and altruism, and he even saw the criteria of the good as undergoing evolutionary transformation.) An exception in the twentieth-century literature is Julian Huxley (Huxley and Huxley; cf. Waddington), who attempted to combine biological, psychological, and historical knowledge in an ethics in which even the role of ethics in human life itself evolved. As against T. H. Huxley's separation of evolution and ethics, he saw man, the gardener, as himself part of nature; his neat garden is itself as much an evolutionary product as the encroaching jungle. Conscience is an early mechanism developing in parent-child relations to hold the child firm till reason matures. Ethics itself moved from an early era in which the need for solidarity was primary to one in which class purposes were dominant; at present its function is to keep open the ways of human survival and conscious advance and control over nature and human development.

A second general position assumed, in various forms, an impassable gulf between *fact* and *value*, the *is* and the *ought*. Description of a situation, including what people desire or seek or value, cannot tell us what is desirable, is worth seeking, or ought to be valued. Philosophical forms of this dichotomy (Moore; cf. Raphael) took the attempt to understand ethical ideas scientifically to be a patent intellectual fallacy. Scientists accepting the dichotomy sharply distinguished means from ends: science could give us means but not ends. The latter had to be furnished separately, whether from religious authority or from individual or group volitional commitment. Positivist philosophies, accepting the dichotomy, analyzed value statements as inherently nonrational emotive expression or persuasion; a morality might be built around procedures of mediation or compromise, or, alternately, uncompromising struggle, but both for them constituted an emotive attitude. In practice, the separation of fact and value or means and ends meant that the scientist as scientist was free to investigate whatever he wanted and was not responsible for the application of his findings. His sole responsibility was to truth. Technology had to get its directives from ends that humans proposed, it had none of its own apart from criteria of efficiency and effectiveness.

The third position rejects both the previous two. It regards the separation of fact and value as a philosophical dogma or at best a program, just as logical positivists had a program for separating theoretical from observational statements. None of these programs actually were realized, and later analyses slowly came to see that absolute dichotomies had been made of what were simply relative distinctions. Thus in any one context one may ask for the full factual picture of the situation and its problems, including people's aims and hopes and aspirations. The decision as to what it is best to do, what ought to be done, what responsibilities participants have, what compromises are acceptable appears in this context as the value judgment determined after the facts are clear. But the grounds for decision and the considerations that would justify it are themselves drawn from the factual picture of people's hopes and fears and ideals, and the lessons of experience about what is probable or attainable.

As against claims that science can furnish definite principles of ethics, the third position argues that contributions of the sciences are piecemeal, that their methods and results exert an influence in diverse ways upon moral principles and moral philosophy (Edel, 1955), and that moral codes no less than sciences are in the making. The influence of science is thus reconstructive rather than simply constructive. Some philosophers hold that all knowledge, especially as it involves action and experiment, includes prescriptive elements; there is thus a continuity of method between science and ethics. Others concentrate primarily on the way in which the results of growing scientific knowledge about humans and their world and history changes the presuppositions on which ethical constructions implicitly rest, much as the discovery of germs replaced the assumption that illness is retribution and so changed moral attitudes to illness (Edel, 1961). So the careful study of different social and historical conditions of life and expressions of human nature helps us decide which psychological and social forms are unavoidable, if any, and which can be developed in the light of growing ideals of the good life. Scientific studies of character and personality refine and help evaluate traditional virtues; for example, differentiating love and dependence, or industriousness and insecure busyness, or anxious pursuit of pleasure and the gratification of the disciplined exercise of powers (Fromm). Studies of social structure and social ideals show how different institutional forms express socio-cultural needs in different ways (for example, in one society private charity provides for the destitute, in another, a governmental welfare system) and so furnish a basis for evaluating institutions in their own complex social settings (Ossowska). Broad historical studies can help us understand the needs and conditions of life that issue in cooperative versus competitive cultures, or intensely striving and success-oriented as against relaxed happiness moralities, or in authoritarian and sternly disciplined as compared with democratic and more flexible experimental moralities. Science thus does not dictate morality but may help guide it by replacing assumptions that incline morality in one direction with growing knowledge that opens up other directions. If it has a general effect on outlook, it is to bring morality itself within the scope of collective evaluation and possible reconstruction.

The twentieth-century impact of technology

Technology, or applied science in all its fields, is the channel through which the greatest scientific influences have been brought to bear on contemporary life, and so in turn on the problems to be faced by morality. Technology has changed the balance of urban and rural life, created artificial environments, unified the globe in communications and economic interdependence. It also makes possible more devastating

wars, widespread pollution, depletion of natural resources, and more inclusive modes of controlling people. For a time, after the development of nuclear energy, there were great hopes that global abundance would replace global scarcity; but by the 1970s, with tremendous growth of population, evidence of pollution and prospective exhaustion of resources, intimations of doomsday have become more frequent.

Some philosophical analyses of technology take it as the means devouring human ends (Ellul): technology mechanizes life and reduces rationality to efficiency; demand for large-scale corporate organization crushes individuality by the need for standardization; every human end that cannot be translated into mass production and economic growth is rejected. The result is the enslavement of mankind to the machine. It need not even be felt as slavery, since the interrelation of means and ends ensures the survival of ends that are adaptable to the powerful means. Hence, Ellul claims, a debased pursuit of material things replaces the nobler ends of earlier times.

Alternative analyses emphasize the wider areas of choice in human affairs now made possible by technology, rather than an overall one-way determinism (Edel, 1974). Blind growth, corporate domination (whether public or private) with consequent individual alienation, impoverished standardization, exaltation of means over ends are all consequences of specific social institutions quite capable of reconstruction to embody rather than thwart human aspirations. Science and technology imply not blind progress but the possibility of human planning and control to overcome basic evils of poverty and war that have been the historical heritage of mankind. Malthusian forebodings are not inevitable, if the nations of the world will cooperate on problems of peace, population, and pollution. Whether such cooperation will be forced by the convergence of impending evils for mankind remains a central question.

Moral problems aided by science

The central problems of morality are not the product of science and technology, but the way in which they are to be faced is closely related to the possibilities and instrumentalities that science and technology afford. Since the Second World War and its global impact upon the overthrow of colonialism, the reaction to Nazi racism, the momentous advance in technology and production, and the rapid strides in global communication, at least the following have emerged as central on the agenda of moral problems: (1) to broaden the moral human community so that everyone counts, achieving a greater equality by removing entrenched discrimination based on color, sex, religion, nationality, class, or other exclusive grouping; (2) to open channels of participation in determining social policy, and opportunities for education and sharing in cultural gains, to all people; (3) to provide basic security in food, shelter, and health care to all; (4) to achieve a higher level of production for all, rather than continue a policy of scarcity and competition for scarce goods; and (5) to project an ideal of individuality that will encourage cultivation of the individual's powers and capacities, and at the same time to project an ideal of community that will overcome widespread contemporary alienation.

These are not speculative ideals, but the ideals of movements and struggles throughout the world. No one of them makes sense except in the prospect of the possibilities that science and technology have opened for human life (Boulding).

Theoretical shifts in moral philosophy

Dominant moral philosophies in the first half of the twentieth century either looked on science as disruptive of ethics or else subscribed to sharp separation of fact and value, which insulated science from contributing fundamental critiques of human ends. Pragmatism stood almost alone in its attempts to develop an ethical theory that would incorporate science and the method of science in its basic procedures. The features that most embody the scientific stance for ethics are: recognition of man as part of nature, continuous with the animal world; appreciation of the thoroughly transactional character between the individual and the environment, including social environment; realization of the constancy of change as a background of nature, life and society, and the consequent insistence that all alleged fixities be reinterpreted as relative stabilities in change; insistence on the purposive and selective character of human experience and thought, and the consequent contextual relevance of human ideas; belief in the applicability of scientific modes of inquiry to all phases of human life. In moral philosophy Dewey, for example, refocused the very notion of a moral situation in the light of the constancy of change. A moral situation is not one in which a person is tempted to deviate from a moral rule (this is

secondary, since he knows there what is right): it is one in which a decision has to be made as to what is right, usually with conflicting claims of rightness. Thus the center of gravity of moral theory is the attempt to use the maximum of our experience and intellectual resources to solve problems that involve action affecting ourselves and others, both in welfare and in selfhood. The body of moral theory at any time is a system of accumulated experience and knowledge, which is constantly subject to critique and correction in the light of subsequent experimental inquiry and experience. For example, distributive principles in the theory of justice take different shapes for changing material and social conditions in different fields of human relations, and the ideal of justice is developed in more concrete terms as our knowledge grows and as fresh institutional devices for its application are discovered. The United Nations formulations of human rights illustrate in detail the growth of possibilities, and such institutions as insurance (a product of statistical science), Medicare, social security, and no-fault insurance illustrate reconstructive imagination. Many questions of bioethics, as general as the proper distribution of health care and as specific as the allocation of dialysis (with consequences of life or death) require an underlying theory of justice.

Such scientific attitudes to morality do not imply that every question can be solved. The individual crises and choices that have figured in existentialist literature are basic in human life, but there is no sharp separation between individual and social ethics. Individual decision starts from a social base: powers and possibilities come from social organization, and many of its problems reflect the social problems. But, more significant, the individual self is a sociocultural and historical product; much of individual alienation is itself a consequence of institutions that divide people, make genuine community difficult or impossible, and impoverish the general quality of life. Autonomy of individual decision, or the development of individuality, is a noble social ideal that aims at enriching, not impoverishing, human community.

The general shift in moral philosophy paralleling the growth of a scientific outlook since the seventeenth century is thus the recognition of humans as active participants in their own making—reflecting the growing areas of control that science in its earlier slow progress and more recently in its accelerated advances has provided for mankind.

Science and the formulation of moral problems

It is sometimes debated whether philosophy is called upon to offer "new answers to old problems," or whether both the problems and the responses are new. This raises the question of what effect scientific advances have on the formulation of moral problems. There are, of course, perennial moral problems in human life that each individual has to face afresh. But there are many for which attempted solutions can only be thwarted if they are thrust into older conceptual frameworks. Technological advances are particularly significant in creating such situations, since the very concepts in terms of which older problems were formulated may themselves alter in meaning. Take, for example, the moral problems generated by the technology of organ transplants. Debates about not taking an organ for transplant till "real death" has occurred are set in terms of a concept of death that is undergoing change; in brief, one may have to choose now between "brain-death" and "heart-death." The debates disguise fears of possible callousness, which are better faced directly as moral problems of human relations, but a new formulation that embodies the advanced scientific knowledge can clearly pose these more lucidly.

Problems of bioethics can be seen as paradigmatic of the changes in morality and moral philosophy that science brings. Such changes are proving especially stimulating to theoretical reflection in morality today for precisely those reasons. They deal with problems that stem from the growth of knowledge and technology. They offer clear instrumentalities of greater control for human well-being, but not without quandaries stemming from traditional moral ideas. They would involve conceptual changes of the types just indicated, and so challenge our *meanings*, yet not without fear that the changes of meaning may hide moral opportunism. Thus they require basic thinking in terms of foundations. They call for sharp distinctions of right and wrong, but reasonable and principled ones governed by appreciation of goods and risks. They are sure to call for changes in older habits of moral interpretation, but in such a way as to preserve continuities and give due place to change. Finally, they deal with problems that cannot be postponed but have to be given an answer now if great values are not to be lost. (In this respect, medicine is as peremptory as judicial decision; even more, since there may be no possibility of appeal to a higher court.)

To a greater or lesser extent most questions of morality in society and its structure, in law, in education, in the development of character, even in formulating the nature of the good life and its quality, face the same problems of reconstruction in a world that has been profoundly altered. Science and technology played a prime role in that alteration. They may not give us moral answers for the new world, but human beings may hope to find answers if adequately equipped with knowledge and if free to engage in reconstruction.

Moral responsibility of science and technology

Influenced by the separation of fact and value, many still regard scientists as responsible only for the pursuit of truth. Recent analyses, no longer bound to the fact-value dichotomy as an inviolable truth, take responsibilities to depend on the state of development of science and its modes of operation and the role of science in the life and well-being of the society (Edel, 1972; Glass). They point to public support of science, large-scale operation of its research processes (often involving human beings in experiment, as well as having dangerous potentials—for example, in nuclear physics and biological research), the dislocating effects of some new discoveries in application as well as the repression of useful applications by entrenched economic interests, the misuse of scientific theories in ideological battles (for example, of genetic theories in supporting racial discrimination), and so on. While the uses and consequences of scientific advance are not always predictable, some responsibility for concern in these areas is taken to be a moral obligation of scientists. Moreover, scientists are increasingly called upon to take a greater part in solving critical problems and should be expected to work toward general improvement in well-being. The detailed shape of scientific and technological responsibilities is seen as a continuing problem of both scientific effort and public policy. While some responsibility would fall on the individual in relation to his work, much would lie in the province of associations of scientists. Perhaps in the long run even the parceling of role obligations may give way to a conception of a common responsibility for the betterment of a common life.

ABRAHAM EDEL

[*Directly related are the entries* ENVIRONMENTAL ETHICS; *and* EVOLUTION. *For discussion of related ideas, see the entries:* BIOETHICS; ETHICS, *article on* THE TASK OF ETHICS; *and* JUSTICE. *For further discussion of topics mentioned in this article, see the entries:* DEATH, DEFINITION AND DETERMINATION OF; HEART TRANSPLANTATION; *and* KIDNEY DIALYSIS AND TRANSPLANTATION. *This article will find application in the entries* CRYONICS; EUGENICS; LIFE-SUPPORT SYSTEMS; MEDICAL ETHICS UNDER NATIONAL SOCIALISM; PRENATAL DIAGNOSIS; RESEARCH, BIOMEDICAL; *and* TECHNOLOGY.]

BIBLIOGRAPHY

BAIER, KURT, and RESCHER, NICHOLAS, eds. *Values and the Future: The Impact of Technological Change on American Values.* New York: Free Press, 1969.

BOULDING, KENNETH E. *The Meaning of the 20th Century: The Great Transition.* New York: Harper Colophon Books, 1965.

BRONOWSKI, JACOB. *Science and Human Values.* 2d ed. New York: Harper Torchbooks, 1965.

BROWN, MARTIN, ed. *The Social Responsibility of the Scientist.* New York: Free Press, 1971.

DARWIN, CHARLES. *The Descent of Man* (1871). Philadelphia: R. West, 1902, ch. 4.

DEWEY, JOHN. *Theory of the Moral Life.* New York: Holt, Rinehart & Winston, 1960. Paperback of John Dewey's and James H. Tufts's *Ethics*, rev. ed., New York: Henry Holt, 1932, pt. 2.

EDEL, ABRAHAM. *Ethical Judgement: The Use of Science in Ethics.* Glencoe, Ill.: Free Press, 1955.

———. *Science and the Structure of Ethics.* Chicago: University of Chicago Press, 1961.

———. "Scientists, Partisans, and Social Conscience." *trans-action,* January 1972, pp. 32–39, 52.

———. "Technology and Morality." *Praxis* 10 (1974): 183–196.

ELLUL, JACQUES. *The Technological Society.* Translated by John Wilkinson. New York: Vintage Books, 1967.

ENGELS, FREDERICK. *Herr Eugen Dühring's Revolution in Science (Anti-Dühring).* Translated by Emile Burns. New York: International Publishers, 1966, pt. 1, chaps, 9–11; pt. 3.

FERKISS, VICTOR C. *Technological Man: The Myth and the Reality.* New York: George Braziller, 1969.

FREUD, SIGMUND. *New Introductory Lectures on Psychoanalysis.* Translated by W. J. H. Sprott. New York: Norton, 1933.

FROMM, ERICH. *Man For Himself.* New York: Rinehart & Co., 1947.

GLASS, BENTLEY. *Science and Ethical Values.* Chapel Hill: University of North Carolina Press, 1965.

HOFSTADTER, RICHARD. *Social Darwinism in American Thought 1860–1915.* Philadelphia: University of Pennsylvania Press, 1945. Rev. ed. New York: George Braziller, 1959.

HUTCHINGS, EDWARD, and HUTCHINGS, ELIZABETH, eds. *Scientific Progress and Human Values.* New York: American Elsevier Publishing Co., 1967.

HUXLEY, THOMAS H., and HUXLEY, JULIAN. *Touchstone for Ethics.* New York: Harper, 1947.

JONAS, HANS. *Philosophical Essays: From Ancient Creed to Technological Man.* Englewood Cliffs, N.J.: Prentice-Hall, 1974.

KROPOTKIN, PETER. *Mutual Aid.* Baltimore: Penguin Books, 1939. New York: New York University Press, 1972.

MOORE, G. E. *Principia Ethica.* Cambridge: Cambridge University Press, 1903, 1959.

OSSOWSKA, MARIA. *Social Determinants of Moral Ideas.* Philadelphia: University of Pennsylvania Press, 1970.

RAPHAEL, D. DAICHES. "Darwinism and Ethics." *A Century of Darwin.* Edited by Samuel Anthony Barnett. Cambridge: Harvard University Press; London: Heinemann, 1958, pp. 334–359.

RAVETZ, JEROME R. *Scientific Knowledge and Its Social Problems.* New York: Oxford University Press, 1971.

"Science and Culture." *Daedalus* 94, no. 1 (Winter 1965).

SPENCER, HERBERT. *Principles of Ethics.* New York: D. Appleton and Co., 1896, vol. I.

VAN MELSEN, ANDREW G. *Science and Responsibility.* Pittsburgh: Duquesne University Press, 1970.

WADDINGTON, CONRAD H. *The Ethical Animal.* Chicago: University of Chicago Phoenix Science Series, 1960.

SCIENCE, PHILOSOPHY OF

See BIOLOGY, PHILOSOPHY OF; HEALTH AND DISEASE, *article on* PHILOSOPHICAL PERSPECTIVES; MEDICINE, PHILOSOPHY OF; REDUCTIONISM.

SCIENCE, SOCIOLOGY OF

Born in the late nineteenth century, but coming of age only in the late 1950s and 1960s, the sociology of science today commands the research attention of an increasing number of sociologists in the United States and Europe. Today the specialty has a distinctive intellectual and professional identity. Robert K. Merton has been the field's leading figure since the publication in 1938 of his now classic work on science, technology, and society in seventeenth-century England. His later work on the ethos of science provided one part of the basic theoretical orientation that has dominated the specialty until today (Merton, 1973).

The sociology of science is curiously self-exemplifying. As a scientific specialty, it exhibits many of the social patterns its own practitioners study in other contexts. It is evolving its own system of stratification, its own arrangements for formal and informal communication, its own politics, its own cognitive and professional identity, and indeed its own conflicts, just as these have become major foci of attention in research by sociologists of science.

Although sociologists of science have attended to the reciprocal relationship between science and other social institutions (Ben-David; Merton, 1938; Salamon), this has not been the primary area of their interest. Since the rapid growth in the 1960s, most theoretical and empirical work has concentrated on the social organization of science itself. Science is viewed as a social community with a distinctive social structure and an identifiable value system. Rather than treat science as a set of individuals working in relative isolation, influenced only by the antecedent ideas produced by other great men and women of science, the sociological angle of vision attempts, among other things, to identify how the value system and social structure of science influence the rate of discovery. the transmission of ideas, the resistance to new knowledge, the disputes over the origin of ideas, and the historical transformations in the cognitive content of science.

Five problem areas account for most of the recent research activity and output by sociologists of science: (1) its ethos, (2) its growth patterns and social stratification, (3) the importance of priority, (4) communications among scientists, and (5) the growth of scientific knowledge.

The ethos of science

For more than thirty years sociologists of science have focused attention on the central values in the scientific community. Robert Merton (1942) first described the complex of values that shaped science as a distinctive enterprise. The ethos of science consists of four basic institutional values or norms:

1. *Universalism* prescribes that scientific contributions be judged according to the degree to which they advance scientific knowledge. Rewards distributed on the basis of race, sex, nationality, religion, or any other personal characteristic violate this value.
2. *Organized skepticism* enjoins scientists to suspend final judgment on discoveries until sufficient data are in hand to judge the validity of scientific work, and it also requires individual scientists to be personally responsible for the material that they claim to be a discovery.
3. *Disinterestedness* is the injunction against self-interest and profiteering from the fruits of a scientist's work. Put positively, it is the commitment of scientists to the growth of the general body of scientific knowledge.
4. *Communism*, or *communality*, as it was later called, refers to the institutional imperative for an open system of communication. Scientists do not have individual rights to their discoveries once they are made.

These components of the cultural structure of science are not simply part of an ethical code for individuals but are seen as functional for the institution of science. Without adherence to these values the development of new, certified scientific knowledge would be significantly impeded.

The articulation of these cultural values, or ethos, proved to have a strong potential for elaboration. Working in much the same mode, there have been theoretical extensions of Merton's ideas (Barber; Hagstrom, 1965; Storer; Zuckerman), and some criticism of them (Mitroff). But even more distinctive is the large number of empirical inquiries that have used this basic complex of values as a point of departure. Studies of the reward and stratification system of science have focused primarily on the value of universalism.

Growth patterns and social stratification

More empirical work has been conducted on the historical growth of science and on its system of social stratification than on any other subject. Sociologists and historians of science have been concerned with charting the number of scientific discoveries made in various epochs as an indicator of the vitality of scientific work, with the overall extended pattern of growth, and with the relationship between growth in personnel and in production of a scientific literature. What has been found thus far? Since at least the seventeenth century science has been growing at an exponential rate (Price; Crane). This general pattern is confirmed by virtually every indicator of growth—number of scientists, number of discoveries published, number of scientific journals, number of citations and their half-life, and so on. The pace of growth is conveyed by the fact that more than half of all scientists who have ever lived are alive today. Indeed, the age of Big Science is here, with its large institutionalized units, such as university departments and laboratories, and its reliance on massive governmental support of scientific resources and facilities. There are, however, some strong indications that the pattern of exponential growth is now leveling off in the United States and probably in other countries as well.

Most scientists are aware that science is a highly stratified institution. Almost any member of the scientific community is aware that the distribution of scientific resources, of power and esteem, is highly skewed. There are few disagreements that science is dominated to a large extent by a relatively small elite. However, there is some disagreement about the bases on which scientific rewards have been distributed. Sociologists of science have been describing the shape of the hierarchy of scientific rewards and discovering the bases on which they are distributed (Zuckerman; Cole and Cole).

Does the scientific social system operate to maximize the universalistic distribution of rewards, or does the system reward scientists on the basis of nonscientific characteristics? As noted, in a meritocratic and universalistic social system, individuals' rewards are based ideally on the quality of their work. The principal functionally relevant criteria for rewards is high-quality performance. That is particularly so in science, but ideally so in most institutions. Individual scientists should become prominent, should receive honors and prizes, and should obtain seats in the best departments of science, because their scientific work is superior to that of others. This turns out to be largely the case.

Limiting the list to eight general conclusions, the following findings are continually supported by empirical inquiries into the reward systems of the physical, biological, and social sciences, and therefore seem increasingly credible: (1) The quality of scientific work, as measured by counts of citations, is the strongest single determinant of various forms of recognition; (2) the sheer bulk of scientists' publications has little influence on rewards above and beyond the quality of those publications; the widespread notion that scientists must "publish or perish" turns out to be a myth; (3) there are few identifiable functionally irrelevant characteristics of scientists, such as race or ethnicity, that affect significantly the allocation of rewards; (4) the quality of research performance is a stronger determinant of peer recognition, esteem, and general prominence within the community than it is in the hiring and promotion of scientists within academic departments; (5) the reward systems are remarkably uniform across a wide variety of fields despite the existence of vastly different cognitive structures; (6) the educational origins and subsequent apprenticeships of scientists play a large role in career mobility and achievement; (7) the reward system operates to reinforce the strong association between the quality and the quantity of scientific research output; (8) the pattern and determinants of rewards are much the same in European science communities as in the United States.

Since social rewards go disproportionately to those who are both scientifically prolific and producers of high-quality work, a relatively small portion of the entire community tends to dominate positions of influence and prestige. Only ten percent of the active research scientists produce about fifty percent of all scientific discoveries. The skewed distributions of productivity and quality have led researchers to ask how many scientists in any historical period contribute significantly to the advance of scientific knowledge through their research. How much does the work of the average scientist, working on relatively minor problems in the obscurity of his laboratory, contribute to the overall development of science? Does his or her work contribute, even if in small measure, to the pathfinding discoveries by the great figures of science—the Newtons, Einsteins, Bohrs? Or is the work of no direct or indirect significance on the growth of science? To study this problem, sociologists have been examining in detail the patterns of intellectual influence in science.

The importance of priority

There is an extraordinary amount of competition in science for priority of discovery. The association of a discovery with a particular person represents property in science. Property rights are established through priority. Nature holds out problems to be solved, and it makes little difference who is the second person to solve those problems. Being first is what counts in terms of scientific recognition. The history of science is punctuated by thousands of priority disputes. Among the more notable were those between Newton and Hooke, Darwin and Wallace, Cavendish and Watt, Freud and Janet. Merton's discussion of priority disputes links them to conflicting values in science (1957). Although scientists are enjoined to humility and to disinterestedness, they are, at the same time, driven to seek recognition of their originality. The association of a discovery with an individual, best seen in cases of eponymous recognition, such as "Boyle's Law," is the scientific community's recognition of the individual's having made an important contribution to science. Consequently, scientists are under great pressure to stake claims to what they take to be their scientific property, to assert their priority of discovery, and, however uncontentious they might be personally, to engage in priority disputes. The difficulty for scientists lies in the disjunction between goals and normatively prescribed means. These structurally induced conflicts are a cause of deviant behavior in science. The incidence of deviance depends both on the rewards at stake and on the structure of opportunities to conform to the norms. Sociologists of science are interested not in psychological sources of deviance that result from cantankerous personalities but in how the social structure of science produces not only strain but the potential for deviance as well. The works of Norman Storer (1966), Jerry Gaston (1973), and Warren Hagstrom (1974) have analyzed competition in contemporary science.

The theoretical framework of the sociology of science has had its strongest impact on the analysis of the ethics of experimentation in its focus on competing scientific values. Bernard Barber and his collaborators have investigated the tension produced by competition for scarce scientific rewards among 337 biomedical research physicians (Sullivan). The essential tension lies in conflicting values: As medical doctors the researchers hold a strong value of humane therapeutic treatment; as scientists they hold the value of establishing priority of discovery. In certain socially structured situations those values compete with each other, creating what Barber calls "the dilemma of science and therapy." Biomedical researchers must continually weigh the actual and perceived risks of experimentation against the possible benefits accruing from the results of experimentation. Further, the need for informed consent from experimental subjects can produce additional conflicts in values (Barber et al.; Katz; Gray). On the one hand, researchers need a sufficiently large sample of subjects whose reactions to the experimental procedures will not be affected by their knowledge of the experiment. On the other, researchers must be concerned with the welfare and personal rights of persons who are potential subjects. In a majority of cases an ethically satisfactory balance can be struck, but in a significant minority ethical standards are compromised in the quest for discovery and priority. Current research is attempting to identify the conditions under which ethical standards are apt to be abandoned and to identify the sources and types of resistance to the introduction of codes of ethics.

Communications among scientists

Sociologists of science have examined in detail two aspects of scientific communications—the patterns of information exchange and the ways communication networks are related to the growth of scientific specialties.

Science has a basically open system of communication. The values of science prescribe that scientific knowledge be public. Secrecy is a violation of this value. Most scientists publish their work in journals that are widely disseminated in libraries open to all who wish to use them. Scientific meetings are generally open. In most fields, so-called invisible colleges are hardly invisible. They represent scientists working on similar problems who exchange ideas through preprints and at informal conferences. Most scientists are willing to send "preprints" of papers to those requesting them. In short, the "invisible colleges" are relatively open to all scientists who wish to join them.

Sociologists of science have been concerned principally with the less formal aspects of communications. They have addressed such questions as: Does the informal communication between scientific "masters" and "apprentices" influence the development of selective tastes for scientific problems and affect the career paths followed by students? Does scientific information diffuse to all corners of the scientific community? Does a scientist's social structural location affect his or her access to information? Does scientific information easily permeate the boundaries of scientific specialties within a field?

Nicholas Mullins, Henry Small, and Belver Griffith, among others, have tried to identify the growth of scientific specialties by focusing on the structure of the communication networks among scientists rather than on the content of scientific innovations. Mullins has developed a stage model of specialty development that has as its principal components the roles of intellectual and social leaders, the role of programmatic statements, the diffusion of group members from centers of activity to the periphery, and the thickening of communication nets with growth (Mullins and Mullins). Griffith and Small have attempted to identify the boundaries of scientific specialties by analyzing networks of citations in scientific journals (Small and Griffith).

The growth of scientific knowledge

The focus by American sociologists of science on the social organization of science has been seen as a congenial first step to understanding how scientific knowledge grows, is codified, and becomes institutionalized. Recently, attention has shifted to the connections between the cognitive and the social structures of the sciences (Zuckerman and Merton; Cole and Zuckerman; Cole). They are considering problems such as the extent to which there is consensus or conflict among scientists in different scientific fields and specialties on problematics, on methods of inquiry, on principal contributors to the growth of knowledge. Differential levels of consensus are then assessed in terms of their potential link to the levels of theoretical codification of the various fields. Much of this work is derivative from earlier work by Thomas Kuhn on scientific revolutions (1962); by Derek Price on parameters of growth (1963); and by philosophers of science such as Karl Popper (1934) and Imre Lakatos (1970).

Are developments built upon a common base or upon a diverse intellectual foundation? How rapidly are new contributions exploited and built upon? How are theory and experimental and empirical research linked, if at all, and how do the linkages change over time? How do foci of attention in scientific specialties shift, and are the shifts related to changes in the intellectual orientations of leading scientists? How long do scientific contributions by leaders continue to be used, and in what ways?

Research is currently attempting to answer some of these queries, particularly the ones that deal with continuities and discontinuities in the growth of scientific knowledge. Thomas Kuhn has suggested that the cumulation of knowledge is uneven, taking place only in periods of "normal science"—when there exists a shared scientific paradigm. Periods of discontinuity occur during revolutionary shifts from one paradigm to another. Some historians and philosophers of science question Kuhn's view of scientific development. Stephen Toulmin and others suggest that there are numerous minor scientific revolutions that cannot be explained by Kuhn's analysis. Sociologists of science have begun to design empirical inquiries to test competing ideas about the extent of continuity in scientific development (Cole). They are developing empirical maps of the cognitive structure of scientific specialties and are analyzing the intellectual linkage between key scientific ideas that existed before and after scientific revolutions.

An intellectual by-product of work on the social and cognitive structure of scientific fields is the production of empirical data that can be used to compare them. It has often been remarked that scientific fields differ in their level of codification—in the extent to which empirical knowledge can be consolidated into interdependent theoretical statements. For example, physics and chemistry are taken to be more highly codified than botany, and the biological sciences are assumed in turn to be more highly codified than their younger sister social sciences. Rather than accept these intuitions as self-evident, sociologists of science have recently turned to empirical inquiries into the level of codification in the sciences. Harriet Zuckerman and Robert Merton have hypothesized that scientists working in more rather than less codified fields are able to reach the research frontiers more rapidly since they will not have to return continually to first principles; are more apt to make important discoveries at an earlier age; and are more likely to receive early institutional recognition for their work (1972). Although work is in its initial phase, preliminary results suggest that there may be more significant variations in the extent of codification within traditional scientific fields than between them. But, as with so many other central problems in the sociology of science, these findings represent only beginnings.

Bioethics and the sociology of science

The sociology of science should be of great interest to those engaged in the study of ethics and of bioethics in particular. A matter of particular interest to bioethics, the use of human subjects in biomedical and behavioral research, has been studied by sociologists (Barber et al.; Gray). By revealing the empirical features of such experimentation, they have shed considerable light on the ethical issues. Ethical questions about truth and deception in reporting research results, the responsibility of researchers for social consequences of discoveries, and the secrecy of the research process for certain endeavors should be discussed with awareness of the actual social structure of scientific research. The impact of technological innovation on medical care has aroused ethical concern. The actual nature of the research process that results in such innovations should be understood in order to evaluate an ethical response to the problem. The effectiveness of government endeavors to review and, to some extent, control the research process, as in the regulation of development of new drugs, is an ethical question that requires considerable empirical information (Fox and Swazey; Swazey). Whether or not there should be public surveillance of the evolution of technology, whether research should be explicitly oriented to solution of public problems, whether regulatory control can be effectively exercised over research, the role scientists should play in public policy—these are ethical questions that can be intelligently discussed only if the discussant understands how scientific knowledge grows and becomes codified and institutionalized.

JONATHAN R. COLE

[Directly related are the entries COMMUNICATION, BIOMEDICAL; MEDICINE, SOCIOLOGY OF; *and* SCIENCE: ETHICAL IMPLICATIONS. *For discussion of related ideas, see:* HUMAN EXPERIMENTATION, *articles on* BASIC ISSUES *and* SOCIAL AND PROFESSIONAL CONTROL; INFORMED CONSENT IN HUMAN RESEARCH; *and* RISK. *This article will find application in the entries* RESEARCH, BIOMEDICAL; RESEARCH POLICY, BIOMEDICAL; TECHNOLOGY, *article on* TECHNOLOGY ASSESSMENT; WARFARE, *article on* BIOMEDICAL SCIENCE AND WAR.]*

BIBLIOGRAPHY

BARBER, BERNARD. *Science and the Social Order.* Foreword by Robert K. Merton. Glencoe, Ill.: Free Press, 1952.

————; LALLY, JOHN J.; MAKARUSHKA, JULIA LOUGHLIN; and SULLIVAN, DANIEL. *Research on Human Subjects: Problems of Social Control in Medical Experimentation.* New York: Russell Sage Foundation, 1973.

BEN-DAVID, JOSEPH. *The Scientist's Role in Society: A Comparative Study.* Foundations of Modern Sociology Series. Englewood Cliffs, N.J.: Prentice-Hall, 1971.

COLE, JONATHAN R., and COLE, STEPHEN. *Social Stratification in Science.* Chicago: University of Chicago Press, 1973.

————, and ZUCKERMAN, HARRIET. "The Emergence of a Scientific Specialty: The Self-Exemplifying Case of the Sociology of Science." *The Idea of Social Structure: Papers in Honor of Robert K. Merton.* Edited by Lewis A. Coser. New York: Harcourt Brace Jovanovich, 1975, pp. 139–174.

COLE, STEPHEN. "The Growth of Scientific Knowledge: Theories of Deviance as a Case Study." *The Idea of Social Structure: Papers in Honor of Robert K. Merton.* Edited by Lewis A. Coser. New York: Harcourt Brace Jovanovich, 1975, pp. 175–220.

CRANE, DIANA. *Invisible Colleges: Diffusion of Knowledge in Scientific Communities.* Chicago: University of Chicago Press, 1972.

FOX, RENÉE, and SWAZEY, JUDITH P. *The Courage to Fail: A Social View of Organ Transplants and Dialysis.* Chicago: University of Chicago Press, 1974.

GASTON, JERRY. *Originality and Competition in Science: A Study of the British High Energy Physics Community.* Chicago: University of Chicago Press, 1973.

GRAY, BRADFORD H. *Human Subjects in Medical Experimentation: A Sociological Study of the Conduct and Regulation of Clinical Research.* Health, Medicine, and Society: Wiley-Interscience Series. New York: John Wiley & Sons, 1975.

HAGSTROM, WARREN O. "Competition in Science." *American Sociological Review* 39 (1974): 1-18.

————. *The Scientific Community.* New York: Basic Books, 1965.

KATZ, JAY, ed. *Experimentation with Human Beings: The Authority of the Investigator, Subject, Profes-* sions, and State in the Human Experimentation Process. New York: Russell Sage Foundation, 1972.

KUHN, THOMAS S. *The Structure of Scientific Revolutions.* Also published as *International Encyclopedia of Unified Science, Foundations of the Unity of Science,* vol. 2, no. 2. Chicago: University of Chicago Press, 1962.

LAKATOS, IMRE. "Falsification and the Methodology of Scientific Research Programmes." *Criticism and the Growth of Knowledge.* Proceedings of the International Colloquium in the Philosophy of Science, London, 1965, vol. 4. Edited by Imre Lakatos and Alan Musgrave. Cambridge: Cambridge University Press, 1970, pp. 91–196.

MERTON, ROBERT K. "Priorities in Scientific Discovery: A Chapter in the Sociology of Science." *American Sociological Review* 22 (1957): 635–659.

————. "Science and Technology in a Democratic Order." *Journal of Legal and Political Sociology* 1 (1942): 115–126. Reprint. *Social Theory and Social Structure.* Rev. ed. Glencoe, Ill.: Free Press, 1957, pp. 550–561.

————. *Science, Technology and Society in Seventeenth Century England.* New York: Howard Fertig, 1970. First published in *Osiris: Studies on the History and Philosophy of Science, and on the History of Learning and Culture* 4, pt. 2 (1938).

————. *The Sociology of Science: Theoretical and Empirical Investigations.* Edited by Norman W. Storer. Chicago: University of Chicago Press, 1973.

MITROFF, IAN I. *The Subjective Side of Science: A Philosophical Inquiry into the Psychology of the Apollo Moon Scientists.* New York: American Elsevier Publishing Co.; Amsterdam: Elsevier Scientific Publishing Co., 1974.

MULLINS, NICHOLAS C., and MULLINS, CAROLYN J. *Theories and Theory Groups in Contemporary American Sociology.* New York: Harper & Row, 1973.

POPPER, KARL R. *The Logic of Scientific Discovery.* Harper Torchbooks. New York: Harper & Row, 1965, 1968. Translation of *Logik der Forschung,* 1934.

PRICE, DEREK JOHN DE SOLLA. *Little Science, Big Science.* George B. Pegram Lectures, 1962. New York: Columbia University Press, 1963.

SALAMON, JEAN-JACQUES. *Science and Politics.* London: Macmillan, 1973.

SMALL, HENRY, and GRIFFITH, BELVER C. "The Structure of Scientific Literatures, I: Identifying and Graphing Specialties." *Science Studies* 4 (1974): 17–40.

STORER, NORMAN W. *The Social System of Science.* New York: Holt, Rinehart & Winston, 1966.

SULLIVAN, DANIEL. "Competition in Bio-Medical Science: Extent, Structure, and Consequences." *Sociology of Education* 48 (1975): 223–241.

SWAZEY, JUDITH P. *Chlorpromazine in Psychiatry: A Study of Therapeutic Innovation.* Cambridge: MIT Press, 1974. One of a series of historical monographs sponsored by the Committee on Brain Sciences, Division of Medical Sciences, National Research Council.

ZUCKERMAN, HARRIET. "Stratification in American Science." *Sociological Inquiry* 40 (1970): 235–257.

————, and MERTON, ROBERT K. "Age, Aging, and Age Structure in Science." *Aging and Society.* Vol. 3: A *Sociology of Age Stratification.* Edited by Matilda White Riley, Marilyn Johnson, and Anne Foner. New York: Russell Sage Foundation, 1972, pp. 292–356.

SCIENCE WRITING AND PUBLISHING
See COMMUNICATION, BIOMEDICAL.

SCREENING
See MASS HEALTH SCREENING; GENETIC SCREENING.

SELF-REALIZATION THERAPIES

Concepts and principles underlying the ethical issues discussed in this entry can be found in the entry BEHAVIOR CONTROL.

Definition

The term "self-realization therapy" evokes a picture of the self imprisoned within the person and needing some help in seeking its full freedom. The development of this quest is aided by techniques that produce strong emotional reactions in a group setting, breaking, as it were, the mold in which the self is imprisoned. The techniques are distinguished from common therapeutic techniques by the fact that they are primarily intended for people with no identifiable distress or deficiencies. They are designed to produce changes, or at least intense experiences, in people who can function in society, but who feel some need for such intense experiences or feelings of change. The rise of these therapies can be dated from 1946 when it was discovered, in a workshop in New Britain, Connecticut, that group interaction, if directed toward the contemplation of its own actions and relationships, can cause an intense emotional experience in the group members (Back).

The purpose of this experience may be autotelic, or it may be part of a future aim; it may be directed toward more efficient group functioning or toward the further development of the individual. The experience may also be generated at different levels of intensity. Thus, such techniques are often used for recreational purposes; some places where these experiences are induced can be called "psych resorts." (Recreation has practically the same literal meaning as self-realization.) Other efforts used as individual therapy may be considered adjuncts to common therapeutic techniques or can be called "therapy for normals." They can also be used as adjuncts to teaching, to improve industrial efficiency, or to train a political action group. Finally, they can be precursors of religious experience, leading to claims of mystical revelations. The possible intense effect of these group experiences leads to ethical questions concerning individual responsibility, social control, and the general aims of intensifying sensations.

Range of techniques

The intense effect of group action has been known for a long time; groups, mobs, and organized movements have been assembled to realize a variety of aims. However, a principle novel to self-realization groups is the deliberate use of feedback: Interaction within the group becomes a topic of activity of the group itself. Group performance and other recent events in the group are analyzed by members; each member recalls his or her own feelings during participation, tries to find the more subtle cues to which each member reacted by distinguishing hidden interpersonal reaction from the ostensible topic of discussion, and finally evaluates everybody's performance.

The attraction of the groups and their propagation came from the discovery that the so-called feedback techniques produce exhilaration, excitement, and usually a positive feeling. Some groups have been used with similar outcomes in the past, but usually in a religious context. Modern self-realization therapy is unique in that it produces emotional effects in groups without resort to an ultimate religious aim, representing a secularization of transcendental experience.

Different centers have emphasized different aspects of the techniques and given different names to them. Groups that mainly try to show the participants how to interact better in working groups, how better to define their roles, are called training groups or T-Groups and were designed by the National Training Laboratory. Groups that mainly emphasize the individual experience and try to intensify it through all kinds of sensual techniques are encounter groups, originally devised by Carl Rogers and adapted at Esalen, California. The Tavistock technique (after the Tavistock Clinic in London) has a purely didactic function: to improve the understanding of group process.

Some groups are not unlike classes, meeting weekly for an hour or so, but most try to make the session an intensive experience by separating it from normal life for a weekend or even for a longer period and keeping it in a special place unlike normal surroundings, frequently a beautiful resort area to emphasize the recreational aspect. Different leadership styles lead to different risks and successes, and different group compositions may lead to different effects on the future interaction of participants. Despite this variety in self-realization techniques, their settings and purposes, they face common ethical problems in responsibility, justification, risk taking, and relation to social values.

Basic ambiguities

The principal ethical problems within all these techniques come from a kind of ambiguity and conflict between the stated aims and actual work. Some difficulties come from the fact that a technique may be either recreation, training, therapy, or experiment; some come from the tension within the session between the professed ideology of concern and caring and the commercial businesslike relationship surrounding it; others arise from the conflict about intellectuality with the emphasis on feeling and the claims of science that it is a resource; and, finally, there is difficulty between the all-embracing claim of spirituality, the regeneration of men, and the quite hedonistic self-centered aim that individual groups are trying to promote.

Assignment of responsibility

The justification for the existence of groups featuring self-realization techniques varies, but there is common agreement that having the experience in itself is necessarily good. Somehow in the process the real self or one's maximum potential are discovered—at least some new insight into one's own functioning can be learned. The self is let out of its cage. However, practically all self-realization groups claim benefits beyond a pleasant experience.

An implicit contract between participant and group leader lies at the center of the many management problems occurring with these groups. The basic model for acquiring group experiences corresponds to a sales agreement. The buyer, the participant in the experience, comes voluntarily, having some idea of what he wants to purchase, and the group leader claims to be selling a specific service. The responsibility for administration of such strong medicine is thus shifted to the buyer.

Let us examine the conditions of the free choice. In many situations it is a quite reasonable assumption. Weekend encounter groups, classroom exercises, and similar enterprises are usually the result of a purely voluntary action on the part of the participants; the enterprise attracts a customer by advertising and other means of publicity.

Some types of self-realization therapy, however, stress the therapeutic more than any other aspect. If that is done, self-realization becomes a medical question, medical ethics would apply, and the basic ambiguity of the service becomes apparent. As it is supposedly unprofessional for medical services to be advertised, any pseudo-psychiatric encounter groups that promise remedies should not be able to advertise; in fact, some newspapers have refused to accept advertisements of such groups. On the other hand, if the encounter service is simply an experience or even, as some of its advocates have claimed, the equivalent of a "singles bar," then there would be no reason to proscribe advertising. If even medical advertising is becoming acceptable, the issue may become moot. However, the question of what services are to be provided to even the most rational customer still remains urgent. Are they educational, recreational, or medical? The selling of a recreational experience can, of course, be justified if the treatment is not actually harmful. On the other hand, if some providers of the service claim that permanent change will occur, then the claim must be examined and also the justification for the change must be established ("Groups").

Ethics of change

There have been several reasons for accepting a policy of changing people. Such a policy can be defended with an appeal to a higher authority. The authority may be either transcendental or a power within the society. Thus the presence of sin and of deviations from religious beliefs has been used frequently as an ethical justification for enforced change. On the other hand, if law is taken as providing a natural base for decision making, either by consensus or by legitimate enactment, then changing people becomes part of the judicial process. Punishment and rehabilitation under statute law are frequently expressed reasons for creating change. However, recognition of a disabling condition is also justification for producing change. The disablement might be sickness or at least a condition labeled as such. Under this rubric drastic change in a person who presents a danger to others as by infection or a psychopath's aggression can be justified even against the individual's will. The justification for personal change can give great power to persons whose positions enable them to define deficiencies.

In the groups that are our main focus, however, no such deficiencies are clearly apparent. The center of the process can be experience itself or the change that the experience is supposed to produce. In the first case, the only outcome is more experience or more self-expression. With the second aim, it is difficult for the consumer really to know what he is getting out of a group experience and equally difficult for the purveyor to express what is really being purveyed. The combination of the two is one of the attractions of self-realization techniques—namely, that some pleasant experience is being sold almost in a recreational way, but the customer is assured also that it is for his own good. The combination is especially valuable for people who feel uneasy in the acceptance of pure enjoyment, those who are affected by a Puritan ethic. The attraction of the whole system in countries deriving from the Puritan ethic—such as the United States, England, and the Scandinavian countries—is striking in this regard.

However, there is another dilemma. If self-realization therapy is effective and can change people without a definite aim derived from higher authority or definition of a deficiency, then there may be some social concern about what is being done. Some of the successes being reported clearly have aroused some questions; even if there are no successes there is still social interest in what is being done. In short, if the experiences given through self-realization techniques do have permanent effects on people, then the question of licensing and social provision might be just as valid as for drugs, for which similar effects are claimed. If it is harmless and purely an experience that is transient, then self-realization is frequently sold under fraudulent claims ("Groups"; Maliver). There is legitimate interest in seeing what kind of lasting effects in the individual are being created. (The social implications are discussed in a separate section below.)

Risks and benefits

Possible benefits have to be measured against the risks. Risk data on self-realization techniques are sparse and controversial. Documented cases report positive effects but also have shown extreme deterioration, breakdowns, and even suicides occurring as a consequence of participation in these kinds of groups (Lieberman, Yalom, and Miles; Maliver; Back). The general ethical problem remains: Can we justify exposing people to risk on a promise of positive effects when the workings of the mechanisms are unknown? Again, answers will depend in great part on the definition. If self-realization is a matter of open free choice, either as recreation or as therapy, informed consent and a guarantee of minimum competence of the practitioner are all that is needed. If the process is part of a training program of an organization, then the relation of the client to the organization itself and the possible benefits to be derived from membership in the organization (such as income) must be considered. However, here one may be frequently doubtful about voluntary participation. There has been controversy over the employer's right to control any part of the private lives or personal behavior of his employees; self-realization programs may interfere with the employees' hard-won right to privacy. Finally, if the procedure is done purely for experimental reasons, then the rules for experimentation with human subjects apply. In this case again, there must be consent; even if it cannot be completely informed, the experimenter has to assume all the risks if there is no immediate benefit offered to the subject. The supposed benefits are assumed to be of social value—value for the general benefit of humanity—only if more knowledge is being obtained. The rules of experimental use are stricter than those of therapy; they reflect an apparent preference in our society for the view that the creation of knowledge is of lower value than individual life (Dyer). Society demands only general control over the qualification and morality of the therapist, while specific control over each step is enforced in experimental use. An assumption of risk and its importance, therefore, would depend on a definition of the procedures, especially whether there is an employer–employee or experimenter–subject relationship or whether there is simply a purchase of an irrelevant but potentially dangerous service (ibid.).

Social control

The question of danger becomes intimately connected with one's outlook on the purpose of self-realization groups and procedures. If they are, as some claim, powerful new techniques able to regenerate and recreate participants, then the dangers must also be taken seriously. If the procedure needs specialized knowledge and great skill, and if risks are involved, then the public has a right to control and certify the practitioners. If practitioners do not understand what they are doing but only know that they have extremely powerful techniques in their hands, then they should be put under the same control as experimenters with human beings. If, on the other hand, the new effort is a harmless pastime—used perhaps to combat boredom—then the only safeguards have to be the general precautions against accidental or purposeful injury.

The evidence needed to make a judgment on this issue is spotty; it has hardly been systematically collected. We know that there is some danger and that some people have been permanently and clearly damaged by exposure to the sessions. We also know that some people have derived benefits, at least by their own definition. There is a great variety of techniques, practitioners, and organizations with a correspondingly great variation in responsibility and skill (Lieberman, Yalom, and Miles). Enough evidence of harm and danger has been shown to warrant some public control over the movement. At their best, techniques have effects similar to those of drugs, in the good and bad sense, and society is as concerned here as with their use. At its worst, it is the legitimation of a confidence game under the doctrine "let the buyer beware."

Social implications

Thus far self-realization therapy has been examined mainly as a question within an accepted framework of self-realization as a worthwhile aim. We have now to consider two related problems that go beyond this therapy and its ostensible purposes. One is the fiction that pictures the group as a self-contained unit in time as well as in space, and the other is the effects that disconfirmation of that fiction may have. The expectation of self-realization therapy is that the group is an end in itself, that there is a here-and-now orientation, and that relations between group and members beyond the experiences themselves are not to be expected. Within the group, however, an atmosphere is set up of trust, of caring, and of mutual sympathy. Members are encouraged to make plans to adjust relationships after the group experience. This is similar to action taken in traditional therapy; however, in that case the therapist has some responsibility for the further action of the patient. There is a contrast between the atmosphere and whole philosophy of mutual care and mutual involve-ment set up within the session and the complete lack of concern that exists once the group is over.

Many casualties of the movement have exposed the great callousness toward individuals who really come to groups for help (Maliver). Some are victims of the belief that the groups are therapy. Patients come to them almost as a last resort and may be deceived by the warm atmosphere. If there is no corresponding assumption of responsibility by the leader and no provision for follow-up, then the letdown is not tolerable and may have extreme consequences. The groups cannot be said to have caused those effects, but they are responsible because of their ambiguous definitions of themselves.

The consequences are different when group members have to stay together after the therapy, as in a working organization. Moreover, if attendance is not voluntary, some actions taken by the group and some interactions that took place are valid only in the group setting but may be carried over to future work. This again has led to many complaints about the legitimacy of setting up these groups in ongoing situations. We have a consistent refusal of groups to assume a definite place within society and to establish mutual links with other institutions.

A final word must be said about the general aims of groups and their place within an ethical system. The general aims of groups, even if they are achieved, are stated in terms of personal enhancement or individual self-expression—goals that are paramount in an individualistic society (Adler). That is one point of view possible as a statement of humanity's ultimate aim, namely, the complete development of each individual. There may be other aims that are just as legitimate: group goals, achievement by a group, achievement within a society by serving human values such as beauty, truth, and spirituality.

Encounter groups do use these terms too, but only in a literal, almost vulgar sense. For instance, trust is used in "trust fall," an exercise in which a person falls backward on another, "trusting" not to be left falling on one's back, i.e., that the other person is not a sadistic practical joker. Trivializing these serious terms is a symptom of the general ethical stance of the movement (Koch). It has a particular view of human destiny, representing an egoistic, self-seeking aim, corresponding to the hedonistic, pleasure-seeking characteristic of the technique.

Conclusion

Self-realization groups may be looked on as a set of institutions within a society. They mirror the problems of how much involvement one can have with another individual and what the legitimate means are to bring about such involvement. The groups are no better or worse than the society that supports them; their problems reflect the ethical dilemmas of society.

KURT W. BACK

[*Directly related are the entries* BEHAVIOR CONTROL; MENTAL HEALTH, *article on* MENTAL HEALTH IN COMPETITION WITH OTHER VALUES; *and* MENTAL HEALTH THERAPIES. *For further discussion of topics mentioned in this article, see the entries:* ADVERTISING BY MEDICAL PROFESSIONALS; *and* RISK. *For discussion of related ideas, see the entries:* INFORMED CONSENT IN MENTAL HEALTH; *and* INFORMED CONSENT IN THE THERAPEUTIC RELATIONSHIP, *article on* CLINICAL ASPECTS.]

BIBLIOGRAPHY

ADLER, NATHAN. *The Underground Stream: New Life Styles and the Antinomian Personality.* New York: Harper & Row, 1972. An evaluation of the social meaning of the therapies, showing how the ethical problems and ideologies have recurred in different times.

BACK, KURT W. *Beyond Words: The Story of Sensitivity Training and the Encounter Movement.* New York: Russell Sage Foundation, 1972. An analysis of the encounter group movement, describing its history, variations, claims, and ethical controversies that have arisen, and discussing the scientific and ethical issues involved.

DYER, WILLIAM G., ed. *Modern Theory and Method in Group Training.* NTL Learning Resources Series. New York: Van Nostrand Reinhold, 1972. Designed as a learning resource for the National Training Laboratory, this book includes essays on leadership style and intervention, design and methods, and ethical issues. The last section, comprising two articles by M. Lakin and W. Dyer, gives an incisive picture of the ethical issues as seen from the classical point of view of T-group technique.

"Groups." *American Journal of Psychiatry* 126 (1969): 823–873. A series of articles looking at self-realization groups from a psychiatric point of view, focusing on the problems of screening, casualties, and leadership responsibilities.

KOCH, SIGMUND. "The Image of Man in Encounter Group Therapy." *Journal of Humanistic Psychology* 11 (1971): 109–128. A discussion of encounter groups as threats to the concepts of human dignity and freedom. A severe but well-reasoned attack.

LIEBERMAN, MORTON A.; YALOM, IRVIN D.; and MILES, MATTHEW B. *Encounter Groups: First Facts.* New York: Basic Books, 1973. A detailed study assessing possible gains, casualties, and justification of encounter groups; stresses the importance of leadership style.

MALIVER, BRUCE L. *The Encounter Game.* New York: Stein & Day, 1973. A documented analysis of current excesses of self-realization groups and their threat to individuals; especially concerned with leadership responsibilities.

SEVENTH-DAY ADVENTISTS

See PROTESTANTISM, *article on* DOMINANT HEALTH CONCERNS IN PROTESTANTISM.

SEX CHANGE

See SEXUAL IDENTITY.

SEX SELECTION or
SEX PREDETERMINATION

See REPRODUCTIVE TECHNOLOGIES, *articles on* SEX SELECTION, ETHICAL ISSUES, *and* LEGAL ASPECTS.

SEX THERAPY AND SEX RESEARCH

I. SCIENTIFIC AND CLINICAL PERSPECTIVES
Sallie Schumacher and Charles W. Lloyd

II. ETHICAL PERSPECTIVES   *Ruth Macklin*

I
SCIENTIFIC AND CLINICAL PERSPECTIVES

The purpose of this article is to analyze the current status of sex therapy and research in the United States and to identify some of the ethical issues involved. Achieving this purpose is difficult because study of sexual behavior is a relatively new area of scientific inquiry with a small body of information, limited and undeveloped theoretical bases, and few organized training or professional development programs.

It has been conservatively estimated that in at least fifty percent of marriages in the United States a serious sexual problem develops at one time or another. Sexual inadequacy affects not only the specific individual involved but his or her spouse and often the basic family structure. Problems of sexual orientation and gender identity often cause distress in families and, sometimes, in society in general. Criminal acts involving sexual behavior are serious problems for society.

Treatment of sexual dysfunction has been attempted for centuries, and therapies have involved innumerable fads and superstitions. The rate of success has apparently been as would be predicted from these nonspecific approaches. Therapeutic methods of today are able to offer help to many patients but still have handicaps. They have evolved since the late nineteenth century and are based on untested, and often untestable, hypotheses. There is little information about the basic physiological mechanisms of human sexual arousal and response and an equal lack of information about possible physiological defects in patients with sexual dysfunction.

The writings of Freud, Havelock Ellis, and Krafft-Ebing at the turn of the century helped generate interest in the study of sex. In the United States the attitudes of the medical profession in 1900 toward professional discussion of sexual matters and dissemination of information to patients are exemplified by the experience of Denslow Lewis (Hollender). Lewis, a gynecologist, presented a paper entitled "The Gynecologic Consideration of the Sexual Act" at a meeting of the American Medical Association in 1899. The paper discussed the importance of sex and the sex education of young women. It was not well received and was rejected for publication in the *Journal of the American Medical Association.*

Sex research

Although clinicians could not comfortably discuss sexual matters among themselves or with patients, there was considerable basic research in the physiology and behavioral aspects of reproduction, research which subsequently increased rapidly (Aberle and Corner; Marshall).

In animals, research methods used to study sexual behavior were observation and experimentation. In the human, the primary method was the use of the sexual survey. Kinsey, et al. (1948, pp. 23–31) summarized nineteen investigations published between 1915 and 1947, which used systematic techniques of questionnaire, interview, and examination of clinical records to obtain information about human sexual behavior. The volumes published by Kinsey and his associates in 1948 and 1953 contain the most comprehensive and scholarly information about sexual behavior in print today. Kinsey's work survived serious problems of acceptance with about ten to fifteen percent of the general population, including a few eminent personages, opposed to the research on "moral" grounds. There was much more criticism of the experimental

design and of the method of presentation of data from the scientific community (Pomeroy, pp. 283–306; 359–372). Now sex research in general is considered socially and morally acceptable by the majority of the scientific community and the informed lay public. A few powerful critics such as Senator Proxmire ("Proxmire Speaks Out") persist.

The widely publicized writings and pronouncements of Masters and Johnson (1966; 1970) provided a powerful stimulus to easing the prejudices and prohibitions on the study of human sexual behavior. Besides influencing the change in attitude toward research in sex, Masters and Johnson also have provided important information about sexual behavior in their observations of peripheral anatomic and physiologic changes that occur in response to sexual stimuli. Perhaps their most important contribution, however, has been the provision of hope of improvement for the person with sexual dysfunction. Their popularization of a direct treatment approach has led to the development of specialized clinics or centers for treatment, serious interest in evaluation of treatment methods, and an increase in continued research in sexual response.

One of the most important areas of sex research, not well-known to the general public, is the area of gender-identity differentiation. During the past twenty-five years, Money and his coworkers have collected and integrated experimental and clinical data from different scientific specialties in the effort to increase understanding of the many determinants of human sexual behavior (Money and Ehrhardt). Many scientists have contributed to this field, and the present level of progress illustrates the benefits of integrating information from the basic laboratory and from clinical observation.

Purposes and types of sex therapy

The purpose of sex therapy is to help people who have problems of sexual dysfunction or of gender identity, or who have committed crimes involving socially unacceptable sexual expression. In general, treatment methods can be grouped in the following categories: (1) psychoanalysis; (2) psychotherapy; (3) behavior therapy; (4) the method of Masters and Johnson; (5) modifications of the Masters and Johnson method; (6) group therapy; and (7) sexual attitude restructuring (SAR).

1. Psychoanalysis is a diversified method of

treatment. However, its basic approach to the clinical understanding of sexual dysfunction remains grounded in Freud's original concepts concerning the dynamic sequence of psychosexual development. Sexual inadequacy is viewed as a symptomatic expression of unresolved conflict originating in certain stages of the individual's psychological development. The therapeutic goal is the resolution of this conflict. Treatment is directed toward the exploration and reorganization of the total personality, rather than limited to direct focus upon a single symptom, such as a specific sexual dysfunction. Psychoanalysis is usually distinguished from psychotherapy in general because it is concerned with problems at a deeper dynamic level and often requires a time commitment of many years.

The literature of psychoanalysis is vast and includes hundreds of publications about the treatment of sexual dysfunction. Because of its broad focus, however, scientific evaluation of the effectiveness of psychoanalysis in reversing sexual symptoms is limited.

2. Psychotherapy may be defined as treatment of emotional and behavioral problems by psychological means. There are many varieties of psychotherapy, and all deal with sexual problems within their own framework. Most forms of psychotherapy are concerned with personality traits and their influence on sexual activity. Most also include reassurance and support, and sex education as needed.

3. Behavior therapy is considered a separate form of psychotherapy because of its emphasis upon specific problem behavior rather than underlying personality conflict. A basic assumption of this approach is that inappropriate behavior is learned and maintained by environmental conditions. Changes in behavior, therefore, can be brought about through reeducative experiences and changes in the environmental situation.

In the behavioral approach to problems of sexual inadequacy, sexual dysfunction is assumed to be the result of learned anxiety and fear associated with sexual performance. The primary technique used to alleviate this anxiety is systematic desensitization. In the desensitization process, anxiety is deconditioned by exposing the patient to graded, anxiety-producing stimuli, either verbal or situational, under conditions of relaxation and acceptance (Wolpe, 1958; 1969). For example, the patient may be instructed to begin sexual activity when positive feelings are present and to terminate activity when feelings of anxiety arise. By avoiding anxiety, positive sexual activities become self-reinforcing.

4. Masters and Johnson advocate an authoritative, educational approach to problems of sexual dysfunction. Their basic premise is that sex is a natural function. They believe that misunderstanding of this natural function, unrealistic cultural demands for effectiveness of performance, and poor communication between sexual partners lead directly to fear of sexual failure, which they consider the major cause of sexual inadequacy.

Masters and Johnson advocate a therapeutic format which consists of: treatment of a sexually distressed couple as a unit, treatment by a male/female therapy team, isolation of the dysfunctional couple from its everyday family and work setting, and participation in the therapy program on a daily basis for a two-week period. Because this approach is not practical for most patients, there are no reports in the literature on the effectiveness of this particular treatment method other than that presented by Masters and Johnson (1970).

5. Other therapists have modified the approach of Masters and Johnson without apparent loss of treatment effectiveness. One major change adopted by almost all practitioners of sex therapy is the treatment of patients within their everyday social setting on a weekly basis. Other modifications include treatment of individuals as well as couples; more extensive biochemical and physiological diagnoses and treatment (Schumacher and Lloyd); treatment by only one therapist; and the integration of sex therapy technique with more traditional psychodynamic therapy (Kaplan; "Panel Highlights").

6. As a specific treatment method for sexual dysfunction, group therapy has been advocated by several therapists. In the most common format patients in the group share the same dysfunction, and group discussion is structured by the leader to include sex education and explanation as well as sharing of experiences by the group members (Barbach). A less successful approach has been group therapy that is more traditional in orientation with the focus on open discussion of the participants' sexual and social problems (Obler).

7. Another approach, originally developed for sex education and now utilized for treatment of sexual dysfunction, revolves around the use

of sexually explicit graphic materials (Bjork-stein). The most widely used model is the Sexual Attitude Restructuring Process (SAR) developed by the National Sex Forum in San Francisco. In this model, participants attend workshops for two to seven days in groups that vary in size from 8 or 10 to 100 or more people. The workshop format includes the explicit portrayal of many styles and kinds of sexual behavior through the use of films, videotapes, and slides in a quiet, relaxed atmosphere. This is followed by large and small group discussions in which feelings and reactions to the visual material are shared and explored.

The rationale of this approach is that most sexual problems are the result of inappropriate emotional and attitudinal factors which produce anxiety about sexual feeling and behavior. Exposure to sexually explicit material initially elicits anxiety in people who have had little exposure to this type of material and limited attitudinal regard for sexual matters. It is thought that, following an audiovisual presentation, open discussion of feelings and attitudes reduces anxiety and leads to the development of more accepting attitudes about sexual behavior. At present there is no definitive information about the value of this approach in the reversal of specific sexual dysfunction.

Effectiveness of sex therapy

Present treatment methods have been found to be comparably effective in reversing sexual dysfunction when used with well-motivated patients who have been selected on the basis of the absence of serious psychological problems (Schumacher). Most of the reported high success in sex therapy has been with this kind of select patient population. Using unselected populations, Cooper (1969) and Johnson (1965) report a lower rate of treatment success. This also has been the experience of Schumacher and Lloyd (1976).

Successful treatment occurs when sexual dysfunction is associated primarily with anxiety, inexperience, and lack of information. When medical factors also contribute to the dysfunction, therapy is more complicated.

Treatment of gender-identity problems has been reported to be successful in alleviating the effects of social stress in individuals who feel the need to live a role that society does not consider appropriate for their phenotypic sex (Green).

Treatment of the sexual offender has not produced sufficiently dramatic results to encourage widespread effort in this direction. The use of steroid preparations, which block the effects of androgen, seems to be of value in men whose offenses are due to excessive sex drive (Laschet).

Ethical issues

Ethical issues involved in sex therapy include confidentiality of information; the need for informed consent of patients entering therapy; the problem of intimacy, particularly sexual intimacy, between patients and therapists; and the standardization of qualifications for sex therapists (Macklin).

In addition to the issues of confidentiality and informed consent, ethical questions related to sex research include: Should research scientists participate in social activism working for changes supported by their findings? Are there some situations in which research findings should be suppressed? Should sex research have as a goal the changing of public attitudes about sex? ("Ethical Issues").

There are also procedural issues in sex research. Two areas of procedural concern related to research in sexual development involve studies of biological sexual differentiation that require the use of human abortuses and investigation of psychological differentiation in children. There is considerable disagreement about the use of even previable abortuses and also about subjecting children to inquiries about their sexual activities.

One final area of ethical concern is that of values and the goals of sex therapy and research. Evidence from the scientific study of sex indicates that people engage in a variety of sexual activities and that there are many uses of sex. However, value judgments about the morality of sexual behaviors are not appropriate for objective science (Reiss). Information by itself cannot resolve specific moral questions, nor can it eliminate all sexual problems. It can, however, increase the data base from which individuals make choices.

It is of ethical concern that the sex therapist or researcher separate his or her own scientific values from personal moral value. The capacity, need, and desire to relate sexually vary greatly among individuals. Learning what one's sexual potential is and how to express it is a developmental and moral task that requires help from many sources and for which there are no short-cuts.

It is evident from this brief discussion of the present status of research in human sexual activity and treatment of various problems in this area that only a beginning has been made. Even so, many difficult ethical problems have surfaced. It is to be predicted that as activity expands in this field, so too will the ethical questions.

SALLIE SCHUMACHER
AND CHARLES W. LLOYD

[*Directly related is the other article in this entry,* ETHICAL PERSPECTIVES. *Also directly related are the entries* HOMOSEXUALITY; SEXUAL BEHAVIOR; SEXUAL IDENTITY; *and* SEXUAL ETHICS. *For further discussion of topics mentioned in this article, see the entries:* BEHAVIORAL THERAPIES; DYNAMIC THERAPIES; *and* SELF-REALIZATION THERAPIES. *See also:* SEXUAL DEVELOPMENT.]

BIBLIOGRAPHY

ABERLE, SOPHIE BLEDSOE DE, and CORNER, GEORGE WASHINGTON. *Twenty-five Years of Sex Research: History of the National Research Council Committee for Research in Problems of Sex, 1922–1947.* Philadelphia: W. B. Saunders Co., 1953.

BARBACH, LONNIE G. *For Yourself—The Fulfillment of Female Sexuality.* New York: Doubleday, 1975. Paperback ed. Anchor Press/Doubleday, 1976.

BJORKSTEIN, OLIVER J. W. "Sexually Graphic Material in the Treatment of Sexual Disorders." *Clinical Management of Sexual Disorders.* Edited by Jon Meyer. Baltimore: Williams & Wilkins Co., 1976, pp. 161–194.

COOPER, ALAN J. "A Factual Study of Male Potency Disorders." *British Journal of Psychiatry* 114 (1968): 719–731.

"Ethical Issues." *Sex Research: Future Directions.* Edited by Eli A. Rubinstein, Richard Green, and Edward Brecher. Proceeding of the Conference held at the State University of New York at Stony Brook, Stony Brook, N.Y., 5–9 June 1974. *Archives of Sexual Behavior* 4 (1975): 459–465. Discussion in a special issue.

GREEN, RICHARD. *Sexual Identity Conflict in Children and Adults.* New York: Basic Books, 1974, pp. 243–245.

HOLLENDER, MARC M. "The Medical Profession and Sex in 1900." *American Journal of Obstetrics and Gynecology* 108 (1970): 139–148.

JOHNSON, J. "Prognosis of Disorders of Sexual Potency in the Male." *Journal of Psychosomatic Research* 9 (1965): 195–200.

KAPLAN, HELEN SINGER. *The New Sex Therapy: Active Treatment of Sexual Dysfunctions.* New York: Brunner/Mazel, 1974.

KINSEY, ALFRED CHARLES; POMEROY, WARDELL B.; and MARTIN, CLYDE E. *Sexual Behavior in the Human Male.* Philadelphia: W. B. Saunders Co., 1948.

———; POMEROY, WARDELL B.; MARTIN, CLYDE E., and GEBHARD, PAUL H. *Sexual Behavior in the Human Female.* Philadelphia: W. B. Saunders Co., 1953.

LASCHET, URSULA. "Antiandrogen in the Treatment of Sex Offenders: Mode of Action and Therapeutic Outcome." *Contemporary Sexual Behavior: Critical Issues in the 1970s.* Edited by Joseph Zubin and John Money. Baltimore: Johns Hopkins University Press, 1973, pp. 311–319.

LAZARUS, ARNOLD A., and ROSEN, RAYMOND C. "Behavior Therapy Techniques in the Treatment of Sexual Disorders." *Clinical Management of Sexual Disorders.* Edited by Jon Meyer. Baltimore: Williams & Wilkins Co., 1976, pp. 148–160.

MACKLIN, RUTH. "Ethics, Sex Research, and Sex Therapy: Masters and Johnson Call a Conference." *Hastings Center Report* 6, no. 2 (1976), pp. 5–7.

MARSHALL, FRANCIS HUGH ADAM. *Physiology of Reproduction.* 3d ed. Edited by Alan Sterling Parkes. London: Longmans, Green & Co., 1956.

MASTERS, WILLIAM H., and JOHNSON, VIRGINIA E. *Human Sexual Inadequacy.* Boston: Little, Brown & Co., 1970.

———, and JOHNSON, VIRGINIA E. *Human Sexual Response.* Boston: Little, Brown & Co., 1966.

———, and JOHNSON, VIRGINIA E. "Principles of the New Sex Therapy." *American Journal of Psychiatry* 133 (1976): 548–554.

MONEY, JOHN, and EHRHARDT, ANKE A. *Man and Woman, Boy and Girl: The Differentiation and Dimorphism of Gender Identity from Conception to Maturity.* Baltimore: Johns Hopkins University Press, 1972.

OBLER, MARTIN. "Systematic Desensitization in Sexual Disorders." *Journal of Behavior Therapy and Experimental Psychiatry* 4 (1973): 93–101.

"Panel Highlights: Modifications of Master-Johnson Sex Therapy Utilize Psychodynamics." *Roche Report: Frontiers of Psychiatry,* October 1976, pp. 1–2.

POMEROY, WARDELL BAXTER. *Dr. Kinsey and the Institute for Sex Research.* New York: Harper & Row, 1972.

"Proxmire Speaks Out on Social Science." *APA Monitor,* May 1975, p. 6.

REISS, IRA I. "Personal Values and the Scientific Study of Sex." *Advances in Sex Research.* Edited by Hugo G. Beigel. A publication of the Society for the Scientific Study of Sex. New York: Harper & Row, Hoeber Medical Division, 1963, chap. 1, pp. 3–10.

SCHUMACHER, SALLIE. "Effectiveness of Sex Therapy." *Progress in Sexology.* Edited by Robert Gemme and Connie Christine Wheeler. Perspectives in Sexuality series. New York: Plenum, 1977, pp. 141–151.

———; and LLOYD, CHARLES W. "Assessment of Sexual Dysfunction." *Behavioral Assessment: A Practical Handbook.* Edited by Michel Hersen and Alan S. Bellack. Pergamon General Psychology series no. 65. New York: Pergamon Press, 1976, chap. 15, pp. 419–435.

WOLPE, JOSEPH. *The Practice of Behavior Therapy.* Elmsford, N.Y.: Pergamon Press, 1969. 2d ed. Pergamon General Psychology series, no. 1. 1973.

———. *Psychotherapy by Reciprocal Inhibition.* Stanford: Stanford University Press, 1958.

II
ETHICAL PERSPECTIVES

Ethical issues in sex research and sex therapy are no different in principle from the moral concerns in other domains of medicine and counseling. Therapist–patient confidentiality, difficulties in gaining informed consent, inappropriate intimacies between therapist and patient, and intrusions of the therapist's personal values head the list of ethical issues in the area of sex therapy. Sex research poses similar ethical problems of informed consent, privacy, and confidentiality; in addition, there are the usual difficulties in assessing risk-benefit equations, as well as the familiar bioethical issues that arise in the case of research on special populations such as prisoners and children.

But in spite of the fact that the moral problems in this area of specialization fall into the same basic categories as bioethical concerns generally, there remains a set of social and psychological factors surrounding sex research and therapy that makes this area somewhat different. These include the facts that open discussion and acknowledgment of sexual dysfunction have only recently become socially acceptable; that there continue to exist taboos in some major religions concerning a variety of sexual practices; and that many people place great importance on adequate or even optimal sexual functioning to an increasing extent. These and related factors make the domain of sex research and therapy a highly charged emotional subject, confronted by considerable skepticism and criticism from without.

The ethical issues identified by those who look upon sex research and therapy from the point of view of a critical outsider are necessarily rather different from the sorts of moral concerns common to most clinical and research practice. It seems appropriate to treat these two sets of ethical issues as comprising (1) general moral considerations and (2) bioethical concerns. After a brief look at the general moral questions surrounding the practice of sex research and sex therapy, this article will focus on the bioethical concerns, drawing on examples from research and therapeutic settings.

General moral considerations

Some basic moral objections. The broadest question put by those who are critical or skeptical of research and therapeutic efforts in the area of human sexuality usually takes the form: Ought there to be any research or therapy conducted in this area at all? Such questions may be motivated by a number of different concerns. Some criticisms of sex research and therapy might stem from a viewpoint holding that the primary purpose of sexual activity is procreation. On this view, the most acceptable form of research on sex would be studies of fertility and infertility, and the main purpose of therapy would be helping married women who have been unable to conceive. A more general and, perhaps, less powerfully motivated criticism arises out of the Western cultural tradition, which has tended to view sexual relations between couples as a wholly private matter. Since sex research and therapy almost always involve open discussion of sexual matters, and may also include observation of couples engaged in intimate sexual behavior, some critics see the entire field as one that violates the social and cultural strictures regarding privacy in the sexual sphere.

Sex as a health priority. There are, in addition, skeptical questions raised about sex research and therapy as yet another instance of too much research on "unnecessary" topics and too much therapy for nondisease states of persons. This sort of objection may be based on beliefs about what research priorities ought to be, since research dollars are a scarce resource that must be allocated carefully and justly; or it may be based on beliefs about what highly trained clinicians ought to be doing, given the numbers of seriously ill or malnourished or handicapped persons in the world. But from whatever source these types of questions may arise, they remain prominent in spite of the fact that sex research and therapy are now well-established investigative and clinical specialties with highly reputable professionals from medicine, the social sciences, and allied health fields as participants.

Public and private morality. Some criticisms of sex research and therapy address issues of "private" as opposed to "public" morality. Examples of these sorts of questions are ones that relate to the use of surrogate partners in sex therapy, masturbation as a therapeutic technique, and treatment of sexual inadequacies in homosexuals. For those whose personal ethical code proscribes sexual relations outside of marriage, the use of surrogate partners in sex therapy would be immoral. It is interesting to note, however, that the use of female surrogates is usually found more acceptable than the use of male surrogates. Whether this is a function of the centuries-old double standard that obtains generally with respect to men and women where sex is concerned, or because a long historical tradition of female prostitution renders acceptable the practice of using female but not male surrogates in sex therapy, it remains the case that this is seen as a genuine moral issue by some but not by others. Similarly, some people continue to view masturbation and homosexual behavior as subject to moral review, while others deny that such practices should be open to moral judgments of any sort. To the extent that disagreement persists about these matters of public and private morality, there will remain some uncertainty about how much of what goes on in sex research and sex therapy is a proper subject for moral discourse, and just which aspects of professional practice should be thought of as morally neutral.

The most significant moral questions are raised by sensitive practitioners within the field of sex research and therapy as well as by outsiders. It is to these questions that the remainder of this article is devoted.

Special bioethical concerns

The ethical issues mentioned in the opening paragraph of this article comprise the bulk of the moral problems in the area of sex research and sex therapy, so in that regard this field is best viewed as a special case of medical practice and research generally, and perhaps psychiatry, clinical and medical psychology, and counseling in particular. But to a greater extent than those more established fields, sex research and therapy are faced with the problem of quack therapists, untrained and methodologically sloppy researchers, and others engaged in profiteering ventures. These difficulties arise in part because of the relative newness of the field—a factor that tends to give rise to abuses easily perpetrated by quacks because no formal licensing or certification procedures as yet exist. Another factor contributing to abuses is the widespread attention devoted to sexual matters in current popular books and in the media. A whole spate of "self-help" books and magazine articles focus on promoting sexual pleasure and improving sexual performance, and even television programs have been known to refer to "performance anxiety" as a cause of impotence in the male. In light of this recent popularization and public emphasis on sexual success, it is not surprising that untrained persons, with a variety of nefarious motives,

have been able to dupe some members of an unsuspecting and vulnerable public. Certification or licensing of sex therapists can do much to alleviate these sorts of abuses, but it should be recalled that every profession suffers a number of unethical practitioners in spite of whatever stringent requirements may exist for authorized practice.

Therapist–patient intimacies. While the practice of sexual relations or other intimacies between a sex therapist and patient is probably the least frequent occurrence among all the activities that give rise to moral review in this field, it has nonetheless attracted much attention among sex therapists themselves and within the psychiatric profession generally (McDonald). Psychoanalytically trained or oriented therapists are quick to point out that engaging in such practices is most likely a manifestation of countertransference on the part of the therapist and does not represent a genuine or promising love relationship on the part of the therapist. In such cases, they hold, while the therapist might not be faulted for deliberately exploiting the doctor–patient relationship in order to seduce a person who is likely to have become dependent on him, still, it is argued, a competent professional ought not allow himself the indulgence of such self-deception as occurs in countertransference. It is possible, however, that a therapist may come to have deep and genuine feelings of love for a patient; in that case, it is usually maintained, the therapist's first responsibility is to terminate the therapeutic relationship.

The conclusions about therapist–patient intimacies drawn by psychoanalytic writers are based on the theoretical precepts of that position and usually rest on presuppositions about the unconscious motivations of patient or therapist or both. But there are other objections to this practice that need not rest on a particular theoretical viewpoint in psychiatry or psychology. These objections point out that the very nature of the therapist–patient relationship places the patient in a particularly vulnerable situation, whether because of a dependency already formed or else because the patient is suffering and holds high expectations for a cure or, at least, relief from intense suffering. It is not merely that the therapist is engaging in "unprofessional" conduct by having sexual relationships with his patient. It is, rather, that such intimacies will most likely not lead to an enduring relationship—an expectation that the patient will probably have

—and so the affair will end not by the therapist's having done good for the patient, but instead by his having done harm. A very few sex therapists appear to hold that, if a therapist's engaging in sexual relations with a patient successfully treats that patient's sexual dysfunction, such activity is not only appropriate but ethically desirable. But since such therapeutic outcomes can rarely be predicted in advance with any degree of precision, most sex therapists overwhelmingly agree that it is morally wrong ever to embark on such a course.

Informed consent. In both sex research and sex therapy, the same requirements for informed consent exist as are found in other research and clinical settings. The special difficulties that arise are found mostly within the area of sex research rather than sex therapy; moreover, the moral problems concerning whether consent is fully informed stem largely from the fact that most of such investigation is a species of social science research rather than from the fact that the subject matter of the research is human sexuality. A considerable amount of social science research essentially involves some sort of deception of the subject, without which the results of the research would be impossible to obtain. An example of this occurred in experiments in which subjects were presented with homosexual stimuli and then falsely told that they had reacted positively to the stimuli in order to assess their reactions to this information. Apart from the ethical issues that stem from the possibility of emotional distress suffered by subjects of such an experiment, there remains the problem of informed consent. It would seem to be impossible, in principle, to gain truly informed consent from subjects who are deliberately deceived about the purpose and nature of research in which they are participants.

Another type of social science research raises a different sort of ethical dilemma of informed consent. This type of investigation is not one in which active deception of volunteer subjects is carried out, but rather one in which observations are made in a natural setting without the knowledge of subjects being observed. In addition to raising ethical problems connected with the need to gain informed consent, this type of research is morally questionable on the grounds that it involves violations of the right of privacy. An example from the field of sex research is the infamous "Tearoom Trade" study, in which the investigator conducted observations of homosexual encounters in a public men's room. Not only

were the behaviors of persons recorded without their knowledge or consent in this phase of the study, but the investigator conducted a second stage of this research on the same subjects. At the time of the initial observations, he took note of the license plates of these persons, then obtained their names and addresses by means of that information, and subsequently interviewed them about their marital and sexual lives. Direct deception was employed in this second stage of the research, in that the investigator informed those whom he interviewed that he was conducting a public survey. Regardless of the fact that all names and addresses were destroyed and the identity of the subjects was not reported, a serious ethical question remains concerning the practice of watching people without their knowledge and recording their behavior without their consent (Humphreys; Warwick).

There are some problems of informed consent that occur in contexts of sex therapy as well as sex research, but instances of outright deception are less frequent in the therapeutic setting. One example is the presumed need for deception in order to evaluate the success of the therapy. One form of sex therapy involves the teaching of "heterosocial skills" to persons who exhibit one form or another of deviant sexual behavior. The heterosocial skill training itself consists of helping the subjects to give appropriate responses to heterosexual stimuli in a natural setting. Evaluation of the success of this form of therapy has included the use of a staged event in which a female, posing as another patient, interacts with the male patient in the therapist's waiting room. The patient's success in acquiring the heterosocial skills taught in the therapy is evaluated in terms of his responses to the woman in the staged event. The rationale for failure to obtain fully informed consent is that the patient's advance knowledge of the possibility of such assessments during the course of therapy is likely to invalidate the evaluation procedure, which is viewed as necessary for determining the patient's progress and the efficacy of the therapeutic techniques themselves.

There is a range of other examples in sex research and therapy where ethical issues of informed consent arise, but these are identical with familiar problems in the larger biomedical domain: the use of placebos, randomization in therapeutic trials, and the use of experimental drugs or other therapeutic techniques, such as sex reassignment, where the success of the outcome for the particular individual may be uncertain. As in the biomedical field generally, it is the responsibility of therapists and researchers to ensure that the consent obtained from patients or subjects is as fully informed and as genuinely voluntary as the nature of the person and the circumstances allow. It is a matter of continuing controversy whether or not prisoners are capable of granting fully voluntary consent —a dilemma that presents problems for research and therapy on criminal sex offenders. Current investigation into the effects of antiandrogens on chronic, aggressive sex offenders is aimed at therapy as well as social control. Researchers contend that prisoners constitute an ideal population for such research and report that criminal sex offenders who hear about such treatments beg for them as relief from the uncontrollable drives from which they suffer. The ethical debate centers on the question of whether those who try to protect prisoners from experimental treatments that may be beneficial, and that the prisoners themselves actively seek, are engaging in an unwarranted form of paternalism. Unlike research on prisoners that is nonbeneficial, experimental drug studies on sex offenders stand to benefit the subjects and may lead to their early release from prison. It is argued that, if such research proves successful, both the prisoners and society at large will be better off.

Confidentiality and privacy. Issues of privacy, while closely related to those of confidentiality, should be kept conceptually distinct. Invasions of privacy occur when a person is observed, listened to, touched, experimented on, filmed, or recorded without his knowledge or consent. Violations of confidentiality take place when a therapist, researcher, or ancillary personnel who have access to data about patients or research subjects reveal that data to some third party. A good example of a situation in which rights of privacy are likely to be violated in the area of sex research is the "Tearoom Trade" investigation discussed earlier in connection with informed consent.

The presumption in favor of maintaining confidentiality with respect to all data about patients and research subjects needs no special moral arguments in the domain of sex research and therapy. There are, however, several considerations that arise out of the sensitivity that most people harbor regarding their sexual lives and the embarrassment that normally follows revelation of such facts to others. First, there is the situation of group therapy. The danger here lies not in the therapist's revealing information about patients, but in the fact that other participants in the group therapy process are not bound by the strict requirements of confidentiality in the way that the therapist himself is. While it is obviously in the interest of every participant in group therapy to keep confidential what is learned about other participants, there seems to be a weaker obligation in this regard than many who enter group therapy might wish. Second, there is the problem in sex therapy where a married person reveals to the therapist intimate details about the marital partner. There is usually no good reason for the therapist to reveal such confidences to others; nevertheless, he may not feel bound by the same professional obligations to the spouse of a patient as he is to the patient himself. Third, there is the problem posed by the use of ancillary personnel in therapeutic contexts. Observation and monitoring often take place during sex therapy, and audio recording and videotaping are not uncommon. These are typically heard or viewed by research assistants and secretaries working in the therapist's office —a fact about which patients may be ignorant before, during, or after the course of therapy. Here again, these office workers may not feel bound by the therapist's duty to keep all information about patients confidential; and the more people who come to know a set of facts about someone, the more likely it is that confidential information will be revealed.

RUTH MACKLIN

[*Directly related are the previous article,* SCIENTIFIC AND CLINICAL PERSPECTIVES, *and the entries* CONFIDENTIALITY; INFORMED CONSENT IN HUMAN RESEARCH; INFORMED CONSENT IN THE THERAPEUTIC RELATIONSHIP; PRIVACY; SEXUAL BEHAVIOR; SEXUAL DEVELOPMENT; *and* SEXUAL ETHICS. *Other relevant material may be found under* PRISONERS, *article on* PRISONER EXPERIMENTATION; THERAPEUTIC RELATIONSHIP; *and* WOMEN AND BIOMEDICINE, *article on* WOMEN AS PATIENTS AND EXPERIMENTAL SUBJECTS.]

BIBLIOGRAPHY

HUMPHREYS, LAUD. *Tearoom Trade: Impersonal Sex in Public Places.* Observations. Chicago: Aldine Publishing Co., 1970.
McDONALD, MARGARET C. "Therapist/Patient Sex—The Veil Is Lifted." *Psychiatric News,* 2 July 1976, pp. 8, 10–11; 16 July 1976, pp. 12–13.
MASTERS, WILLIAM H.; JOHNSON, VIRGINIA E.; and KOLODNY, ROBERT C., eds. *Ethical Issues in Sex Research and Sex Therapy.* Boston: Little, Brown & Co., 1977.
WARWICK, DONALD P. "Tearoom Trade: Means and Ends in Social Research." *Hastings Center Studies* 1, no. 1 (1973), pp. 27–38.

SEXUAL BEHAVIOR

The technologies of biology and medicine have helped shape new attitudes about what is valuable in sexual matters and have also contributed to the therapies by which people may now seek to fulfill otherwise frustrated sexual obligations. Furthermore, recent changes in attitudes toward sexual behavior have created a new spectrum of ethical problems. This entry analyzes the technological, social, and historical factors that have resulted in a new ethos concerning the nature of ethical problems dealing with sex.

Few subjects in the entire history of Western thought have done as thorough an "about face" in public acceptability at all levels as has that of sexual behavior in the twentieth century. The "sexual revolution" has been so rapid and so massive, at least in the United States and the wealthier European democracies, that its social and ethical implications cannot yet be documented very thoroughly. No one can say precisely how much this "revolution" has taken hold or how long it may last. It has been accelerating, however, since the Second World War. The background for it rests both in the biological sexual peculiarities of human beings and in conflicting cultural forces that have shaped Western sexual norms through the Victorian era. The first part of this article, therefore, will briefly discuss those factors which constituted the background for the sexual revolution.

The Victorian period can be considered the Age of Repression with respect to sexuality (London, 1973), but the groundwork was then laid for the sexual revolution by medical and other scholars, who made sexual behavior into a legitimate subject of professional interest. From the end of the last century until the end of the Second World War was a period for the spreading acceptability of sexual interest among respectable people, with growing belief in the right to sexual satisfaction in marriage. Since then, the interaction of favorable publicity and facilitating technology has created an explosion of sexual activity and, corollary to it, great changes in norms of sexual conduct, sexual attitudes, and attitudes toward marriage and the family.

Part two will deal with the weapons of sexual revolution (the publicity of sex, the technology of sex), part three with the ensuing changes in contemporary norms for sexual behavior, and part four with some contemporary problems and long-range implications connected with them.

Background for the sexual revolution

Biological background of sexual behavior. Human sexual behavior is the product of long experience in physical contact and social training, starting with that between mothers and infants and continuing until maturational processes have directed the playful explorations of children into the lustful aims of adolescence and adulthood. Even then, sexual activities vary more with what people have *learned* than with any species-common biological traits. Even the objects of sexual activity are learned, and sexual aims may vary widely within a single individual. That sex impulses are "natural" but sex acts are not is the primary biological fact of human sexual behavior.

Another essential biological fact distinguishes human sexual behavior from that of other species: Humans do not have a rutting season or an estrus cycle to force their sexual interests into narrow seasonal or cyclic patterns. Human females are potentially receptive to sexual advances at any time; human males are potentially interested in sex at all times. In effect, this gives us a higher sex drive than other animals. For them, adult life has sexual seasons; for us, it *is* the sexual season.

In the absence of seasonal limitations, the great advantages in learning ability of humans guarantee that sexual motives, in the broadest sense, pervade our lives. Rapid *conditionability* and the depth of human *memory* capacity conspire to ensure that our sex drive attaches our emotions deeply to sexual objects, shapes our acts toward the satisfaction of that drive through them, and renews our interest in those objects over a long time. Freud may have overstated the uniqueness of sexual motives in behavior, but not their ubiquity. And Harlow's empirical studies of primates have convinced most observers that adult sexuality depends on the preparatory physical contacts of infancy.

Cultural forces in human sexuality. Culture actualizes human sexual biology and regulates it among people who live together, weaving sexual patterns into a social fabric. The short-range consequences of sexual motivation for interpersonal relationships and the long-range effects on family structure, property distribution, and the organization of power in social groups make sexual conduct the target of regulation in any society. Sometimes this regulation has worked through religious rituals and restrictions; at other times it has been controlled by secular regulatory agencies. In general, sex has been subject to both religious and secular authorities, generally reinforcing one another. All societies, evidently, have always practiced some kind of regulation over some aspects of sexual behavior. The permitted and prohibited practices across all cultures have been as varied as the variety of sexual practices possible. Homosexuality, prostitution, bestiality, relations between blood relatives or nonrelatives, masturbation, and abstinence have all been prohibited, tolerated, required, ignored, and punished at different times by different societies under different conditions for different reasons. All of these, and virtually all other sex acts, have been considered sacred, profane, natural, perverse, healthful, diseased, blessed, cursed, abominable, and virtually all other values. All sexual behavior is *acculturated,* despite its firm rooting individual urges, longings, and fears. Religious institutions are among the chief sources of acculturation, so we may look to the varying religious beliefs and values of most societies as a primary source of sexual norms and values.

Sexual norms of Judaism and Christianity. The "Judeo-Christian" tradition, as it is glibly called, consists of many traditions extant over more than three millennia, and often at odds with each other. Different sexual norms and values are implicit in different biblical stories and precepts. Even so, by the advent of Christianity there were general norms of sexual behavior within Judaism that legitimized sexual pleasure within marriage, independently of its procreative function (e.g., a husband was legally obligated to give his wife sexual pleasure regularly), and disapproved of virtually all other sexual behavior, with objections ranging from distaste to condemnation.

Christianity absorbed most of the sexual prohibitions of Judaism, but with a critical change in attitude—marriage was not to be the joyous expression of the sexual impulse, but merely an alternative to the perdition that would otherwise follow its unleashing. In the traditional Christian ideal as it evolved, love was pure to the degree that it was disembodied or, better still, in firm renunciation of lust.

Victorian love.   Against this background, the ideals of romantic love blossomed in Europe. Romanticism lifted woman from the role of satanic agent or temptress into an ideal figure but, in so doing, unsexed her. The apotheosis of romantic love depicted the object of purest love united with the object of the only legitimate sexual aim, in matrimony. The marriage ideal was that of blissful happiness between two people who would create a loving Christian family, revolving around the tender devotion of wife and mother. She would, of course, be chosen by an ardent and devoted suitor, and would respond to him, if she requited his feelings.

This blend of courtship, housekeeping, and propagation became the Victorian ideal of love (Hunt, 1959). It had already become popular late in the eighteenth century (Victoria was crowned in 1837) and was dominant by the latter part of the nineteenth. However, the role of sexuality in this scheme was always ambiguous.

The Victorian wife was to be sweet-tempered, docile, adoring, and utterly subservient to her husband, who was to dominate the relationship in all respects. Neither admitted to any sexual feelings, and the more "pure" their love, the less lustful it was presumed to be. Wifely modesty required the wearing of copious garments, never exposing the body naked (not to physician, not to husband), never naming body parts or functions, and never showing passion in the sex act. By and large, the husband reciprocated in modesty and language, and did his "connubial duty" quickly and silently.

Masturbation, then considered a serious disease, was called "the secret vice" (Engelhardt). Homosexuality was an unspeakable perversion. Prostitution was rampant in Victorian England, and London became the pornography capital of the world. Women, in most medical opinion, did not masturbate unless they were quite demented and did not have sexual passions at all if they were quite well. At best, sex was for procreation only, and the more silently it was used, even for that, the better. It was against this repression that the "sexual revolution" took place.

The weapons of sexual revolution

Two determinants of the sexual revolution offer useful means of tracking its progress, assessing its current status, and identifying some of its major social and ethical implications. These are the *technology* of sexual convenience and safety and the *publicity* that describes sexual conduct and attitudes. The publicity surrounding sex popularizes it, indexes its acceptability and, willy-nilly, promotes what it surveys. The technology of sex becomes known through the publicity, which leads to its widespread use. Technology's use, in turn, fosters its improvement, as it makes it easier for people to express their sexuality safely. This expression is then publicized and, by acknowledging sex without condemning it, tends to validate it socially. The full circle etches the social change into the public consciousness.

The publicity of sex. A century ago, the publicity of sex consisted of a professional literature, written by physicians for each other, and a popular literature, with pornography at one extreme and sermonics at the other. There was no journalism on the subject, nor any scholarly literature. By the turn of the century that had changed greatly; it has continued changing at an accelerating rate.

Professional sex literature was greatly influenced by the publication of Richard von Krafft-Ebing's *Psychopathia Sexualis* in 1886. Written for other physicians, its descriptions of sexual behavior reverted to Latin. Though his views were advanced for the times, Krafft-Ebing still devoted extensive space to discussion of masturbation, which he thought reflected a "hereditary taint." A more general scholarly work of perhaps even greater influence was Havelock Ellis's seven-volume *Studies in the Psychology of Sex,* the first volume of which appeared in 1901. Its explicit descriptions of sexual behavior were in plain English.

The most important intellectual break with Victorian sexuality came in the psychoanalytic theory of Sigmund Freud, whose central thesis argued that the primary psychological motivation of human beings, from childhood on, is sex. Psychoanalytic theory was not widely accepted in medical or psychiatric circles for more than a generation, and then not comfortably. But its slow advance, both through the practice of psychoanalysis, with its emphasis on the sexual motifs in people's personal histories, and through the intellectual interest it stimulated outside of psychiatry, eventually made it the most effective advertisement for sexual awareness.

The immediate predecessor of contemporary professional sexual publicity is the monumental work of Alfred Kinsey and his collaborators at Indiana University, surveying male (1948) and female sexuality (1953) among Americans. A biologist by training, Kinsey established a sexual studies institute and ran the most elaborate surveys done until then with great scientific care, publishing his results in two long scholarly monographs.

Both books were immediate bestsellers. They offered contemporary information about the general public, not about social deviants. Readers learned two main things from them: first, that forbidden sex was far more practiced than had been realized—people discovered that they were not the only ones who masturbated or who had had homosexual experiences; second, of shockingly positive interest, was the discovery that talking about sex was easier than anyone had ever realized. The Kinsey publications, despite some criticism of them on both scientific and ethical grounds, signaled the intellectual finish of sexual puritanism in this society. We may mark the date at 1950. Since then, changes in the publicity of sex have occurred at an accelerating pace.

By 1959 a court decree had rescued D. H. Lawrence's *Lady Chatterley's Lover* from designation as "hard-core pornography," and in the decade that followed sexually explicit literature became widely available. It ranged from Ralph Ginzburg's art-book magazine, *Eros,* first published in 1962, through drugstore paperbacks of pornographic classics such as *Fanny Hill* and *Autobiography of a Flea.*

By 1970 sexually explicit films had graduated from 8-millimeter silent movies shown in the back rooms of bordellos into hard-core pornography, both heterosexual and homosexual, shown in commercial theaters and advertised in daily newspapers. In some cities, there were also open presentations of live "sex shows." *Deep Throat,* perhaps the best known of these films, was reviewed at length in such major U.S. magazines as *Time* and *Newsweek.*

In 1967 the U.S. Congress created a commission to investigate the effects of pornography on the public. Its majority findings, made public in 1970, argued that the government should not legislate the restriction of sexually explicit material to adults because it lacked evidence that pornography was harmful. The publication of such material has exploded since then. Its availability virtually everywhere today is one index of how radically the perspective of the entire society has changed toward sexual behavior.

The technology of sex. As publicity about sex raises interest in exploring it, technology provides the opportunity to pursue those interests. A major technological contribution in the United States to free sexual behavior was the invention of the automobile, a readily available, low-cost, mobile bedroom. It satisfied a vital prerequisite for sex relations in Western society, the need for *privacy,* probably an even more important constraint on sex than fear of pregnancy or damnation.

The most important technological impetus toward freer sex, of course, has been improvement in contraceptive methods. Primitive contraceptives have been around for millennia, but the modern diaphragm, intrauterine devices, and "the pill" have become efficient contraceptives only since 1960. Part of their significance lies in the fact that these devices, for the first time in history, placed the control of pregnancy in the hands of women (London, 1977). The repression of sexuality has been historically allied with the subjugation of women. Women's economic independence and education are at least as important in the sexual revolution as the technology of contraception.

Improved technology makes it possible to indulge the sexual appetites that increased publicity now says are commonplace. The result of more sexual activity, in turn, is more public interest in it, and more desensitization to variants of it, which ultimately produces striking shifts in norms of conduct and of attitude.

Contemporary sexual norms

Contemporary normative changes.   The content of contemporary normative changes and their pervasiveness cannot be measured very precisely, but the attempts by scientific survey at pinpointing these changes have been good enough, even at their worst, to give some important indications of what has happened. The most important data on these changes come from Morton Hunt's report of the Playboy Foundation's 1972 effort "to resurvey the territory mapped out in 1948 and 1953" by the Kinsey reports. An independent *Redbook* magazine survey of 1975, reported by Robert and Amy Levin, offers corroboration of Hunt's careful work.

The forefront of normative changes in sexual behavior apparently is to be found among educated, urban people of at least moderate means. They popularize important social changes, index their acceptability, and legitimize them. Their sexual behavior may not reflect that of the general population so much as predict it.

If the *Playboy* study is accurate, then in only two decades between Kinsey and Hunt there was a dramatic change in the norms of sexual behavior (Kinsey, 1948, 1953; Hunt, 1974). People became more permissive sexually than they had ever been, young people most; sexual behavior became more varied; and the ages at which people admitted to beginning certain sex acts was lower. In every age group, ninety percent of respondents agreed that "sex is one of the most beautiful parts of life."

In the *Playboy* survey, more than eighty percent of both sexes felt strongly that the male should not always be the partner to initiate sex. Sixty to eighty-four percent of males approved of premarital sex for men and forty-four percent approved of it for women. Females were only slightly less permissive. Fifty-nine percent of males and forty-three percent of females thought that premarital sex improved the likelihood of stable and happy marriage. A Roper poll in the 1940s had found that sixty-four to seventy-two percent of a national sample felt that men should require virginity in the girls they marry, while less than half of the *Playboy* respondents felt that way. Recent attitudes were also much more liberal toward homosexuality, toward masturbation, and toward legalizing prostitution, abortion, and no-fault divorce. Almost one-third of men and one-fifth of women in Hunt's report did not oppose mate swapping. Three-quarters or more of both sexes approved of oral–genital and anal–genital contacts. Fifty to ninety percent said they were sexually aroused by pornography, four times as large as Kinsey's figures for women and double those for men.

Kinsey found that over a quarter of unmarried males had not had intercourse by the age of twenty-five, but Hunt found only about three percent. There was an even greater increase in premarital intercourse among females. In Kinsey's sample, one-third had had intercourse by age twenty-five, but in Hunt's report, over two-thirds had done so. Among women married before age twenty-five, Kinsey found forty-two to forty-seven percent had had premarital intercourse, while Hunt found eighty-one percent. "The double standard," Hunt concludes, has apparently "been relegated to the scrap heap of history."

There has also been a great increase in sexual variation. Only forty percent of Kinsey's married men had ever kissed their wives' genitals, but sixty-three percent of Hunt's sample had done so within the past year. Only forty percent of Kinsey's sample had ever been fellated by their wives, but fifty-eight percent of Hunt's sample had been within the year. Kinsey offered no data on anal intercourse (he said it was too rare to collect statistics on), but Hunt found that about twenty-five percent of married couples under age thirty-five use anal intercourse occasionally.

Hunt also found that sex acts with animals were less common than among Kinsey's sample, and homosexuality was apparently no more common. Hunt also found that only two percent of married males and less than two percent of married females had ever done wife swapping, and most of those only rarely. He also found a moderate increase in *covert* extramarital affairs among men under twenty-five since Kinsey's day, but a big increase for women under twenty-five, though still lower than the male level of activity.

The apparently accelerating differences in the generation from Kinsey to Hunt are also seen in the *Redbook Magazine* 1975 survey of 100,000 female readers (Levin and Levin). Among married women, oral–genital contact is practiced by eighty to ninety percent of women at all ages (younger ones more), half have had anal intercourse, ninety percent initiate lovemaking sometimes (sixty percent initiate it at least half the time), and almost three-quarters have masturbated with varying frequency since marrying. Ninety percent of all married respondents under twenty-five had had premarital intercourse, and the rate accelerated steadily among women married since 1964. Thirty percent of all respondents have had extramarital sex relations, and among the most likely to have extramarital affairs are those whose premarital sex activities started earliest, those who have been married longest, and those who work full time. Kinsey found only nine percent of wives under twenty-five had extramarital affairs; *Playboy* and *Redbook* found twenty-five percent. *Redbook* found mate swapping among less than four percent of its respondents (compared to just under two percent of Hunt's female sample) and homosexual contacts among four percent of married women (Kinsey reported three percent), but among ten percent of separated, divorced, or widowed females.

Neither the *Playboy* nor the *Redbook* survey concluded that these permissive changes indicated casual attitudes toward sex or unhappy marriages. Hunt points out that his respondents are highly selective of both sex acts and sex partners and regard sexual behavior as very important emotionally rather than merely sensual gratification. Robert Levin notes that, while sexual satisfaction is highly correlated to satisfaction with marriage among his respondents, half or more of those women who have outside affairs also report satisfaction, sexually and otherwise, with their marriages. Add the fact that both males and females masturbate much more

than they used to, and Hunt's conclusion that there is simply less guilt about sex of all kinds nowadays seems justified; more people have experimental attitudes, permitting them to do things once forbidden without wounding their consciences or their marriages.

Some of the differences between survey results may reflect differences in sampling procedures, but even accounting for them the general interpretation of increased permissiveness would still hold. The changes reported since Kinsey are too consistent and too correlated with permissive changes in laws governing sex to be seen as anything other than indices of widespread and genuine change in the United States.

Some of the changes in reportage may not signify so much changes in actual behavior as changes in people's willingness to admit to things they may have been doing all along. Such admission still indicates enormous changes in attitudes and when such changes become public knowledge, they pique public interest. Interest then stimulates experimentation, and attitude change yields behavior change. If the behavior is gratifying, it can then become normative. Sexual experimentation seems to gratify a number of people, some of whom are more public about it than they would have been previously.

The display of sexual permissiveness. The 1970 report of the U.S. Congressional Commission on Obscenity and Pornography released a flood of sexual publicity. "Even in respectable literary works, descriptions of sex acts . . . included scenes . . . of such explicitness that Lady Chatterley seemed second cousin to Heidi. . . . Historically unprintable words were, by 1970, being freely used in respectable books . . . and in late 1972, the magisterial Oxford English dictionary . . . included the word fuck in its long awaited supplement" (Hunt, 1974). The trend toward sexual explicitness soon spread to "teaser" literature (*Playboy* started showing pubic hair in 1972), to movies, and to television, and has continued what seems to be a linear expansion. *High Society*, the photographically elegant, sexually explicit, formal equivalent of *Playboy*, began publication in 1976. Then too began *Mary Hartman, Mary Hartman*, the nighttime television soap opera, which dealt explicitly with adultery, homosexuality, impotence, and so forth—a generation away from daytime soap operas, which treated the same themes by innuendo rather than illustration.

Pornographic movies such as *Deep Throat* best illustrate the phenomenon involved, because they are the most public possible demonstration of interest. Such movies had long existed, but in the 1970s they began to be publicly displayed, publicly commented on, and publicly viewed. *Deep Throat* grossed more than 30 million dollars worth of ticket sales through 1974, according to Hollywood's *Daily Variety* and was viewed principally by an educated, wealthy audience, who likely learned about the movie from *Time* magazine and attended it with sweethearts, spouses, and casual dates. Nothing testifies better to normative acceptability than casually public behavior.

The same process that has desensitized guilt and anxiety about public prurient interests has supported more and more public pornographic displays. Thus, in most liquor stores in Los Angeles and on many street racks one can buy an array of pornographic picture newspapers, titled *Ecstasy, Pulse, Throb, Hump,* and *Finger,* whose content ranges from very explicit photographic displays of professional models in varied sexual acts, with accompanying stories, to advertisements for liaisons, dirty movies, and stimulating devices.

More important still is the fact that the main sellers are ostensibly "reader written" magazines, such as *Love,* which consist largely of dirty pictures sent in by readers of themselves, ostensibly filmed at home and accompanied by personal stories. The magazines award free subscriptions for such tantalizing pictures and stories.

The most significant display of permissiveness, however, comes not in such "shadow" material but in the most legitimate arenas of public discussion—newspapers, respectable magazines, radio, television, films, and theater. In an already permissive atmosphere, once secretive deviance now becomes public defiance of earlier constraints, and a demand for recognition and acceptance. The present status of homosexuality evidences the success of such demands.

Homosexuality: a case study in contemporary change. Kinsey estimated that less than two percent of women and four percent of men were exclusively homosexual, with thirteen percent of males predominantly homosexual for at least three years. Subsequent surveys suggest that he overestimated and that the actual incidence of homosexuality has not increased since his time.

What has changed are taboo public attitudes toward homosexuality and the willingness of homosexuals to admit their sexual orientation and demand its acceptance. In 1953 the U.S. government was officially denying classified jobs

to suspected homosexuals because of their susceptibility to blackmail. In September 1975 an Air Force sergeant was the cover figure on *Time* magazine because he provoked a discharge from service in order to make a court test of the military's ban on homosexuals. In 1973 Hunt estimates there were 600 homosexual organizations and publications in the United States; in 1975 by *Time's* estimate, there were 800 gay groups and 4,000 gay bars. The *Advocate,* a national newspaper for homosexuals, claimed a circulation of 60,000 by 1976. If the actual incidence of homosexuality is the same as a generation ago, then these facts are convincing indices of its changed acceptability. The surveys concur. Kinsey reported general hostility towards homosexuality, while Hunt reports that nearly half of *Playboy* respondents believe it should be legalized. In fact, eleven states, according to *Time,* had repealed their antisodomy laws by 1975.

The second step in acceptability is public acknowledgement. This has come in the willingness of several large corporations, and of the U.S. Civil Service Commission, to hire admitted homosexuals. Also, homosexuals have lobbied at political conventions, demanded their own facilities on some college campuses, established their own churches, and sought court action to legalize homosexual marriage.

Further legitimation of homosexuality was its removal from the realm of pathological behavior. In 1973 the American Psychiatric Association officially decided that homosexuality was not, per se, "a psychiatric disorder," implying that there was nothing wrong with homosexuals who did not want to change their condition.

The final validation is the refusal to treat those who do not want to give up homosexuality. Some thoughtful professionals are now arguing that it is unethical to agree out of hand to change the sexual preferences even of homosexuals who want them changed (Davison), though this is clearly a minority opinion.

Thus homosexuality has passed from a criminal act, widely distasteful to the general public, through the role of pathological condition, and now seeks the social status of acceptable and unremarkable difference, like race and gender and age, which, as such, should not disqualify people from most public functions or from *any* public approval. Whether it should be seen in this way is paradigmatic of the main social and ethical problem of contemporary sexual behavior—perspective on the permissible.

Problems of contemporary sex

Acts are simply acts, as Aldous Huxley notes, until one starts talking about them, thinking about them, abstracting about them. Then they become ethical problems. So it has been with sex. Two generations ago, people wondered if they were doing the right thing. Now, they wonder if they are "doing the thing right." The shift in word order reflects the shift in the character of social attitudes toward sex.

The definition of all problems surrounding sex is now visible largely as a matter of perspective. Homosexuality, for instance, is widely regarded as not damaging psychologically. And were it damaging, it is still unclear that anything should be done to stop it—marriage, at least for women, is demonstrably more damaging both mentally and psychologically (Tavris and Offir). What makes sex ethically problematic is the moral conflict of contemporary norms with traditional ones; what makes it socially problematic is its effect on other behavior.

Since about 1960 sexual mores have been becoming increasingly permissive—so quickly that most adults in the 1970s were raised to more conservative standards than they practiced. Some conflict results. People's sexual expectations have been turned up, as it were, but their anxiety and guilt continue to operate from more conservative platforms then their behavioral expectations. The moral anxiety produced by this ambivalence has behavioral consequences in symptoms that have been classical since Victorian times and were probably even more widespread then: frigidity and vaginismus in women; secondary impotence and premature ejaculation in men.

Younger people, though raised with more permissive sexual standards, may have the same behavior problems resulting, ironically, from *performance* anxiety rather than *moral* anxiety. Increased expectations, such as the notion that women are entitled to expect orgasmic satisfaction from sex, places a burden of skill, if not of artistry, on young males, which they often fear, and a burden of expectation on young females that, unmet in their early sex encounters, leaves them as nonplussed as their partners. Since sex education in America lags far behind sexual action, the results of performance anxiety also help populate the sex therapy clinics.

Sex therapy. No one knows if sexual dysfunctions are more or less common today then they used to be, but the allowable public display of sexual interest and concern certainly lets them be confessed and cured more openly. Modern sex therapy became widespread since 1959 largely through the work of William Masters and Virginia Johnson, especially *Human Sexual Inadequacy*. It is estimated that there are now about four thousand sex therapy clinics in the United States. Some of the treatments used are simple variants of conventional interview psychotherapy, in which the substance of treatment is talk alone. Others, however, involve varying degrees of physical contact between sex partners. In some instances clinics may provide a *sexual surrogate*, that is, a therapist who treats the patient by performing as a sex partner in some indicated therapeutic sequence. Some critics of this practice consider surrogates prostitutes. This fallacious pejorative misses the main ethical issue involved, namely, that sex acts in the therapeutic encounter may be improper practice, taking the doctor too deeply into the life of the patient, violating the privileged, hence private, experience that the conventional wisdom has always labeled therapy. The issue is the normative status of sex.

The same question arises more subtly in ordinary psychotherapy. Some psychotherapists have sex relations with some patients and rationalize it on technical grounds that it is good for the patient and on moral grounds that there is nothing wrong with it (Shephard). The practice, still mostly unadvertised, is evidently becoming common. It does not quite parallel the evidently widespread phenomenon of physicians' having sex with their medical patients. The latter is practiced as a secret vice; the former is rationalized as a secret virtue. If so, it cannot remain secret for long. Will it, then, still emerge as virtue? Perhaps so.

The unknowns of sexual transition. Whether we are talking about sex therapy, homosexuality, extramarital relations, sex education, or sex in prisons and other public institutions, the same issue is joined: that of the limits of the sexually permissible. Our Western society no longer has a firm ethical base, as it may once have had in its dominant religious traditions, for limiting sexual legitimacy to the marriage bed. And as the repressive lid comes off of sexuality, the impetus to broaden the limits of what is permissible continues to grow, while the grounds for arguing restraint decrease. The U.S. Supreme Court refuses to discuss the subject altogether, dismissing it with the legal device of "community standards" as the proper basis for sexual norms. Appeals to mental or physical health as rational bases for curbing any kind of pleasure seeking have provided no platforms of much convincing value to anyone. It is plain that there is some real cost in human misery created by increasing sexual freedom, as there has been by restricting it, but there is no way to balance one misery against another and argue clearly what the general welfare concerning sex might be. The ethics of sex has always been anchored to the traditions and aspirations of society. Contemporary Western society has broken with the traditions that contained sexuality and has not established aspirations that might hope to contain it. What has been evolving, since midcentury, has been a virtual "norm of transition," in which an ever bolder libertarian ethic of individual conduct presses against an ever weaker normative ethic of social restraint.

No one knows what the limits of sexual permissiveness will be, nor how pervasive the changed norms of sexual behavior will be, nor what their indirect effects will be. Homosexuality and sexual dysfunctions, as we have seen, are more widely acknowledged than they were, but they also may be more prevalent. Certainly, every kind of heterosexual conduct is more permissible now than a generation ago. With the technology of sex developing rapidly, even making transsexual surgery practical, and women's status changing to destroy systematically double standards of sexual conduct, there is reason to think that the sexual revolution presages the sexual norms of American society in the twenty-first century. A complacent view might say that sex will become a socially accepted medium of casual recreation. A less optimistic view would worry that the changes possibly could ravage society.

Sex, family, and crime.   There are some unhappy social changes correlated with the sexual revolution. Striking increases in the incidence of divorce and of violent personal crime have accompanied the changes in sexual behavior among Americans. There may be no causal relation between them, but sociologist Philip Rieff, citing the Roman Empire as example, argues that the unlimited expression of sexuality is inevitably correlated with a general social acceptance of violence (Rieff).

Even if sex is not directly implicated in violent crime, it may well be connected with decaying family life. If norms are the social expression of individual character, and if the development of character, with its conservative restraints on individual expressiveness, depends on children's identification with the behavioral and ethical models of their parents, then stable families are the key to a society in which normative restraints operate effectively. In the United States in 1975, the number of divorces actually exceeded the number of marriages, and in 1976, in Washington, D.C., the number of children born out of wedlock exceeded the number born to married women. These figures reflect long-term trends, the result of which is that more and more children in this country are being raised by from one to many parents in homes whose occupants change a good deal. In a society where norms are already in such flux, the effect on character can only be more unstabilizing. Permissive sexual norms contribute something to these trends by making extramarital sex more acceptable than it was, thus increasing the availability of new partners, and by making sexual frustration into legitimate grounds for dissatisfaction with marriage.

The de-moralization of sex.   It is also unclear whether sex will long remain a topic for ethical concerns of any kind in our society. That it should not be is unthinkable to some people. But in the long view of human society, and the shifting ethical concerns that have marked change in it, many such changes have occurred. Many people once responded to food in the same terms of temptation and sin with which their children may still be treating sex. But how many Jews today, whose grandparents abhorred eating forbidden foods, think twice about buying non-kosher meat, or about eating it with butter? And how many young Catholics, devout in all other respects, even remember that, when they were small, they ate no meat on Fridays?

If sexual norms were to follow a similar course, then common attitudes and behavior connected with it, like those that predominate today with food, might become matters of preference, of health and manners, not of religion and morals. Some people choose diets for their ostensible impact on health—shellfish and pork are as forbidden now to some people because of cholesterol as they were to others because of divine proscription. And the ritual aspects of health food faddery, with vitamin munching, preservative deprecation, and organic-food apotheosizing may have the same saving quality for them as the religious control of food ever did.

Health could become the kind of rationalization for free sexual conduct as it is for food selection. Indeed, health is the transitional justification still used for sexual *restriction* by people whose religious traditions of sexual conduct could not be justified for them from the religious proscriptions alone. So—masturbation was once bad for you because God forbade it, and then was bad for you because it made you crazy; then it was not *so* bad for you, but it was unhealthy to be preoccupied with it—now, says the obverse side of the same argument, it is good for you because it relieves sexual tensions and frustrations, thereby freeing you of their gratuitous burden. Other things in the canon of sexual prohibitions and restrictions have run the same course, and still others doubtless will. Some physicians today tell males with prostate trouble that increasing the frequency of sexual relations will improve their condition. Some health moralists (and their publishers) have discovered that sex is strenuous exercise, exercise is good for the heart, lungs, and disposition—so more sex, maybe more athletically, makes you healthier. It is not hard, once this door is opened, to stretch the point to all kinds of activity (including rape and mugging). Especially once the distinction between physical health and mental health is blurred, as perhaps it often should be, and the distinction between individual health and society's health grows similarly indistinct, the possibilities of permissible, even laudable, sexual variety grow even greater. They include things like the public practice of group sex, of homosexuality, perhaps even of incest. Indeed, there is already a literature on the last, let alone pornography on incest. Might the argument that it is good for families to do things together, and that nothing could be more intimate, and therefore wholesome, than family sex play, sound less strange in another generation than it does now? Just as Morton Hunt reports highly permissive attitudes toward aspects of sex that Kinsey could not even ask about a generation earlier, the next generation's survey may be full of questions and answers about things that barely crossed Hunt's mind.

Even with permissiveness run rampant by freeing sex from religious restrictions and endorsing it with hygienic fervor, however, we may not find ourselves in a social milieu where "anything goes." For there are always manners to pattern important social interactions, and there may be some potential limits on sex dictated by them. People who feel no religious restrictions on their eating habits still do not generally stuff themselves to bursting and certainly do not engage publicly in every kind of eating behavior.

Sex, like all appetites, also has some limits.

And like all appetite indulgences, some ways of satisfying it are more likely to be socially approved than others. The most important characteristics of sex may finally be that it is so deeply intertwined with affection and that it is still the chief human instrument for making progeny, and these may suggest some limits on its exercise, though they do not reveal the contents of those limits. The question, finally, is the extent to which sex will remain an important social interaction rather than become a merely urgent, or even whimsical, personal indulgence. Its ethical implications and its social importance are obverses of each other.

PERRY LONDON

[*Directly related are the entries* SEX THERAPY AND SEX RESEARCH, *article on* SCIENTIFIC AND CLINICAL PERSPECTIVES; SEXUAL DEVELOPMENT; *and* SEXUAL ETHICS. *Other relevant material may be found under* POPULATION ETHICS: RELIGIOUS TRADITIONS, *articles on* ROMAN CATHOLIC PERSPECTIVES *and* PROTESTANT PERSPECTIVES; *and* WOMEN AND BIOMEDICINE, *article on* WOMEN AS PATIENTS AND EXPERIMENTAL SUBJECTS. *See also:* HOMOSEXUALITY.]

BIBLIOGRAPHY

DAVISON, GERALD C. "Homosexuality: The Ethical Challenge." *Journal of Consulting and Clinical Psychology* 44 (1976): 157–162.

ELLIS, HAVELOCK. *Studies in the Psychology of Sex.* 7 vols. Philadelphia: F. A. Davis Co., 1901–1928.

ENGELHARDT, H. TRISTRAM, JR. "The Disease of Masturbation: Values and the Concepts of Disease." *Bulletin of the History of Medicine* 48 (1974): 234–248.

FREUD, SIGMUND. "Three Contributions to the Theory of Sex." *The Basic Writings of Sigmund Freud.* Translated and edited by A. A. Brill. New York: Modern Library, 1938, bk. 3, pp. 553–629.

"Gays on the March." *Time,* 8 September 1975, pp. 32–37, 43.

GILDER, GEORGE F. *Sexual Suicide.* New York: Quadrangle Books, 1973.

GOLDBERG, BEN ZION. *The Sacred Fire: The Story of Sex in Religion.* Garden City, N.Y.: Garden City Publishing Co., 1930.

HARLOW, HARRY FREDERICK; McGAUGH, JAMES L.; and THOMPSON, RICHARD F. *Psychology.* San Francisco: Albion Publishing Co., 1971.

HUNT, MORTON M. *The Natural History of Love.* New York: Alfred A. Knopf, 1959.

———. *Sexual Behavior in the 1970s.* New York: Dell Publishing Co., 1974.

KINSEY, ALFRED CHARLES; POMEROY, WARDELL B.; and MARTIN, CLYDE E. *Sexual Behavior in the Human Male.* Philadelphia: W. B. Saunders Co., 1948.

———; POMEROY, WARDELL B.; MARTIN, CLYDE E.; and GEBHARD, P. H. *Sexual Behavior in the Human Female.* Philadelphia: W. B. Saunders Co., 1953.

KRAFFT-EBING, RICHARD VON. *Psychopathia Sexualis: A Medico-Forensic Study* (1886). Translated by F. J. Rebman. New York: Pioneer Publications, 1939.

LEVIN, ROBERT J. "The Redbook Report on Premarital and Extramarital Sex: The End of the Double Standard?" *Redbook,* October 1975, pp. 38, 40, 42, 44, 190, 192.

——, and LEVIN, AMY. "Sexual Pleasure: The Surprising Preferences of 100,000 Women." *Redbook,* September 1975, pp. 51–58.

LONDON, PERRY. *Behavior Control.* 2d ed. New York: New American Library, 1977.

——. "The Future of Psychotherapy." *Hastings Center Report* 3, no. 6 (1973), pp. 10–13.

MASTERS, WILLIAM H., and JOHNSON, VIRGINIA E. *Human Sexual Inadequacy.* Boston: Little, Brown & Co., 1970.

RIEFF, PHILIP. *Fellow Teachers.* New York: Harper & Row, 1973.

SHEPHARD, MARTIN. *The Love Treatment: Sexual Intimacy between Patients and Psychotherapists.* New York: P. H. Wyden, 1971.

TAVRIS, CAROL, and OFFIR, CAROLE. *The Longest War: Sex Differences in Perspective.* New York: Harcourt, Brace, Jovanovitch, 1977.

United States, Commission on Obscenity and Pornography. *The Report of the Commission on Obscenity and Pornography.* Introduction by Clive Barnes. A New York Times Book. New York: Bantam Books, 1970.

SEXUAL DEVELOPMENT

More than any other modality of experience, sex expresses the human being's dual identity as organism and as person. On the one hand, it is an episodic desire, necessary to the survival of the species and correlated with measurable physiological processes; on the other, it is inextricably tied to the human need for intimacy and in this respect is subject to many psychological vicissitudes. Mature sexuality is the synthesis of a psychobiological activity grounded in the body and a distinctively human activity grounded in consciousness and culture.

As scientists our focus will be on the psychological aspects of sexual development. As moral philosophers our concern will be not with the rightness or wrongness of any sexual behavior, nor with the wisdom of any pedagogical practice, but with the ways in which, under favorable circumstances, the human infant becomes an adult who is capable of having and of generating values in any significant sense and of bestowing value on others. Our thesis is that these capacities emerge out of, or are inextricable from, the processes which we shall trace in our discussion of sexual development.

This suggests that the study of sexuality is one way of investigating the central problem of moral philosophy, the relationship between fact and value: between the body and consciousness, between a human being as a part of nature and as the evolving subject of principled action and commitment.

We begin with the assumption that at no stage in growth are an individual's values simply the passive impress of others. Both specific values and more pervasive valuational attitudes —for example, whether one is authoritarian or liberal, rigidly moralistic or flexible, suspicious or trusting—are consequences of interactions that developmentally begin with the infant's inherent capacities for pleasure and pain, curiosity and disinterest. As the child grows, value judgments about what is "good" and "bad," "beautiful" and "ugly," are among the inevitable and increasingly complicated ways of organizing experiences of oneself and the world. What these experiences are will vary with the individual's needs and stage of development.

We take valuing, then, to be a way of structuring experience which is inherent in the human organism. We do not deny that the values of others by which a child is educated will have a profound effect on all aspects of its evolution; but we assert that the thrust toward a coherent system of values must be understood in terms of the maturational process itself.

Freud and psychosexual development

Sigmund Freud was the first psychologist to articulate a theory of psychosexual development that sees it as continuous with processes that begin in infancy. Puzzled by the fact that in human beings sexuality cannot be identified with procreative behavior—as it is still by many behavioral scientists—Freud was looking for an invariant as the common factor in genital sexuality, sexual foreplay, the so-called perversions, homosexuality, hysterical symptoms, and the masturbatory activities of children.

Freud's solution was to identify sexuality with distinctive processes of tension and pleasure located in any body zone (Freud, 1905). In thus assimilating sexuality to sensuality, he was able to explain why it is that sexual significance infuses the most diverse experiences; for the fact that sensual pleasure is not restricted to the genitals but is educed through the child's earliest modes of interaction with the environment accounts for the ways in which ultimately sexual pleasure is locked into other complicated forms of learning and behavior (Klein). The mouth and the anus, for example, which Freud considered to be the earliest erogenous zones, are not only mucous membranes generously supplied with nerve endings but, as primary routes to the world, they are also the foci of major informational systems.

Because, as Freud recognized, human sexuality is so interwoven with other forms of experience, it is impossible to trace a single developmental line. To focus the discussion, therefore, we begin by defining the nature of the complete sexual act from which we can infer the paths that lead to it (Ruddick). Whether "maturity," like "health," is itself a value term is a difficult question. The essential characteristics of a complete sexual act or experience are: (1) It is a relationship initiated by and through mutual desire, that is, it is an act involving two (or possibly more) persons, recognized by each other to be such, and each responsive to the desire which he or she perceives in the other. An analysis of the concept of "perversion" reveals it to apply to acts that violate this condition (Nagel). (2) It is pleasurable in and of itself. (3) It has the rhythm of tension and release, experienced specifically in the genitals, though characteristically the entire body of the other is the object of one's desire and the experience is one of progressive embodiment in which one's own self is taken over by one's body.

The most important developmental paths implied here are interrelated: the integration of the body as a source of pleasure into the sense of self, the capacity for mutuality with other people and the processes of separation and differentiation, or separation and individuation. In general, the sense of one's self as separate from others evolves out of a reliable cognitive development in which the child learns to differentiate and accurately describe objects in space, and a less reliable cognitive–emotional development which in the same movement yields the concept of "person" and the ability to love. While love and sex can occur independently of one another, we take sexuality to be the richer category, since the complete sexual act presumes the ability to love, though the reverse is not the case.

The earliest years

The body yields the infant's first pleasure, its first intimacy, and the experiences from which it simultaneously constructs its self and reality. In the beginning the infant "lives and loves with its mouth" (Erikson, 1950, chap. 2). It is there that its experiences of frustration and gratification, of love and loss, are localized. Through its mouth it first learns about its own capacity to

incorporate, to spit out, to bite, and to destroy.

How the child meets and is encouraged by its environment to meet these experiences affects the way in which it understands later experiences, for the body is not only the first object of a child's thoughts about what might and what ought to be; it also provides the schema by which its thinking is structured. "Devouring," "eating," "being nourished by," "taking in," become metaphors for any act in which one expands one's self in some way, and are the literal content of many fantasies about what may happen in an interpersonal experience. Later they form part of the imagery with which the older child tries to understand adult sexuality.

The infant's hunger is satisfied through an experience that brings it close to the person or persons who are responsible for its care. How promptly and reliably they answer the infant's needs, the feelings and attitudes which they subtly convey in the way they hold and handle it, tell the infant whether or not the world can be trusted. At the same time, the infant begins to acquire a sense of its own ability or inability to summon its caretakers, a sense of adequacy which is the basis for its later confidence and self-reliance. Thus in his various accounts of the evolution of personal identity and of the autonomous self, Erikson speaks of the earliest period as the time in which the healthy child begins to acquire a "basic trust" in itself and the world.

This "oral" period (approximately the first two years) coincides with the first phases of the separation–differentiation process, which is well under way in the healthy child by the end of the third year (Mahler). Some psychologists have posited an initial stage of symbiotic fusion in which the infant has no sense of itself as differentiated from the environment and, in particular, from its mother; others have claimed that the capacity for relationship to objects, to some degree perceived as such, exists from the outset (Guntrip). But there is general agreement that the capacity for self-consciousness develops along with the recognition of another as a person with a life of his or her own.

Essential to this recognition is the cognitive sequence that Piaget outlines in describing the child's early construction of reality (Piaget). In its first months, the child's universe consists of impressions that begin to be recognizable but that have no substantial permanence or spatial organization. By the ninth or tenth month it begins to endow its perceptions with permanence, though the degree of permanence they have is a function of its own eye movements or seeking behavior. The child of this age does not "find" the object; its actions allow it to exist. Between the tenth and the eighteenth months its pictures have begun to become objects in the sense that it regards them as permanent individual substances. And between the sixteenth and the eighteenth months it begins to achieve "object constancy": The object is freed from the subject, that is, from the child's perceptions and actions, is regarded as independent of its will, as enduring in space and time, and as remaining identical to itself wherever it is. The child can now comprehend its own body as a single entity, even though unable to see all of it, and to understand that as an object it has no priority in space. In becoming less egocentric, the child has begun to acquire the capacity to see objects as separate from itself.

The sequence just reviewed seems to be less subject to the vicissitudes of early childhood than the processes which lead to the child's sense of other *persons* as separate from itself in a quite different sense. The crucial factor in this recognition is a relationship with a mother or mothering figure in the first year and a half of the child's life who will be empathic both to the child's primary need for intimacy (Bowlby), and to the child's early impulses to do things for itself. Without such a relationship the child is likely to feel a degree of frustration and rage which precludes basic trust, and to attempt to extract from other people the obedience to its needs without which it feels helpless and impotent (Modell, chaps. 2 and 3). With such a relationship, it is able to move through different kinds of attachment, beginning with the pleasure the eight-month-old baby feels for its mother, whom it now recognizes as "mother" and as special. The separation anxiety that the year-and-a-half-old feels out of its deeper love and the greater recognition of its mother's independence is followed by the three-year-old's ability to integrate into its picture of her both the good and the bad—the fact that she is need-gratifying and need-frustrating—and to tolerate longer periods of absence from her (Winnicott).

At first able to feel securely related to its mother only when she is holding it, the child acquires the capacity to feel just as securely related when she is away and learns to be alone without feeling isolated. At first related to her through her capacity to satisfy its specific wants, the child becomes related to her as another whole self. It is from these beginnings that the healthy child will grow into an adult capable of caring about and identifying with the needs of another, curious about and responsive to the person underneath the skin, and able to be excited about the entirety of that person's body as an expression of its developing self, rather than by an isolated part of it (Kernberg, "Barriers").

From two to four

The child's increased ability to move around on its own with a new control over its sphincter muscles, among others, and the adult world's responses to a creature who begins to have the capacity to inflict real damage on objects and other small people, means that new demands are being made of it, for which its own greater self-control makes it ready. Freud designated this the anal period, partly because the most recurrent subject of parental demands in Western culture is where, when, and how the child will urinate and defecate. Elimination is thus apt to be at the center of conflicts about dependence and autonomy, which the child is suffering in any case.

Important developments in a child's gender identification occur in this period. Though the sense of one's self as male or female is learned primarily through the responses of others in the first year and a half of life (Money, Hampson, and Hampson), it is in its second and third years that it begins to acquire a sense of masculinity or femininity as part of its psychological self-image (Stoller). What traits and values a child learns to correlate with its gender depends, of course, on its parents and its culture. But whatever these variations, there is evidence that the moral and characterological development of every child is to some extent guided by its gender and by its own early propensities to structure its experience egocentrically and in terms of sexual stereotypes. That is, the child classifies men and women according to sex-roles that accord prestige, competence, or goodness to each sex on the basis of certain qualities and tends to schematize its own interests and values in ways that are consistent with its gender identity (Kohlberg, 1966). Whether and to what extent the child will eventually outgrow these sexual stereotypes depend on further cognitive developments and on the quality of its interpersonal relationships.

As the first category to which the young child learns to assign itself, gender is another important variable in the processes of separation and individuation. In any society in which children of both sexes are cared for primarily by women, the female child is encouraged to feel about the person to whom she is closest, "I am like her," whereas the boy senses that he is unlike her. As a result, the girl may begin life with a surer sense of who she is, though by the same token she may later have a more difficult time differentiating herself from her mother. And while the physical signs of masculinity are evident to the boy as soon as he has the cognitive ability to register them, the girl will have to wait many years before her gender identity is confirmed (Mead).

Four to six

Whether or not the Oedipus complex as described by classical psychoanalysis is a cross-cultural phenomenon is still the subject of much debate. But interpreted in its broadest sense, it refers to the extraordinary fact that in the same period of development, every child experiences specific sexual feelings and fantasies, some of which the child is inevitably forbidden to act out, and realizes that it is not the member of a dyad only (mother and child) but of a group. The child begins to comprehend generation and generations, sex, and death: that sexuality is a most intimate experience from which it is excluded at present by its own immaturity; that it will outgrow its parents; that there is a larger scheme of things than its nursery and one in which persons of different ages and gender perforce play different roles.

The universality of the sexual taboos—though they may vary in nature from society to society —to which children in this period are subject may be a function of the biological fact that human beings are dependent for a much longer time than any other species. In consequence, periods of increased gonadal activity and sexual interest are periods in which the child would normally turn for gratification first toward its parents as the persons who have excited its sexual curiosity and to whom it feels the closest. Spontaneous expression of such desires, however, would threaten not only the social fabric, but the development of the child as well, since the family is the unit from which the child must to some degree become independent.

If the long dependency of the human child is in these ways the source of its most painful conflicts, it is also the soil that nourishes its most distinctively human capacities—for manipulating complex symbol-systems, for creativity of all kinds, for self-consciousness, and for moral thought (Hallowell, Part I). In fact, Freud traced the erection of the superego to the end of the Oedipal period: From now on, he said, the child makes certain values and inhibitions its own and so becomes an authority to itself, particularly with regard to specific sexual and aggressive behaviors (Freud). However, since on our analysis moral character is a function not of the superego but of ego strength in general— that is, of all the intellectual and emotional qualities that allow for communication with an external world of events and people—the moral significance of such a change, assuming that it takes place, is questionable.

Adolescence

In adolescence—roughly the period between twelve and sixteen—the child experiences the greatest period of physical growth and development since its first years. As a culturally molded transition from childhood to adulthood, adolescence takes its cue from these bodily changes and prepares the child for its life decisions about work, sex, and love, each of which crucially challenges the child's gender and role identifications.

The small child's self-delight, the sense of coming into possession of its body, which the adolescent reexperiences, makes the child at the same time newly vulnerable to shame and to conflicts about independence. Childhood conflicts with the mother as the vigilant violator of physical autonomy are reawakened, conflicts which boys typically handle with a studied contempt for women, and girls with a frantic attempt to attach themselves to a boy or to a "masculine" activity. Both boys and girls, furthermore, are subject now to intense fears about the damage their bodies will suffer sexually and about their own power to inflict damage (Blos, 1962).

But the self-preoccupation, the push toward independence, and the greater emotionality that are characteristic of adolescence reflect not only the power of the past and the anatomical changes of puberty, but also the fact that adolescence marks another stage in cognitive development as well. There is a fresh discovery of the self because the category of subjectivity has taken on a new dimension. Prior to age twelve, for example, the child experiences anger "because the parents are bad"; it does not see its anger as something arising within, which may or may not have an adequate base in present reality. The adolescent, on the other hand, is more aware of emotions as one's own.

This sharper delineation between "subject" and "object," "mine" and "other," is yet another phase in the process of separation and individuation, which we followed earlier. To pick up Piaget's scheme once again: From approximately the second to the fifth year, the child's view of the world is animistic and magical. In its thinking about reality it makes no distinction in the kinds of explanations it offers for human and nonhuman behavior, confuses apparent or imagined events with real events, and objects and perceptual appearances of qualitative and quantitative change with actual change. From the fifth to the seventh year, the child begins to make the transition to "concrete logical thought," which manifests itself with regard to dreams, for example, as the awareness that dreams are not real, that they are not seen by others, and that in some sense they are internal (Kohlberg and Gilligan).

"Concrete logical thought" is a stage that all children reach; not all go on, however, to acquire the cognitive competence of adolescence in which the child is able to reason about reasoning itself, to isolate variables when it is trying to consider alternative explanations, to examine the consistency of its beliefs, to be able to accept hypothetical premises and to appreciate that problems can be self-centered entities solved by specific rules, to be able to evaluate the rightness and wrongness of an act in a way that takes account of motive and particularity of circumstance.

The emergence of this cognitive competence may be dependent on biological changes in the central nervous system which are catalyzed by experiences confronting the adolescent with phenomena inconsistent with his existing beliefs. Sexuality is one of these—for the adolescent has to reconcile the obvious pleasure of sexuality with whatever moral beliefs he or she has previously accepted about it. And moral beliefs in general are another. Thus the adolescent who reaches this stage is a natural philosopher (Kohlberg, 1971), whose own thought processes push toward self-examination, logical consistency, and flexibility of moral principles. Whether or not the adolescent goes beyond his or her ability to see that the moral quality of an action is dependent on the circumstances, to articulate a moral view which takes certain values and ideals as absolutely valuable, is another of the choices peculiar to this period. But

only someone who has at least reached adolescence is in a position to do so.

Thus because of this cognitive–emotional development, the adolescent is not only more preoccupied with the body than the prepubescent child but also able to appreciate how extraordinary it is as the locus of the person yet not identical with it, as having a mind of its own to which one can yield or attempt to master. More aware of subjectivity, the developing adolescent understands its implications: that no two people ever see the world in the same way, that the body of another is as intimately related to that person's self as is one's own to oneself, that to force, humiliate, or invade the body is therefore to attempt the same violations on the body's person. There develops a deeper capacity for experiencing guilt and a greater ability to commit oneself to friendships, activities, and ideas. And out of a greater sense of aloneness one is also able to feel a transcendence of oneself toward others, to nature, and to society (Kernberg, "Mature Love"). Sexually, the adolescent is becoming capable of a caring relationship that is respectful both of the accessibility of the body and the relative inaccessibility of the person, and able to identify with another without losing one's own sense of self.

The fact that a person is becoming ready for such a relationship, however, does not mean that he or she is already there. The physical developments of puberty—which are occurring progressively earlier in the West (Tanner)—do not guarantee a comparable psychological development but may be the instigating factors. And life in the highly technological societies may be making the integrating work of adolescence more difficult than ever (Blos, 1971).

We have omitted explicit reference in our chronology to the years of middle childhood—the so-called latency period—and to those following adolescence, in the first case because the relevant developments—primarily cognitive—have been indicated under the heading "adolescence"; and, in the second, because questions are raised about the meaning of "development" in general that are beyond the scope of this article. The position (maintained by Erik Erikson, in particular) that sexual development continues past the childbearing years and into old age is certainly implied by the belief (1) that the end point of all biological development is not some particular maturational achievement, but simply death itself; and is suggested by the belief (2) that in its psychological aspects, sexuality must be understood in terms of a structure of needs, motives, and concerns which may be independent of reproduction. Our own position is that while the various stages of life may call for different orientations toward one's own sexuality, and therefore may be part of a continuous process of change and personal growth, the concept of "development" should be reserved for those processes in which new aptitudes are acquired, and in a phase-specific way. We do not know of any such developments in the sexual life of human beings past the stage of young adulthood that do not represent simply the ability to use in various kinds of situations the maturity we have already described.

Conclusions: sexual maturity and moral agency

The maturation of the capacities for empathy, for accepting the separateness of one's self and respecting the different perspective of another, presumes a relatively high degree of emotional and intellectual development and is the distinctive mark of both sexual and moral maturity.

All adults prefer some things to others, impose on themselves, more or less erratically, some set of rules, experience some degree of shame or guilt, and carry around with them admonishing voices and images. In this sense, all adults have values. But to the degree that they are inhibited in their capacities for pleasure, deep emotional investments, and reflective thinking, or are torn by conflicts that prevent them from allowing their needs, fantasies, and experiences to modify one another, they cannot evolve a system of values which is coherent both in itself and with their own desires and abilities.

The criteria for moral agency are the capacities for choice and for knowing what one is doing. In the sense in which it is used here, choice is the ability to deliberate between alternative courses of action and to act in accordance with the outcome of one's deliberations. It requires, in turn, the capacities to withstand frustration, to think about the relevant facts and possibilities, to remember and anticipate, to tolerate ambiguity and resolve ambivalence. To a large extent, to say that one is acting with some knowledge or self-consciousness assumes that the self refers to a person, that is, to one whose needs, desires, values, and identifications form a fairly integrated whole; that it is possible for the self to understand the implications of and envision the consequences of what one is doing, and to distinguish between doing (or

action in the world) and fantasy. When the action in question involves other persons, as moral decisions characteristically do, then knowledge of the nature of the action is inseparable from feeling, since knowing that a body evinces pain-behavior, for example, is not the same as knowing that a person feels pain. The latter requires having felt pain oneself and being able to identify with the pain of another.

It would be stretching the concept of sexual development to claim that it is the ground for all the capacities involved in moral agency. We claim less. Beginning with a definition of the "complete sexual act," according to which bodily desire and a relationship of mutuality with another person are central, we have argued that: (1) Sexuality in human beings is so locked into forms of learning which are essential to moral development that it is inextricable from them; and (2) sexual development is the ground for one of the central lines of moral development, namely the capacity for valuing another organism as a person. Our analysis implies that any consistent pattern of sexual behavior that is intentionally depersonalizing, either to one's own self or to another, signifies a failure of sexual development.

MARCIA CAVELL AUFHAUSER

[*For further discussion of topics mentioned in this article, see the entries:* ADOLESCENTS; PERSON; SEXUAL BEHAVIOR; *and* SEXUAL IDENTITY. *Also directly related are the entries* SEX THERAPY AND SEX RESEARCH; *and* SEXUAL ETHICS. *For discussion of related ideas, see:* SOCIALITY.]

BIBLIOGRAPHY

BIEBER, I. "Bisocial Roles of Childhood Sexuality." *Sexuality and Psychoanalysis.* Edited by E. T. Adelsen. New York: Brunner Mazel, 1975, pp. 161–175.

BLOS, PETER. "The Child Analyst Looks at the Young Adolescent." *Daedalus* 100 (1971): 961–978.

———. *On Adolescence: A Psychoanalytic Interpretation.* New York: Free Press of Glencoe, 1962.

BOWLBY, JOHN. *Attachment and Loss.* Vol. I: *Attachment.* New York: Basic Books, 1969.

ERIKSON, ERIK H. "The Life Cycle: Epigenesis of Identity." *Identity, Youth, and Crisis.* New York: W. W. Norton & Co., 1968, pp. 91–141; see especially pp. 91–134. All of Erikson's works bear on the relationship between moral and psychosexual development, notably *Childhood and Society* and "The Roots of Virtue."

———. *Childhood and Society.* New York: Norton, 1950.

———. "The Roots of Virtue." *The Humanist Frame.* Edited by Julian Huxley. New York: Harper & Brothers, 1961, pp. 145–165. Erikson divides the life cycle into eight stages, each marked by a particular kind of identity crisis and an emergent virtue or valuational attitude. These are: trust vs. mis-trust (the 'oral' period); autonomy vs. shame and doubt (the 'anal' period); initiative vs. shame and guilt (the 'oedipal' period); industry vs. inferiority (latency); identity vs. identity confusion (adolescence); intimacy vs. isolation (young adulthood); generativity vs. stagnation (maturity); integrity vs. despair (old age).

FREUD, SIGMUND. "Civilization and Its Discontents (1929)." *Standard Edition of the Complete Psychological Works of Sigmund Freud.* Translated by James Strachey. London: Hogarth Press, 1953–, vol. 21, pp. 57–145.

————. "Introductory Lectures on Psychoanalysis (1916–1917)." *Standard Edition,* vol. 16, lectures 20 and 21, pp. 303–339.

————. "On Beginning the Treatment (Further Recommendations on the Technique of Psychoanalysis I) (1913)." *Standard Edition,* vol. 12, pp. 121–144. See especially pp. 123–134.

————. "Three Essays on the Theory of Sexuality, (1905)." *Standard Edition,* vol. 7, pp. 123–245.

GUNTRIP, HENRY J. S. [HARRY GUNTRIP]. *Psychoanalytic Theory, Therapy, and the Self.* New York: Basic Books, 1971.

HALLOWELL, A. IRVING. "Culture, Personality, and Experience." *Culture and Experience.* New York: Schocken, 1967, pp. 2–110. Originally published in 1955.

KAGAN, J. "A Conception of Early Adolescence." *Daedalus* 100 (1971): 997–1012.

KERNBERG, OTTO F. "Barriers to Falling and Remaining in Love." *Journal of the American Psychoanalytic Association* 22 (1974): 486–511.

————. "Mature Love: Prerequisites and Characteristics." *Journal of the American Psychoanalytic Association* 22 (1974): 743–768.

KLEIN, GEORGE S. "Freud's Two Theories of Sexuality." *Clinical–Cognitive Psychology: Models and Integrations.* Edited by Louis Berger. Englewood Cliffs, N.J.: Prentice-Hall, 1969, pp. 136–181.

KOHLBERG, LAWRENCE. "A Cognitive–Developmental Analysis of Children's Sex-Role Concepts and Attitudes." *The Development of Sex Differences.* Edited by Eleanor E. Maccoby. Stanford: Stanford University Press, 1966, pp. 82–173.

————, and GILLIGAN, CAROL. "The Adolescent as a Philosopher: The Discovery of the Self in a Postconventional World." *Daedalus* 100 (1971): 1051–1086.

MAHLER, MARGARET S. *On Human Symbiosis and the Vicissitudes of Individuation.* The International Psycho-Analytical Library, no. 82. New York: International Universities Press, 1968.

MEAD, MARGARET. "The Ways of the Body." *Male and Female.* New York: William Morrow & Co., 1949, pp. 51–160.

MODELL, ARNOLD H. *Object Love and Reality.* New York: International Universities Press, 1968. See chaps. 2, 3, and 4.

MONEY, JOHN; HAMPSON, JOAN G.; and HAMPSON, JOHN L. "Imprinting and the Establishment of Gender Role." *Archives of Neurology* 77 (1957): 333–336.

NAGEL, THOMAS. "Sexual Perversion." *Moral Problems.* 2d ed. Edited by James Rachels. New York: Harper & Row, 1975, pp. 3–15. Negel's article, like Ruddick's listed below, provides good bibliographical guides to the philosophical literature on sex.

PIAGET, JEAN. *The Construction of Reality in the Child.* Translated by Margaret Cook. New York: Basic Books, 1954.

RUDDICK, SARA. "On Sexual Morality." Rachels, *Moral Problems,* pp. 16–34. Our definition of "the complete sex act" is similar to, though not identical with, Ruddick's.

STOLLER, ROBERT J. *Sex and Gender.* New York: Science House; London: Hogarth, 1968.

TANNER, J. M. "Sequence, Tempo and Individual Variation in the Growth and Development of Boys and Girls Aged Twelve to Sixteen." *Daedalus* 100 (1971): 907–930.

WINNICOTT, DONALD WOODS. *The Maturational Process and the Facilitating Environment.* New York: International Universities Press, 1965.

SEXUAL ETHICS

The relevance of sexual ethics for bioethics consists most generally in the concern of both for human bodily behavior. Like other issues in bioethics, questions of sexuality have entailed questions of the body's relation to the whole person, moral standards for rational intervention in physical processes, and norms for the overall health of the individual and society. More specifically, ethical evaluations of sexual behavior have at times included claims that some sexual behavior is sick (as, for example, when homosexuality has been considered an illness) and claims that some sexual behavior leads to sickness (as, for example, when masturbation has been thought to have medical consequences). Bioethical questions regarding contraception, sterilization, abortion, venereal disease, sex therapy and sex research, and genetics are directly concerned with sexuality. Not surprisingly, health professionals both in the past and in the present have frequently found themselves called upon as counselors with regard to sexual matters.

To the extent that ethical reflection on sexuality can provide a helpful context for issues in bioethics, an overview of sexual ethics is called for. The present state of sexual ethics cannot be assessed without understanding something of its historical antecedents and their more immediate contributions to contemporary theory and practice. It is also necessary to understand in some degree the sources of the widespread contemporary challenge to traditional sexual ethics. This article will limit its concern to Western traditions of sexual ethics (the most systematic of which have been religious). It will begin with a historical overview, consider next those factors which have rendered traditional norms problematic, and finally focus on central issues that now engage ethical reflection on the sexual life of human persons.

The Jewish tradition

Earliest Hebrew moral codes were simple and without systematic theological underpinnings. Like other ancient Near Eastern legislation, they prescribed marriage laws and prohibited adultery, rape, and certain forms of prostitution, incest, and nakedness. In contrast to neighboring Eastern civilizations, Hebrew belief in a god who is beyond sexuality led to a kind of desacralization of sex. Human sexuality was sacred only insofar as marriage and fertility were part of the plan of a creator God. Such a view of sexuality, however, set the stage for a positive valuation that endured despite later tendencies toward negative asceticism.

Marriage and procreation. The injunction to marry is central to the Jewish tradition of sexual morality. Marriage is a religious duty, affirmed by all the codes of Jewish law (Feldman, p. 27). Two elements in Judaism's concept of marriage account for many other important laws regarding sexuality. The first is the perception of the command to procreate, at the heart of the command to marry. The second is the patriarchal model upon which the Jewish notion of marriage is institutionally based. These two elements help explain prohibitions against adultery and regulations regarding divorce, prostitution, polygamous marriage, and concubinage. Thus, for example, biblical law considered adultery primarily a violation of a husband's property rights. With minor modifications this was true also of talmudic and post-talmudic law. Further, polygamy and concubinage were accepted for a long time as a solution to a childless marriage. Prostitution was forbidden as idolatrous, but no legislation ever applied to the use of female slaves. Early in the tradition, custom recognized an almost unlimited right on the part of the husband to divorce his wife. Later the rabbis introduced various restrictions but did not abolish the right. The obvious double standard for men and for women which marked much of this legislation did not hinder, and in some cases helped, the fulfillment of the law of procreation. It was, moreover, in accord with the subordinate status of women in relation to men. These laws do not by themselves, however, give an adequate picture of traditional Jewish sexual morality.

Sex and the marital relationship. In fact, monogamous, lifelong marriage always stood as the ideal context for sexuality. As the centuries passed, that ideal came to be emphasized more and more. It took precedence even over the command to procreate. Gradually polygamy or divorce and remarriage were less and less accepted as remedies for childless marriages. Concern for the value of the marital relationship in itself finally overruled both as options. In the talmudic period monogamy became the custom as well as the ideal, and polygamy later disappeared entirely in Europe. The rabbis came to teach that neither unilateral nor mutually agreed-upon divorce was required or even always justified as a solution to barrenness in a wife. As the tradition developed, moreover, the moral tide ran against concubinage, and prostitution was more and more proscribed as a matter of conscience if not of law (Borowitz, p. 47).

A conflict between the marital relationship and the command to procreate, then, could be resolved in favor of the relationship. The fabric of the relationship has always been of great concern in the Jewish tradition. While the core of the legal imperative to marry is the command to procreate, marriage has also always been considered a duty because it conduces to the holiness of the partners. Holiness here refers more to the opportunity for channeling sexual desire than to companionship and mutual fulfillment, but the latter are clearly included in the purposes of marriage and are an expected concomitant result. Now it is the element of holiness in the Jewish concept of marriage that has proved decisive in determining questions of fertility control. Contraception is allowed for the sake of preserving the existing marriage relationship when a new pregnancy would be harmful either to the wife or to the welfare of existing children (Feldman, pp. 42–53). It is morally preferable to abstinence because it is the husband's duty to promote the happiness and holiness of his wife through uniting with her in sexual union.

Unnatural sex acts. Judaism traditionally has shown a concern for the "improper emission of seed." Included in this concern are proscriptions of masturbation and homosexual acts. Both are considered unnatural, beneath the dignity of humanly meaningful sexual intercourse, and indicative of uncontrolled and hence morally evil sexual desire (Epstein, pp. 134–147). The source of these prohibitions seems to be more clearly the historical connection between such acts and the idolatrous practices of neighboring peoples than the contradiction between sexual acts and the command to procreate. Indeed, the minimum criterion for "proper emission of seed" is the mutual pleasure of husband and wife, not the procreative intent of their act of intercourse (Feldman, p. 104).

Contemporary efforts to articulate a Jewish position on questions of sexual morality involve efforts to draw forth as yet unexplicated directions within the tradition and to correct perceived deficiencies in the tradition. Thus, for example, in a tradition where marriage has been the ideal context for sexual activity, contemporary questions of premarital sex are nonetheless not yet settled (Borowitz, p. 50). And contemporary concern to equalize the relation between women and men encounters the factor of male dominance, which has characterized sexual relationship from the beginning of Jewish history.

Ancient Greece and Rome

General attitudes. Attitudes toward sexual behavior differed significantly between the ancient Greeks and Romans. In comparison with Rome, the Greeks seem to have had a balanced, humane, refined culture in which sexuality was accepted as an integral part of life. Sensuality and reason were harmonized in a kind of idealized virtue of the whole person. Rome, too, accepted sex as a natural part of life, but the refinement of Greek culture was missing.

Marriage for both Greeks and Romans was monogamous. In ancient Greece, however, no sexual ethic confined sex to marriage. Human nature was generally assumed to be bisexual, and polyerotic needs especially of the male were easily accepted. Hence, there was what some have referred to as sexual polygamy within marital monogamy. Monogamous marriage in Rome, on the other hand, was the foundation of social life. In fact, the institutionalization of marriage, through the development of marriage laws, was thought to be of central importance in the achievement of Roman civilization.

Both Greece and Rome were male-dominated societies, and a double standard was obvious in regard to sexual morality. Divorce was an easy matter in ancient Greece, but for a long time it was available only to husbands. In Rome, while there was apparently no divorce at all for a period of five hundred years, later a husband could divorce his wife for adultery and a variety of other sometimes trivial reasons. Both Greek and Roman brides but not bridegrooms were expected to be virgins. The only women in Greece who were given some equal status with men

were a special class of prostitutes, the *hetairae*. Wives had no public life at all, though they were given the power to manage the home. In the Roman household, on the contrary, the husband had an entirely free hand. Indeed, perhaps nowhere else did the ideal of *patria potestas* reach such complete fulfillment. Outside the home, husbands could also consort freely with slaves or prostitutes. Adultery was not proscribed so long as it was not with another man's wife. Fidelity was required of wives, however, primarily in order to secure the inheritance of property by legitimate children. Though by the first century A.D. women in Rome achieved some economic and political freedom, they could never assume the sexual freedom traditionally granted to men.

Homosexuality was accepted in both Greek and Roman culture. Indeed, the Greeks incorporated societal attitudes toward relationships between men into their most highly developed philosophies of interpersonal relations. Both Plato and Aristotle assumed that the ideal of human friendship was possible only between men. In Plato's *Symposium*, the unequal relationship between a man and a woman could never give rise to the mutual pursuit of higher than sensual goods. Aristotle, in his *Nicomachean Ethics* (1158b), could only list the friendship between husband and wife among the lesser forms of friendship that exist between those who are not equal.

Greek and Roman philosophical appraisals of sex. The ethical theory of Greek and Roman philosophers was clearly influenced by the cultural mores of their time. The reciprocal impact of the theory upon the mores is less clear than its later influence upon Jewish and Christian thought. Overall it must be said that Greek and Roman philosophy contributed to subsequent distrust of sexual desire and negative evaluation of sexual pleasure. The Pythagoreans in the sixth century B.C. advocated purity of the body for the sake of culture of the soul. The force of their position was felt in the later thinking of Socrates and Plato. Though Plato moved from the general hostility to pleasure, which marks the *Gorgias*, to a careful distinction between lower and higher pleasures in, for example, the *Republic, Phaedo, Symposium*, and *Philebus*, sexual pleasure continued to be deprecated as one of the lower pleasures. Above all Plato wanted to unleash, not to restrain, the power of eros, which could move the human spirit to union with the greatest good. If bodily pleasures could be taken up into that pursuit, there was no objection to them.

But Plato thought, finally, that the pleasure connected with sexual intercourse diminished quantitatively the power of eros for higher things.

Aristotle, like Plato, distinguished between lower and higher pleasures, placing the pleasures of touch at the bottom of the scale. He was sufficiently more this-worldly than Plato to caution moderation rather than transcendence, however. He never conceived of the possibility of equality or mutuality in relationships between men and women (and opposed Plato's design for this in the *Republic* and *Laws*). The highest forms of friendship and love, and of happiness in the contemplation of the life of one's friend, had no room for the incorporation of sexual activity and even less room than Plato for the possible nurturing power of erotic love.

Of all Greek philosophies, Stoicism had the greatest impact on Roman philosophy and on the early formation of Christian thought. Philosophers such as Seneca, Musonius Rufus, Epictetus, and Marcus Aurelius taught a strong doctrine of the power of the human will to regulate emotion and of the desirability of such regulation for the sake of inner peace. Sexual desire, like the passions of fear and anger, was in itself irrational, disturbing, liable to excess. It needed to be moderated if not eliminated. It could never be indulged for its own sake, but only if it served some rational purpose. The goal of procreation provided that purpose. Hence, even in marriage, sexual intercourse was morally justified only when it was engaged in for the sake of procreation.

The Greco-Roman legacy to Western sexual ethics contained, somewhat ironically, little of the freedom and imagination of sex life in ancient Greece. The dominant themes picked up by later traditions were suspicion and control, elimination, or severe restriction. This may have been largely due to the failure of both the Greeks and the Romans to integrate sexuality into their best insights into human relationships. Whether such an integration was in principle a possibility remained an unanswered question in the centuries that followed.

Christian traditions

Like other religious and cultural traditions, the teachings within the Christian tradition regarding human sexuality are complex, subject to multiple outside influences, and expressive of change and development through succeeding generations of Christians. Christianity does not begin with a systematic code of sexual ethics.

The teachings of Jesus and his followers, as recorded in the New Testament, provide a central focus for the moral life of Christians in the command to love God and neighbor. Beyond that, the New Testament offers grounds for a sexual ethic that (1) values marriage and procreation on the one hand and celibacy on the other; (2) gives as much importance or more to internal attitudes and thoughts as to external actions; and (3) affirms a sacred symbolic meaning for sexual intercourse yet both subordinates it as a value to other human values and finds in it a possibility for evil.

Stoic and Gnostic influences on Christian understandings of sex. Christianity emerged in the late Hellenistic Age when even Judaism with its strong positive valuation of marriage and procreation was influenced by the dualistic anthropologies of Stoic philosophy and Gnostic religions. New Testament writers as well as the Fathers of the Church found a special appeal in Stoic doctrines of the mind's control of body and of reason's effecting detachment from all forms of passionate desire. Stoicism, though this-worldly in itself, blended well with the early Christian expectation of the end of the world. More important, it offered a way of rational response to Gnostic devaluation of marriage and procreation.

Gnosticism was a series of religious movements that deeply affected formulations of Christian sexual ethics for the first three centuries (Noonan, pp. 78–136). Combining elements of Eastern mysticism, Greek philosophy, and Christian belief, the Gnostics claimed a special "knowledge" of divine revelation. Among other things, they taught that marriage is evil or at least useless, primarily because the procreation of children is a vehicle for forces of evil. That led to two extreme positions in Gnosticism—one that opposed all sexual intercourse and hence prescribed celibacy, and one advocating every possible experience of sexual intercourse so long as it was not procreative.

What Christian moral teaching sought in order to combat both Gnostic rejection of sexual intercourse and Gnostic licentiousness was a doctrine that incorporated an affirmation of sex as good (because part of creation) but set serious limits to sexual activity (and hence provided an order for sexual emotion). The Stoic doctrine of justification of sexual intercourse by reason of its relation to procreation served both of those needs. The connection made between sexual intercourse and procreation was not the same as the Jewish affirmation of the importance of fecundity, though it was in harmony with it. Christian teaching could thus both affirm procreation as the central rationale for sexual union and advocate virginity as a praiseworthy option for Christians who could choose it.

With the adoption of the Stoic norm for sexual intercourse, the direction of Christian sexual ethics was set for centuries to come. A sexual ethic that concerned itself primarily with affirming the good of procreation and thereby the good of otherwise evil sexual tendencies was, moreover, reinforced by the continued appearance of antagonists who played the same role the Gnostics had played. No sooner had Gnosticism begun to wane than, in the fourth century, Manichaeanism emerged. And it was largely in response to Manichaeanism that Augustine formulated his sexual ethic—an ethic which continued and went beyond the Stoic elements already incorporated by Clement of Alexandria, Origen, Ambrose, and Jerome.

The sexual ethics of St. Augustine and its legacy. Augustine argued against the Manichaeans in favor of the goodness of marriage and procreation (*On the Good of Marriage*), though he shared with them a negative view of sexual desire as in itself a tendency to evil. Because evil was for him, however, a privation of right order (and not an autonomous principle), it was possible to reorder sexual desire according to reason, to integrate its meaning into a right and whole love of God and neighbor. That was done only when sexual intercourse had the purpose of procreation. Intercourse without a procreative purpose was, according to Augustine, sinful (though not necessarily lethally so). Marriage, on the other hand, had a threefold purpose: not only the good of children, but also the goods of fidelity between spouses (as opposed to adultery) and the indissolubility of their union (as opposed to divorce). Augustine wrote appreciatively of the possibility of love and companionship between persons in marriage, but he did not integrate a positive role for sexual intercourse.

In his writings against the Pelagians (*Marriage and Concupiscence*) Augustine tried to clarify the place of sexual desire in a theology of original sin. Although for Augustine original sin was a sin of the spirit (the sin of prideful disobedience), its effects were most acutely seen in the chaos experienced when sexual desire wars against reasoned choice of higher goods. Moreover, the loss of integrity in affectivity (the effect of original sin) is, according to Augustine,

passed on from one generation to another through the mode of procreation wherein sexual intercourse always interferes with self-possessed reason and will. Augustine's formulation of a sexual ethic held sway in Christian moral teaching until the sixteenth century. There were a few Christian writers (for example, John Chrysostom) who raised up the Pauline purpose for marriage—that is, as a remedy for incontinence. Such a position hardly served to foster a more optimistic view of the value of sex, but it did offer a possibility for moral goodness in sexual intercourse without a direct relation to procreation. From the sixth to the eleventh century, the weight of Augustine's negative evaluation of sexuality became even more burdensome. Following the premise that sexual intercourse can be justified only by its relation to procreative purpose, the Penitentials (manuals providing lists of sins and their prescribed penances) detailed prohibitions of adultery, fornication, oral and anal sex, contraception, and even certain positions for sexual intercourse according as they were departures from the procreative norm.

The rise of the courtly love tradition and new forms of mystical ideologies in the twelfth century presented a new challenge to the procreation ethic. Once again the meaning of sexuality in relation to marriage and procreation was questioned, and Christian moral theory reacted by renewing its commitment to Augustine's sexual ethic. In theology, Peter Lombard's *Sentences* led the way in renewing the connection between concupiscence and original sin, so that sexual intercourse within marriage demanded once again a procreative justification. In church discipline, this was the period of Gratian's great collection of canon law, and canonical regulations were shaped with the rigorism dictated by a sexual ethics that held all sexual activity to be evil unless it could be excused under the rationale of a procreative purpose.

While the tradition became more and more emphatic in one direction, nonetheless other directions were being opened. A few voices (for example, Abelard and John Damascene) continued to argue that concupiscence does not make sexual pleasure evil in itself, and that sexual intercourse in marriage can be justified by the intention to avoid fornication. The courtly love tradition, while it served to rigidify the opposition, nonetheless also introduced a powerful new element in its assertion that sexuality can be a mediation of interpersonal love (Rougement, p. 65).

The teaching of Aquinas. Thomas Aquinas came on the scene in the thirteenth century at a time when rigorism prevailed in Christian teaching and church discipline. His massive and innovative synthesis in Christian theology did not offer much that was new in the area of sexual ethics. Yet there was a clarity regarding all that was brought forward from the tradition that made Aquinas's own participation important for the generations that succeeded him. Christian moral teaching as he understood it included a disclaimer regarding the intrinsic evil of sexual desire. Moral evil is always and only tied up with evil moral choice and not with spontaneous bodily tendencies or desires. Yet there is in fallen human nature, as the result of original sin, a loss of order in natural human tendencies. All emotions are good insofar as they are ordered according to reason; they become evil when they are freely affirmed in opposition to reason's norm.

Aquinas offered two grounds for the procreative norm of reason, which the tradition had so far affirmed. One was the Augustinian argument that sexual pleasure always, in the fallen human person, hinders the best working of the mind. It must, then, be brought into some accord with reason by having an overriding value as its goal. No less an end than procreation can serve to justify it (*Summa Theologiae* I-II, 34 1 ad 1). But secondly, reason does not merely provide a good purpose for sexual pleasure. It discovers that purpose through the very facts of the biological function of sexual organs (*Summa Theologiae* II-II, 154, 11; *Summa Contra Gentiles* III, 122, 4 and 5). Hence, the norm of reason in sexual behavior is not only the conscious intention of procreation but the accurate and unimpeded physical process whereby procreation is possible. So important is this process that whether or not procreation is in fact possible (that is, whether or not actual conception can take place—as it could not in the case of the sterile), it is sufficient that the process of intercourse be complete and there be no intention to avoid procreation. If *per accidens* generation cannot follow, nonetheless the intercourse is in its *essence* justifiable.

It was the procreative norm for sexual intercourse that provided specific moral rules to govern, either directly or indirectly, a variety of sexual activities and relationships. In addition to a general proscription of anything that produces sexual pleasure for its own sake (not justified by the purpose of procreation), Aquinas argued from the assumption that sexual intercourse would be procreative to considerations of the morality of instances of intercourse from the standpoint of the progeny that might result. Thus, for example, he argued against fornication and adultery on the grounds that they injure a child born of the union by not providing a responsible context for its rearing. He argued against divorce because the children of a marriage need a stable home in order to grow into the fullness of life. He considered sexual acts that could not meet the requirements of the biological norm for heterosexual intercourse immoral because there was no way in which they could be procreative. And he opposed contraception not only because it was in intention nonprocreative but because it constituted an injury against an unborn child and/or the human species (Fuchs, p. 181).

Aquinas's treatment of marriage contained only hints of possible new insights regarding the relation of sexual intercourse to marital love. He worked out a theory of love as a passion that had room in it for an assertion that sexual union can be an aid to interpersonal love (*Summa Theologiae* II-II, 26, 11), and he had the bare beginnings of a theory of marriage that opened it to the possibility of maximum friendship (*Summa Contra Gentiles* III, 123). Indeed, some Thomistic scholars assert that a closer analysis of Aquinas's texts shows that he broke with Augustine's theory of procreative sex and fully justified marital intercourse as an expression of the good of fidelity. In so doing he rejected only *anti*procreative marital intercourse (Parmisano, pp. 650–660; Grisez, pp. 9–11).

Fifteenth-century justifications of nonprocreative sex. Though what had crystallized in the Middle Ages canonically and theologically would continue to influence Christian moral teaching into the indefinite future, the fifteenth century marked the beginning of significant change. Finding some grounds for opposing the prevailing Augustinian sexual ethic in both Albert the Great and in the general (if not the specifically sexual) ethics of Thomas Aquinas, writers such as Denis the Carthusian began to speak of the possible integration of spiritual love and sexual pleasure. Martin LeMaistre, teaching at the University of Paris, argued that sexual intercourse in marriage is justified for its own sake; that is, sexual pleasure can be sought precisely as sexual pleasure, as the opposite of the pain experienced in the lack of sexual pleasure. When it is enjoyed thus it contributes to the general well-being of the persons involved. The influence of LeMaistre and others was not such as to reverse the Augustinian tradition, but it weakened it. The effects of the new theories of human sexuality were felt in the important controversies of the sixteenth-century Reformation and Counter Reformation within Christianity.

Reformation teaching on sex. Questions of sexual behavior played a significant role in the Protestant Reformation. The issue of clerical celibacy, for example, was raised not just as a matter of church discipline but as a question intimately tied into doctrinal controversies over nature and grace, original sin, sacramental theology, and ecclesiology. Martin Luther and John Calvin were both, paradoxically, deeply influenced by the Augustinian tradition regarding original sin and its consequences for human sexuality. Yet both developed a position on marriage that was complementary to, if not in opposition with, the procreative ethic. Like Augustine and the Christian tradition that followed him, they affirmed marriage and human sexuality as part of the divine plan for creation, and therefore good. But they shared Augustine's pessimistic view of fallen nature in which human sexual desire is no longer ordered as it should be within the complex structure of the human personality. The cure for disordered desire that Luther offered, however, was not the one put forth by Augustine. For Luther, the remedy was marriage; for Augustine, it was celibacy. And so the issue was joined over a key element in Christian teaching regarding sexuality. Luther, of course, was not the first to advocate marriage as a remedy for unruly sexual desire. But he took on the whole of the Christian tradition in a way that no one else had, challenging theory and practice, offering not just an alternative justification for marriage but a view of the human person that demanded marriage for almost all Christians (*The Estate of Marriage*). Sexual pleasure itself, then, in one sense needed no justification. The desire for it was simply a fact of life. It remained, like all the givens in creation, a good so long as it was channeled through marriage into the meaningful whole of life (which included above all, for Luther, the good of offspring). What there was in it that was a distraction from the "knowledge and worship of God," and hence sinful, had to be simply forgiven, as did the inevitable sinful elements in all dimensions of human life (*A Sermon on the Estate of Marriage*).

Calvin, too, saw marriage as a corrective to otherwise disordered desires. But Calvin went beyond that in affirming that the greatest good of marriage and sex is the mutual society that is formed between husband and wife (*Commentary on Genesis*). Calvin thought that sexual desire is more subject to control than did Luther, though whatever fault remains in it is "covered over" by marriage (*Institutes of the Christian Religion* 2, 8, 44). He worried that marriage, while it is the remedy for incontinence, could nonetheless be itself a provocation to "uncontrolled and dissolute lust."

The converse of both Luther's and Calvin's teaching regarding marriage was their opposition to premarital and extramarital sex less out of a concern for irresponsible procreation than out of a belief that sexuality not restrained by the marriage bond was wholly disordered. So concerned was Luther to provide some institutionally tempering form to sexual desire that he preferred a second marriage to adultery (yet so inevitable did he consider the need for sexual activity that he allowed adultery for either a husband or wife whose spouse was impotent or frigid). Both Luther and Calvin were opposed to divorce, though its possibility was admitted in a situation of adultery or impotence. Overall, every sexual moral norm was influenced by the belief that any sex outside the forgiving context of marriage was sinful. Hence, Calvin unquestioningly opposed homosexuality and bestiality along with adultery and fornication (though he followed the scholastics in considering the first two a violation of nature).

Post-Reformation developments. In the four centuries following the Reformation, development occurred, of course, in Christian attitudes and theory regarding sexuality. Yet the fundamental directions of both Roman Catholic and Protestant thought changed surprisingly little before the twentieth century. Even now, basic norms and patterns of justification for norms affirmed by Augustine and Aquinas, Luther and Calvin, remain intact for many Christians despite the radical challenges put to them in recent years. The fundamental struggle in each of the Christian traditions through the centuries has been to modulate an essentially negative approach to sexuality into a positive one, to move from the need to justify sexual intercourse even in marriage by reason of either procreation or the avoidance of fornication to an affirmation of its potential for expressing and effecting interpersonal love. The difficulties in such a transition are more evident in the efforts of the churches to articulate a new position than in the writings of individual theologians.

In Roman Catholicism. During and after the Reformation, new developments in the Roman Catholic tradition alternated with the reassertion of the Augustinian ethic. Though the Council of Trent became the first ecumenical council to treat of the role of love in marriage, it also reaffirmed the primacy of the procreative ethic and reemphasized the superiority of celibacy. The move away from the procreative ethic by sixteenth-, seventeenth-, and eighteenth-century Roman Catholic theologians proved to be primarily a move to lean like Luther and Calvin in the direction of justifying marriage for the sake of continence. In the seventeenth century Jansenism reacted against a lowering of sexual standards and brought back the Augustinian connection between sex, concupiscence, and original sin. The nineteenth century stagnated in a manualist tradition that never moved beyond Alphonsus Liguouri's eighteenth-century attempt to integrate the Pauline purpose of marriage with the purpose of intercourse. Then came the twentieth century with the rise of Roman Catholic theological interest in personalism and the move on the part of the Protestant churches to accept birth control.

It was the issue of contraception that served once again to focus Roman Catholic teaching firmly on the procreative ethic. In 1930 Pius XI responded to the Anglican approval of contraception by reaffirming in his encyclical letter, *Casti Connubii,* the full rationale for the procreative ethic (Pius XI). At the same time, he gave approval for the use of the rhythm method for restricting procreation, an approval that Pius XII reiterated in an address to midwives in 1951 (Pius XII). Theologians such as Bernard Häring, Josef Fuchs, John Ford, and Gerald Kelly began to move cautiously in the direction of allowing sexual intercourse in marriage without a procreative intent and for the purpose of fostering marital union.

The change in Roman Catholic moral theology from the 1950s to the 1970s was dramatic. The wedge introduced between procreation and sexual intercourse by the acceptance of the rhythm method joined with new understandings of the totality of the human person to support a radically new concern for sexuality as an expression and cause of married love. The effects of this theological reflection were striking in the Vatican II teaching on marriage. Here it was affirmed that the love essential to marriage is uniquely expressed and perfected in the act of sexual intercourse (Second Vatican Council). Although the Council still held that marriage is by its very nature ordered to the procreation of children, it made no distinction between the primary and secondary ends of marriage. Nonprocreative marital intercourse thus was accepted by the Catholic community. This was recognized by Paul VI in his encyclical *Humanae Vitae* in 1968, although at the same time he insisted that contraception is immoral. The debate continues between those who reject contraception and those who believe that acceptance of nonprocreative purposes for marital intercourse entails acceptance of contraception. For some, a distinction between *non*procreative and *anti*procreative behavior mediates the dispute.

In Protestantism. In the meantime, twentieth-century theological reflection on sexual behavior has developed as dramatically in the Protestant communities as in the Roman Catholic. After the Reformation, Protestant sexual ethics continued to affirm heterosexual marriage as the only acceptable context for sexual activity. Lutheran pietism and Calvinistic Puritanism continued to justify sex in marriage only as a corrective to disordered sexual desire or as a means to procreation of children (Cole, p. 162). Except for the differences regarding celibacy and divorce, sexual norms in Protestantism looked much the same as those in the Roman Catholic tradition. Nineteenth-century Protestantism was little influenced by the unconventional sexual attitudes of Romanticism (with the exception of perhaps Schleiermacher), and it shared the cultural pressures of Victorianism. But in the twentieth century Protestant thinking was deeply affected by historical studies that revealed the early roots of Christian sexual norms (Bailey, 1959), biblical research that questioned direct recourse to explicit biblical sexual norms (Baltensweiler, p. 145), and new philosophical anthropologies and psychoanalytic theories.

It is difficult, of course, to trace one clear line of development in twentieth-century Protestant sexual ethics, or even as clear a dialectic as may be found in Roman Catholicism. The fact that Protestantism in general was less dependent from the beginning on the procreative ethic may have led it almost unanimously to a much easier acceptance of, for example, contraception. The Anglican Lambeth Conference in 1930 marked the beginning of new official positions on the part of major Protestant churches in this regard.

Protestant theologians from Bonhoeffer to Barth, Brunner to Reinhold Niebuhr, Thielicke to Ellul, have concurred with this change.

The fact that Protestant sexual ethics has more frequently been based on a biblical rather than a natural law ethic may account for its earlier (than Roman Catholic) willingness to favor the civil rights of homosexuals. This would not account as easily for the fact that a number of Protestant churches and theologians have suggested a new position on the morality of homosexuality as well. In 1963 a group of Quakers published a formal essay in which a general sexual ethic of mutual consent did not rule out homosexual relationships as a Christian option (Heron). The Lutheran theologian Helmut Thielicke (pp. 269–292) and the Anglican Derrick S. Bailey (1955) have both advocated a new openness to the needs of the homosexual at least for the pastoral concern of the churches. On the other hand, Karl Barth called for "protest, warning, and conversion," because homosexuality violates the command of God (1961), and the Luthern Church, Missouri Synod, condemned homosexuality in 1973 as "intrinsically sinful."

Overall, Protestant sexual ethics is moving to integrate an understanding of the human person, male and female, into a theology of marriage that no longer deprecates sexual desire and sexual pleasure as primarily occasions of moral danger. For the most part, the ideal context for sexual intercourse is still seen to be heterosexual marriage. Yet questions of premarital sex, homosexuality, masturbation, and new questions of artificial insemination, genetic control, and in vitro fertilization are being raised by Protestant theologians in Protestant communities.

Relativization of norms

The long story of the contemporary challenge to traditional sexual norms can be made short by noting seven factors that have contributed to the shaking of the ethical foundations.

1. Historical contingency. The very disclosure of the history of sexual norms has revealed the historical contingency of their sources and foundations. To see that a procreative ethic rose as much from Stoic philosophy as from Sacred Scripture has caused questions to arise concerning its validity for Christians. To recognize that important traditional norms have been subject to a double standard of application makes problematic the assumption that the norms are grounded in human nature.

2. New knowledge about sexuality. The introduction of new "factual" knowledge has contradicted previously held beliefs about the meaning and potentiality of human sexuality. Thus, for example, new biological knowledge about the reproductive process has ruled out any norms built on the mistaken belief that the male sperm is the only active principle in human procreation. Moral rules regarding, for example, the dorsal position for sexual intercourse have fallen before more accurate knowledge of the way in which conception takes place. Arguments for the "unnaturalness" of certain sexual activities based either implicitly or explicitly on the belief that animals do not engage in them have been largely undercut by the growing evidence that higher forms of animals do, in fact, masturbate, perform sexual acts with members of the same sex, etc. Finally, many would argue today that the "facts" of the situation in which persons live out their sexuality have changed significantly with the advent of technology that can separate procreation from sexual intercourse and promiscuity from physical disease.

3. Cultural variations. Anthropological studies have testified that there are large variations between cultural groups regarding patterns of sexual behavior. What may be considered deviant in Western society is found to be permitted and even socially accepted in other societies. One report, for example, shows that in forty-nine out of seventy-six societies studied, homosexual activities of one kind or another are considered normal for certain members of the community (Ford and Beach, p. 130). Masturbation appears among both sexes in almost every society anywhere studied. There are no consistent norms for premarital or extramarital sex. Such information has tended to relativize for many persons the norms which they had previously assumed were universally adhered to by all persons with any insight into human nature.

4. Behavioral studies. Similarly, surveys of sexual behavior such as those made by Alfred Kinsey and Morton Hunt have caused many persons to be skeptical about the importance of sexual norms that are not adhered to by large portions of the society in which they live. This may have no meaning in itself for the validity of sexual norms, and indeed the studies have been roundly criticized for the assumptions on which they proceeded and the conclusions to which they have led. Nonetheless, even the suggestion that, for example, ninety-five percent of the male population in the United States, and seventy percent of the female population, engage in autoerotic acts has inevitably raised questions about past teachings regarding the evil consequences of masturbation.

5. Women's awareness of sexuality. The rise in self-consciousness among women has had an extraordinary effect on the way in which women perceive the meaning of sexual norms. Women's growing awareness of the dissonance between past teachings regarding their nature and role on the one hand and their own experience of themselves and their possibilities on the other has become a key source of insight for challenging laws and structures, attitudes, and patterns of behavior. The sobering experience of recognizing the long centuries of failure of vision that allowed sexism to flourish in spite of the best moral insights of their traditions has made many women dubious of the validity of almost all past moral teachings regarding sex. They have come to know firsthand the irrationality of sexual taboos, whereby, as Freud commented in regard to beliefs about the defilement associated with menstruation, pregnancy, and childbirth, "it might almost be said that women are altogether taboo" (Freud, 1918, p. 75). Their consequent struggle to overcome the fears that taboos engender has become a struggle to find new freedom from past norms for sexuality. Further, both men and women have come to question the adequacy of moral norms that arose in a context where equality and mutuality were not a possibility in relations between them (Rainwater, p. 204).

6. Psychoanalytic theory. The emergence of psychoanalytic theory has brought with it new perceptions of the meaning and role of sexuality in the life of each person. Whatever the final validity of, for example, Freud's insights, they have broken upon the modern world with a force that has swept away for many persons the foundations of traditional sexual morality. Luther's assertion of the inevitability of sexual desire and activity in every ordinary human life has found support in Freud's theory of sexuality (Freud, 1905). But now the power of sexual need and desire is not the result of sin but a natural drive, importantly constitutive of the dynamism at the base of the human personality. What for years could be understood as an effort to order sexuality according to rational purposes now must be understood in terms of repression (Freud, 1908). Where sex goes awry, there is psycholog-

ical illness, not moral evil. What is called for in response to a new form of determinism is not forgiveness but medical treatment. And overall, negative taboos that limit sexual expression must give way to a freedom in sexual activity that alone will allow health and well-being in individuals and a new order and creativity in society.

But psychoanalytic theory, like the other sources of challenge to traditional sexual ethics, raises as many questions as it answers. Even as Freud argued for liberation from sexual taboos and from the hypocrisy and sickness they entailed, he nonetheless maintained the need for sexual restraint. The move from undifferentiated sexuality to genital sexuality (in the service of procreation) and the move from the pleasure principle to the reality principle were affirmed as necessary to the existence of the individual in society and to the progress of civilization as a whole. Such moves imply, however, a reintroduction of sexual norms. Those norms, in turn, are subject to critique by new theories of sexuality joined with theories of economics and politics and radical projections of wholly nonrepressive, nongenitally oriented persons and societies (Marcuse, pp. 197–221).

7. Developments in modern philosophy. Psychoanalytic theory, then, was not alone in introducing new ideas about sexuality. Philosophy, too, has both mirrored changing patterns of sexual behavior and gradually offered new ways of conceptualizing and justifying these patterns. Seventeenth- and eighteenth-century philosophers continued to argue in favor of traditional forms of monogamous marriage and against anything that threatened those forms. Thus, Rousseau's *La Nouvelle Heloise* deplored the faults of conventional marriage, but strongly opposed divorce and marital infidelity. Hume, in his "Of Polygamy and Divorces," insisted that all arguments finally lead to a recommendation of "our present European practice with regard to marriage." Immanuel Kant, too, ultimately defended traditional sexual mores and institutions, though he introduced in his *Lectures on Ethics* a strong justification for marriage not in terms of procreation but in terms of altruistic love.

The late eighteenth century and the nineteenth century, however, showed clearly the growing break of philosophy with religious traditions regarding sexuality. The strong naturalism of Schopenhauer and Nietzsche paved the way for more radical theories of sexuality as an instinct without norms. The feminism of Mary

Wollstonecraft, Charles Fourier, and John Stuart Mill offered new ways of understanding sexual relationships. The charge of Marx and Engels that the institution of monogamous marriage was based on capitalist economics provided a radical critique of traditional sexual institutions.

Such an intellectual history, along with the work of Freud and sexual psychologists like Richard von Krafft-Ebing and Havelock Ellis, provides a background for twentieth-century sexual theory. On the one hand, philosophers like Jean-Paul Sartre and Maurice Merleau-Ponty, Bertrand Russell and Ortega y Gasset, Solovyev and Bordyaev attempt to reconstruct a meaning for human sexuality in general on new understandings of interpersonal love. On the other hand, philosophers like John MacMurray, Joseph Margolis, Richard Wasserstrom, Frederick Elliston, and R. M. Hare debate the need for and nature of norms regarding specific issues of monogamous marriage, adultery, homosexuality, and abortion (Baker and Elliston).

Contemporary ethical reconstruction

Those who are serious about specifying a sexual ethic that takes account of contemporary challenges to traditional ethics may gain insight from recent attempts at evolutionary analyses of Western views of sexuality. Thus, for example, in 1964 the French philosopher Paul Ricoeur noted three major stages in the development of sexual morality in the Western tradition as a whole (Ricoeur, 1964; Richardson). The beginning, according to Ricoeur, was marked by the identification of sexuality with the sacred. Through myth, ritual, and symbol, sexuality was incorporated into a total understanding of the cosmos, of life and death, of the gods of both heaven and earth. Then, in a second stage, with the rise of the great religions, sexuality and the sacred were separated. The sacred was now identified as transcendent, "celestial" not "earthly," separate and untouchable. Sexuality was hence demythologized, its meaning limited to but a small part of a total order. Thus arose the principle: Sexuality has meaning only as a function of procreation. Its boundaries were charted by the institution of marriage, its power restrained by discipline, and its expression governed by an ethic of justice rather than a lyricism of life. To the extent that sexuality, in this second stage, threatened to break out of its limited realm, it was feared and condemned. But a third stage emerges with the contem-

porary concern to free once more the power and beauty of sexuality for the whole of human life. Freud's lessons regarding the suffusion of the personality by sexuality have not gone unheard, and new understandings of the person plead for a new understanding of sexuality as language for the newly discovered sacred, spiritual-carnal realm of the interpersonal. Yet the power of sexuality is elusive, not inexhaustible as Freud thought, and subject to a sense of the absurd.

Ricoeur's evolutionary analysis, however inchoate, offers a background for outlining three possible steps in the formulation of an adequate contemporary sexual ethic. Within these three steps it is also possible at least to note some of the varied efforts already made in the formulation of such an ethic.

1. Dissociation of sex from symbols of defilement. Ricoeur wrote that sexuality is mysteriously tied up with Western symbolism of evil—tied up with it in a way that keeps human sexual life at a level of moral development far below the supposed justice ethic of stage two. In this analysis, the Greco-Hebraic history of the consciousness of evil is characterized by three moments—a sense of defilement, of sin, and of guilt. The sense of defilement is a pre-ethical, irrational, quasi-material sense of "something" that infects by contact (Ricoeur, 1967, pp. 25–46). A sense of sin, however, is a sense of betrayal of a covenant, of a rupture in a relationship. And guilt is the subjective side of sin. It is characterized primarily by a consciousness of the evil use of liberty, of a freely chosen rupture in a relationship.

The import of all this for sexual morality is that historically sexuality appears as paradigmatic of the experience of defilement, and the sense of defilement is not easily left behind in the moral development of either the individual or a people. There remains in the implicit consciousness of persons and the collective unconscious of a people an inarticulate but persistent connection between sexuality and evil. Advanced notions of justice in bonds between persons have not yet fully penetrated personal relations precisely as sexual. Hence, the first step in the formulation of a contemporary sexual ethic must be to move sexuality more completely from the realm of the pre-ethical to the ethical by refining the meaning of justice in its regard.

2. Introduction of principles of justice. Justice, of course, can have many meanings. If it is taken to mean affirming persons and groups of persons according to their concrete reality—according to the claims that their actual and potential reality places upon others—then the formulation of principles of justice depends upon an interpretation of the reality of persons. Now it is clear that contemporary efforts to develop a new sexual ethic are to a great extent based on new interpretations not only of human sexuality but of the human person. Thus, for example, new emphases on the element of freedom in the complex structure of the person give rise to norms for sexual behavior that place greater emphasis on the need for the free consent of both sexual partners. Similarly, new understandings of the nature and role of women give rise to norms of equality and mutuality in sexual relations between women and men.

The fundamental principle of respect for persons is not itself, of course, a new principle in either philosophical or religious ethics. It can be argued that it has functioned within Jewish and Christian ethics from the beginning (as the central meaning of the command to love one's neighbor). It was formulated explicitly in philosophical ethics at least by Kant. Its role in sexual ethics, however, has clearly grown in contemporary times. A new cry, for example, has arisen demanding that Christianity's traditional rejection of a double standard be visible in practice as well as in theory. And eighteenth-century philosophical arguments for marriage as the way to a mutual surrender that alone prevents the reduction of persons to mere means (and not ends in themselves) have attracted attention not heretofore accorded them (Baker and Elliston, pp. 8–10). Whatever the confusion and uncertainty in efforts to formulate a contemporary sexual ethic, some things at least are clear: that is, that sex should not be used (even in marriage) in a way that exploits, objectifies, or dominates either women or men; that rape, violence, or any harmful use of power against unwilling victims is never justified; that sex insofar as it is procreative must continue to be responsible in relation to offspring.

New perceptions of the reality of persons, and of the role of sexuality in human life, are at the heart of current ethical debate regarding contraception, masturbation, and homosexuality. What were previously dismissed out of hand as perversions of human sexuality are more likely to be regarded as quite natural—if human nature is understood to be essentially open to sexual expression in any intense relationship (Nagel); as more or less virtuous as they are more or less mutual, active, and integrated into the whole of human personhood—and not as they are more or less procreative or complete as physiological processes (Ruddick); or as, at worst, fixations at a not yet ideal level of psychosexual development (Freud, 1905, pp. 51–52).

Just as the general ethical principle of respect for persons has come to play a key role in contemporary sexual ethics, so, too, have other general ethical principles such as the principle of fairness, and principles of truth-telling and promise keeping (Atkinson, pp. 59–62; Wasserstrom). Thus, for example, adultery may be judged morally unacceptable on grounds of fairness, fidelity to promises, and a proscription of deception. Struggles to find measures of justice or injustice focus on questions of whether or not individuals are harmed and the common good is promoted. There is a strong tendency to place sexual ethical issues in the context of human rights—whether they have to do with personal justice claims of wives and husbands in relation to one another or more general claims of individuals and groups against social and legal oppression (Great Britain).

Special consideration continues to be given to the development of an ethics of procreative sex. Concern to maintain the traditional position that only sex with a procreative intent (or at least with an intent that is compatible with not closing off the possibility of procreation) is justified now tends to modulate into concern for discerning proportionate reasons for letting go one value (procreation) when it cannot be had without the loss of a prior value (conjugal love, or the welfare of existing children) (McCormick, 1971; 1973, pp. 77–92). Stronger arguments are being made, however, for holding together procreation and conjugal sex. Unlike traditional arguments, they lead not to the conclusion that if there is sex it must be procreative, but rather to the conclusion that if there is procreation it must be within the context of conjugal love (Ramsey, 1967; Russell, pp. 76–77, 129; Roach). Such arguments attempt to establish norms that assure both just care of offspring and the continued personalization of the process of procreation. They oppose arguments that attempt to justify procreation through artificial insemination by a third party donor, or through nonsexual means altogether, or through procreative sex that is not also an expression of conjugal love (Fletcher, pp. 164–165).

It is not an easy task to introduce considerations of justice into every sexual relation and the evaluation of every sexual activity. Critical questions remain unanswered, and serious disagreements are all too frequent, regarding the reality of persons and the meaning of sexuality. As continuing philosophical debates about sexual norms attest, what is harmful and what helpful to individual persons and societies is not always clear. What moral options for sexual behavior can exist outside the institution of marriage without threatening the institution is still debatable (Bertocci). Which sexual activities contribute to and which prevent the integration of sexuality into the whole of human life is not in every case evident (Rubenstein, p. 114).

3. Enhancement of sexuality. Perhaps the central insight from contemporary ethical reflection on sexuality is that norms of justice cannot have as their whole goal to set limits to the power and expression of human sexuality. Sexuality is of such importance in human life, and in interpersonal relationships, that it needs to be freed, nurtured, and sustained, as well as disciplined, channeled, and controlled. Indeed, an agent-centered ethic (as opposed to an act-centered ethic) now takes up with radically new seriousness the development of sexuality into what is traditionally called a theory of virtue.

Affirmation of sexuality as morally enhancing demands more than the mere assertion that sexuality is good whether procreative or not. In the past, sexual desire was suspect because of what was thought to be its power to distract and cloud the mind. What is being maintained in the present is that sex not only need not be distracting but, indeed, may enable a concentration of powers so that the deepest and most creative springs of action are tapped close to the center of personal life. What is denied is precisely the Platonic (and, in a way, the Freudian) notion that the power of eros is so structured that it can be freed for personal and cultural creativity only to the extent that it leaves behind the specifically sexual sphere.

On the other hand, hardly any ethicist argues today that sex necessarily leads to creative power in the individual or to depth of union between persons. Sexual desire left to itself is not even able to sustain its own ardor. In the past, persons feared that sexual desire would be too great; in the present the rise in impotence and sexual boredom makes persons more likely to fear that sexual desire will be too little. There is growing general evidence that sex is neither the indomitable drive that Luther thought it was nor the primordial impulse of early Freud-

ian theory. When it was culturally repressed, it seemed an inexhaustible power, underlying other motivations, always struggling to express itself in one way or another. Now that it is less repressed, it is easier to see other complex motivations behind it, and to recognize its inability in and of itself to satisfy the affective yearning of human persons (Russell, p. 128; Freud, 1912, pp. 66–68; Løgstrup, pp. 70–93). More and more theorists are coming to the conclusion that sexual desire without interpersonal love leads to disappointment and a growing meaninglessness. The other side of that conclusion is that sexuality is an expression of something beyond itself. Its power is a power for union and its desire a desire for intimacy.

The third step in the formulation of a contemporary sexual ethic is, then, discernment of the ways in which an ethic of justice can discipline sexuality precisely in order to prevent it from contributing to a general personal apathy. Though the institutionalization of sex runs the risk of taming the power of sex to the point of great loss, it nonetheless also offers a way finally to preserve that power. Sexual institutions, of course, like any other, must be reexamined in every age in the light of new insights into persons. Sexuality as language, so contemporary philosophy suggests, must become more true as well as more free.

MARGARET A. FARLEY

[*Directly related are the entries* SEX THERAPY AND SEX RESEARCH; SEXUAL BEHAVIOR; SEXUAL DEVELOPMENT; *and* SEXUAL IDENTITY. *For further discussion of topics mentioned in this article, see the entries:* ABORTION; CONTRACEPTION; HOMOSEXUALITY; *and* STERILIZATION. *Other relevant material may be found under* JUDAISM; PROTESTANTISM; *and* ROMAN CATHOLICISM. *For discussion of related ideas, see:* REPRODUCTIVE TECHNOLOGIES, *article on* ETHICAL ISSUES.]

BIBLIOGRAPHY

ATKINSON, RONALD F. *Sexual Morality.* New York: Harcourt, Brace & World, 1965.
BAILEY, DERRICK SHERWIN. *Homosexuality and the Western Christian Tradition.* New York: Longmans, Green & Co., 1955. Reprint. Shoe String Press, 1975.
———. *Sexual Relation in Christian Thought.* New York: Harper & Brothers, 1959. London ed. titled *The Man–Woman Relation in Christian Thought.*
BAKER, ROBERT, and ELLISTON, FREDERICK, eds. *Philosophy and Sex.* Buffalo, N.Y.: Prometheus Books, 1975.
BALTENSWEILER, HEINRICH. "Current Developments in the Theology of Marriage in the Reformed Churches." *The Future of Marriage as Institution.* Edited by Franz Böckle. Concilium: Theology in the Age of Re-

newal, vol. 55. New York: Herder & Herder, 1970, pp. 144–151.

BARTH, KARL. *Church Dogmatics.* Edited by G. W. Bromiley and T. F. Torrance. Vol. 3, pt. 4: *The Doctrine of the Word of God.* Translated by A. T. Mackay, T. H. L. Parker, Harold Knight, Henry A. Kennedy, and John Marks. Edinburgh: T. & T. Clark, 1961, p. 166.

BERTOCCI, PETER A. "The Human Venture in Sex, Love, and Marriage." Wasserstrom, *Today's Moral Problems,* pp. 218–233, especially p. 220.

BOROWITZ, EUGENE B. *Choosing a Sex Ethic: A Jewish Inquiry.* Hillel Library Series. New York: Schocken Books, B'nai B'rith Hillel Foundations, 1969.

BOUSQUET, GEORGE HENRI. *L'Ethique sexuelle de l'Islam.* Rev. enl. ed. Islam d'hier et aujour'hui, vol. 14. Edited by R. Brunschvig. Paris: G. P. Maisonneuve & Larose, 1966. 1st ed., 1953, titled *La Morale de l'Islam et son ethique sexuelle.*

COLE, WILLIAM GRAHAM. *Sex in Christianity and Psychoanalysis.* New York: Oxford University Press, 1955.

CURRAN, CHARLES E. "Sexuality and Sin: A Current Appraisal." *Sex: Thoughts for Contemporary Christians.* Image, D324. Edited by Michael J. Taylor. Garden City, N.Y.: Image Books, 1973, chap. 7, pp. 104–121.

EPSTEIN, LOUIS M. *Sex Laws and Customs in Judaism.* New York: Block Publishing Co., 1948. Reprint. Ktav Publishing House, 1967.

FELDMAN, DAVID M. *Marital Relations, Birth Control, and Abortion in Jewish Law.* New York: Schocken Books, 1974.

FLETCHER, JOSEPH F. *Situation Ethics: The New Morality.* Philadelphia: Westminster Press, 1966.

FORD, CLELLAN S., and BEACH, FRANK A. *Patterns of Sexual Behavior.* Foreword by Robert Latou Dickinson. New York: Harper & Row, 1951.

FREUD, SIGMUND. " 'Civilized' Sexual Morality and Modern Nervousness (1908)." *Collected Papers,* vol. 8, chap. 2, pp. 20–40.

———. *The Collected Papers of Sigmund Freud.* Edited by Philip Rieff. Vol. 8: *Sexuality and the Psychology of Love.* New York: Collier Books, 1963.

———. "The Most Prevalent Form of Degradation in Erotic Life (1912)." *Collected Papers,* vol. 8, chap. 4, pt. 2, pp. 58–70.

———. "The Taboo of Virginity (1918)." *Collected Papers,* vol. 8, chap. 4, pt. 3, pp. 70–86.

———. *Three Essays on the Theory of Sexuality* (1905). Translated and edited by James Strachey. New York: Discus Books, 1971. Reprint. Basic Books, 1976.

FUCHS, JOSEF. *Die Sexualethik des heiligen Thomas von Aquin.* Cologne: J. P. Bachem, 1949.

Great Britain, Committee on Homosexual Offences and Prostitution. *The Wolfenden Report: Report of the Committee on Homosexual Offenses and Prostitution* (1957). Introduction by Karl Menninger. New York: Stein & Day, 1963.

GRISEZ, GERMAIN G. "Marriage: Reflections Based on St. Thomas and Vatican Council II." *Catholic Mind,* June 1966, pp. 4–19.

HERON, ALASTAIR, ed. *Towards a Quaker View of Sex: An Essay by a Group of Friends.* London: Friends Home Service Committee, 1963. 2d rev. ed. 1964.

KIEFER, OTTO. *Sexual Life in Ancient Rome.* New York: AMS Press, 1975. Reprint of 1934 ed.

LØGSTRUP, KNUD E. C. *The Ethical Demand.* Translated by Theodor I. Jensen. Philadelphia: Fortress Press, 1971.

McCORMICK, RICHARD A. "Current Theology: Notes on Moral Theology: April–September, 1970: (Situations of Conflict)." *Theological Studies* 32 (1971): 80–97.

———. "Current Theology: Notes on Moral Theology: April–September, 1972." *Theological Studies* 34 (1973): 53–102.

MARCUSE, HERBERT. *Eros and Civilization: A Philosophical Inquiry into Freud.* Humanitas: Beacon Studies in Humanities. Boston: Beacon Press, 1966.

MEAD, MARGARET. *Male and Female: A Study of the Sexes in a Changing World.* New York: William Morrow, 1949. Paperback ed. 1975.

NAGEL, THOMAS. "Sexual Perversion." *Journal of Philosophy* 66 (1969): 5–17.

NOONAN, JOHN T., JR. *Contraception: A History of Its Treatment by the Catholic Theologians and Canonists.* Cambridge: Harvard University Press, Belknap Press, 1965.

PARMISANO, FABIAN. "Love and Marriage in the Middle Ages." *New Blackfriars* 50 (1969): 599–608, 649–660.

PIUS XI. "Casti Connubii." *Acta Apostolica Sedis* 22 (1930): 539–592. Translated as "On Christian Marriage." *Catholic Mind* 29 (1931): 21–64.

PIUS XII. "His Holiness Pope Pius XII's Discourse to Members of the Congress of the Italian Association of Catholic Midwives, Castel Gandolfo, Monday, 29th October, 1951." *Catholic Documents: Containing Recent Pronouncements and Decisions of His Holiness Pope Pius XII,* no. 6, 1952, pp. 1–16.

RAINWATER, LEE. "Marital Sexuality in Four 'Cultures of Poverty'." *Human Sexual Behavior: Variations in the Ethnographic Spectrum.* Edited by Donald S. Marshall and Robert C. Suggs. Studies in Sex and Society. New York: Basic Books, 1971, chap. 7, pp. 187–205.

RAMSEY, PAUL. "The Case of the Curious Exception." *Norm and Context in Christian Ethics.* Edited by Gene H. Outka and Paul Ramsey. New York: Charles Scribner's Sons, 1968, chap. 4, pp. 67–135.

———. "Responsible Parenthood: An Essay in Ecumenical Ethics." *Religion in Life* 36 (1967): 343–354.

RICHARDSON, HERBERT W. *Nun, Witch, Playmate: The Americanization of Sex.* New York: Harper & Row, 1971.

RICOEUR, PAUL. *The Symbolism of Evil.* Translated by Emerson Buchanan. Religious Perspectives, vol. 17. Edited by Ruth Nanda Anshen. New York: Harper & Row, 1967.

———. "Wonder, Eroticism, and Enigma." *Sexuality and Identity.* Edited by Hendrik M. Ruitenbeek. A Delta Book. New York: Dell Publishing Co., 1970, pp. 13–24. Original appearance in English. *Cross Currents* 14 (1964): 133–141.

ROACH, RICHARD R. "Theological Trends: Sex in Christian Morality." *Way* 11 (1971): 148–161.

ROBINSON, PAUL A. *The Modernization of Sex: Havelock Ellis, Alfred Kinsey, William Masters, and Virginia Johnson.* New York: Harper & Row, 1976.

ROUGEMONT, DENIS DE. *Love in the Western World.* Translated by Montgomery Belgion. Rev. ed. Garden City, N.Y.: Doubleday/Anchor Books, 1957.

RUBENSTEIN, RICHARD L. *Morality and Eros.* New York: McGraw-Hill Book Co., 1970.

RUDDICK, SARA. "Better Sex." Baker, *Philosophy & Sex*, pp. 83–104.

RUSSELL, BERTRAND. *Marriage and Morals*. New York: Horace Liveright Publishing Corporation, 1929.

Second Vatican Council. "Pastoral Constitution on the Church in the Modern World." *The Sixteen Documents of Vatican II and the Instruction on the Liturgy*. Boston: St. Paul Editions, 1962, pp. 511–625, especially chap. 1, sec. 49, pp. 563–564. *Gaudium et Spes*.

THIELICKE, HELMUT. *The Ethics of Sex*. Translated by John W. Doberstein. New York: Harper & Row, 1964.

WASSERSTROM, RICHARD. "Is Adultery Immoral?" Wasserstrom, *Today's Moral Problems*, pp. 240–252.

———, ed. *Today's Moral Problems*. New York: Macmillan Co., 1975.

WYNN, JOHN CHARLES, ed. *Sexual Ethics and Christian Responsibility: Some Divergent Views*. New York: Association Press, 1970.

SEXUAL IDENTITY

There are many medical, psychological, philosophical, and ethical issues concerning sexual identity and sexual orientation—for example, in reference to homosexuality and transsexualism. The problems have long been hidden by the facile assumption that, quite simply, "boys will be boys and girls will be girls." However, serious studies of sexual identity have barely begun. Scientific study can be measured in decades; sexual psychology is less than a century old; and the philosophy of sex, although broached by Socrates, might still be said to be in its infancy.

In more detail, the credos of the facile assumption are these: There are two sexes without gradations—distinct biological types—each with its consequent psychological attributes, "normal" behavioral stereotypes and social roles, and a "natural" attraction for those of the "opposite" sex. The interplay of these various aspects of sexuality, according to the glib assumption, is singularly to have "intercourse." There may be accompanying desires—to have children, to prove a point, or to improve one's social standing. And there may be considerable "foreplay." But sex qua sex is simply sexual intercourse, whether embellished or completed or not.

In different cultures, within different theories, and among various individuals, one finds many divergent conceptions of male and female, of masculinity and femininity as sex roles, of sexual relations and attractions, and, in short, of sexual identity. As Kinsey insisted in 1948, sexuality is a continuum, and the various dimensions and degrees of sexuality do not always function in harmony. Biological males may play feminine roles; biological females may play masculine roles. Masculine males can be attracted to other males; feminine females to other females. Some girls act like boys; some boys dress like girls. Some want so much to be like the other that they have operations to effect just such a change. In a word, boys will not always be boys, nor girls always girls.

In any discussion of sexual identity it is important to remember that the concern is not merely with classification but with *self*-conception or *self-identity* as well. The problems of sexual identity, however they are tied to biological complexities or psychosocial circumstances, are always problems of how a person sees himself or herself and how he or she will and *ought* to relate to other people. Consequently, the questions of sexual identity immediately become *ethical* problems as well.

For clarity, the various dimensions of sexual identity can be grouped into four categories: (1) *biological sex:* male or female physiology and anatomic structure; (2) *gender identity:* the internalized psychosocial and cultural stereotypes of masculinity and femininity; (3) *sexual orientation:* sex roles as the external expression of gender identity, sexual aims, and choice of sexual objects (who or what attracts and excites a person, and what he or she wants to do with/ to them or have done by them); and (4) *sexual ethics:* ethical attitudes toward sex in general (What are its purpose and its functions in human life? Consequently, what sexual aims and objects are normal? Which are perverted? Which moral? And which immoral? Or are these questions even appropriate?).

Biological sex

It has too long been assumed that all levels of sexual identity depend solely on biological structures. In fact, however, it is becoming increasingly evident that even the biological distinction between males and females is far more complex than the traditional definition based on configuration of the external genitals.

John Money, director of the Johns Hopkins Gender Identity Clinic, and many of his collaborators have contributed to the growing body of information concerning sexual process development by studying intersexed people, individuals who show discordance *within* the components of their biological sex (i.e., they possess either or both the internal and the external sexual organs of each sex, or their sexual organs may be in contrast with their chromosomal makeup).

Money has suggested that our chromosomal sex, whether we possess the Y chromosome or not, is simply the first step in the biological unfolding of our sexual morphology (Money and Ehrhardt; Money, Hampson, and Hampson; Money and Tucker). The process of structural differentiation creating the internal and external sexual and reproductive organs for both sexes appears to be dependent upon critically timed events that occur during fetal development. These events, which are a function of gonadal release of androgenic hormones or the absence of such release, set the stage for the development of sex organs and also seem to create sexual differences in the sensitivity of the brain to circulating sex hormones. The brain differences will apparently mediate adult sexual behavior and perhaps even create some of the earlier behaviors, such as aggression, which are differentially exhibited by girls and boys (Maccoby and Jacklin).

In one of his earlier works, Money identifies five categories of biological sex (Money, Hampson, and Hampson). The categories are: (1) chromosomal configuration (XX or XY), (2) gonadal sex (presence of ovaries or testes), (3) hormonal sex (androgen or estrogen dominance), (4) internal reproductive structure, and (5) external genitalia.

With each stage dependent upon the satisfactory outcome of the previous stages, the possibility exists that either environmental or genetic factors may interrupt or alter the unfolding process to create sexual anomalies in which there remain some structural components of both sexes within the same person.

Gender identity

Just as the complexities of our biological sex have only recently been appreciated, there is also a growing understanding of the interaction between our physiology and the cultural prescriptions and proscriptions that define our gender role behavior. Though many have viewed gender identity merely as an inevitable extension of our biological sex, it has become increasingly evident that much of our so-called femininity or masculinity is the result of culturally accepted roles and expectations.

Money has reported that children to whom a sex is assigned at birth that is different from their chromosomal sex, grow up in all likelihood with a gender identity that conforms to their assigned sex rather than their chromosomal sex (Money and Ehrhardt). Social learning theorists (Gagnon and Simon; Mead) suggest that the identification at birth by doctor or parent—simply on the evidence of the child's genital formation—may be the most significant labeling that the child will ever receive. For accompanying the label is a collection of beliefs about sex and gender behavioral differences reflecting cultural definitions of what is proper for boys and girls or men and women to act like, aspire to, dress in, play with, think about, etc. These differences in cultural expectations create differences in treatment from which the child develops his/her own sense of gender identity (Sanders).

Money, Hampson, and Hampson have credited the cultural impact on gender specific behavior in this way: "A gender role is not established at birth, but is built up cumulatively through experiences encountered and transacted —through casual and unplanned learning, through explicit instruction and inculcation, and through spontaneously putting two and two together to make four and sometimes, erroneously, five" (p. 285).

A summary of research on the origins of psychological sex differences suggests that there are broad differences in the socialization of children of each sex: "Boys seem to have more intense socialization experiences than girls. They receive more pressure against engaging in sex-inappropriate behavior, whereas the activities that girls are not supposed to engage in are much less clearly defined and less firmly enforced. Boys receive more punishment and probably more praise and encouragement" (Maccoby, p. 348).

While some investigators believe that reward and punishment by such socializing agents as parents and teachers create the appearance of gender differences in the behavior of children (Sears et al.), others (Kohlberg) believe that the child, once recognizing his or her biological sex, begins to copy the behavior of others of the same sex, acquiring sex role behavior through an imitative process based on a recognition of sex differences.

In contrast to the usual pattern of sexual identity development are the comparatively few cases of people who show significant discordance between one of the components of their sexual identity and the other two. Perhaps the best known sexual identity variation is homosexuality, a categorization applied to individuals whose sexual orientation is toward members of the same sex but whose gender identity is consistent with their biological sex.

Transvestism, in distinction, may be viewed as the sexual identity mix in which gender identity is the inconsistent component. There are some men who simply wish to dress like women on occasion, thrilled at the idea of being accepted as women but delighting in the knowledge that their biological maleness is retained. Further, the true transvestite, as has been reported by Karlen, while often having only a mild interest in coitus, emphatically claims to be heterosexual in orientation. Curiously, transvestism is a variation of male sexual identity only and has rarely, if ever, been associated with women.

Finally, there are people (usually men, but sometimes women) whose entire gender identity and sexual orientation are in such conflict with their biological sex that they believe they will be satisfied with nothing less than alteration of their anatomy to resolve this inconsistency. These are people who are considered transsexual and who desire sex change operations to express their "true nature." Such operations succeed in harmonizing the former discord between biology and gender identity.

Finally, analysis of the bulk of evidence on the origins of gender differences and on the acquisition of sex-specific types of behavior supports the conclusion that biological predispositions may contribute to the types of behavior appropriate in an environment that encourages the acquisition of such behavior. Yet the latter may be acquired even in the absence of biological determinants through selective reinforcement by the adults who care for the child and through imitative modeling by the child.

Sexual orientation

Medical aspect of sexual orientation. The degree to which biological mechanisms alone determine our sexual object choice is as unclear as the complex biological influences on gender identity. Most scientists in this field seem unwilling to commit themselves too strongly to either the nature or the nurture side of the controversy. Is our choice of sexual partner simply one more bit of sex-appropriate behavior that is learned through social indoctrination, or is there a biological mechanism that triggers our eroticism?

In an effort to resolve the issue, some researchers are looking for possible physiological (hormonal and anatomic) differences between people who maintain nonstandard (so-called deviant) sexual orientations compared to those who are in conformity with the norm, while others are attempting to delve into the early childhood experiences of people to search for the social supports for development of either standard or nonstandard sexual practices.

There has been tenuous support for the decisive role of hormones in determining sexual object choice. Some researchers, such as Money, believe that the same fetal hormones that organize the dimorphic sexual structures also influence the organization of brain structures that affect sex appropriate behaviors, including sexual orientation. Others, e.g., Ingebord Ward, have found that female rats, whose mothers were injected with testosterone during pregnancy, and who also received testosterone shortly after birth, showed masculine appearances in their external genitalia and expressed significantly more masculine behavior such as aggression as well as more mounting and thrusting behavior toward other females. While Dr. Ward is careful about stretching her conclusions to explain human sexual behavior, her work does suggest that hormones may play a neurological organizing role in creating sexual object choice.

Studies of hormonal levels and sexual object choice in humans are less clear in identifying the connection. Some investigators have shown that testosterone level may be quantitatively lower among homosexual men as compared to heterosexual men (Kolodny et al.); others find no difference (Money and Ehrhardt; Greene). However, even the conclusive correlation of low testosterone level with homosexuality will not immediately establish a hormonal source for sexual object choice since lower testosterone levels also are associated with high levels of stress (Rose et al.), a state which may characterize many homosexual men and women given the negative view of society toward homosexual acts.

Psychological view of sexual orientation. Freud believed that sexual object choice resulted from an identification with the same sex parent and the internalization of social standards regarding sexual activity. Those events occurred, he observed, through the process of satisfying biologically focused needs within a supportive, but not too permissive, family structure. Much of the clinical research in studies of sexual orientation has dealt with the origins of homosexuality, and the studies have followed the basic tenet of

Freudian theory by examining the early parent–child relationship.

One of the better-known studies concerning the origins of homosexuality was made by a psychoanalyst, Irving Bieber, who compared the early family histories of male homosexual patients with the histories of male heterosexual patients. According to Bieber, homosexuals show similar family patterns typically characterized by dominant mothers and passive fathers (Bieber et al.). Other investigators (e.g., Bene, "On the Genesis . . . Female," "On the Genesis . . . Male") find that a poor relationship between children and their fathers is the most critical antecedent condition for a homosexual life-style. Whether from the psychoanalytic perspective or from a social learning model, which stresses that children fail to learn which is the appropriate sex partner for them (Mischel; Greene), there is considerable evidence to suggest that parents play an essential role in establishing the child's psychosexual health and feelings of sexual adequacy. There is still no conclusive evidence, however, that it is the parents who "create" a homosexual child.

Homosexuality is but one of a great many variations in sexual orientation. People are sometimes attracted to animals (zoophilia), to young children (pedophilia), to corpses (necrophilia), and to various inanimate objects and particular parts of people (fetishism). Furthermore, the varieties in sexual aim are even far more elaborate than the variations in object choice. The many embellishments of intercourse are well enough known. But once research begins to explore those more-than-mere embellishments, which are frequently known as perversions (though virtually every sexual activity has been labeled "perverse" by some people), it is evident that science has gone beyond purely clinical considerations and has firmly committed itself to an ethics of sexuality. (The scientific term, "paraphilia," glosses over the ethical views inherent in "perversion.") Voyeurism, exhibitionism, sadism, and masochism, within certain severely restricted limits, may occur in "normal" behavior (wearing a bikini; going to a burlesque; a "love bite" on the shoulder). But when such activities replace "normal" sex, when people inflict severe pain on their sexual partners (perhaps even without his or her consent), an ethical judgment is in order.

Sexual ethics

What is "normal" sexuality? The once prevalent paradigm of the two-minute-male-superior-ejaculation bout is no longer so generally accepted. Yet it must still be asked, and without the arrogance that usually accompanies the pride of "liberation," how far from that model we have in fact moved. Furthermore, we must not give in too quickly to the modern "all-stops-out" sense of liberation, as if "anything goes" (at least between consenting adults). If sex was too long too restricted, it does not immediately follow that it must henceforth be without any restrictions whatsoever. Rape, for example, is clearly over the ethical limits of sexual expression. Rape is not only perverse but immoral, since it does not require the consent of the raped. But there have long been laws, and most states and countries have them still, which hold that a man cannot, legally or logically, rape his wife no matter how explicit her lack of consent. Is seduction also over the limits? What of causing pain by mutual consent? What of fetishism, bestiality, or even masturbation? It is evident that the ethics of sex depends upon far more than a few simple rules of morality and etiquette. What constitutes "normal" versus "perverse" sexuality, and what is considered moral or immoral in sex, depends upon our overall conception of sex—What is its purpose? What function should it play in human life? Is it merely a biological "necessity" or one of the true joys of human existence? Is it merely nature's way of continuing the species, or is it primarily a source of aesthetic inspiration and an expression for the more spiritual emotions?

We are now into the philosophical questions of sexuality. Though philosophers have often avoided the subject, the perseverance of certain public philosophies has been a vital determinant of sexual attitudes in general. In particular, we can distinguish four general conceptions of sex, four different models or ideal types, in terms of which "normalcy" and "perversion," "morality" and "immorality" have been defined.

The reproduction model. For two thousand years, the harsher side of the Old Testament and the Christian theological tradition have viewed sex as primarily procreative, a means to conceiving children, i.e., with the dominant value placed on procreative effect and procreative intent, while avoiding all excessive sensuality. In accordance with "God's will" and his "natural law," sex was seen, among other perspectives, as a dutiful function between husband and wife. Sexual intercourse may also be an expression of love, but within this model its romantic, erotic, and protracted pleasures are trimmed away. For conception to occur, it is necessary for the male to ejaculate; therefore male orgasm, in the biologically appropriate place, is morally acceptable. Female orgasm, however, and female pleasure in general have dubious procreative function. It is usually thought to be an indifferent by-product; in excess, it is a perversion. So, too, with prolonged foreplay and any sexual activity that does not culminate in the conditions required for conception. Homosexuality, needless to say, is out of the question. So are all other forms of "wasting of seed," such as masturbation. The concept of procreation already has religious connotations. The reproduction model may persist, however, outside of any religious context, for example, in Darwinian or Aristotelian appeal to preserve the species. Within the reproduction model, sex for the purpose of having children becomes the ideal: Mutual pleasure and even expressions of love become of secondary importance. It is only with the addition of further demands, for example, that sex must provide mutual fulfillment, that we would insist that sex is more than a means of having children, even between a man and a woman who have that intention as well.

The pleasure model. The pleasure model might also be called the "liberal" model, since it is distinctively a reaction against the conservative reproduction model. We might also call it the "Freudian" model, in order to give homage to the person most responsible for its dominance in contemporary society. For it was Freud, in his *Three Contributions to the Theory of Sex*, who argued for sexuality as enjoyable for its own sake, not as a means to any other end, whether natural or divine. In Freud's theory, the pleasure model rested on a male-dominated biological foundation, a "discharge" model where sexual pleasure has its origins in the release of tension or *catharsis*. Of course, the tensions are not merely physiological; they also arise from complexes of ego-needs and identifications with various sexual "objects," usually (but not always) other people. Thus he distinguished (as we still distinguish) between merely physical gratification and "physical satisfaction." But the key to the model, and the cornerstone of most contemporary sexual ethics, is the idea that sex ought to be pleasurable. "Good" sex is that which provides maximum mutual pleasure; "bad" or mediocre sex is that which fails to satisfy either or both partners. But notice that, once the reproduction model has been rejected, there are no longer the same restrictions on either the objects or the obvious aims of sexual activity. Homosexuality is no longer "a perversion of sex";

at most (and even this is questionable), it is a less prevalent set of sex partner preferences. Sexual activities that will not result in conception are no longer secondary, and sex that is conscientiously *prevented* from resulting in undesired conception becomes the norm. And even masturbation, on the pleasure model, becomes a paradigm of acceptable sexuality, even if it lacks the dimension of *shared* sexual enjoyment. (This had been denied, for example, even by Krafft-Ebing writing several years before Freud.)

The metaphysical model. Despite the prevalence of the pleasure model today, much more is usually demanded of sexuality than mere pleasure, even mutual pleasure. People demand "meaningful" relationships. The metaphysical model provides just this sense of "meaning." The metaphysical model is the paradigm of romantic love, the idea that two people were "made for each other." We might also call this the "platonic" model, since its classic expression appears in Plato's *Symposium* ("platonic love," despite our current usage of that term, was not sexless in the least). It is the view of two half-souls joining together to form a unity. Christianity takes up this notion in its conception of marriage, though its use of the metaphysical model is sometimes confused by its concurrent stress on the reproduction model. And pleasure, according to the metaphysical model, is no longer the purpose of sex, although it will inevitably and desirably be its accompaniment. But sex without love, no matter how enjoyable, is to be rejected on this model. If it is not "perverse" or "immoral" it will at least be meaningless. And the meaning of a relationship is what is primary for the metaphysical model.

The communication model. Sex is often "meaningful" without love. Sometimes those "meanings" are demeaning, as in the extremes of a sado-masochistic relationship. But what is one to say of the many varieties of sexual activity that are aimed neither at reproduction, nor at pure pleasure, nor at expressions of romantic love? What of those relationships that seem to thrive on domination and pain? And what of those many tender encounters that, nonetheless, make no pretenses of love? To explain such aspects of sexuality, a fourth model is in order (Solomon, 1974). It views sex as *communication*, as a physical form of expression of one's emotions and attitudes for other people. It is a language—a body language—whose vocabulary consists of touches, gestures, and physical positions. It may be an expression of domination and submission; it may be an expression of respect, fear, tenderness, anger, admiration, worship, concern, and (of course) love as well. In the 1940s Jean-Paul Sartre defended a truncated version of this model in his classic, *Being and Nothingness*. He interpreted all sexuality as the expression of conflict, a war for domination and freedom. But what is communicated in sex is surely not this alone, nor is it always this at all.

The communication model shifts the emphasis in sexuality from the more physical and sensual aspects of reproduction and pleasure to interpersonal roles and attitudes and their expressions. In this it resembles the metaphysical model, with the emphasis broadened from expressions of love alone to expressions of all emotions and attitudes. Thus Sartre's model is clearly a communication model, but it is also too narrow, viewing only the more conflict-ridden and competitive interpersonal attitudes and neglecting attitudes of love and respect. Certain sexual positions and activities, for example, are visibly more expressive of domination–submission, or equality and respect, or resentment and fear, or shyness and timidity, and, according to the communication model, these nonverbal expressions are what is essential to sexuality, not merely a secondary "expression." This does not mean, however, that other sexual aspects are excluded. The intention to impregnate a woman, for example, is a most important expression of certain male–female attitudes (for example, in several of Norman Mailer's novels). Pleasure is quite obviously an important aspect of the communication model, but pleasure for its own sake is not. Pleasure, both the giving and the receiving of it as well as the sharing of it, is vital to the communication of many emotions. But pain may be important as well, and the infliction of small amounts of pain as well as the endurance of certain moderate discomfort is familiar as a means of expression in sex. What marks the communication model from the three more traditional models is its emphasis on expression of interpersonal emotions and attitudes. These expressions are recognized by the other models, but not as essential and primary.

But now it is evident that the answers to such questions as, "What is normal sex?" and "What is perverse?" become immensely complicated. On a strict reproduction model of sexuality, normal sex is whatever minimal erotic activity is necessary to promote conception (with an appropriate person—normally one's marital partner). All else is either irrelevant or immoral. On the pleasure model, whatever gives pleasure (to consenting adults) is "normal" and acceptable. Perversions of this model provide pain instead of pleasure, ignore the pleasures of the other person, or produce pleasures in a manner that is, in the longer run, harmful. On the metaphysical model, normalcy is sex as an expression of mutual love. On the communication model, what is "normal" becomes extremely complex, for one must view the emotions being expressed and the entire psyche of the people involved to make any intelligent judgment. Would there be perversions on this model? Perhaps any form of deceit would be (just as lying is a "perversion" of verbal communication). And masturbation, while not exactly perverse, would surely be less than wholly sexual (just as talking to oneself is less than a whole conversation).

Conclusion: the problem of normalcy

So long as biological specifications and sexual intercourse alone defined sexuality, "normalcy," as opposed to "perversion," could be easily defined. Males were equipped with certain obvious features, and females were differently equipped with equally obvious sexual features, and "normal" sex was intercourse between male and female. But as more was learned about the complexities of chromosome configuration and the biology of sex, the distinction between male and female—although usually still clear enough—became increasingly difficult. With the possibility of transsexual operations, the distinction approaches a legal-conceptual crisis, which has not yet been resolved. Are the defining characteristics of maleness and femaleness to be retained from ancient times in terms of obvious external characteristics? Or are less changeable aspects, such as chromosomal configuration, to be the determining factor? The second choice has the advantage of permanence but the disadvantage of contradicting the gender identity of a great many people whose lives are not wholly determined by their genetics. And as soon as one adds the necessary concerns of psychology to the medical considerations, the traditional view of "normalcy" becomes a Pandora's box of problems.

Gender identity and sexual orientation are largely based on, but not wholly determined by, biological sexual characteristics. Accordingly, any attempt to discuss the ethical category of "normalcy" depends not only upon increasingly complex biological considerations but even more complicated subjective and psychological considerations as well. Of the various cases and models we have considered, not a single one would be accepted as "normal" in every society and by everyone. Moreover, a pure instance of an ideal type or model is probably nowhere to be found; not even the most pious proponent of a religiously oriented reproductive view would deny the desirability of love, pleasure, and emotional expression in sex, nor would the most enthusiastic hedonist deny the desirability of reproduction (on at least some occasions), and, perhaps, love and communication also. And when these four models of sexuality are integrated with the matrix of possibilities that are to be found in the various combinations of gender identity and sexual orientation (and, in the most extreme cases, transsexual biological operations), the result is an enormous number of sexual life-styles, desires, and activities, every one of which would be insisted upon as "normal," at least according to some people.

How does one decide what is "normal" and what is not? In one sense, "normal" simply means "statistically predominant," and there are still many people who would insist on this as a proper definition. But it is clear that, in ethical contexts, "normal" means something else as well, namely "correct." But in an area where most behavior is private and involves only consenting adults, the relevance of statistics is easily challenged. Furthermore, what is statistically predominant in one portion of a population may be relatively rare in a larger domain; and what is prominent or even universal in one society may be rare and considered "perverted" in another. If sexual normalcy includes subjective preferences and psychological as well as biological considerations, then any definition of sexual normalcy will necessarily give priority to certain preferences and models over others. But which ones? The traditional religious standards? The more modern "anything-between-consenting-adults" attitude? The current "local standards" criterion (assuming it can be made clear how small a domain is "local"—a home or a block or a town or a state)?

The problem of "normalcy," then, becomes a dilemma. It begins with a built-in ambiguity between "statistically dominant" and what ethically ought to be. The first is easily enough ascertained, assuming either truthful informants or extremely inquisitive investigators. But the second, the quest for what ethically ought to be, cannot help but arise from within a particular psychological, cultural, and personal setting,

thereby presupposing many of the norms and attitudes that are supposedly to be investigated. In other words, the distinction between sociological description and ethical considerations becomes hopelessly blurred as soon as it is one's own sexual activities and values that are in question. If norms are culturally defined, and if biological considerations are not sufficient for a definition of normalcy, then all of the questions of sexual identity and normalcy versus perversity are left without definitive answers and without objective standards for providing such answers, except within an already well-defined community. But the delineation of such a community is precisely what is at stake in the quest for normalcy. A community of homosexuals will have persuasive and personally satisfying reasons in the defense of the normalcy of their sexual preferences. A traditional family in the Christian tradition will have its authoritative and personally conclusive reasons for its sexual mores. A person who has had a transsexual operation will provide, in the name of all of those who have also had or would like to have such operations, a set of urgent considerations that provide ample justification for his/her extreme nontraditional concerns.

The result of these moral complexities is not the rejection of the ethical quest, nor even the abandonment of the concepts of "normalcy" and "perversion." What emerges is a very complex matrix of models and considerations all of which must be taken into account, with the understanding that sexual ethics and sexual identity, as well as the concepts of "normalcy" and "perversion," are variously tied to these different models and considerations, not something "above" them to be defined without reference to them. In other words, what is needed in the quest for sexual ethics is a great deal of appreciation for diversity and complexity. It is with this appreciation for diversity and complexity that the contemporary quest begins.

ROBERT C. SOLOMON AND
JUDITH ROSE SANDERS

[For further discussion of topics mentioned in this article, see the entries: CONTRACEPTION; HOMOSEXUALITY; NATURAL LAW; RELIGIOUS DIRECTIVES IN MEDICAL ETHICS; SEXUAL BEHAVIOR; SEXUAL DEVELOPMENT; and SEXUAL ETHICS. This article will find application in the entries REPRODUCTIVE TECHNOLOGIES, articles on SEX SELECTION, ARTIFICIAL INSEMINATION, SPERM AND ZYGOTE BANKING, and ASEXUAL HUMAN REPRODUCTION; and WOMEN AND BIOMEDICINE. Other *relevant material may be found under* ABORTION, *article on* CONTEMPORARY DEBATE IN PHILOSOPHICAL AND RELIGIOUS ETHICS; EMBODIMENT; GENETIC ASPECTS OF HUMAN BEHAVIOR, *article on* MALES WITH SEX CHROMOSOME ABNORMALITIES (XYY AND XXY GENOTYPES); POPULATION ETHICS: ELEMENTS OF THE FIELD; POPULATION ETHICS: RELIGIOUS TRADITIONS; *and* SEX THERAPY AND SEX RESEARCH. *See also:* MAN, IMAGES OF; *and* STERILIZATION.]

BIBLIOGRAPHY

BAKER, ROBERT, and ELLISTON, FREDERICK, eds. *Philosophy and Sex.* Buffalo: Prometheus Books, 1975.

BENE, EVA. "On the Genesis of Female Homosexuality." *British Journal of Psychiatry* 111 (1965): 815–821.

————."On the Genesis of Male Homosexuality: An Attempt at Clarifying the Role of the Parents." *British Journal of Psychiatry* 111 (1965): 803–813.

BIEBER, IRVING; DAIN, HARVEY J.; DINCE, PAUL R.; DRELLICH, MARVIN G.; GRAND, HENRY G.; GRUNDLACH, RALPH H.; KREMER, MALVINA W.; RIFKIN, ALFRED H.; WILBUR, CORNELIA B.; and BIEBER, TOBY B. *Homosexuality: A Psychoanalytic Study.* New York: Basic Books, 1962.

FREUD, SIGMUND. *Three Contributions to the Theory of Sex.* New York: Dutton, 1962.

GAGNON, JOHN H., and SIMON, WILLIAM. *Sexual Conduct: The Social Sources of Human Sexuality.* Chicago: Aldine Publishing Co., 1973.

GREENE, R. *Sexual Identity Conflict in Children and Adults.* New York: Basic Books, 1974.

KINSEY, ALFRED CHARLES; POMEROY, WARDELL; and MARTIN, CLYDE E. *Sexual Behavior in the Human Male.* Philadelphia: W. B. Saunders Co., 1948.

KOHLBERG, LAWRENCE. "A Cognitive–Developmental Analysis of Children's Sex-Role Concepts and Attitudes." *The Development of Sex Differences.* Edited by Eleanor E. Maccoby. Stanford: Stanford University Press, 1966, pp. 82–173.

KOLODNY, ROBERT C.; MASTERS, WILLIAM H.; HENDRYX, JULIE; and TORO, GELSON. "Plasma Testosterone and Semen Analysis in Male Homosexuals." *New England Journal of Medicine* 285 (1971): 1170–1174.

MACCOBY, ELEANOR EMMONS, and JACKLIN, CAROL NAGY. *The Psychology of Sex Differences.* Stanford: Stanford University Press, 1974.

MEAD, MARGARET. *Sex and Temperament in Three Primitive Societies.* New York: William Morrow & Co., 1935.

MISCHEL, WALTER. "Sex-Typing and Socialization." *Carmichael's Manual of Child Psychology.* 2 vols. 3d ed. Edited by Paul H. Mussen. New York: John Wiley & Sons, 1970, vol. 2, pp. 3–72.

MONEY, JOHN, and EHRHARDT, ANKE A. *Man and Woman, Boy and Girl: The Differentiation and Dimorphism of Gender Identity from Conception to Maturity.* Baltimore: Johns Hopkins University Press, 1972.

————; HAMPSON, JOAN G.; and HAMPSON, JOHN L. "Hermaphroditism: Recommendations Concerning Assignment of Sex, Change of Sex, and Psychologic Management." *Bulletin of the Johns Hopkins Hospital* 97 (1955): 284–300.

————, and TUCKER, PATRICIA. *Sexual Signatures: On Being a Man or a Woman.* Boston: Little, Brown & Co., 1975.

NAGEL, THOMAS. "Sexual Perversion." *Journal of Philosophy* 61 (1969): 5–17.

ROSE, ROBERT M.; BOURNE, PETER G.; POE, RICHARD O.; MOUGEY, EDWARD H.; COLLINS, DAVID R.; and MASON, JOHN W. "Androgen Responses to Stress: II. Excretion of Testosterone, Epitestosterone, Androsterone, and Etiocholanolone during Basic Combat Training and under Threat of Attack." *Psychosomatic Medicine* 31 (1969): 418–436.

SANDERS, JUDITH ROSE. "Parental Sex Preference and Expectations of Gender-Appropriate Behavior in Offspring." M.A. thesis, Brooklyn College, 1974.

SARTRE, JEAN-PAUL. *L'Être et le néant: Essai d'ontologie phénoménologique.* Bibliothèque des idées. Paris: Gallimard, 1943.

SEARS, ROBERT RICHARDSON; MACCOBY, ELEANOR E.; and LEVIN, HARRY; in collaboration with LOWELL, EDGAR L.; SEARS, PAULINE S.; and WHITING, JOHN W. M. *Patterns of Child Rearing.* Illustrated by Jean Berwick. Evanston, Ill.: Row, Peterson, & Co., 1957.

SOLOMON, R. C. "Sex and Perversion." Baker, *Philosophy and Sex,* pp. 268–287.

————. "Sexual Paradigms." *Journal of Philosophy* 71 (1974): 336–345.

SHOCK THERAPY, ELECTRIC
See ELECTROCONVULSIVE THERAPY.

SITUATION ETHICS
See ETHICS, *article on* SITUATION ETHICS.

SMOKING

Tobacco smoking, especially cigarette smoking, has become increasingly recognized as a health concern. Studies cited in publications of the United States Department of Health, Education, and Welfare relate smoking to several serious conditions: (1) Cigarette smoking is one of the major risk factors contributing to the development of coronary heart disease; (2) smoking is an important cause of chronic bronchitis and pulmonary emphysema; (3) cigarette smoking has been clearly identified as a major cause of lung cancer; (4) some relationship between cigarette smoking and peptic ulcer disease has been established; (5) smoking during pregnancy may contribute to a higher stillbirth rate (U.S. DHEW). With the recognition that smoking constitutes a health risk has come renewed awareness of smoking as a moral issue.

Long before the scientific evidence on the dangers of smoking began to accumulate, there were serious objections raised by some to the use of tobacco. The Evangelical United Brethren, Quakers, Salvation Army, Mennonites, Mormons, Seventh-Day Adventists, and other religionists have consistently objected to the use of tobacco, not only because it is injurious and a needless waste of time but also because it is incompatible with an ethical belief in simplicity of life and a religious belief that smoking does not show respect for the body as a temple of the Holy Spirit. The use of tobacco has often been associated with a type of worldliness that the religious person should overcome in the pursuit of perfection.

Most religious and ethical traditions have insisted that, since life is good, each person has a moral obligation to take reasonable care of his or her own health. Smoking would be acceptable provided it did not significantly harm health and provided it did not lead to neglect of other responsibilities. Relaxation and enjoyment are legitimate needs. The use of tobacco to meet these needs is wrong only if it is immoderate or unreasonable (Ford, pp. 366–369).

With the increasing evidence that tobacco smoking is, in fact, harmful to health, the primary focus in the ethical analysis of smoking today is on the implications of one's duty to preserve one's own health and not to endanger the health of others. Ethical dilemmas arise in the realization that this duty may sometimes be in conflict with other important values, such as the need for relaxation and the importance of conforming to one's own personal life-style. Questions relating to the ethics of smoking can be described as they relate to the following dimensions of the question: (1) the individual and his or her own health, (2) the health (or rights) of nonsmokers, and (3) the public policy on smoking.

In the case of the individual and his or her responsibility to preserve health, the question is one of the proper balance between that responsibility and the right to risk health in the pursuit of other human values. Ethical reflection on the benefits and risks of smoking requires some sort of a ranking of goods; it requires a decision about how important bodily health is compared to tranquility and enjoyment.

Smoking, as it affects the health of others, poses several types of ethical questions. Many would hold that the pregnant woman has no right to smoke when she may be endangering the health of her unborn child. Do nonsmokers have rights not to be exposed to unnecessary risks and inconveniences caused by smokers? Perhaps the most important ethical issue regarding smoking and the health of others concerns the growing, selling, and advertising of tobacco products. Some of the values in conflict here are the needs of persons in tobacco farming, in-

dustry, and sales to earn a living and the obligation not to lead people into practices that are harmful to health. The issue is complicated by the fact that it is difficult to know how much of the demand for tobacco products is created by the suppliers.

One of the most important public policy questions regarding smoking is the use of taxation power. Heavy taxation of tobacco products to discourage smoking or to provide additional health care funds without burdening nonsmokers might be considered a proper expression of the government's role in protecting public health, or it might be considered excessive coercion of private choice of life-style. It has been argued that it is much more difficult for governments to protect the public from the dangers of tobacco if tobacco taxation constitutes a significant source of revenue (Friedman). Other public policy questions include the extent and type of advertising permitted, public support of research into the effects of smoking, and the manner in which the public is educated on smoking as a public health issue.

LEONARD J. WEBER

[*For further discussion of topics mentioned in this article, see the entries:* HEALTH AS AN OBLIGATION; *and* PROTESTANTISM, *article on* DOMINANT HEALTH CONCERNS IN PROTESTANTISM. *Also directly related are the entries* FETAL–MATERNAL RELATIONSHIP; *and* PUBLIC HEALTH. *Other relevant material may be found under* DRUG USE; RIGHTS; RISK; *and* SOCIALITY.]

BIBLIOGRAPHY

FORD, JOHN C. "Chemical Comfort and Christian Virtue." *American Ecclesiastical Review* 141 (1959): 361–379.
FRIEDMAN, KENNETH MICHAEL. *Public Policy and the Smoking–Health Controversy: A Comparative Study.* Lexington, Mass.: D. C. Heath & Co., Lexington Books, 1975.
National Research Conference on Smoking Behavior, 2d, University of Arizona, 1966. *Studies and Issues in Smoking Behavior.* Edited by Salvatore V. Zagona. Tucson: University of Arizona Press, 1967.
United States, Department of Health, Education, and Welfare, Public Health Service, Health Services and Mental Health Administration. *The Health Consequences of Smoking.* DHEW Publication no. (HSM) 73–8704. Washington: Government Printing Office, 1973.

SOCIAL MEDICINE

Social medicine has been a concern within the professional community for a much briefer time than ethics. We have the Hippocratic Oath, dating back several thousand years. Thoughtful physicians, through the centuries, have contributed their own glosses on this Oath as to the physician's responsibility to a patient in his professional practice. None of these has attempted to evoke a sense of moral responsibility for *society*. The physician's role has been chiefly seen as a *personal* one. Whether the "prayer" of Maimonides, the Chinese traditional "commandments and requirements," or the more modernized codification of ethical principles for physicians, it is for the most part the one-to-one relationship that is elucidated in medical ethical principles. True, since the Second World War, from the shocking evidence of physician participation in grisly genocidal activities, new ethical statements (Declarations of Geneva, Helsinki, etc.) have been drafted to place physician behavior in a social context; but they nevertheless remain codifications of ethical behavior of a physician toward a particular patient.

Origin and meaning of social medicine

What is social medicine? What does it have to do with the question of medical ethics and the role of the physician? The origin of the term itself is relatively easy to describe. The origin of the concept is a little more difficult to set forth.

Changes in characteristic social attitudes among physicians grew slowly. The Industrial Revolution brought about such far-reaching changes in the lives of most people that care of the sick forced physicians increasingly to address themselves to larger matters than simply their relationship with an individual patient. They began to see that to take care of an individual patient it was necessary to do something with society as well. The early nineteenth century saw the beginning of a transformation of the physician's role (Rosen, 1948; 1949); the pathologist Rudolf Virchow, noting the victimization of the poor and helpless in the face of an epidemic, decided he had to take *political* action. He joined a political party and edited a radical medical–political newspaper whose masthead read "The physician is the natural attorney of the poor" (Terris).

While the term "social medicine" itself was first used by Guérin in 1846, it did not achieve wide use or stimulate scholarly study until the twentieth century, when Alfred Grotjahn published his *Soziale Pathologie*, and René Sand, *Vers la Médecine Sociale*. These works, among others, established the importance, or perhaps even the predominance, of social factors in disease causation, maintenance, and cure, leading

to the development of a whole field understood in this way. Thus, while a more traditional ethic imposed a discipline upon a physician in connection with his responsibility to a patient or to other physicians, social medicine, concerned as it is with the relationship between health and the conditions of society, imposed on him an added discipline of responsibility to society (Sand; Grotjahn).

When it was recognized that certain kinds of illnesses need not occur but could be prevented, the field of preventive medicine arose. As it was discovered that many of the causative agents were social in nature, social medicine embraced preventive medicine and included efforts to prevent disease not only in an individual but in whole communities. Through these processes it became clearly established that, for health and disease, there was an interface between society and medicine, not just between the doctor and a patient. The family itself, the home, the work place, the environment, and other social conditions played a part in whether or not a person became sick, how long he was sick, whether he recovered, and even if medical care and health services were available.

Early social medicine moved from helping the doctor make a better diagnosis or offer better treatment (an approach to clinical problems) to helping the medical profession recognize social factors that were pathological or therapeutic in society (an approach to public health). In its most recent interpretation, social medicine has also come to mean influencing the doctor's frame of mind as a professional, so he will recognize the need to modify social factors (in effect, an approach to social reform) (Ryle, 1948; 1949).

Social medicine, therefore, is the stage of ethical involvement *beyond* the doctor–patient relationship. Benefit to all patients ensues as a result of broad social action. Social medicine recognizes and aims to combat disease-causing factors within the social structure, whether they are sociological or psychological, economic or political, chemical or biological.

Social medicine as an ethical model

Physicians who would engage in the field of social medicine must therefore concern themselves with a wide variety of problems, disciplines, and factors that would in other times (or perhaps even today to most physicians) be considered outside the proper concerns of the profession of medicine.

The narrower view of the physician's responsibility actually served to restrict the physician from full consideration even of an individual patient. Once a person is recognized as a social creature, the physician must be broadly enough educated to recognize the total needs of a patient's life. The traditional physician, for example, never saw himself intervening to attack a social situation that might be contributing to the patient's illness or obstructing recovery. The medical profession as a whole has rarely taken any vigorous action to promote improved housing, nutrition, or educational opportunities, nor to combat racism, discriminatory practices, or the inequities and inadequacies of the medical delivery system and its distribution or availability.

The added ethical considerations included in social medicine may still relate to the improvement of the condition of an individual patient but not necessarily to the application of therapeutic modalities to that individual. Social medicine sees the ethical responsibility of the physician as the obligation to take steps to change or transform necessary pathogenic situations in order to protect society—of which the particular patient for whom he bears responsibility is a part.

It should be clear, then, that the full-scale practice of social medicine may place a physician in serious opposition to many powerful forces in society, not excluding the majority membership of his own profession. The penalties for taking moral positions in times of confused values are fairly heavy. In such times a physician adopting such a position may find the usual penalties increased by both the social and professional opprobrium visited upon him.

In their mildest efforts, physicians who undertake the practice of social medicine will face resistance if they attempt to utilize their professional role for the improvement of pathogenic social situations like inadequate nutrition or malnutrition; accidents and disease that befall those who live in inadequate housing; unsafe working conditions; environmental hazards or decayed neighborhoods; or polluted air and water. Since many of these factors are the result of neglect commonly visited upon the poor, the physician who seeks to modify such situations will find that he must act to eliminate poverty itself and to reverse the powerlessness of the poor to change the environment which accompanies poverty. The physician must perforce take a *political* position, even initiate political action, in pursuing this end.

Environmental health. An even larger step would have to be taken by a physician, as a responsibility of social medicine, when he recognizes the potent and often baleful influence of industry on the health not only of its workers but of the community in which the industry is located. There is more and more recognition that a great deal of cancer is environmental in origin, and the commonest such environment is the work place (Stellman and Daum, pp. 5–10). Accidents, very largely the result of inadequate safety measures, dangerous work places, and careless or callous disregard for safety standards, result in thousands of deaths and millions of injuries to which American workers are subject (Scott, pp. 1–4). Further, the effluent of factories poisons rivers, lakes, and air, contributing to chronic morbidity and increased mortality.

In these instances, the social medicine specialist, a physician with social concern, may find that political action is unwelcome since the community is torn between its need for the jobs provided by the industrial presence and the fear of its lethal qualities. In some communities the answer has been to keep the factory—the lethal factory—rather than run the risk of unemployment, poverty, and starvation without it.

A complex range of social action will be required to modify this situation since it touches upon the paradox of democratic capitalism: How can the government allow free rein to profit making while protecting the citizenry from destructive exploitation?

Medical care systems. The social medicine specialist would have to agitate for change and improvement in the structure of the medical care system since, as it currently operates, it is discriminatory in terms of both access and quality against the poor, the geographically isolated, and the marginally self-supporting workers. The dizzying inflation of medical costs has bankrupted families and barred access to medical care for many others. The disorganization of the medical care system contributes to these inequities and causes higher costs and poorer quality. What role should the physician play?

If access to medical care is dependent upon ability to pay, is there an ethical imperative for the physician to oppose ability to pay as a condition for service? Should not physicians demand that medical care be without cost to everyone at the time of service? In our society, profit making is not considered unethical, and at first glance there would seem to be no reason why medical care should be dealt with differently from other social services. But when it becomes clear that ability to pay interferes with appropriate access to and quality of medical care the matter takes on a different coloration. And whether or not the physician profits personally from the delivery of medical care, the profit motive clearly tends to operate against the best interests of the patient. Official reports as well as the shocking stories in the press about the scandalous treatment of old people confined to nursing homes makes this obvious. The profit motive too often leads not only to cutting corners on services and short weights in food or supplies, but to substitutions of less qualified staff, elimination of necessary services, and waiver of safety measures and protection of the helpless inhabitants. Aside from the corrupt financial dealings it encourages in such cases, profit making prevents and obstructs the best care and the provision of alternatives to institutional care. A physician cannot insulate himself morally from the mistreatment of old people in nursing homes nor from the exploitation of patients in the entrepreneurial mechanics of the drug industry.

A corollary to this is the ethical question raised by the high incomes of certain physicians and their penchant for investment in drug industry stocks, in private proprietary hospitals, and in other profit making enterprises in the health field. Such physicians ignore bioethical principles based on sociomedical concepts.

Responsibility of the profession. In addition to this question of the individual physician's ethics in financial dealings that may compromise patients' best interests, there is the associated question of the physician's responsibility for taking action when he observes any unethical or unprofessional behavior on the part of a colleague. If a physician knows about the poor quality of a particular nursing home he visits, even if his particular patient is not touched by it, is he required to take steps to correct the situation? Legal steps? Professional steps? Or even more narrowly, if he knows of a colleague who does not and cannot carry out his obligations as a physician adequately because he is incompetent by reason of training, age, illness, or addiction—what does he do about it? He has an ethical responsibility to call attention to these facts by reason of his own professional ethical standards.

The physician is asked to make a difficult choice, as a citizen and as a doctor. Social medicine as an ethical model imposes an obligation on the physician to serve his patient by serving all patients. In another sense, it could be said that social medicine requires that the physician act as if he were personally and individually responsible for what his profession does. He must act not only as an individual but as a member of the profession. That profession, in turn, is expected to adopt an attitude of social support for all groups in society that require special attention, advocacy, and care. The profession is being asked to act toward society as the individual physician is asked in traditional ethical statements to act toward an individual patient.

But, for many of the demands, professional medical action is not the answer. The requirements are for social change and political action, e.g., nutrition for the children of the poor or occupational safety measures. The profession is then expected to adopt the role of advocate, to plead the case, agitate, and make representation to state and federal legislatures.

In some situations the physician may very well be torn between social concern and his livelihood. A physician who works for an industry whose work processes may be resulting in disease or death to workers or community jeopardizes his job by taking a stand against his employer or the industry of which his employer is a part. If he takes a public position he endangers his own working life; if he does not, he is involved in complicity and endangers the lives of countless others. As we learn more of the etiology of cancer and the powerful role played in the causation of cancer by environmental factors, a physician cannot be expected ethically to keep silent when the work situation is carcinogenic. By his silence he threatens the lives of the workers in the plant, citizens in the surrounding community, perhaps even distant populations.

Other examples of this dilemma of dual responsibility can be given. In wartime, a physician's responsibility to care for the wounded is only a part of his job. He also has a responsibility to his government to restore the wounded to action as quickly as possible. His decision as to which patient to treat has to take into consideration which one can be returned to duty most quickly. In an extreme case, he would be expected to let a seriously wounded soldier die in order to save the life of one less seriously wounded who was able to return more quickly to action. And if there were enemy wounded, more seriously hurt, when would their turn be?

In peacetime, the situation of some employed physicians may parallel that of the wartime front line doctor. A physician may be expected to minimize injury or disease reports in order to reduce the employer's financial commitment. That's his "job," as the employer sees it, that for which he was hired. Is the physician's "job" to put the patient's interests first, or the interests of the employer who pays his salary?

In traditional medical-ethical concepts, the physician is seen as an independent actor, or at best acting as a member of a professional group, but still as an individual. He is challenged to see himself as reacting to an internal demand of "medical ethics," and not to a law, or public requirement. In combining social medical concepts with these more individualistic ethical principles there comes a point where political action is required, because the action needed has no purely professional component. For this purpose, and for the physician to be effective, an educated and knowledgeable constituency is required to provide the necessary support for the political social action. The doctor, as a concerned and knowledgeable citizen, ought to undertake a public educational role. Discussing the dangers of smoking, though, is hardly enough. He ought also to discuss the economics of the tobacco industry and what can be done to correct that. If there is an industrial hazard that needs correction, he ought to advise not only on the danger but on means for correcting it.

It is clear, nonetheless, that for a physician to discharge his social medical responsibilities in complex areas, he would be much more effective as a part of a group larger than the medical profession alone. Social medicine asks that the physician be part of a "health profession" rather than of a medical profession exclusively. More than twenty years ago, Sir Theodore Fox talked about "the Greater Medical Profession," converting the medical empire into a commonwealth, as he put it (Fox). The imperious necessities of the times make it clear that to respond ethically to social needs is to act in concert with all others in and out of the health field for the protection of the health of all the people.

So the physician is asked to play a role in public education on health matters as a member both of his medical organization and of the larger health organization of which he is a part. And that educational activity is expected to offer political as well as medical grounds for action. When the matters touched upon, like carcinogenic substances, are clearly medical, the physician may be more likely to take personal sociopolitical action, or move his whole professional group and organization to such action. When it comes to more broadly social and less clearly medical and professional matters, such as poverty and racism, the obligation upon the physician may remain that of a socially concerned citizen, but the likelihood and opportunity for corporate professional action will diminish.

In the bioethical sense, it is hard to justify a hierarchy of ethical principles—"more ethical" or "less ethical" matters. If one accepts the fact that ethical behavior requires a personal commitment to social action to change *all* circumstances and instances that cause disease or obstruct treatment, it is difficult to introduce a calibration of judgment as to which of these matters is "necessary" for the physician to attack while others are less so.

And when one accepts a social base for ethical medical behavior, it is logical to ask why so few physicians have taken such positions and why so little is heard or spoken of this matter in discussions of medical ethics. Medical education is doubtlessly at fault since the emphasis in medical education in the past fifty years has been on technical skills that must be acquired by the physician in order to perform adequately and in the modern sense, in diagnosis and treatment. Again, the continuing emphasis on the one-to-one relationship between doctor and patient, strongly supported by technical and technological underpinnings, has drawn attention away from the moral and ethical aspects of the physician's social role.

Recently, in the spate of observations on modern China, the slogan "Serve the People" has been offered as a paramount example of Chinese medical philosophy and medical ethics (Sidel and Sidel). It establishes social medicine as the source of ethical principles for physicians' behavior. While the concept of community medicine in the latest revision of the British National Health Service (Great Britain, DHSS), and the proposal for national policy in the Canadian government publication *A New Perspective on the Health of Canadians* (Canada, DNHW) also express the intention, it is fair to say that the Chinese model is still the only one that demands social responsibility as an aspect of the physician's ethical behavior.

Social medicine in medical education

It might not be amiss to ask whether a philosophy similar to that of the Chinese might not be included in the education of physicians in the United States and other Western countries as well, so that we will recognize and accept this social role as well as the personal patient-oriented role. Medical education should include not only the technical, laboratory, and clinical models of what a physician can do, must know, and must be able to deal with, but should also give the budding physician an opportunity to recognize the various social circumstances—industrial, neighborhood, legislative, administrative—which play a part in the production of disease or influence medical care. Not all physicians will be motivated to undertake administrative or nonclinical medical roles. The majority must continue to be personal physicians; but it is inevitable that exposure to these other factors, as important components of medical education, will influence physicians' ideas as to what their responsibilities are and how these responsibilities can be discharged (Silver). It should be emphasized that this teaching cannot then be relegated to a relatively minor place in the curriculum. The various elements must be significantly featured and presented as of equal prestige and dignity with the clinical and laboratory departments which occupy the larger part of the student's time and shape his career values.

Given a student who has been exposed to these perspectives, as a practitioner he is bound to recognize a wider and more definitely social role. The likelihood will be that many more questions will be raised among students regarding the need for social action in health matters with the result that a great deal more leadership by the medical profession will in the future be offered to the community, to the legislatures, and to society as a whole.

Conclusion

Early medical ethics was largely restricted to the concept of a physician–patient dyad. Social relationships of pathogenic factors were unknown or ignored. In recent years it has become clearer that the social aspects of the prevention, causation, maintenance, or cure of disease cannot be adequately dealt with in the one-to-one relationship. Expanded notions of the physician's responsibility based on these social factors ought, then, to be included in modern medical ethics statements. The physician should learn to recognize and articulate social demands for change in situations that are harmful to patients (citizens) and not simply deal with problems as they arise in his patient. To this end, he must know more about the social situations in which disease occurs, or which contribute to

disease, adopt an advocacy role in pursuing change, and join with other health workers in assuring appropriate social action for correction. In addition to the Hippocratic Oath, the prayer of Maimonides, the Declarations of Helsinki and Geneva, and the like, in which physicians bind themselves to serve a patient honorably and ethically, it is suggested that service to society also be demanded from physicians as an ethical commitment. Social medicine deserves an integral place within a more traditional medical ethics.

George A. Silver

[*Directly related are the entries* Environmental Ethics, *article on* environmental health and human disease; Poverty and Health; *and* Public Health. *For discussion of related ideas, see the entries:* Food Policy; Health Care, *article on* health-care system; Medical Profession, *article on* medical professionalism; Racism, *article on* racism and medicine; *and* Medicine, Sociology of. *Other relevant material may be found under* Aging and the Aged, *article on* health care and research in the aged; Drug Industry and Medicine; Health and Disease, *article on* philosophical perspectives; Medical Education; Sociality; Therapeutic Relationship, *articles on* contemporary sociological analysis *and* contemporary medical perspective; *and* Warfare, *article on* medicine and war.]

BIBLIOGRAPHY

Canada, Department of National Health and Welfare. *A New Perspective on the Health of Canadians; A Working Document.* Ottawa: 1974.

Cochrane, A. L. *Effectiveness and Efficiency: Random Reflections on Health Services.* London: Nuffield Provincial Hospitals Trust, 1972.

Fox, T. F. "The Greater Medical Profession." *Lancet* 2 (1956): 779–780.

Great Britain, Department of Health and Social Security. *National Health Service Reorganization: England.* Cmnd. 5055. Her Majesty's Stationery Office, 1972.

Grotjahn, Alfred. *Soziale Pathologie.* Berlin: A. Hirschwald, 1912.

McKeown, Thomas, and Lowe, C. R. *An Introduction to Social Medicine.* 2d ed. Oxford: Blackwell Scientific Publications, 1974.

Rosen, George. "Approaches to a Concept of Social Medicine." *Milbank Memorial Fund Quarterly* 26 (1948): 7–21.

———. "In the Age of Enlightenment." *Social Medicine: Its Derivation and Objectives.* Edited by Iago Galdston. New York: Commonwealth Fund, 1949, pp. 13–29.

———. "What is Social Medicine? A Genetic Analysis of the Concept." *Bulletin of the History of Medicine* 21 (1947): 674–733.

Ryle, John A. "The Modern Concept of Social Medicine." *Practitioner,* no. 961 (1948), pp. 5–10.

———. "Social Pathology." *Social Medicine: Its Derivation and Objectives.* Edited by Iago Galdston. New York: Commonwealth Fund, 1949, pp. 55–75.

SAND, RENÉ. "The Advent of Social Medicine." *The Advance to Social Medicine.* London: Staples Press, 1952, pp. 507–589.

SCOTT, RACHEL. *Muscle and Blood.* New York: Dutton, 1974.

SIDEL, VICTOR W., and SIDEL, RUTH. *Serve the People.* New York: Josiah Macy, Jr., Foundation, 1973. Paperback ed. Boston: Beacon Press, 1974.

SILVER, GEORGE A. "The Teaching of Social Medicine." *Clinical Research* 21 (1973): 151–155.

STELLMAN, JEANNE M., and DAUM, SUSAN M. *Work Is Dangerous to Your Health.* New York: Vintage Books, 1973.

TERRIS, MILTON. "Concepts of Social Medicine." *Social Service Review* 31 (1957): 164–178.

SOCIAL WORK

See MEDICAL SOCIAL WORK.

SOCIALITY

The question of human sociality has implications that pervade the entire spectrum of bioethics; it governs the context within which bioethical issues are raised. The answers to questions about the definition of "disease," medical care as a right, and the social responsibilities of physicians, to name but a few, vary greatly depending on whether one sees human beings as fundamentally social or as individuals for whom society is a matter of convention. This article will examine the concept of sociality in some dominant contemporary schools of philosophical thought, as well as its implications for bioethics.

The question of human sociality

It was not until the seventeenth century, with social contract theorists such as Hobbes and Locke, that the question of man's sociality was raised for extended discussion. Plato, for example, has Socrates ask the question rhetorically in Book I of *The Republic,* and his interlocutor, Glaucon, simply accepts it as a premise that "no man is self-sufficing." Aristotle, in Book I, chapter 2 of his *Politics,* begins with the same assumption and is not embarrassed by doubts as to its validity.

This is understandable, since in the context of ancient and feudal social systems, man's relationship to society was explicit and necessary. Social cohesion made human sociality a truism. But, with the disintegration of the feudal order and the ascendancy of the market economy, social relations began to take on a form that reflected the possibility of considering man as primarily individual.

Those philosophers who hold the social contract theory, or some variation of it, consider this theory to be the liberation of man from a deficient form of civilization. They consider the issue of sociality to be a new and more sophisticated philosophical question—a question indicating a substantial step forward in political and social theorizing.

On the other hand, philosophers of the Hegelian–Marxist tradition consider the question profoundly ideological because, they say, it in no way reflects, and in fact *veils,* the real interdependence of humanity, an interdependence that has increased rather than decreased with the development of market society. Likewise, they would contend that virtually everything one might say about man as qualitatively distinguishable from other animals presupposes society. Culture, language, self-consciousness, historicity, and the like presuppose society, and the ability to raise the question of man's sociality begs the question itself.

Furthermore, modern philosophers and sociologists like Schutz, Berger, and Luckmann have held that the very ideas we have of reality are socially based, and that human consciousness is itself a social product. Thus they reassert in a modified form the core of what Hegel demonstrated in the beginning of the *Phenomenology of Spirit,* i.e., that any attempt even to name, let alone describe, a sheer particularity involves terms and concepts that are invariably universal.

If this is true, then the so-called determination of individual needs—the basis for the exchange relationship and therefore of contracts—is socially derived, and the alleged primacy of the discrete individual is a fiction. The Hegelian–Marxists would even go so far as to deny the validity of the very idea of private interest; the content of every private interest, they would say, is socially defined and historically developed, so the determination of needs and interests must always extend beyond an analysis of the individual. As Marx wrote:

The point is rather that private interest is itself already a socially-determined interest, which can be achieved only within the conditions laid down by society and with the means provided by society; hence it is bound to the reproduction of these conditions and means. It is the interest of private persons; but its content as well as the form and means of its realization, is given by social conditions independent of all [Marx, p. 156].

In spite of this, the contract theorists might claim, there is ample evidence in modern society of man's competitiveness, aggressiveness, self-centeredness, and anarchic behavior, all of which is mitigated only through contracts whose validity is upheld by the state. If we are to be realistic, they would say, we must accept the contractual model as the only alternative to chaos. The notion of the *free individual* is the legitimizing basis of individual rights.

Yet the notion of the free individual is open to interpretation. The Hegelian–Marxists have held that real freedom is socially developed and is not constituted by liberty in the abstract but by conformity to laws that express man's fundamentally social nature. The so-called free individual of contract theory is in fact imprisoned by his own individuality, cut off from the exercise of his sociality, an exercise possible only through cooperation. Immediately as one takes any action at all he is determining himself concretely in the world, and it is only insofar as one's actions are unhindered that he is *actually* free.

But unhindered action requires social cooperation. No one lives in the world alone, not even a hermit, and each person's ability to act depends upon a level of technical expertise that is socially derived. Sociality and freedom are therefore coextensive, and the Hegelian–Marxists would claim that this fact makes the idea of a so-called free *individual* incomprehensible. The duties of the individual toward society are in a profound sense the duties of the human being toward himself.

Implications for bioethics

What, then, are the implications for bioethics of each side of this question?

Implications of the contractual view. Recent social contract theorists of varying sorts, like Rawls and Nozick, would locate medical care completely within the realm of contractual relations. They would treat issues like doctor–patient relations, malpractice, the right to medical care, the medical definition of "person," etc., entirely under a contractual social model. Thus their answer would have to conform to the limits of the marketplace. The social origins of the "commodities" exchanged could not be considered, because exchange relations abstract from the qualitatively different histories of their objects and because all parties to a contract are considered abstractly equal.

There are limitations to the contract model.

For example, some issues other than those mentioned above could not even be raised within this context, because the language used in their formulation is social in a sense that far over-reaches the contract relationship. Questions about the connection between life-style and disease, for example, or between environmental conditions and epidemiology simply surpass the limits of the market, as does the comparison of the notion of medical "care" with the notion of medical "service."

For instance, the position of the most extreme modern contract theorists, exemplified by Robert Nozick, holds that there is some original, unexplained private entitlement to resources that forms the basis of all subsequent contractual relationships, and that each property-holder enters into the initial exchange completely free and equal with those with whom he does business. The doctor–patient relationship, as all other relationships, would be seen in this light to have developed out of a random series of exchanges and would have no special priority or uniqueness in comparison with any other exchange of commodities. The patient is simply buying services similar to those offered by an expert mechanic, and there are no social obligations on either part except those agreed to specifically in the contract. The issue of the right to medical care, on this view, is a moot question, because, in a system where everything is a commodity, nobody has a *right* to anything; all commodities are bought and sold. Malpractice would come under the dictum caveat emptor, and the social origins of the physician's expertise would be ignored.

A more moderate contract view, such as the one expressed by John Rawls, grounds the social contract in an ahistorical principle of justice-as-fairness and, while basing society on the "free, rational individual," holds that the principles of their association are "the principles that free and rational persons concerned to further their own interests would accept in an initial position of equality as defining the fundamental terms of their association" (p. 11).

While each person is looking after his own private interests, he nonetheless has a lowest-common-denominator notion of justice-as-fairness that grounds his consent to the social contract and therefore can appeal to an eternal principle when judging particular relationships within a market society. Thus issues like medical care as a right can be discussed in terms of the fair distribution of resources, although medical care itself cannot be considered a relationship that transcends the exchange of resources.

In other words, the *fairness* of particular exchanges can be discussed, but the validity of limiting medical care to an exchange context cannot. The principle of fairness, although meant to be an attempt to mitigate the blind individualism of private entitlement, abstracts from the exchange process and thus *presupposes* that entitlement. It does not alter the limits imposed by this view on the discussion of medical care and therefore does not allow for the possibility of considering medical care as a social resource rather than a private one.

Implications of the noncontractual view. In contrast, the noncontractual view of human society, expressed most vigorously by the Hegelian–Marxist tradition, can analyze the context of bioethical problems as well as the particular problems themselves. Not only can particular exchange relationships be called into question, but the validity of exchange itself as a so-called external form can be scrutinized. The possibility of regarding medical care as a fundamentally *human* relationship—one of direct assistance and cooperation for the maintenance of values *not* capable of exchange—can be raised under this perspective, along with the corresponding claim that perhaps many of the problems arising out of the exchange context of bioethics stem from the fact that something is being treated as a commodity that cannot and should not be.

On this view, the right to medical care is a live issue, and if the question "Is medical care a right?" is answered affirmatively, the necessity of socialized medicine is implied. Since man is considered *fundamentally* social, there is no problem about certain social restraints and requirements being placed upon individual physicians and the medical community as a whole; their necessity is taken for granted.

Aside from these obviously social issues, questions seemingly internal to medical practice can be interpreted differently depending upon one's view of human sociality. Clearly, if one wishes to investigate the social nature of certain diseases, for example lung cancer, one needs to take seriously the objective, empirical dependence of human beings upon their environment, and furthermore, of that environment upon social conditions that affect it fundamentally. The social basis of advertising—e.g., private profit—and the socialization of personal habits through advertising—e.g., by cigarette commercials—can be taken more or less seriously depending on how one wants to view human choice.

If, as the contract theorists would have it, each person enters into every relationship and every action with his own private interests and his choice intact, then the effect of cigarette ads on personal behavior resulting in lung cancer is only indirectly causal, i.e., a nuisance that can be ignored. If, however, one agrees with the theory that holds that the content of private interest is socially defined, and that advertisements are central to the creation of that definition, then the treatment of lung cancer must extend to the banishment of cigarettes and their commercials as well as to surgery and radiation therapy.

Conclusion

The final verdict on this discussion is not yet in and may, in fact, be unavailable to philosophical reflection alone. However, one might make a provisional judgment based on how each position addresses the questions raised by social forces developing outside as well as within the context of medical care.

From the foregoing analysis it is clear that each position described takes some questions seriously and leaves others aside. Yet, regardless of which view one holds, it seems that the majority of bioethical issues presuppose a social nexus and have to be discussed in terms of the real relations between people. If those relations are simply contractual, or contractual within an overriding idea of justice, then a variety of bioethical questions are rendered moot. But if those relations are viewed from a perspective that takes human sociality as a fact, that sees human beings to be intrinsically social in the production and reproduction of their lives, then the only moot question is that of human sociality itself.

MICHAEL GORDY

[*This article will find application in the entries* HEALTH CARE, *articles on* RIGHT TO HEALTH-CARE SERVICES *and* THEORIES OF JUSTICE AND HEALTH CARE; MEDICAL MALPRACTICE; *and* SMOKING. *For discussion of related ideas, see the entries:* FREE WILL AND DETERMINISM; OBLIGATION AND SUPEREROGATION; *and* THERAPEUTIC RELATIONSHIP, *articles on* SOCIOHISTORICAL PERSPECTIVES *and* CONTEMPORARY MEDICAL PERSPECTIVE. *Other relevant material may be found under* JUSTICE.]

BIBLIOGRAPHY

BERGER, PETER L., and LUCKMANN, THOMAS. *The Social Construction of Reality: A Treatise in the Sociology of Knowledge.* Garden City, N.Y.: Doubleday, 1966.
HEGEL, GEORG WILHELM FRIEDRICH. *Hegel's Philosophy of Right.* Translated by T. M. Knox. Oxford: Clarendon Press, 1942.
———. *The Phenomenology of Mind.* Translated by J. B. Baille. London: S. Sonneschein & Co.; New York: Macmillan Co., 1910.

HOBBES, THOMAS. *Leviathan, Parts One and Two.* Introduction by Herbert W. Schneider. The Library of Liberal Arts, no. 69. Indianapolis: Bobbs-Merrill, 1958.

LOCKE, JOHN. *The Second Treatise on Government.* The Library of Liberal Arts, no. 31, Political Science. Indianapolis: Liberal Arts Press, 1952.

MARX, KARL. "The Chapter on Money." *Grundrisse: Foundations of the Critique of Political Economy (Rough Draft).* Translated with a foreword by Martin Nicolaus. Baltimore: Penguin Books, 1973, pp. 115–238.

————, and ENGELS, FRIEDRICH. The *German Ideology: Part One, with Selections from Parts Two and Three, together with Marx's 'Introduction to a Critique of Political Economy'.* Edited and with an introduction by C. J. Arthur. New York: International Publishers, 1970.

NOZICK, ROBERT. *Anarchy, State and Utopia.* New York: Basic Books; Oxford: Basil Blackwell, 1974.

RAWLS, JOHN. *A Theory of Justice.* Cambridge: Harvard University Press, Belknap Press, 1971.

SCHUTZ, ALFRED, and LUCKMANN, THOMAS. *The Structures of the Life-World.* Translated by Richard M. Zaner and H. Tristram Engelhardt, Jr. Northwestern University Studies in Phenomenology and Existential Philosophy. Edited by John Wild. Evanston: Northwestern University Press, 1973.

SOCIOBIOLOGY

See GENETIC ASPECTS OF HUMAN BEHAVIOR; EVOLUTION; BIOLOGY, PHILOSOPHY OF; POPULATION POLICY PROPOSALS, *article on* GENETIC IMPLICATIONS OF POPULATION CONTROL.

SOCIOLOGY OF MEDICINE

See MEDICINE, SOCIOLOGY OF.

SOCIOLOGY OF SCIENCE

See SCIENCE, SOCIOLOGY OF.

SOVIET UNION

See MEDICAL ETHICS, HISTORY OF, *section on* EUROPE AND THE AMERICAS, *article on* EASTERN EUROPE IN THE TWENTIETH CENTURY. *See also* APPENDIX, SECTION I, OATH OF SOVIET PHYSICIANS.

SPAIN

See MEDICAL ETHICS, HISTORY OF, *section on* EUROPE AND THE AMERICAS, *article on* WESTERN EUROPE IN THE TWENTIETH CENTURY.

SPERM BANKING

See REPRODUCTIVE TECHNOLOGIES, *articles on* SPERM AND ZYGOTE BANKING, ETHICAL ISSUES, *and* LEGAL ASPECTS.

SPIRITUAL HEALING

See MIRACLE AND FAITH HEALING.

STERILIZATION

I. MEDICAL ASPECTS   *Louis M. Hellman*
II. ETHICAL ASPECTS   *Karen Lebacqz*
III. LEGAL ASPECTS   *Jane M. Friedman*

I
MEDICAL ASPECTS

Introduction

The surgical techniques for sterilization are based on the interruption of continuity of the fallopian tubes in the female and of the vas deferens or sperm ducts in the male, thus preventing the passage of the egg or the sperm. While male sterilization procedures are fairly uniform, there are different techniques in the female. These operative techniques, developed principally in the early part of this century, were initially performed for medical reasons, although occasionally for eugenic reasons. In 1940 an important observation was made by Eastman that sterilization after eight viable pregnancies would reduce maternal mortality and that it could be safely and easily performed within several days of delivery. As sterilization gained in popularity, prerequisites for the operation, such as age of mother and number of live births, were rapidly eroded and replaced by the voluntary decisions of the patient and her physician. Similarly, male sterilization, which formerly required multiple consultations, is now done virtually on request of a patient who has given informed consent to the procedure. Gone too is the legal requirement for the spouse's consent in most instances.

Sterilization is any operation the primary purpose of which is to render an individual incapable of reproducing. Therapeutic sterilization is done to prevent a future pregnancy that because of an existing medical condition would be life-threatening to the mother or her fetus. Nontherapeutic sterilization is done primarily to avoid having children for other than medical reasons. Medically indicated procedures in which sterility is an unavoidable outcome do not fall under these definitions.

While the extent of sterilization in the United States is unknown, the operation is becoming very popular. There is a growing acceptance of vasectomy, at least among middle-class white males. It has been estimated (Westoff) that one partner in one out of six married couples between the ages of twenty and thirty-nine has had a sterilization operation. In 1974 there were 326,000 tubal ligations performed for women aged fifteen to sixty-four in the United States (unpublished data). Sterilization is becoming the most popular form of contraception among couples desiring no additional children. The increasing demand for this form of contraception is highlighted by a fifty percent rise between 1965 and 1970.

Sterilization in the male

Men can be sterilized by the procedure of bilateral vasectomy. In this operation, the vas deferens or sperm ducts are occluded or cut. The procedure is safe and relatively simple compared to sterilizations in women. It usually is done on an outpatient basis and takes about twenty minutes.

Vasectomy is performed under local anesthesia injected just below the skin into the scrotum. The surgeon makes a small cut (about one-half inch) on each side of the scrotum or a single midline cut. The sperm ducts are then easily reached and severed. The scrotal incision is sutured, leaving an invisible scar.

Sterility is not immediate after vasectomy. Live sperm may be present in the distal part of the sperm ducts for up to several months, depending on the frequency of ejaculation. It is for this reason that vasectomized men must submit semen samples for microscopic analysis until tests confirm the absence of live sperm, hence sterility. Most medical problems associated with vasectomy are minor. Some pain, swelling or bruising may be expected in the days immediately following the operation. In rare cases, an infection will set in and require medical attention.

Another rare medical phenomenon has been reported in which vasectomized men later developed antibodies against their own sperm protein. There is no evidence that this phenomenon is associated with pathology of any kind.

Very few vasectomized men have been noted to complain about such problems as impotence, decrease in sexual desire, or a feeling of loss of masculinity. Studies have shown that such complaints may be virtually eliminated through proper preoperative counseling.

If a man is unsure about ending his reproductive capacity or has doubts about vasectomy, he should not have the operation. A man undergoing vasectomy should consider it to be an irreversible procedure even though recent reports indicate that the sperm ducts may be rejoined surgically and fertility restored.

Finally, there are cases in which fertility is restored spontaneously. The growing back of the cut ends of the sperm ducts is possible, even years later, but this is rare.

Sterilization in the female

Tubal sterilizations involve interrupting the continuity of the fallopian tubes, thereby preventing the union of egg with sperm. The most common method of tubal sterilization is the "Pomeroy operation." In this procedure a section in the midpart of the tube is elevated, tied at its base with an absorbable suture, and cut. When the suture is absorbed, the severed ends separate and are covered with peritoneum (internal membrane) thus totally occluding each tube. Most other methods of transecting the fallopian tubes do not have the success rate (ninety-nine percent) of this simple procedure, nor are they as easily repairable should a reversal of the sterilization be desired.

The fallopian tubes can also be approached through the vagina, and either the Pomeroy ligation or removal of the fimbriated ends of the tubes can be accomplished. The morbidity associated with the vaginal method is somewhat higher than the very low morbidity of two to four percent associated with the abdominal approach. Mortality is also considered to be somewhat higher with the vaginal approach. The operating times for these traditional sterilizing procedures should not exceed twenty minutes.

More recently, endoscopic procedures for tubal sterilization have gained in popularity. These include laparoscopy, culdoscopy, and hysteroscopy. They hold great promise for accomplishing female sterilization without major surgery and costly hospitalization. In performing the laparoscopic operation, gas is introduced to distend the abdomen, and the laparoscope is inserted through a very small incision made to infuse the gas. Through the same or a second small incision, a cautery forceps is inserted. The uterus is then manipulated so that the tubes can be visualized, grasped, and obstructed by use of the cauterizing forceps. Usually the patient may go home after several hours. The morbidity associated with laparoscopic sterilization is difficult to estimate but may be as low as one or two percent. Accidents with cauterization, while infrequent, can be serious if the bowel is burned. Recently, clips or rings have been used to block the tubes offering less hazard than cauterization, but effectiveness has not yet been ascertained. There are many large series of laparoscopies where no pregnancies have occurred following the operation. The mortality may be as low as 14 per 100,000 procedures.

While laparoscopic sterilization can be performed in about fifteen to thirty minutes, it requires considerable training of the gynecologist, and the instruments used are expensive, costing between $2,500 and $3,500. Because the operation can be performed on an outpatient basis, however, the cost to the patient is much less than for abdominal sterilizations.

Another endoscopic technique involves the insertion of the culdoscope through the vagina. After distension of the abdomen, each tube is drawn out through the vaginal incision and blocked either by ligation or by the application of Tanteleum clips. This operation requires less anesthesia than the laparoscopic operation and produces no visible scars. However, it also requires special training. Previous pelvic adhesions and obesity can make this operation difficult if not impossible. The failure rate for culdoscopic sterilization is equivalent to that for vaginal ligation using the Pomeroy method. With a single Tanteleum clip, failure rates have been greater than two percent, and there is a high incidence of ectopic pregnancy. Failure rates can be reduced if two clips are used in each tube.

Hysteroscopic techniques for female sterilization are now under study in a number of countries. In this procedure a hysteroscope is inserted into the uterus filled with dextrose solution. Cauterization is then performed at each uterotubal junction resulting in the blocking of each tube. The failure rate of this procedure is considerably greater than the two previously mentioned procedures, and this method must be considered experimental.

Hysterectomy is the surgical removal of the uterus. It is often the recommended procedure in certain types of pathological conditions, such as cancer or other tumors. Recently, however, there has been an increasing trend toward hysterectomy for contraceptive sterilization. The operation is often justified with evidence that twenty to thirty percent of women sterilized by simpler methods develop gynecologic problems. This proportion, however, is probably no greater than in the population at large, thus may not be sufficient argument for elective hysterectomy and its risks. The operation is complex and costly in both hospital and surgeon fees. The morbidity may be as high as twenty percent; the mortality, as much as four times greater than for tubal sterilizations. Such risks make hysterectomy a drastic procedure to effect contraception which can be more simply accomplished.

Informed consent

Informed consent to sterilization means voluntary acceptance and assent to the sterilization operation with full understanding of the intent, the operative procedures, anticipated recovery time, attendant discomforts and risks, expected benefits, and expected outcome of, as well as alternatives to, the surgery. Failure of the operation to sterilize, though rare, is considered a risk. The benefits of sterilization are explained in such a way as to enable the patient to weigh them against the discomforts and risks before deciding to request and consent to the operation.

All oral and written explanations about the procedure must be in the primary language of the candidate for sterilization. Furthermore, consent must be truly voluntary and free of coercion. The patient must have freedom to withdraw a decision at any time prior to the operation. The intent of the procedure is explained as the permanent termination of fertility. While there are operations that may restore fertility after certain types of sterilizations, the patient must be told that the procedure must be considered to have a permanent effect.

The attendant discomforts as well as known risks to the health and well-being of the patient are to be stated. Anything the patient is apt to feel is to be accurately described.

Alternatives to sterilization are the available temporary methods of birth control. The patient is told that he or she has the option of choosing temporary methods to limit fertility and that there are sterilizing procedures for the opposite sex. The patient must be given ample opportunity to ask questions, and adequate answers must be supplied. Only when the above elements are presented to and understood by the patient can truly informed consent be obtained.

Sterilization procedures must be an integral part of sound medical care and practice at all times and in all places, requiring the highest medical standards and most complete and competent services available before, during, and after surgery.

Extreme care should be given to the motivational and educational preparation of patients with an adequate lead-time before surgery. Such patients must fully understand that voluntary sterilization is a final step in a series of available contraceptive measures.

LOUIS M. HELLMAN

[Directly related are the other articles in this entry, ETHICAL ASPECTS *and* LEGAL ASPECTS. *For discussion of related ideas, see the entries:* CONTRACEPTION; INFORMED CONSENT IN THE THERAPEUTIC RELATIONSHIP; *and* RISK.]

BIBLIOGRAPHY

Advances in Voluntary Sterilization. Proceedings of the Second International Conference, Geneva, Switzerland, 25 February–1 March 1973. Edited by Marilyn E. Schima, Ira Lubell, Joseph E. Davis, Elizabeth Connell, and Dennis W. K. Cotton. Amsterdam: Excepta Medica; New York: American Elsevier Publishing Co., 1974.

EASTMAN, NICHOLSON J. "The Hazards of Pregnancy and Labor in the 'Grande Multipara'." *New York State Journal of Medicine* 40 (1940): 1708–1712.

HELLMAN, L. M. and PRITCHARD, J. A., eds. *Williams Obstetrics.* 14th ed. New York: Appleton-Century-Crofts, 1971.

RICHART, RALPH M., and PRAGER, DENIS J., eds., *Human Sterilization.* Springfield, Ill.: Charles C. Thomas, 1972.

ROBITSCHER, JONAS, ed. *Eugenic Sterilization,* Springfield, Ill.: Charles C. Thomas, 1973.

WESTOFF, CHARLES F. "Changes in Contraceptive Practices among Married Couples." *Toward the End of Growth.* A Spectrum Book. Introduction by Charles F. Westoff. Englewood Cliffs, N.J.: Prentice-Hall, 1973. Based in part on the 1970 National Fertility Study, supported by the Center for Population Research of the National Institute for Child Health and Human Development under contract with the Office of Population Research, Princeton University.

WORTMAN, JUDITH. "Vasectomy: What are the Problems?" *Population Reports,* ser. D, no. 2, January 1975, pp. (D–25)–(D–39).

ZIEGLER, FREDERICK J., et al., *Vasectomy: Current Research in Male Sterilization.* New York: MSS Information Corporation, 1973.

II
ETHICAL ASPECTS

Sterilization is the deprivation, usually by surgical means, of one's ability to procreate. While sterilization can be temporary or permanent, this article will follow the general trend of ethical discussion and focus primarily on permanent loss of capacity. Sterilization may be voluntary, involuntary, or compulsory.

This article will be divided according to the various purposes of sterilization; sterilization may be done for (1) therapeutic, (2) contraceptive, (3) eugenic, (4) social, or (5) punitive reasons—reasons that are not necessarily exclusive of each other.

Therapeutic sterilization

The official Roman Catholic view begins from two premises. First, sterilization is a form of mutilation. It is therefore governed by the principle of "totality," which allows the removal of an organ only to save one's life or promote bodily integrity. Second, the generative organs exist for the good of the species and may not simply be subordinated to the good of the individual. The principle of totality is therefore modified by the principle of double effect according to which sterilizing operations are permissible only when interference with the generative function is an unintended or "indirect" effect; "direct" sterilization undertaken to limit generativity is never permissible. Thus, the official position of the Roman Catholic Church accepts only therapeutic and not contraceptive sterilization.

In the most conservative interpretation, removal of a scarred uterus that will endanger a woman's life in a future pregnancy is not permissible, since the organ does not threaten her unless she becomes pregnant—i.e., it threatens her only in its generative capacity. The sterilization is thus "direct" and immoral. Decisions about sterilization depend on the physician's assessment of the immediacy of danger. In this conservative Catholic view, all other uses of sterilization are rejected.

In contrast, John C. Ford and Gerald Kelly have argued that a scarred and weakened uterus may be considered a pathological organ and removed under the principle of totality (pp. 328–329). They thus broaden the definition of "therapeutic" sterilization to include not only instances of clear and present danger but also clear and future danger. Joseph Fletcher and other Protestant ethicists accept this broader definition of "therapeutic" sterilization.

Contraceptive sterilization: limited

Many Catholic, Protestant, Jewish, and Hindu spokespersons accept not only therapeutic sterilization but also some contraceptive sterilization.

Contemporary Catholic views. Bernard Häring argues that "totality" includes not only physical but spiritual health, including those "essential relationships" that constitute the context of well-being (Häring, pp. 56–57). Thus sterilization is permissible to save the "totality" of a marriage. (By extension, a man whose wife's life is threatened by future pregnancy could be sterilized.) Charles Curran argues that, since sterilization is distinguished from other mutilation because it is contraceptive, it should be judged under the broadening acceptance of stewardship over one's bodily functions (Curran, pp. 197–198). Rosemary Reuther asserts that in condoning the "rhythm" method of contraception, the Church opens the door to other means of contraception (including sterilization) since there is no obvious moral difference between temporal and spatial barriers to procreation. E. R. Baltazar notes that human marriage is "naturally" divided into a period of procreativity followed by a period of preservation; if the "marriage act" is understood as the totality of the marriage, prohibitions against interference in the procreative possibility of "the act" would not prevent use of contraception or sterilization at some point (Baltazar, pp. 159–172). Finally, Häring, Curran, and others argue that the decision rests ultimately with the individual's conscience rather than simply with Church teaching (Häring, pp. 37–38; Curran, p. 210). They do require reasons commensurate with the seriousness of a permanent intervention in a fundamental faculty, but they nonetheless accept some contraceptive sterilization.

Traditional Protestant views. Protestants argue that all means of contraception, including "rhythm," intervene in "natural" processes; thus there is no absolute rule for choosing among means (Barth, p. 273; Thielicke, p. 214). Further, many Protestants give primary importance to the *unitive* over the procreative function of sexuality; thus methods of contraception that undermine unity (e.g., prolonged abstinence) are rejected (Barth, p. 269; Bonhoeffer, p. 178). If sterilization is medically approved, it is morally permissible and becomes a question of conscience, according to *The Book of Resolutions of the United Methodist Church* (United Methodist Church, Program Council, p. 41).

However, willingness to have children is essential to marital fellowship (Thielicke, p. 205; Bonhoeffer, p. 176). Sterilization is not generally condoned in the absence of any children (Thielicke, pp. 205–206). Its acceptability depends on specific justifying reasons including serious illness, probability of genetic abnormality, or severe financial hardship. Its permanence mandates caution—hence, the "age-parity" rule, in which permissibility of sterilization is a function of the woman's age and the number of living children (Lader, p. 3). The possibility of reversible sterilization (or of sperm banking or in vitro fertilization) might induce broader acceptance of sterilization among Protestants and Catholics alike, although Paul Ramsey argues that if the reasons for bearing no children or no additional children are sufficiently grave, reversibility is not requisite and sterilization may be morally obligatory (1970, pp. 43–44).

Jewish views. Judaic law and practice have generally been opposed to all forms of castration and sterilization. The opposition to any tampering with the organs of generation is rooted both in the Hebraic view that it is a stringent obligation to fulfill the commandment, "Be fruitful and multiply," and in an abhorrence of radical interference with the order of nature, which is the product of a wise and loving God.

In orthodox and conservative Judaism, the only leniency is in regard to a woman. She was formerly permitted to take the "cup of roots," believed to render her sterile, if she was in fear of the pain of childbirth or in danger from childbirth. The "cup" was permitted because it did not directly damage the genital organs and also because the primary responsibility to "be fruitful and multiply" applied to the man. While the cup of roots is not known to modern medicine, contemporary sterilization techniques may also be acceptable, because they do not interfere with the normal manner of intercourse or with the course of the semen.

Reformed Judaism permits sterilization of women when health is involved and effective consent is given. The woman may use sterilization if childbearing would be dangerous to her or if the procreative commandment has been fulfilled. The unitive function of sexuality is sufficiently important so that contraception is preferable to abstinence.

Hindu views. Non-Western religions have not generally developed specific literature on the ethical acceptability of sterilization. In response to the introduction of government-supported programs of sterilization in India, however, some reflection has emerged regarding the ethical acceptability of sterilization in the Hindu tradition.

While there are no specific doctrinal objections to sterilization in Hinduism, there are pragmatic reasons for accepting only limited contraceptive sterilization. An Indian couple needs at least one surviving son and one daughter to fulfill their religious obligations. Moreover, impairment of health, fear of loss of children through accident, possibilities of sexual promiscuity, and the disgrace to a sterilized man whose wife becomes pregnant are offered as objections to sterilization (Mandelbaum, pp. 99–102). Thus, although sterilization has advantages over certain other forms of contraception, it is not acceptable to many Hindus until their families are established or there are strong reasons to prevent future childbearing, e.g., the disgrace to a grandmother who becomes pregnant (ibid., pp. 83–84).

Contraceptive sterilization: unlimited

Some Protestants have joined humanists and others in urging removal of age-parity formulas and approving unlimited availability of contraceptive sterilization. The primary justification offered is the prevention of worldwide disaster and protection of the "quality of life" (United Methodist Church, *Book of Discipline*, p. 89). The aesthetic superiority of sterilization over other forms of contraception and its permanence and dependability are also proffered as justifications. Finally, it is argued that sterilization promotes individual well-being through spontaneity in intercourse.

To those utilitarian arguments are added arguments about individual rights. The right to control one's body is a major tenet of feminist support for voluntary sterilization: Anselma dell'Olio argues that discrimination against women in political and economic spheres results from biological subjugation and can be righted only by reasserting control of one's own body. All forms of birth control should be available to women; however, vasectomy is the preferred contraceptive means because it is "easy, fast, safe, efficient, and cheap" (dell'Olio, pp. 38–39).

Spokespersons from the Judeo-Christian tradition do not generally accept the notion that one's body is one's own to control completely. Although such representatives might share a concern for population limitation, they are therefore reluctant to support unlimited sterilization as a means to that end. A different, pragmatic objection has been offered by one Hindu scholar, who argues against unlimited sterilization of Hindus on grounds that a reduced population will weaken their position vis-à-vis Moslems in India (Hendre).

Some go so far as to advocate economic penalties to induce sterilization or various forms of compulsory contraceptive sterilization (Lader, p. 252; Berelson, p. 2). Loss of individual freedom is justified by the gains of "sanity and survival" for society at large. Rights of future generations are also used as justification, but the overriding concern is survival of the species. Such proposals are unacceptable not only to spokespersons from the Judeo-Christian tradition but also to those who stress individual freedom.

Eugenic and social sterilization

Contemporary arguments for compulsory contraceptive sterilization resemble earlier arguments for eugenic and social sterilization.

E. S. Gosney and Paul Popenoe of the "Human Betterment Foundation" justified sterilization "(1) if mental disease and defect are a menace to the state, (2) if they are perpetuated by heredity, and (3) if sterilization seems to be the most effective means of dealing with them" (Gosney and Popenoe, p. 116). The good of the whole justified the sacrifice of individual freedom; eugenic sterilization was part of a "planned society," in which the physician protected the interests of the state. Jonas Robitscher notes that women were the usual targets of such proposals (Robitscher, p. 5).

Most eugenicists rejected widespread voluntary contraceptive sterilization, for fear that "good" people would fail to reproduce. Their interest was solely the sterilization of "defectives." Yet they hesitated to advocate compulsory sterilization directly, lest the eugenics movement lose credibility. Many compromised by allowing "proxy consent" on behalf of defectives or by arguing that release from a mental institution should be contingent upon sterilization.

Religious objections were dismissed as not appropriate in a "scientific" age. Sterilization was defended as cheaper and more effective than other proposed means to reach eugenic goals (e.g., lifelong institutionalization or a ban on marriage between defectives). When opponents charged that knowledge of heredity was not accurate enough to predict which children would become burdens to the state, eugenicists responded that, although the children of "degenerates" might be genetically normal, the environment in which they would be raised would be subnormal; thus where "eugenic" indications were not sufficient, they were supplemented by "social" arguments.

Lack of scientific basis has discredited arguments for eugenic sterilization. A few advocates remain—e.g., Joseph Fletcher and Glanville Williams—but most philosophers, theologians, and physicians oppose any eugenic sterilization other than a strictly voluntary one. Compulsory sterilization is rejected (1) as a violation of individual rights, and (2) as a dangerous precedent. Those Protestants who allow consent of the guardian for sterilization of a mentally retarded person often require stringent additional review (Thielicke, p. 224). Many Catholics, while rejecting compulsory eugenic sterilization, would allow "indirect" sterilization of a mentally retarded woman where the primary purpose is suppression of menstrual bleeding for one who is not able to take care of her own hygiene (Curran, p. 202). Further, many Catholic scholars would justify direct sterilization in the case of a retarded girl who could become pregnant because someone might take advantage of her—arguing that *prohibited* direct sterilization can apply only to voluntary sexual acts (ibid., p. 201).

In the face of public opposition, the "Human Betterment Foundation" has become the "Association for Voluntary Sterilization."

A renaissance of interest in compulsory sterilization for social reasons is reflected in the recent introduction into state legislatures of proposals, aimed largely at women who have borne children out of wedlock, requiring sterilization as a condition for receipt of welfare payments or child custody (Paul, p. 78). Such proposals are justified on grounds that they will reduce welfare costs and lower illegitimacy rates.

Counterarguments include pragmatic objections (e.g., that illegitimacy rates will scarcely be affected) and religious and moral objections (e.g., that abridgment of a fundamental freedom is not justified by the good of the whole). Objections have also been raised on grounds that such proposals are discriminatory since they affect largely poor or black populations (Gullattee, p. 92). All such proposals have thus far been defeated.

Several publicized cases indicate that women may also be unknowingly and involuntarily sterilized during childbirth or abortion by physicians acting without legal sanction (Rosoff). Such involuntary sterilization would be rejected by most religious and philosophical spokespersons.

Punitive sterilization

Julius Paul classifies involuntary or conditional social sterilization as "punitive" sterilization, since it appears to involve a mixture of public defense and private punishment (Paul, p. 82). Some persons have advocated sterilization as a punishment for crime or antisocial behavior, particularly for rape and other sex crimes. The physician performing such punitive sterilization becomes the agent of the state in exercising its penal functions.

Some Catholic theologians have defended punitive sterilization on grounds that the steril-

ization is not "direct" since the intended effect is punishment and the contraceptive effect therefore "indirect" (as reported in Curran, pp. 99–100). Protestant theologians Joseph Fletcher and Paul Ramsey suggest that there might be limited cases in which punitive sterilization is justifiable, on analogy with the right of the state to take life or the need to restrain the subject, but they urge caution (Fletcher, p. 169; Ramsey, 1956, p. 1199).

However, the mainstream of Catholic, Protestant, and Jewish thought opposes all punitive sterilization. The eugenicists also oppose it—in part for pragmatic reasons, lest it give sterilization a bad name, but in part as a matter of principle. Some also consider it a perversion of the proper role of the physician. Today there is less support for punitive sterilization than for any other form.

Conclusions

Contemporary religious and philosophical views on sterilization are in flux. While opposition to compulsory sterilization still runs high, pressure for voluntary sterilization has increased. Future directions of the flux will depend on (1) changes in underlying conceptions of the meaning and purpose of sexuality, for example, the relative weight given to the unitive and procreative functions of sexuality; (2) concern for the implications of world population growth and its effect on the "quality of life"; (3) increasing sensitivity to the possibilities of abuse of sterilizing operations, as highlighted in the public outcry over the involuntary sterilization of mildly retarded young women; and (4) credence given to feminist and other claims for the right to control one's own body.

KAREN LEBACQZ

[For further discussion of topics mentioned in this article, see the entries: CONTRACEPTION; EUGENICS; HINDUISM; JUDAISM; POPULATION ETHICS: ELEMENTS OF THE FIELD, *article on* ETHICAL PERSPECTIVES ON POPULATION; *and* POPULATION ETHICS: RELIGIOUS TRADITIONS, *articles on* ROMAN CATHOLIC PERSPECTIVES *and* PROTESTANT PERSPECTIVES. *Also directly related are the entries* POPULATION ETHICS: ELEMENTS OF THE FIELD, *article on* NORMATIVE ASPECTS OF POPULATION POLICY; *and* POPULATION POLICY PROPOSALS, *article on* COMPULSORY POPULATION CONTROL PROGRAMS. *Other relevant material may be found under* FUTURE GENERATIONS, OBLIGATIONS TO; PRISONERS, *article on* MEDICAL CARE OF PRISONERS; REPRODUCTIVE TECHNOLOGIES, *article on* ETHICAL ISSUES; *and* SEXUAL ETHICS.]

BIBLIOGRAPHY

BALTAZAR, E. R. "Contraception and the Philosophy of Process." *Contraception and Holiness: The Catholic Predicament.* Introduction by Thomas D. Roberts. New York: Herder & Herder, 1964, pp. 154–174.

BARTH, KARL. *Church Dogmatics.* 4 vols. Vol. 3: *The Doctrine of Creation.* 4 pts. Edited by G. W. Bromiley and T. F. Torrance. Translated by A. T. Mackay, T. H. L. Parker, Harold Knight, Henry A. Kennedy, and John Marks. Edinburgh: T. & T. Clark; New York: Charles Scribner's Sons, 1961, pt. 4.

BERELSON, BERNARD. "Beyond Family Planning." *Studies in Family Planning,* no. 38 (1969), pp. 1–16.

BONHOEFFER, DIETRICH. *Ethics* (1949). Edited by Eberhard Bethge. Paperback ed. New York: Macmillan Co., 1965.

CURRAN, CHARLES E. "Sterilization: Exposition, Critique and Refutation of Past Teaching." *New Perspectives in Moral Theology.* Notre Dame, Ind.: Fides Publishers, 1974, pp. 194–211. Original appearance. "Sterilization: Roman Catholic Theory and Practice." *Linacre Quarterly* 40 (1973): 97–108.

DELL'OLIO, ANSELMA. "A Feminist Case for Vasectomy." Lader, *Foolproof Birth Control,* pp. 38–40.

"The Family in Contemporary Society: From an Anglican Report." *Christian Ethics and Contemporary Philosophy.* Edited by Ian T. Ramsey. New York: Macmillan Co., 1966, pp. 340–381. The Lambeth Report.

FELDMAN, DAVID M. *Birth Control in Jewish Law: Marital Relations, Contraception, and Abortion as Set Forth in the Classic Texts of Jewish Law.* New York: New York University Press; London: University of London Press, 1968.

FLETCHER, JOSEPH. "Sterilization: Our Right to Foreclose Parenthood." *Morals and Medicine: The Moral Problems of the Patient's Right to Know the Truth, Contraception, Artificial Insemination, Sterilization, Euthanasia.* Boston: Beacon Press, 1960, chap. 5, pp. 141–171.

FORD, JOHN C., and KELLY, GERALD. *Contemporary Moral Theology.* Vol. 2: *Marriage Questions.* Westminster, Md.: Newman Press, 1964.

GOSNEY, EZRA SEYMOUR, and POPENOE, PAUL. *Sterilization for Human Betterment: A Summary of Results of 6,000 Operations in California, 1909–1929.* Publication of the Human Betterment Foundation, Calif. New York: Macmillan Co., 1929.

GULLATTEE, ALYCE. "The Politics of Eugenics." Robitscher, *Eugenic Sterilization,* pp. 82–93.

HÄRING, BERNARD. *Medical Ethics.* Edited by Gabrielle L. Jean. Notre Dame, Ind.: Fides Publishers, 1973.

HENDRE, SUDHIR. *Hindus and Family Planning: A Socio-Political Demography.* Bombay: Supraja Prakashan, 1971.

JAKOBOVITS, IMMANUEL. *Jewish Medical Ethics: A Comparative and Historical Study of the Jewish Religious Attitude to Medicine and Its Practice.* New York: Philosophical Library, 1959.

KALLEN, HORACE M. "An Ethic of Freedom: A Philosopher's View." *New York University Law Review* 31 (1956): 1164–1169.

LADER, LAWRENCE, ed. *Foolproof Birth Control: Male and Female Sterilization.* Boston: Beacon Press, 1972.

MANDELBAUM, DAVID G. *Human Fertility in India: Social Components and Policy Perspectives.* Berkeley: University of California Press, 1974.

PAUL VI. "Humanae vitae." *Acta Apostolicae Sedis* 60 (1968): 481–503. Translated as "Humanae Vitae (Human Life)." *Catholic Mind,* September 1968, pp. 35–48.

PAUL, JULIUS. "The Return of Punitive Sterilization Proposals: Current Attacks on Illegitimacy and the AFDC Program." *Law and Society Review* 3 (1968): 77–106.

RAMSEY, PAUL. *Fabricated Man: The Ethics of Genetic Control.* Yale Fastback, no. 6. New Haven: Yale University Press, 1970.

————. "Freedom and Responsibility in Medical and Sex Ethics: A Protestant View." *New York University Law Review* 31 (1956): 1189–1204.

ROBITSCHER, JONAS, ed. *Eugenic Sterilization.* Springfield, Ill.: Charles C. Thomas, 1973.

RUETHER, ROSEMARY. "Birth Control and the Ideals of Marital Sexuality." *Contraception and Holiness: The Catholic Predicament.* Introduction by Thomas D. Roberts. New York: Herder & Herder, 1964, pp. 72–91.

ROSOFF, JEANNIE I. "Sterilization: The Montgomery Case." *Hastings Center Report* 3, no. 4 (1973), p. 6.

THIELICKE, HELMUT. *The Ethics of Sex.* Translated by John W. Doberstein. New York: Harper & Row, 1964.

United Methodist Church. *The Book of Discipline of the United Methodist Church.* Edited by Emory Stevens Bucke. Nashville, Tenn.: United Methodist Publishing House, 1972.

————, Program Council. *The Book of Resolutions of the United Methodist Church.* Nashville, Tenn.: United Methodist Publishing House, 1972.

WILLIAMS, GLANVILLE L. *The Sanctity of Life and the Criminal Law.* Foreword by William C. Warren. James S. Carpentier Series of Lectures, 15th, 1956. New York: Alfred A. Knopf, 1957, 1970.

III
LEGAL ASPECTS

Sterilization, for purposes of this discussion, is a permanent deprivation of one's reproductive capacity. When the government becomes involved in the sterilization process, two types of legal problems can arise: (1) The state might attempt to compel an unwilling person to submit to sterilization (this assertion of state power will be hereafter referred to as compulsory or involuntary sterilization). (2) The state might attempt to prohibit or impose conditions on sterilizations of persons who desire to submit to the procedure, hereafter referred to as voluntary sterilization.

The first section of this article will explore the issue of the state's power, under the U.S. Constitution, to subject persons (usually "mental incompetents") to *compulsory* sterilization. The second section is devoted to a discussion of four current issues surrounding *voluntary* sterilizations. The latter problems will be presented in an international context, but with an emphasis on U.S. federal and state law.

Compulsory sterilization of "incompetent" adults and minors

Compulsory sterilization laws have historically been proposed by those who advocate the practice of eugenics—the improvement of human stock through the manipulation of heredity. Many eugenicists believe that the state can, indeed should, use its police power to prevent certain persons from procreating. In the 1920s in the United States there was a strong interest in the compulsory eugenic sterilization of a wide range of "socially inadequate" persons, including the blind, the deaf, and the homeless (Kindregan, p. 1405). The influence of those advocating such measures declined sharply in the 1930s, when their notions of national purity became associated in the public mind with the Nazi ideal.

However, compulsory sterilization laws still exist in many countries and in twenty-one states of the United States (Friedman, p. 131). Typically these measures are aimed solely at "mentally incompetent" adults and minors. The rationale behind such legislation is twofold. First, it is presumed that mentally disabled parents are incapable of taking care of their children. Second, it is believed that mental retardation is inherited and that society has an independent interest in preventing the birth of "defective" offspring.

In a few states the compulsory sterilization laws are extremely extensive in their coverage. For example, at the present time (1976) in Oregon a "Board of Social Protection," consisting of physicians and mental health workers, is empowered to order the sterilization of any person if his or her procreation would produce children "who have an inherited tendency to mental retardation or mental illness," or "who would become neglected or dependent children as a result of the parent's inability by reason of mental illness or mental retardation to provide adequate care" (Oregon Revised Statutes). A 1961 opinion of the Oregon Attorney General contains a list of persons who were, as of that date, candidates for compulsory sterilization. Among those were:

Feeble-minded, insane, epileptic, habitual criminals, incurable syphilitics, moral degenerates or sexual perverts, who are, or, in the opinion of the institution heads, are likely to become menaces to society . . . [and] persons convicted of committing or attempting to commit the crimes of sodomy . . . or . . . an act of sustained osculatory relations with the private parts of any person, or permitting such relations.

The constitutionality of compulsory sterilization measures was sustained in 1927 by the U.S. Supreme Court in the landmark case of *Buck* v. *Bell.* Justice Oliver Wendell Holmes, who wrote the opinion of the Court, explained why such laws were a social necessity: "It is better for all the world, if instead of waiting to execute degenerate offspring for crime, or to let them starve for their imbecility, society can prevent those who are manifestly unfit from continuing their kind. . . . Three generations of imbeciles are enough."

Subsequent to *Buck,* many state courts have been called upon to decide the validity of compulsory sterilization laws. Several have declared the laws unconstitutional, but their decisions were based on procedural inadequacies within the statute. Every state appellate court that has faced the issue of the substantive constitutionality of the statutes has concluded that compulsory sterilization laws are valid (Friedman, p. 131).

For example, in 1976 the North Carolina Supreme Court unanimously upheld the constitutionality of a 1974 state law that provided for mandatory, involuntary sterilization of "mentally incompetent" persons (In re *Joseph Lee Moore*). Under the terms of that statute, the candidate for sterilization was protected by stringent legal safeguards including the right to counsel, a hearing, and an appeal. The plaintiff, a moderately retarded minor, argued that the law was unconstitutional in that it denied equal protection of the law, violated the due process clause, was vague and arbitrary, and constituted cruel and unusual punishment. In rejecting those claims, the court stated: "Our research does not disclose any case which holds that a state does not have the right to sterilize an insane or a retarded person, if notice and hearing are provided, if it is applied equally to all persons, and if it is not prescribed as a punishment for a crime."

The North Carolina court, much like the U.S. Supreme Court fifty years earlier, noted that the state had an interest in curtailing reproduction by persons incapable of taking care of their children and an independent interest in preventing the birth of prospective "incompetent" offspring. The court characterized those interests as "compelling."

If the issue of compulsory sterilization should once again reach the U.S. Supreme Court, the result of that potential case is unpredictable. On the one hand, *Buck* v. *Bell* has never been expressly overruled. Indeed, as previously mentioned, *Buck* has been followed by every *state* appellate court that has considered the issue. On the other hand, during the fifty years subsequent to *Buck*, the U.S. Supreme Court has repeatedly recognized a constitutional right of "procreational privacy." That doctrine might cast serious constitutional doubt on the continuing validity of compulsory sterilization laws.

That the right to procreate might be a right of constitutional dimension was first recognized by the U.S. Supreme Court in 1942, in the case of *Skinner* v. *Oklahoma*. In that case the Supreme Court invalidated a statute that provided for the compulsory sterilization of persons who had been convicted two or more times of certain classes of felonies, but expressly excluded those convicted of "white collar" felonies, such as embezzlement. The Court did not hold that compulsory sterilization was unconstitutional per se, but only that it was a denial of equal protection to subject larcenists but not embezzlers to a compulsory cessation of their procreational capacity: "When the law lays an unequal hand on those who have committed intrinsically the same quality of offense and sterilizes one and not the other, it has made as invidious a discrimination as if it selected a particular race or nationality for oppressive treatment."

Both the majority and concurring opinions were also influenced by the lack of scientific evidence regarding the inheritability of criminal traits; and both opinions also clearly recognized that "undoubtedly a state may, after appropriate inquiry, constitutionally interfere with the personal liberty of the individual to prevent the transmission by inheritance of his socially injurious tendencies."

Thus, *Skinner* actually seemed to strengthen, rather than undermine, the notion that compulsory sterilization laws, if applied equally to those with genetically transmissible "socially injurious tendencies," are constitutionally permissible. On the other hand, Justice Douglas, writing for the majority, did refer to the right to procreate as "a basic liberty" and "one of the basic civil rights of man."

Although *Skinner* struck down a law that prevented certain people from procreating, the decision was used as authority for the invalidation of laws which, in effect, promoted procreation. In *Griswold* v. *Connecticut* (1965), the U.S. Supreme Court held unconstitutional a Connecticut statute that forbade the use of contraceptives. Citing *Skinner*, the Court held that the statute had a "maximum destructive impact upon [the marital] relationship" and that the privacy of that relationship was protected by the specific guarantees of the Bill of Rights.

Several years later, the Supreme Court made it clear that the right to procreate or not to procreate extended to unmarried as well as married individuals. *Eisenstadt* v. *Baird* (1972) invalidated a Massachusetts law that forbade distribution of contraceptives to unmarried persons. In holding that contraception was a fundamental right and that it therefore must be equally available to married and unmarried persons, the Court stated: "If the right of privacy means anything, it is the right of the *individual*, married or single, to be free from unwarranted governmental intrusion into matters so fundamentally affecting a person as the decision whether to bear or beget a child."

Finally, in invalidating the Texas antiabortion statute in *Roe* v. *Wade* (1973), the Supreme Court concluded that "the right of personal privacy includes the abortion decision, but . . . this right is not unqualified and must be considered against important state interests in regulation."

These decisions indicate that there is a constitutional right to procreate, to refrain from procreation, and to terminate a pregnancy. These rights are not absolute, however, and may be abridged if the state can advance an interest that is "sufficiently compelling."

The question that thus emerges is whether the state has a compelling interest in preventing the birth of offspring who are likely to be mentally disabled, and whether the compulsory sterilization of potential "incompetent" parents is an appropriate means for the achievement of that goal. While currently (1976) binding U.S. Supreme Court and state appellate court decisions have upheld the state's power to compel sterilization of mental incompetents, the issue of compulsory sterilization by the federal government or by institutions receiving federal funds was resolved in a contrary manner by a U.S. federal trial court. In 1974, in *Relf* v. *Weinberger*, the federal district court for the District of Columbia held, inter alia, that

. . . federally assisted family planning sterilizations are permissible only with the voluntary, knowing, and uncoerced consent of individuals competent to give such consent. . . . No person who is mentally incompetent can meet these standards.

Citing the aforementioned "procreational

privacy" cases, the court reiterated that individuals have a right "to be free from unwarranted governmental intrusion into matters so fundamentally affecting a person as the decision whether to bear or beget a child. *Involuntary sterilizations directly threaten that right."* (Emphasis added.)

The Department of Health, Education, and Welfare has appealed portions of this ruling, and at this writing (1976) the matter is before a court of appeals.

In sum, the issue of the validity of compulsory sterilization of mental incompetents is currently in doubt. The *Relf* decision has enjoined the federal government from providing funds for the sterilization of any person who (1) has been judicially declared mentally incompetent or (2) is in fact legally incompetent, under applicable state law, to give informed consent to the performance of such an operation. The state governments, however, apparently do have the constitutional power to subject mentally incompetent persons to compulsory sterilization.

Voluntary sterilization

Voluntary sterilization procedures give rise to at least four discrete legal issues: (1) Can an *"incompetent" person* (either adult or child) give legally sufficient "informed consent" to a voluntary sterilization? (2) Can a mentally *competent minor* give legally sufficient "informed consent" to a voluntary sterilization? (3) Can the state or state-assisted hospitals proscribe sterilizations for mentally *competent adults?* (4) In those jurisdictions permitting voluntary sterilization, what are the conditions that must be fulfilled before a *competent adult* may be sterilized?

Can an incompetent person (either adult or child) give legally sufficient "informed consent" to a voluntary sterilization? As previously discussed, the United States district court in the *Relf* case has held that all incompetent adults and minors are incapable of giving "knowing, and uncoerced consent" to a "voluntary sterilization." The court further noted that "the consent of a representative, however sufficient under state law, [cannot] impute voluntariness to the individual actually undergoing irreversible sterilization."

This matter has been appealed by the Department of Health, Education, and Welfare (DHEW); for DHEW desires to promulgate regulations under which persons who have been adjudicated mentally incompetent can be "voluntarily" sterilized. Those proposed DHEW regula-

tions would permit sterilization of a mentally incompetent person subsequent to certification by an "interviewer" that the patient (1) has requested the operation, (2) appears to understand the nature of it, and (3) has consented to it. The proposed regulations require additional and similar certifications by a physician and a review committee. In the event that the person is institutionalized, the proposed regulations further require the approval of a state court.

Can a mentally competent minor give legally sufficient "informed consent" to a voluntary sterilization? In the United States sterilization of minors is generally prohibited by state statute. As a matter of federal law, the *Relf* case proscribes the federally funded sterilization of persons who are minors under state law. In addition, DHEW has imposed a moratorium on all sterilization, either voluntary or involuntary, of persons who are under the age of twenty-one. However, DHEW is free to lift the ban at any time and to follow the *Relf* decree which allows state law to determine age-related eligibility for sterilization.

Many other countries also impose minimum age requirements on candidates for voluntary sterilization. Apparently there is a virtual universality of belief that young persons must be protected from making far-reaching, irreversible decisions that they are likely to regret later in life. The actual age of eligibility appears to range from eighteen, e.g., in Denmark and many states of the United States, to twenty-five, e.g., in Austria (Pilpel, p. 108).

Can the state or state-assisted hospitals proscribe sterilizations for mentally competent adults? Despite the increasing popularity of sterilization as a form of birth control, several countries currently prohibit competent adults from being voluntarily sterilized under any circumstances. For example, in Italy and Turkey a heavy monetary fine and up to two years' imprisonment are imposed on both the person performing the procedure and the person consenting to it (ibid., p. 109).

In the United States there are no statutes that actually prohibit voluntary sterilization. However, under a 1974 federal statute hospitals and other medical facilities that receive federal funds are permitted to assert a "religious belief" or "moral conviction" against performing sterilization or abortion procedures (Church Amendment). In 1975 the United States Court of Appeals for the Ninth Circuit sustained the validity of that law, holding that a Roman Catholic hospital could refuse to perform sterilizations, even though that hospital received federal funds and had the only maternity department in the city where the plaintiff could secure a tubal ligation at the time of her caesarean delivery (*Taylor* v. *St. Vincent's Hospital*). Despite the fact that this decision was squarely in conflict with a decision rendered by a different U.S. Court of Appeals (*Doe* v. *Charleston Area Medical Center*; cf. *Hathaway* v. *Worcester City Hospital*), the U.S. Supreme Court declined to review the matter. The result of the Supreme Court's inaction is that hospitals receiving federal funds in some parts of the country are required to perform voluntary sterilizations while federally funded hospitals in other parts of the country are permitted to refrain from performing the procedure on the grounds of religious or moral conviction.

In those jurisdictions permitting voluntary sterilization, what are the conditions that must be fulfilled before a competent adult can be sterilized?

Waiting period. The most universal precondition to the voluntary sterilization of competent adults is the waiting period. Designed to ensure that this irreversible decision is reached after careful deliberation, the actual time period appears to range from three days (U.S. federal regulation) to thirty days (e.g., New York City and the State of Virginia).

At least one country has a *maximum* waiting period. In Denmark a sterilization may not be performed *more* than six months after its authorization (Pilpel, p. 108). To ensure that there has been no change of mind, renewed consent must be obtained after this time period has elapsed.

Minimum number of children. In some countries a woman is not eligible for sterilization unless she has already given birth to a certain number of children. The requisite number appears to range from one (Singapore) to five (Panama) (ibid., pp. 108–109). There appear to be no such laws in the United States. However, in some states (e.g., Virginia) women who have not given birth to a child are subjected to a longer waiting period than those who have already borne at least one child.

Other conditions. In addition to the preconditions of a waiting period and a minimum number of children, several countries impose conditions relating to proof of economic or social hardship, e.g., Denmark and Sweden; spousal consent, e.g., Denmark, Singapore, and Japan; and governmental supervision of the procedure, e.g., Czechoslovakia, Denmark, and Singapore (ibid., pp. 107–109).

Conclusion

While governmental involvement in the sterilization process has given rise to a number of legal problems, the principal current issue involves the type of legal protection to be given to mentally incompetent persons. The two polar alternatives are represented by *Buck* v. *Bell*, in which the U.S. Supreme Court upheld the compulsory sterilization of "mental incompetents" and *Relf* v. *Weinberger*, in which a federal trial court enjoined all federally funded sterilizations of mental incompetents, including those procedures that are purportedly voluntary and uncoerced.

While the notion of compulsory eugenic sterilization is objectionable to many, it is arguable that *Relf* goes farther than is necessary to solve the problem of potential coercion. Surely, not all sterilizations of "mental incompetents" are the products of undue pressure. Perhaps the procedure should be made available to persons who are sexually active, unable to care for a child, and capable of giving voluntary informed consent to the permanent deprivation of their reproductive capacity. In such cases the interest of the individual and the interest of the state are identical, and it is difficult to ascertain what interests are being protected by making it impossible for such a person to obtain this permanent form of birth control. On the other hand, those who support the *Relf* decision argue that "mental incompetents" are a class of extremely vulnerable persons, and that they are simply incapable of giving informed consent and of withstanding coercive pressures. Therefore, it is argued, it is not possible to make sterilization available to the mentally incompetent and, at the same time, to ensure that all such sterilizations are truly voluntary.

JANE M. FRIEDMAN

[*For discussion of related ideas, see the entries:* ABORTION, *article on* LEGAL ASPECTS; CONTRACEPTION; EUGENICS; GENETICS AND THE LAW; INFORMED CONSENT IN MENTAL HEALTH; INFORMED CONSENT IN THE THERAPEUTIC RELATIONSHIP; *and* REPRODUCTIVE TECHNOLOGIES, *article on* LEGAL ASPECTS. *Other relevant material may be found under* MENTALLY HANDICAPPED; POPULATION POLICY PROPOSALS, *article on* COMPULSORY POPULATION CONTROL PROGRAMS; PRIVACY; *and* PUBLIC HEALTH.]

BIBLIOGRAPHY

ARTICLES

FERSTER, ELYCE ZENOFF. "Eliminating the Unfit—Is Sterilization the Answer?" *Ohio State Law Journal* 27 (1966): 591–633.

FRIEDMAN, JANE M. "Legal Implications of Amniocentesis." *University of Pennsylvania Law Review* 123 (1974): 92–156.

GIANNELLA, DONALD. "Eugenic Sterilization and the Law." *Eugenic Sterilization.* Edited by Jonas B. Robitscher. Springfield, Ill.: Charles C. Thomas, 1973, pp. 61–81.

KINDREGAN, CHARLES P. "State Power over Human Fertility and Individual Liberty." *Hastings Law Journal* 23 (1972): 1401–1426.

MATOUSH, WILLIAM R. "Eugenic Sterilization: A Scientific Analysis." *Denver Law Journal* 46 (1969): 631–656.

PAUL, JULIUS. "The Return of Punitive Sterilization Proposals: Current Attacks on Illegitimacy and the AFDC Program." *Law and Society Review* 3 (1968): 77–106.

PILPEL, HARRIET F. "Voluntary Sterilization: A Human Right." *Columbia Human Rights Law Review* 7 (1975): 105–119.

COURT OPINIONS

Buck v. Bell. 274 U.S. 200. 71 L. Ed. 1000. 47 S. Ct. 584 (1927).

Doe v. Bellin Memorial Hospital. 479 F. 2d 756 (7th Cir. 1973).

Doe v. Charleston Area Medical Center, Inc. 529 F. 2d 638 (4th Cir. 1975).

Douglas v. Holloman. Civil No. 76 Civ. 6 (U.S.D.C., S.D.N.Y.).

Eisenstadt v. Baird. 405 U.S. 438. 31 L. Ed. 2d 349. 92 S. Ct. 1029 (1972).

Griswold v. Connecticut. 381 U.S. 479. 14 L. Ed. 2d 510. 85 S. Ct. 1678 (1965).

Hathaway v. Worcester City Hospital. 475 F. 2d 701 (1st Cir. 1973).

In re Joseph Lee Moore, no. 72 (N.C., 29 January 1976).

Jackson v. Norton-Children's Hospitals Inc. 487 F. 2d 502 (6th Cir. 1973).

Relf v. Weinberger. 372 F. Supp. 1196 (D.C. D.C. 1974).

Roe v. Wade. 410 U.S. 113. 35 L. Ed. 2d 147. 93 S. Ct. 705 (1973).

Skinner v. Oklahoma. 316 U.S. 535. 86 L. Ed. 1655. 62 S. Ct. 1110 (1942).

Taylor v. St. Vincent's Hospital. 523 F. 2d 75 (9th Cir. 1975).

Taylor v. St. Vincent's Hospital. No. 75-759, 44 U.S.L.W. 3492 (1976).

Ward v. St. Anthony Hospital. 476 F. 2d 671 (10th Cir. 1973).

STATUTES

Church Amendment to the Health Programs Extension Act of 1973, 42 U.S.C. sec. 300a-7 (1974), Pub. L. 93–348, Title II, sec. 214, 12 July 1974, 88 Stat. 353.

Or. Rev. Stat. sec. 436.

MISCELLANEOUS

Opinion of the Attorney General of the State of Oregon, Number 5158 (Feb. 2, 1961).

STRIKE, PHYSICIAN'S RIGHT TO
See MEDICAL PROFESSION, *article on* ORGANIZED MEDICINE.

SUBJECTIVISM
See ETHICS, *articles on* NON-DESCRIPTIVISM *and* OBJECTIVISM IN ETHICS.

SUFFERING
See PAIN AND SUFFERING.

SUICIDE

Introduction

Nature and incidence of suicide.   A 1974 World Health Organization estimate indicates that in the reporting nations at least 1,000 persons kill themselves every day (Brooke). During 1975 in the United States, 27,000 deaths were reported as suicide, a rate of 12.6 per 100,000 (United States). Suicide is usually ranked as the tenth cause of death in the general population. It is among the first five causes of death for white males from ten to fifty-five years of age and the second cause of death for white males aged from fifteen to nineteen. Rates tend to reflect suicides in males, since the ratio of male to female suicide is about 2.5 to 1. The male suicide rate is consistently higher at all ages, but the trend may be toward increases in female suicide. Among white males suicide increases directly with age, while rates for white females increase until ages forty-five to sixty-four and then decrease slightly. Statistics used to establish suicide rates by race are even less accurate than those for the population as a whole. (In all likelihood, young black suicides occur at the same rate or above those of young whites, and above age forty-five below those of whites of the same age.) Married people have the lowest suicide rates. Completers and attempters of suicide are usually considered in separate but overlapping groups. Among the attempters there are usually three times as many females as males. A suicide attempt may be regarded as a communication, a "cry for help," to persons important to the attempter. Of those who attempt suicide, one to two percent complete suicide during each of the subsequent years when followed for a decade. The attempters most likely to complete suicide are usually older, male, divorced, widowed or single, abusers of alcohol or drugs, and physically or mentally ill.

Underreporting is common and varies with the criteria used for ascertaining suicide, the competence in medicine and law of persons responsible for completing the death certificate, the mechanisms used for collecting vital statistics, and the social and cultural attitude of the community in which the event occurs. So the social meaning of suicide in a given group is not adequately reflected by such figures (Douglas). For, unlike most causes of death, suicide may stigmatize the survivors as well.

Suicide has been recorded throughout man's history. The term suicide, which was first used in the seventeenth century to designate "self-killing," is usually meant to convey a self-decreed, self-intended, wished-for death. Definitions of suicide tend to vary with the social approval or disapproval of suicide and with different assessments of motives leading to the act of suicide. A life-style may even be regarded as "suicidal." Since the degree and awareness of a person's intention in any behavior followed by death may vary, Shneidman has suggested the classification of all deaths in terms of the intentioned, subintentioned, or unintentioned role of the individual in his own demise (1970).

Farberow views suicide in the perspective of self-destructive conditions, which vary historically and culturally in relative degree of importance. This leads to two ways of understanding suicide: (1) social or institutional suicide and (2) individual or personal suicide (Farberow). Social or institutional suicide implies that the suicide rate is a social product with social explanations, which supposedly do not rely on an awareness of intentions. Thus Durkheim concluded that suicide occurs when a person knows he will die from his own action, and that the rate of suicide varies with the social integration into society and the regulation by that society of social groups of which the individual forms a part.

To try to predict which persons are most susceptible to suicide, Durkheim used the following categories. (1) *Egoistic suicide.* A lack of meaningful social interaction subjects members of a society to personal isolation. For example, a single person who has few close personal friends is a greater risk for suicide than a married individual. (2) *Anomic suicide.* A lack of participation in the societal structure may occur when a person is deprived of position, wealth, spouse, etc. (3) *Altruistic suicide.* In the third, but minor, category social integration is actually excessive, and so suicide, as, e.g., in *harakiri*, becomes an honorable and socially encouraged action under certain circumstances (Durkheim).

The individual involved in such relationships with his group and society may be studied by a variety of concepts elaborated since Durkheim, e.g., status integration, the values and sentiments of the group, personal attitudes, the meaning(s) of the situation to the suicide, social-psychological variables such as internal restraint and frustration-aggression, and social mobility.

But since social forces alone cannot predict or explain the individual suicides, a psychological approach must be used. Freud viewed the causes of suicide as mechanisms involving the breakdown of ego defenses and the release of increased destructive, instinctual energy. Among these mechanisms are loss of love objects, aggression directed toward an introjected love object, narcissistic injury, overwhelming affect, and a setting of one part of the ego against the rest. Less dependent on the supposition of a death instinct is the adaptational concept of a failure to alter the environment and the inability to adapt to this failure, resulting in a retroflection of rage in which the object for punishment becomes oneself. (Identification with a hated object may still occur.) Suicidal intent may reflect negative feelings about oneself and one's world along with helplessness and hopelessness; and, particularly among the aged, suicide may be seen as a release.

Menninger, in a classic statement embodying the issues concerning the complexity of the suicidal act, regards suicide "as a peculiar kind of death which entails three internal elements: the element of dying, the element of killing, and the element of being killed" (Menninger, p. 24). Many likely suicides, however, wish neither to die nor to kill themselves; rather, they wish to interrupt intense anxiety and see no other way than to interrupt their lives. In the reconstruction of personal histories of suicides, ambivalence is found. Often contingent factors, such as the availability of a gun, seem crucial to carrying out the act. Impulse plays a major role. Such factors make it difficult to judge "intentionality" since an impulsive, contingent decision may occur either after intense planning or under acute stress, without such planning. Under acute stress, the person may be influenced to carry out his or her ideas by the immobilization of a person who might interrupt the attempt, the loss of interest of others, and the passive, or even the active, collusion of others, individually or collectively. It is possible to drive another person to suicide. Thus the degree to which a given act of suicide is a voluntary or compulsive behavior is difficult to evaluate. Although the person who commits suicide is no longer diagnosed as psychotic on the basis of the act itself, the possibility of making a "rational" decision to commit suicide is still debated. Brandt argues that suicide may be rational from the person's point of view in certain circumstances, but only when such a decision follows exhaustive examination of other options (Brandt).

Suicide is not a disease, for suicide is a form of behavior influenced by historical, cultural, social and personal relationships, and no single psychological, social, or medical theory suffices for its understanding and prevention (Perlin and Schmidt, p. 147).

Suicide as an ethical question. Suicide has become an important topic of discussion in recent medical ethics for three reasons. First, contemporary psychological and sociological studies of suicide raise serious moral questions, especially concerning the morality of suicide prevention. Second, developing medical technologies have transformed the process of dying into one that seems undesirable to many people, and suicide may present a way to avoid the pains and indignities of that process. Third, much modern analysis of medicine stresses the importance of patient freedom and patient rights, especially the right to refuse treatment. Yet refusal of lifesaving treatment and suicide may appear indistinguishable to those who hold certain ethical positions. We do not suggest that such distinctions are unimportant, but we will simply adopt a usage in which suicide denotes intentional self-destruction. The term in English often carries a connotation of moral disapproval as well, but we mean to use it in a strictly descriptive sense.

Obligations prohibiting suicide

There seems to be general agreement that obligations to other human persons are relevant to the morality of any decision for or against suicide. In contrast, two other types of obligation are more controversial. Some authors have claimed that we have obligations to ourselves; they then argue that suicide may (although it need not always) represent a violation of our duties to ourselves. Again, some writers claim that we have obligations to God that prohibit suicide in some (if not all) circumstances; other writers either deny the existence of God or deny that persons have obligations to him that are

distinguishable from their obligations to finite persons. In the former case theological arguments are meaningless; in the latter case they are redundant. We shall try to show something of the diversity of answers to questions of obligation to be found in Western discussions of the morality of suicide.

Obligations to other people. Many Western writers have held that obligations to other people make acts of suicide immoral. This stress goes back at least to Aristotle, who claimed that suicide was unjust to other Athenians (Aristotle). Thomas Aquinas reaffirmed the point: Each human being is part of some social group. In killing myself I injure the group by depriving it of whatever contribution (economic, psychological, political, or religious) I could make. Moreover, my act may offend the members of the group who view suicide as immoral on other grounds. Suicide deprives the group of resources and affronts its sensibilities (Thomas Aquinas II-II, 64, 5).

While the force of these arguments as practical counsels is hard to deny, it seems clear that they do not yield an exceptionless prohibition on suicide. It is not difficult to point to cases, especially in the context of contemporary medicine, in which an act of suicide would represent an honoring, rather than a default, of obligations to others, and suicide is not always perceived as offensive, even in the West. Moreover, as Hume, the Stoics, the Epicureans, and other writers have pointed out, it is not obvious that a community's legitimate claims on an individual are unlimited. Real obligations to others need not be unqualified or exceptionless obligations. Therefore, an act of suicide that avoids a hideous life, yet admittedly harms or offends others in some ways, need not always be thought of as an unjust act.

On the other hand, the modern psychological and sociological study of suicide (Stengel; Durkheim) suggests that suicide stems from a breakdown of community. The person who commits suicide is often someone who has been inadequately loved and cared for, who is isolated. Responsibility for the breakdown may lie with the individual person, the family, or society more generally; but it seems clearly the case that obligations *to* suicidal persons are, as a clinical issue, prior to the obligations *of* those persons.

Obligations to oneself. Despite his generally antisuicide view, Aristotle held that suicide cannot be an injustice against the self. His claim was based on the idea that it is impossible to treat oneself unjustly, since an injustice is an act done to oneself against one's will. Suicide, however, is a voluntary human action. Therefore, it cannot be *unjust* to the actor. One and the same act (the suicide) cannot be both voluntary and against one's will (Aristotle).

Aquinas, in contrast, appealed to the natural tendencies of the self. He held that life is a natural good, that persons have a natural instinct for life, and, therefore, that we have an obligation to preserve our own lives. A prohibition on suicide is part of natural law (Thomas Aquinas II-II, 64, 5). He supplemented this with the suggestion that self-destruction is a violation of charity to God. Against him, of course, it may be contended that persons have other instincts as basic as the instinct for self-preservation—instincts that may lead to decisions for self-destruction. And it is not obvious that morally binding rules can be inferred from descriptions of natural fact.

Although Kant's discussion of the morality of suicide may have a naturalistic ingredient, it is of special interest as an attempt to argue for a prohibition on modern, secular terms; he does this by concentrating on duties to one's rational self. Kant did not deny that an act of suicide might violate obligations to other persons, or that sacrifice of life might be a requirement of duty. Thus he did not mean for his argument to be comprehensive or exceptionless. Kant's sole concern was with the relatively narrow issue of what might be called self-interested self-destruction.

His argument is based on his fundamental moral principles. One of them is the idea that any morally right choice must be based on a universalizable maxim or rational moral policy. Such a policy is one that could be adopted by anyone in the same, or essentially similar, circumstances as the actor. An obvious requirement of a universalizable policy is that it be self-consistent. But if the reason for a given suicide is that "care for myself requires destruction of myself," then this basic principle is incoherent. Love for self is not a consistent reason for destruction of the self. Some policy choices leading to self-destruction may be moral, but those in which self-interest is the *reason for* the self-destruction cannot be. One cannot consistently both affirm and deny the legitimacy of self-interest (Kant, p. 39).

A serious difficulty with this argument is associated with ambiguity of a central term in the moral policy at issue. That term is "self-love" or "self-preservation." In order for Kant's argument to work, these terms must be interchangeable and must mean something like "commitment to maximize length of life." That commitment is obviously, and trivially, inconsistent with a policy of self-destruction. A broader definition of self-love, however, will include a desire for personal growth and excellence. From self-love one wants the best, as much as the longest, life possible. Kant's assumption that "love of life" and "self-preservation" are identical conceals the very issue that is pressing today.

Whatever their philosophical merits, it remains true that both the naturalistic and the Kantian consistency arguments play a role in contemporary discussion of the morality of suicide. While suicide is not in itself evidence of mental disease or disorder, it is the case that suicide and attempted suicide are more prevalent among persons who have been in psychiatric treatment or, retrospectively, can be shown to have been in need of such treatment. Thus a concept of "natural mental health" has some implications as we interpret suicidal acts and consider the morality of suicide prevention. Second, clinical interaction with a suicidal individual may well involve direct or subtle use of a commonsense version of the Kantian argument: an appeal to the inconsistency between self-destruction and the patient's real desire for and interest in happiness may often be therapeutically indicated.

Religious obligations

Eastern views. In the religious traditions nurtured on the Indian subcontinent, Vedic and even early Upanishadic literature oppose self-destruction. This opposition continued in the Dharmashastric (legal) tradition. However, the later Upanishads admit that the *sannyasin* who has already attained insight into reality may fittingly choose to die through drowning, starvation, fire, or some other heroic act. Consistent with this, later Hinduism and Jainism permit, even commend, a kind of passive ascetic self-destruction in which a person accepts death from hunger or starvation. The holy person ceases to beg for food and allows death to come. Moreover, self-destruction from devotion to a deity has been commended in theistic Hinduism. Generally, however, Indian traditions oppose active forms of self-destruction. This is most vivid in Jainism, in which the taking of any life is viewed with revulsion.

Indian Buddhism began with an opposition to suicide. Early Buddhist teachings insist that release from the world of *dukkha* (or suffering) comes primarily through a changed attitude toward the self and the world. External ascetic practices, of which passive self-destruction may be an example, are misguided ways to find release. Yet, in developing Buddhist tradition, suicide was seen as compatible with the life of an *arahat* (or saint); self-renunciation to the point of voluntary choice of death is highly respected in many Mahayana traditions.

Two kinds of self-destruction have been sanctioned in East Asian traditions. Although suicide for honor or vengeance was approved, in China male self-destruction was generally opposed since a man's highest duty was to preserve himself for his family. Female self-destruction, in contrast, was praised in more cases, e.g., when a woman killed herself to avoid violation of her deceased husband's rights. As in India, this sutteeism became quite widespread. It was opposed by Imperial Decree in 1729, but fashionable public acts of suttee continued at least until the late nineteenth century. In Japan *harakiri* (or *seppuku*) was originally sanctioned as an alternative to some forms of dishonorable death, but it has developed into a general technique for clearing one's name. The forty-seven Ronin, who committed *harakiri* in 1703 after having avenged their unjustly slain master, are revered throughout Japan, and the *harakiri* of the author Yukio Mishima in 1970 and, to a lesser extent, the suicide of Nobel Prize author Kawabata Yasunari in 1972 attracted worldwide attention. Although Japanese suicide rates are not unusually high, the Japanese preoccupation with suicide is obvious.

Western views. The Bible contains neither an explicit word for suicide nor an explicit prohibition of the act. In the Hebrew Bible Saul and his armor bearer fall on their swords (1 Sam. 31:3–5), Ahitophel hangs himself after the failure of his political intrigue (2 Sam. 17:23), and Zimri burns himself to death after the failure of his attempt to take the throne of Israel (1 Kings 16:18 f.). Samson prays to die with the Philistines he kills as he topples their temple (Judg. 16:23–31). In the New Testament Judas is presented as a suicide (Matt. 27:4–5; cf. Acts 1:13). Yet in none of these cases is there the suggestion that the persons are bad, or fail to live up to obligations, *because* they have committed suicide. The moral quality of the acts of Saul and his armor bearer is at worst ambiguous; Samson's action seems meritorious.

On the other hand, one can see in these documents bases from which a prohibition of suicide could be (and was in fact) inferred by later Jewish and Christian writers. If suicide is the appropriate form of death for Ahitophel, Zimri, and Judas, it is so because of the seriousness of their moral wrongdoing. Both the sixth commandment (Exod. 20:13) and the penalty for the shedding of human blood (Gen. 9:5–6) suggest an opposition to suicide. So does the notion of God's sovereignty over human life found throughout the Bible, especially in such passages as Genesis 1–3, Romans 14:7–12, and 1 Corinthians 6:19.

This idea—that human beings have limited sovereignty over their own lives—took on great cultural force from its inclusion in the teaching of the Western religions. Developing Jewish traditions condemned suicide, taking as the key text not the prohibition on murder in the Decalogue but that on shedding human blood in Genesis 9:5 f. Sacrifice of one's own life was allowed only as a last resort to avoid committing one of the cardinal sins of adultery, murder, or idolatry. Death was better than betrayal of the name of God (and thus many medieval European Jews died rather than be forced into apostasy); but it is God, not human persons, who is the Lord of Life and Death. A Jew may not take his life to avoid profaning the Sabbath; burial ritual for someone who commits suicide is greatly abbreviated.

Similarly in Islam (a monotheistic religion of the Western type) we find no explicit statement on the subject in the Koran, although Sura 3:139 ("It is not given to any soul to die, save by the leave of God, at an appointed time.") has been taken as the grounds for a prohibition against suicide. Reinforced by *hadith* (traditions) telling of the Prophet's refusal to bury someone who had committed suicide, this prohibition was included in the *Sunna* (customary law) of the Muslim community.

This same theme of the incongruence between God's sovereignty and suicide was also developed apart from any biblical traditions. In Plato's *Phaedo* (61–62) Socrates concedes that there are times when a person would be better off dead. Why not act oneself to bring about this state of affairs? The prohibition of such action is based on the fact that persons are "possessions" of the gods. Just as I would be wronged by the theft of one of my possessions (such as my cattle), so gods are wronged when one of their possessions is taken. Personal authority over one's own life is limited by the prior sovereignty of the gods; suicide represents a usurpation of power.

Building on these religious and philosophical bases, much Christian thought elaborates these arguments. For instance, Thomas Aquinas claimed that suicide is not only an offense against self and society; it is also a violation of God's sovereignty. People belong to God who is their creator, and suicide is somewhat analogous to theft. A thief steals my property, and in suicide I steal God's. "Because life is God's gift to man . . . whoever takes his own life sins against God, even as he who kills another's slave, sins against that slave's master" (Thomas Aquinas II-II, 64, 5). Thomas goes on to appeal to God's explicit statements in the Bible, but the core of his argument seems to be that suicide runs counter to the creator's general interest in human life and flourishing. In fact, some twentieth-century theologians have based their opposition to suicide on a revised version of this theological argument. With Aquinas, they argue that suicide is wrong because it is an inappropriate response to God's *gift* of life. Suicide is an act of ingratitude, a failure to recognize that God is the "owner" of human life (Barth, p. 402). Ultimately, they claim, a prohibition of suicide makes sense only in the context of Western monotheism. In that context suicide is an act of hubris, a usurpation of power.

A fundamental criticism of all these religious arguments was made by David Hume in his posthumously published essay *On Suicide*. Hume argued that, *if* God is the creator of the world, his will must be expressed in *all* events. God's will "appears not immediately in any operation, but governs everything by those general and immutable laws which have been established from the beginning of time." The lives of men "are subjected to the general laws of matter and motion" and it is "no encroachment on the office of Providence to disturb or alter these general laws." To say the contrary would absurdly imply that lifesaving actions violate God's will. "When I fall upon my own sword . . . I receive my death equally from the hands of the Deity as if it had proceeded from a lion, a precipice, or a fever." If all events equally reflect God's will, then suicide *cannot* be a departure from that will.

It seems plausible to suggest that the prior commitments which differentiate the views of religious from nonreligious moralists will continue to affect their views on the obligations involved in moral decisions about suicide. This need not mean that self-consciously Judeo-Chris-

tian writers will be "conservative" while others are "liberal," but the notion of obligations to God complicates the religious moralists' arguments in various ways. Speaking very generally, these obligations will suggest that some suicides that violate no duties to self or others are, nevertheless, wrong as unfaithful to God. The extent of this class of cases may not be great, but its predictable existence suggests that the morality of suicide is a normative issue in which the validity or invalidity of religious ethics has concrete implications.

The moral character of persons who commit suicide

Assessment of the character of a person who commits or attempts suicide is a second distinguishable kind of moral judgment. These assessments are, of course, related to obligations of persons, but the issues must be separated. For instance, one might want to say that a particular act of suicide represented a failure to live up to obligations to others *and* that it was an act of a brave person. Generally, acts based on misunderstanding or misjudgment may nevertheless be free and, in a sense, praiseworthy acts. Moreover, some suicidal behavior may be involuntary, and such self-destructive human behavior does not count as human *moral* action.

As might be expected, we can see a spectrum from severe to lenient judgments on the question of virtue in the history of Western morals. The most liberal tradition began with some Stoic and Epicurean writers, reemerged in nineteenth-century Romanticism, and has been defended by writers of various philosophical and literary persuasions ever since. Its main tenet has been an association of human virtue with self-determination. The good person is the one who controls his or her own destiny. Suicide, as an act of human self-control in the face of fate or misfortune, is a noble act.

The most conservative tradition began with Aristotle, who claimed that the motive in suicide is not noble. Suicide reveals cowardice. "[T]o kill oneself as a means of escape from poverty, or disappointed love or bodily or mental anguish is the deed of a coward rather than a brave man" (Aristotle). This same conservative view reappeared in Christian theology sanctioned by the authorities of Augustine and Aquinas. So endorsed, it led to draconian ecclesiastical and civil penalties for suicide and attempted suicide.

A median position, however, has not been lacking. Despite the antisuicide arguments of

Phaedo and *Laws*, in the latter dialogue Plato argued that suicide is not blameworthy if it is done because of legal requirements (i.e., as the form of death penalty imposed by the state), "under the compulsion of some painful and inevitable misfortune," or because one suffers from "irremediable and intolerable shame" (*Laws* 9, 873). Thus he would excuse many more acts of suicide than Aristotle. Twentieth-century theological writers have held that it is very difficult to determine whether a given act of suicide was an act of loving "self-giving" or of unfaithful "self-taking" (Barth, p. 410). "It is only if the action is undertaken exclusively and consciously out of consideration for one's own person that self-killing becomes self-murder" (Bonhoeffer, p. 126). The notion of suicide as an unforgivable sin has few, if any, defenders in contemporary moral theology.

A more subtle view of this moderate type is called for by contemporary medical realities. Generalized judgments that persons who commit suicide are brave or cowardly distort our moral sensibility. One wants to praise the chooser of death in the face of some medical adversities and to fault those who make the same choice in other situations.

Obligation to prevent suicide

Here we shall discuss the obligations of other persons to individuals who may attempt or commit suicide. Does morality require one to prevent others from committing suicide?

Conflicting principles. In traditional societies and at some earlier stages in Western history suicide prevention would not have appeared as a separate moral issue. In different social and historical contexts it has been possible to be certain that some particular action is wrong, prohibited, and therefore to be prevented by others; other actions are right, allowable, and therefore not to be interfered with. Thus one could speak of a liberty for "rational" suicide.

Two facts make it impossible today to adopt this point of view on suicide intervention. The first of these is the moral pluralism of Western society. Acts of self-destruction will be described and evaluated differently by different people, probably on the basis of their education in diverse (more or less organized) communities of moral discourse. If Western societies at the end of the twentieth century agree on basic moral principles, these are quite abstract and general. If perception, description, and evaluation of acts of self-destruction lead to little consensus, it is even more difficult to come to consensus on the morality of interference with such acts.

Second, this general problem of pluralism is made unusually vexing in the case of suicide intervention because of a possible conflict among the moral principles that we do share. We usually assume that we have some obligation to secure the physical welfare of other persons. Furthermore, many would say that our obligations to others involve something more than respect for their physical welfare. Thus, people often feel obligations to aid in the moral growth or character development of others. This obligation to nurture the moral self of another person may be especially important when there are special kinds of relationships (e.g., familial, professional) between the persons involved. Both kinds of obligation to the welfare of others suggest an obligation to interfere with suicidal acts, for those acts are not only physically destructive but, even if virtuous at the moment, they foreclose the possibility of continued moral growth.

On the other hand, we have long assumed that personal liberty is a necessary condition for human dignity. When a long life will be continually shattered by pain, the free choice of a short life can sensibly be described as one for the greater physical good. And moral growth or character development cannot occur unless choices are freely made by the subject. Therefore, we can provide neither the good life nor virtue for others, if we do not allow them liberty. This liberty need not be unlimited, especially when its exercise affects the welfare of others, but it would seem that it should involve the liberty to commit suicide, at least in some cases. In sum, our obligation to meet the needs and secure the welfare of persons justifies intervention; our obligation to respect the liberty of others requires noninterference. On the whole, Western societies have given preference to the first of those conflicting obligations. The rationale for such a choice has varied. For a long time it was religious; more recently it has been secular. Views making liberty more central, however, have not been lacking. Thomas Szasz has defended them with great force in this century. According to Szasz, disease of a suicidal individual is "nonexistent," and therefore that individual should not be coerced into therapy any more than a diabetic. Moreover, suicide is an action primarily affecting the self, so the public cannot properly interfere with it. Denials of this principle, he suggests, are based on an unjustifiable assumption that all suicidal acts are irrational (Szasz, pp. 7–17).

Against this, many respond with considerations such as these: They note the higher incidence of suicide among those persons who are plausibly thought to be mentally ill (Perlin and Schmidt; Stengel) and that persons who intend to commit suicide often still wish very much to live. The act of suicide is "an all-or-none action," but it reflects "a complicated, undecided internal debate" (Shneidman, Farberow, and Litman, p. 430). The question for the psychiatrist is not simply how to respect the free choice of the individual: What the individual wants is usually ambiguous, and the apparent choice of an act of suicide conceals an ambivalent situation in the personality. Also, the suicidal person may be under the strain of a temporary crisis and act impulsively. The dilemma for psychiatric medicine, then, is: Which part or component of the self is the physician required to respect? Exhortations to respect integrity (and freedom) run into problems when the self is fragmented.

For example, persons in the process of committing suicide are often under the influence of drugs or alcohol; under such circumstances, intervention would seem reasonable. Indeed, some persons who commit suicide simply wish to reduce or interrupt anxiety and do not wish to die at all. If a person is driven to suicide by an intense compulsion, intervention would seem morally required—and likely to be carried out by antipaternalists and paternalists alike.

Programs for intervening in and preventing suicide are difficult to evaluate. Concern has been expressed that the threat of intervention may in fact precipitate suicide among some groups, such as the aged (Sainsbury). Thus suicide prevention techniques must always be based on a multiple-etiology, multiple-determinant mode of suicide. For example, in the clinically depressed hospitalized subgroups, the knowledge of psychopharmacological measures for the treatment of manic–depressive illness may be essential. And among the lonely and isolated aged out in the community, a "befriending" outreach program may reduce the suicide rate far more effectively than hospitalization and/or medication. Thus there are limits to the type and degree of intervention. The effectiveness of suicide prevention centers and psychiatric clinics seems to be related not only to services actually rendered but also to the network of related care and to the known availability of help when needed (even if not used). The effect of suicide prevention centers is difficult to evaluate; the reporting of suicide, the time period under study, the "sui-cidal" dispositions of clients contacting a given center, the matching of control populations—all create problems for the investigator. However, one study has found that communities in Great Britain that had Samaritan suicide prevention services were likely to have decreased suicide rates after initiation and maintenance of those programs (Bagley).

Issues requiring attention. Obviously the debate over the morality of suicide intervention, as that over the morality of suicide itself, will continue. It appears that this debate should include attention to at least these issues:

1. *The actual histories of persons who commit or attempt suicide* either because of poor health or for some other reason. Important evaluation of suicidal acts apart from their biographical and social context is impossible.

2. *The general social-psychological roots of suicide.* Although there has been much discussion about matters of classification, scholars since Durkheim have continued to note that suicide may reflect excessive isolation and loneliness, on the one hand, or loss of selfhood in excessive commitment and dependence, on the other. Insofar as society finds suicide intervention plausible, that far it should feel obliged to attack the problem at the root. If suicide prevention is not to be merely palliative, it must involve an attack on more general forms of malaise within society. At the same time, by not intervening directly the community may seem not to care and may thereby facilitate the action of would-be suicides. Thus the circumstances of intervention may vary and may defy being fully captured in "formal" guidelines for prudential good judgments.

3. *The overall role of psychiatric medicine.* If mental illness is, as Szasz suggests, a "myth," then intervention in suicide is only one of the many unjustified interferences with liberty perpetrated by psychiatry. As psychopharmacology increases the power to alter mental states, we will need to reach more clarity about the legitimate role of professionals in the mental health field.

4. *The relationship between the morality and the legality of suicide intervention.* In the case of suicide, it is probable that there are occasions when one should be morally, but not legally, required to prevent the act. Thus law and morality diverge. Yet our legal commitments to respect both life and liberty would seem to have a moral foundation. Jurisprudential and philosophical

1626 SUICIDE

discussion of this issue should clarify the role of law in suicide prevention and intervention.

DAVID H. SMITH AND
SEYMOUR PERLIN

[*Directly related are the entries* DEATH AND DYING: EUTHANASIA AND SUSTAINING LIFE; LIFE, *article on* VALUE OF LIFE; NATURAL LAW; RIGHT TO REFUSE MEDICAL CARE; *and* RIGHTS. *For further discussion of topics mentioned in this article, see:* MEDICAL ETHICS, HISTORY OF, *section on* SOUTH AND EAST ASIA, *articles on* PREREPUBLICAN CHINA, CONTEMPORARY CHINA, JAPAN THROUGH THE NINETEENTH CENTURY, CONTEMPORARY JAPAN: MEDICAL ETHICS AND LEGAL MEDICINE, INDIA, *and the section on* EUROPE AND THE AMERICAS, *article on* MEDIEVAL EUROPE: FOURTH TO SIXTEENTH CENTURY. *For discussion of related ideas, see the entries:* MENTAL HEALTH, *article on* RELIGION AND MENTAL HEALTH; *and* WOMEN AND BIOMEDICINE, *article on* WOMEN AS PATIENTS AND EXPERIMENTAL SUBJECTS.]

BIBLIOGRAPHY

ARISTOTLE. *Nicomachean Ethics.* 1138A. Translated by J. A. K. Thomson as *The Ethics of Aristotle: The Nicomachean Ethics Translated.* Classics series. London: George Allen & Unwin, 1953; Baltimore: Penguin Books, 1955, bk. 5, chap. 11, pp. 147–149.

AUGUSTINE. *Augustine.* Vol. 6: *The City of God: Books I–VII.* Translated by Demetrius B. Zema and Gerald G. Walsh. Introduction by Étienne Gilson. The Fathers of the Church: A New Translation, vol. 8. Edited by Roy Joseph Deferrari. New York: 1950, bk. 1, chaps. 16–17, 20–22, 25–27; pp. 45–47, 52–55, 59–62.

BAGLEY, CHRISTOPHER. "The Evaluation of a Suicide Prevention Scheme by an Ecological Method." *Social Science and Medicine* 2 (1968): 1–14.

BARTH, KARL. *Church Dogmatics.* Vol. 3: *The Doctrine of Creation.* Edited by G. W. Bromiley and T. F. Torrance. Translated by A. T. Mackay, T. H. L. Parker, Harold Knight, Henry A. Kennedy, and John Marks. Edinburgh: T. & T. Clark, 1961, pt. 4, pp. 400–414.

BEAUCHAMP, TOM L., and PERLIN, SEYMOUR, eds. *Ethical Issues in Death and Dying.* Englewood Cliffs, N.J.: Prentice-Hall, 1978.

BONHOEFFER, DIETRICH. *Ethics.* Translated by Neville Horton Smith. Edited by Eberhard Bethge. New York: Macmillan Co., 1955.

BRANDT, R. B. "The Morality and Rationality of Suicide." Perlin, *Handbook,* chap. 3, pp. 61–76.

BROOKE, EILEEN M., ed. *Suicide and Attempted Suicide.* Public Health Papers, no. 58. Geneva: World Health Organization, 1974.

CHORON, JACQUES. *Suicide.* New York: Scribner, 1972.

DOUGLAS, JACK D. *The Social Meanings of Suicide.* Princeton: Princeton University Press, 1967.

DURKHEIM, ÉMILE. *Suicide: A Study in Sociology.* Translated by John A. Spaulding and George Simpson. Glencoe, Ill.: Free Press, 1951.

FARBEROW, NORMAN L. "Cultural History of Suicide." *Suicide in Different Cultures.* Edited by Norman L. Farberow. Baltimore: University Park Press, 1975, chap. 1, pp. 1–15.

HILLMAN, JAMES. *Suicide and the Soul.* New York: Harper & Row, 1964.

HOLLAND, R. F. "Suicide." *Moral Problems: A Collection of Philosophical Essays.* Edited by James Rachels. New York: Harper & Row, 1971, pp. 346–359.

HUME, DAVID. "On Suicide." *The Philosophical Works of David Hume.* 4 vols. Boston: Little, Brown & Co., 1854, vol. 4, pp. 535–546.

KANT, IMMANUEL. *Fundamental Principles of the Metaphysic of Morals.* Translated by Thomas Kingsmill Abbott. Library of Liberal Arts. Indianapolis: Bobbs-Merrill, 1949.

LITMAN, ROBERT E. "Sigmund Freud on Suicide." Shneidman, *Essays in Self-Destruction,* chap. 15, pp. 324–344.

———, and TABACHNICK, NORMAN D. "Psychoanalytic Theories of Suicide." *Suicidal Behaviors: Diagnosis and Management.* Edited by H. L. P. Resnik. Boston: Little, Brown & Co., 1968, pp. 73–82.

MARIS, RONALD. "Sociology." Perlin, *Handbook,* chap. 5, pp. 93–112.

MENNINGER, KARL. *Man against Himself* (1938). A Harvest Book. New York: Harcourt, Brace & World, n.d., especially p. 24.

PERLIN, SEYMOUR, ed. *A Handbook for the Study of Suicide.* New York: Oxford University Press, 1975.

———, and SCHMIDT, CHESTER W., JR. "Psychiatry." Perlin, *Handbook,* chap. 8, pp. 147–163.

PLATO. *Laws.* Translated by Benjamin Jowett as "Laws." *The Dialogues of Plato.* 2 vols. New York: Random House, 1937, vol. 2, pp. 407–703. See especially chap. 9, 865A–875B; pp. 610–619.

———. *Phaedo.* Translated by Benjamin Jowett as "Phaedo." *The Dialogues of Plato.* 2 vols. New York: Random House, 1937, vol. 1, pp. 441–501.

PRETZEL, PAUL. "Philosophical and Ethical Considerations of Suicide Prevention." *Bulletin of Suicidology,* July 1968, pp. 30–38.

ROCKWELL, DON A., and O'BRIEN, WILLIAM. "Physicians' Knowledge and Attitudes about Suicide." *Journal of the American Medical Association* 225 (1973): 1347–1349.

SAINSBURY, PETER. "Community Psychiatry." Perlin, *Handbook,* chap. 8, pp. 147–163.

SHNEIDMAN, EDWIN S., ed. *Essays in Self-Destruction.* New York: Science House, 1967.

———; FARBEROW, NORMAN L.; and LITMAN, ROBERT E. *The Psychology of Suicide.* New York: Science House, 1970.

SILVING, HELEN. "Suicide and Law." *Clues to Suicide.* Edited by Edwin S. Shneidman and Norman L. Farberow. New York: McGraw-Hill, 1957, chap. 9, pp. 79–95.

SINGER, MARCUS GEORGE. *Generalization in Ethics: An Essay in the Logic of Ethics with the Rudiments of a System of Moral Philosophy.* New York: Alfred A. Knopf, 1961, pp. 311–318.

STENGEL, ERWIN. *Suicide and Attempted Suicide.* Pelican Book, no. A704. Baltimore: Penguin Books, 1964.

STEPPACHER, ROBERT C., and MAUSNER, JUDITH S. "Suicide in Male and Female Physicians." *Journal of the American Medical Association* 228 (1974): 323–328.

SZASZ, THOMAS S. "The Ethics of Suicide." *Antioch Review* 31 (1971): 7–17.

THAKUR, UPENDRA. *The History of Suicide in India: An Introduction.* Delhi: Munshi Ram Manahar Lal, 1963.

Thomas Aquinas. *Summa Theologiae.* II-II 26,4; 64,5. Translated by Fathers of the English Dominican Province as "The Order of Charity: Whether out of Charity, Man Ought to Love Himself More than His Neighbor," and "Of Murder: Whether It Is Lawful to Kill Oneself." *Summa Theologica: First Complete American Edition.* 3 vols. Vol. 2: *Containing Second Part of the Second Part, QQ. 1–189 and Third Part, QQ. 1–90, with Synoptical Charts.* New York: Benziger Brothers, 1947, question 26, art. 4, pp. 1297–1298; question 64, art. 5, pp. 1468–1470.

United States; Department of Health, Education, and Welfare; Public Health Service; Health Resources Administration; National Center for Health Statistics. "Provisional Statistics: Annual Summary for the United States, 1975, Births, Deaths, Marriages, and Divorces." *Monthly Vital Statistics Report* 24, no. 13 (1976), table 8, p. 25; table 9, p. 26. (HRA)76-1120.

SUPEREROGATION AND OBLIGATION
See Obligation and Supererogation.

SURGERY

The ethical problems encountered by surgeons, both individually and as collective members of a specialized area of medicine, are by and large those faced by most physicians engaged in modern medical diagnosis and treatment. A subset of surgeons, those involved in clinical research, also must grapple with the ethical problems devolving from their double role as physician-investigators. In that dual role they have a joint responsibility: both to care for patient-subjects and to perform upon them research that, on the one hand, may not directly influence their clinical condition and, on the other, given the uncertainties and risks inherent in research, could harm them.

This article will first discuss ethical aspects of the role of the surgeon and then will touch on some of the most difficult and troublesome ethical issues confronting surgeons and surgeon-investigators, including those surrounding (1) informed consent, (2) the design and conduct of clinical trials, (3) disclosure of diagnosis and prognosis, and (4) decisions concerning the prolongation or termination of treatment. We shall also consider why those types of ethical problems appear to have some special characteristics and nuances in surgery, related to the role of the surgeon and the demands and setting of his work.

Ethical aspects of the surgeon's role

The professional role of the surgeon centers upon his unique license to invade the living human body, trying to cure or ameliorate a disease, anomaly, or injury by correcting, repairing, or removing a part of that body. The fact that this must usually be done when the patient is unable to communicate because of general anesthesia raises special issues, which will be discussed below. Partly in the interests of efficiency and safety, the surgeon's role traditionally has been oriented toward a high degree of autonomous functioning, toward making and carrying out often on-the-spot, solo decisions about which course of action he or she should pursue for the patient under his or her surgical care.

In his immediate work environment the surgeon is vested with a high degree of responsibility and attendant prestige. He is likely to be the explicit or implicit head of any team with which he works; his opinions are commonly sought by others on the team, and in that role he frequently acts as the final decision maker if a consensual decision is not readily attained. For the surgeon, the role of "head of the team" in turn raises ethical questions about the degree to which he is, or should be, responsible for making decisions on behalf of the team and is, or should be, responsible for the actions of those working under him.

These traditional aspects of "being a surgeon" have increasing import as surgeons are called upon to make decisions about the preoperative, operative, and postoperative care of a large percentage of hospitalized patients. For, particularly in urban settings, hospitalized patients are in increasing numbers surgical patients; some seventy percent of the patient population at Boston's Massachusetts General Hospital, for example, undergo a surgical procedure. Often invoking group statistics, the surgeon must make a fundamental medical and ethical decision about each of those individual patients: Given the fact that surgical treatment, by and large, is acute and expensive, what should the chance of "success" be to make it worthwhile to recommend a given procedure for a given patient?

Ethical issues in surgery

Informed consent. In reaching and acting upon a decision, surgeons, like other physicians and physician-investigators, are ethically and legally bound to obtain informed, voluntary consent from their patients prior to performing a diagnostic, therapeutic, or experimental procedure. The informed consent transaction involves the giving of information by the surgeon about the patient's disease, the proposed intervention and its attendant risks, and alternative procedures; the receipt and "processing" of this information by the patient; and the patient's subsequent decision to undergo or not to undergo the procedure. The requirements of the informed consent transaction as codified in ethical codes, laws, and regulations, are often difficult to execute in the reality of physician–patient or investigator–subject interactions.

With respect to informed consent for surgical procedures, one rarely discussed variable that may compound the difficulties of the surgeon's obtaining informed, voluntary consent is the meaning to the patient of "being operated on." Particularly in the case of major operations, and given the mystique surrounding certain vital organs such as the heart and the brain, the prospect of having one's body "cut open" may, whether seen as actual or symbolic, evoke a spectrum of fears and anxieties that will probably affect the patient's ability to comprehend objectively the information conveyed by the surgeon, and consequently the patient's ability to decide rationally whether or not to undergo the procedure in question.

Surgeons responsible for the training of residents need to resolve a particularly sensitive aspect of the generic problem of how much information should be conveyed to their patients. That is, can the surgeon ethically delegate the performance of an operation to a resident without the explicit informed consent of the patient? At a minimum the senior surgeon has a responsibility to explain to his patient that, in a teaching hospital, an operation commonly is performed by a team, of which he is the head, with different doctors assisting with various parts of the surgical procedure. If, however, a resident or other physician is to perform the operation, with the senior surgeon merely assisting or supervising, that fact should be disclosed to the patient. For, as stated by the American Medical Association, "to have another physician operate on one's patient without that patient's consent, and without his knowledge of the substitution, is a fraud and deceit and a violation of a basic ethical concept."

Another aspect of the consent transaction that frequently poses an ethical dilemma for the surgeon is that, while he is operating, he may find it advisable, in his professional judgment, to perform some unanticipated surgery. In this situation, he must decide unilaterally whether or not to proceed when the unconscious patient cannot consent.

Clinical trials. A second set of ethical issues confronting surgeons is in the area of clinical research and concerns the design and evaluation of investigative studies. In the past twenty years, methods for conducting controlled clinical trials have been developed, using such techniques as random assignment, control groups, quantitative measures of change, and advanced statistical measurements. Those techniques have been applied predominantly to the evaluation of drug therapies. A few innovative surgical procedures have been subjected to the types of concurrent-controlled trials now common for clinical pharmacological research. They include the use of sham controls, feasible because of low risk, to evaluate the efficacy of bilateral internal mammary artery ligation for coronary insufficiency, and current randomized trials of mastectomy procedures and of coronary artery bypass surgery for certain classes of patients with ischemic heart disease. Most surgical procedures, however, are evaluated by less formal methods, involving retrospective case analyses and the use of the patient-subject as his own control. There are a number of medical, ethical, and sociological reasons why the evaluative procedures commonly employed in clinical pharmacological research are so different from those employed in surgical research. For example, it is considered more difficult, medically and ethically, to use a surgical patient-subject as a control, performing a sham operation (namely, performing all parts of the operation except the actual corrective procedure) or using procedure "B" when a surgeon-investigator believes that a sham procedure (or "B") is probably less efficacious than procedure "A" in the treatment of a life-threatening condition. The rule of evaluating each case on its own merits, many surgeons would argue, is also common in surgery because both regular and investigative surgical interventions are inherently different from pharmacological interventions. An operation is more apt to be employed "when all else has failed" or on an emergency basis, and the surgeon, more than other physicians, is likely to have to improvise on the spot because of the patient's revealed condition. And yet, establishing the true efficacy of certain operative procedures may demand the courage to apply the randomized trial approach, at least to the extent of employing or not employing a given operation for a group of similar patients on a strictly randomized basis.

The absence of rigorously developed evaluative data on the efficacy of many procedures, coupled with the high costs of modern, technologically complex surgical care and—as some would argue—the monetary advantage to the surgeon, has helped to generate what many see as the central ethical (and economic) issue in surgery today, that of "unnecessary" surgery. The push to resolve the debate about "necessary" versus "unnecessary" surgery is one force that may impel more systematic clinical trials to determine the efficacy of both innovative and established (but poorly evaluated) surgical procedures. While there are sharp differences of opinion about both the definition and the extent of "unnecessary" surgery, the potential for abuse of the surgeon's license to "invade" the body is a problem that must be dealt with ethically as well as by regulatory means.

Truth-telling in surgery. Decisions about the disclosure of diagnosis and prognosis to patients, particularly those with critical or terminal conditions, pose troublesome ethical issues for surgeons, issues that bear on how the informed consent transaction is to be handled. Although the matter of disclosure is a much debated one in medicine, particularly with respect to the terminally ill patient, relatively little quantitative or qualitative research has been done on this ethically complex subject. The literature has indicated that most decisions about disclosure of terminal illness depend on the personal preferences and judgments of individual physicians; that a family member, rather than the patient, is often first informed about the latter's grave condition; that many ostensibly uninformed patients nonetheless are aware of their terminal prognosis; and that more patients than are informed apparently would prefer to be told their diagnosis and prognosis.

Those findings suggest the medical and ethical uncertainties and ambiguities that surgeons, as well as other physicians, must resolve, in light of the patient's right to know, as they decide how much information to convey to each patient, and when, concerning his or her condition and its proposed treatment. For example, surgeons must balance the patient's legal and moral rights to self-determination, including the right to be informed of the possible risks attending a surgical procedure and the right to refuse treatment, with their judgments about the medical and psychological consequences to the patient of full disclosure. However, both the methods and the purposes of evaluating these medical and psychological consequences are in need of considerable examination, to reduce intuition or guesswork on the surgeon's part.

Prolongation and termination of treatment. A final example of difficult-to-resolve ethical issues in surgery is that of whether or not to intervene surgically and, if so, when to prolong and when to terminate treatment. Both in the operating room and in the postoperative intensive care unit, the proliferation and increasing technological sophistication of mechanical assistance devices that can sustain cardiac, respiratory, and other vital functions have increased the frequency and difficulty of making treatment decisions.

A critical event in a patient's course is reached when the physician recognizes the possibility that the patient's condition probably has reached an irreversible or terminal stage. In such a situation, physicians and other medical staff are faced with two medically and ethically difficult questions. First, can one firmly establish that an individual patient's case is judged "hopeless" and, if so, by what criteria? Second, after such a judgment has been made, should all "curative" efforts be withdrawn in favor of simply palliative measures? Are there circumstances in which all efforts to prolong life should be ended?

In reaching such decisions, physicians must weigh and balance often conflicting personal, professional, and societal norms and values. Thus, for example, the humanitarian motivation that prescribes the alleviation of pain and the prevention of suffering may impel a physician toward deciding against prolonging a terminally ill patient's treatment, while a conviction on the part of a physician or a member of the patient's family that the life of each individual is sacred may influence him toward prolonging life as long as possible.

Conclusion

The types of ethically complex and troublesome problems confronting surgeons, illustrated by the examples we have presented, are encountered by many physicians and physician-investigators; but surgeons, by virtue of their medical roles, grapple with particularly urgent problems under conditions that are often unique. Recent scientific and technological developments have made the challenges more demanding, and the ethical training of surgeons that would enable them to perform optimally under those circumstances has not always kept pace. The surgeon, of all modern practicing medical professionals, may often be faced with problems demanding the greatest resources for their solution, under conditions of training and practice that make shared decisions difficult but not necessarily impossible to accomplish.

JUDITH P. SWAZEY AND
PAUL S. RUSSELL

[*For further discussion of topics mentioned in this article, see:* INFORMED CONSENT IN HUMAN RESEARCH; INFORMED CONSENT IN THE THERAPEUTIC RELATIONSHIP; *and* TRUTH-TELLING. *Also directly related is* DEATH AND DYING: EUTHANASIA AND SUSTAINING LIFE, *article on* ETHICAL VIEWS. *Other relevant material may be found under* MEDICAL ETHICS, HISTORY OF, *section on* EUROPE AND THE AMERICAS, *article on* MEDIEVAL EUROPE: FOURTH TO SIXTEENTH CENTURY.]

BIBLIOGRAPHY

American Medical Association, Judicial Council. "Substitution of Surgeon without Patient's Knowledge or Consent." *Opinions and Reports of the Judicial Council.* Chicago: 1971, pp. 6–7.

American Surgical Association. "Statement on Professional Liability, September 1976." *New England Journal of Medicine* 295 (1976): 1292–1296.

BRIM, ORVILLE G., JR.; FREEMAN, H. E.; LEVINE, S.; and SCOTCH, N., eds. *The Dying Patient.* New York: Russell Sage Foundation, 1970.

BUNKER, JOHN P.; BARNES, BENJAMIN; and MOSTELLER, FREDERICK. *Costs, Risks, and Benefits of Surgery.* New York: Oxford University Press, 1977.

———, and BROWN, WILLIAM, JR. "The Physician-Patient as an Informed Consumer of Surgical Services." *New England Journal of Medicine* 290 (1974): 1051–1055.

CAPRON, ALEXANDER M. "Informed Consent in Catastrophic Disease Research and Treatment." *University of Pennsylvania Law Review* 123 (1974): 340–438.

COYNE, PATRICIA S. "May I Cut In? Unnecessary Surgery in America." *Private Practice* 7, no. 11 (1975), pp. 12–19.

CRANE, DIANA. *The Sanctity of Social Life.* New York: Russell Sage Foundation, 1975.

EMERSON, RALPH. "Unjustified Surgery: Fact or Myth?" *New York State Journal of Medicine* 76 (1976): 454–460.

FOX, RENÉE C., and SWAZEY, JUDITH P. *The Courage to Fail: A Social View of Organ Transplants and Dialysis.* Chicago: University of Chicago Press, 1974.

FREUND, PAUL ABRAHAM, ed. *Experimentation with Human Subjects.* The Daedalus Library. New York: George Braziller, 1970.

HAUCK, WALTER W., JR.; BLOOM, BERNARD S.; McPHERSON, C. KLIM; NICKERSON, RITA J.; COLTON, THEODORE; and PETERSON, OSLER L. "Surgeons in the United States: Activities, Output, and Income." *Journal of the American Medical Association* 236 (1976): 1864–1871.

KELLY, GERALD A. *Medico-Moral Problems.* St. Louis: Catholic Hospital Association, 1958, pp. 254–257.

McCARTHY, EUGENE G., and WIDMER, GERALDINE W. "Effects of Screening by Consultants on Recommended Elective Surgical Procedures." *New England Journal of Medicine* 291 (1974): 1331–1335.

NICKERSON, RITA J.; COLTON, THEODORE; PETERSON, OSLER L.; BLOOM, BERNARD S.; and HAUCK, WALTER W., JR. "Doctors Who Perform Operations: A Study on In-Hospital Surgery in Four Diverse Geographical Areas." *New England Journal of Medicine* 295 (1976): 921–926, 982–989.

NOLEN, WILLIAM A. *The Making of a Surgeon.* New York: Pocket Books, 1972.

———. *A Surgeon's World.* Greenwich, Conn.: Fawcett World Library, 1972.

OKEN, DONALD. "What to Tell Cancer Patients: A Study of Medical Attitudes." *Journal of the American Medical Association* 175 (1961): 1120–1128.

PARROTT, MAX H. "Elective Hysterectomy." *American Journal of Obstetrics and Gynecology* 113 (1972): 531–540.

United States, Congress, House of Representatives, Committee on Interstate and Foreign Commerce, Subcommittee on Oversight and Investigations. *Cost and Quality of Health Care: Unnecessary Surgery, Report.* 94th Cong., 2d sess., January 1976. Subcommittee Print.

VEATCH, ROBERT M. *Death, Dying, and the Biological Revolution: Our Last Quest for Responsibility.* New Haven: Yale University Press, 1976.

WILLIAMS, LAWRENCE P. *How to Avoid Unnecessary Surgery.* Los Angeles: Nash Publishing Corporation, 1971.

SWEDEN

See MEDICAL ETHICS, HISTORY OF, *section on* EUROPE AND THE AMERICAS, *article on* WESTERN EUROPE IN THE TWENTIETH CENTURY.

SWITZERLAND

See MEDICAL ETHICS, HISTORY OF, *section on* EUROPE AND THE AMERICAS, *article on* WESTERN EUROPE IN THE TWENTIETH CENTURY.

T

TAOISM

Taoism is one of the traditional "three religions" of China (the *san-chiao:* Taoism, Confucianism, Buddhism) that traces its heritage back to the semihistorical figures Lao-tzu and Chuang-tzu at the end of the Eastern Chou period (ca. fourth to third centuries B.C.). Taoism, however, is a label that must be used in a loose bibliographical sense since it ordinarily embraces a whole gamut of philosophical, mystical, esoteric, and liturgical phenomena not easily unified under any single ideological or ethical framework. In fact, it has been common to distinguish between a classical Taoist naturalistic and elitist "philosophy" (*tao-chia*) associated with early literary texts (especially the *Lao-tzu* or the *Tao-te Ching* and the *Chuang-tzu*) and later "religious" or sectarian movements (*tao-chiao*) involving either esoteric traditions seeking "immortality" or ecclesiastical traditions providing for the spiritual needs of the community.

More recent scholarship tends to see this as a too facile and artificial dichotomy and suggests that, while there are real differences, there is also a general thematic continuity underlying the multiple strains of Taoist tradition (Welch, 1969–1970, pp. 108–129). It is most significant that the general ideological and ethical continuity of Taoist tradition seems at least partly to be rooted in a "medicinal" concern for maintaining and prolonging human health and life (*sheng*). But the task of delineating the nature of Taoist thought in relation to Chinese medical ethics must take three factors into consideration: (1) the overall and deep-seated sympathy between Taoism and the motivations, goals, and methods of traditional Chinese medicine; (2) syncretistic changes in the ethical motivations particular to different aspects of Taoist history; and (3) Taoism's failure to generate an independent ethical code and, consequently, the diffuse traditional mixture of Taoist and Buddhist ideas within an ethical superstructure that was basically Confucian.

While all three factors must be taken into account, it should be emphasized that the most basic general ethical value implicit throughout Taoist tradition is the tendency to understand salvation in the biomedical sense of health and the qualitative improvement and prolongation of human life (Yü, pp. 81–87). Indeed, the very idea of life or health, including as it does both physical and spiritual dimensions, evokes an archaic aura of religious meaning—that the fullness of life is supranormal by conventional standards—and symbolically is closely linked with a generalized Taoist notion of the mystic and religious, individual and social, salvational goal of reestablishing harmony with the cosmic life principle of the Tao.

For Confucianism the Tao (literally "way, path, to direct or guide") is seen as a rational and moralistic standard of hierarchically graded social harmony (the Chinese term *tao-te* means "moral philosophy"); but for Taoism the universal principle of the Tao is, above all, the mysterious biological and spiritual life rhythm or order of nature. This is an "order" that cannot be evaluated rationally or according to human ethical standards.

Whereas Confucianism tends to understand

the Tao as the rationally appropriated pattern of harmony between man and society, Taoism centers its philosophical and religious concerns on the need for the extrasocietal "healing" reunification of individual human life and the cosmic life current known as the Tao. Throughout its history, therefore, Taoism is primarily associated with the methods of *yang-sheng* (or *wei-sheng*) which can be translated as the mystic and ritual techniques of "cultivating and preserving life" (Needham, 1970, pp. 342–343).

The biomedical connotation of *yang-sheng* is somewhat muted in the earliest Taoist texts, but by the time of the Former Han dynasty (206 B.C. to A.D. 8) Taoism was a vast health cult where perfect health and longevity were the most important tokens of sainthood (*hsien*ship). Thus, the various esoteric arts of later Taoism (especially the alchemical tradition) can in many cases be seen as specialized aspects of the overall Taoist medicinal and this-worldly concern for reestablishing a harmony between man and nature.

Traditional Chinese medicine thus fundamentally reflects this same soteriological concern; for medicine was always directed toward the healing of the human condition and the returning of individual human life to its natural course. From the broadest perspective, the traditional Chinese medical system might be viewed as a secularized variety of the mystic life-nurturing arts of *yang-sheng*. Knowing and living a natural life—following the Tao—is the secret of both health and sagehood. As the most ancient Chinese medical text (A.D. 100?), *The Yellow Emperor's Inner Classic* states, "Those who follow Tao, the Right Way, can escape old age and keep their body in perfect condition. Although they are old in years they are still able to produce offspring" (Veith, p. 100).

In addition, the contemporary historian of Chinese science, Joseph Needham, maintains that in Taoism the roots of an early Chinese scientific and empirical tradition are found. In Needham's view this is especially true as regards early speculations concerning biology and medicine, for the Taoist, like the physician, has an ethical obligation to act on his desire for improving human life and to promote an empirical knowledge of the natural order of the Tao. In contrast to Confucianism, Taoism was seemingly always an artisan's tradition closely related to the experimental, diagnostic, and therapeutic methods of Chinese medicine. In this way, Needham describes Taoism as a kind of "experimental mysti-

cism," which sought pragmatic medical techniques, along with and symbolically coupled with its religious techniques of meditation and ritual, for reestablishing a harmony of body and spirit, man and nature (Needham, 1956, pp. 86–89; 1970, pp. 263–293). It should be noted, however, that despite Needham's reputation and authority this is still something of a premature and overly beguiling generalization that requires further analysis and documentation.

Taoism and the history of Chinese medicine

The specific historical relationship between Taoism and traditional Chinese medicine goes back to the earliest periods of Chinese tradition before the formation of separate Taoist and Confucian movements. In this archaic period (ca. first millennium to the sixth century B.C.) it is clear that medicine (*i*) was etymologically and ideologically linked to some form of shamanism (generally associated with the term *wu*) which was, in turn, one of the most important roots of the Taoist tradition (Needham, 1956, pp. 132–139).

By the time of Confucius in the sixth century B.C. there is a tendency to distinguish between a class of secular physicians and a class of religious functionaries like the shamans. This culminates in the first and second centuries B.C. with the crystallization of the orthodox "great tradition" of Confucianism and a separate secular medical tradition not specifically bound to Taoist tradition. But in comparison to the more wholly secularized Hippocratic tradition of medicine in ancient Greece, there was still a close association between medical theory and religion. This is indicated during this period by the role of the *fang-shih*, who were magicians, technologists, and physicians associated with the so-called Huang-Lao (Huang-ti or the Yellow Emperor and Lao-tzu) Taoist tradition. Even more important, *The Yellow Emperor's Inner Classic* of medicine roughly dates to this period and is strongly imbued with values from the early Taoist classics (Needham, 1970, pp. 265–274).

The continuing relationship is also suggested by the fact that the legendary Yellow Emperor is traditionally the patron saint of Taoism and the founder of the classical medical tradition. Moreover, the mythology of the Yellow Emperor is specifically connected to those archaic shamanic traditions most closely identified with the origins of both Taoism and medicine.

The outcome of this development is that, while medicine was taken into the mainline

Confucian tradition as the "benevolent art" for promoting the social values of filial piety (*hsiao*), Chinese medicine was never wholly identified with orthodox Confucian tradition. It is perhaps best, therefore, to think of a continuity between a classical—more secular and rational—medical tradition represented by the *ju-i* (also *tai-fu* or *liang-i*) Confucian physicians and a more clearly religious folk tradition of common practitioners (*yung-i*) and itinerant healers (*ch'uang-i* or *ling-i*). In Chinese history there is no absolute dichotomy between these two levels in terms of the general theory and ethics of medical practice; and, most significantly, Taoism seemed to act as the primary mediating agent (Nakayama and Sivin, pp. xx–xxvi; pp. 206 f.).

Medicine, like Taoism itself, always tended to straddle the classical and folk, orthodox and heterodox polarities of Chinese tradition. Therefore, even when described in Confucian terms as the "benevolent art," medicine was never seen as a quite proper occupation for a Confucian scholar-gentleman. In fact, much as Taoism traditionally functioned as a refuge for the retired or failed Confucian bureaucrat, so also was medicine seen as a legitimate Confucian calling only as an avocation, or upon retirement or failure to pass the civil service examinations.

Thus while classical medical practice and theory were officially identified with Confucianism, Taoism was always an underlying factor, even periodically resurfacing (especially during the T'ang dynasty, A.D. 618 to 907, and the Sung dynasty, A.D. 960 to 1126) as the single most important influence on medicine. Furthermore, many of the most famous physicians of the classical medical tradition were closely associated with Taoist tradition—for example, Ko Hung (third century), T'ao Hung-ching (fifth century), Sun Ssu-miao (seventh century), Wang Ping (eighth century), Ma Chih (tenth century), and Wang Huai-yin (tenth century).

Taoism and the traditional moral order

Traditional Chinese medicine can be said to be intimately linked with the general Taoist concern for promoting life, health, and longevity; but Chinese biomedical ethics cannot be exclusively identified with Taoism, because early Taoist antisocial individualism and ethical relativism denied the validity of any absolute moral standards. Even more important is the generally diffuse and eclectic nature of Chinese religious, philosophical, and ethical tradition. Given the ultimate hegemony of Confucianism in traditional China, Taoism and Buddhism failed to develop independent ethical codes and were essentially absorbed into the conventional moral order structured on the Confucian social values of benevolence (*jen*) and filial piety (*hsiao*) (Yang, pp. 278–293).

The ethical basis of traditional Chinese medicine must, therefore, be seen as a syncretistic blend of (1) the predominantly Confucian values of benevolence and filial piety, (2) the Buddhist ideas of universal compassion (*karuna*), karmic retribution, and the ideal of the *boddhisattva* or "returned Buddha" who vows to help all men, and (3) the Taoist passion for the preservation of individual life and its emphasis on "natural" behavior (i.e., the principle of *wu-wei*), which leads to a disinterested tolerance and open acceptance of the multifarious ways of man and nature.

Classical Taoism and the *Inner Classic* of medicine

The early Taoism of Lao-tzu and Chuang-tzu may be generally described as a particular kind of nature mysticism. Starting with the basic premise that the fulfillment of human life, both biologically and spiritually, only comes through the harmonious relationship between man and the impersonal natural life rhythm of the Tao, Taoism is, above all, concerned with the way of thought and action necessary for a "natural" life.

At the core of this idea is a mythic remembrance of a "golden age" when man was intrinsically in tune with nature and lived a long and healthy life. With the rise of the artificial constraints of civilization man lost sight of his primary relatedness with nature and, in effect, suffered a fall from the condition of paradise. The real disease of the human condition (and the fundamental understanding of disease in Chinese medicine) is, therefore, the disequilibrium between man and nature; and the Taoist methods of *yang-sheng* are essentially conceived as mental and physical techniques for restoring man to that primordial life-giving condition of solidarity with cosmic life (Needham, 1956, pp. 107–130).

It should be emphasized that this idea of the fall of man is in stark contrast to the Judeo-Christian ideas of original sin since early Taoism is fully committed to the view that the individual person is the only agent for reestablishing the primordial condition of health and longevity. Whereas in Western religious tradition ethical values are generally centered in the desire to overcome the problems of this life in an other-worldly transcendence after death, Taoism (and Chinese thought in general) tends to emphasize a more positive attitude toward the ultimate sacrality of this world, this human life (Gruman, pp. 9–37).

The golden age idea and its basic standard of "naturalness" and health is extremely important since it also forms the basis for the theory and practice of medicine found in the ancient medical text known as *The Yellow Emperor's Inner Classic*. In this most important of all Chinese medical treatises, the ideological and ethical motivation for the practice of medicine is to a great extent colored by these Taoist concerns. Thus, the *Inner Classic* is not so much a secular textbook for the physician but a semimystical essay on the practical methods of healing the fallen condition of man, methods of restoring man to a condition that approximates the condition of paradise. Disease is a soteriological problem that is consequent on man's being "negligent of the laws of nature" (Veith, chap. 1, p. 97).

The "superior physician" must, therefore, know the ways of applying the natural healing power of the Tao. He must follow the Tao in order to be able to help others. Here the meaning of "following the Tao" is particularly linked to the key ethical idea of *wu-wei*—literally "non-action," but more accurately the idea of "natural," "spontaneous," or "disinterested" action. The methods for returning to the Tao, the methods of *yang-sheng*, seem to imply meditation techniques leading to an egoless state of mystic identification with nature; but they also involve a special way of acting in the world. *Wu-wei* is that special kind of behavior which flows spontaneously from the individual's inner psychic nature in perfect harmony with his body and the cosmos. *Wu-wei* is behavior that is in congruence with the spontaneity and vitality, the *tzu-jan*, of the Tao as the creative and life-sustaining principle of nature. Negatively this means that the Taoist must avoid a life of ambition and struggle; or as the *Chuang-tzu* says: "Do not fall prey to the fidget and fuss of thoughts and scheming" (Watson, chap. 23, p. 250).

Wu-wei does not mean, however, a complete passivity or a total withdrawal from social life but rather unselfish action that gives rise to the positive values of kindness, sincerity, and tolerance (Lao-tzu, chap. 49, p. 186). There is a close connection between acting with *wu-wei* and human health since only by "yielding" in life, by being humble and egoless, can one "be preserved whole" (ibid., chap 22, p. 139).

Needham also makes the interesting if not wholly demonstrable assertion that the principle of *wu-wei* is the basis for a protoscientific drive in Taoism. Man must learn to be totally open and receptive to the mysterious order of nature; and, consequently, acting in and knowing the world cannot be predetermined by any absolute standards of truth (Needham, 1956, pp. 71–74). In its extreme sense this negates much of the "tolerance" associated with *wu-wei* and can amount to a kind of extreme ethical relativism since potentially the Taoist is a Frankenstein who puts pure knowledge of nature ahead of any humane considerations (cf. *Tao-te Ching*, chap. 5, where it is said that the sage is essentially ruthless or "nonbenevolent"). In fact, there were problems along these lines in later Taoist tradition such as the overly enthusiastic use of deadly mercury-based elixir drugs (Needham, 1970, pp. 316–339); but ultimately the implicit principle that action must be ethically neutral is tempered both by the overriding Taoist concern to preserve human life and by the syncretistic adoption of the Confucian ideas of benevolence and filial piety as corollaries to *wu-wei*.

For the *Inner Classic* the principle of *wu-wei* is a cardinal principle for the physician since it is implied that he must emulate the Taoist sage by following the methods of self-cultivation used by the ancients of the golden age; and with the practice of *wu-wei* comes physical and spiritual health and a prolongation of life. Being with the Tao himself, the physician is in a position selflessly to help others return to a harmony with nature. It is possible that this idea becomes inculcated in the classical medical tradition as the basic principle that a physician practices medicine gratis and never as a means to fame and personal reward. Ordinarily this is explained as deriving from the Confucian idea of benevolence, but in the *Inner Classic* it also seems to be linked to the Taoist idea of *wu-wei*.

In the *Inner Classic*, then, the ideal physician cannot be described solely in Taoist terms, but there is very much of an element of Taoist mysticism emphasizing the importance of self-cultivation (such as meditation), a concern for the quality and prolongation of human life (*yang-sheng* cultivation), and the selfless application of the methods of healing (principle of *wu-wei*). The physician's method is thus a pragmatic art of healing intrinsically related to the more immediately mystical and spiritual goals of Taoism which stressed the importance of an extrarational or intuitive knowledge of the ways of the Tao. Medicine in this sense always includes a moral or even sacred dimension, which may be one reason why a specific legalistic code of medical ethics was not generated.

This is not to say that in the *Inner Classic* there are not already certain "maxims of the art of healing." Aside from interdictions against neglectful and careless practice and avoiding surgical operations that violate the integral unity of the body, one of the most characteristic maxims seen in the *Inner Classic* and most of later Chinese medicine is the importance attributed to preventive medicine. In the *Inner Classic* it is a principle specifically rooted in the golden age theory, since "the ancient sages did not treat those who were already ill. They instructed those who were not ill" (Veith, p. 105; Needham, 1970, pp. 370–378). Of course, the meaning behind this reference is that while one should try to emulate the preventive practices of the ancient sages, the present age was a time of decay (in fact, sickness and disease are the primary manifestations of a "fall"), and it was necessary to deal medically with the disharmony and disease of human nature.

In his introduction to the *Inner Classic*, written in A.D. 762, Wang Ping, the Taoist physician and master "who opens up mysteries," summarized most of these principles by stating that

. . . the superior physician wishes to give to men the hope of prolonging their lives; and to clarify matters for the students; and to make the highest Tao prevail; and to keep in continuous existence the highest principles, so that after a thousand years the people shall know that the wisdom and kindness of the great sages were without limits [Veith, p. 85].

Esoteric Taoism

The biomedical significance of *yang-sheng* becomes even more intense in later centuries (especially after the second century A.D.) with the prominence given to all sorts of specialized techniques (alchemy, macrobiotics, sexual hygiene, medical gymnastics, etc.) devoted to the quest for perfect health and "immortality" (the condition of the Taoist holy man or saint known as the *hsien*). The idea of the *hsien* differs considerably from the more limited and naturalistic ideals seen in classical Taoism but it also seems clear that the idea of the *hsien* must be qualified as a kind of this-worldly "material immortality"

of body and spirit essentially reflecting an extreme elaboration on the earlier idea of the prolongation and qualitative transformation of human life. In this way *hsien*ship may be said to be implicit in the earlier classical texts and does not represent a totally foreign religious or supernaturalistic ideology (Gruman, pp. 28–39).

These esoteric traditions come closest to what Needham intends by his description of Taoism as a protoscientific "experimental mysticism" since the therapeutic repertory of traditional Chinese medicine is greatly influenced by the efforts of the Taoists in seeking methods and compounds for the healing transformation of the human condition. The alchemical tradition (*fu-lien*: in both its "outer, or *wai-tan*" [laboratory], and "inner, or *nei-tan*" [physiological], sense) is especially important in this regard and might be thought of as basically an experimental soteriology concerned with the preparation of the medicine or elixir of long life (Needham, 1974, pp. 71–126; Lu, pp. 68–84).

There were aberrant, wildly superstitious, and even dangerous aspects in this tradition, but it was also an important motivating factor in the broadening of medical knowledge and the elaboration of specific pharmacological techniques. For example, Taoist alchemists had pioneered in the use of iatro-chemical compounds and endrocrinological techniques (including the preparation of sex hormones) (Needham, 1970, pp. 294–377).

These esoteric movements tended at first to accentuate the asocial quest of the individual adept for the status of the *hsien*, who was beyond the constraints of the mundane world; but by the third century Confucian influence had largely socialized the quest for *hsien*ship and made it contingent upon ethical behavior and the helping of others.

The best example of the Taoist quest for *hsien*ship as syncretistically conditioned by the Confucian social consciousness and the Buddhist idea of meritorious good works is seen in the writings of the famous fourth-century alchemist and physician Ko Hung. By this time Taoist ethics are conceived on the basis of the principle that the "three religions are one."

When we examine the moral injunctions of the various teachings, we find all of them agreeing that those desiring fullness of life must strive to accumulate goodness, win merit, be kind and affectionate to others, practice the Golden Rule, love even the creeping things, rejoice in the good fortune of others and commiserate with their sufferings, help those in distress, aid the poor, harm no living thing, utter no curses, look upon success and failures of others as their own, not be proud, not vaunt themselves, not envy their betters, and conceal no evil intentions with flattery. In this way, they become men of exalted character and receive good fortune from Heaven. Their undertakings are sure to be successful, and they can seek geniehood [*hsien*ship] with hope of success [Ware, p. 116].

The Taoist Church

Along with the more individualistic esoteric practices, Taoism also developed, under Buddhist influence, an ecclesiastical and monastic tradition (such as the "Heavenly Masters" sect) during the Six Dynasties period (third to sixth century A.D.). In church Taoism the basic goals of health, longevity, and *hsien*ship are still present but the mechanism of attainment is dependent upon communal and liturgical acts colored by the Buddhist ideas of the devotion to savior gods (*boddhisattva*) and the performance of good works according to the karmic law of retribution (Maspero, 1967, pp. 43–57).

In this tradition there is a real sense of sin (primarily indicated by sickness and disease) as a transgression of divine sanctions and an elaborate hierarchical and moralistic structure of reward and punishment in multiple heavens and hells. While this strongly contrasts with the earlier naturalistic cosmology of classical Taoism, it should be noted that the divine realm was not completely transcendental in nature and was still considered part of the cosmic order.

The idea of doing meritorious good works also stressed the basic Taoist values of cultivating and protecting human life. This is clearly seen in the early-second-century text known as the *T'ai-p'ing ching* (*Classic of the Great Peace*), which emphasized the meritorious nature of sexual reproduction and strongly condemned abortion and infanticide (Yü, p. 86). Taoism, in all its various forms, tended to look with extreme abhorrence on the unnatural termination of any form of human life.

Later moral treatises claimed by religious Taoism, such as the eleventh-century *T'ai-shang kan ying p'ing* (translated by Legge, 1891, pp. 235–246, as the *Tractate of Actions and Their Retributions*), continue this concern for the preservation of life but are also basically expressive of the traditional moral order defined by Confucian values and in general may be described as compendiums of universal folk belief without any intrinsic Taoist origin or affiliation.

Along with Buddhism, the Taoist monastic and church tradition is especially significant in stressing social health care as a meritorious good work expected of all the faithful. Thus, Taoist texts specifically list the care of orphans and the protecting of men from sickness and premature death as meritorious acts. In fact, rather than being promoted by a Confucian sense of social service, hospitals, orphan care, and community quarantine procedures were linked to the activities of the Taoist and Buddhist monasteries during the Six Dynasties period (Needham, 1970, p. 277; Demiéville). The root of this concern for community health care would seem to be most strongly influenced by the Buddhist idea of universal compassion (*karuna*), but in Taoism this idea could be interpreted as an aspect of the selfless kindness and concern for human health extended to all persons in the practice of *wu-wei*.

The idea of morally good works related to the Taoist and Buddhist theory of retribution is the ethical principle most directly influencing the practice of medicine. From the seventh century on, medical codes influenced by Taoism and Buddhism specifically mention karmic retribution as one of the most important factors in controlling professional neglect and selfish conduct (Lee, pp. 124–129). Of course, the criterion as to what determines a meritorious act is basically expressive of the traditional moral order, and retribution is present as a mechanism of supernatural enforcement.

All of the above elements are best exemplified by the work of the seventh-century alchemist, recluse, and physician Sun Ssu-miao. His book, the *Ch'ien chin fang* (*The Thousand Golden Prescriptions*), sets out the first specific code of medical ethics in Chinese tradition; and, while generally reflecting the traditional moral order and heavily inculcated with the Mahayana idea of the *boddhisattva*, who must vow to help all men attain salvation, it is also clear that the ideal of the Chinese physician was at least partially modeled on the idea of the Taoist sage seen in classical Taoism and the *Inner Classic* of medicine.

In Sun Ssu-miao's work the theory of retribution is ascribed to Lao-tzu, and medicine is described, as in the *Inner Classic*, as a difficult and sacred art that requires the guidance of the Tao in order to understand the "mysterious points." The superior physician (*ta-i*), therefore, uses intuition and scholarship, "mastering all the medical literature and working carefully and tirelessly." The superior physician is honest and selfless in the practice of his art: "He should look upon the misery of the patient as if it were his own" (Lee, p. 123; Unschuld).

Conclusion

Given the diffuse and syncretistic nature of religion and philosophy in China, Taoism cannot be strictly identified as the basis for Chinese medical ethics. In a very broad sense, however, Taoism and Chinese medicine are closely linked in their mutual concern for the arts of cultivating and preserving human life. The important point is that human health must be approached holistically as a problem encompassing the total psychosomatic makeup of man in relationship to nature. The Tao or "right way" of Chinese medicine is fundamentally, therefore, an ethics that seeks to know and follow the natural law. But the Tao as natural law is a law without a lawgiver or revealed absolute standards; each individual has to evaluate the naturalness, or life-preserving nature, of an action. There is a deontological imperative here, because not knowing or not following the Tao is a definitional aspect of individual sickness and social disorder.

To sum up: (1) The traditional ethics of medical practice is most strongly influenced by Confucian values, but the underlying ideal of the "superior physician" is strongly colored by the idea of the Taoist sage. (2) The ethics of health care is related to the Confucian social consciousness but was stimulated by the Buddhist theory of compassion and retribution. Taoism is mainly supportive of Buddhism in this respect. (3) Characteristic of the Taoist contribution is the emphasis placed on the medicinal context of meaning surrounding the tradition of mystic and alchemical techniques of self-cultivation and the nurturing of human life (*yang-sheng*). In a sense, the Taoist is a physician by definition since he intimately knows and lives the Tao. Knowing the principle of life gives him the personal potency (*te*) and selfless motivation (*wu-wei*) to bring others back to bodily and spiritual health.

NORMAN J. GIRARDOT

[For further discussion of topics mentioned in this article, see the entries: BUDDHISM; CONFUCIANISM; DEATH, articles on EASTERN THOUGHT, WESTERN PHILOSOPHICAL THOUGHT, and WESTERN RELIGIOUS THOUGHT; MEDICAL ETHICS, HISTORY OF, section on SOUTH AND EAST ASIA, articles on GENERAL HISTORICAL SURVEY and PREREPUBLICAN CHINA; and THERAPEUTIC RELATIONSHIP. Also directly related are the entries ENVIRONMENT AND MAN, article on EASTERN THOUGHT; ETHICS, articles on DEONTOLOGICAL THEORIES and THEOLOGICAL ETHICS; MIRACLE AND FAITH HEALING; and NATURAL LAW. Other relevant material may be found under BIOLOGY, PHILOSOPHY OF; HEALTH AND DISEASE; LIFE; and SCIENCE: ETHICAL IMPLICATIONS.]

BIBLIOGRAPHY

DEMIÉVILLE, PAUL. "Byo." *Hobogirin: Dictionnaire encyclopédique du bouddhisme d'après les sources chinoises et japonaises.* Edited by Paul Demiéville. Tokyo: Maison franco-japonaise, 1929–. Fasc. 3: *Bussokuseki-Chi.* Paris: Librairie d'Amérique et d'Orient, Adrien Maisonneuve, 1937, pp. 245–265.

GRUMAN, GERALD J. *A History of Ideas about the Prolongation of Life.* Transactions of the American Philosophical Society, vol. 56, pt. 9. Philadelphia: 1966. Excellent comparative survey of Taoist and Western philosophical, religious, and medical thought concerning the idea of the prolongation of life. Should also be consulted for its helpful bibliographies.

KALTENMARK, MAX. *Lao Tzu and Taoism.* Rev. ed. Translated by Roger Greaves. Stanford: Stanford University Press, 1969. Concise and readable introduction to Taoist tradition by one of the leading European scholars.

LAO-TZU. *The Way of Lao Tzu.* Translated, with introductory essays, comments, and notes by Wing-tsit Chan. Indianapolis: Bobbs-Merrill, 1963. One of the best and most reliable translations of the *Tao-te ching* with extensive background and textual notes.

LEE, T'AO. "Medical Ethics in Ancient China." *Bulletin of the History of Medicine* 13 (1943): 268–277. Reprint. *Chinese Medical Journal* 61 (1943): 123–131. Discussion of Sun Ssu-miao as well as most of the later traditional codes of Chinese medical ethics. English translation of texts unreliable and sometimes misleading. The original Chinese version of this article is listed below under Li T'ao.

LEGGE, JAMES, trans. *The Sacred Books of China: The Texts of Tāoism.* Pt. 2: *The Writings of Kwang-zze, Books XVIII–XXXIII, The Thāi-Shang: Tractate of Actions and Their Retributions, Appendixes I–VIII.* The Sacred Books of the East, vol. 40. Edited by F. Max Müller. London: Clarendon Press, 1891. Reprint. Delhi: Motilal Banarsidass, 1966.

LI T'AO. "Chung-kuo ti i-hsüeh tao-te kuan" [Chinese medical ethics]. *Chung-hua i-hsüeh tsa-chih* [Chinese medical journal] 27 (1941): 679–688. This journal carries the English title *National Medical Journal of China and the Tsinan Medical Review.* There is a brief English abstract with the title "Medical Ethics in China," by T'ao Lee.

LU, GWEI-DJEN. "The Inner Elixir (Nei Tan); Chinese Physiological Alchemy." *Changing Perspectives in the History of Science.* Edited by Mikulas Teich and Robert Young. Boston: D. Reidel Publishing Co.; London: Heinemann, 1973, pp. 68–84. Important article on the alchemical practice of *yang-sheng* as "redemptive hygiene."

MASPERO, HENRI. "Les Procédés de 'nourrir le principe vital' dans la religion taoïste ancienne." *Journal asiatique* 229 (1937): 177–252, 353–430. Classic study of the Taoist idea of *yang-sheng* and its relation to medical theories of anatomy and therapy.

———. *Mélanges posthumes sur les religions et l'histoire de la Chine.* Vol. 2: *Le Taoïsme.* Paris:

Presses Universitaires de France, 1967. Most important for its discussion of the Taoist Church tradition.

NAKAYAMA, SHIGERU, and SIVIN, NATHAN, eds. *Chinese Science: Explorations of an Ancient Tradition.* Cambridge: MIT Press, 1973. See especially the article by William C. Cooper and Nathan Sivin, "Man as a Medicine," pp. 203–272. The annotated bibliography is also a valuable reference source.

NEEDHAM, JOSEPH. *Clerks and Craftsmen in China and the West.* London: Cambridge University Press, 1970. Especially important for the essays "Medicine and Chinese Culture," pp. 263–293, and "Hygiene and Preventive Medicine in Ancient China," pp. 340–378.

————. *Science and Civilisation in China.* Vol. 2: *History of Scientific Thought.* London: Cambridge University Press, 1956. Monumental and controversial work on the history of Chinese science. The section on Taoism is most stimulating with regard to medicine. Valuable also for the exhaustive bibliographies.

————. *Science and Civilisation in China.* Vol. 5: *Chemistry and Chemical Technology.* Pt. 2: *Spagyrical Discovery and Invention: Magisteries of Gold and Immortality.* London: Cambridge University Press, 1974. Significant for its stimulating comparative discussion of Chinese and Western alchemy.

SIVIN, NATHAN. *Chinese Alchemy: Preliminary Studies.* Cambridge: Harvard University Press, 1968. Translation and discussion of Sun Ssu-miao's alchemical work. High standards of scholarship and reliability.

UNSCHULD, PAUL ULRICH. *Medizin und Ethik: Sozialkonflikte im China der Kaiserzeit.* Münchener ostasiatische Studien, vol. 11. Wiesbaden: F. Steiner Verlag, 1975.

VEITH, ILZA. *The Yellow Emperor's Classic of Internal Medicine.* Berkeley: University of California Press, 1966. Only available translation of the *Inner Classic, Huang-ti nei ching,* but should be used cautiously because of the generally flawed translations. Veith's translation of the title of this work as the classic of "internal medicine" is particularly inaccurate and misleading.

WARE, JAMES R., ed. and trans. *Alchemy, Medicine, and Religion in the China of A.D. 320: The Nei P'ien of Ko Hung.* Cambridge: MIT Press, 1966. Translation of Ko Hung's important alchemical work, the *Pao p'u tzu.* Ware's translations are sometimes eccentric and must be used with caution.

WATSON, BURTON, trans. *The Complete Works of Chuang Tzu.* New York: Columbia University Press, 1968. Excellent translation of the Taoist classic.

WELCH, HOLMES H. "The Bellagio Conference on Taoist Studies." *History of Religions* 9 (1969–1970): 107–136. Important survey of recent developments in Taoist studies.

————. *Taoism: The Parting of the Way.* Boston: Beacon Press, 1966. Along with Kaltenmark, the best general and nontechnical introduction to Taoism.

YANG, CH'ING-K'UN. *Religion in Chinese Society.* Berkeley: University of California Press, 1967. Excellent treatment of the diffuse nature of Chinese religion and ethics from a sociological point of view.

YÜ, YING-SHIH. "Life and Immortality in the Mind of Han China." *Harvard Journal of Asiatic Studies* 25 (1964–1965): 80–122. Important study on the significance of the idea of life in Chinese thought in general and Taoism in particular.

TEACHING OF MEDICAL ETHICS

See MEDICAL ETHICS EDUCATION.

TECHNOLOGY

I. PHILOSOPHY OF TECHNOLOGY   *Carl Mitcham and Jim Grote*

II. TECHNOLOGY AND THE LAW   *Laurence H. Tribe and Kenneth M. Casebeer*

III. TECHNOLOGY ASSESSMENT   *LeRoy Walters*

I

PHILOSOPHY OF TECHNOLOGY

Philosophy of technology is the attempt to give an ordered account of the nature and meaning of technology, i.e., the making and using of artifacts. A key figure in the development of the notion of a philosophy of technology distinct from the philosophy of science is Friedrich Dessauer (1881–1963). The philosophy of science generally assumes one of two forms. The first is an analysis of the structure and validity of scientific knowledge in general; the other focuses on specific theories, e.g., Copernican astronomy, Darwinian evolution, in order to speculate about the nature of the universe and man's place in it. For Dessauer both approaches fail to deal with the question of the power of scientific-technical knowledge, which has become through modern engineering a new form of making. Dessauer's *Philosophie der Technik* (1927) is an attempt to explain, in Kantian terms, the source of the power of this knowledge, and to reflect on the ethical implications of its application. He argues that the autonomous, world-transforming power of modern technology points toward a transcendental reality, and that the human exercise of that power places man in union with the creative activity of God.

The growing influence of Dessauer's work and of other European reflections on technology—notably Martin Heidegger's analysis of the technological attitude toward the world, Jacques Ellul's study of technological society, and various theories about the meaning of artificial intelligence—can be seen reflected in successive *Proceedings* of the International Congresses of Philosophy.

The more recent genesis of the philosophy of technology in the United States is usually dated from two events. First, in March 1962, at the Center for the Study of Democratic Institutions in Santa Barbara, California, the Encyclopaedia

Britannica Conference on the Technological Order took place. Ellul's *The Technological Society* was published in English shortly afterward (1964). Second, in the Summer 1966 issue of *Technology and Culture* appeared a set of papers on the theme "Toward a Philosophy of Technology." This symposium included contributions by Lewis Mumford, one of the outstanding historians and social critics of technology, as well as by a group of philosophers who have since come to be recognized among the leading English-language philosophers of technology: Joseph Agassi, Mario Bunge, and Henryk Skolimowski. Since then the frequency and importance of scholarly developments in this area can be measured by the publication of the comprehensive *Bibliography of the Philosophy of Technology* (Mitcham and Mackey, 1973), the appearance of several anthologies (e.g., Mitcham and Mackey, 1972), and the launching of the first journal in the field in 1977: *Philosophy and Technology: An Annual Compilation of Research*.

Metaphysical analyses

Against the background of this development, philosophical analyses of technology can be divided into four basic categories. From a metaphysical or theoretical perspective, technology can be viewed (1) as object, (2) as knowledge, (3) as process, or (4) as volition.

1. Technology as object. The theory that identifies technology with particular artifacts such as tools, machines, electronic devices, or consumer products, may be described as the commonsense view. Developed philosophically, it involves a classification of technological objects into various types of artifacts. Franz Reuleaux, for instance, organizes machines into classes according to the varieties of motion they employ. His contemporary Ernst Kapp, in *Grundlinien einer Philosophie der Technik* (1877)—the first book to bear the title "philosophy of technology" —approaches the subject from an anthropological standpoint. After extensive comparisons between human anatomy and technological inventions, he concludes that weapons and tools are essentially projections of human organs: the hammer an extension of the fist, clothing an extension of body skin and hair, etc.

The notion of technological objects as projections of the human body has become the most widely adopted theory about the metaphysical status of artifacts—that is, about the kind of

reality artifacts have. Marshall McLuhan, for instance, in *Understanding Media: The Extensions of Man* (1964) suggests that, just as mechanical technology extends the body, so electronic media extend the nervous system. This is also the theory of technology incorporated in a synthetic organ or prosthetic device—where a creation of bioengineering functions not simply as an extension but as a vital replacement for some defective human organ.

2. Technology as knowledge. Heidegger, however, argues that the synthetic use of nature is possible only when materials are first made "available" or "in supply" by abstraction from all particularity and definiteness. In contrast to the flesh of the body or the wood and stone of traditional artifacts, prosthetic devices are fabricated out of highly indefinite plastics and powered by abstract chemical or electrical energies. For Heidegger, modern artifacts are made possible by a special kind of consciousness or comportment toward nature, what he calls "the provoking, setting up disclosure of the world." Ultimately technology is to be understood not as a kind of object but as a comprehensive attitude toward the world. Indeed, it is the same attitude toward the world that manifests itself practically in technology that is manifested theoretically in modern science. This latter understanding of modern science as a kind of theoretical technology is also well argued in some of the work of Hans Jonas (1959, 1971).

The more common conception of technology as knowledge is, however, that technology is applied science. This is the position of most scientists and engineers and is given detailed philosophical articulation by Mario Bunge. For Bunge modern technology develops when the rules of prescientific crafts, originally discovered by trial-and-error methods, are replaced by the "grounded rules" of technological theories. In essence, technological theories are "scientific theories of action." For example, prior to the nineteenth century, most medical practice relied on rule-of-thumb experience. Since then the development of modern medicine has involved the progressive grounding of medical practice in the sciences of anatomy and physiology.

3. Technology as process. Another alternative to the idea of technology as object is contained in the theory of technology as process or activity, the basic assumption of socioeconomic studies of technology. In sociological analyses technology is usually identified with technique. Jacques Ellul, in his study *The Technological Society*, specifically rejects any identification of technology with technological objects such as machines. Instead, modern technology is defined as a kind of action, one whose fundamental characteristic is the rational pursuit of efficiency. Ellul's definition has roots in Max Weber's observation that there are techniques of every conceivable human activity—from prayer and thought to education, politics, artistic production, and performance. The problem for a sociologist is to explain what Harold Lasswell terms "technicalization." Traditional techniques, note Lasswell and Kaplan in *Power and Society* (pp. 50–51), were "hedged about sanctions" and therefore "included in the social order"—i.e., "the pattern of mores and countermores institutions." In traditional society animals could be eaten only if butchered in a ritually prescribed manner. In modern social behavior, however, techniques have ceased "to be treated or symbolized as subject to sanctions." At best they are subject to calculations of total efficiency, as in contemporary programs of technology assessment. Technicalization is thus the transformation "from involvement with mores and countermores to expediency alone." Contemporary attitudes toward abortion, euthanasia, and capital punishment are often grim examples of this development.

4. **Technology as volition.** Finally, some thinkers have argued that the status of technology is best revealed not through objects, knowledge, or action, but through will or volition. This is the position of the Canadian philosopher George Grant:

All descriptions or definitions of technique which place it outside ourselves hide us from what it is. This applies to the simplest accounts which describe technological advance as new machines and inventions as well as to the more sophisticated which include within their understanding the whole hierarchy of interdependent organisations and their methods. Technique comes forth from and is sustained in our vision of ourselves as creative freedom, making ourselves, and conquering the chances of an indifferent world [Grant, p. 137].

This modern notion that man makes himself, or wills what he is to become, has serious practical consequences in the biomedical field. Genetic counseling, followed up by abortion when necessary, is designed to keep the spontaneity of nature from interfering with an individual's self-creative volition.

Ernst Jünger, José Ortega y Gasset, and Lewis Mumford also argue that technology is essentially a matter of the will. For Jünger, technology is the "mobilization of the world through the *Gestalt* of the worker." For Ortega, technology is created whenever any self-image seeks worldly realization. In Mumford's historical analysis, technology emerges when man subordinates his traditional polytechnical activities of craft, religious ritual, and poetry to a monotechnical pursuit of physical power—something that first happened, he thinks, about five thousand years ago in Egypt with the construction of pyramids and in Assyria with the creation of large standing armies.

Ethical issues

Despite its logical priority, it is not theoretical analysis but ethical concern that has dominated the philosophy of technology. This dominance of ethical and political problems obtains in part because of the modern emphasis on practice over theory; in part it reflects the pressing nature of the problems themselves. Thus the ethical analysis of modern technology can conveniently be sketched as a series of reactions to specific problems.

Alienation. The first crisis of modern technology, historically speaking, involved the Industrial Revolution and the problem of alienation. At the basis of modern technological making lies the idea that the world as it is given does not provide a suitable home for man; rather man must construct one for himself. The problem is that man does not immediately find himself at home in the world he creates and, because of his initial commitment, is highly sensitive to alienation in a variety of social forms. The two most radical critiques of alienation are Romantic and socialist in their foundations.

The Romantic critique focuses on how modern technology alienates the individual from feelings and sentiments, as manifested in relationships with nature, the past, or other men and women. This is caused, according to the Romantic mind, by a one-sided development of rationality. Romanticism thus views technology as an extension of reason and proposes to enclose it within a larger affective life. In contrast, Karl Marx, representing the socialist critique of alienation, explicitly conceives of technology as an organ projection. Thus he focuses on the separation of man from control over the products of his labor, as is found in an economy based on money and the "fetishism of commodities." To meet this problem the socialist argues for a comprehensive restructuring of society ordered toward worker control of the means of production.

In biomedical practice the increasing use of technological instruments and rationalized systems of diagnosis has raised the problem of alienation in the form of questions about depersonalization of health-care techniques and organizations. Responses to such depersonalization often exhibit characteristically Romantic or socialist features. A typically Romantic response is to propose the situating of diagnostic techniques within a larger humanistic framework of beautiful buildings and a pleasant environment. One typically socialist response seeks to give patients direct control over their own health-care institutions.

War.   A second ethical issue has arisen concerning technology and war. About the relationship betwen war and technology there are two beliefs: (1) Technology makes war unnecessary and so horrible that it becomes unthinkable; and (2) man will always go to war; technology just makes it more horrible. Prior to 1914–1919, the first belief prevailed in popular thought. The trauma of the First World War was not just the fact that it was the most technologically destructive war up to that time; its main historical force was to shatter the internal confidence of a culture. As a result, intellectual criticism of technological civilization turned into a pessimistic reassessment of man's tendency, contrary to all rational self-interest, to direct immense destructive powers against himself. Yet, because technological power is not readily renounced, recognition of the deep potentiality for evil brings about a new and unqualified desire to master or overcome it. This desire was stimulated even more forcefully by the Second World War and the technological practice of genocide, the invention and use of the atomic bomb, and the subsequent cold war spread of nuclear weapons. Ideals of human brotherhood and peace, which in the past could remain as moral exhortations not necessarily realized in deed, became necessities of the present, lest man obliterate himself from the face of the earth.

The prospects for social and genetic engineering engender similar demands. In the last ten years the progressive refinement of conditioning techniques and sophisticated drug therapies has created behavior control technologies of immense potential power. The corresponding development of recombinant DNA technology proffers the opportunity to extend this power to the very creation of human life. With such power the possibilities for evil use further increase the need for the practice of high ethical ideals.

Technological change.   In conjunction with studies of how technology affects personal alienation and alters the character of warfare, there have been many investigations of such related subjects as bureaucracy, urbanization, increased public leisure and mobility, secularization, automation and the second industrial revolution, new forms of communication media (telephone, radio, TV, computers), the effects of these media on international relations, education, privacy, etc. Today a distinct discipline called science policy studies even analyzes how political or governmental action influences scientific and technological development, and vice versa. Since World War I, however, historians and sociologists have more and more tried to generalize about the relationship between technology and society as a whole. One early instance is William F. Ogburn's description of a "cultural lag" between technological development and social change; more recently a number of universities have established special institutes, such as the Harvard Program on Technology and Society (1964–1972), to focus on this general question.

Growing out of such general empirical studies has come a third ethical issue of technology. In light of the fact that technology alters the social order (and is not easily restricted in its development), philosophical questions arise about what changes in moral action and attitude are required by and for an ethical evaluation of technological change. One of the earliest attempts to deal with this type of question is part of Henri Bergson's *The Two Sources of Morality and Religion* (1932). Bergson, following upon his distinction between "closed" and "open" societies, differentiates static, myth-making religions from dynamic, mystical ones. Then he argues that the constricting vices of industrial civilization can be corrected only by a revival of mysticism, which is at once ascetic (against luxuries) and charitable (for eliminating inequalities).

Until recently Bergson's suggestions have been viewed with skepticism as historically unrealistic. (Contemporary interest in Oriental religious practices may now give pause to this judgment.) And the search for historically real possibilities has, generally speaking, led in two different directions. One calls for a modification of the self-image of man dominant in advanced industrial society. This is illustrated in radical form by the Marxist criticism of technological consumption to be found in thinkers such as Herbert Marcuse or C. B. Macpherson, who argue for a more self-creative idea of man. Moderate forms of the same approach call for the social redefinition of work or higher economic valuations on service and educational activities in order, e.g., to meet the problems of automation and extended leisure. A second approach, in contrast, calls not so much for the modification of basic instincts and volitions as for some increase or intensification of knowledge and intelligence.

This second view, if any, is characteristic of advanced industrial society itself, with its commitment to large-scale educational institutions and activities. The ethical difficulty, from this perspective, is not with what men aim for or wish to do but with what they know about how to get there and do it. Emmanuel G. Mesthene argues that technology, by creating new physical possibilities for human action, is a means for human liberation. The necessary price of liberation is that man not accede to the widespread fear that technology creates an unintelligible or ungovernable world; instead, one must affirm its essential intelligibility, striving especially to understand how technology affects society. Technology, far from undermining human values, simply requires that they be exercised or pursued more intelligently. This, it might also be noted, has been a leading response to those social changes fostered by advances in biomedical technology—e.g., the availability of oral contraceptives affects sexual behavior in ways that need to be more fully understood.

Pollution and ecological issues. One aspect of technological change that has become specially prominent in recent years concerns pollution and the energy crisis. Because of its importance, it may even be said to constitute a fourth ethical issue of technology. As a biomedical problem of the health and safety of man, pollution once again drives a wedge of necessity into the need either for changes in the human self-image or for more comprehensive knowledge—or both. At the same time it extends man's moral concern beyond his own personal interest. As a bioethical issue, pollution has engendered the science of ecology and a new awareness of man's responsibilities toward the natural world and future generations, as has been forcefully argued by Jonas (1973, 1976). It has also raised questions in the minds of social scientists such as Robert Heilbroner about the limits of industrial growth and the long-range adequacy of democratic forms of government.

Conclusion

This development of the ethical analysis of technology may be reviewed as follows. Technological crises have provoked a series of specific moral reactions. Each response, because it focused on some particular aspect of technology, has articulated a theme that needs to be related to others and tested by generalization. One likely generalization would be that technological action progressively increases human moral responsibility. By the practical power of its objects, knowledge, and processes technology creates problems that demand immediate response in terms of what has traditionally been called heroic virtue. The central moral issue thus becomes: Does this demand more from man than he is naturally capable of? Or is it possible that technology itself can aid man in making his required response by means of what Alvin Weinberg has called a "technological fix"? Such questions can adequately be approached only through a comprehensive understanding of the nature and meaning of making and using. Such an understanding will necessarily be quite theoretical in character and involve careful delineation of the various material, cognitive, active, and volitional elements of technology. It is against this background of an emerging philosophical account of technology that the problems of bioethics, as the most recent ethical issue of technology, might helpfully be appraised.

CARL MITCHAM AND JIM GROTE

[*Directly related are the entries* BIOETHICS; *and* RIGHTS, *article on* SYSTEMATIC ANALYSIS; *and the two subsequent articles in this entry. For further discussion of topics mentioned in this article, see the entries:* ENVIRONMENTAL ETHICS; LIFE-SUPPORT SYSTEMS; *and* WARFARE, *article on* BIOMEDICAL SCIENCE AND WAR. *For discussion of related ideas, see the entries:* BIOLOGY, PHILOSOPHY OF; MEDICINE, PHILOSOPHY OF; *and* SCIENCE: ETHICAL IMPLICATIONS.]

BIBLIOGRAPHY

BERGSON, HENRI LOUIS. *The Two Sources of Morality and Religion.* Translated by Ruth Ashley Audra and Cloudesley Brereton, with the assistance of W. Horsfall Carter. London: Macmillan; New York: Henry Holt & Co., 1935. Translated from *Les Deux sources de la morale et de la religion.* Paris: Librairie Félix Alcan, 1932.

BORGMANN, ALBERT. "Orientation in Technology." *Philosophy Today* 16 (1972): 135–147.

BUNGE, MARIO. "Action." *Scientific Research.* Vol. 2: *The Search for Truth.* Studies in the Foundations, Methodology and Philosophy, vol. 3/II. New York: Springer-Verlag, 1967, chap. 11, pp. 121–250.

———. "Cybernetics and the Philosophy of Technical Science." *Proceedings of the XIVth International Congress of Philosophy: Vienna, 2nd to 9th September 1968.* Vienna: Herder, 1968, vol. 2, colloquium 6, pp. 477–614. Contains papers by Adam, Agassi, Cardone, Dreyfus, Granger, Greniewski, Kleyff, Kotarbiński, Mays, Mazur, Ostrowski, Serres, Skolimowski, Titze, Tondl, and Tuchel.

DESSAUER, FRIEDRICH. *Philosophie der Technik: Das Problem der Realisierung.* Bonn: Friedrich Cohen, 1927.

———. *Streit um die Technik.* Frankfurt am Main: J. Knecht, 1956. 2nd ed. 1958.

ELLUL, JACQUES. *The Technological Society.* Translated by John Wilkinson. Introduction by Robert K. Merton. New York: Alfred A. Knopf, 1964. Originally published in French as *La Technique ou l'enjeu du siècle.* Paris: Librairie Armand Colin, 1954.

GRANT, GEORGE PARKIN. *Technology and Empire: Perspectives on North America.* Toronto: House of Anansi, 1969.

HEIDEGGER, MARTIN. "Die Frage nach der Technik." *Vorträge und Aufsätze.* Pfullingen: Günther Neske, 1954, pp. 13–44.

HEILBRONER, ROBERT L. *An Inquiry into the Human Prospect.* New York: W. W. Norton & Co., 1974.

JONAS, HANS. *Philosophical Essays: From Ancient Creed to Technological Man.* Englewood Cliffs, N.J.: Prentice-Hall, 1974.

———. "The Practical Uses of Theory." *Social Research* 26 (1959): 127–150. Comments by Solomon E. Asch, Erich Hula, and Adolph Lowe, pp. 151–166. Reprint. *The Phenomenon of Life: Toward a Philosophical Biology.* New York: Harper & Row, 1966, 8th essay, pp. 188–210.

———. "Responsibility Today: The Ethics of an Endangered Future." *Social Research* 43 (1976): 77–97.

———. "The Scientific and Technological Revolutions: Their History and Meaning." *Philosophy Today* 15 (1971): 76–101. Reprint in new version with new title. "Seventeenth Century and After: The Meaning of the Scientific and Technological Revolution." Jonas, *Philosophical Essays,* chap. 3, pp. 45–80.

———. "Technology and Responsibility: Reflections on the New Tasks of Ethics." *Social Research* 40 (1973): 31–54. Reprint. Jonas, *Philosophical Essays,* chap. 1, pp. 3–20.

KAPP, ERNST. *Grundlinien einer Philosophie der Technik: Zur Emtstehungsgeschichte der Cultur aus neuen Gesichtspunkten.* Braunschweig: G. Westermann, 1877.

KASS, LEON R. "The New Biology: What Price Relieving Man's Estate?" *Science* 174 (1971): 779–788.

LASSWELL, HAROLD DWIGHT, and KAPLAN, ABRAHAM. *Power and Society: A Framework for Political Inquiry.* New Haven: Yale University Press, 1950; London: Routledge & Kegan Paul, 1952.

McDERMOTT, JOHN. "Technology: The Opiate of the Intellectuals." *New York Review of Books,* 31 July 1969, pp. 25–35. Critique of Mesthene and the idea that social problems can have technological solutions.

McLUHAN, HERBERT MARSHALL. *Understanding Media: The Extensions of Man.* New York: McGraw-Hill, 1964.

MARCUSE, HERBERT. *One-Dimensional Man: Studies in the Ideology of Advanced Industrial Society.* Boston: Beacon Press, 1964.

MESTHENE, EMMANUEL G. *Technological Change: Its Impact on Man and Society.* Cambridge: Harvard University Press, 1970.

MITCHAM, CARL, and MACKEY, ROBERT, eds. *Bibliography of the Philosophy of Technology.* Chicago: University of Chicago Press, 1973. A comprehensive annotated bibliography covering comprehensive philosophical works, ethical and political critiques, religious critiques, and metaphysical and epistemological studies.

———, and MACKEY, ROBERT, eds. *Philosophy and Technology: Readings in the Philosophical Problems of Technology.* New York: Free Press, 1972. Contains essays divided into five categories: conceptual issues, ethical and political critiques, religious critiques, existentialist critiques, metaphysical studies. Authors included: Skolimowski, Bunge, Mumford, Ellul, Mesthene, Macpherson, Junger, Ortega, Dessauer, Jonas, etc. Select annotated bibliography.

MOSER, SIMON. "Toward a Metaphysics of Technology." *Philosophy Today* 15 (1971): 129–156. The most extensive review of European thought on this subject available in English.

MUMFORD, LEWIS. *The Myth of the Machine.* 2 vols. Vol. 1: *Technics and Human Development.* Vol. 2: *The Pentagon of Power.* New York: Harcourt Brace Jovanovich, 1967, 1970. Mumford's *magnum opus.* Vol. 1 is an extended critique of the definition of man as a tool-using animal. Vol. 2 analyzes the closed circle of technological rationality.

———. *Technics and Civilization.* New York: Harcourt, Brace & Co., 1934. A classic historical analysis.

RAPP, FRIEDRICH, ed. *Contributions to a Philosophy of Technology: Studies in the Structure of Thinking in the Technological Sciences.* Theory and Decision Library, vol. 5. Edited by Gerald Eberlein and Werner Leinfellner. Boston: D. Reidel Publishing Co., 1974. Epistemological papers from the *Technology and Culture* symposium "Toward a Philosophy of Technology" with works by European engineers and other thinkers. Annotated bibliography.

REULEAUX, FRANZ. *The Kinematics of Machinery: Outlines of a Theory of Machines.* Translated and edited by Alexander B. W. Kennedy. London: Macmillan & Co., 1876.

SKOLIMOWSKI, HENRYK. "Technology and Philosophy." *Contemporary Philosophy: A Survey.* Vol. 2: *Philosophy of Science.* Edited by Raymond Klibansky. Florence: Nuova Italia Editrice, 1968, pp. 426–437.

STOVER, CARL F., ed. *The Technological Order: Proceedings of the Encyclopaedia Britannica Conference.* Foreword by William Benton. Detroit: Wayne State University Press, 1963. Original appearance. *Technology and Culture* 3, no. 4 (1962), pp. 380–658.

WEINBERG, ALVIN M. "Can Technology Replace Social Engineering?" *Bulletin of the Atomic Scientists,* December 1966, pp. 4–8. Original presentation of the concept of a "technological fix." Other works on this topic listed in Mitcham and Mackey, 1973, p. 45.

II
TECHNOLOGY AND THE LAW

Many bioethical issues focus on health-related technologies—such as those dealing with life-support, genetic intervention, reproductive methods, behavior control, and environmental quality—and the legal principles and processes that affect their use. This article will deal with the ways in which law and biomedical technology have interacted and might yet interact in the future.

Most analyses of the interaction between law and technology treat technology as an independent variable. By focusing on an emerging technique, such as amniocentesis or artificial organ transplantation, such analyses typically assume that the technique will be used and ask what the legal system might do about the problems and possibilities thereby created. There is virtue in such analysis but little virtue in not going farther. For, however complex the processes by which it does so, the legal system determines not only how a technique will be deployed but whether it will be developed at all.

Means and ends in law and technology

We begin with the classic distinction between means and ends, between instruments for the attainment of objectives and the objectives sought. Both "law" and "technology" can be conceived in terms that bridge this duality: Both can be conceived as tools for implementing a given set of social or physical purposes, or as expressions of a society's inner character and embodiments of its ideals. Analyses of the law-technology interaction can convey the full sweep of relevant considerations only if one always remembers that tools—whether social, conceptual, or physical—always possess this double aspect.

This duality has an important dynamic aspect. Over time, the decision to deploy a set of tools, legal or technological, profoundly alters the society in which those tools are used. The very patterns of wants, needs, and aspirations that motivate technological and legal choice—far from being fixed in time or determined by an invariant human nature—are in part the products of prior choices. By shaping the experiences available to its members and structuring their relationships to one another, a society that pursues one technological path rather than another does more than distribute gains and losses; it also takes a step in the continuing process of determining what people value and what they seek to avoid—in effect defining, over time, what *counts* as a "gain" and what counts as a "loss."

The distinctiveness of current biomedical options. Perhaps the dominant characteristic of modern society is the reality that the dynamic of means and ends has become an arena for deliberate social choice (Ferkiss). The industrial technologies of the past several centuries have increasingly represented intentional alterations in the conditions of life and culture. Perhaps even more important than the physical technologies of production and transportation have been the conceptual technologies of market structure and bureaucratic organization—technologies that have made it impossible to continue perceiving economic reality as determined by an invisible hand rather than chosen by increasingly visible processes of decision. What was once "given," including the basic body of law governing who may do what with technologies, has become very much the subject of debate and deliberate reflection (MacPherson).

This historical process is irreversible, in that a phenomenon, having become an object of choice, cannot recede into the realm of the inevitable. But the directions in which the process moves are far from inexorable. For example, having embraced technologies increasingly committed to intervention in the reproductive process, such as amniocentesis, a society is not fated to support or even tolerate all forms of genetic engineering. Although the discovery of potential interventions such as sex determination irreversibly places certain aspects of reproduction and evolution in the realm of choice, that reality need not in itself lead to a rejection of the normative premise that individual identity contains an irreducible element of chance. One may decide to *affirm* such a premise by choosing *not* to do something—cloning, perhaps—even after it has become scientifically thinkable and technically feasible.

The case for such an affirmation may be strongest in the context of biomedical techniques that, like psychosurgery or direct determination of an unborn person's genetic characteristics, impinge on the very core of the human condition. Such techniques threaten to redesign what humanity *is* and to alter perceptions of what it *should be,* potentially undermining the very concept of persons as unique entities, consciously shaping their own choices and hence entitled to resist external manipulation of their lives (Jonas).

Even an incompletely substantiated fear that the very essence of humanity is at stake plausibly justifies public intervention to end certain narrowly defined biomedical procedures. Indeed, this may be required even if the maximum permissible response to most technological choices would be a more measured and moderate form of regulation. For example, recombinant-DNA-molecular research plainly poses tangible risks of the global spread of uncontrollable disease. But, since even that awful development can be evaluated in terms of a framework of values that would remain intact, it is likely that an acceptable accommodation of the risks and benefits of such research will involve a compromise between uncontrolled pursuit and total restraint. However, when the anticipated consequence entails a fundamental change in the value framework itself, for example, by directly altering what it means to be human, the very notion of accommodation among affected values is incoherent. Any intermediate choice—like limiting the number of occasions on which one carries out such a procedure—probably represents the worst of both worlds. Far from being an option that respects each affected interest and norm, it may violate them all. The only meaningful choice in such a case is the all-or-nothing choice of allowing the procedure and accepting the value consequences that follow, or forbidding it and preventing the value experiment altogether. A "little cloning," like a little knowledge, may be the worst alternative of all.

Values at stake in the degree and timing of legal intervention. A fundamental distinction must be made between forbidding a precisely identified procedure and seeking to cut off the prospect of its development by terminating an entire avenue of biomedical research. Among possible objections to the latter choice are the following. First, each avenue of research is likely to have too many promising and indeed life-enhancing offshoots to permit necessarily speculative concerns to carry the day in a controversy over an outright ban. Second, the difficulty of implementing such a prohibition without an almost unimaginable level of global cooperation will counsel against the very attempt. Third, governmental efforts to reinforce prevailing conceptions and values against the feared onslaught of new technology invariably pose difficult problems for a society committed to freedom of belief and expression (Tribe, 1975, p. 1316).

These problems cannot be wholly avoided even by a totally laissez-faire stance, since the sorts of technologies here contemplated may themselves compromise the idea of freedom. At the same time, to ignore free inquiry while limiting research in the name of preserving freedom seems a perverse policy indeed. These tensions are likely to be minimized when public choice seeks to *slow* the pace of development in order to give educational and other efforts time to deflect the apprehended deformation of values. Such attempts aim to show how the values in question—human dignity or freedom—may be defensible even after technology renders them vulnerable. The tensions will be at a maximum when public policy either pretends that no choice is presented or, at the other extreme, aims beyond moratorium or deceleration and toward total prohibition. The prospect of unacceptable dehumanization is thus most likely to be met defensibly by measures designed to assure that change occurs incrementally, only after the educational and cultural climate has been prepared for its advent, and at a rate that facilitates a wise choice of which particularly egregious interventions should be banned altogether.

Against this central background, it is useful to canvass more particularly the variety of legal devices available to effect a desired level of public control with respect to science and technology.

The taxonomy of legal technique

It is useful to distinguish among alternative models or methods of legal intervention by identifying the central focus of each. Legal techniques may center upon (1) particular technological tools or practices; (2) the incentives affecting choice of a particular technology; (3) specified values or areas of concern upon which various technologies or incentives might impinge; and (4) the institutional and conceptual structures through which decisions are made.

Technology-centered legal intervention. In its simplest and most direct form, law intentionally intervenes in research, development, or technological application by directing some act or omission in those processes. Characteristically, a directive may vary in form from mandating quite specific uses of technology to promulgating universal rules requiring that a technology or technologies be used in accordance with such rules or not at all.

As early as the research stage, a development may be subjected to specific legal prohibitions in the belief that later controls may be more difficult to enact and enforce as the developing technology gathers momentum and becomes surrounded by vested interests (National Academy of Sciences). But even when scientists voluntarily adopt codes of self-limitation, as in research on manipulation of genetic codes, those who urge early control confront the age-old argument that basic scientific investigation must remain untrammeled. Put in so stark a form, that argument must be rejected if controls at any stage are to be justified. If there is a "clear and present" danger that research involving the transplantation of DNA would unleash a global epidemic, for example, the case for coercive governmental action is as strong at that point as it would be if the same danger were associated instead with the application of an already developed technology. The timing of legal control should depend not on the phase of development of the technology to be regulated but on the justification offered for legal intervention. Justification on the basis of immediate consequences demands the same form of response whether the intervention comes early or late in the technique's history; it matters little whether an action imminently threatening the ecosphere is labeled "basic research" or an "application." But an intervention justified by the alleged need to avoid the first in a series of steps in an irreversible slide to some future disfavored state or some abhorrent change in values ought to be cast in a form that forecloses the fewest options, which may well depend on the time at which the law acts. In this respect it may matter a great deal whether an action only remotely and speculatively threatening is at the experimental or the application end of development.

Regardless of justification, when the dangers are less certain or fundamental, the argument for relatively uninhibited research or development becomes more compelling. When that is the case, law characteristically intervenes not by outlawing certain procedures altogether but by mandating the institution of a sequence of safeguards as those procedures are developed for more widespread use. Typically, as in the case of food and drug regulations in the United States, such safeguards entail required investigations in subhuman species, compulsory monitoring of effects in human users, and the sharing of the information thereby generated with a regulatory authority.

After a technology has been widely disseminated, the law may intervene by licensing its users and regulating the conditions under which it may be used—as in the case of even routine medical procedures and the prescription of drugs and devices. A particularly common form of regulation at this stage is the rationing of a technology—either by limiting the total quantity of its use, as in the case of certain pesticides, like DDT, or by allocating its availability among competing users, as in the case of television channels, renal dialysis, and organ transplantation. For each model of allocation—from a lottery to a market to a bureaucracy—there is a corresponding legal model of control.

A further form of regulation requires compensation for those injured by a technique's use. If the coverage, beneficiaries, and benefits are correctly tailored, a technique's introduction need not adversely alter the preexisting distribution of resources. Without compensation, the user of the technology imposes part of the costs of its use on those injured, in effect transferring relative wealth from the latter to all beneficiaries of the technique. Compensation requirements also ensure that an incentive is maintained for minimizing hazards associated with the technique's use.

Finally, if the notion of "law" is taken to include governmental action generally, then an increasingly frequent form of direct "legal" intervention is governmental expenditure. Patterns of this form of intervention vary from private research subsidized through public organizations like the National Institutes of Health to public competition with private industry through such governmental organizations as the proposed U.S. Federal Energy Corporation. In nations or fields of inquiry where most research resources are channeled through government agencies, the effect of specific prohibitions can be approximated by controlling the quantity of funds allocated to a given area or project, or by tying the receipt of support—in an area like fetal research —to the observance of certain preconditions.

Incentive-centered legal intervention. Law may intervene by changing economic incentives instead of intervening directly in technological choice. Whether by rewarding innovation or investment-oriented activity (through patents, tax credits, or other special incentives) or by imposing effluent charges, side-effects taxes, or other devices for internalizing the costs associated with various developments, law can alter the boundaries of technological choice without mandating that specific options be adopted or avoided. Such incentives can occasionally be utilized to accomplish the same objective as direct legal commands, and at times with greater efficacy. In the environmental area, for example, it is sometimes politically and technically impossible for the legal system to converge upon the specific levels of environmental discharge that should be accepted from particular sources, but quite feasible to achieve agreement as to the total level of pollution to be tolerated. In such cases, charging each source for its effluents until the desired aggregate level is reached represents a substitute for telling each source how to behave. Periodic adjustments of the level of the effluent charge can be continued until the community feels comfortable with the balance struck between the polluting technology's use and the quality of its environment, even though an attempt to mandate the precise technological conduct required to strike that balance would rest on blind guesswork.

More commonly, the idea of incentive modification is associated with an even less centralized model of decision—one in which even the aggregate result to be achieved, e.g., the total level of pollution, is not agreed upon collectively but represents instead the summation of individual choices. In this mode of choice, individuals govern their own actions with a view to the per-unit "cost" society has agreed to impose on the adverse effect (e.g., the effluent) in question. Whether collective choice in a given context is more fruitfully directed to the question of aggregate effects (the overall environmental goal to be achieved) or to the issue of unit effects (the degree of harm to be attributed to individual actions that affect the environment) will determine which form of incentive modification is preferred.

Value-centered legal intervention. Law may also intervene by identifying values to protect. Such intervention focuses on effects but centers neither on a specific technology nor on a specific set of incentives, concentrating instead on conditions thought to be worth preserving against any technology or other activity, however motivated. The examples of wildlife preserves and legally enforceable zones of personal privacy should suggest the range of possibilities.

Although the focus may be on physical "zones" or "areas," the real point always concerns underlying values. When a legal system structures or affects a community's choice between building a dam and saving a wildlife area from inundation, for example, law and technology alike not only affect the degree to which existing regions are preserved and wants realized, but also alter the set of experiences available to the community whose legal system is involved. A decision to preserve rather than inundate may enhance the value attached to wildlife and nature, just as an alternative decision to dam might enhance the value attached to the productive use of natural resources. In either case, what starts as a zoning-off of physical territory ends as a reconstruction of values and ideals.

Institutionally or conceptually centered intervention. Finally, law may operate at a truly systemic level, redefining the steps that must be taken or the groups that must be represented before certain actions may go forward. Legislation might require environmental impact statements to precede specified governmental choices, or a court decision might insist on the representation of interests otherwise lacking voices of their own —interests as varied as those of mountain streams, mute children, or unborn generations. Procedural interventions of this sort need be committed to no particular goal apart from full and careful deliberation in the development and deployment of technologies. On occasion, however, legal procedures may serve to assure that the opportunity to be heard is more pointedly targeted to the ventilation of possible risks. Thus, especially in basic medical research or experimentation, decision making can be structured so as to maximize the impact of dissenters' "early warnings"—through guarantees of confidentiality; through third-party public hearings or audits; and through guarantees of due process before one is dismissed, passed over in promotion, or denied governmental benefits.

More generally, the legal structure often shapes dispute-resolution proceedings by favoring various substantive outcomes through evidentiary rules setting burdens of proof, determining admissibility of evidence, or deciding what privileged relationships to protect even at the cost of concealing potentially relevant information.

Law may also operate through the legitimation of wholly new categories of discourse—categories like "brain death" or "fetal viability"— which suggest possibilities, evoke associations, and signal dangers that might otherwise have been obscure.

Comparison of available legal approaches

Although a detailed "recipe" for matching legal means with various technological contexts or social ends is both beyond the scope of this article and beyond the reach of current understanding, it is possible to venture several generalizations. For instance, there is a natural, though not inevitable, connection between technology-centered legal intervention and the centralization of choice. Whereas a legal change in the incentives affecting individual decisions tends to disperse decision-making responsibility, specific directives issued to particular technologies represent a more centralized exercise of power. In choosing between more and less centralized approaches, one must have recourse first to highly pragmatic criteria—e.g., (1) whether the relevant technology is too dynamic to make centralized choice truly responsive; (2) whether the relevant information is too inaccessible to central decision makers for directives to be intelligently framed; and (3) whether the need for predictability and uniformity of outcomes grows so great, or the problem of transforming the relevant values into common denominators so intractable, as to make collectively derived rules of thumb preferable to case-by-case analysis. Second, one must also be guided by basic principles—e.g., whether the problem is one for which justice demands uniformity; and whether it is one in which political morality commands participatory and pluralistic rather than centralized administrative choice.

Moreover, there is a natural, though again not inevitable, connection between the regime of incentive modification and the goal of maximizing the aggregate satisfaction of existing individual wants. Although both spending and taxation can be used to alter such wants, the devices of cost and benefit internalization (e.g., imposing effluent fees in terms of the costs thought to be associated with each additional contribution of a pollutant) essentially increase the likelihood that existing wants will be measured in the calculus of choice. Whenever government does not feel bound to honor aggregate individual desires, either for paternalistic reasons (distrusting the capacity of the chooser or the context of the choice) or for evolutionary reasons (feeling determined to shape the development of preferences over time), the internalization of costs or of benefits is an inherently inappropriate technique. For example, a legal system would typically forbid outright certain medical experiments on children, prisoners, or dying patients (rather than simply making the experimenter pay the subject an adequate price for participation) for a blend of reasons: The system may be designed to avoid a world in which poorer experimental subjects can more readily be tempted; there may be reason to mistrust the subjects' capacity for intelligent choice in the circumstances; there

may be a wish to affirm the symbolic proposition that some aspects of life are pearls beyond price; or a desire may exist to prevent the gradual deformation of public consciousness and preference from a posture that attaches great value to life and bodily integrity to a position that regards these as readily interchangeable with other commodities.

A feature common to legal intervention of the first three types (technology-centered, incentive-centered, and value-centered) is that, in order to be workable, each must be targeted with substantial specificity at a relatively narrow range of phenomena. A statutory mandate to halt all genetic experimentation, to pay a tax equal to all the damages done by one's technological activities, or to respect privacy generally would be so sweeping as to represent either a source of total paralysis or, more likely, an exhortation too vague to have much operational significance. When a legal order sets itself the task of making changes so general while avoiding the extremes of both paralysis and abstraction, it must almost invariably proceed by redefining the structures through which decisions are made or the categories in terms of which decisions are expressed —by invoking, in short, the fourth model of legal intervention.

Such restructuring, both institutional and conceptual, cannot be understood either as purely instrumental—a means to some specified end— or as wholly intrinsic—an end in itself and an expression of a point of view. Requiring the filing of bioethical impact statements, for example, both alters the probability that human values will be preserved in experimental settings and represents a commitment to a decision-making process thought to be significant in itself. To alter slightly a familiar allusion, even an experimental subject knows the difference between being kicked and being tripped over, and a community that worries about such subjects is different in kind from one that does not—even in the unlikely event that both finally cause the same unconsented injuries.

The realm of conceptual structuring is not always neatly separable from that of institutional design. Opting in favor of institutional representation for the nonhuman, for example, may contribute to a conception that a mountain or a seashore has intrinsic needs and can make moral demands on our designs, since the very experience of treating places and things with respect may create conceptual possibilities beyond our present capacities. Conversely, society may discover in the articulation of conceptual possibilities and in thinking the formerly unthinkable that new institutional arrangements seem at first plausible and in the end necessary (Stone; Tribe, 1974, pp. 1345, 1346). There is also a major role for legal-technological reconceptualization quite apart from particular institutional embodiments. To illustrate, research involving organ transplantation led to pressures that the concept of "brain death" was in part invented to meet, just as changes in the social role of women generated needs that the concept of "fetal viability" was in part designed to satisfy. Neither concept automatically produced altered norms of behavior; it remained possible to insist that the fact of a mechanically induced heartbeat would render wrong the use of a human body for "spare parts," just as it remained possible to maintain that government may forbid the termination of pregnancy even before the viability of the fetus would permit its protection without involuntary use of anyone's body. Both positions remained possible—but each probably became less likely. The intersection of law and technology, by creating new categories of discourse, altered the reality within which human choice continued to operate, and in terms of which social and governmental decisions continued to be made.

A new reality, it must be stressed, does not merely add options to the old. In every case, it subtracts options as well. To think of a "natural birth" once reproduction has been charged with technological possibility is to invoke an image we are increasingly incapable of experiencing. And once one has perceived and named the choice between "unplugging the machinery" and letting it run on, one cannot easily recreate the world in which no such choice existed—however successfully "natural death" legislation might reflect the desire of some to live without the intervention such a choice represents.

That people may, and indeed must, *choose* what they are to become may once have seemed an abstraction, since such a "choice" was made by a barely visible process of accretion over the course of many generations. But the technological options to which law must visibly address itself today may work changes so rapid and profound that the social capacity to decide whether to embrace them may be as tightly constrained as the need to make such decisions is inescapable. In such circumstances, there can be no escape from a choice between at least two fundamentally different postures toward the techno-

logical order. The first embraces technological imperatives as blessings, reasoning that the dead hand of the past has no legitimate claim to judgment over the unfolding values of the future. The second, even while it may avoid the Luddite extreme of a full-bodied "return to nature," rejects claims of any technological imperative as Faustian temptations, insisting that humanity, as expressed in our law and history and literature, speaks with a voice—albeit muffled and ambiguous—that it is our duty to heed. The essence of the second posture is not opposition to all technology-induced change or the freezing of historically received norms and principles, but the subjection of change to critique and control through a body of principles which, though changing, retains its essential continuity (Tribe, "Technology Assessment").

Laurence H. Tribe and
Kenneth M. Casebeer

[*Directly related are the other articles in this entry, and the entries* Genetics and the Law; Research, Biomedical; Research Policy, Biomedical; *and* Science: Ethical Implications. *For further discussion of topics mentioned in this article, see the entries:* Abortion, *articles on* Contemporary Debate in Philosophical and Religious Ethics *and* Legal Aspects; Death and Dying: Euthanasia and Sustaining Life, *article on* Professional and Public Policies; Environmental Ethics, *articles on* Environmental Health and Human Disease *and* Questions of Social Justice; Human Experimentation; Life-Support Systems; Organ Transplantation, *articles on* Sociocultural Aspects *and* Ethical Principles; Psychosurgery; *and* Reproductive Technologies. *See also:* Law and Morality; *and* Warfare, *article on* Biomedical Science and War.]

BIBLIOGRAPHY

[The following entries illustrate the range of literature considering the general relation of law to technology. To avoid overlap with other articles, few examples of specific legal responses to particular technologies are included, nor are all entries equally recommended.]

Ackerman, Bruce A.; Rose-Ackerman, Susan; Sawyer, James W., Jr.; and Henderson, Dale W. *The Uncertain Search for Environmental Quality.* New York: Free Press, Macmillan Publishing Co., 1974.

Calabresi, Guido. *The Costs of Accidents: A Legal and Economic Analysis.* New Haven: Yale University Press, 1970. An optimistic treatment of structuring market incentives to internalize costs and benefits.

Carroll, James D. "Participatory Technology." *Science* 171 (1971): 647–653.

Ferkiss, Victor. *The Future of Technological Civiliza-*

tion. New York: George Braziller, 1974. An illuminating treatment of the need for social control of technological development.

Harvard University, Program on Technology and Society. *Harvard University Program on Technology and Society: 1964–1972: A Final Review.* Cambridge: 1972. A useful general survey.

JAFFE, LOUIS L. "Law as a System of Control." *Experimentation with Human Subjects.* Edited by Paul Abraham Freund. New York: George Braziller, 1970, pp. 197–217. An excellent general introduction.

JONAS, HANS. *Philosophical Essays: From Ancient Creed to Technological Man.* Englewood Cliffs, N.J.: Prentice-Hall, 1974.

LEDERBERG, JOSHUA. "The Freedoms and the Control of Science: Notes from the Ivory Tower." *Southern California Law Review* 45 (1972): 596–614. Advocating freedom of inquiry and the need to limit control of research accordingly.

MACPHERSON, C. B. "Democratic Theory: Ontology and Technology." *Political Theory and Social Change.* Edited with an introduction by David Spitz. New York: Atherton Press, 1967, pp. 203–220.

National Academy of Sciences. *Technology: Processes of Assessment and Choice.* Washington: Committee on Science and Astronautics, United States House of Representatives. Government Printing Office, 1969. Useful for its comparison of different modes of evaluation and control.

STONE, CHRISTOPHER D. "Should Trees Have Standing? —Toward Legal Rights for Natural Objects." *Southern California Law Review* 45 (1972): 450–501.

"Symposium: Technology Assessment." *George Washington Law Review* 36 (1968): 1033–1149.

"Symposium: The Implications of Science-Technology for the Legal Process." *Denver Law Journal* 47 (1970): 549–552.

TRIBE, LAURENCE H. *Channeling Technology Through Law.* Chicago: Bracton Press, 1973. The standard case-reference book in this field.

———. "Technology Assessment and the Fourth Discontinuity: The Limits of Instrumental Rationality." *Southern California Law Review* 46 (1973): 617–660. A general treatment that examines both law and technology as dependent variables, with examples.

———. "Ways Not to Think about Plastic Trees: New Foundations for Environmental Law." *Yale Law Journal* 83 (1974): 1315–1348. On the relationship between processes of choice and philosophies of value in the technology–environment context. Response to a critical view of this article: "From Environmental Foundation to Constitutional Structures: Learning from Nature's Future." *Yale Law Journal* 84 (1975): 545–556.

III

TECHNOLOGY ASSESSMENT

The concept of technology assessment

Technology assessment is "the systematic study of the effects on society that may occur when a technology is introduced, extended, or modified, with special emphasis on the impacts that are unintended, indirect, and delayed" (Coates, 1971, p. 225). A relatively new concept, the phrase "technology assessment" seems to have been employed for the first time in a 1966 report of a subcommittee of the United States House of Representatives (U.S., Congress, House, Committee on Science and Astronautics, pp. 27–28). By 1969 a scholarly literature on the topic had begun to develop. In 1971 an International Society for Technology Assessment was founded, which began, in turn, to publish a quarterly journal, *Technology Assessment,* in 1972. By the late 1970s an international group of academicians from numerous fields, including physics, engineering, economics, law, and the policy sciences, was devoting substantial attention to the topic of technology assessment.

There is no single universally accepted methodology for performing technology assessments. However, the most detailed programmatic essay on the question of methodology lists seven major steps to be taken in the performance of any comprehensive assessment (The following enumeration is adapted from Jones, p. 26):

1. Define the assessment task: establish the scope of the inquiry.
2. Describe relevant technologies: outline the state of the art in the major technology being assessed as well as in related technologies.
3. Develop state-of-society assumptions: identify and describe the major nontechnological factors influencing the development and application of the relevant technologies.
4. Identify impact areas: list the societal characteristics that will be most influenced by the application of the assessed technology.
5. Prepare preliminary impact analysis: trace and integrate the various specific impacts of the assessed technology upon society.
6. Identify possible action options: develop and analyze various programs for obtaining maximum public benefit from the assessed technologies.
7. Complete impact analysis: analyze the degree to which each action option would alter the specific societal impacts (listed in step 5) of the assessed technology.

In step 1 the assessor decides whether to attempt an assessment of all anticipated social consequences of a technology or whether to perform a more restricted assessment, limited to a specific time period, type of impact, or affected social group. Step 2 describes the current state of the technological art, outlines technological breakthroughs required for further development, surveys related technologies that might contribute to the advancement of the assessed technology, and attempts to project the future state of the art and magnitude of use for the technology.

Step 3 is perhaps the most difficult aspect of any technology assessment. In this step the assessor seeks to paint a reasonably accurate picture of the society of the future, with which the technology of the future will interact. Thus, the assessor must anticipate the values of the future society (Baier and Rescher), as well as its demographic, economic, political, and environmental characteristics. A major shift in a society's value system could, for example, either accelerate or retard the development of a particular technology.

Steps 4 and 5 identify the general and specific impacts that can be anticipated when the assessed technology and the society of the future interact. In the latter step the assessor seeks to determine what social groups will be affected by a technology, how they will be affected, and what the likelihood, timing, magnitude, duration, diffusion, sources, and potential controllability of such effects will be.

In step 6 the society again emerges as an active participant, seeking to develop options that would modify the social impact of the assessed technology and to reduce if not eliminate technological consequences that are judged to be negative. Among these options are changes in the allocation of research and development funds and other financial incentives (including taxes), legislation, executive regulation, judicial action, mass-media publicity, and education. Finally, step 7 revises the projections of step 5 in the light of action options considered in step 6 (Jones).

Technology assessment and the biomedical fields

The earliest efforts to perform systematic technology assessments were concentrated in six major areas: transportation, energy, natural resources, communications, food production, and the environment (Coates, 1975, p. 6; U.S., Congress, House, Commission on Information and Facilities, pp. 108–109). Of these areas, the first four are most closely related to the disciplines of physics and engineering; the last two, food production and the environment, include significant biological components but are not directly related to biomedical technologies.

As major technology assessments were being undertaken in the nonbiomedical fields noted above, a modest literature on technology assessment in the biomedical fields began to develop, particularly in the United States. This literature included the following studies:

1969: a forecast of future developments in the biomedical fields and their potential social impacts (Gordon and Ament)

1971: a survey of numerous biomedical technologies, which employed technology-assessment categories (Kass)

1973: an extensive assessment of the totally implantable artificial heart (U.S., National Heart and Lung Institute)

1975: a detailed assessment of four biomedical technologies: in vitro fertilization, sex preselection, anti-aging techniques, and behavior control (National Research Council)

1976: an overview of nine biomedical candidates for further assessment, for example, polio and rubella vaccines and renal dialysis (U.S., Congress, Office of Technology Assessment)

1977: "a comprehensive study of the ethical, legal, and social implications of advances in biomedical and behavioral research and technology" (U.S., National Commission for the Protection of Human Subjects).

A brief review of two of these studies will serve to illustrate the diversity of approach in assessments of biomedical technology, as well as to indicate some of the conclusions reached in early assessments. In 1972 and 1973 a major biomedical technology assessment was performed by the Artificial Heart Assessment Panel of the National Heart and Lung Institute, National Institutes of Health. The panel—comprising experts in medicine, law, ethics, and the social sciences—examined the state of the art and the potential implications of a future medical device: the totally implantable artificial heart.

In its state-of-the-art review the panel surveyed available data concerning the construction and activation of the artificial heart. If the necessary biomaterials could be developed for the construction of a satisfactory heart, the question of an appropriate power source would remain to be solved. The panel considered two alternative power sources, batteries and nuclear energy; it concluded that, on balance, a battery-powered artificial heart would pose fewer hazards to the recipient, the recipient's family, and the society at large.

The panel considered two major types of implications of the artificial heart: implications for the individual recipient and implications for society. For the individual the panel noted that the recipient's quality of life with an implanted artificial heart would be a primary concern. Use of this novel device might also raise new questions about the definition of death and the prolongation of life. For example, would a refusal to have one's battery-powered heart recharged constitute an act of suicide? The social implications of the artificial heart would be primarily those of high initial cost (perhaps $25,000 per implantation), much of which would probably be borne by public funds; the need for expanded special-care facilities; and the potential spinoff effects of this device for general improvements in the care of cardiac patients.

In addition to considering the state of the art and the implications of the artificial heart for the individual and society, the panel explored two ethical issues that cannot readily be related to the seven-step technology assessment methodology outlined above: issues in research and early clinical trials with the artificial heart and issues in the allocation of this rather expensive new device. The allocation question, in turn, raised issues of macroallocation (the fraction of society's resources to be devoted to the artificial heart) and microallocation (the appropriate mechanism for the selection of recipients). Perhaps the panel's discussion of these ethical issues can most appropriately be considered an exercise in identifying possible action options (step 6)—in this case action options that would avoid the potential impact of injustice in the production and distribution of the artificial heart (U.S., National Heart and Lung Institute).

In 1973 an ad hoc interdisciplinary committee of the National Research Council—the Committee on the Life Sciences and Social Policy—compiled a detailed assessment of four biomedical technologies or powers: "in vitro fertilization and related technologies," "choosing the sex of children," the "retardation of aging," and "modifying human behavior" (National Research Council, p. vii). The committee's study, published in 1975, was entitled *Assessing Biomedical Technologies: An Inquiry into the Nature of the Process* (ibid.).

In its detailed discussion of the four biomedical case studies, the committee applied the following categories of analysis to each technology: stage of development, scale of use, relation to other technologies, ease of monitoring and control, reversability, nature and scope of social consequences, and implications for decision making. These categories roughly parallel the seven-step methodology outlined in the preceding section. However, relatively little attention was paid to step 3 (developing state-of-society assumptions); step 6 (the development of action options) received heavy emphasis in the committee's concern for monitoring and control, reversibility, and decision making at various levels.

The report's treatment of in vitro fertilization and related technologies illustrates its method of assessing biomedical technologies. After surveying the current state of the reproductive art and the likely scale of its use by society, the committee presented several scenarios which depict potential future developments. Embryo transfer could be accomplished in three ways, according to the report: (1) An embryo derived from the fertilization of the wife's ovum by the husband's sperm could be transplanted into the wife's uterus for gestation and delivery; (2) an ovum donor could provide the ovum to be fertilized by the husband's sperm, and the resulting embryo could then be transferred to the wife; or (3) a third female party could provide the "surrogate womb" in which the genetic offspring of the husband and wife would be developed. In the laboratory, products of in vitro fertilization could be employed at an early stage for research on the causes of congenital defects or at a later stage for research on the feasibility of extrauterine gestation.

The committee briefly considered the likely effect of these potential developments on the practice of medicine, societal attitudes toward sex and reproduction, and the potential offspring of the new techniques. In discussing the implications of in vitro fertilization for decision making, the committee questioned whether patients and medical professionals, acting privately, are the appropriate persons to introduce such potentially far-reaching innovations. Accordingly, the committee recommended that consideration be given to vesting decision-making authority in various other groups, for example, medico-scientific review bodies, interdisciplinary public committees, legislators, the courts (through the appointment of guardians for the unborn child), or the public at large through participation in open forums.

The introduction to the committee's report indicates that, in addition to considering the question of technology's consequences, the committee also wished to address broader, more philosophical questions about biomedical technologies (National Research Council, p. 3):

What ends should these new technologies serve? What ideas about the nature of human beings and about the good for them underlie these technological efforts? What values should govern public and private choices? Do the scientific conceptions of nature and of human beings provide an adequate basis for deciding what ought to be done with the new technologies? If they do not, what alternative or additional views could be invoked to serve this purpose?

None of the seven steps in the technology assessment method seems to address these questions. Indeed, as the committee's report conceded, the committee itself was not able to pursue these questions in its assessment of four biomedical technologies.

An appraisal of technology assessment

The technology-assessment methodology outlined in the first section of this article includes both descriptive (or predictive) and prescriptive (or evaluative) components. Insofar as the assessor of technology is able to avoid bias in perception and explication, he or she can carry through the initial three steps of an assessment without resort to evaluative judgments. However, if in steps 4 and 5 the assessor goes beyond an enumeration of consequences to a discussion of "risks," "benefits," or "positive and negative consequences," he or she has ceased to be purely descriptive (Lowrance, pp. 75–79). Even if evaluation can be avoided in steps 4 and 5, step 6 (the identification of possible action options) almost inevitably involves the making of value judgments, for the assessor seeks to discover alternatives that will maximize the benefits and minimize the harms produced by the technology.

The value-laden character of technology assessment suggests, in turn, a further question: What is the relationship of technology assessment to traditional value-oriented fields, like law and ethics? Insofar as law is process- rather than outcome-oriented, it approaches decision making in a way that differs radically from the method of technology assessment. Indeed, Laurence Tribe, a constitutional lawyer, has argued

that technology assessment, in its emphasis on outcomes and impacts, tends to minimize "soft" (that is, nonquantifiable) variables. In Tribe's view technology assessment, unless complemented by other methods of evaluation, may become an exercise in "instrumental rationality" (Tribe).

Ethically, it seems clear that the intellectual roots of technology assessment—as of the social and policy sciences general—are firmly grounded in the utilitarian tradition of ethics (Walters, pp. 679–680). Thus, it focuses primary attention on the consequences or effects of human action rather than on the virtues of moral agents (as in virtue theories of ethics) or on an action's accordance with a moral rule (as in deontological theories). However, the value theory of technology assessment, unlike Bentham's simple pleasure-pain calculus, seems highly sophisticated, taking into account a complex variety of economic, demographic, political, environmental, and other consequences.

As a method closely akin to the utilitarian mode of ethical reasoning, technology assessment is subject to some of the standard objections that nonutilitarians have raised against utilitarianism. Can various types of consequences—for example, economic and environmental consequences—be compared, or are they incommensurable? If various types of consequences are compared, what factor or consideration will serve as the common denominator? Finally, if multiple individuals reach different conclusions concerning the balance of harms and benefits, can their divergent assessments be harmonized into a single collective judgment?

The foregoing comments are intended to characterize the method of technology assessment and to identify some of the potential limits of the method. It remains to acknowledge the past achievements and future promise of technology assessment. Perhaps the most important contribution of technology assessment has been to broaden and lengthen the perspective from which technological developments are viewed. Unlike traditional cost-benefit analyses, which have tended to focus on the immediate economic or institutional consequences of a technology for those developing it, technology assessment requires the consideration of a broad range of effects on numerous social groups in the near and distant future. Thus, technology assessment provides an alternative to the fatalistic view that whatever can be done will be done and to an uncritical technological optimism which asserts that whatever can be done should be done. In sum, technology assessment constitutes a highly useful and important approach to the evaluation of present and future biomedical technologies.

LeRoy Walters

[*Directly related are the other articles in this entry:* PHILOSOPHY OF TECHNOLOGY *and* TECHNOLOGY AND THE LAW. *Other relevant material may be found under* ETHICS, *articles on* DEONTOLOGICAL THEORIES, TELEOLOGICAL THEORIES, *and* UTILITARIANISM; *and* SCIENCE: ETHICAL IMPLICATIONS.]

BIBLIOGRAPHY

BAIER, KURT, and RESCHER, NICHOLAS, eds. *Values and the Future: The Impact of Technological Change on American Values.* New York: Free Press, 1969.

BROOKS, HARVEY, and BOWERS, RAYMOND. "The Assessment of Technology." *Scientific American* 222, no. 2 (1970), pp. 13–21.

COATES, JOSEPH F. "Technology Assessment and Public Wisdom." *Journal of the Washington Academy of Sciences* 65 (1975): 3–12.

——. "Technology Assessment: The Benefits . . . the Costs . . . the Consequences." *Futurist* 5 (1971): 225–231.

GORDON, THEODORE J., and AMENT, ROBERT H. *Forecasts of Some Technological Developments and Their Societal Consequences.* IFF report, no. R–6. Middletown, Conn.: Institute for the Future, 1969.

HETMAN, FRANÇOIS. *Society and the Assessment of Technology: Premises, Conceptions, Methodology, Experiments, Areas of Application.* Paris: Organization for Economic Co-operation and Development, 1973.

JONES, MARTIN V. *A Technology Assessment Methodology.* 7 vols. Vol. 1: *Some Basic Propositions.* MTR 6009. Washington: MITRE Corporation, Washington Operations, 1971.

JONSEN, ALBERT R. "The Totally Implantable Artificial Heart." *Hastings Center Report* 3, no. 5 (1973) pp. 1–4.

KASS, LEON R. "The New Biology: What Price Relieving Man's Estate?" *Science* 174 (1971): 779–788.

LOWRANCE, WILLIAM W. *Of Acceptable Risk: Science and the Determination of Safety.* Los Altos, Calif.: William Kaufman, 1976.

National Academy of Sciences, Panel on Technology Assessment. *Technology: Processes of Assessment and Choice: Report of the National Academy of Sciences.* Report to the Committee on Science and Astronautics, U.S. House of Representatives, July 1969. Washington: Government Printing Office, 1969. Committee Print.

National Research Council. Committee on the Life Sciences and Social Policy. *Assessing Biomedical Technologies: An Inquiry into the Nature of the Process.* Washington: National Academy of Sciences, 1975.

TRIBE, LAURENCE H. "Technology Assessment and the Fourth Discontinuity: The Limits of Instrumental Rationality." *Southern California Law Review* 46 (1973): 617–660.

United States, Congress, House, Commission on Information and Facilities. *The Office of Technology Assessment: A Study of Its Organizational Effectiveness.* House Document, no. 94–538. Washington: Government Printing Office, 1976.

——; Congress; House; Committee on Science and Astronautics; Subcommittee on Science, Research, and Development. *Inquiries, Legislation, Policy Studies Re: Science and Technology, Review and Forecast, 2d Progress Report.* 89th Cong., 2d sess., 1966. Washington: Government Printing Office, 1966. Committee Print.

——, Congress, Office of Technology Assessment. *Development of Medical Technology: Opportunities for Assessment.* Washington: Government Printing Office, 1976.

——, National Commission for the Protection of Human Subjects. *A Comprehensive Study of the Ethical, Legal and Social Implications of Advances in Biomedical and Behavioral Research and Technology.* A report prepared by the New Jersey Institute of Technology and Policy Research. Bethesda, Md.: 1977. Available through National Technical Information Service.

——, National Heart and Lung Institute. *The Totally Implantable Artificial Heart: Economic, Ethical, Legal, Medical, Psychiatric and Social Implications.* Report by the Artificial Heart Assessment Panel. DHEW Publication, no. (NIH) 74–191. Bethesda, Md.: National Institutes of Health, 1973.

WALTERS, LEROY. "Technology Assessment and Genetics." *Theological Studies* 33 (1972): 666–683.

TELEOLOGICAL ETHICS
See ETHICS, *article on* TELEOLOGICAL THEORIES.

TEST TUBE FERTILIZATION
See REPRODUCTIVE TECHNOLOGIES, *articles on* IN VITRO FERTILIZATION, ETHICAL ISSUES, *and* LEGAL ASPECTS.

THEOLOGICAL ETHICS
See ETHICS, *article on* THEOLOGICAL ETHICS.

THERAPEUTIC RELATIONSHIP

I. HISTORY OF THE RELATIONSHIP
Pedro Laín Entralgo

II. SOCIOHISTORICAL PERSPECTIVES
Samuel W. Bloom

III. CONTEMPORARY SOCIOLOGICAL ANALYSIS
David Mechanic

IV. CONTEMPORARY MEDICAL PERSPECTIVE
Eric J. Cassell

I
HISTORY OF THE RELATIONSHIP

We give the name "therapeutic relationship" to the link established between an individual (the patient) and another individual or group (the healers), with the aim of curing or relieving the disease suffered by the former. Our problem is to describe as exactly as possible the various forms this relationship has assumed throughout history.

The empirico-magical stage

Ever since records have existed concerning the treatment of the sick, we may distinguish the following four chief forms: (1) the spontaneous or instinctive, (2) the empirical, (3) the magico-religious and (4) the scientific. In all periods of history, all of these forms have had their practitioners. The mother who holds her feverish child on her lap, embracing him to protect him from the cold air, illustrates the first form, *spontaneous* or *instinctive* help. The second form, *empirical* help, consists in using a remedy merely because it has provided some relief in similar cases, that is to say, without asking oneself why the remedy has those particular healing qualities. Medicine owes some very important discoveries simply to therapeutic empiricism. The treatment of wounds from firearms, discovered by chance by Ambrosio Paré (c. 1510–1590), the introduction of quinine into the Western world, and Jenner's vaccination against smallpox are three superb examples. Generically speaking, in *magico-religious* treatment both healer and patient believe that the cure is due to the action of "supernatural" or "divine" powers available for the purpose. In some cases the curative effectiveness of these powers would depend on "who" uses them (medicine man, shaman, witch doctor, etc.), in others on "how" they are applied (magic ritual), and in others again upon "where" the cure takes place (in localities "singled out" or "favored" for their healing powers—some shrine, island, or spring).

Since scientific treatment in the strict sense began in Greece in the fifth century B.C., we can definitely state that from the origin of the human race and for 2,500 years the therapeutic relationship was empirico-magical in character, with either the "empirical" or the "magical" element of the healing process more or less dominant, according to circumstances. It is known that in the most highly developed pre-Hellenic cultures of ancient Egypt, China, and India, a form of medicine existed in which strictly "magical" or magico-religious elements were minor compared to the empirical and theoretical. However, a careful study of these three methods of understanding and practicing the care of the sick would reveal to some extent attitudes of the doctor that can only be called "magical" and that, above all, show a lack of intellectual and methodical principles capable of correcting these attitudes and initiating a way toward purely "scientific" medicine. That explains why, in spite of their respective merits, ancient Egypt, China, and India have reached nothing but dead ends in the world's development of medicine.

The ancient scientific stage

As Aristotle taught, treatment of the sick is scientific ("technical") in the strictest sense when it depends on the knowledge of "why" it is being done, "what" is being done, and by what means it takes effect (in other words, "what" is the disease, "what" remedy is being used, and by "what" therapeutic procedure it is administered). Thus the healer's ability to cure does not depend on the agent who applies the remedy, nor on the ceremony accompanying its application, nor on the privileged place where the cure takes place, i.e., not on a magical "who," "how," or "where," but on a series of "whats" concerning the illness and its remedy.

Taking as their starting point the most important cosmological idea of the pre-Socratic philosophers—the idea of *physis* or "nature"—the group of physicians, the Aesclepiades, known as "Hippocratics," originated the technical concept of illness a whole century before Aristotle had formulated the conceptual definitions just mentioned. Consequently, a doctor would try to cure his patient, or alleviate his pain, in the rational or scientifically definitive knowledge of the "nature" of man, of illness in general, of the special disease he was treating, and of the remedy being used—while at the same time having the knowledge and skill to perform everything required by the treatment. I do not mean to say that Hippocratic medicine—apart from its inevitable deficiencies—was free from some serious errors and superstitious practices; but I am affirming that it already contained various principles: the notion of *physis* as the basis of all technical knowledge, the concept of medicine as *téchne iatriké*, the idea of a method of knowing whose first rule is the attentive sensory examination of the patient's body—as a result of which defects and errors would be gradually corrected.

From Hippocrates to Galen (A.D. 130?–200?), that is to say while the ancient view of technical medicine remained in force, the therapeutic relationship can be described under the following heads:

Basis of the therapeutic relationship. Ideally considered, this basis is *philanthropia,* or the "love of man," because, according to a famous saying, "where there is love of man, *philanthropia,* there is love of the art (of healing) *philotechnia*" (Hippocrates, *Praec.* L, IX, 258). Of course, this saying belongs to a later, post-Stoic period; but the study of much earlier medical texts, such as the *Epidemias,* gives grounds for the belief that the "Hippocratics," as they were called, practiced *philanthropia* before the word was invented. In any case, the "love of man" of ancient Greece was the same as "love of nature," of the divine *physis,* as is specifically and individually realized in the name given to the subject in question: *physiophilia.* It is not necessary to add that other less noble interests, such as love of money and thirst for fame, in practice often obscured this ethical and technical ideal of "physiological philanthropy" as the basis of the therapeutic relationship.

Diagnostic aspect of the relationship. As scientific and effective "knowledge" was the first premise of the technical concept of medicine, the therapeutic relationship required—as it has of doctors since—that the Greek physician should reach a diagnosis by rational means. During the period in the history of medicine here called "ancient scientific," this diagnostic activity appears to have consisted of (1) a fourfold desire to discover whether the illness is determined by an insuperable and necessary cause (*kat'ananken*) or by some controllable contingency (*katà tychen*); to identify the typical form (*tropos, eidos*) of the suffering; to determine its causes, both remote and immediate (*aitia, prophasis*); and to establish a well-founded prognosis; (2) a series of exploratory maneuvers (*anamnesis,* study of the surroundings, examination of the patient's body by means of sight, touch, hearing, smell, and taste); and (3) adequate inductive reasoning (*logismos*).

Curative aspect of the relationship. After some deliberation, the therapeutic activity of the Greek doctor was subjected to the following rules: (1) to help the patient, or at least do him no harm (Hippocrates, *Epid.* I, L. 11, 634); (2) to refrain from interfering if the illness were incurable and

inevitably mortal, because in that case the doctor, by intervening, would commit the sin of *hybris,* or rebellion against an edict of the divine and sovereign *physis;* and (3) insofar as possible, to attack the cause of the disease therapeutically. Diet, drugs, surgery, and to a lesser degree "psychotherapy" were the four great healing methods of ancient medicine.

Ethical and social aspects of the therapeutic relationship. One must avoid the common error of seeing the Oath contained in the *Corpus Hippocraticum* as the ethical code of Greek medicine; in all probability it was not in force outside the Pythagorean order (Edelstein). However, it is possible to trace the outline of the medical ethics and social medicine of the ancient Greeks. Its structure was as follows: (1) the doctor's duties to his patient: to help or not to harm, to abstain from the impossible, to adjust his fees to the patient's income. (2) Duties toward other doctors: The ideal principle of regarding his colleague as a brother (Hippocrates, *Praec.* 4, IX, 258) was very frequently infringed by the competitiveness of which doctors of antiquity are so often accused (Edelstein). (3) Duties toward himself: A doctor should take care of his personal appearance and behave in a manner that would be called "beautiful and good" (Hippocrates, *Med.* L, IX, 204). To serve nature through his skill (Hippocrates, *Epid.* I, L. 11, 636) should be his paramount principle; (4) Duties to society: Though clearly stated by Plato (*Republic, Laws*), these are given much less importance in strictly medical writings; in any case (Plato, the Hippocratic treatise *On diet*), it is certain that there was "medicine for the rich" and "medicine for the poor" in the ancient world.

Christianity and the therapeutic relationship

The propagation of Christianity was not motivated by the need to reform the conduct of doctor to patient, insofar as this conduct could be held as technical, but because the medical technique prevailing at the time had been created by pagans. Because the Christian concept of love was relatively new, Christ's religious message influenced both the problem and the form taken by the therapeutic relationship in various ways.

Could the pagan medical technique have been accepted without more ado by Christians? Out of excessively vehement opposition to paganism, some of them—Tatian the Assyrian and Tertullian, for instance—gave a negative answer to this question. But the good sense of others prevailed in the end; and thus, from the fourth century to the increasingly strong anti-Galenism of the sixteenth and seventeenth centuries, the medicine of Christian peoples—such as Byzantium and medieval Europe—showed a progressive intellectual effort to relate the art of healing, inherited from ancient Greece and culminating in the work of Galen, to the Christian world view.

One can note the novelty of the Christian concept of love and its decisive effect on the form taken by the therapeutic relationship. When this was the direct, pure expression of the evangelical message—in other words, before the time when Constantine's edict led to the primitive Christian communities' becoming involved with the civil power—the following were the chief features of its structure:

Ideal basis of the therapeutic relationship. We are no longer facing love of *physis* or universal "nature," as individualized in the sick man, but confronting his unique "persona" as a "neighbor" (parable of the good Samaritan). Moreover, in helping an ailing neighbor, one is helping Christ (Matt. 25:39–40).

The therapeutic relationship as help. Herein lie the most significant new developments in primitive or pre-Constantinian Christianity. (1) In the assistance given to the sick man there should be no "natural limits," thus putting an end to the Hellenic imperative to refrain from therapy in cases of "necessarily" mortal or incurable disease. Here, although there is no place for therapeutic technique, the patient can always be helped by spiritual advice. (2) The egalitarian nature of treatment: No difference should be made between Greeks and barbarians, free men and slaves, friends and enemies. (3) The necessity of giving free help: Within a community governed by the principle that possessions are shared (see the texts of the Acts of the Apostles), the basic motive of help for the sick was charity, not only on the part of the doctor but also on the part of other people (widows acting as nurses, later on "deaconesses"). The Greek doctor would give free treatment in exchange for some favor received or to acquire prestige in his town (Hippocrates, *Praec.* L. IX, 258); the Christian doctor should give his help free on principle. (4) Such practices of the Christian religion as prayer and extreme unction were incorporated into the care of the sick.

The medieval scientific stage

After Constantine's Edict of Milan (A.D. 312), the links between Christianity and the civil power became increasingly strong, and this gave rise to public awareness that the Christian life, such as was led outside the new conventual communities, was losing at least some of its original purity. This is shown by a brief examination of the two main politico-social forms of Christianity, during the historical period that we call the Middle Ages, in the Byzantine Empire and Medieval Europe. Exigencies of space allow no more than a mention of the third great cultural ambit of the Middle Ages: the world of Islam.

Therapeutic relationship in Byzantium. The theocratic fusion between the Christian religion and civil power has never been stronger than in the Byzantine Empire; never has religious error or heresy been more methodically and sternly treated as "political crime." From this are derived the two main characteristics of the therapeutic relationship in Byzantine society: its doctrinal basis and its importance as help. The doctrinal basis of the therapeutic relationship in the Byzantine world was essentially the result of a juxtaposition that never turned out well. On the ethical plane, Byzantine medicine went on accepting and proclaiming the Christian concept of helping the sick; on the technical plane it accepted in principle everything described by the Greeks as "practical," and refused to acknowledge (as pagan and evil) the basic "theoretic" concepts of Hippocratic-Galenic medicine—for example, the notion of *physis* as "divine" and the denial or negation of a personal, spiritual God, creator of the world and transcending it. The doctors of Byzantium did not succeed in connecting the dogmas of their Christian faith with the scientific and philosophic basis of Hellenic *téchne iatriké*.

The most important contribution made by Byzantine Christianity to medical care was the creation of hospitals to treat poor invalids; among them was the famous "hospital city" of Caesarea, founded about the year 370. (Earlier institutions did not strictly deserve the name of "hospitals.") In those institutions there were specialists, male and female nurses, surgeons, assistant doctors (*parabalani*), and servants. Charity was the ruling principle in their activity; but that did not prevent the distinction between "medicine for the rich" and "medicine for the poor" from being clearly observed in Byzantium. And finally, we must mention the magical and pseudoreligious cures, which particularly attracted poorer patients.

The therapeutic relationship in medieval Europe. The historical period we call the Middle Ages covers the millennium between the invasion of

Rome by the Germanic races and the conquest of Constantinople by the Turks in 1453, and is far from uniform in character—suffice it to compare the life surrounding a feudal castle in the ninth century with that of a Flemish or Italian town in the fifteenth. It is shown also by the gradual changes in the therapeutic relationship throughout this period.

Doctrinal basis of the therapeutic relationship. Two chief aspects must be distinguished—the technical and the ethical. Until the School of Salerno became famous (in the eleventh and twelfth centuries) and the later scholastic medicine of the thirteenth to fifteenth centuries was flourishing, medieval medicine hardly deserves the term "technical" or scientific in the strict sense. Mainly practiced by monks ("monastic medicine") either inside or outside monasteries, it was based solely on a certain amount of experience and the extremely scanty remains of ancient learning that had survived the destruction of the Roman Empire.

There was a marked change with the beginning of the twelfth century: Secular doctors with professional degrees became more common; from the time of Roger of Sicily in 1140 Graeco-Arab learning began to spread from Salerno, or from Toledo, and became truly "technical" medicine, an authentic *ars medica*. By means of the intellectual resources provided by the theology and philosophy of the period, the scholastic European doctors of the thirteenth and fourteenth centuries achieved something not attained by Byzantine medicine; they systematically adapted Hippocratic and Galenic thought to the needs of the Christian faith.

From the ethical point of view, medieval medicine continued to base itself ideally on the Christian concept of aid for the needy and sick—ideally because in practice the pressure of economic interest was not uncommon, nor, sometimes, free from corruption.

Diagnostic aspect of the therapeutic relationship. Though it had become impoverished and schematized in comparison with that of ancient Greece, the diagnostic relationship between doctor and patient—examination and establishment of "genus" and "species" of the affliction observed—remained much the same. Two techniques gained prominence and were gradually perfected: examination of the urine (*uroscopia*) and taking of the pulse. There were also two doctrinal guidelines to help the doctor pass from clinical experience to reasoning, treatises that systematically described the different species of disease (*de passionibus, de affectionibus*) and the didactic descriptions of individual cases of disease (*consilia*).

Curative aspect of the therapeutic relationship. From a technical standpoint the Middle Ages added little that was new to the treatment of the sick as taught by Greek and Arab doctors. Diet, the use of drugs, surgery, and "psychotherapy"—with a Christian orientation—remained the principal methods of treatment. As to theory, the chief concept of Galenic therapy, the "symptom" (*endeixis*), became latinized and scholasticized under the name of *insinuatio agendi*. On the other hand, the problem arose of how to harmonize "technical" requirements derived from the Galenic concept of symptoms with the "moral" rules imposed by the Christian idea of man: the bond between *ars* and *caritas*. However, medieval physicians did not succeed in solving this delicate human problem coherently or systematically.

Ethical and social aspects of the therapeutic relationship. As to principles and ideals, medieval medical ethics are as faithfully Christian as the society to which they belong; but individual and social realization of this sincere Christianity was very different from that prevailing in pre-Constantine communities. Various reasons contribute to this: (1) the avarice of many clerical and secular doctors: "Doctor, do not be afraid of asking good fees from the rich," writes Lanfranc in the thirteenth century; (2) the growing interference of the civil power in regulating doctors' duties by means of ordinances—not only relating to the healer's technical behavior, but also sometimes to his religious conduct—infringement of which was punished; (3) the frequent critico-burlesque attitude of society toward the doctor's greed for gain or lack of skill (John of Salisbury's *Metalogicus* and Petrarch's *Invectivae*); and (4) the marked difference between "medicine for the rich" and "medicine for the poor"—in monasteries, the distance separating the *infirmarium* from the *hospitale pauperum*; in cities the even greater gap between the treatment of those in power—politicians or churchmen, nearly all of whom had their own private doctors—and the almost purely religious treatment given to the unfortunates in hospital beds. Not everything in the Christian Middle Ages was in fact Christian.

Modern scientific stage: Christian modernity

It is a platitude to say that the "modern world" began with the Renaissance or even in the fifteenth century. However, a thorough study of the various characteristics of this modernity—

greater knowledge of classical antiquity, importance of worldly matters, new conceptions of science, rationalization of life, awareness of historical progress—clearly shows the roots of all these developments to be already present in the transition from the thirteenth to the fourteenth century, when the voluntarism and nominalism of Franciscan thought (e.g., William of Occam, 1285?–1349?) began to influence European culture. When man's freedom (and hence his creative ability) was seen as his chief similarity to God, the idea of "natural" and "necessary" limitations to man's scientific and technical capacity with regard to the cosmos disappeared in principle, and the human mind began to entertain the idea of "indefinite progress." Science and modern techniques took their first steps, in the belief that knowledge of the sensible world consisted in creating abstract symbols—they would soon be called mathematical symbols—by means of which the external world could be understood and dominated. Many years had to pass, however, for these germinal concepts to be converted into strong, widespread social customs. Only in the secularized society of the eighteenth through the twentieth century would a great tree have grown from the tiny seed of the fourteenth century.

Two periods must be distinguished in the history of the modern Euro-American world: in the first, from the fifteenth to the second half of the eighteenth century, by far the largest proportion of society were still nominally Christians, although the form of their religion, whether Catholic or Protestant, was growing away from that of the Middle Ages; in the second, the nineteenth and twentieth centuries, society was becoming secularized.

Basis of the therapeutic relationship.   Whether Catholic or Protestant, the modern Christian doctor still saw the injunction to give charitable help to those in need as the basic ideal of his healing activity: He thought of Paracelsus, he remembered the ritual oath taken by newly graduated French doctors in front of the altar of Nôtre Dame. But the diversity of religions in Europe and America, and the growing esteem both for the reality of worldly values and for increasing civil power led to two new features in this ideal: (1) greater respect for the personal religious life of the patient; and (2) an increasing and sharper separation between the spiritual and material worlds, the latter being known and governed by the beginnings of modern science and the technology founded upon it. Two examples of this spiritual–material separation will

suffice: Boerhaave's teaching of the distinction between the mind and the body (*De distinctione mentis a corpore*) and Hoffmann's significant anthropological contrast between the physical (*cor corporale*) and the spiritual (*cor spirituale*).

Diagnostic aspect of the therapeutic relationship. The principle of understanding nature in order to master it (Francis Bacon, Descartes) gained strength in modern society and led to the physician's concern to make diagnoses that were objectively correct. Very briefly, the following are the chief characteristics of the diagnostic aspect of the therapeutic relationship during this period. (1) Understanding of the disease being treated became more individualized, as was very clear in the form taken by case histories, i.e., Montanus, Boerhaave, etc. (2) Numerical measurement gradually began to figure in examinations, leading to the first use of instruments such as watches and thermometers. (3) Diagnosis was increasingly used to guess at the existence of an anatomic lesion, which could be proved by an autopsy, i.e., Lancini and Albertini, Boerhaave, Morgagni. (4) A more lively and objective interest was evinced in the influence of the social environment on the disease, i.e., Paracelsus, Ramazzini, Johann Peter Frank.

Curative aspect of the relationship.   The spread and strength of the modern scientific mentality required a doctor who wished to keep up with his times to validate by experimentation the efficacy of the remedies he used. On the other hand, awareness of man's power over natural phenomena demanded a constant increase in the number and curative scope of those remedies. Paracelsus thought that every natural substance could be an efficacious medicament, if only convenient means of using it could be discovered; God had disposed the world thus, when he created it, and this the inquiring and inventive intelligence of the doctor should be able to make plain. Consequently, the doctor no longer saw himself as a "servant of nature by means of his skill," as in ancient Greece, but also during the Middle Ages in a Christian interpretation of the words as the true "collaborator of God." Whether Paracelsists or not, the most eminent doctors of the fifteenth to eighteenth centuries made use more or less consciously of this concept of therapeutic activity. But at the same time there was increasing distrust of the healing qualities assumed to belong to many of the remedies traditional practice had recommended.

The main therapeutic methods were still the four employed in Hippocratic medicine: diet (adapted to new ways of life), cure by drugs (enriched by various new medicines), surgery (whose technique had advanced considerably, from Paré to Cheselden, Pott, and Hunter), and, on a distinctly lower plane, psychotherapy, whose later triumph would be unconsciously heralded by Mesmer at the end of the eighteenth century. The separation of healers into "doctors" (or "physicians") and "surgeons" was daily becoming more clear.

Ethical and social aspects of the relationship. Since both doctor and patient were Christians, it was natural for the former to find his ethical principles in those of the Christian life; but at the same time, since the creation and rational order of the world had become more important in men's eyes, it was also natural for the form in which these principles were individually and socially realized to change to some extent. There should have been, and indeed there was, a relationship between religion and medicine that was both theoretical and practical. As religion was concerned with the life of the spirit and medicine with the life of the body (or what human knowledge tells us about the cosmos), the scientist and the physician did their best to discover and establish points of direct communication between those two worlds. In regard to theory, such communication was guaranteed by the "harmony" between Holy Writ and science, as for example, in Valles's *Sacra philosophia* (sixteenth century) and Hoffmann's *Dissertatio theologico-medica* (eighteenth century). Naturally, such communication and the bridge establishing it had to take a different form on the practical level. There the communication gave rise to "medical deontology," a collection of ethical precepts that were to be respected in the healer's technical activity. Examples of both early and mature forms of them are to be found in certain parts of the *Quaestiones medico-legales* of Zacchia (1621–1635) and the *Embriologia sacra* of Cangiamilla (1758).

Between the fifteenth and the seventeenth centuries, and therefore during the ancien régime, the bourgeois structure of society in Europe and America was being developed, and three distinct strata began to emerge: the "upper classes" (aristocrats, magnates of Church and state, rich merchants), the "middle classes" (artisans, officials, and members of various professions), and the "lower classes" (laborers, the poor). Parallel strata could be observed in medical care. Ill persons of the upper classes were looked after in their luxurious homes and had a monopoly on more expensive treatments (one need only think

of the distribution of quinine in the seventeenth century). The lower classes still went to hospitals for the poor, although during the eighteenth century those were altered or completely rebuilt on a larger scale. But the care of the sick inside those hospitals was far from acceptable (as to dirt, parasites, smell), as can be seen from denunciations by some socially and philanthropically sensitive doctors, like Tenon in 1788 and Howard in 1789. Nor was the medical care of the middle classes entirely satisfactory.

Modern scientific stage: secularized modernity

The process of secularizing society advanced at progressive speed during the nineteenth and twentieth centuries. Certainly there were still many Christians in the cities of Europe and America, but their individual and social style of living, their habits, were affected by this secularization; and it was in the eighteenth century that distinct groups came to be known as "intellectuals" and "aristocrats," and later (from the second half of the nineteenth century), a class came to be known as "proletarian."

Combined with this increasing secularization of behavior, we find that in the nineteenth century life was becoming more technical, and in consequence of the industrial revolution an urban proletariat made its appearance. Submissive at first, the proletariat afterward organized itself as the "workers' movement" and asserted its rights more effectively, so that in one way or another it has decisively contributed to shaping the social scene of our own century. How was the therapeutic relationship to be interpreted in this secularized world, part bourgeois, part proletarian?

Doctrinal basis of the relationship. As had been the case ever since Hippocratic medicine, this basis had two essential aspects, one ethical, the other scientific or technical. (1) From an ethical standpoint, the ideal motive of medical care of the sick was "philanthropy," the feelings and the rules of conduct in which Christian charity were secularized. But modern philanthropy was radically different from the Hippocratic form (which had as its ultimate goal the divine *physis*, or universal nature), in that it was concerned with the "individual persona" of the patient—although the doctor's theory of man might not be formally "personalist." During the nineteenth and twentieth centuries many doctors have been "naturalist" in theory (in their scientific concept of man's nature) and "personalist" in practice (in their therapeutic relation with the patient). Not until

Marxist socialism did there appear a philanthropy based on the notions of "social or civil nature" and "state of nature." (2) From a scientific point of view, the ideal basis of medical care was the concept of medicine as the application of pure natural science. "Medicine should be natural science—in other words, what the second half of the nineteenth century understood as natural science—or it will be nothing" was the oracular saying of Helmholtz. The sick man was *scientifically* considered as a fragment of the cosmos, acted on by biological evolution and governed by the laws of physics and chemistry. Scientifically, because in practice nearly all doctors obeyed the rule of Bérard and Gluber, *Guérir parfois, soulager souvent, consoler toujours* (heal sometimes, relieve often, always console). This does not of course preclude the usual corruption of the medical profession—desire for gain, thirst for social prestige—often contaminating that philanthropic and scientific ideal.

Diagnostic aspect of the relationship. The diagnostic relationship with the patient now conformed to the following principles: (1) The patient was seen, above all, as an individual, capable of being rationally understood. (2) This understanding was increased by means of the instrumental aids to clinical examination (stethoscope, sphygmograph, ophthalmoscope, chemical analysis, X-rays, etc.). (3) The disease was scientifically understood by applying rules that were anatamoclinical (diagnosis of anatomical lesions), physiopathological (diagnosis of disorders typical of the functional and material processes of life), or etiopathological (diagnosis of external causes, microbes, poison, etc., of the diseased process); or the doctor could try to coordinate these three approaches. (4) Neurosis, whose frequency increased from the second half of the nineteenth century as a result of industrial civilization, was understood by natural scientific medicine by reference to anatomoclinical (Charcot) or physiopathological rules (German practice since Frerichs and Traube). (5) To sum up, the diagnosis was, or tried to be *at the same time* natural-scientific and individualist.

Curative aspect of the relationship. When medicine was considered as applied natural science, the doctor's powers of healing (by experimental pharmacology, surgery enhanced by the development of anesthesia and antisepsis, synthesis of new drugs, serum therapy, vaccination, etc.) were progressively and wonderfully increased. Moreover, giving broad social expression to that which was merely a slight and theoretical germ

at the end of the thirteenth century and the beginning of the fourteenth, the doctor finally freed himself from the Hellenic concept of "natural force" (*ananke physeos*) and began to think of man as not being, in principle, subject to diseases that were mortal or incurable "of necessity." What could not be cured today might well be curable tomorrow. In fact, the doctor ceased being "the servant of nature by means of his skill" and became instead her "guardian, master, and sculptor."

Alongside dietetics, now scientifically regulated, increasingly rich therapy by drugs, and increasingly effective surgery, the psychotherapeutic element in treatment was acquiring more importance through several different methods and interpretations. In the history of this renewed importance of psychotherapy, the most distinguished names are those of the Englishmen Tuke, Carpenter, and Hughes Bennet, the Frenchmen Charcot and Bernheim, and, above all, Sigmund Freud, whose work had already reached maturity at the start of the First World War in 1914.

Ethical and social aspects of the relationship. Something has already been said about medical ethics in the society of the nineteenth and twentieth centuries. Like the society to which it belonged, this ethic became more secular, as is shown by the different attempts to codify it, beginning with Percival's in 1803. From an ethical and social point of view, medical care was a service purchased at different prices or given free to the poor in hospitals supported by charity and inspired by the new philanthropy. The poor received medical care as a gift.

The sick were cared for in three different ambits. (1) *Hospitals* were supported by charity, the state, municipality, or church. Here the patient was one of two things to his doctor: either an object that could be scientifically understood and modified combined with a human being who was unknown and indifferent (if the doctor was a cold and matter-of-fact man), or an object that could be scientifically understood and modified, combined with a person suffering and in need of compassion (if the doctor was a man of feeling and carried out the rule of Bérard and Gluber). (2) *The patient's own home.* For the "family doctor," as he is called, the patient visited at home was an object that could be scientifically understood and modified, combined with a well-known person—a friend. (3) *The doctor's private consulting room.* Here the patient was, according to circumstances, either an object that could be scientifically understood and modified, combined with a person to whom the therapist was indifferent (purely "scientific" doctors); an object that could be understood and modified combined with a person who paid the fees asked (doctors dominated by desire for gain); or an object that could be understood and modified, combined with a friend in need of compassion (generous, sympathetic doctors). These three ambits, with certain exceptions, correspond to the three strata into which the bourgeois and proletarian society of the age are divided, and to the three socioeconomic methods of providing medical care: "medicine for the rich" (private consulting rooms for specialists), "medicine for the middle classes" (attendance in their homes), and "medicine for the poor and proletarians" (charitable hospitals).

The injustice of this social organization of medicine becomes flagrant and untenable when the proletariat becomes conscious of its right to health and proper medical care, and when, one may add, medical treatment is both efficient and expensive.

Since the second half of the nineteenth century there has been a visible rebellion against this injustice with its politico-social and clinical aspects. Since Turner Thackrah in 1831, Chadwick in 1842 and Villermé in 1840, some doctors have denounced the terrible effects on health of industrial poverty; and workers' movements have included the right to put an end to this painful and unjustifiable situation in their programs for social reform. The great vogue of *Friendly Societies* in the United Kingdom between 1800 and 1875, the institution of the *zemstvo* system in tsarist Russia in 1867 after the liberation of the serfs, and the creation of *Krankenkassen* in Germany by Bismarck (1882–1884) are examples of the first medical results of the proletarian rebellion.

Among the clinical results of this rebellion may be counted the increase in neurotic forms of illness, which were direct consequences in some cases of social injustice and maladjustment. The "introduction of the subject in medicine" (von Weizsäcker's term), that is to say, the methodical study of the patient as an individual, both in diagnosis and treatment (penetration of hospitals by Freudian psychoanalysis and psychosomatic medicine), as well as social pathology and medical sociology (Grotjahn and various English authors), constitutes the response of scientific medicine to the clinical rebellion of the sick against the medical care of the nineteenth century.

To the ordinary man as well as to the doctor of today, the present period begins with the First World War. From that point on the historian of yesterday must defer to the chronicler of the present day.

PEDRO LAÍN ENTRALGO
[*translated by* Frances Partridge]

[*While all the articles in this entry are relevant, see especially the article* SOCIOHISTORICAL PERSPECTIVES. *For further discussion of topics mentioned in this article, see the entries:* CARE; DEATH AND DYING: EUTHANASIA AND SUSTAINING LIFE, *article on* HISTORICAL PERSPECTIVES; HEALTH AND DISEASE; HOSPITALS; *and* MIND–BODY PROBLEM. *See also:* MEDICINE, PHILOSOPHY OF. *For discussion of related ideas, see:* MEDICAL ETHICS, HISTORY OF, *section on* PRIMITIVE SOCIETIES; *and section on* EUROPE AND THE AMERICAS, *articles on* MEDIEVAL EUROPE: FOURTH TO SIXTEENTH CENTURY *and* CENTRAL EUROPE IN THE NINETEENTH CENTURY.]

BIBLIOGRAPHY

BAAS, KARL. "Uranfänge und Frühgeschichte der Krankenpflege." (*Sudhoffs*) *Archiv für die Geschichte der Medizin* 8 (1915): 146–164.

BALINT, MICHAEL. *The Doctor, His Patient, and His Illness.* London: Pitman Medical Publishing Co., 1957. *The Doctor, His Patient, and the Illness.* Foreword by Maurice Levine. New York: International Universities Press, 1957. 2d ed. rev. and enl. London: Pitman Medical Publishing Co., 1964.

BLUM, RICHARD H.; SADUSK, JOSEPH; and WATERSON, ROLLEN. *The Management of the Doctor–Patient Relationship.* New York: McGraw-Hill, Blakiston Division, 1960.

CHRISTIAN, PAUL. *Das Personsverständnis im modernen medizinischen Denken.* Schriften der Studiengemeinschaft der Evangelischen Akademien. Tübingen: Mohr, 1952.

EDELSTEIN, LUDWIG. *The Hippocratic Oath: Text, Translation, and Interpretation.* Supplements to the Bulletin of the History of Medicine, no. 1. Baltimore: Johns Hopkins Press, 1943. Reprint. *Ancient Medicine: Selected Papers of Ludwig Edelstein.* Edited by Owsei Temkin and C. Lilian Temkin. Baltimore: Johns Hopkins Press, 1967, pp. 3–63.

FIELD, MARK G. *Doctor and Patient in Soviet Russia.* Foreword by Paul Dudley White. Russian Research Center Studies, no. 29. Cambridge: Harvard University Press, 1957.

HIPPOCRATES. *Epid.* I, L. II, 634. Littré, *Oeuvres complètes d'Hippocrate,* vol. 2, pp. 634–637. *Epidēmiōn* A. Translated as "Epidemics I," Jones, *Hippocrates,* vol. 1, second constitution, par. 11, 11. 10–12, pp. 164–165.

———. *Epid.* I, L. II, 636. Littré, *Oeuvres complètes d'Hippocrate,* vol. 2, pp. 636–637. *Epidēmiōn* A. Translated as "Epidemics I," Jones, *Hippocrates,* vol. 1, second constitution, par. 11, 11. 13–14, pp. 164–

165. According to Littré the reference to "nature" does not occur in all recensions.

————. *Med.*, L. IX, 204. Littré, *Oeuvres complètes d'Hippocrate*, vol. 9, pp. 204–207. *Peri iētrou.* Translated as "The Physician," Jones, *Hippocrates*, vol. 2, chap. 1, pp. 310–313.

————. *Praec.*, L. IX, 258. Littré, *Oeuvres complètes d'Hippocrate*, vol. 9, pp. 258–263. *Parangeliai.* Translated as "Precepts," Jones, *Hippocrates*, vol. 1, pars. 6–7, pp. 318–323.

————. *Reg.*, L. VI, 466. Littré, *Oeuvres complètes d'Hippocrate*, vol. 6, pp. 466–663. *Peri diaitēs.* Translated as "Regimen" [On diet], Jones, *Hippocrates*, vol. 4, pp. 224–447.

JONES, W. H. S., trans. *Hippocrates*. 4 vols. The Loeb Classical Library. Edited by E. Capps, T. E. Page, and W. H. D. Rouse. London: William Heinemann; New York: G. P. Putnam's Sons, 1923–1931. Greek and English.

LAÍN ENTRALGO, PEDRO. "La Asistencia médica en la obra de Platón." *Marañón y el enfermo.* Madrid: Revista de Occidente, 1962, pp. 90–135.

————. "El Christianismo primitivo y la medicina." *Historia universal de la medicina.* 6 vols. Vol. 3: *Edad media.* Barcelona: Salvat Editores, 1972, pp. 1–7.

————. *La Curación por la palabra en la antigüedad clásica.* Madrid: Revista de Occidente, 1958. Edited and translated by L. J. Rather and John M. Sharp as *The Therapy of the Word in Classical Antiquity.* New Haven: Yale University Press, 1970.

————. *Doctor and Patient.* Translated by Francis Partridge. World University Library. London: Weidenfeld & Nicholson; New York: McGraw-Hill, 1969.

————. *Enfermedad y pecado.* Medicina de hoy. Barcelona: Ediciones Toray, 1961.

————. *La Medicina hipocrática.* Madrid: Revista de Occidente, 1970.

————. *La Relación médico-enfermo: Historia y teoría.* Madrid: Revista de Occidente, 1964.

————. *Sobre la amistad.* Collección Selecta, no. 40. Madrid: Revista de Occidente, 1972.

LITTRÉ, ÉMILE, ed. and trans. *Oeuvres complètes d'Hippocrate: Traduction nouvelle avec le texte grec en regard, collationné sur les manuscrits et toutes les éditions; accompagnée d'une introduction, de commentaires médicaux, de variantes et de notes philologiques; suivie d'une table générale des matières.* 10 vols. Paris: J. B. Baillière, 1839–1861. Reprint. Amsterdam: Adolf M. Hakkert, 1961.

NUTTING, MARY ADELAIDE, and DOCK, LAVINIA L. *A History of Nursing: The Evolution of Nursing Systems from the Earliest Times to the Foundation of the First English and American Training School for Nurses.* 4 vols. New York: G. P. Putnam's Sons, 1907–1912. Title varies. Translated by Agnes Karll as *Geschichte der Krankenpflege: Die Entwicklung der Krankenpflege-Systeme von Urzeiten bis zur Gründung der ersten englischen und amerikanischen Pflegerinnenschulen.* 3 vols. Berlin: D. Reimer, 1910–1913.

ORR, DOUGLAS W. "Transference and Countertransference: A Historical Survey." *Journal of the American Psychoanalytic Association* 2 (1954): 621–670.

PARSONS, TALCOTT. "Illness and the Role of the Physician: A Sociological Perspective." *American Journal of Orthopsychiatry* 21 (1951): 452–460.

PITTENGER, ROBERT E.; HACKETT, CHARLES F.; and DANEHY, JOHN J. *The First Five Minutes: A Sample of Microscopic Interview Analysis.* Ithaca, N.Y.: Paul Martineau, 1960.

RITTER-RÖHR, DOROTHEA, ed. *Der Arzt, sein Patient, und die Gesellschaft.* Edition Suhrkamp, no. 746. Frankfurt: 1975.

ROF CARBALLO, J. *Urdimbre afectiva y enfermedad: Introducción a una medicina dialógica.* Colección Hombre y mundo. Barcelona: Editorial Labor, 1961.

SNYDER, WILLIAM U., and SNYDER, B. JUNE. *The Psychotherapy Relationship.* New York: Macmillan Co., 1961.

SZASZ, THOMAS S. "Scientific Method and Social Role in Medicine and Psychiatry." *Archives of Internal Medicine* 101 (1958): 228–238.

VALABREGA, JEAN-PAUL. *La Relation thérapeutique: Malade et médicin.* Nouvelle bibliothèque scientifique. Paris: Flammarion, 1962.

WEISS, GEORG. "Die ethischen Anschauunger im Cropus Hippokraticum." (*Sudhoffs*) *Archiv für die Geschichte der Medizin* 4 (1910): 235–262.

ZBOROWSKI, MARK. "Cultural Components in Responses to Pain." *Journal of Social Issues* 8, no. 4 (1952), pp. 16–30.

II

SOCIOHISTORICAL PERSPECTIVES

Although the healing art is older than the physician, the doctor's role has been, for sociology, the centerpiece of the therapeutic relationship (Sigerist). Other helping roles—the nurse, social worker, and various "allied health professionals"—have received attention, but historically it is the therapist as a professional in modern society who has interested the sociologist most, and medicine is seen as the archetypal profession.

The literature on the doctor–patient relationship by many distinguished sociologists illustrates the major theoretical paradigms of the past fifty years: structural functionalism, structural-conflict theory, and neo-Marxism. The result has been a changing portrait of both doctor and patient—from a dominantly psychological perspective of "a pure person-to-person relationship" as Sigerist wrote in 1931, to a sharp turn when the social system frame of reference was introduced, shifting the analysis to the social roles of therapist and client. Their roles were interpreted as "functional" components of society. Within this framework of cultural socialization, the doctor's achieved high level of expertise was described as essential to modern scientific health care, and, as a consequence, medical education was spotlighted. The medical school was seen as the principal source of attitudes and values as well as training in skills and knowledge. That approach enhanced the physician's image of awesome technological accomplishment and heroic personal attributes, while the patient was relegated to a subordinate, fragile state in which the only requirements were to be motivated to get well and to consult the physician toward that end. Perhaps inevitably, there was a reaction to those images and to the underlying approach that was thought to have spawned them. The "monopoly of dominance" replaced "technological achievement" as the more popular view of the doctor; the patient came to be viewed as "exploited" by the physician as much as or more than he was victimized by the primarily organic forces of illness. The doctor and patient became antagonists, each from a separate world, and their adversary relationship was described as "a clash of perspectives" instead of a balanced interdependent system.

In this changing approach, sociological thought has run parallel to the public's attitude to the medical profession. The sociologists' picture of the physician, at first cautious and respectful, reflected the high peak of public prestige and trust that allocated to doctors the privilege of virtually complete autonomy as "high priests in the temples of science" (Churchill). That pedestal was not to be an easy resting place, however. Physicians fell into a lion pit of public exhortation, government regulation, and legal attack.

The implications for the ethical standards of medicine have been profound. After centuries of struggle to win the right to take risks under conditions of uncertainty (Fox, 1957), in "the best interests of their patients," doctors now find themselves confronted by a fresh demand for accountability. The responsibility that was once assumed in trust is increasingly subject to the formal controls of various forms of peer review and medical audit.

The concern of this historical article is to sketch the models of the doctor–patient relationship as they have been developed by sociology as a background for the ethical questions raised about the therapeutic relationship.

Origins of the system model

Lawrence J. Henderson, a distinguished physician-scientist, first conceptualized the doctor–patient relationship as "a social system" (Henderson, "Physician and Patient"). From 1930 until almost two decades after the Second World War, the social system concept was the keystone of functionalist theory, and one of the foremost ideas in American sociology.

The essence of the social system formulation is that human relationships can be described in regularities of pattern, that such patterns of social behavior are based in cultural expectations about the social roles of the group participants, that the fundamental process of behavior is communication, and that the dynamic which maintains the integrity of the system is homeostasis (social equilibrium). The central theme of functional system theory was that the whole was not the sum of its parts, but rather that change in any part alters simultaneously the character of the whole system.

Henderson first applied system theory in the physiological study of the blood, building upon the model of the phase-rule of Willard Gibbs in the explanation of physicochemical systems. Henderson's work, published in 1907, established him as one of the outstanding biologists of his time. His reputation was based on more than the elegance of his theory: He was able to apply simultaneous equations to the data of the physiological laboratory as verification of the theory. Not until mid-career did Henderson turn to sociology, and with Vilfredo Pareto (1848–1923) as his inspiration, he attempted to apply system theory to social relationships. As his prime example, he studied the doctor–patient relationship.

When Henderson turned his attention to more general questions about human behavior, he seemed only to be following the pattern of his earlier scientific work. Pareto's efforts to work out a mathematical formulation for a system of economic equilibrium in society had a natural appeal for Henderson. Much as Henderson had made his reputation by finding a mathematical method for the Gibbs model, Pareto used indifference curves to formulate equations of economic equilibrium. Pareto, like Henderson, came into the social sciences late in life, after education in mathematics and physical science and twenty years of experience as a practicing engineer.

Henderson's descriptions of the doctor–patient relationship were eloquent, but his analysis lacked the clarity of his work in biological science. He *was* passionately concerned. The doctor, he was convinced, could damage a patient as much with a misplaced word as with a slip of his scalpel. But his social science, built as it was upon analogies that were primarily mechanical or physiological, did not go very far beyond a direct translation of the general propositions of the system model as derived from the physical sciences into the terms of interpersonal relationships.

The Parsonian model

It remained for Talcott Parsons to carry forward Henderson's discussion of the doctor–patient relationship as a social system and to give it full expression as part of sociological theory (Parsons, pp. 428–479). The premises of the Parsonian model include the following: (1) The problem of health is "intimately involved in the *functional prerequisites* of the social system"; too low a general level of health or too high an incidence of illness is dysfunctional; (2) sickness and health are significant themes of culture; (3) health care is a social role relationship between a helping agent and a person needing help; (4) the social roles of the health-care relationship are a patterned sector of culture and thus *learned* sequences of behavior. From these premises Parsons constructed ideal types of sick role and professional role. The former is characterized as a type of social deviance that, though involuntary, must be controlled to prevent the abuse that is inherent as a threat to the society because of the psychological rewards of the legitimized dependency of illness. The professional role combines healing that is oriented to help the patient and social control as the agent of society. Within this framework, the sick role is temporary, undesirable, and basically disruptive socially. The professional is a technical expert who legitimizes the claim to illness and is responsible for returning the sick person to his normal role in society.

Criticisms of Parsons's views are of two distinct types. One is intellectual, challenging his theoretical premises and argument (Freidson, 1961, 1970). The other is political, interpreting the work of both Henderson and Parsons as a conservative political response to the historical events of the early 1930s (Gouldner, p. 149).

The theoretical criticism of the model focuses on Parsons's emphasis on the asymmetry, professional dominance–client dependence, in the therapeutic situation and the distancing effect of the role attributes of the professional. Parsons is interpreted as a defender of the technical elitism of the modern professional. His patients must be "controlled" lest they take advantage of the privileges of the sick role to prolong dependency; his physicians must be "protected" from over-involvement emotionally with their patients. The consequences, the criticism asserts, are not just to explain a role asymmetry based upon the achieved technical expertise of the professional but to label the passive dependent patient and the expert doctor, the one needing control and the other protection.

Behavioral implications of organic symptoms

The next important step in developing a model of the doctor–patient relationship was by Szasz and Hollender. It was closely related to but not directly based upon the Parsonian formulation that the "state of the organism as a biological system" is related to the social system of medical practice. Szasz and Hollender, both physicians, saw more extensive implications of organic systems for behavior. Their model of the doctor–patient relationship is based on a three-fold typology of behavior patterns determined by the organic nature of the illnesses involved: (1) activity–passivity, (2) guidance–cooperation, and (3) mutual participation. Again, as in Parsons, dependence–independence is the primary behavioral variable. As Szasz and Hollender point out, if a patient is in a coma, there is no question about the nature of the required doctor's role: He must take charge. If, on the other hand, the patient has a chronic illness like diabetes, then the implications are very different: The patient must be an active partner involved in his own treatment. If, therefore, the doctor learns to act as a dominant, controlling figure, essentially authoritarian, and uses this style under all conditions, he is bound to fail when he enters a situation with a patient in which mutual participation and not the active–passive interaction is required (Szasz and Hollender).

During the decade of the 1950s, a variety of efforts to extend the range and deepen the meaning of the Parsonian model were undertaken. The viewpoints of psychoanalysis, anthropology, and small group laboratory research were among those represented. In the same spirit, attempts were made to explicate the theory with reference to other relevant social contexts. The problem became one of integrating these diverse contributions to the explanation of the therapeutic relationship as a social system, and this too was attempted (Bloom).

Fox, more than any other sociologist, used the Parsonian model to interpret what she defined as the moral dilemma of the clinical investigator, whose dual responsibility is to care for patients at the same time as he conducts research upon them (Fox, 1959). Especially when patients are ill with diseases not well understood or not within the easy therapeutic control of modern medicine, the main problem of the physician and patient, Fox asserted, is to cope with the stressful experience of "uncertainty" (ibid., p. 27). Her early research on doctors and patients in a metabolic ward anticipated the ethical conflicts that grew to such intensity later in connection with organ transplantation, hemodialysis, and other breakthrough technological procedures of recent years. Throughout her work, the perspective leads to emphasis on the "courage" of the professional who is willing to undertake "adventures into the unknown" (Fox and Swazey). Her "courage to fail" hypothesis is clearly the heir of Parsons's approach to the ethics of medicine, but it is not shared by several more skeptical students of the medical profession (Freidson, 1970; Waitzkin and Waterman).

The conflict model

The continuity that links all of the work cited up to this point was broken abruptly with the appearance of studies by Freidson (1961), Mechanic and Volkhart (1961), and Zola (1966). The critique of the social system analysis was explained by Freidson as follows: (1) The Parsons model sees the doctor–patient relationship from too limited a perspective, most essentially that of the physician; it does not pay attention to the varying expectations of all members of the "role-set" (Merton), including the patients (or more inclusively his lay associates), and the nurses and other persons involved in the process of treatment; (2) moreover, expectations are presented by Parsons as though they are the primary influence on actual behavior; they are only an ideal standard against which actual behavior is judged; (3) influence does not inhere in the expectation but in the position of the person holding it; only from the structure of the situation and the limits imposed by that situation can one weigh the possibility of an expectation's being met; (4) most important, the functional model ignores the necessity of conflict in human relationships. Insofar as each person, the professional and the patient, seeks from the other to gain his own terms, there is conflict.

The doctor–patient relationship, Freidson concluded, is most effectively analyzed within a framework of *a clash of perspectives*. In other words, it represents the encounter between two distinct social systems, and not a functionally contained, homeostatic system in itself.

Freidson develops his own model from a revision of the Parsonian conception of illness as deviance. Parsons saw illness as a biological state with social implications and consequences. For Freidson it is the reverse: The physician defines illness. "Medicine's monopoly includes the right to create illness as an official social role. . . . It is a part of being a profession to be given the official power to define and therefore create the shape of problematic segments of social behavior: the judge determines what is legal and who is guilty, the priest what is holy and who is profane, the physician what is normal and who is sick" (Freidson, 1970, p. 37). Thus Freidson articulates the basic sociological position underlying the "labeling theory" of Szasz and Scheff in their analyses of mental illness, and he extends that position in his own discussion of chronic illness. He classifies deviant roles according to the qualities attributed to them, seeing the individual patient as someone to whom something happens, who is then labeled by others and pressed to behave in a particular expected way quite independently of his own motives or desires (ibid.).

In the history of sociological theory as it has been applied to the study of medicine, Freidson played the key role in the assertion of conflict between groups as the assumptive framework for analysis. His work coincided with the revolutionary changes of a period in the recent history of the United States when all the most basic values of the society were weighed against the consequences of racial discrimination, poverty, and war. However, Freidson conducted his challenge within the traditional boundaries of scholarship, avoiding identification with any specific political ideology.

The critique by neo-Marxism

A distinctly new direction, though based on similar premises to those of Freidson's structural analysis, was taken by Waitzkin and Waterman in 1974 and Navarro in 1975. Their model is Marxist, and the doctor–patient relationship is, in their view, a "typical collectivity" within the institution of medicine—a social institution that can be understood only as part of a sociopolitical structure. In the United States, they argue, medicine is organized for profit, reflecting the normative principles of a capitalist society. Therefore, although the need for good health to maintain the system creates a certain "ambiguity" about the right to health, the tension between profit and good health has persisted. The one group exploits the other. Only in this way, they assert, can the persistent maldistribution of health services favoring wealthy patients be explained. They go on to document the structure of the growing industries that provide health services and produce medical products, together with the increasingly concentrated distribution of profit among certain small groups of physicians, a documentation that has challenged the ongoing scholarly debate.

Conclusions

A sharp polarization of interpretation about the ethical behavior of physicians emerges from the history of sociological ideas. The earlier point of view is in the tradition of individualism, interpreting behavior as a social psychological process determined by the learned values which individuals carry with them into social encounters. In a second and different view, material technologies and organizational constraints dominate the therapeutic relationship. No one can question the fact of the changes that, over half a century, have occurred in both the technology and the organization of health care. The bureaucratization of medicine is already far advanced, creating a situation in which both doctor and patient meet together less as independent individuals than as members of groups. The resulting formalization of the relationship is bound to alter the emotional quality of the exchange and the nature of responsibility and accountability for those involved.

The polar differences of theory have been identified with equally divergent ideological positions. There are signs, however, of a plateau in the intensity of dialogue, while a new spirit of empirical research asserts itself in the effort to describe and understand the therapeutic relationship.

SAMUEL W. BLOOM

[*Directly related are the other articles in this entry, and the entry* HEALTH AND DISEASE, *articles on* A SOCIOLOGICAL AND ACTION PERSPECTIVE *and* PHILOSOPHICAL PERSPECTIVES. *For discussion of related ideas, see the entries:* MENTAL ILLNESS, *article on* LABELING IN MENTAL ILLNESS: LEGAL ASPECTS; PATERNALISM; *and* SOCIALITY. *Other relevant material may be found under* MEDICAL EDUCATION; MEDICAL PROFESSION, *article on* MEDICAL PROFESSIONALISM; MEDICINE, SOCIOLOGY OF; *and* POVERTY AND HEALTH, *article on* POVERTY AND HEALTH IN THE UNITED STATES.]

BIBLIOGRAPHY

BLOOM, SAMUEL W. *The Doctor and His Patient: A Sociological Interpretation.* Paperback ed. with new introduction. New York: Macmillan Publishing Co., Free Press, 1965.
CHURCHILL, EDWARD D. "The Development of the Hospital." *The Hospital in Contemporary Life.* Edited by Nathaniel W. Faxon. Cambridge: Harvard University Press, 1949, chap. 1, pp. 1–69.
FOX, RENÉE C. *Experiment Perilous: Physicians and Patients Facing the Unknown.* Glencoe, Ill.: Free Press, 1959.
———. "Training for Uncertainty." *The Student Physician: Introductory Studies in the Sociology of Medical Education.* Edited by Robert K. Merton, George G. Reader, and Patricia L. Kendall. Cambridge: Commonwealth Fund, Harvard University Press, 1957, pp. 207–241.
———, and SWAZEY, JUDITH P. *The Courage to Fail: A Social View of Organ Transplants and Dialysis.* Chicago: University of Chicago Press, 1974.
FREIDSON, ELIOT. *Patients' Views of Medical Practice: A Study of Subscribers to a Prepaid Medical Plan in the Bronx.* New York: Russell Sage Foundation, 1961.
———. *Profession of Medicine: A Study of the Sociology of Applied Knowledge.* New York: Dodd, Mead & Co., 1970.
GOULDNER, ALVIN W. *The Coming Crisis of Western Sociology.* Studies in the Series on the Social Origins of Social Theory. New York: Basic Books, 1970.
HENDERSON, LAWRENCE J. *Pareto's General Sociology: A Physiologist's Interpretation.* Cambridge: Harvard University Press, 1935, 1937. Reprint. New York: Russell & Russell, 1967.
———. "Physician and Patient as a Social System." *New England Journal of Medicine* 212 (1935): 819–823.
MECHANIC, DAVID, and VOLKART, EDMUND H. "Stress, Illness Behavior, and the Sick Role." *American Sociological Review* 26 (1961): 51–58.
MERTON, ROBERT K. "The Role-Set: Problems in Sociological Theory." *British Journal of Sociology* 8 (1957): 106–120.
NAVARRO, VICENTE. "Social Policy Issues: An Explanation of the Composition, Nature, and Functions of the Present Health Sector of the United States." *Bulletin of the New York Academy of Medicine* 51 (1975): 199–234.
PARSONS, TALCOTT. *The Social System.* Glencoe, Ill.: Free Press, 1951.
SCHEFF, THOMAS J. *Being Mentally Ill: A Sociological Theory.* Observations. Chicago, Ill.: Aldine Publishing Co., 1966.
SIGERIST, HENRY E. "The Physician and His Environment (1931)." *Henry E. Sigerist on the Sociology of Medicine.* Edited by Milton I. Roemer. New York: MD Publications, 1960, pp. 3–8.
SZASZ, THOMAS S. *The Myth of Mental Illness: Foundations of a Theory of Personal Conduct.* New York: Harper & Row, Hoeber Medical Division, 1961.
———, and HOLLENDER, MARC HALE. "A Contribution to the Philosophy of Medicine: The Basic Models of

the Doctor–Patient Relationship." *A.M.A. Archives of Internal Medicine* 97 (1956): 585–592.

WAITZKIN, HOWARD, and WATERMAN, BARBARA. The *Exploitation of Illness in Capitalist Society.* Bobbs-Merrill Studies in Sociology. Indianapolis: 1974.

ZOLA, IRVING KENNETH. "Culture and Symptoms—An Analysis of Patients' Presenting Complaints." *American Sociological Review* 31 (1966): 615–630.

III
CONTEMPORARY SOCIOLOGICAL ANALYSIS

While the elaboration of medical science and technology increases the focus on technical aspects of patient care, the social role of the physician remains most basically that of a sustaining professional—one that must be responsive to a wide variety of human problems that cause distress and limit social functioning (Mechanic, 1968). Particularly in the case of practitioners of first contact, problems they must deal with are conditioned less by their own conceptions and training and more by social patterns and environmental events that trigger help-seeking processes and choices of practitioners.

Much of the attractiveness of primary medical care is that it remains one of the few social institutions in society that deal with people's problems with minimal evaluation of the individual's "moral worth." Moreover, medicine has sufficient legitimacy to provide acceptable explanations that excuse failures in social performance or that justify the release of the patient from community and family obligations (Parsons). Many persons who are failing in their social obligations may find medicine a valuable ally in rendering assistance and maintaining self-esteem and in protecting themselves against social sanctions even when the cause of their problem may not be strictly "medical." With increased social and geographic mobility, kinship and neighborhood supports are progressively weaker, and social roots in modern society are relatively shallow. Many institutions such as religion, traditionally important sources of assistance, have lost some of their capacity to provide sustenance, and thus the sustaining functions of medicine have become especially important. Increasingly, problems that were dealt with informally by kin and neighbors are handled by professional practitioners, and the wide range of personal problems reflects not only disease and dysfunction but also the cumulation of life stresses, failures in coping with life problems, and the need for social support.

A traditional concept of the physician's role is that his relationship with the patient is an implied contractual one in which he uses his special expertise and competence as agent for the patient. Implicit in such a contract is that the physician can be trusted to treat the patient's health needs and interests as central, thus minimizing the need for the patient to be defensive or to withhold information. Both the status of the physician and the ethical bases of his practice facilitate the patient's willingness to put his health in the hands of the physician with little demand for detailed explanations or monitoring of the physician's decisions. This is not to imply that physicians have always conformed to these ethical mandates or that patients have generally been docile, but only that the physician's authority has been assumed to be part of the ordinary understanding of relationships between physicians and patients and their respective responsibilities. The structure of the contract has tended to increase not only the physician's technical authority, but also his "moral" influence (Frank).

Much of the character of doctor–patient contracts has customarily depended on a continuing association and mutual knowledge. Trust in the physician has, to some extent, been nurtured by the continuity of care, and with time patients' dependence on particular physicians grew. In recent times a great deal has occurred to erode such trust, despite the fact that more resources of high quality and potentiality for effective intervention are available to individuals than ever before. In part, with the growth of knowledge and technology and higher levels of education among the public, many physicians have difficulty in maintaining credible claims to special status and judgment. Increasingly, physicians are recognized as having a limited expertise despite the fact that the boundaries of medical intervention and practice have continued to grow, encompassing problems that in past eras were under the authority of law, religion, and the family (Mechanic, 1973). The expanding domain of medicine in light of the growing sophistication of clients produces new strains and uncertainties for the practitioner that tend to erode his authority and perhaps his confidence as well.

With increasing specialization, a more segmented pattern of delivery of medical care, and greater geographic mobility of the public, continuity of care and the more primary social relationship usually associated with continuing contact have also become less common. As the physician directs his attention more to specialized technical functions and neglects the concerns of the whole person, his ability to build moral as compared with technical authority is very much restrained. Authority that stems from a limited technical expertise is more fragile and susceptible to challenge or attack for error than deeper, more personal relationships. It has been suggested that among the factors responsible for growing malpractice litigation are the impersonality of doctor–patient relationships and the erosion of the physician's moral authority (Blum).

A variety of ethical and organizational dilemmas have confounded the simplicity of the traditional model. With the growth of mass communication and the availability of much information on physicians and medical practice, expectations concerning the character of medical care and what it should be are influenced as much from without as from within. No longer is any relationship insulated from the continuing flow of information about appropriate treatment, new drugs, and ethical conflicts. Also, with the growing organizational basis of medicine, physicians are less likely to have a simple defined loyalty to the patient, but, rather, are subjected to a complex set of conflicting loyalties that require them to balance the interests of patients against such other interests as economic efficiency, the functioning needs of the organization, research, and teaching. Physicians are more likely than ever before to be faced with incentive structures that make it organizationally and personally disadvantageous to serve as exclusive advocate of the patient. Finally, the practice of medicine—because of both its growing domain and its technological capacities—confronts both doctor and patient with enormous ethical choices on which the population as a whole has widely differing views. It is increasingly likely that doctor and patient will face serious conflicts in these ethical domains, and such possibilities put increased strain on the relationship and create new occasions for conflict and criticism.

Patients have responded to these conditions with uncertainty. While they bring a great range of problems to the physician, they are insecure as to his expertise in many of these areas. While they have very high and often unrealistic expectations, they are also skeptical and frequently critical. While they desire a trusting relationship, they are frequently untrusting and demand greater representation, information, and voice in decision making. Obviously, patients and doctors vary a great deal, and there are no simple

generalizations that adequately describe the variability that is evident. What can be said, however, is that there is at present ambivalence in the public mind as to the appropriate role of medicine and the proper stance of the physician. This uncertainty reflects the substantial changes that science has brought to the public concerning the manner in which medicine is perceived, organized, and practiced. The rapidity of scientific and technological development in medicine and social and cultural change, in general, have left medicine in a quandary concerning its roles and responsibilities in modern society, and uncertain and divided as to its most appropriate organizational framework.

The epidemiology of help-seeking and therapist–patient relationships

Except in such limited spheres as institutional psychiatry, where care may be provided to an involuntary patient, most relationships between doctors and patients are voluntarily initiated by the patient because he or she anticipates that the likely benefits outweigh the costs of seeking care. The willingness to seek care for any problems is conditioned by the social and cultural background of the patient, the patient's faith in medical care, and the nature of the barriers to seeking assistance (Mechanic, 1968). The most common problems seen in first-contact medicine are also generally found in segments of the populations who receive no treatment, suggesting that the social and environmental conditions in initiating the care process may be as important as the specific complaints presented. Symptoms and problems are commonplace in populations (White, Williams, and Greenberg). Individuals attempt to assess the meaning of their distress in light of their social and cultural propensities, and to appraise varying alternatives for coping with their problems (Mechanic, "Social Psychologic Factors"). The decision to seek care and the particular types of assistance sought depend on complex attribution processes in which the person makes an informal assessment of the nature of the problem, its likely cause, and its possible outcomes. Help is more likely to be sought when the problem interferes in some significant way with the person's life routines by restricting valued activities. Although we have limited data on alternative routes of help-seeking, there is sufficient evidence to suggest that a variety of therapists and social agencies deal with some of the same problems. Seeking care is a selective process in which people often search for practitioners who share their frames of reference and who are socially and culturally compatible (Kadushin). Thus doctors, psychologists, clergy, and social agencies come to have an overlapping clientele. Frequently, however, patients will present problems so as to make them compatible with the type of practitioner consulted. Depending on the circumstances, the same problem may be construed as a medical, social, or moral problem, and often the first task of the therapist is to come to some acceptable understanding with the patient as to the appropriate frame of reference (Balint).

The practice of medicine—unlike psychiatry, psychology, counseling, or social work—is viewed by physicians more as a scientific activity and thus less as one in which the patient's values or life perspectives should be important variables. The explicit definition of the relationship states that it is neutral in respect to the patient's worth or social status, whatever the empirical realities might be. Thus, patients who bring problems to physicians are likely to be constrained in the manner in which they present their problem, usually anticipating that symptoms are one of the prices of admission to the encounter. While some patients who have highly developed psychological and problem vocabularies may be able to break out of such stereotypical presentations, the typical patient will often present a variety of vague or "trivial" symptoms as a way of justifying being there (Mechanic, "Social Psychologic Factors"). Although such symptoms may be characteristic of a generalized distress related to life problems, patients frequently feel uncomfortable in addressing the problems in these terms, or they may be incapable of recognizing the true source of their distress because of cultural inhibitions and previous socialization. There is considerable evidence that much of illness seen in primary medical care is associated with life situations and problems that affect both the occurrence of symptoms and the pursuit of medical care (Dohrenwend and Dohrenwend).

Physicians, in part because of the nature of their training and in part because of the demands of medical practice, face the difficult task of carefully assessing the patient's problem and determining its appropriate management within a limited time period. The physician thus tends to focus on disturbing symptoms and organizes taking a case history, the physical examination, and clinical investigation in a search for underlying conditions explaining the patient's symptoms. Both the logic of the diagnostic approach and the pressure of the patient queue direct the physician to categorical problems rather than to the patient's total life situation. Patients whose problems are obviously complicated by psychosocial issues or sociocultural complexities cause difficulties in relation to the physician's total responsibilities, because such patients take a great deal of time and attention with uncertain evidence that desired outcomes can be achieved. It is much easier to treat the symptoms of such patients than to undertake the time-consuming, uncertain, and often frustrating course of using the therapeutic contact as an exploratory and educational relationship. Although the problem is somewhat different in the hospital context, many of the same considerations prevail, and physicians find it more expedient to work on the patient than to treat the relationship with the patient as a means of educational participation and change (Duff and Hollingshead; Cartwright).

In focusing on the patient's symptoms and disease, the physician can proceed in a manner relatively independent of the patient and his social and psychological identities. As long as he remains within this framework, the object is the identification of deviations from a baseline defined by the absence of symptoms and their correction, and the physician for the most part does not have to cope with the complexities of the patient's viewpoints, his special social characteristics and life situation, and his unique preferences. Thus, the physician can proceed relatively independently in ordering tests, evaluating the patient, and suggesting how the problem can be managed. One consequence, however, is that medical practice is characterized by frequent disruptions in communication and in achieving mutual understanding, and patients frequently either fail to understand the physician's advice or choose to ignore it (Ley and Spelman). Given the frequent failures of implementation, following careful and expensive evaluations, it is not apparent that what appears expedient in practice is cost-effective in outcome.

An alternate model of therapist–patient interaction is an educational one, based on the assumption that, aside from emergency treatment, much of the assistance of long-term value to the patient depends on his willingness to come to terms with his own behavior and problems in his life. While the physician may have technical expertise that the patient lacks, he perceives that effective long-term management depends as much on assisting the patient to understand his own health problem as it does on any unilateral actions taken by the physician. In this context, there is far more choice for the patient to exercise his options and to share in treatment situations. To the extent that the patient becomes actively involved in his own care, and to the extent that medical management is approached within the larger context of the patient's job, family, and community situation, it becomes more possible to select those interventions of medical utility that are also consistent with the patient's social situation and ethical needs.

The elaboration of therapeutic relationships

While the most common models of medical practice and medical ethics envisage one physician and one patient, therapeutic relationships have become greatly elaborated in recent decades, making such models less relevant to empirical reality. In the usual hospital situation, and increasingly in ambulatory medical settings, medical services are provided either by a team or by a loosely coordinated collection of health personnel. The elaboration of the relationship results from the growing complexity of care and associated specialization, desires to achieve greater productivity and economies through rearranging care functions among varying levels of personnel, and the practicalities of establishing organizational timetables and the scheduling of manpower utilization.

The elaboration of medical care, if well-organized, can increase the technical potential of care, but frequently it also results in inflexible and unresponsive relationships with patients (Freidson). Whether bureaucratic organization itself, the technical priorities of physicians in salaried situations free of client controls, or poor organizational arrangements are the major cause, the fact is that patients treated in such settings often feel that a sense of warmth and concern for their problems is lacking (Mechanic, *Public Expectations*). As the medical services needed become more complex, such patients are faced with a bewildering array of personnel attuned to their special functions, with often no one particularly responsible to the person as a whole. Such segmentation of care may inhibit the patient from raising questions or expressing fears and anxieties, and often results in failures to clarify mistaken perceptions and understandings. It may also strip the patient of a sense of personal dignity and worth, and indirectly may retard his capacity to overcome his problem.

The elaboration of care further confronts medical organizations with strategic problems of coordination. As more people participate in the patient's care, responsibility is more difficult to define, communication among medical personnel may break down, and patients may be given conflicting and confusing information about their problems. Errors in assessment and management of the patient may result because of communication failures or low morale among personnel. But elaboration of care may have even more basic consequences for the provision of humane care, for as each type of personnel directs attention to its special technical function, the comfort of the patient becomes secondary. The priorities are usually technical, and perhaps properly so. But we have yet to really understand the negative consequences of treating illness as a technical in contrast to a humane function (Howard and Strauss). While such actions as rooming a nervous patient suffering from a heart attack with a dying cancer patient may be seen simply as a housekeeping function, it may have devastating effects on the cardiac patient's morale and recuperation. Controlled clinical trials of patients with heart attacks who were treated at home and in a hospital, which show some advantage for home treatment, should give us cause to reflect on the role of care environments on illness (Mather et al.; Cochrane).

The problem is less the elaboration of care and more the priorities that govern it. The trend toward growing organization and specialization of function in recent years has been encouraged more for reasons of professional interest (Stevens) and efficiency (Mechanic, *Public Expectations*) than for the purpose of enhancing patient care. The priorities that have shaped therapeutic encounters have not been patient-centered ones, and we have developed some horrendous organizational practices in the process. But organizations can be humane if they reward humane behavior and if they treat patient concerns and comfort as important. This requires a clear concept of who is responsible for the patient's care as a whole and a willingness to weigh the advantages of one or another seemingly efficient practice against the total consequences for the patient, not only as a machine but as a moral actor who seeks to maintain a sense of dignity and self-esteem.

DAVID MECHANIC

[*Directly related are the other articles in this entry, and the entries:* CARE; HEALTH AND DISEASE, *article on* A SOCIOLOGICAL AND ACTION PERSPECTIVE; HEALTH CARE, *articles on* HEALTH-CARE SYSTEM *and* HUMANIZATION AND DEHUMANIZA-

TION OF HEALTH CARE; MEDICINE, SOCIOLOGY OF; *and* SOCIAL MEDICINE. *Other relevant material may be found under* MEDICAL MALPRACTICE; MEDICAL PROFESSION, *article on* MEDICAL PROFESSIONALISM; PATERNALISM; PATIENTS' RIGHTS MOVEMENT; *and* RIGHTS, *article on* RIGHTS IN BIOETHICS.]

BIBLIOGRAPHY

BALINT, MICHAEL. *The Doctor, His Patient, and the Illness.* New York: International Universities Press, 1957.

BLUM, RICHARD. *The Management of the Doctor–Patient Relationship.* New York: McGraw-Hill, 1960.

CARTWRIGHT, ANN. *Human Relations and Hospital Care.* Boston: Routledge & Kegan Paul, 1964.

COCHRANE, A. L. *Effectiveness and Efficiency: Random Reflections on Health Services.* London: Nuffield Provincial Hospital Trust, 1972.

DOHRENWEND, BARBARA S., and DOHRENWEND, BRUCE P., eds. *Stressful Life Events: Their Nature and Effects.* New York: Wiley-Interscience, 1974.

DUFF, RAYMOND S., and HOLLINGSHEAD, AUGUST B. *Sickness and Society.* New York: Harper & Row, 1968.

FRANK, JEROME. *Persuasion and Healing.* Baltimore: Johns Hopkins Press, 1961. Rev. ed. 1973.

FREIDSON, ELIOT. *Patients' Views of Medical Practice.* New York: Russell Sage Foundation, 1961.

HOWARD, JAN, and STRAUSS, ANSELM, eds. *Humanizing Health Care.* New York: Wiley-Interscience, 1975.

KADUSHIN, CHARLES. *Why People Go to Psychiatrists.* New York: Atherton Press, 1969.

LEY, P., and SPELMAN, M. S. *Communicating with the Patient.* London: Staples Press, 1967.

MATHER, H. G., et al. "Acute Myocardial Infarction: Home and Hospital Treatment." *British Medical Journal* 3 (1971): 334–338.

MECHANIC, DAVID. "Health and Illness in Technological Societies." *Hastings Center Studies* 1, no. 3 (1973), pp. 7–18.

———. *Medical Sociology: A Selective View.* New York: Free Press, 1968.

———. *Public Expectations and Health Care.* New York: Wiley-Interscience, 1972.

———. "Social Psychologic Factors Affecting the Presentation of Bodily Complaints." *New England Journal of Medicine* 286 (1972): 1132–1139.

PARSONS, TALCOTT. *The Social System.* New York: Free Press, 1951.

STEVENS, ROSEMARY. *American Medicine and the Public Interest.* New Haven: Yale University Press, 1971.

WHITE, K. L.; WILLIAMS, T. F.; and GREENBERG, B. G. "The Ecology of Medical Care." *New England Journal of Medicine* 265 (1961): 885–892.

IV

CONTEMPORARY MEDICAL PERSPECTIVE

Concepts of the therapeutic relationship have undergone evolution, particularly during this century. The conventional, idealized view of the physician simply attending to the sick patient has been altered and transformed by the awareness that this interaction is a complex personal relationship occurring within a social matrix. Conceptual understanding requires knowledge not only of what both doctor and patient bring to the relationship, but also of what social norms and forces are acting on the two.

However, it is the presence or possibility of serious illness that governs the genesis of a therapeutic relationship. Whether the doctor is caring for a person who has fallen ill or is looking after a well patient and fostering the bond of trust between them in anticipation of possible sickness, the phenomenon of illness remains the central point around which the relationship is built.

The phenomenon of illness

Whatever the cause, from fractures to cancer, the sick person undergoes a specific set of events that characterize the experience of illness. The sick person suffers a series of symptoms—alien body sensations and a loss of normal function occurring in a body he only poorly understands. He is disconnected from his normal world by his symptoms (from inability to walk to sensory deprivation), by external forces such as hospitalization or avoidance by others, and by his loss of interest in things and in persons.

The well individual functions with a sense of indestructibility that acts to deny the possibility of injury or death; the sick person is threatened with loss of his own sense of indestructibility. Further, in illness the ability to reason is weakened in the patient and cognitive function can be qualitatively impaired. Normal thought continually strives to comprehend the world, but the significance of events is often beyond the grasp and scope of the sick.

Perhaps the most powerful factor in the illness syndrome is the fact that the sick person must endure the loss of his sense of his own ability to control himself, his body, and his world. Maintaining control over oneself is so deep a human need that one might see all the other phenomena of illness as doing harm not only in their own right, but doubly so as they reinforce the sick person's perception that he is no longer in control (Cassell, 1976, pp. 25 ff.).

It should be understood that in any given instance of a doctor–patient interaction the extent to which these factors are operative may vary markedly. The degree to which the sick person loses his sense of his own indestructibility, becomes disconnected, finds his reasoning insufficient, and loses his control of self and of world varies with the severity of the sickness and the patient's perception of illness, as well as other personality and social factors. The patient may be entirely well, as in a preventive medical examination, or catastrophically ill following a heart attack. But however well or ill the patient is, the individual interaction with the physician takes place within a framework informed, at least in part, by past, present, or the possibility of future illness. The events in the set described above, which occur in illness, derive their force by their interplay with the personalities of both the patient and the physician, as well as the setting in which the interaction takes place.

The personality of the patient is of real import because features of illness such as the loss of control or the sense of disconnection may be better tolerated or, conversely, be more threatening to one individual than to another. It is for this reason that, in terms of the care of patients, the disease that causes an illness cannot be truly understood without the physician's understanding of the person in whom the disease occurs. The personality of the doctor is of concern insofar as individual physicians deal better or worse with some or all of the phenomena of illness. In seeking a therapeutic relationship, then, a patient—in addition to looking for a technically competent practitioner—is searching for a physician who is prepared to attend to personal factors that are or will be of serious consequence in his illness (Balint).

The setting in which the relationship takes place also influences how forcefully certain aspects of illness will operate. Impersonal versus personal settings and attitudes, high technology versus low technology settings—all have both positive and negative effects.

The physician in the therapeutic relationship

With the view of illness described above in mind, it is necessary to see what the doctor and the patient each bring to the therapeutic relationship aside from their personalities. The physician brings technical expertise drawn from training and experience. The technical knowledge includes not only the technical skills involved in the treatment of the patient but also the system of reasoning, knowledge, cares, and concerns by virtue of which medicine and society bring order into and remove mystery from the manifestations of illness. It is more important that the doctor's explanations be culturally consonant than that they be true, since

all explanations of illness as well as role relationships between doctor (healer) and patient are related to the belief system of the culture in which they occur (Ackerknecht). This is underscored by the fact that explanations of illness for most of the world's history and in most cultures have proved inadequate or false with the passage of time and the progress of scientific inquiry, despite the fact that they served their function while extant.

While technical expertise is part of the doctor's manifest contribution known to all participants, the physician also brings healing skills of which neither he nor the patient may be aware, particularly in Western scientific medicine. The healing factors, which are also of personal, moral concern for the patient, are necessary for dealing with those aspects of the illness syndrome identified above. The high social status accorded physicians in this society (and healers in almost all groups) allows them to replace the ill person's loss of social connection with their own connectedness. Physicians and clergy travel between the world of the well and the world of the sick and the dying. The physicians' own often overdeveloped sense of invulnerability and their patients' frequent attribution to them of exaggerated power over illness help supplant the sick person's loss of the sense of omnipotence. In addition, the doctor's rational system of explanations reinforces the patient's system of reason so that the mysteries of illness are again contained. Reflect, in this aspect, on how important it is that the patient's illness have a name, since the word is often seen as containing the thing (Laín Entralgo, 1970). The disease concepts of Western medicine can be seen in this light as a highly useful and effective conceptual structure. Finally, the physician serves as an alternative mode of control for the patient, restoring some balance to the relationship of the person with his body, as well as with the outer world.

The physician also brings to the relationship access to other parts of the medical care system such as medical specialists, drug prescriptions, diagnostic treatment facilities, hospitals, or other institutions. This function has become increasingly important in the highly technical and specialized medical care world of modern Western cultures. The social and moral functions of physicians have been much discussed in recent years with special attention paid to their ability to provide access to and legitimate the sick role, without which the patient cannot assume the special position assigned to the sick in this and other societies (Parsons). The importance of this function is illustrated by the change in the status of the alcoholic, as alcoholism has changed from being a moral problem to being an illness as well. Part of the same function is the ability of the physician to legitimate or even enforce the reentry of the sick person to the healthy world. This role is exemplified by the success of the rehabilitation movement since the Second World War in having society consider the physically disabled as healthy. The doctor also carries a legal mantle, shown by his sole right legally to pronounce death, as well as a host of certification functions. Finally, physicians, more than most, are expected to be honest, objective as well as empathetic, trustworthy, kind, and gentle.

It has been pointed out that physicians also serve a quasi-missionary function, which seems to compel them to convert their patients to their own standards for health and moral beliefs (Balint). This educational process may, when extreme, apply to all aspects of the patient's life, but it certainly applies to matters connected with health or sickness. Attitudes toward drug use, exercise, and cigarette smoking are obvious examples. Less apparent to both doctor and patient but no less important are basic beliefs about sickness and its causes and about attitudes toward the body. Each episode of illness for which the patient sees the physician provides the doctor with an opportunity to transmit his own beliefs. For one, it is that illness must be borne in passive silence; for another, the opposite. One doctor may transmit the attitude that the body is full of dangerous, hidden mysteries that may strike at any time, while another teaches that the body is a mutable friend. In this aspect of the relationship as in others, the patient is not merely a passive recipient. The patient may reject the lesson and the physician with it. Indeed, the patient may be teacher. Physicians are exposed to wide variations in human behavior, mostly because their daily confrontation with illness and their experience in treating a variety of persons inevitably shape their lives, their work, and their moral beliefs.

The patient in the therapeutic relationship

The patient brings to his relationship his need, manifested by the symptoms of his disease. As part of the process of socialization, starting in infancy, individuals in any group become aware of the acceptable mode in which symptoms must be expressed and aware of those problems which warrant the care of the doctor (Cassell, 1976). The patient also brings to the transaction a desire to get better as part of his social responsibility. Patients are expected to be honest and trusting in the relationship as well as to provide physical access to their person in a manner not usually accorded strangers. Finally, of course, the patient provides monetary reward to the doctor.

The patient, acting as client, also exercises powerful controls over both the form and substance of the physician's act. The patient may exercise this control through a self-determined referral system in which he seeks consultation on his own from more highly trained specialists if he perceives his illness to be beyond the competence of his primary physician. By questioning the diagnosis or treatment, he may cause his own physician to seek consultation, broaden the range of diagnostic tests, force hospitalization, or merely increase the time spent in his care. Such demands may be explicit but are more often made by the continued presentation of his symptoms to the physician. Client demand may induce physicians as a group to change what is considered proper practice. The rapid introduction of the Papanicolaou cervical smear ("Pap smear") into the routine examination was due as much to patient demand as to professional education. Of greater importance to ethical issues are currently increasing client demand for full explanations of diagnosis and treatment, for protection of the rights of patients and experimental subjects, and for a right to determine the care of the dying. In part, the modern patient has been able to increase his role in determining the nature of his care because of widespread and increasing knowledge among laymen about science and recent medical advances. In this sense, the patient becomes an intellectual partner in his own care. If his demands are perceived as excessive by the physician, however, the patient may diminish the bond of trust that holds the physician to him. Increasing fear of malpractice actions is the opposite face of the patient's desire for autonomy, and such fears also diminish the trust between physician and patient. Although the word *client* is used to refer to the patient, it should be seen as applying also to the patient's family and to the wider community.

Two views of the relationship: social implications

The elements of the therapeutic relationship described above lead to a picture of the interaction that is different in emphasis from that described by social scientists over the past few decades. Following Talcott Parsons's lead, or in reaction to it, social scientists have tended to see the doctor–patient relationship in terms of social roles, role conflicts, or power conflicts within the role model (Parsons and Fox). Their view of medicine has inevitably been *technico-social,* whereas that described above is a *technico-personal* view of the doctor–patient interaction. There are several reasons for the disparity of these two views, and the reasons are important to understanding the relationship. In the technico-social view, the sick person is seen simply as a well person with a disease, rather than as qualitatively different, not only physically but also socially, emotionally, and even cognitively. Indeed, the disease model is so widely accepted that the facets of illness described above, apart from the disease that caused them, have been insufficiently studied. When it is not understood that the relationship between doctor and patient is an important part of the process of returning to health, and it is believed that the physician's role in the care of the sick is primarily the application of technology for cure, then health can be seen as a commodity. In its most radical form, that view of medicine suggests that a surgeon performing an appendectomy is not different from a cabinet-maker building furniture, and the product (health), as well as the doctor–patient relationship itself, can be described in the usual economic or market terms. The more usual derivation of the technico-social view of medicine is that health is believed to be primarily the result of medical care (Winkelstein). More recently, as preventive medicine has been widely accepted, health is also thought to be the result of preventive care. In both instances access to health is seen as access to care. Such commodity views of medicine are true only to a limited degree. The healthy in a population are primarily those who have never been seriously ill. Indeed, epidemiologic evidence makes it clear that health is related far more to behavioral, social, and environmental factors than to medical care. Most medical care, then, is properly seen as illness care, not health care.

Therefore, the two views of the therapeutic relationship, primarily personal and primarily social, rest on differing views of the nature and source of health and the function of medical care. Two developments of modern society may tend to widen the divergence of these beliefs rather than effecting a necessary amalgam. The first, supporting the technico-social view, is the increasing use of the technology of medicine, paraprofessionals, and nonmedical personnel—which suggests that the involvement of physicians is either not necessary or even wasteful. The second, supporting the technico-personal view, is the increasing size of the aging population with its great burden of disease and disability. Here and in the chronic and incurable diseases that increasingly fill the disease picture of modern societies, patients and society are better served by a medicine resting on a basic understanding of the personal nature of the therapeutic relationship. This is underscored by recently highlighted problems in the care of the dying resulting from overzealous application of technology in the absence of sufficient personal and moral human understanding.

It seems important, however, that both major views of the therapeutic relationship be better studied and understood. To deny the importance of a wide social view of medicine would be to deny what could be gained from a much wider dissemination and utilization of modern medical technology. On the other hand, to deny the intimately personal nature of illness and the ethical as well as technical function of physicians as healers is to force medicine increasingly into a technological mold whose benefits may be many, but whose cost in human terms is also high. The care of the sick, whatever technology may be involved, ultimately arises from bonds among humans based in conscience, moral values, and the knowledge of the right.

Conclusion

The viewpoint of someone considering ethical issues in medical care will be greatly influenced by his perspective on the therapeutic relationship. The question of paternalism on the part of physicians and the related issue of the autonomy of the sick cannot be discussed without some reference to the respective characteristics and roles of the doctor and the sick person. If the sick person is regarded merely as a normally well person with a disease, and the doctor–patient relationship is looked at in mechanistic technico-social terms (a view Parsons did not hold, since he recognized the importance of the psychological issues involved), then ethical problems within medicine can be examined in the same light as ethical issues in politics. If the technico-personal perspective is followed and the sick person is seen as a wholly dependent creature having no autonomy because of his illness, then ethical issues in medicine can be looked at in the same light as the parent–child relationship. Both views are oversimplifications, which, moreover, miss an essential element in the therapeutic relationship—variation with time and situation. The complexity of the relationship—and part of the problem it poses for ethical analysis—derives not only from the number of variables present (social, technical, psychological, and economic) but from the fact that the doctor–patient relationship is not a thing but a process. As such, change is a key element: change over time in the same illness episode, change from episode to episode, change deriving from different modes of medical care delivery, and even change that comes from treatment by different types of medical specialists. It is precisely the complexity and variability of the therapeutic relationship that pose a challenge to ethical analysis.

ERIC J. CASSELL

[*While all the articles in this entry are relevant, see especially the articles* SOCIOHISTORICAL PERSPECTIVES *and* CONTEMPORARY SOCIOLOGICAL ANALYSIS. *For discussion of related ideas, see the entries:* CARE; HEALTH AND DISEASE, *articles on* A SOCIOLOGICAL AND ACTION PERSPECTIVE *and* PHILOSOPHICAL PERSPECTIVES; *and* PATERNALISM. *See also:* AGING AND THE AGED, *articles on* SOCIAL IMPLICATIONS OF AGING *and* HEALTH CARE AND RESEARCH IN THE AGED; INFORMED CONSENT IN THE THERAPEUTIC RELATIONSHIP; MEDICAL MALPRACTICE; MEDICAL PROFESSION, *article on* MEDICAL PROFESSIONALISM; RIGHT TO REFUSE MEDICAL CARE; RIGHTS, *article on* RIGHTS IN BIOETHICS; *and* TRUTH-TELLING. *See* APPENDIX, SECTION I, MEDICAL ETHICS: STATEMENTS OF POLICY DEFINITIONS AND RULES (BRITISH MEDICAL ASSOCIATION); *and* SECTION IV, AMERICAN OSTEOPATHIC ASSOCIATION, *and* AMERICAN PSYCHOLOGICAL ASSOCIATION.

BIBLIOGRAPHY

ACKERKNECHT, ERWIN HEINZ. *Medicine and Ethnology: Selected Essays.* Edited by Hans Huldrych Walser and Huldrych Martin Koelbing. Baltimore: Johns Hopkins Press, 1971.
BALINT, MICHAEL. *The Doctor, His Patient, and the Illness.* New York: International Universities Press, 1957.
CASSELL, ERIC J. "Disease as a Way of Life." *Commentary*, February 1973, pp. 80–82.
———. *The Healer's Art: A New Approach to the Doctor–Patient Relationship.* J. B. Lippincott Co., 1976.
———. "Preliminary Explorations of Thinking in Medicine." *Ethics in Science and Medicine* 2 (1975): 1–12.
FREIDSON, ELIOT. "Client Control and Medical Practice." *Patients, Physicians, and Illness: A Sourcebook in Behavioral Science and Health.* 2d ed. Edited by E. Gartly Jaco. New York: Free Press, 1972, pp. 214–221.
LAÍN ENTRALGO, P. *Doctor and Patient.* Translated by Frances Partridge. New York: McGraw-Hill Book Co., 1969.
———. *The Therapy of the Word in Classical Antiquity.* Edited and translated by L. J. Rather and John M. Sharp. New Haven: Yale University Press, 1970.
MAGRAW, RICHARD M. *Ferment in Medicine.* Philadelphia: W. B. Saunders, 1966.
PARSONS, TALCOTT. *The Social System.* New York: Free Press, 1951.
———, and FOX, RENÉE. "Therapy and the Modern Urban Family." *Journal of Social Issues* 8, no. 4 (1952), pp. 31–44.
WILSON, ROBERT N., and BLOOM, SAMUEL W. "Patient–Practitioner Relationships." *Handbook of Medical Sociology.* 2d ed. Edited by Howard E. Freeman, Sol Levine, and Lee G. Reeder. Englewood Cliffs, N.J.: Prentice-Hall, 1972, pp. 315–339.
WINKELSTEIN, WARREN, JR. "Epidemiological Consideration Underlying the Allocation of Health and Disease Care Resources." *International Journal of Epidemiology* 1 (1972): 69–74.

THERAPEUTIC RELATIONSHIP, INFORMED CONSENT IN

See INFORMED CONSENT IN THE THERAPEUTIC RELATIONSHIP.

THERAPIES, DYNAMIC

See DYNAMIC THERAPIES.

THERAPIES, MENTAL HEALTH

See MENTAL HEALTH THERAPIES.

THERAPIES, SELF-REALIZATION

See SELF-REALIZATION THERAPIES.

THERAPY AND VIOLENCE

See VIOLENCE AND THERAPY.

THERAPY, ELECTROCONVULSIVE

See ELECTROCONVULSIVE THERAPY.

THERAPY, GENETIC

See GENE THERAPY.

TOBACCO
See SMOKING.

TORTURE
See PRISONERS, *article on* TORTURE AND THE HEALTH PROFESSIONAL; WARFARE, *article on* BIOMEDICAL SCIENCE AND WAR.

TOTALITY, PRINCIPLE OF
See ORGAN TRANSPLANTATION, *article on* ETHICAL PRINCIPLES.

TRANSFUSION, BLOOD
See BLOOD TRANSFUSION.

TRANSPLANTATION
See ORGAN TRANSPLANTATION; KIDNEY DIALYSIS AND TRANSPLANTATION; HEART TRANSPLANTATION.

TRANSSEXUAL SURGERY
See SEXUAL IDENTITY.

TREATMENT REFUSAL
See RIGHT TO REFUSE MEDICAL CARE.

TRIAGE or TRIAGE MEDICINE
See RATIONING OF MEDICAL TREATMENT; JUSTICE; ENVIRONMENTAL ETHICS, *article on* QUESTIONS OF SOCIAL JUSTICE.

TRUTH-TELLING

I. ATTITUDES   *Robert M. Veatch*
II. ETHICAL ASPECTS   *Sissela Bok*

I
ATTITUDES

What information ought to be transmitted in medical relationships is among the most controversial issues in medical ethics. This article will review the range of attitudes held by lay people and medical professionals about such transmission. The question arises in a wide variety of contexts: whether the dying patient should be told of a bleak prognosis; how quickly the parents of a newborn genetically afflicted infant should be told by a physician-researcher of a small, unproved risk of a side effect with an experimental drug; whether the government should withhold information that might deter some citizens from participating in a national public health program such as an immunization campaign if it believes the public health will suffer from the decreased participation.

Ethical judgments about these questions will depend in part upon ethical norms: whether the objective is to produce the most happiness, protect individual rights, or follow general moral rules such as a prohibition against lying under certain circumstances. They will depend also upon beliefs about relevant facts. If one believes that the goal of the medical professional ought to be to benefit the patient, then it will make a great difference whether disclosing a bleak diagnosis is seen as psychologically disturbing or a relief from the anxiety of not knowing one's condition.

The normative ethical debate is the subject of the article following this one. The present article will address attitudes expressed by lay people and health-care professionals. It is often difficult to determine whether differences in these attitudes can be accounted for by differences in ethical norms or whether they are the result of disagreement about the consequences of a disclosure. Two people may disagree about telling a dying patient about a prognosis because, even if they both agreed disclosure would make the patient uncomfortable, one believes that the criterion should be making the patient comfortable while the other believes the criterion should be protecting the patient's autonomy to consent to treatment.

Information about attitudes on medical disclosure has been gathered primarily by social science survey researchers. The quality of the information varies. Furthermore the interpretation of the responses is open to debate. Some argue that one cannot immediately conclude that, because patients say they want to be told something, they really do want to be told that information or, more critically, they would want to be told it at a critical time such as prior to an operation or when they are terminally ill. On the other hand, reinterpretation of responses is exceedingly difficult. It is dangerous to attempt to translate expressed attitudes to "what an individual respondent really believes." No adequate method demonstrated to be valid has ever been devised. What is presented here is a review of attitudes as expressed. While taking these expressed attitudes completely at face value is questionable, reinterpretations are even more so. At least when there are important differences in expressed attitudes, it seems reasonable to assume that those differences reflect some real underlying views. Attitudes of lay people, both patients and healthy individuals, will be reviewed first; following that, attitudes of health-care professionals will be discussed.

Attitudes of lay people

Information about terminal illness. The paradigm case of medical truth-telling is whether to disclose information about diagnosis and prognosis to a terminally ill patient. Often the question is addressed in terms of the cancer patient. Kelly and Friesen surveyed three groups of lay people, all outpatients of university-affiliated hospitals. During the course of interviews with 100 cancer patients they determined that 89 preferred knowing about having cancer, while 6 said they would rather not know. When the question was put more generally, 73 said that they thought people in general should be told, while 4 thought they should not. The remainder were indefinite or thought it was an individual matter (Kelly and Friesen, p. 824).

Since the responses of these cancer patients could be interpreted as being influenced by the patient's knowledge of his cancer, Kelly and Friesen also asked a group of 100 noncancer patients. For that group Kelly and Friesen report that 82 said they wanted to be told while 14 said they did not. Finally they asked a group of 740 patients being examined in a cancer detection center. In that group 729 or 98.5 percent said they wanted to be told of the cancer diagnosis.

Other surveys have produced similar results. Branch found that 88 percent of a group who did not have cancer would prefer to be told of their condition should cancer develop. Samp and Curreri found that 81 percent of a group made up of both patients and nonpatients held that if a patient has cancer he or she should be told this fact while 11 percent said such a patient should not be told. A survey by *Medical World News* of 183 people ages fifty to eighty-six indicated that 80 percent said they would want to be told.

The British data are somewhat more varied. A study of 1,200 women in the Manchester area by Paterson and Aitken-Swan in 1953 asked, "Do you think a doctor should tell a person frankly when he is sure she has cancer?" They found that 40 percent said he should, 34 percent said he should not, and 26 percent were listed as "do not know." Aitken-Swan and Easson, in a study of British patients, used interview techniques to discover indirectly the nature of the patient's

reaction to the consultant's explanation. They reported initial patient responses for males and females. Among males 61 approved, while 1 disapproved and in 9 cases the findings were inconclusive; 23 were recorded as denying they had been told. Among females they reported that 92 approved, 17 disapproved, 21 denied having been told, and in 8 cases the results were inconclusive. The precise basis for classification was not reported, though in several cases the excerpts from the interviews are cited. For 41 patients the study was repeated two and a half years later. Little variation was found: 3 of the 32 who originally approved of being told now were reported as disapproving, while 2 of 5 who originally disapproved now were reported as approving. Their overall findings were that two-thirds of the group preferred to know what was wrong and 7 percent claimed to have been upset by the knowledge of their diagnosis.

Thus in spite of the differences in the respondent's condition, the precise wording of the questions, and the date of the survey, the studies indicate that lay people report consistently and by a significant margin that they want to be told of such a diagnosis.

Only one recent British study suggests a potentially contrary conclusion. McIntosh found that, among 74 patients hospitalized in a ward for the treatment of malignant diseases in a Scottish teaching hospital, 88 percent either knew or suspected that they had a malignant tumor at admission to the ward. He reported that "the great majority of them had no wish to augment that knowledge." The interpretation of this finding is difficult because the author never reports the basis of the finding, nor does he report the questions asked that led to this conclusion (making it impossible to know the basis of the author's conclusion), and because the finding is that the patients who already knew or suspected their condition did not desire to augment their knowledge. How this finding relates to the findings of the other studies that such individuals have a desire to know of their condition in the first place is not clear.

Other information. At this time there are no comparable attitudinal surveys about what lay people would want to know about nonterminal medical conditions, participation in medical research, participation in surgery, and formation of governmental public health policies. The increased amount of activity focusing on the issues of informed consent and patients' bills of rights suggests a similar interest on the part of lay people, but data are not available specifically confirming this. Among the questions to be addressed are: Do lay people have attitudes different from those of health professionals about how much information must be disclosed for consent to be informed? Do research subjects desire to be told only about potential risks and benefits of an experiment, or would they want to know about even nonrisky research—research where amputated limbs, human placentas, or bodily wastes were to be used, for instance? Recent American court cases such as *Cobbs* v. *Grant* recognize that it is still an open question whether the lay person would reasonably want to know a piece of information even if the consensus of the medical profession is that the information should not be disclosed. The implication may be that the American courts are beginning to hold open the possibility that lay people and medical professionals may differ on the question of what information must be disclosed for consent to be reasonably informed.

Health-care professionals

Physicians. Determining the attitudes of physicians about how much information should be transmitted to their patients is at least as complex a task as that of determining the views of lay people. Traditionally physicians have been committed to professional secrecy for its presumed therapeutic as well as other benefits. There is impressionistic evidence that physicians, at least in Western culture, are often reluctant to disclose information. The stated grounds are often that the information may be upsetting to the patient. Beginning in the 1950s there have been some American survey data to support that impression.

Fitts and Ravdin in a study published in 1953 questioned a sample of 444 physicians from eight specialty groups practicing medicine in Philadelphia County, Pennsylvania. There are some problems with the data—specialty groups were not represented in proportion to their presence in the county and 18 percent did not respond or responded with answers not complete enough to be analyzed. Nevertheless the responses give us some picture of the attitudes of this group of American physicians. In tabulating what Philadelphia physicians tell cancer patients they reported that 3 percent say they always tell, 28 percent say they usually tell, 57 percent that they usually do not tell, and 12 percent that they never do (Fitts and Ravdin, p. 902).

Oken asked a similar question of physicians in a study published in 1961. He asked 219 members of the staff of the Departments of Internal Medicine, Obstetrics–Gynecology, and Surgery of Michael Reese Hospital in Chicago; he received and tabulated 193 replies. Of the total group 88 percent said they followed a usual policy of not telling. They were subdivided into 9 percent of the total sample who said they never told, 47 percent who did not tell with rare exceptions, 29 percent who said they occasionally made exceptions to the policy of not telling, and 3 percent who said they often made such exceptions. Among those who said they followed a usual policy of telling, 4 percent often made exceptions, 5 percent occasionally did, 3 percent very rarely did, and none said they never made exceptions to the policy of not telling. The breakdown by specialties revealed variations that will be discussed below.

It has been suggested that attitudes of physicians are changing rapidly and that physicians in the 1970s would be more willing to disclose terminal cancer diagnoses. Rea, Greenspoon, and Spilka, in a study published in 1976 of 151 physicians in ten medical specialties, found that "39 percent expressed some degree of negativity toward informing these patients of their condition" (Rea, Greenspoon, and Spilka, pp. 293–294). Only 22 percent would refuse outright to tell a dying patient who is functioning well that he or she is terminal. For 30 percent, age of the patient was not a factor. Another 33 percent are least hesitant with patients over sixty-five and 30 percent are least hesitant with patients under eighteen (ibid., p. 294). The researchers attempted to determine the role of the family in deciding what should be disclosed. They found that 37 percent would primarily honor the wishes of the family; 9 percent would tell the patient what he wants to know regardless of the family's decision, and the remainder would leave their options open by coordinating with the family what the patient would be told (ibid., p. 295).

Differences among specialties. Not only are there apparent differences among physicians in general, specialties seem to have characteristic patterns as well. Fitts and Ravdin's data show dramatic differences by specialty (see table, page 1680).

For Oken's group the differences were not as dramatic. For internists 10 percent would follow the usual policy of disclosing; for surgeons the percentage was 12 percent; for generalists it was 24 percent (Oken, p. 1123).

	ALWAYS TELL OR USUALLY TELL
Dermatology-Syphilology	94%
Psychiatry-Neurology	60%
Surgery	41%
Academy of General Practice	30%
Nonspecialty groups	25%
Internal medicine	21%
Obstetrics–Gynecology	19%
Radiology	12%

Source: William T. Fitts, Jr., and I. S. Ravdin, "What Philadelphia Physicians Tell Patients with Cancer," *Journal of the American Medical Association* 153 (1953) 902. Copyright 1953, American Medical Association. Reprinted by permission of the publisher.

The study by Rea, Greenspoon, and Spilka reports a statistically significant difference among the ten specialties studied in judgments of the percentage of terminal patients that can be told of their condition. Oncologists—that is, cancer specialists—were the highest (84 percent), but the other percentages are not reported.

Other health-care professionals. There is relatively little information about the attitudes of other health-care professionals on the disclosure of medical information. Traditionally other health-care professionals—nurses, social workers, pharmacists, and other medical personnel—have been trained to leave final judgments about information transmission to the physician. This can sometimes create morally difficult situations, because the nurse, social worker, or even the orderly may be asked for information that he or she knows when the physician has adopted a policy of nondisclosure. There is reason to believe that these health professionals do not always share the views of the physician community. One survey of American nurses reading the magazine *Nursing 75* generated 15,430 responses (Popoff). Since they were self-selected respondents to a journal there are problems in knowing if there are biases. Nevertheless, the responses are informative. In response to the question, "When should a patient with a terminal illness be told that he is dying?" 60 percent said "as soon as possible after diagnosis," while 21 percent said only when he asks, and 2 percent said never. Another 16 percent said slowly, over an extended period of time, as illness progresses (ibid., p. 23). Nurses seem convinced that patients know about their terminal illness. They were asked, "When physicians have refused to tell your patients that they were dying, how many of these patients nevertheless clearly knew of and referred to their impending death?"

Although 24 percent said they had not cared for enough dying patients to estimate, 14 percent of the total group said less than 25 percent, 34 percent said up to 75 percent, and 23 percent said up to 90 percent. The moral dilemma of the nurse who feels that a patient ought to know his condition but also feels that the physician's instructions must predominate is seen in the response to the question, "When a patient who has a terminal illness bluntly asks you if he is dying and his physician does not want him to know, what do you usually do?": 1 percent would tell him, 2 percent would lie, saying they did not know, and 1 percent would reassure him that he is not dying, just ill. Some 14 percent would tell him that only the physician can answer the question. The vast majority would neither directly lie nor refuse to answer: 81 percent would "ask why he brought up the question, try to get him to talk about his feelings"; 1 percent more would avoid the question and try to distract him.

It seems clear that nurses differ among themselves on what patients should be told. Their views as a group may differ from those of the patient population they serve and the physicians and other health professionals among whom they must work. The moral dilemma for one in the nursing role is not only the basic dilemma of what to do when truth-telling seems to conflict with doing what will benefit the patient, but also one of what to do when the nurse sees behavior that, though justified by the traditional line of authority, he or she finds morally unacceptable.

Ethical implications

It seems likely that lay people, physicians, and other health-care professionals hold a wide range of attitudes about what information ought to be disclosed. Several moral dilemmas are posed by the differences, and several differences might account for them. The most basic question is, What, if anything, justifies withholding information potentially meaningful or useful to a patient or other decision maker? For family members, physicians, or other health-care professionals there is an additional moral question: What should be done when my judgment about what ought to be done conflicts with the patient's, and what is my responsibility for finding out what the patient's attitude is prior to beginning a medical relationship? Individual physicians, nurses, and patients will disagree about the relevant facts of a case as well as the more fundamental ethical principles of truth-telling even if there are no systematic differences from one of those groups to another. If it is the case that physicians as a group have a different attitude about truth-telling from that of patients, then there is still another ethical problem. In cases where the individual cannot be asked whether a diagnosis should be disclosed—in the case where one is trying to decide whether it is moral to disclose a terminal diagnosis, for instance—appeal might be made to the consensus view of the professional group. That is often a procedure for deciding which information must be transmitted for consent to be adequately informed in cases involving research or surgery. If, however, the consensus of the professional group reflects a special set of attitudes that are not shared by the patient, then the procedure would seem to be inadequate.

What accounts for differences among attitudes? The possible difference among medical specialties can be accounted for in several ways. In some cases the difference may be a function of the role of the physician; radiologists, for instance, are not likely to be primary care givers. In other cases it can be a function of the likelihood of successful treatment. Cancers of the skin have a high rate of effective treatment. This may explain the willingness of dermatologists to disclose. Another reason for the difference in attitudes may be that different individuals emphasize different consequences of disclosure or evaluate those consequences differently. Physicians may emphasize medical consequences of disclosure (such as fear that frightening a surgery patient with the risks of the surgery might deter him from the surgery) or the psychological consequences (such as anxiety and fear). Some patients may be concerned about the consequences for their families, business, or personal future planning. They may be concerned about religious preparation for dying. If different consequences are emphasized, or if the consequences are evaluated differently, then different attitudes about truth-telling may be plausible.

The relatively high rate for psychiatrists of willingness to disclose found by Fitts and Ravdin is provocative. Since psychiatrists would be expected to see relatively anxious and disturbed patients who would be likely to be upset at disclosure, one might expect them to be inclined against disclosure, especially if they believed the psychological impact would be negative. If psychiatrists are a specialty group with special skills necessary to evaluate the psychological impacts of disclosure, then their relative willingness to disclose in comparison with other physicians

may suggest that some other physicians tend to overestimate the harm done by disclosure. Several studies (Feifel; Schulz and Aderman) suggest that physicians tend to have uniquely high fear of death and that "most terminal patients suffer no permanent negative consequences if they are informed tactfully about the true nature of their illnesses" (Schulz and Aderman, p. 11). If an individual has high or low fear of death and then asks himself what the impact would be on another of disclosure of terminal illness, he may systematically misjudge the impact by appealing to his own high or low death fear.

Relatively few studies have been done to document harm or lack thereof from disclosures. Ralph Alfidi attempted to determine if patients would refuse angiographic procedures (a rather risky but important diagnostic test for measuring circulatory function). He explained in detailed written consent forms a large number of serious risks, expecting to prove that patients would refuse the angiography. Instead, out of a total of 232 patients (receiving two somewhat different forms) only 4 patients refused the procedure, and in one of those cases, when the patient's chart was examined, the physician found "questionable indications" for an angiogram and made no effort to change the patient's mind. The vast majority appreciated receiving the information, regarded it as useful, and indicated they would not have preferred to have had the information withheld.

Still another possible explanation for differences in attitudes is that some individuals or groups may prefer what they take to be indirect or gradual communication. Indirect communication including more subtle nonverbal ways of communicating is advocated by some as a more humane form of disclosure. All would agree that there are means of communicating that are unnecessarily blunt and insensitive. Yet the argument for indirect communication raises ethical problems as well (May; Veatch, p. 228). Sometimes it may simply be a rationalization for noncommunication. At least the problem is raised: How willing should one be to run the risk of misunderstood communication in order to attempt to be more humane? If indirect communication is defended on consequentialist grounds, then the same problems of errors in evaluating the consequences will arise in deciding the ethics of indirect communication as in evaluating more direct disclosure. If, on the other hand, one is making a moral argument that is not based on consequences, then it should make no difference whether the communication is direct or indirect, provided it conveys the message effectively.

Even if individuals dealing with similar kinds of cases with treatment potential are evaluating the same consequences, and are evaluating them in the same way, it is still possible that they may have different views on the ethics of truth-telling and withholding information. In that case it is likely that they are using different ethical principles. Differences in ethical norms about the duty to prevent harm, the duty to protect patient autonomy, and the right of the patient to consent to treatment could lead to different judgments about disclosure even if the evaluations of the impacts of the disclosure were similar.

ROBERT M. VEATCH

[*Directly related are the entries* INFORMED CONSENT IN THE THERAPEUTIC RELATIONSHIP; NURSING; PATERNALISM; SURGERY; *and* THERAPEUTIC RELATIONSHIP, *article on* CONTEMPORARY MEDICAL PERSPECTIVE.]

BIBLIOGRAPHY

AITKEN-SWAN, JEAN, and EASSON, E. C. "Reactions of Cancer Patients on Being Told Their Diagnosis." *British Medical Journal* 1 (1959): 779–783.

ALFIDI, RALPH J. "Informed Consent: A Study of Patient Reaction." *Journal of the American Medical Association* 216 (1971): 1325–1329.

BRANCH, C. H. "Psychiatric Aspects of Malignant Disease." *CA: Bulletin of Cancer Progress* 6, no. 3 (1956), pp. 102–104.

FEIFEL, HERMAN. "The Function of Attitudes toward Death." *Death and Dying: Attitudes of Patient and Doctor.* Group for the Advancement of Psychiatry, vol. 5, Symposium no. 11. New York: 1965, chap. 5, pp. 632–641.

FITTS, WILLIAMS T., JR., and RAVDIN, I. S. "What Philadelphia Physicians Tell Patients with Cancer." *Journal of the American Medical Association* 153 (1953): 901–904.

KELLY, WILLIAM D., and FRIESEN, STANLEY, R. "Do Cancer Patients Want to Be Told?" *Surgery* 27 (1950): 822–826.

McINTOSH, JIM. "Patients' Awareness and Desire for Information about Diagnosed but Undisclosed Malignant Disease." *Lancet* 2 (1976): 300–303.

MAY, WILLIAM F. "The Sacral Power of Death in Contemporary Experience." *Social Research* 39 (1972): 463–488.

OKEN, DONALD. "What to Tell Cancer Patients." *Journal of the American Medical Association* 175 (1961): 1120–1128.

"Over 65: Most of the Aged Want MD to Tell Them If They're Due to Die." *Medical World News,* 11 December 1970, p. 32a.

PATERSON, RALSTON, and AITKEN-SWAN, JEAN. "Public Opinion on Cancer: A Survey among Women in the Manchester Area." *Lancet* 2 (1954): 857–861.

POPOFF, DAVID, and *Nursing75.* "What Are Your Feelings about Death and Dying? Part I." *Nursing* 5, no. 8 (1975), pp. 15–24.

REA, M. PRISCILLA; GREENSPOON, SHIRLEY; and SPILKA, BERNARD. "Physicians and the Terminal Patient: Some Selected Attitudes and Behavior." *Omega* 6 (1975): 291–302.

SAMP, ROBERT J., and CURRERI, ANTHONY R. "A Questionnaire Survey on Public Cancer Education Obtained from Cancer Patients and Their Families." *Cancer* 10 (1957): 382–384.

SCHULZ, RICHARD, and ADERMAN, DAVID. "How the Medical Staff Copes with Dying Patients: A Critical Review." *Omega* 7 (1976): 11–21.

STANDARD, SAMUEL, and NATHAN, HELMUTH, eds. *Should the Patient Know the Truth?: A Response of Physicians, Nurses, Clergymen, and Lawyers.* New York: Springer, 1955.

VEATCH, ROBERT M. "She'll Be Happier If She Never Knows: The Patient's Right and Obligation to Have the Truth." *Death, Dying, and the Biological Revolution: Our Last Quest for Responsibility.* New Haven: Yale University Press, 1976, chap. 6, pp. 204–248.

II
ETHICAL ASPECTS

Communication enters into all human relationships, and all communication can be more or less truthful. What is spoken and left unsaid between health professionals and their patients is often of crucial importance insofar as it pertains to illness, well-being, at times even survival. Under this rubric fall many questions of confidentiality, access to records, informed consent, and others, which are discussed separately in this encyclopedia.

The primary concern of this article is with truthfulness and deception in therapeutic relationships. How much information should be given to patients and their families? Should a physician lie to a dying patient? To what extent should one physician answer questions honestly about a fellow physician's incompetence or fraud? And, quite apart from conscious deception of others, how should health professionals cope with the problems of error and self-deception in diagnosis, for instance, or in relying on different kinds of medical treatment?

These questions of truth and deception have been debated for centuries in medical practice and writings. A very wide latitude in behavior has always existed, from the quacks and purveyors of false remedies to the conscientious health professional who worries whether *any* method of communication can sufficiently inform a patient.

Ethical dilemmas in truth-telling

The major early oaths and codes are silent on the subject of what physicians should tell patients. To be sure, these documents often refer to the confidentiality with which information provided by patients should be treated; but there is no reference to honesty *toward* patients. The Declaration of Geneva (Etziony, p. 89), adopted in 1948 by the World Medical Association, is similarly silent on the subject.

The Code of Ethics of the American Medical Association of 1847 even endorses some forms of deception by stating that the physician has a sacred duty "to avoid all things which have a tendency to discourage the patient and to depress his spirits" (par. 4). The current Principles of Medical Ethics adopted by the same organization in 1957 (Ten Principles) bypass the question altogether, thus leaving the matter of informing patients up to the physician. As a result, patients are often given only that amount of information believed to be in their best interests.

It is at this point that we strike at the roots of the reluctance to recommend truthfulness. For there are many times when doctors judge that the best interests of patients will *not* be served by informing them of their conditions. At such times a dilemma exists which is acutely felt by some, though still ignored by many health professionals. On the one hand, lying to a patient goes against the basic moral principle of veracity and against the patient's right to make informed choices. Yet telling the truth, on the other hand, can at times seem harmful and not in the patient's best interests. The concern for curing and helping someone may then appear to run counter to the desire to be completely open. This is especially the case when patients are so affected by their illness or their medication as to be more dependent on those who care for them than usual, perhaps even seriously depressed.

Physicians, moreover, are acutely aware of the uncertainties of diagnosis and prognosis. They know how hard it is to give meaningful and correct answers to questions regarding health and illness. They also know that disclosing their uncertainty or their pessimistic prognosis can reduce those benefits which depend upon faith and the placebo effect. They dislike being the bearers of uncertain or bad news as much as anyone else. Sitting down to discuss an illness with a patient truthfully and sensitively may take much-needed time away from other patients. For all these reasons, physicians and other health professionals often prefer not to be bound by codes or rules that might limit their ability to suppress, delay, and even distort the information about their patients' conditions.

But the right of patients to be adequately informed is now increasingly being pressed by health consumers and regulatory agencies alike. Thus the recent Patient's Bill of Rights, published by the American Hospital Association, states that the patient has the right to receive information concerning his diagnosis, treatment, and prognosis, except when not medically advisable, in which case the information should be made available to an appropriate person in his behalf ("Statement").

The argument behind such a position is that, when information of this kind is denied or distorted, patients are no longer in a position to make informed choices concerning their health. Whether or not to enter a hospital, whether or not to have surgery, whether or not to put one's affairs in order as a prelude to dying—these most personal choices can then no longer be made by patients on the basis of the best available information. And patients, as consumers of medical care, are less willing than in the past to entrust the choice to the physician. This reduced trust stems in part from publicity given to the high levels of unnecessary surgery, hospitalization, and expensive or risky procedures. In part, it stems also from a growing change in the relationship of physician to patient from a paternalistic one to that of a partnership in which decision making is shared. And shared information is regarded as basic to shared decision making.

The issues of truth-telling in medical relationships, however, are not always so clear cut as to permit an obvious conflict to arise between the right to straightforward information concerning health and the motive to deceive based on what is most conducive to recovery. Very often, it is hard to know what constitutes truth-telling in the first place.

Truth-telling and deception

There are many false statements that are not intentionally deceptive. In medicine, as in all fields of knowledge, erroneous statements are often made in the belief that they are true. Useless or harmful remedies are prescribed; operations not known to be helpful are performed. Diagnostic techniques are employed that cannot give correct information. But unless the health professional knows that these are inappropriate, they are not intentionally deceptive.

In other ways, too, communication between doctors and patients can be interfered with or can fail to be understood without intentional deception on the part of the speaker. The speaker can be inarticulate, for example, or the listener too fatigued or emotionally wrought up to listen carefully. There can also be unexpected interferences with what is spoken, by noise or by other messages. Or a message can be so complex and filled with details, as in the bedside use of medical jargon, that the listener fails to comprehend or to get a clear picture of what is at stake.

It is important to take these unintentional factors of deception into account and to distinguish them carefully from what is purposely done or said to deceive or confuse. Only when communication is intended to mislead is there an *ethical* problem concerning transmission of information. For among the innumerable sources of error, one such source is clearly the human agent, receiving and providing information: deflecting, withholding, or distorting it. What is thus purposefully done to manipulate information reaching others constitutes the intricate variations on the theme of deception.

Intentional deception takes place when there is a flow of information between at least two persons, such that the information is believed by the transmitter to be misleading to the recipient and is intended to mislead. Such deception may be verbal, as when dying patients are told they will recover. We speak, then, of lies. But deception is often nonverbal, and conveyed instead by gestures or false visual cues; even by silence, as in situations where a clear risk ought to be pointed out.

These factors are all present in clear-cut cases of deception. When a child lies out of fear of the dentist's drill, or a physician falsely reports having treated 500 welfare patients, the magnitude of intentions and effects differs, and therefore also our evaluation of such acts differs, but there is no disagreement about the presence of deception as such. In other cases, however, there are doubts as to whether there has even been deception in the first place. This is so because the above-mentioned factors of communication, belief, and intention can be present to a greater or lesser degree.

Human beings constantly receive information from a number of sources—other persons, objects, their own bodies, the environment. Messages between human beings can be intentionally deceptive, and even truthful statements can deceive. A message can be couched in words impossible for a listener to understand, or spoken so rapidly that the listener is confused. Patients often have such experiences when doctors and medical students discuss their condition on rounds. Doctors, like lawyers and bureaucrats, often fail to make themselves understood. At times the resulting deception is intentional, at other times merely clumsy or based on a failure to understand the level of comprehension of the listeners.

A vexing problem in considering the factor of intentionally deceptive communication is that of distinguishing between *omission* and *commission*. Some argue that, if one remains silent, there is no communication and therefore no intentional deception, even if others turn out to be misled. In this way, many excuse themselves from responsibility for mishaps befalling others of which they could have given warning by arguing that silence cannot be deceptive.

But if two human beings are in a relationship such that communication under certain circumstances is known to be expected by both, then the lack of explicit communication is deceptive. When company physicians intentionally fail to inform employees that they are handling materials that can give them cancer, for instance, the employees are deceived intentionally, even though no actual lie may have been spoken. On the other hand, two persons who, on a subway for instance, happen to be next to each other but not in such a binding relationship are in a very different situation, where silence is not in any sense deceptive. In this way, a doctor who subjects a patient to a dangerous experiment with a new drug without informing the patient of its risks or asking for consent is deceiving the patient by remaining silent on these matters. But a doctor who sits across the aisle in a subway from someone whose skin has an easily curable condition but fails to communicate this fact is in no way acting deceptively.

To sum up: On the one hand, uttering a falsehood is always deceptive. Omitting to provide information, on the other hand, is deceptive only where one person is silent knowing that another will draw a false inference from that silence. Immense complexity enters into the evaluation of any lie as soon as one begins to consider the nature of what is omitted, the proportion of the total message which it constitutes, and its relevance to the listener.

Debates among moral philosophers

From antiquity on, philosophers and religious thinkers have debated issues having to do with deception and truth-telling. They have generally regarded truthfulness as fundamental to the existence of trust among human beings, and therefore as an indispensable trait for individuals to strive for. Aristotle expressed this sense of the inherent preference for truth over lying by saying, in the *Nicomachean Ethics*, that falsehood is in itself mean and culpable, and truth noble and full of praise.

Truth, then, is generally regarded as preferable if not indispensable, and deception as something that, at the very least, stands in need of justification. All, therefore, agree that the burden of proof rests on those who wish to defend instances of deception. The major dividing line separates those who believe, with Kant, that there can be no sufficient justification for lying and those who believe that there are times when deception can be justifiably undertaken. Those who subscribe to the latter view, when asked to give examples of justifiable lies, often point to times when they believe it is right for physicians to deceive their patients.

Thus Plato argued that falsehood should be available to physicians as "medicine" for the good of patients, but not to laymen who should have no part of it (Plato). Then, by analogy, the rulers of a city should also be able to lie to citizens for the public good. Sidgwick similarly argued that lies to invalids and children could be warranted by the best interests of those thus deceived (Sidgwick, p. 316).

The most subtle and illuminating account of all the complex forms of duplicity may well be that given by Augustine. He argues that all lies should be avoided, even the mildest ones, because they are forbidden by God. Not even to preserve chastity or life itself ought lies to be told. Nor should Christians lie to heretics in order to draw them out of hiding. But Augustine admits being troubled in situations where the truth would deal a cruel blow to an innocent person. He qualifies his prohibition of lies by holding that some lies, though never justifiable, are more excusable than others, thus providing some flexibility for desperate situations. Moreover, certain forms of concealment are permitted, but never by means of falsehood (Augustine).

Aquinas treats truth and lying in the *Summa Theologiae* with frequent references to Augustine's works. He divides lies into three kinds: officious lies, told for the well-being and convenience of someone; jocose lies, told in fun; and mischievous lies, told in malice. The last kind constitutes the gravest sin (Thomas Aquinas). He also takes up the distinction first made by Aristotle in the *Nicomachean Ethics* between lies that go beyond the truth, and constitute boasting, and lies that stop short of the truth, belonging to irony. Truth itself is then seen as a mean between the two.

For Aquinas, as for Augustine, certain lies that intend great good are less serious than the others. Nevertheless, both counsel against all lies, holding them to be unnatural since they go against the very purpose of communication, which is to convey truth.

While excluding lies, Aquinas permits concealment, as did Augustine, and distinguishes from lying the truthful statement intended to awaken false meanings in others. This distinction gave rise to a vast controversy in the centuries to follow. Much was at stake for those who believed that certain statements, if characterized as lies, could cause speakers to suffer eternal damnation, whereas if held *not* deceptive could have no such horrible consequences, while permitting a comfortable latitude in behavior. By omitting the intention to deceive from the definition of lying, some scholastics came to regard a whole panoply of deceptive statements not as lies, but as statements made with "mental reservations." Thus a culprit, asked whether he had broken somebody's window, could answer "no," according to these thinkers, so long as he made the mental reservation that he meant "no, not last year," or "no, not with an axe."

The same reasoning has been used in medicine, even very recently. Thus McFadden (pp. 388–413) argues that doctors and nurses can answer, when asked by a feverish patient to know his temperature, that it is normal, making the mental reservation that the temperature is normal for that patient's physical condition. He holds that when a permissible mental reservation is made, the speaker does not deceive the questioner. Rather, the questioner places a hasty interpretation on the words he hears and thus misleads himself.

In a powerful but brief article, Kant ("On a Supposed Right") took a distance from these and other compromises about lying. Using a well-known scholastic example of a murderer asking for the whereabouts of his victim, Kant argued that even then a lie would be a breach of the duty of veracity that is owed to all people. Elsewhere, in the *Metaphysics of Morals*, he held that in telling a lie a man throws away, even annihilates, his dignity as a man. Looking back at the distinction made by Aquinas between lies that harm others and other lies, Kant stated that lies are reprehensible whether or not they harm others, since they degrade the liar himself. Jeremy Bentham (pp. 205–223) disagreed sharply with Kant on this issue. If there could be a falsehood without any harmful effects, he argued, it could not possibly constitute an offense either to others or to the liar. He went on to say, however, that in practice there is scarcely any pernicious effect that falsehoods do not produce; in practice, therefore, his policy toward lying might not differ substantially from that of Kant.

But it is important to see that consequences determine the evaluation of a lie for Bentham, whereas this is not so for Kant. The utilitarian position in moral philosophy, expounded by Bentham, was elaborated and defended by many. Thus Sidgwick took for granted that certain lies are necessary, such as those told to invalids if dangerous shocks can thereby be avoided. And he stated that the way to decide whether or not a lie is allowable is to weigh the gain of any particular deception against the imperilment of mutual confidence involved in all violation of the truth. But this process of weighing gains and losses, which is advocated by all utilitarians, runs into great problems in actual application. It is hard enough to make such estimates for one person; but to make them for several, as must needs be done in all cases of deception, which are by definition interpersonal, is well nigh impossible except in the simplest of cases.

Several philosophers in this century have shown how one might go beyond the Kantian position (which allows for no moral conflict once truthfulness is at stake, and which they therefore regard as discordant with our moral intuition), and also beyond the utilitarian position (with its problems of application and its assumption that there is nothing inherently valuable about truthfulness apart from its consequences). Ross, in *The Right and The Good*, argues that there is a *prima facie duty* of fidelity, which includes that of veracity, but that such a duty can conflict with other *prima facie duties*, such as that of "not injuring others," or that of "beneficence." And Warnock, in *The Object of Morality*, similarly stresses the possibility of conflict among duties. He states that the four virtues of nonmaleficence, beneficence, justice, and veracity are required if things are not to go quite

so badly among human beings as they otherwise might, given the nature of the human predicament. But there can be no assurance that these will always work together; at times they may even be in such a conflict that no good solution exists.

Medicine and truth-telling

Moral philosophers, then, disagree about whether there can be any exceptions to a policy of truth-telling, and, if there are to be exceptions, what these might be. Among those who hold that there *are* exceptions, there is agreement on the point that a lie to save someone from imminent harm is the most clear cut of these exceptions. This is precisely the view taken by many physicians who advocate lying or withholding the truth from patients. Physicians may be bound to uphold moral principles, according to this view, but the most important of all moral principles is to "do no harm." If physicians find themselves in situations where information is of a saddening, sometimes of a frightening and even harmful nature, they should be able to temper the truth, perhaps to alter it.

Thus Dr. Oliver Wendell Holmes advised young physicians in his *Medical Essays* (p. 398), to deceive the sick and the dying in their own best interests, holding that the face of a physician, like that of a diplomatist, should be impenetrable. Nature is a benevolent old hypocrite, he argued, who cheats the sick and the dying with illusions better than any anodynes.

Indeed, lies to the dying have come to seem the prototype for such benevolent deception. Three distinct arguments support such a position. In the first place, it is clear that perfect information can never be given on any subject to anyone. As a result, a number of writers have supported Henderson's conclusion that any information given would be imperfect, and that there is therefore no possible clear distinction between true and false information in medicine (Henderson). This argument shows a confusion between the dimensions of completeness and accuracy of information. It is clearly an absurdity in most walks of life to say that, because complete information is impossible, erroneous information can be justified.

The second argument often made by practitioners is that patients do not in fact *want* information of a depressing kind; that they resist it, fail to understand it, or forget it when it is provided. While it is doubtless clear that many cope with such information with some degree of resistance, there is growing evidence to contradict the notion that patients do not want it at all; the great majority of patients want to be told of critical illness, and their most consistent complaint is that they are kept in the dark, not informed, sometimes lied to (Waitzkin and Stoeckle). Tolstoy provides an unforgettable portrait of a man thus deceived in *The Death of Ivan Ilych;* the story is pervaded by his sense of terror and despair, of inadequate knowledge and occasional hope, of anger at the refusal of family and physicians to help him cope with his life's hardest struggle. It provides a vivid response to the complacent view that dying patients know about their condition without needing anybody to discuss it with them.

Fletcher has argued, in *Morals and Medicine,* that not only should doctors provide truthful information even to patients who do not ask for it, but even patients who give every overt sign of refusing to want to deal with such information should be confronted with it. And a physician should consider himself entitled to ask to withdraw from a case if a patient persists in this refusal. Many doctors would disagree with such a way of dealing with patients who need their help and who are unable to assimilate truthful information. They argue that the patient's wish to be spared such information should be respected, especially if it is overtly expressed.

The third argument for altering the truth holds that the patient's right to know must be balanced against the risk of harm that the knowledge might bring about. Perhaps a patient will suffer a cardiac arrest or wish to commit suicide on receiving painful news. Perhaps he may simply cease to struggle, and thus not seize the small chance of recovery. The principle of the "therapeutic privilege" upholds the doctor's legal right to withhold information from patients in cases where it would clearly be deleterious to the health of patients. But this privilege has been sharply limited by the courts, and commentators have argued that it ought not to be based, as is now the case, on the standards of other physicians in the community (Fried, p. 22). Certainly this privilege cannot be interpreted so broadly as to permit physicians to deceive patients "for their own good" as a general practice.

Conclusion

Most philosophers and physicians agree that some balance between veracity and the harms it can bring must at times be struck. There are great differences in practice, however, which stem in part from the divergent ways in which truth is defined, in part also from what is and is not seen to be actually harmful. In medical activities ranging from the care of the terminally ill to the everyday prescription of placebos (Bok), the problems of truth-telling and deception are pervasive. They expose basic differences of point of view as to what is owed to human beings.

SISSELA BOK

[*Directly related are the entries* HUMAN EXPERIMENTATION, *article on* BASIC ISSUES; INFORMED CONSENT IN HUMAN RESEARCH, *article on* ETHICAL AND LEGAL ASPECTS; *and* INFORMED CONSENT IN THE THERAPEUTIC RELATIONSHIP, *article on* LEGAL AND ETHICAL ASPECTS. *Also directly related is the other article in this entry,* ATTITUDES. *Other relevant material may be found under* PATIENTS' RIGHTS MOVEMENT; RIGHT TO REFUSE MEDICAL CARE; RIGHTS; *and* THERAPEUTIC RELATIONSHIP. *See also:* CONFIDENTIALITY; ORTHODOXY IN MEDICINE; *and* PATERNALISM. *See* APPENDIX, SECTION I, PRINCIPLES OF MEDICAL ETHICS (AMERICAN MEDICAL ASSOCIATION); *and* SECTION III, A PATIENT'S BILL OF RIGHTS.]

BIBLIOGRAPHY

ARISTOTLE. *Nicomachaen Ethics.* 4, 7, 1127.

AUGUSTINE. "De mendacio" [Lying], "Contra mendacium" [Against Lying]. *St. Augustine.* Vol. 14: *Treatises on Various Subjects.* The Fathers of the Church: A New Translation, vol. 16. Edited by Roy J. Deferrari. New York: Fathers of the Church, 1952, pp. 45–110, 111–179.

BENTHAM, JEREMY. "Division of Offenses." *An Introduction to the Principles of Morals and Legislation* (1823). Hafner Library of Classics, no. 6. New York: 1948, chap. 16, pp. 204–308.

BOK, SISSELA. "The Ethics of Giving Placebos." *Scientific American* 231, no. 5 (1974), pp. 17–23.

CABOT, RICHARD CLARKE. "Team-Work of Doctor and Patient through the Annihilation of Lying." *Social Services and the Art of Healing.* New York: Moffat, Yard & Co., 1909, pp. 116–170.

DAVIES, EDMUND. "The Patient's Right to Know the Truth." *Proceedings of the Royal Society of Medicine* 66 (1973): 533–536.

ETZIONY, M. B., ed. *The Physician's Creed.* Springfield, Ill.: Charles C. Thomas Publishers, 1973.

FLETCHER, JOSEPH FRANCIS. "Medical Diagnosis: Our Right to Know the Truth." *Morals and Medicine: The Moral Problems of: The Patient's Right to Know the Truth, Contraception, Artificial Insemination, Sterilization, Euthanasia.* Foreword by Karl Menninger. Princeton: Princeton University Press, 1954. Paperback ed. Boston: Beacon Press, 1960, pp. 34–64.

FRIED, CHARLES. *Medical Experimentation: Personal Integrity and Social Policy.* Clinical Studies, A North-Holland Frontiers Series, vol. 5. Edited by A. G.

Bearn, D. A. K. Blank, and H. H. Hiatt. New York: American Elsevier Publishing Co., 1974.

HARROD, R. F. "Utilitarianism Revised." *Mind* 45 (1936): 137–156.

HENDERSON, L. J. "Physician and Patient as a Social System." *New England Journal of Medicine* 212 (1935): 819–823.

HOLMES, OLIVER WENDELL. "The Young Practitioner." *The Writings of Oliver Wendell Holmes.* 13 vols. Riverside ed. Vol. 9: *Medical Essays 1842–1882.* Boston: Houghton, Mifflin & Co., 1891, pp. 370–395, especially pp. 388–389.

KANT, IMMANUEL. "On Lying." *The Doctrine of Virtue: Part II of the Metaphysics of Morals and the Pref. to the Doctrine of Law.* Translated by Mary J. Gregor. Foreword by H. J. Paton. New York: Harper & Row, 1964. Reprint. Philadelphia: University of Pennsylvania Press, 1971, pp. 92–96.

————. "On a Supposed Right to Tell Lies from Benevolent Motives." *The Critique of Practical Reason and Other Writings in Moral Philosophy.* Translated by Lewis White Beck. Chicago: University of Chicago Press, 1949, pp. 346–450.

LUND, CHARLES C. "The Doctor, the Patient and the Truth." *Annals of Internal Medicine* 24 (1946): 955–959.

McFADDEN, CHARLES JOSEPH. *Medical Ethics.* 6th ed. Foreword by Fulton J. Sheen. Philadelphia: F. A. Davis Co., 1967. First edition published in 1946 under the title *Medical Ethics for Nurses.*

MEYER, BERNARD C. "Truth and the Physician." *Bulletin of the New York Academy of Medicine* 45 (1969): 59–71.

PEMBERTON, L. BEATY. "Diagnosis: Ca: Should We Tell the Truth?" *Bulletin of the American College of Surgeons,* March 1971, pp. 7–13.

PLATO. *Republic.* 389B–389D.

PIAGET, JEAN. "Adult Constraint and Moral Realism." *The Moral Judgment of the Child.* Translated by Marjorie Gabain. Glencoe, Ill.: Free Press, 1948, chap. 2, pp. 104–194.

"Principles of Medical Ethics of the American Medical Association." *Journal of the American Medical Association* 164 (1957): 1119–1120.

ROSS, WILLIAM DAVID. *The Right and the Good.* Oxford: At the Clarendon Press, 1930, pp. 19–22.

SIDGWICK, HENRY. "Classification of Duties—Veracity." *The Methods of Ethics.* London: Macmillan & Co., 1909, pp. 312–319. Reprint. New York: Dover Publications, 1966.

"Statement on a Patient's Bill of Rights." *Hospitals,* 16 February 1973, p. 41. "Affirmed by the Board of Trustees, Nov. 17, 1972."

THOMAS AQUINAS. *Summa Theologiae.* II–II 40,3.

TOLSTOY, LEO. "The Death of Ivan Ilych." *Great Short Works of Leo Tolstoy.* Introduction by John Bayley. Translated by Louise Maude and Aylmer Maude. A Perennial Classic, no. 3071. New York: Harper & Row, 1967, pp. 245–302.

WAITZKIN, H., and STOECKLE, J. D. "The Communication of Information about Illness: Clinical, Sociological, and Methodological Consideration." *Psychosocial Aspects of Physical Illness.* Edited by Z. J. Lipowski. Advances in Psychosomatic Medicine, vol. 8. Edited by J. Bastianns et al. New York: S. Karger, 1972, pp. 180–215.

WARNOCK, GEOFFREY JAMES. "Moral Virtues." *The Object of Morality.* London: Methuen & Co., 1971, chap. 6, pp. 71–93.

UV

UNITED STATES

See MEDICAL ETHICS, HISTORY OF, *section on* EUROPE AND THE AMERICAS, *articles on* INTRODUCTION TO THE MODERN PERIOD IN EUROPE AND THE AMERICAS, BRITAIN AND THE UNITED STATES IN THE EIGHTEENTH CENTURY, NORTH AMERICA: SEVENTEENTH TO NINETEENTH CENTURY, *and* NORTH AMERICA IN THE TWENTIETH CENTURY.

UTILITARIANISM

See ETHICS, *articles on* TELEOLOGICAL THEORIES *and* UTILITARIANISM.

VIOLENCE AND THERAPY

The meanings of "violence"

In ordinary usage, "violence," which has the same Latin root as "vehemence," means "excessive use of force," and since each person's idea of excess tends to differ the application of the term to various situations is, essentially, a subjective matter. So, in order to introduce the degree of objectivity demanded by their discipline, for the purposes of their work scientists have redefined "violence" in terms of "aggression"—not aggression in the ordinary English sense of unprovoked attack, nor the peculiarly American conception of aggressiveness as self-assertion, but rather the relatively objective notion developed for the study of animal behavior in which an animal is held to act aggressively if it inflicts, attempts to inflict, or threatens to inflict, a harm or damage to an animal or something closely identified with an animal. So "violence"

was redefined as intraspecial aggression; thus an act of violence is an act of intraspecial aggression, and a violent person is one who is performing or who is predisposed to perform such acts. Or, to put the point differently, when a scientist uses the expression "human violence" he is talking about human beings inflicting, attempting to inflict, or threatening to inflict a harm or damage to a human being (including himself). Now this conception of human violence is quite different from the lay conception. Ordinarily, we tend to distinguish between violent crimes, such as rape or murder, and nonviolent crimes such as embezzlement. No such distinction can be made among victimed crimes on the scientific conception of human violence, for on the scientific view forging a signature is as truly an act of violence as assault or genocide. Despite the oddness of some aspects of the scientific usage, I shall be using the term "violence" in its scientific sense throughout this article.

Classical medicine and the control of violence

Classically, the Hippocratic physician was constrained by his moral obligations to his guild and to his patient, and by the limits of his expertise. His primary moral obligation was defined by the principle of patient benefit, the principle that, to use the words of the classical Oath, the physician is to "follow that system of regimen which, according to my knowledge and ability, I consider for the *benefit* of my *patients.*"

His expertise was limited to discovering, preventing, ameliorating, or curing the *diseases* or disorders of his patients. Benefit, disease, and patient were thus the sine qua non for the applicability of classical medical models. And so, if any of these should prove to be inapplicable to the violent—i.e., if the violent cannot be benefited, if they have no disease, if they are not patients—then, for the classical physician, violence would not be a matter of medical concern; in other words, the classical medical model would be inapplicable to violence. And, of course, there are innumerable acts that are violent, in the scientific sense, but that no one would hold to be a matter of sickness or disease. Consider surgery, a physically damaging intrusion into the body. As a damaging intrusion, the act qualifies as intraspecial aggression, and hence as violence in the scientific sense of the term. Yet, surely, a surgeon performing an appendectomy would not ordinarily be thought of as sick or pathologically violent. Hence the violence of the surgeon provides us with a paradigm of nonpathological violence—violence unassimilable to a medical model. By way of contrast, the rage of hydrophobics provides a paradigm of medically assimilable violence. Hydrophobia, or rabies, is the result of an infection of the spinal column and brain—a disease—that causes rage, which in turn frequently leads to involuntary attacks on others and typically impels the victim voluntarily to accept the role of patient. Here we have the contrast between violence assimilable to the classical model—rabies, with its disease, healing, and patient—and violence unassimilable to the classical model—the surgeon, who is neither diseased nor a patient, and who cannot benefit from medical attention.

Unfortunately, most violence falls somewhere between the paradigms of pathology and nonpathology established by rabies and surgery. Consider the case of a continual handwasher who has worn his fingers rather close to the bone. If the handwasher, unlike the typical hydrophobe, but like the surgeon, does feel himself to be suffering from an illness and so does not voluntarily assume the role of patient, but nonetheless seems to be involuntarily compelled to self-destruction, should his self-directed violence be assimilated to a medical model? Should a physician *force* the handwasher to accept the role of patient against the handwasher's wishes? There are, as it turns out, four patterns of answers given to this question, four positions on the assimilability of nonparadigmatic violence to medical models: (1) ultratraditionalism, (2) conservatism, (3) liberalism, and (4) ultraliberalism.

Ultratraditionalism

Within traditional Hippocratic–Galenic medicine there was no objective scientific criterion for determining which organic states should be recognized as symptoms or as abnormal. Rather, classical medicine was built on a model of individual self-determination of symptoms. Symptoms are self-discovered anomalies that impel the sick into the physician's hands as volunteered patients. Pathology is simply those abnormal states capable of causing symptoms; thus pathology is parasitic on symptomology. Hence, it would appear that, within classical medicine, unless a patient acknowledges a symptom as such, he cannot be said to be in a pathological condition.

If one is to retain the traditional model of classical medicine, one cannot regard the continual handwasher, or any other violent person, as suffering from a pathological condition or as a patient unless he himself recognizes his handwashing as symptomatic. It follows, argue the ultratraditionalists, that save in those relatively few cases where the violent themselves regard their violence as pathological, violence is unassimilable to traditional medical models (Szasz, 1961).

Conservatism

In reply conservatives provide a slightly different reading of classical medicine and focus rather sharply on the rabies case. They note that, even when no aid was requested, the physician could aid the rabies victim if the physician believed that by doing so he was satisfying the principle of patient benefit by acting in the patient's interest. It is, the conservatives argue, "the physician's duty to help those who are in no position to recognize the fact that they are in need of help." Thus, if it is reasonable to view the handwasher's continual handwashing as a symptom of a disease, the Hippocratic principle of patient benefit obligates the physician to treat the handwasher as a patient, even if the "patient" is in no position to recognize that he is sick and to volunteer for the role of patient.

Consider another case. Suppose that a hemodialysis patient, knowing the fatal consequences of discontinuing treatment, requests that his treatments be discontinued nonetheless. Here we have a case where, unlike the case of the person so raving or so debilitated that he cannot request help, the patient seems to come to a deliberate, albeit suicidal, decision. Can a Hippocratic physician override such a decision?

Suppose that the physician had clear evidence that the patient's suicidal inclinations were caused by a depressive state attendant upon his uremia or some other condition caused by his illness. Would he not, then, have evidence that it was not the patient's decision but rather the disease's so to speak? And if the uremia were reversible, does not the Hippocratic physician's obligation to the principle of patient benefit obligate him to treat this patient, just as it obligates him to treat the severely debilitated and the rabid, despite the patient's request that treatment be terminated?

Szasz and other ultratraditionalists would claim that the conservative argument is meaningless nonsense. To have a disease is to be in an abnormal condition that can or will cause states that the patient himself will accept as symptoms. Clearly the hemodialysis patient does not accept his desire to commit suicide as a symptom, nor does the handwasher view his behavior as symptomatic; hence, on the classical model, those behaviors cannot be viewed as pathological. Absent pathology, absent the rationale for medical intervention. Hence, neither the handwasher's nor the dialysis patient's case can be assimilated to the classical model. Moreover, ultratraditionalists argue, it would be a mistake to liberalize the model in order to accommodate cases such as these; for, however humane the motivation for liberalization might be, the institutionalization of such humanitarianism is unworkable, since in practice there is no way of ensuring that the conservative is not imposing his own alien ideals upon the patient (Szasz, 1970).

Most conservatives recognize this danger and seek the liberalization of the classical model, believing that they can guard against abuses. Vernon Mark and Robert Neville have, in fact, attempted to develop safeguards for the medical treatment of nonparadigm cases of violence to ensure that the operative interests in treatment are those of the patient. They argue that nonparadigmatic cases of violence are assimilable to a conservative interpretation of the classical medical model only if the violence is caused by a determinate abnormality of the type that would be recognized as pathological in noncontroversial cases (Mark and Neville). On this criterion, while pathology in general remains parasitic upon symptomology, the pathology of the instant case is not. It is independent not only of the patient's determination of what counts as a symptom (and so is useful in cases where the patient cannot or will not recognize his symp-

toms as such) but also of the physician's valuation of what should count as a symptom (and here lies its value as a response to the ultratraditionalist fear that the physician will impose his values on the patient). The criterion can act as a constraint both on the subjective biases of the physician and the disease-induced incompetency of the patient by appealing to the neutral standard of general recognition of pathology in noncontroversial cases. So, just as the Hippocratic physician's decision to treat the nonconsenting rabies victim or debilitated patient is legitimate, even obligatory on the principle of patient benefit—since *in general,* when competent, people recognize this condition as pathological and seek treatment—similarly, if the continual handwasher can be determined to be suffering from a lesion of the brain or from some other condition that would be recognized as pathological in noncontroversial cases, the Hippocratic physician can and should treat him.

The strength of the Mark–Neville criterion is to be found not only in its appeal to generality but in its requirement of determinate pathology. For, as the criterion is stated here, and as Mark and Neville use it in their writings, it is applied only to cases where the condition deemed pathological can be distinguished from the anomalies held to be symptomatic. Disease cannot be postulated, causality may not be hypothesized, an anomaly cannot be transubstantiated into a symptom simply by dubbing it a "syndrome"; the causal relationship must have been discovered. And the insistence on determinate causality is important, because it inhibits the propensity to utilize the medical epithet and the medical institution as a mechanism of social control. Without such a check any deviant could be recruited into a medical model if the society regarded his deviation as "sick." Thus a society of warriors might regard Ghandian pacifists as suffering from "hypoaggressive syndrome," while a society of pacificists might regard those who played football as "hyperaggressives." But any such medicalization of nonviolence or violence is impermissible on the Mark–Neville criterion, even if there is virtually universal agreement that the behavior in question is sick, for unless a cause for this behavior has been discovered, and unless there is also a consensus that, in noncontroversial cases, this cause is pathological, even universally despised behavior is unassimilable to a medical model.

If the requirement of determinate pathology is one of the strengths of the Mark–Neville criterion, it is also a severe limitation. For, while pathology of the brain may be detected by X-ray even in asymptomatic cases, nonphysiological psychopathology cannot even be detected by anything as definite as a shadow on a negative of an X-ray, and it is virtually undetectable in the absence of symptoms. Thus, either the criterion will have to be read as ruling out the possibility of treating nonparadigmatic cases of violence on a nonphysiological psychiatric model, or it will have to be weakened to accommodate the notion of psychopathology. The work of many psychiatrists, while not addressing the Mark–Neville criterion directly, seems to be involved with the specification of criteria of pathology that would create a version of the Mark–Neville test liberalized to meet the special problems of psychiatry (these psychiatrists are referred to as *liberals*).

Liberalism

Typically, liberal conceptions of psychopathology are premised on a conception of the *normal* psychophysical organism as purposively self-maintaining, or homeostatic. And so any psychophysical state that threatens homeostasis (e.g., uremia, which induces suicidal depression) is *abnormal* and hence pathological. On one interpretation of this view,

. . . expressions of violence may be regarded as psychopathological only when they are expressive of abnormal development or impairment of function of the *individual* superego and ego. One may discern at least five patterns of maldevelopment: (1) Insane, deficiency in brain growth leading to mental retardation may determine individual inability to absorb leading values from the family and culture systems which lead to the internalization of rage; (2) emotional deprivation . . .; (3) harsh childhood repression by parent or school; (4) reaction formation hostile ideology; (5) superego deficit [Kolb, p. 314].

Kolb's five patterns of maldevelopment seem to provide objective criteria for determining the existence of psychopathology. Thus, if we suspect that an individual is violent because of superego deficit and we discover that he was reared under conditions inimical to the formation of a superego, then, presumably, we would have the same type of grounds for regarding the violence in question as pathological as a neurologist would have if he discovered that an episodically violent patient had a brain tumor.

But are these grounds comparable? Is a childhood history the equivalent of a shadow on an X-ray negative? Has the liberal an objective constraint equivalent to the Mark–Neville criterion? Can he really assure the ultratraditionalist or the conservative that he is acting in the real interests of his patient rather than the interests that he, or society, has foisted on his patient? Consider the following case. A pathologist informs the executive staff of a medical center that the vast preponderance of total mastectomies performed by a certain member of the surgical staff are remarkable in that, on examination, the breasts removed are usually found to be healthy. Acting on this information the executive staff examines the clinical records and discovers that, as they interpret the clinical data, those mastectomies were uncalled for. They interview the surgeon in question and find that his philosophy of surgery is basically, and rather crudely, "when in doubt, cut it out." They also discover that the surgeon was raised by a large-breasted stepmother and has a history of childhood repression and emotional deprivation. Thus, a liberal psychiatrist might well argue, applying Kolb's criteria for psychopathology, that the surgical violence in question would appear to be an expression of deficient control by the superego. Hence the surgeon ought to be required to undergo psychiatric treatment.

Now this, of course, is just the sort of case that the ultratraditionalist and the adamant conservative is apprehensive about: the case where a deviant might be motivated to be deviant for legitimate reasons and yet find his deviance medicalized, and his position stigmatized. How can the liberal protect the right to be different if he accepts his liberalized criteria for medicalizing violence?

Ultraliberalism

There are two answers a liberal might make. He can argue that no criterion is foolproof, and therefore one must ensure that they are employed not by fools but by tolerant and humane people of good will—people who, in the case of the surgeon, might argue that the surgeon be dismissed officially (since the medical center did not accept his practices as legitimate) and unofficially recommend that he see a psychiatrist to determine for himself whether his reasons for such extensive surgery was medical or psychopathological. Such a liberal might argue that, while his criteria are, no doubt, subject to abuse, the inhumanity of denying the psychopathologically violent the treatment they need and deserve is far greater than the dangers inherent in the possible abuses of the criterion.

Another liberal, the *ultraliberal* (most prominently, Karl Menninger), might remind us that, when the psychopathologically violent do not receive the treatment they deserve they are treated as criminals and punished. And since such punishments serve neither to protect the public nor to compensate the victims, they are in effect more criminal than the crimes that are said to deserve them. Consider the case of the surgeon. Doesn't the public deserve to be protected against unwarranted surgery? And isn't it more humane to treat the surgeon in question (if he is found to be sick) than to fire him, or, in the extreme case, to jail him for assault and battery or fine him for negligence?

The ultratraditionalist answer to this question is "No." For he would note that the liberal and the ultraliberal criterion for the assimilability of violence to a medical model is so weak that it has permitted the assimilation of the very paradigm of nonassimilable violence, surgery; and if the paradigm of unassimilable violence can be assimilated, then surely any act of violence could be "properly" regarded as a medical matter. He would object that to allow this is to violate the Hippocratic tradition by giving others the right to determine our symptoms and our health, and since the values governing health are our ideals for our minds and bodies, they are too significant, too deep, too personal to be given into the hands of others. If others determine whether our violence is healthy, then they decide the significance of defiance, of defense, of resistance, of rebellion, and even of death. They have the power to turn protest into lunacy, disobedience into madness, and rebellion into raving. If we are to decide the meaning of our own lives, then we must determine our own standards of health, and so we must preserve the classical medical model in its most traditional form.

Conclusion

Notice that the pivotal point on which the arguments for the four positions turn is the balance between the duty to heal the sick and the obligation to respect autonomy. Thus the ultratraditionalist is unwilling to allow *any* attrition of individual autonomy, no matter the cost in the suffering of the sick; while the ultraliberal is unwilling to allow any of the sick to remain untreated, no matter the cost in the attrition of individual autonomy. Conservatism and liberalism are essentially attempts to achieve the benefits of each of the extreme positions without

sacrificing either autonomy or healing by developing relatively objective criteria for distinguishing between pathological and nonpathological violence. So, while in part the issue is purely normative, i.e., a matter of values (whether autonomy is preferable to the relief of suffering), in part the issue is whether or not the proposed objective criteria for pathology are valid. There is, moreover, a nonmedical dimension to the controversy; for, unlike the legal systems of Eastern Europe, the preservation of individual autonomy lies at the heart of Western jurisprudence. And some legal constraints are designed to prevent physicians from overriding the wishes of their patients. Most prominent among them is the requirement that medical treatment is permissible only when a patient or his guardian has given his informed, voluntary consent to be treated. So the effectiveness of the law, too, must be weighed in the balance.

Where does the balance stand in actual medical practice? Our laws tilt toward ultraliberalism (since most states permit the civil commitment of persons who are dangerous either to themselves or to others); psychiatric practice tends toward liberalism; and nonpsychiatric medicine is more comfortable with conservative or even ultratraditional models. Each group tends to weigh the balance differently. The purpose of this article was not to determine how, ultimately, our society or any area of medicine, should resolve these issues, but rather to indicate the sort of considerations being weighed, and the rationale underlying the balancing.

ROBERT BAKER

[*Directly related is* HEALTH AND DISEASE. *Other relevant material may be found under* INFORMED CONSENT IN THE THERAPEUTIC RELATIONSHIP; MENTAL ILLNESS; *and* THERAPEUTIC RELATIONSHIP. *See also:* RACISM, *article on* RACISM AND MENTAL HEALTH. *For discussion of related ideas, see:* MEDICAL ETHICS, HISTORY OF, *section on* EUROPE AND THE AMERICAS, *article on* ANCIENT GREECE AND ROME.]

BIBLIOGRAPHY

CARTHY, J. D., and EBLING, F. J. *The Natural History of Aggression.* Institute of Biology, Symposia, no. 13. New York: Published for the Institute of Biology by Academic Press, 1964.

CLEMENTE, CARMINE D., and LINDSLEY, DONALD B. *Aggression and Defense: Neural Mechanisms and Social Patterns: Proceedings of the Fifth Conference on Brain Function, November 1965, Sponsored by the Brain Research Institute.* UCLA Forum in Medical Sciences, no. 7, Brain Function, vol. 5. Berkeley: University of California Press, 1967.

Delgado, José M. R. *Physical Control of the Mind: Toward a Psychocivilized Society.* World Perspectives, vol. 41. New York: Harper & Row, 1969.

Eleftheriou, Basil E., and Scott, John Paul. *The Physiology of Aggression and Defeat: Proceedings of a Symposium Held during the Meeting of the American Association for the Advancement of Science in Dallas, Texas, December 1968.* New York: Plenum Press, 1971.

Frazier, Shervert H., ed. *Aggression: Proceedings of the Association, December 1 and 2, 1972, New York, N.Y.* Research Publications, Association for Research in Nervous and Mental Disease, vol. 52. Baltimore: Williams & Wilkins, 1974.

Gunn, John. *Violence in Human Society.* People, Plans and Problems Series. Newton Abbot, England: David & Charles, 1973.

Jones, Howard Mumford. *Violence and Reason: A Book of Essays.* New York: Atheneum, 1969.

Kolb, Lawrence C. "Control of Violence." Frazier, *Aggression,* chap. 17, pp. 313–318.

Lorenz, Konrad. *On Aggression.* Translated by Marjorie Latzke. Foreword by Julian Huxley. London: Methuen Co., 1966.

Mark, Vernon H., and Ervin, Frank R. *Violence and the Brain.* New York: Harper & Row, 1970.

————, and Neville, Robert. "Brain Surgery in Aggressive Epileptics: Social and Ethical Implications." *Journal of the American Medical Association* 226 (1973): 765–772.

Menninger, Karl. *The Crime of Punishment.* The Isaac Ray Award Lectures, 1963–1966. New York: Viking Press, 1968.

Montagu, Ashley, ed. *Man and Aggression.* New York: Oxford University Press, 1968.

Rochlin, Gregory. *Man's Aggression: The Defence of the Self.* Boston: Gambit; London: Constable & Co., 1973.

Singer, Jerome L., ed. *The Control of Aggression and Violence: Cognitive and Physiological Factors.* Personality and Psychopathology, no. 10. New York: Academic Press, 1971.

Storr, Anthony. *Human Aggression.* New York: Atheneum; London: Penguin Press, 1968.

Szasz, Thomas S. *The Manufacture of Madness: A Comparative Study of the Inquisition and the Mental Health Movement.* New York: Harper & Row, 1970.

————. *The Myth of Mental Illness: Foundations of a Theory of Personal Conduct.* New York: Hoeber-Harper, 1961.

VIVISECTION

See Animal Experimentation.

WXZ

WARFARE

I. MEDICINE AND WAR — *E. A. Vastyan*
II. BIOMEDICAL SCIENCE AND WAR — *Victor W. Sidel and Mark Sidel*

I
MEDICINE AND WAR

"When wounded, enemies become brothers" has been an axiom of the most elementary international law in all epochs. A similar recognition —that humanity's most basic bond is a bond of common vulnerability—lies at the root of the esteem accorded the physician, the privileges granted him, and the obligations he assumes. That recognition foreshadows, as well, the ethical problems and conflicts inherent in the relations of medicine and war.

Many of the earliest documents attest to the antiquity of the intertwined relationships between the medical and the martial arts—and to the tensions between them (Friedman). Hebraic contributions to military hygiene demonstrated sound principles of preventive medicine. Hippocrates urged that "he who would become a surgeon should join an army and follow it," recognizing war as an important school for surgery. And by the fourth century B.C., in *The Art of War,* Sun Tzu noted that it was forbidden to injure a previously wounded enemy and urged humane care for captives. Thus, while medical knowledge has long been regarded as important to the conduct of war, war has also been a resource for the advancement of medical skills; while ethics has expressed concern for a restraint to war's cruelty and mitigation of its ravages, war has also tested the force of practicable medical ethics.

Ethical conflicts and tensions occur wherever the practice of medicine and the practice of war intersect. Such intersections stretch back to antiquity, but this article will be chiefly concerned with more modern developments, for, as armies have become more dependent upon technology, they have also become more dependent upon medical technology. As medical skills have grown increasingly important to any war effort, the physician's conflict between military duty and medical duty has increased as well.

Conflicting obligations

As a member of the military forces of a nation, the military physician has been charged through the centuries with a major mission: "Conserve the fighting strength." As a member of the medical profession, and part of an age-old tradition of healing, the physician obligates himself morally to all the sick and all the wounded. The conflict between the physician's military role and his ethical obligations constitutes our chief focus.

Perhaps history's most ironic melding of conflicting claims and obligations lay with the Knights Hospitallers of St. John of Jerusalem, a religious order founded in the eleventh century, responsible for building the first known institutional hospital. With a sworn fealty to "Our Lords the Sick," the Knights defended their hospitals against "enemies of the Faith," becoming the first organized military medical officers. "Not 'non-combatants' they, but warring physicians who could strike the enemy mighty blows, and yet later bind up the wounds of that same enemy along with those of their own comrades" (Hume). Fighting in retreat from Jerusalem to Rhodes to Malta, they built hospitals and cared for the sick and needy until evicted from their small island empire by Napoleon.

New organizations and codes

When supply trains were made possible by improved roads and transport in the eighteenth century, the resultant development of modern warfare techniques and the almost concurrent dramatic increase of medical technology made strategic deployment of medical resources an imperative of warfare. Deplorable medical care during the American Revolution caused bitter political conflicts over the management of hospitals and general health care for soldiers. The alarming death rate from disease during the Crimean campaign forced a governmental crisis in Britain, resolved only by the mission of Florence Nightingale. Through the dramatic changes and effective care she worked among the sick and wounded, and, aided by her troop of thirty-eight well-educated and competent women, she laid the foundation for the modern profession of nursing. Her work led, as well, to the founding of the Sanitary Commission, a forerunner of the Red Cross societies which soon began to appear throughout the world. These gained an international standing through the work of a Swiss banker, Henri Dunant, who became the first recipient of the Nobel Peace Prize for his dramatic account of the carnage in the Battle of Solferino between Italian and Austrian forces, *Un Souvenir de Solferino*. Coupled with Dunant's zeal to ameliorate suffering during that war, the book led directly to an international conference in 1863 and the founding of the International Red Cross and its national affiliates. In turn, Dunant's work and that assemblage led to the first Geneva Convention of 1864; fourteen signatory nations pledged themselves to regard the sick and wounded, as well as medical and nursing staffs, as neutrals on the battlefield. Specific immunities and privileges were accorded the military physician; specific duties and obligations, regardless of those laid upon him by military necessity, were likewise to be clarified, outlined, and codified. Such provisions were to become the heart of that series of documents which became basic in the development of international law.

Two events in America, almost simultaneous to the conferences at Geneva, influenced future codifications and applications of international law and its bearing on medicine. During the Civil War, through a series of fortuitous influences, Francis Lieber, a German-born philosopher-lawyer-historian, was commissioned by the Union commander to draft a code of regulations for armies in the field. The resultant "Lieber Code" was promulgated in May 1863 as General Orders No. 100 by the Union Army and became the foundation for the international conferences at the Hague and Geneva, which met in 1899, 1907, 1929, and 1949 to modify the agreements first made in 1864. Those agreements, which codified as well the special status of medical personnel in wartime, are still basic documents of international law.

The plea of "superior orders"

Related to such developments, too—though the Lieber Code was not invoked at the time—was the 1865 trial of Captain Henry Wirz, the only such trial consequent to the Civil War. Wirz, a physician who had served as commandant of the infamous Confederate prison at Andersonville, Georgia, was charged with a series of offenses alleging inhumane regard for prisoners under his charge. His plea of "superior orders," as mitigating the negligences of duty with which he was charged, raised issues that were to be important to the Nuremberg trials after the Second World War. That plea was disallowed, and Wirz was convicted and sentenced to be hanged.

Twenty-three German physicians were tried in December 1946 by the Nuremberg war crimes tribunal on charges relating to experiments conducted by them upon human beings. Besides experimentation related to sterilization techniques, cold-water survival, decompression, and heteroplastic transplantation, German physicians had participated in mass programs of euthanasia of persons with chronic mental illness. Like Wirz, they raised the defense of "superior orders," but the Nuremberg tribunal also discarded superior authority as a defense. Commenting editorially at the time of the trial, the *Journal of the American Medical Association* decried such a total breakdown of medical tradition and castigated the profession for its failures. "Perhaps the most serious of all is the failure of German medical organizations and societies to express in any manner their disapproval" ("Brutalities of Nazi Physicians").

Contrasted to the experience in Germany, and reinforcing the editorial's position, had been the wartime history of medical care in the Netherlands. Dutch physicians resisted all efforts of Nazi coercion, beginning with the seemingly innocuous "first order" of the Reich Commissar, which called medical care "a public task," implying that it was entirely under his control. Declaring the order unacceptable, Dutch physicians were threatened with a loss of license; in response, they surrendered their licenses en masse, quit signing birth and death certificates, and continued to see patients in secret. Their resistance continued even after one hundred Dutch physicians were arrested and deported to Nazi death camps. Throughout the war not a single Dutch physician participated in euthanasia or nontherapeutic sterilization.

Geneva: a clarifying of obligations

Such precedents had a strong influence on the Geneva Conference of 1949. While the first conference there in 1864 had resulted in a relatively simple document—which set forth a common recognition of the neutrality of medical personnel, acknowledged the need for their common protection in time of battle, and agreed upon rules for the protection and exchange of wounded personnel—the revisions agreed upon in 1949 went far beyond. Agreed to at that time by sixty nations, the 1949 conventions were declared binding upon all nations according to "customary law, the usages established among civilized people . . . the laws of humanity, and the dictates of the public conscience."

Under the conventions, medical personnel are singled out for certain specific protections, by an explicit separation of the healing from the wounding roles. Medical personnel and treatment facilities are designated as immune from attack; captured medical personnel are to be promptly repatriated. Certain specific obligations are likewise laid upon medical personnel:

1. Declared as "noncombatants," medical personnel are forbidden to engage in or be parties to the acts of war.

2. The wounded and sick—both soldier and civilian, both friend and foe—shall be respected, protected, treated humanely, and cared for by the belligerents.

3. The wounded and sick may not be left without medical assistance, and only urgent medical reasons authorize any priority in the order of their treatment.

4. Medical aid must be dispensed solely on medical grounds, "without distinctions founded on sex, race, nationality, religion, political opinions, or any other similar criteria."

5. No physical or moral coercion shall be exercised against protected persons (civilians), in particular to obtain information from them or from third parties.

Such duties are imposed clearly, permitting no exceptions, and given priority over all other considerations.

Thus the Geneva Conventions formalized the recognition that, while professional expertise merits special privileges, it likewise incurs very specific obligations, legal as well as moral. Such issues were once again cast into the foreground during the hostilities conducted by the United States in Vietnam.

Captain Howard B. Levy, M.D., a reluctantly conscripted dermatologist, during the final months of his tour of duty in the U.S. Army refused to give medical training to Special Forces ("Green Beret") medical aidmen being trained for guerrilla warfare in Vietnam. For this refusal he was charged with one of the most serious breaches of the Uniform Code of Military Justice: willfully disobeying a lawful order. Tried by a general court martial in 1967, Levy admitted his disobedience. Training the aidmen, he said, violated his ethical principles. His defense contended that Special Forces aidmen were specific agents of military objectives; that they were combat troops first and medical personnel only secondarily; and that they used medicine primarily as weaponry.

He did not argue that aidmen used medicine to kill directly, as did the Nazi physicians, but to kill in more subtle ways. He charged that aidmen used medicine to win the allegiance of the native population. Once the aidmen gain the people's confidence, Levy's defense contended, their real purpose became clear—to serve as an entry for other Special Forces to move in and conclude their military–political mission, to which everything else, including medical care, became incidental. His defense contended that aidmen functioned as full-fledged combat troops in carrying out their mission and that the use of such troops was a clear violation of the Geneva Conventions.

Though Levy was supported by expert medical witnesses in his contentions, the law officer of the court declared them irrelevant to the issue of whether Levy had disobeyed a lawful order. A court of combat officers—all his senior in rank and none physicians—convicted him of three charges and sentenced him to three years at hard labor. None of Levy's appeals was successful.

U.S. government policies in Vietnam

Levy's defense allegations would have been strengthened had there been available at the time of trial a series of documents that later emerged from investigations conducted by the Senate Subcommittee on Refugees (U.S. Senate). While commending individual physicians and medical programs for providing desperately needed medical care to civilians, the Subcommittee aimed sharp criticism at the *policies* under which American government assistance was being provided. The Subcommittee called attention to official policies that urged the use of medical assistance as the most potent weapon in the Army's arsenal of psychological warfare, a tool "to win the hearts and minds" of a civilian populace. "High-impact" and high-visibility medical practices were encouraged and became a form of political and psychological triage. Medicine's new role, moreover, was not only accepted by the military-medical leadership, but it became a major mission of the Army Medical Services: "The real objective is to do those things which have a sharp impact upon the people *now* in order to convince them that their government is trying to help them and thus contribute to an early end to the war" (Humphreys).

Old questions posed anew

From the time of the warring physicians of the Knights of Malta during the Middle Ages, the role of military physicians has evolved through agreed-upon neutral status in 1864 to the specific designations and obligations of the Geneva Conventions of 1949. The ethical tensions attendant upon the military physician's duties, although obviously not resolved, were nevertheless recognized in the legal codifications. The weight of such laws rests clearly on the side of professional duty—on the side of a recognized and now legally required primary obligation—to the sick and wounded, friend and foe alike, civilian as well as soldier.

But the Levy case and the issue of American medical policies in Vietnam demonstrate clearly how difficult it is for ideals, ethical principles, and law itself to prevail in times of war. That such principles and laws are not consistently respected becomes, as Levy's defense contended, more and not less reason for their strict observance, by the medical profession if not by the leaders of its governments.

Levy's case clearly demonstrated that when it takes an act of courage to act on conscience and ethics, a system of self-censorship is inevitably fostered. At what point should the physician dissent openly from his government's policy? And if he does dissent, placing his professional conscience above what he believes is unconscionable behavior, what is there to protect and defend his decision? Dutch physicians, during the Second World War, decided that it is the first, although slight, step away from principle that is the most important one. The *Journal of the American Medical Association* editorial regarding the Nazi physicians suggested that the silence of a profession deserves castigation even more than the silence of the individual. Are professional societies ready to defend their colleagues who are arbitrarily treated for invoking their professional ethics?

While the Vietnamese conflict engendered many acts of dedication by physicians, policy decisions at the highest levels determined what resources were to be provided and how they were to be utilized. Those operations were seen as "stability operations . . . assailing latent or incipient turbulence," seeking military and political objectives, and utilizing medical programs to achieve those objectives (Neel). Ethically, an overriding duty for any professional is to foresee and forestall the risks to which his superior knowledge makes him privy. It takes little prescience to foresee the dangers to the profession of medicine—and to humanity—if the traditions and laws that claim clear and special obligations from the military physician continue to crumble before the demands of "military necessity."

E. A. Vastyan

[*For further discussion of topics mentioned in this article, see the entries:* Hospitals; Human Experimentation, *articles on* history *and* basic issues; Medical Ethics under National Socialism; Nursing; *and* Women and Biomedicine, *article on* women as health professionals. *Also directly related are the entries* Codes of Medical Ethics; *and* Prisoners. *See* Appendix, Section I, declaration of geneva.]

BIBLIOGRAPHY

"The Brutalities of Nazi Physicians." *Journal of the American Medical Association* 132 (1946): 714–715. Editorial.

Dulles, Foster Rhea. *The American Red Cross: A History.* New York: Harper & Brothers, 1950.

FRIEDMAN, LEON, ed. *The Law of War: A Documentary History.* 2 vols. Foreword by Telford Taylor. New York: Random House, 1972.

GARRISON, FIELDING HUDSON. *Notes on the History of Military Medicine.* Washington: Association of Military Surgeons, 1922. Reprinted from the *Military Surgeon,* 1921–1922.

GLASSER, IRA. "Judgment at Fort Jackson: The Court-Martial of Captain Howard B. Levy." *Law in Transition Quarterly* 4 (1967): 123–156.

GOLDWYN, ROBERT M., and SIDEL, VICTOR W. "The Physician and War." *Ethical Issues in Medicine: The Role of the Physician in Today's Society.* Edited by E. Fuller Torrey. Boston: Little, Brown & Co., 1968, pp. 323–346.

HUME, EDGAR ERSKINE. *Medical Work of the Knights Hospitallers of Saint John of Jerusalem.* Foreword by Ludovico Chigi-Albani. Preface by Aldo Castellani. Baltimore: Johns Hopkins Press, 1940. First appearance, in part. *Bulletin of the Institute of the History of Medicine, Johns Hopkins University* 6 (1938): 399–466, 495–613, 617–819.

HUMPHREYS, JAMES W., JR. "The A.I.D. Medical Mission in Vietnam." *Military Medicine* 133 (1968): 200–207.

MITSCHERLICH, ALEXANDER, and MIELKE, FRED. *Doctors of Infamy: The Story of the Nazi Medical Crimes.* Translated by Heinz Norden. Statements by Andrew C. Ivy, Telford Taylor, and Leo Alexander. A note on medical ethics by Albert Deutch. New York: Henry Schuman, 1949. A translation of *Das Diktat der Menschenverachtung.*

NEEL, SPURGEON. "The Medical Role in Army Stability Operations." *Military Medicine* 132 (1967): 605–608.

United States, Department of Defense, Army Department. *The Law of Land Warfare: July 1956.* Field Manual FM Series 27–10. Washington: Government Printing Office, 1956.

———, Senate, Committee on the Judiciary, Subcommittee to Investigate Problems Connected With Refugees and Escapees. *Civilian Casualty, Social Welfare and Refugee Problems in South Vietnam: Hearings: 91st Congress, 1st Session, Part 1, June 24 and 25, 1969.* Washington: Government Printing Office, 1969. Also pertinent are the hearings and reports issued by this subcommittee from 1965–1972.

VASTYAN, E. A. "Warriors in White: Some Questions about the Nature and Mission of Military Medicine." *Texas Reports on Biology and Medicine* 32 (1974): 327–342.

II

BIOMEDICAL SCIENCE AND WAR

Scientists of every nation have usually been called upon in time of war to play a role in the preparation for it or in the conflict itself. Archimedes used his skills on behalf of the Tyrant of Syracuse in preparation for war against the Romans; Leonardo designed fortifications for the Duke of Milan; and Galileo calculated trajectories of projectiles for the Grand Duke of Tuscany. Chemists who developed explosives and poison gases in World War I, physicists who developed nuclear weapons in World War II, and biomedical scientists and physicians who worked on biological weapons and herbicides are examples in the twentieth century.

At the same time, however, there have been numerous examples of scientists who refused to work on the development of weapons of war. During the Crimean War the British government consulted the noted physicist Michael Faraday on the feasibility of the development of poison gases; Faraday responded that it was entirely feasible, but that it was inhuman and he would have nothing to do with it (Russell). Other scientists, such as Alfred Nobel, have participated in the development of weapons, or in scientific advances that led to weapons, and then tried in some way to prevent the wars in which the weapons might be used.

The ethical issues that lie behind the decision of any scientist—including biomedical scientists—to participate or not to participate are part of the broader issues of the responsibility of the scientist for the social consequences of his or her work (Bernal; Brown). This article will outline the wide spectrum of views on the nature of that responsibility and will focus specifically on the views regarding the responsibility of the biomedical scientist and the physician. Discussion is limited to the ethical issues related to the use of applied biomedical science and technology (for both of which we shall use the general term "science") in the development and testing of weapons of war. The ethical issues involved in the actual use of such weapons (i.e., the ethics of various forms of or reasons for warfare) are beyond the scope of this article; the ethical issues related to the role of the scientist in basic research and to the role of the physician and of clinical care in warfare are covered in other articles.

Social responsibility of the scientist

At one end of the ethical spectrum is the view that the scientist has no responsibility at all for the consequences of his or her scientific work. This argument was stated, for example, by the sociologist Lundberg and his colleagues in 1929:

> It is not the business of a chemist who invents a high explosive to be influenced in his task by considerations as to whether his product will be used to blow up cathedrals or to build tunnels through the mountains [Merton].

This view of the "amorality" of science and the lack of responsibility of the scientist followed in part from the assumptions (1) that scientific progress was the road to human perfection and (2) that science was "an autonomous force working for man's welfare in contrast to the disruptive force of politics" (Gilpin, pp. 26–27).

For the special case of work on what was clearly intended to be a weapon of war, the "amoral" view was stated by Professor Louis Fieser, leader of a team of Harvard University scientists who developed napalm—jellied gasoline used as an incendiary weapon—during World War II. When asked in 1967 about the use of napalm in that war and later in Vietnam, he said that he felt free of guilt:

You don't know what's coming. That wasn't my business. That is for other people. I was working on a technical problem that was considered pressing. . . . I distinguish between developing a munition of some kind and using it. You can't blame the outfit that put out the rifle that killed the President. I'd do it again, if called upon, in defense of the country ["Napalm Inventor"].

The assumptions of the "moral neutrality" of the scientist and of any scientific finding's invariably leading to progress were increasingly challenged in the 1930s and 1940s. The use to which science was put by Nazi Germany, at that time the world's leading scientific nation, shocked many scientists who saw that use as inhuman. The potential for destructiveness inherent in the development of controlled nuclear fission (and later fusion) further weakened the notion of scientific neutrality. J. Robert Oppenheimer wrote, for example, in 1949, "the physicists have known sin" and, in 1956, "we did the Devil's work" (Reid). The founding of the *Bulletin of the Atomic Scientists* and of the Federation of American Scientists after World War II reflected this moral concern (Jungk).

Some scientists resolved what they indeed saw as an ethical dilemma by focusing on "duty to their country." For example, the German, later American, rocket scientist Wernher von Braun wrote in a letter in 1968:

While right from the beginning I deeply deplored the war and the misery and suffering it spread all over the world, I found myself caught in a maelstrom in which I simply felt that, like it or not, it was my duty to work for my country at war [Reid, p. 105].

Dr. Theodor Rosebury, who worked on biological weapons during World War II, explained his participation by saying that, although there was an ethical question involved, crisis circumstances expected to pass in a limited time required that he act. "We were fighting a fire, and it seemed necessary to risk getting dirty as well as burnt," he later wrote (Rosebury, 1963, p. 514).

Rosebury's view contrasts sharply with Fieser's and goes much farther than von Braun's. It explicitly recognizes the ethical conflicts involved in such work but permits some higher ethical principle—the imperative of defending one's country or of helping to destroy what is seen as evil—to decide in favor of producing the weapons.

Other scientists who recognized an ethical dilemma in work on weapons resolved it in a different fashion, by arguing that their work was itself designed to reduce the possibility that war could occur, or at least to reduce its devastation. For example, Dr. Knut Krieger, while working on chemical and biological weapons in the 1960s, argued in defense of his work on "nonlethal" weapons by asserting that the research would lead to decreased fatalities: ". . . if we do indeed succeed in creating incapacitating systems and are able to substitute incapacitation for death it appears to me that, next to stopping war, this would be an important step forward" (Reid, p. 315).

Paradoxically, other scientists view their work as contributing to the lessening of the devastation of war by producing even more horrible weapons. Although this argument has been used most strongly for nuclear weapons, as early as 1892 Albert Nobel defended his development and production of dynamite: ". . . on the day that two army corps can mutually annihilate each other in a second, all civilized nations will surely recoil with horror and disband their troops" (ibid., p. 19).

A more modern expression of the same concept—that scientific weapons research would lead to a lessening of the possibility of war—was given in 1958 by Professor Hans Bethe, a physicist who had worked on the hydrogen bomb. He argued that scientists who help in the research on such weapons should be closely involved with the policy decisions on their development. The scientists, he said, must preserve the precarious balance of armament which would make it disastrous for either side to start a war. Wrote Bethe, "Only then can we argue for and embark on more constructive ventures like disarmament and international cooperation which may eventually lead to a more definite peace" (Bethe, p. 428).

Along with the scientists who feel on moral

grounds—the reduction of the killing of war— that they *should* participate in weapons research there are of course those who on precisely the same grounds believe that they *should not* participate. For example, Dr. Theodor Rosebury, who felt during World War II that his work on the development of biological weapons, although "dirty," could be morally justified because of the special circumstances, shortly after the end of the war refused any further participation in such work.

The most extreme and all-encompassing expression of the view of the responsibility of scientists to refuse to participate is provided in an oath proposed by one of the participants in the 1962 Pugwash Conference on Science and World Affairs, one of a series of meetings of scientists from different countries to discuss problems of disarmament and world peace: "Under no circumstances shall I work for war, neither directly nor through any advice. Only those who take the same oath shall be admitted to my laboratory and to any learned societies of which I am a member" (Magat, p. 124). The Society for Social Responsibility in Science cites the following among its principles that scientists should adhere to:

To foster throughout the world a . . . tradition of personal moral responsibility for the consequences for humanity of professional activity, with emphasis on constructive alternatives to militarism; to embody in this tradition the principle that the individual must abstain from destructive work and devote himself to constructive work, according to his own moral judgment; to ascertain . . . the boundary between constructive and destructive work, to serve as a guide for individual and group decisions and action . . . [Bry and Doe, p. 913].

Along with the decision whether or not to participate, there is another potential ethical responsibility of the scientist that is often stressed, particularly by those who feel that the "pure," as contrasted to the "applied," scientist also has this responsibility. Scientists are often in a unique position to warn the public of specific dangers that special knowledge permits them to perceive earlier or more clearly than do others. Debate arises, however, on whether scientists "should simply state the facts" (which in itself involves deciding which facts, and how and where they are presented) or should take a public position on a course of action to which they have been led by analysis of the "facts." Since the prestige of the scientist in most societies often lends considerable weight to such

statements, and since often there are elements of the analysis that lie outside the special expertise of the scientist as a scientist, the propriety of public policy statements by scientists has at times been questioned; on the other hand, silence by scientists on urgent public policy issues in which they have relevant technical information has also been questioned as a possible evasion of moral responsibility. The problem of how to avoid arrogating to scientists undue power to influence social decisions while at the same time maintaining their responsibility for the consequences of their work is still unresolved.

Thus we see a spectrum of views among scientists on their ethical responsibilities in relation to the development of weapons of war: complete denial of moral responsibility for the consequences of any scientific work; responsibility to do their country's bidding whatever the consequences; responsibility to work for the reduction of war and its devastation but paradoxically, in the eyes of some by working on certain weapons, and in the eyes of others by refusing to work on them; and responsibility to inform and/ or to lead public opinion on policies related to the weapons.

Social responsibility of the physician

Narrowing the focus from a consideration of the work of all scientists in the development and testing of weapons to a look at the more specific case of the physician, the question that first arises is whether it is useful to view certain ethical responsibilities as peculiar to that social role or whether it is "elitist" and possibly self-defeating to assert that there is a special form of "medical ethics" (Rosebury, 1949, pp. 192–193). While the physician shares the moral responsibilities of all scientists, and indeed of all people, the physician may have special additional ethical responsibilities because of the role of the physician in preserving life. There has usually been a feeling in relation to work on weapons of war that the physician's role was a singular one. For example, Rosebury described the views of the physician's role at Fort Detrick in the work on biological weapons: "There was much quiet searching discussion among us regarding the place of doctors in such work . . . a certain delicacy concentrated most of the physicians into principally or primarily defensive operations" (Rosebury, 1963, p. 514).

Rosebury goes on to point out, however, that work on weapons can never be exclusively defensive and that the distinction is quite arbitrary; in biological weapons defense, for example, it is often necessary to conceptualize new types of agents that might be used offensively, and often to produce them, in order to design a defense against them. In addition, a number of special aspects of biological weapons have been cited as raising special ethical problems in their development, namely (1) the likelihood of their being used specifically against noncombatants; (2) their unpredictability, with the possibility that vast unintended damage to both combatants and noncombatants would be caused; and (3) their potential genocidal quality (Sidel). Some physicians have felt, however, that it is entirely ethical—in fact, that it is their responsibility—to continue to work on biological weapons, particularly the defensive aspects (Crozier).

Another example of the conflict in the role of the physician was seen in the debate on the testing of chemical weapons. The Surgeon General of the U.S. Public Health Service headed a committee to develop guidelines for safety in open-air testing of nerve gas after an accident in Utah led to the death of 6,400 sheep; the Surgeon General testified in congressional hearings in 1969 that open-air testing which followed the newly developed committee guidelines was unlikely to cause harm and should be permitted. Other physicians, including one of the authors of this article, testified at the same hearings that there was no way of assuring safety in open-air testing and criticized the Surgeon General for using his office and his authority as a physician to legitimize continuing testing (U.S. Congress). The U.S. Department of Health, Education, and Welfare was involved in biological warfare research ("U.S. Health Service") and is reported as continuing to be involved in determinations such as the quantities of biological warfare research materials that are acceptable in the United States under the terms of the 1972 biological warfare convention now signed by 111 of the world's nations. Thus the U.S. equivalent of a national "department of health" appears to be concerned not only with public health but also with biological warfare policies.

What is seen as the special responsibility of physicians in these areas is based largely on what is felt to be a special ethical responsibility, due to the special power of the physician, not to do harm (*primum non nocere*). Although a very small percentage of U.S. medical students now swear to the Hippocratic Oath, this code is often cited as the source of the special responsibility:

"I will use treatment to help the sick according to my ability and judgement, but never with a view to injury and wrongdoing. Neither will I administer a poison to anybody even when asked to do so, nor will I suggest such a course."

Comments by professional medical groups often support this view of the special responsibility of the profession. For example, the Code of Ethics in Wartime of the World Medical Association states: "It is deemed unethical for doctors to weaken the physical and mental strength of a human being without therapeutic justification, and to employ scientific knowledge to imperil health or destroy life" (Liberman, Gold, and Sidel, p. 300). Presumably this special proscription on doctors (as compared to others) is necessary because of the doctor's special skill and special opportunities to do harm. Some physicians have carried this principle so far as to urge that physicians refuse on principle to play any role at all in war or in the preparation for it (Joules, pp. 7–10).

A few physicians have taken the public position of absolute refusal on the grounds of "medical ethics" to participate in any aspect of the preparation for all wars or for a specific war; one example during the Vietnam War was that of Dr. Howard Levy, who refused to train U.S. Army combat troops in health techniques. Many physicians have, however, taken the position that the physician or biomedical scientist has a special responsibility—no matter how "just" the war—to call public attention to the dangers of war to the human race and specifically of the dangers of the development, testing, stockpiling, and potential use of nuclear, chemical, or biological weapons. One example during the Vietnam War was that of Dr. Howard Levy, who refused to train U.S. Army combat troops in health tech-weapons.

Continuing controversies

Although many of the controversies described thus far no longer appear current, the fundamental issues continue to arise in new, often less clear-cut, forms. For example, recent issues include the continuation of atmospheric testing of nuclear weapons by relatively poor nations that have only recently developed a nuclear capability; the evaluation by physicians under contract to the U.S. Department of Defense of the effect of radiation on terminal cancer patients in order to evaluate potential nuclear weapon effects ("Medical Center"); and the biological warfare implications, in addition to other potential public health hazards, of DNA recombinant molecular research (Lederberg; Lappé; Lappé and Morison). Brown, Commoner, Klaw, Lappé, Lederberg and others have in recent years discussed some relevant issues of the social responsibilities of all scientists and of biological scientists in particular (Klaw; Brown).

It appears in general that the decision by the biomedical scientist to use his or her scientific knowledge in the development or testing of war weapons depends on two possible approaches. Some will make the decision based on whether more or less harm or good will be done by the participation or by the refusal to participate, by silence or by taking a public position on the issues. Others will make the decision regarding participation in the development and testing of weapons principally on the basis of values to which they have a prior commitment—such as life, peace, and human solidarity. Often decisions are at variance according to whether stress is placed on doing immediate harm to individual human beings or on doing harm to a larger cause, with the result that many individuals will be harmed or benefited. Much depends on the response to even more fundamental ethical questions: Is killing and maiming justified by participation in a "just" war? Is singling out the physician or the scientist for special ethical responsibilities deeply moral, or is it—as a manifestation of "elitism" at one pole or of "antiscientism" at the other—profoundly immoral?

While the role of the physician seems to be more defined and circumscribed by tradition than is that of the biomedical scientist, both can find precedents and arguments offered to justify any decisions. At root the decisions rest, as ethical decisions for all people rest, on personal and societal views of the responsibilities of people toward each other.

VICTOR W. SIDEL AND MARK SIDEL

[*Directly related are the entries* CODES OF MEDICAL ETHICS; PRISONERS; *and* TECHNOLOGY. *Also directly related is the other article in this entry,* MEDICINE AND WAR.]

BIBLIOGRAPHY

BERNAL, JOHN DESMOND. *Science in History.* London: C. A. Watts & Co., 1954.

BETHE, HANS A. Review of *Brighter than a Thousand Suns. Bulletin of the Atomic Scientists* 14 (1958): 426–428.

BROWN, MARTIN, ed. *The Social Responsibility of the Scientist.* New York: Free Press, 1971.

BRY, ILSE, and DOE, JANET. "War and Men of Science." *Science* 122 (1955): 911–913.

CROZIER, DAN. "The Physician and Biologic Warfare." *New England Journal of Medicine* 284 (1971): 1008–1011.

GILPIN, ROBERT. *American Scientists and Nuclear Weapons Policy.* Princeton: Princeton University Press, 1962.

GOLDWYN, ROBERT M., and SIDEL, VICTOR W. "The Physician and War." *Ethical Issues in Medicine: The Role of the Physician in Today's Society.* Edited by Edwin Fuller Torrey. Boston: Little, Brown & Co., 1968, pp. 323–346.

JOULES, HORACE, ed. *The Doctor's View of War.* London: G. Allen & Unwin, 1938.

JUNGK, ROBERT. *Brighter Than a Thousand Suns: A Personal History of the Atomic Scientists.* Translated by James Cleugh. 1st American ed. New York: Harcourt, Brace & Co., 1958.

KLAW, SPENCER. *The New Brahmins: Scientific Life in America.* New York: William Morrow & Co., 1968.

LAPPÉ, MARC. "The Human Uses of Molecular Genetics." *Federation Proceedings* (Federation of American Societies for Experimental Biology) 34 (1975): 1425–1427.

———, and MORISON, ROBERT S., eds. *Ethical and Scientific Issues Posed by Human Uses of Molecular Genetics. Annals of the New York Academy of Sciences* 265 (1976): 1–208.

LEDERBERG, JOSHUA. "Remarks by Joshua Lederberg, Professor of Genetics, Stanford University, for Informal Discussion at the Conference of the Committee on Disarmament, Geneva, August 5, 1970." *Congressional Record,* 91st Cong., 2d sess., 1970, 116, pt. 23: 31395–31396.

LIBERMAN, ROBERT; GOLD, WARREN; and SIDEL, VICTOR W. "Medical Ethics and the Military." *New Physician* 17 (1968): 299–309.

MAGAT, MICHEL. "Some Remarks Concerning the Responsibility of Scientists." *Scientists and World Affairs.* Pugwash Conference on Science and World Affairs, 10th. London: 1962, pp. 123–126.

"Medical Center in Cincinnati Defends Whole-Body Radiation in Cancer Care." *New York Times,* 12 October 1971, p. 24.

MERTON, ROBERT K. *Social Theory and Social Structure.* Rev. and enl. ed. Glencoe, Ill.: Free Press, 1957, p. 543, fn. 22.

"Napalm Inventor Discounts 'Guilt': Harvard Chemist Would 'Do It Again' for the Country." *New York Times,* 27 December 1967, p. 8.

REID, ROBERT WILLIAM. *Tongues of Conscience: Weapons Research and the Scientists' Dilemma.* New York: Walker & Co., 1969.

ROSEBURY, THEODOR. "Medical Ethics and Biological Warfare." *Perspectives in Biology and Medicine* 6 (1963): 512–523.

———. *Peace or Pestilence: Biological Warfare and How to Avoid It.* New York: Whittlesey House, 1949.

RUSSELL, BERTRAND. *Facts and Fiction.* New York: Simon & Schuster, 1962.

SIDEL, VICTOR W. "Medical Ethics." *CBW: Chemical and Biological Warfare.* Edited by Steven Rose. London Conference on CBW. London: George G. Harrap & Co., 1968; Boston: Beacon Press, 1969, pp. 172–180.

"U.S. Health Service Aided Army on Poison Weapon." *New York Times,* 18 September 1975, pp. 1, 26.

United States, Congress, House of Representatives, Sub-committee on Government Operations. *Environmental Dangers of Open-Air Testing of Lethal Chemicals: Hearings Before a Subcommittee.* 91st Cong., 1st sess., 20 and 21 May 1969.

WESTERN EUROPE

See MEDICAL ETHICS, HISTORY OF, *section on* EUROPE AND THE AMERICAS, *article on* WESTERN EUROPE IN THE SEVENTEENTH CENTURY.

WOMEN AND BIOMEDICINE

I. WOMEN AS PATIENTS AND EXPERIMENTAL
   SUBJECTS   *Malkah T. Notman*
                               and Carol C. Nadelson
II. WOMEN AS HEALTH PROFESSIONALS
                            Carol C. Nadelson
                            and Malkah T. Notman

I
WOMEN AS PATIENTS AND EXPERIMENTAL SUBJECTS

Many of the ethical issues in patient care and biomedical research affect men and women in the same manner. However, at present there is widespread discussion about the meaning, role, and functions of women—a discussion that has many value overtones—and the outcome of that discussion has an important bearing on the ethics of the relationship between the physician and the woman patient and between the experimenter and the woman subject. Hence it is altogether fitting to discuss these questions here. Yet any attempt to deal with these ethical problems is necessarily dependent not only on an assessment of the therapeutic and experimental relationships, but of women. We rely on important studies, but these studies can only *describe,* not *prescribe* the status of women. This article offers more of a descriptive explanation of ethical dilemmas involving women, rather than a prescriptive statement on what women and women's relationships *ought* to be. Emphasis is placed on current views in North American and European cultures—views that may not be relevant to other cultures or even to all segments of modern Western cultures. As to its scope, this article examines (1) general aspects of the relationship between physicians and female patients, (2) specific problems in the health care of women, and (3) some questions raised by research involving women as subjects.

General aspects of the therapeutic relationship

Sociologists have noted that "professional dominance" frequently characterizes the relationship between health-care providers and their patients. When female patients receive health care from physicians, who are usually male, they are subjected to a kind of double dominance, the one professional, the other sexual. Miller and Mothner note that women have generally been the nondominant group in an unequal relationship between the sexes (Miller and Mothner). A large literature in psychology and sociology documents that norms of behavior and social roles for women have tended to support more compliant, dependent, and passive orientations in relationships with men. Broverman et al., in a study of mental health norms for men and women patients as defined by male and female therapists, found that women are seen as normal if they are obedient, dependent, easily influenced, not self-confident, and emotional (Broverman et al.). These stereotyped social roles are reflected in the expectations and responses of women as patients. They influence what the physician, who is usually a man, expects when caring for a woman. The physician may approach her with advice, commands, directions, or decisions rather than including her as a partner or collaborator in the plan for her care. The relationship takes on the quality of a parent–child interaction rather than a partnership.

Women, on the other hand, often perceive themselves in a way consistent with this view; they may appear to be naive, compliant, and childlike. This parent–child model can result in lack of adequate expression of their concerns and wishes and consequently cause failure in providing or obtaining proper information or care. At times of crisis and in gratitude for being helped, the patient may overlook the depreciation implicit in this paternalistic pattern. The dependent, compliant response of the woman patient can affect her adaptation to the illness by interfering with active mastery, an important part of the process of recovery from trauma and illness.

A second problem in the relationship between female patient and male physician is the potential for sexualization of the relationship because of the intimate nature of the interaction where private information and body parts are exposed. The statistical incidence of sexual contact between physicians and patients is obviously difficult to document, but recurring complaints before ethics committees attest to its prevalence. Although some physicians discuss the "therapeutic" role of sex, most judge it exploitative and unethical. There have been recent discussions of the issues and efforts at implementation of ethical principles involving sexual activity between doctor and patient. These are hampered by secrecy and the patient's dependency on the doctor (Dahlberg; Marmor).

Women patients who have learned to handle many of their relationships with men by sexualization bring these responses into the patient–doctor relationship. They may use coping mechanisms that appear to be seductive in response to the anxiety induced by their feelings or their illness. This apparent seductiveness may be unconscious on the part of the patient who may also not be aware of her anxiety; it may be perceived as seductive by a doctor who may be particularly vulnerable because of his own life circumstances such as loneliness, disappointment in his career, or stresses in his relationships. These problems may lead him to respond inappropriately to a patient who enhances his feelings of importance and effectiveness or who is sexually appealing. Sexualization of a relationship may be brought by the patient or the doctor into almost any relationship regardless of age or appropriateness.

Specific problems in health care of women

Reproductive decisions. A major category of ethical consideration arises from the special characteristics of women's bodies and their reproductive roles. Since decisions made about childbearing, contraception, sterilization, and surgery involving reproductive organs have profound social consequences, the autonomy of the woman in deciding these questions has been a matter of intense public debate.

Historically and economically women have generally not been in a position to achieve their own goals, and they have not conceptualized these as distinct from the goals and values of family and society. Decisions about medical or surgical procedures which have an impact on sexuality and childbearing have often been made by the physician on the basis of his or her assumptions about the patient's best interest. Such decisions may reflect personal values of the physician although they may be presented as purely medical problems. For example, a gynecologist may assume that a patient would not want more children after she reaches thirty-five and that she does not want to expose herself to the risk of having a defective child by becoming pregnant after age forty. However, many women want to make that choice and assume the risk themselves.

A clinical example illustrates this problem. Mrs. A., a thirty-five-year-old married woman with two small sons, aged seven and five, developed heavy periods. Her gynecologist diagnosed uterine "fibroids," nonmalignant tumors, which may lead to excessive menstrual bleeding. Noting her age, he suggested a hysterectomy for relief of her symptoms. Mrs. A. was depressed and anxious about cancer, which she associated with the "tumors." She was unable to tell the gynecologist her previous thoughts about having a third child and her wishes for a girl, because the gynecologist seemed so dubious about a woman having children after age thirty-five. She could not openly question the gynecologist's decision nor ask about alternatives and thus agreed to the surgery. His recommendation might have been altered had she communicated her concerns.

Hysterectomy. Hysterectomies are the second most common gynecological procedure in the United States (Bunker). There has been considerable debate about the appropriate indications and the justification for the procedure. Some gynecologists have called the uterus after childbearing a "useless organ," disregarding the emotional meaning of the uterus and bodily intactness for the self-image of women. There is evidence that hysterectomy is followed by depression more frequently than are other surgical procedures. The difficulty of establishing rigid uniform criteria for performing a hysterectomy is well known. However, the arbitrariness of the decision is implied by a Canadian study where a 32.8 percent drop in the total number of hysterectomies done in Saskatchewan occurred when review committees were formed to examine indications for the procedure (Dyck et al.).

The ambiguity of the indications has led to accusations that hysterectomies are done as practice for surgeons, especially on poorly educated women who are not fully informed about the alternatives (Scully). On the other hand, some women who are themselves ambivalent about contraception or for whom contraception causes conflict with religious beliefs or cultural practices may seek a hysterectomy essentially for contraceptive purposes, generally not an accepted indication.

Certain gynecological conditions, such as severe pelvic pain where no organic pathology is found, have unclear etiology and are often the expression in physical sensations of other conflicts. The patient may then press the doctor for surgery, which does not really relieve the underlying problems and may set in motion a series of further physical and psychological complications (Castelnuovo-Tedesco and Krout). The surgeon's interest in performing the procedure may then be supported by the patient's pressure, and it becomes difficult to sustain the long-range goal of addressing the underlying causes of the symptoms. In this case, if a hysterectomy is performed, an unexpected depression might well be the result.

Contraception. Developments of new contraceptive methods in the past two decades have had a profound impact on women's lives and families by making effective control of reproduction much closer to a reality. *Today* most research is on contraceptive techniques for women, and most widely available new contraceptives have been for women. Although new contraceptive techniques offer control to those most vulnerable to the hazards of pregnancy, they also expose women to the risks and side effects of new drugs and methods whose long-term consequences will not be determined for many years. Recent reports have demonstrated that these long-term problems can occur. Indeed some problems can arise very quickly as in the case of the Dalkon Shield, an intrauterine device that was marketed for several years. Subsequently substantial evidence was compiled which indicated that uterine infections and maternal deaths were caused in some cases. The Dalkon Shield has been withdrawn after the evidence implicating this device became quite impressive.

Diethylstibestrol (DES) was given in the past to pregnant women to prevent spontaneous abortions. Daughters of women taking DES are now known to risk developing precancerous changes of the vaginal epithelium and in some cases carcinoma as well. Here, too, the greater vulnerability of women to an unpredictable long-term hazard of medication arises from their reproductive roles.

Sterilization, involuntary and voluntary. In some places, laws have permitted sterilization of women who have been considered socially undesirable or psychologically deviant or retarded. The justification for this practice has been two-fold: (1) the protection of the individual, e.g., a mentally retarded girl who is sexually active and may be exploited; and (2) the protection of society against reproduction by "unfit" individuals. Compulsory sterilization statutes have been punitive and discriminatory rather than based on scientific evidence. The conditions considered indications for sterilization, such as psychosis, criminality, and retardation, have not been clearly defined. Furthermore, no genetic basis for many of these conditions has been established. Permission for sterilization procedures was either not obtained or obtained from patients or guardians under pressure and without the patient's full awareness of the implications of the procedure. For minors, the decisions have been made by social agencies or physicians. Many patients have been black, poor, and uneducated, and thus vulnerable (*Relf* v. *Weinberger*).

Changes in patient populations have brought into focus other aspects of sterilization. The young woman who seeks sterilization raises important ethical and clinical issues for the physician. The physician may be aware that the woman may change her mind in the future. He or she may be reluctant to perform an irreversible procedure that may be self-destructive to the patient. However, the few studies that do exist indicate that at least for some women the motivation for childlessness may be deeply rooted and consistent with other desires.

A small study of women in their early twenties who had never been pregnant or had a child and who were seeking voluntary tubal ligation, found that the wish for childlessness was based on negative feelings toward children, on feelings that they had limited capacity to be mothers, and on the desire to be independent. The researcher noted the importance of assessing the character of the decision-making process to determine that there has been no outside pressure and no major internal psychological conflicts (Lindenmayer). One might raise an ethical question about the importance of obtaining the agreement of both partners if the woman is married or involved in a stable relationship.

Kaltreider and Margolis, in a San Francisco study of women under age thirty who had decided never to have children, found a strong internal psychological motivation in those electing tubal ligations. A history of family disruption, fear of motherhood, and dislike of children also characterized this group. The authors suggested that for this group "the choice to be barren was multidetermined, persistent over time," and in agreement with other aspects of their psychological functioning.

Abortion.   In the past decade abortion has become legally available to an increasing number of women. The 1973 U.S. Supreme Court decision made abortion a legal procedure in the United States within limits of time and the circumstances under which it could be performed. The decision then became the responsibility of the pregnant woman and her physician. Even those intimately involved, such as her husband or, for minors, parents, are not legally able to change the decision. These conditions, however, are not necessarily honored in the attitudes and prejudices toward a woman who seeks an abortion. Women are expected to exert sexual controls—and thus an unwanted pregnancy is still linked with sinfulness—yet the woman is held more responsible than the man for unfortunate outcomes.

Some physicians refuse to perform abortions on the grounds of their moral convictions, and indeed they cannot be expected to act against them. However, problems are at present created by the refusal of some hospitals to perform abortions and the limitation of funds for the procedure. These policies discriminate against women with limited mobility and finances. Where abortions are unavailable to recipients of welfare or to patients in a specific geographic area, it is the poor and neediest women who are most affected.

Abortion has been practiced for centuries, and illegal abortions with greater hazards increase in the face of restrictive laws (Callahan). One must be particularly concerned about the health and welfare of the woman with an unwanted pregnancy who may be unable to care for a child and would put herself at risk by seeking an illegal abortion.

Childbirth.   Many changes have taken place in obstetrical practice in the direction of greater involvement by the pregnant woman and her family. The diminished use of anethesia, the increase in "natural" or prepared childbirth, greater participation of fathers in childbirth classes and their presence during labor and in delivery rooms—all of these are somewhat more widely practiced today than twenty years ago. Home births have seen a revival. However,

significant problems remain. Many patients feel uninformed and unable to communicate with their doctors; the impersonality of the hospital and frequent lack of support for the mother have also caused distress. On the other hand, home delivery raises many ethical problems about responsibility toward the child: Obstetricians have been penalized for assisting at them on grounds of unethical disregard for the welfare of the child.

Pregnancy and childbirth can be stressful experiences (Bibring and Valenstein), and problems are intensified by the increased emphasis on the technical aspects of obstetrics and the sacrifice of humanistic attitudes. In the relationship between the pregnant woman and her obstetrician, the potential for her to be dependent increases the likelihood that the physician will respond in an authoritarian manner.

Other issues in somatic health

Menstruation.   Many myths exist about menstruation and its effects, causing stereotyping and prejudiced reactions to menstruating women. The existence and basis of behavioral and mood fluctuations with phases of the menstrual cycle have been debated for years. On the grounds that they were too strongly affected by cyclic changes, women were considered unsuitable for important positions. Although many women experience no changes premenstrually, for others the days before each period are characterized by irritability, lability, or depression. These symptoms disappear with the onset of the menstrual period.

Premenstrual tension has been said to be responsible for various types of social behavior and psychological phenomena. Crimes committed (Morton et al.; Dalton), suicide attempts, misbehavior of schoolgirls, psychiatric admissions in emergency rooms, and visits to clinics (Sommer; Koeske) have been related to the premenstrual period. A number of studies of suicidal attempts (Mandell and Mandell; MacKinnon, MacKinnon, and Thomson) have indicated that a majority occurred in the bleeding phase of the cycle. Self-reports of functioning during the menstrual cycle indicate that a small percentage of women feel that their judgment and mental faculties are impaired to some extent, particularly in the premenstrual phase of the cycle.

Sommer, in a review of studies of cognitive and perceptual-motor behavior in relation to menstruation, points out methodological problems in much of the research. The problem of determining the hormonal status of the subjects, the selection bias toward women with regular cycles, the use of self-reports, and the combination of objective with subjective data complicate evaluation of results. Many studies have not been replicated, and correlational studies do not clearly indicate relationships between cause and effect. A majority of studies using objective performance measures failed to demonstrate significant cyclic fluctuation in performance.

Sommer concludes that cyclic effects are seen where the demands of the social milieu and the woman's own expectations predict them: "Where social-psychological expectations of menstrual debilitation are altered, the effect disappears." Menstrual variations may reflect responses of the individual to personal and social expectations, identification with important women in her life, or somatic expressions of a wide variety of feelings about herself, her femininity, and her body. Observation of family patterns in menstrual responses indicate a strong tendency for girls to repeat the patterns of their mothers in their premenstrual reactions, dysmenorrhea, and the extent of morbidity around the menstrual period. Although recent electroencephalograms and other data (Vogel, Broverman, and Klarber) suggest possible cyclic effects to be further studied, the premenstrual syndrome and menstrual fluctuations often become the inappropriate basis for stereotyping women's behavior.

Menopause. Recent endocrinological and social-psychological data (Bart and Grossman; McKinley and Jefferys) indicate that many misconceptions have existed about the nature and extent of the symptomatology directly ascribable to the menopause. In a review of endocrinological data, Perlmutter states that there are multiple disorders that have been ascribed to the changing hormonal balance and equated with menopause which may not be due to these imbalances (Perlmutter).

Research on menopause suffers from methodological problems, such as relying on case histories, clinical impressions, or analyses of data from selected samples of women under the care of gynecologists or psychiatrists. Those studies which are more reliable show that "psychosomatic and psychological complaints were not reported more frequently by so-called 'menopausal' than by younger women" (McKinley and Jefferys).

Vasomotor instability, manifested as hot flashes, flushes, and excess of perspiration, has been one of the consistent symptoms accompanying menopause. Such phenomena are present in a large number of women, up to seventy-five percent reporting some degree of symptomatology (Perlmutter; Reynolds). McKinley and Jefferys in a review of symptoms of women aged forty-five to fifty-four found that hot flashes and night sweats are "clearly associated with the onset of a natural menopause and that they occur in the majority of women." The other symptoms investigated—headaches, dizzy spells, palpitations, sleeplessness, depression, and weight increase—showed no direct relationship to menopause.

Not only are many symptoms attributed to menopause not necessarily biological, but menopause itself may not be as central to the midlife crisis for women as has previously been thought (Bart and Grossman; Neugarten et al.). The cessation of menses and the accompanying endocrine changes may be less critical than the reaction to menopause as a signal of aging and the awareness that a phase of life has ended. For many women there are concomitant changes in social role at that time with the loss of their status as mothers and the disruption of a network of important social relationships.

The stereotyping of menopause as the determining diagnostic entity for midlife depression or midlife stress has led to premature decisions for estrogen replacement treatment, with insufficient attention to social, family, or psychiatric conditions, or to the possible deleterious effects of estrogen. Estrogen therapy has been widely used for menopausal symptoms. Although the only symptoms clearly related to estrogen deficiency are the "hot flashes" (Jones, Cohen, and Wilson), estrogens are given for a wide variety of other symptoms for which their results are less predictable, e.g., symptoms that are probably psychogenic or the result of social phenomena. Therapy with estrogens would be considered simply useless and wasteful except for the fact that recent data indicate a strong possibility of carcinogenicity and bloodclotting (Ziel and Finkle).

Mastectomy. Recent articles have questioned the efficacy of radical mastectomy as the treatment of choice for breast cancer (Tishler, 1978). Modified radical surgery, simple mastectomy, and even "lumpectomy" for malignancy are performed with good results. For some women, the knowledge that a disfiguring operation is not inevitable has made it easier to seek medical attention for breast masses. For surgeons, the resistance to abandoning an established treatment is compounded by the difficulty in acknowledging patients' reactions to the mutilating aspect of the surgery. When patients demand a procedure other than one the doctor is used to, he or she may defend the accepted practice. The controversy about whether post-mastectomy plastic surgery is necessary or indicated has been cited as an expression of the insensitivity of medicine and of insurance companies to the psychological needs of women (Gifford).

Rape. Women who have been raped face a number of prejudices. They have been blamed, disbelieved, and criticized by society. Health professionals have often shared these social attitudes, warding off their own anxiety and their own sense of vulnerability and helplessness by a variety of mechanisms such as withdrawal, denial, disbelief, or blaming the victim. Such mechanisms may be adaptive to those employing them but are not helpful to the rape victim. Indeed, such responses by professionals accentuate the dehumanizing aspect of the experience.

Since they may be looked on as the perpetrators rather than the victims of the crime, women who have been raped have frequently been reluctant to seek medical care or to report the attack. The tendency to blame rape victims results in their receiving poor medical care, creating a disparity between them and victims of other aggressions or disasters. Professionals have shared the popular view that the victim was acting out conscious or unconscious sexual fantasies, and therefore was not "really" a victim. Thus, she could not expect to receive the empathy and understanding usually extended to people in crisis (Notman and Nadelson, 1976).

Rape is a violent crime which is often misperceived as a sexual experience with consequent guilt feelings of the victim. The possibility of serious harm or death exists, and the victim's prime concern is to protect herself from injury. The absence of consent is crucial to the definition of rape. In the past in order to prove the absence of consent the rape victim had to demonstrate signs of struggle. Current laws are changing to acknowledge threat of violence as sufficient.

In the rape victim's experience with physicians any harshness, criticism, or humiliation is perceived as if it were a repetition of the trauma of the rape. The physician is in a dual role here, since the doctor who first sees the rape victim is in a position of collecting evidence for possible prosecution. Sensitivity to the patient's condition may be in conflict with the need for complete information. The availability of women as caregivers has been particularly important to many rape victims during the crisis phase of their reaction, when they may be frightened or mistrustful of men.

Mental health issues. Women have generally been considered more vulnerable than men to a variety of emotional symptoms and mental illnesses. The actual incidence of mental illness is difficult to evaluate, because definitions of mental illness and concepts of symptomatology vary widely. The criteria of mental health and illness vary with social class, cultural group, and historical context. They are also different for women and men.

The Brovermans and their co-workers documented these variations in a study which indicated that both men and women therapists had different criteria for mental health for men and women. Clinicians' concepts of a mentally healthy mature man are similar to their concepts of a mentally healthy adult; their concepts of a mature mentally healthy woman differ from ideas about adult health and are more similar to those for a child—e.g., healthy women are seen as being more submissive, less independent, less adventurous, more sensitive to being hurt, less aggressive and competitive, etc. These concepts reflect social stereotypes and also represent normative values regarding women that still persist to some degree. The value differences become important in judging the mental health of a woman who is not behaving in a conventional way. The differentiation between psychopathology and deviance is particularly relevant for women patients who have complained that psychotherapists, often male, have supported traditional values rather than offering genuine help (Chesler).

Despite the evidence that there is variability in criteria for mental illness and that many symptoms go unreported, it seems clear that greater numbers of women than men turn to mental health facilities. Gove and Tudor found that women show a greater prevalence of mental illness than men. More mentally ill women than men are treated in general hospitals, as well as in psychiatric outpatient facilities and by private practitioners. Depression is more common in women, by a consistent ratio, cross-culturally (Weissman and Klerman).

Although suicide rates indicate that more men commit suicide, more women than men make attempts (Stengel; Farberow and Schneidman). Farberow and Schneidman found that sixty-nine percent of attempted suicides in the United States were women and seventy percent of completed suicides were men.

Married women make up the largest group of mentally ill women. The major difference in rates of mental illness between men and women is found among married men and women, with married men doing better and single women doing better (Weissman and Klerman; Gove and Tudor). Contrary to popular expectations marriage would seem to offer men some protection against mental illness and to make women more vulnerable. Additional data from many sources indicate that the group of women most vulnerable to symptoms are young married women with small children (Bernard).

Chesler has charged that women are labeled mentally ill when they cannot perform the service and maintenance functions of wife and mother. Another explanation may lie in the demands of the maternal phase of life, in which women are responding to the stresses of social isolation, particularly from other adults, the physical and emotional fatigue of dealing with small children, and the strain of being confronted with the primitive impulses and feelings stirred up in parents by their young children.

Recommendations for change. The health-care system is in the process of change in a number of directions. Changes have started to be implemented in authority and hierarchical relationships. The entrance of paraprofessionals, many of whom are women, may dilute the strict division into a doctor–patient hierarchy. The increasing importance and responsibility of the nurse-practitioner, the nurse, and the community mental health worker are potential examples of this trend. Placing women in positions of authority does not, of course, automatically reduce authoritarian issues, but where women are patients, the potential for identification with the patient is greater. The entrance of significantly more women into medicine will have an impact that has thus far not been possible to assess.

Challenges to the authority and exclusive expertise of the physician have come from the consumer movement, self-help groups, and the women's movement. The idea that professionalism is always crucial for good care has been questioned. Women are encouraged to examine and understand their bodies, and to have a strong voice in decisions about their own care (Boston Women's Health Book Collective).

Professionals have expressed concern about the dangers that the lack of knowledge and expertise might introduce when vital decisions are to be made. An assessment of the risks as well as the reasons for professional rigidity is important. An example of effective collaboration is seen in the area of natural childbirth where there have been some major changes. The totally passive, anesthetized patient is not as much the rule as it was. The patient participates in a collaborative way, and the results have been generally positive.

Women as experimental subjects

Informed consent. A central value in our society is the individual's freedom to determine his or her own thoughts and actions within broad social limits (Katz). Guttentag stresses the importance of a relationship of partnership, mutual trust, and confidence between experimenter and experimental subject and the significance of the "inner freedom" necessary to volunteer to be a subject. By this he means the capacity to understand information and make a true choice. Informed consent, a crucial issue for all research, has "become the most important, most complex and most confused concept in medical ethics" (Redlich and Mollica).

When women are experimental subjects their freedom may be diminished by the authority relationships discussed above. A woman subject is frequently vulnerable because of the parent–child dynamics of her relationship with the doctor. The agreement to participate in an experiment may be influenced by her perception of the experimenter as possessing "superior" knowledge and authority, a perception that may be entirely without supportive evidence. Agreement is thus given by a person who appears to be willing but may not be able to make an objective or considered decision.

Choice of research areas. Inequalities in power and in access to decision making influence the kinds of research done. The relative lack of research on certain gynecological problems, such as nonsurgical treatment of uterine "fibroids," has been cited as reflecting the lack of interest of researchers, who are primarily male, in women's concerns and in developing treatment alternatives that are more considerate of women's needs.

Contraceptive research has raised several ethical dilemmas. The development of effective reversible contraceptives for women has proceeded more quickly than the development of similar techniques for men, possibly reflecting prejudices about which sex should bear responsibility for contraception, but perhaps reflecting as well the pressure from women for gaining reproductive control (Bremmer and deKretzer).

An often quoted example of an ethically unacceptable study is one conducted by Goldzieher in Texas on Mexican-American women. The aim was to study the side effects of contraceptive pills (Katz). One group of women was given pills; another group was given placebos and a vaginal cream known to the investigators to be a less effective contraceptive. The latter group of women believed they were protected, but some did become pregnant. The ethical problems arise from the deceit, the misuse by the investigators of the trust of the subject, and the impossibility of their having given informed consent. They were exposed to risks that far outweighed the benefits to be derived from their participation in the study.

In research on oral contraceptives, long-term cumulative data have often demonstrated a deleterious effect or hazard which was initially understated. Katz traces the successive reports of serious side effects since the 1957 studies in Puerto Rico. Although some problems later proved unconnected with pill usage, other important ones emerged. Action to limit indications and to notify potential users of risks was taken slowly and reluctantly. For example, the American Medical Association initially protested the Food and Drug Administration regulation requiring a warning on pill containers (ibid., pp. 785–788).

Conclusion

Social changes have brought about alterations in the relationship between men and women. Simultaneously, a new awareness on the part of patients and research subjects has fundamentally effected their relationships with health-care providers and biomedical researchers. In the future the combination of these changes promises to bring into being a new pattern of relationships in which a genuine partnership exists between physician or researcher and female patient—one in which the woman's autonomy and maturity are respected as she receives needed health care or participates in the search for new biomedical knowledge.

MALKAH T. NOTMAN
AND CAROL C. NADELSON

[*Directly related is the other article in this entry,* WOMEN AS HEALTH PROFESSIONALS. *For further discussion of topics mentioned in this article, see the entries:* ABORTION; CONTRACEPTION; INFORMED CONSENT IN HUMAN RESEARCH; INFORMED CONSENT IN THE THERAPEUTIC RELATIONSHIP; MENTAL ILLNESS, *articles on* DIAGNOSIS OF MENTAL ILLNESS *and* LABELING IN MENTAL ILLNESS: LEGAL ASPECTS; PATERNALISM; STERILIZATION; SUICIDE; SURGERY; *and* THERAPEUTIC RELATIONSHIP. *For discussion of related ideas, see:* HEALTH CARE, *article on* HUMANIZATION AND DEHUMANIZATION OF HEALTH CARE. *See also:* DRUG INDUSTRY AND MEDICINE; HUMAN EXPERIMENTATION, *articles on* BASIC ISSUES *and* SOCIAL AND PROFESSIONAL CONTROL; MEDICINE, SOCIOLOGY OF; SEX THERAPY AND SEX RESEARCH, *article on* ETHICAL PERSPECTIVES; *and* SEXUAL IDENTITY.]

BIBLIOGRAPHY

BART, PAULINE B., and GROSSMAN, MARLYN. "Menopause." *Women and Health* 1, no. 3 (1976), pp. 3–10.

BERNARD, JESSIE SHIRLEY. *The Future of Marriage.* New York: World Publication Co., 1972.

BIBRING, GRETE L., and VALENSTEIN, ARTHUR F. "Psychological Aspects of Pregnancy." *Clinical Obstetrics and Gynecology* 19 (1976): 357–371.

Boston Women's Health Book Collective. *Our Bodies, Ourselves: A Book by and for Women.* 2d ed., rev. and exp. New York: Simon & Schuster, 1976.

BREMMER, WILLIAM J., and DE KRETZER, DAVID M. "The Prospects for New, Reversible Male Contraceptives." *New England Journal of Medicine* 295 (1976): 1111–1117.

BROVERMAN, INGE K.; BROVERMAN, DONALD M.; CLARKSON, FRANK E.; ROSENCRANTZ, PAUL S.; and VOGEL, SUSAN R. "Sex Role Stereotypes and Clinical Judgments of Mental Health." *Journal of Consulting and Clinical Psychology* 34 (1970): 1–7.

BUNKER, JOHN P. "Elective Hysterectomy: Pros and Cons." *New England Journal of Medicine* 295 (1976): 264–268.

CALLAHAN, DANIEL J. *Abortion: Law, Choice and Morality.* New York: Macmillan Co., 1970.

CASTELNUOVO-TEDESCO, PIETRO, and KROUT, BOYD M. "Psychosomatic Aspects of Chronic Pelvic Pain." *Psychiatry in Medicine* 1 (1970): 109–126.

CHESLER, PHYLLIS. *Women and Madness.* New York: Avon, 1972.

COPE, OLIVER. *The Breast: Its Problems, Benign and Malignant.* Boston: Houghton & Mifflin, 1977.

DAHLBERG, CHARLES CLAY. "Sexual Contact between Patient and Therapist." *Contemporary Psycholanalysis* 6 (1970): 107–124.

DALTON, KATHARINA. *The Premenstrual Syndrome.* Springfield, Ill.: Charles C Thomas, 1964.

DYCK, ARTHUR J. "Procreative Rights and Population Policy: Freedom, Compulsion, and Context." *Hastings Center Studies* 1, no. 1 (1973), pp. 74–82.

DYCK, FRANK J., et al. "Effect of Surveillance on the Number of Hysterectomies in the Province of Saskatchewan." *New England Journal of Medicine* 296 (1977): 1326–1328.

FARBEROW, NORMAN L., and SCHNEIDMAN, EDWIN S. "Statistical Comparisons between Attempted and Committed Suicides." *The Cry for Help.* Edited by Norman L. Farberow and Edwin S. Schneidman. Foreword by Robert H. Felix. New York: McGraw-Hill Book Co., 1965, pp. 19–47.

"FDA Investigating IUD's after Deaths Reported." *FDA Drug Bulletin,* July 1974. Unpaginated.

GIFFORD, SANFORD. "Emotional Attitudes toward Cosmetic Breast Surgery: Loss and Restitution of the 'Ideal Self'." *Plastic and Reconstructive Surgery of the Breast.* Edited by Robert M. Goldwyn. Boston: Little, Brown & Co., 1976, pp. 103–121.

GOLDWYN, ROBERT M. "Reconstruction after Mastectomy." *Archives of Surgery* 110 (1975): 246. Editorial.

GOVE, WALTER R., and TUDOR, JEANNETTE F. "Adult Sex Roles and Mental Illness." *Changing Women in a Changing Society.* Edited by Joan Huber. Sociology: Women's Studies. Chicago: University of Chicago Press, 1973, pp. 50–73. Also, *American Journal of Sociology* 78 (1973): 812–835.

GUTTENTAG, OTTO E. "Ethical Problems in Human Experimentation." Torrey, *Ethical Issues in Medicine,* pp. 195–226.

HILBERMAN, ELAINE. *The Rape Victim.* New York: Basic Books, 1976.

JONES, HOWARD W., JR.; COHEN, EUGENE J.; and WILSON, ROBERT B. "Clinical Aspects of the Menopause." *Menopause and Aging: Summary Report and Selected Papers from a Research Conference on Menopause and Aging, May 23–26, 1971, Hot Springs, Arkansas.* Edited by Kenneth J. Ryan and Don C. Gibson. DHEW Publication no. (NIH) 73-319. Bethesda, Md.: Public Health Service, National Institute of Child Health and Human Development, 1973, pp. 2–4.

KAHANA, RALPH J. and BIBRING, GRETE L., "Personality Types in Medical Management." *Psychiatry and Medical Practice in a General Hospital.* Edited by Norman Earl Zinberg. New York: International University Press, 1964, pp. 108–123.

KALTREIDER, N. B., and MARGOLIS, A. G. "Childless by Choice: A Clinical Study." *American Journal of Psychiatry* 134 (1977): 179–182.

KATZ, J. ed. *Experimentation with Human Beings: The Authority of the Investigator, Subject, Professions, and State in the Human Experimentation Process.* New York: Russell Sage Foundation, 1972.

KOESKE, RANDI DAIMON. "Premenstrual Emotionality: Is Biology Destiny?" *Women and Health* 1, no. 3 (1976), pp. 11–14.

LENNANE, K. JEAN, and LEANNANE, R. JOHN. "Alleged Psychogenic Disorders in Women—A Possible Manifestation of Sexual Prejudice." *New England Journal of Medicine* 288 (1973): 288–292.

LINDENMAYER, JEAN-PIERRE. Quoted in "More Young, Childless Women Seek Surgical Sterilization." *Roche Report: Frontiers of Psychiatry,* 15 June 1976, pp. 5–6.

McKINLEY, SONJA M., and JEFFERYS, MARGOT. "The Menopausal Syndrome." *British Journal of Preventive and Social Medicine* 28 (1974): 108–115.

MacKINNON, I. L.; MacKINNON, P. C. B.; and THOMSON, A. D. "Lethal Hazards of the Luteal Phase of the Menstrual Cycle." *British Medical Journal* 1 (1959): 1015–1017.

MANDELL, ARNOLD J., and MANDELL, MARY P. "Suicide and the Menstrual Cycle." *Journal of the American Medical Association* 200 (1967): 792–793. Clinical note.

MARMOR, JUDD. "The Seductive Psychotherapist." *Psychiatry Digest* 31, no. 10 (1970), pp. 10–16.

"Maternal Death and the IUD." *Lancet* 2 (1976): 1234.

MILLER, JEAN BAKER, and MOTHNER, IRA. "Psychological Consequences of Sexual Inequality." *American Journal of Orthopsychiatry* 41 (1971): 767–775.

MORTON, J. H.; ADDITON, H.; ADDISON, R. G.; HUNT, L.; and SULLIVAN, J. J. "A Clinical Study of Premenstrual Tension." *American Journal of Obstetrics and Gynecology* 65 (1953): 1182–1191.

NADELSON, CAROL C., and NOTMAN, MALKAH. "The Woman Physician." *Journal of Medical Education* 47 (1972): 176–183.

NEUGARTEN, B. L.; WOOD, VIVIAN; KRAINES, RUTH J.; and LOOMIS, BARBARA. "Women's Attitudes towards the Menopause." *Middle Age and Aging: A Reader in Social Psychology.* Edited by Bernice Levin Neugarten. Chicago: University of Chicago Press, 1968, pp. 195–200.

NOTMAN, MALKAH, and NADELSON, CAROL C. "The Rape Victim: Psychodynamic Considerations." *American Journal of Psychiatry* 133 (1976): 408–413.

———, and NADELSON, CAROL C., eds. *The Woman Patient.* 2 vols. New York: Plenum Press, 1978.

PERLMUTTER, JOHANNA. "Temporary Symptoms and Permanent Changes." *The Menopause Book.* Edited by Louisa Rose. Information House Books. New York: Hawthorn Books, 1977, pp. 18–34.

REDLICH, FRITZ, and MOLLICA, RICHARD F. "Overview: Ethical Issues in Contemporary Psychiatry." *American Journal of Psychiatry* 133 (1976): 125–135.

Relf v. Weinberger and National Welfare Rights Organization v. Weinberger. 372 F. Supp. 1196 (D.C.D.C. 1974).

REYNOLDS, S. R. M. "Physiological and Psychogenic Factors in the Menopausal Flush Syndrome." *Psychosomatic Obstetrics, Gynecology, and Endocrinology, Including Diseases of Metabolism.* Edited by William S. Kroger. Foreword by J. P. Greenhill. A Monograph in the Bannerstone Division of American Lectures in Gynecology and Obstetrics. Edited by E. C. Hamblen. American Lecture series, Publication no. 499. Springfield, Ill.: Charles C Thomas, 1962, pp. 618–628.

SCULLY, DIANA. "Hysterectomy." Paper presented at a panel on Women as Gynecological Patients at the American Psychiatric Association Annual Meeting, Toronto, Canada, May 1977. To appear as part of a book on obstetrics and gynecology by Scully to be published by Houghton Mifflin in 1979.

SOMMER, BARBARA. "The Effect of Menstruation on Cognitive and Perceptual-Motor Behavior: A Review." *Psychosomatic Medicine* 35 (1973): 515–534.

SORENSON, ROBERT C. *Adolescent Sexuality in Contemporary America: Personal Values and Sexual Behavior Ages Thirteen to Nineteen.* Introduction by Paul

Moore, Jr. Note by Jiri Nehnevajsa. New York: World Publishing Co., 1973. The Sorenson Report.

STENGEL, ERWIN. *Suicide and Attempted Suicide.* Rev. ed. Pellican Book, no. A704. Baltimore: Penguin, 1969.

TISHLER, SIGRID. "Breast Disorders." Notman, *The Woman Patient,* vol. 1, chap. 17.

TORREY, EDWIN FULLER, ed. *Ethical Issues in Medicine: The Role of the Physician in Today's Society.* Boston: Little, Brown & Co., 1968.

VOGEL, WILLIAM; BROVERMAN, DONALD M.; and KLARBER, EDWARD L. "EEG Responses in Regularly Menstruating Women and in Amenorrheic Women Treated with Ovarian Hormones." *Science* 172 (1971): 388–391.

WEISSMAN, MYRNA M., and KLERMAN, GERALD L. "Sex Differences and the Epidemiology of Depression." *Archives of General Psychiatry* 34 (1977): 98–111.

ZIEL, HARRY K., and FINKLE, WILLIAM D. "Increased Risk of Endometrial Carcinoma among Users of Conjugated Estrogens." *New England Journal of Medicine* 293 (1975): 1167–1170.

II
WOMEN AS HEALTH PROFESSIONALS

To those who are ill, the road back to health is best traveled when both nurturing and healing are the concerns of those responsible for medical care. Women have always been caretakers in their role as homemakers and mothers. The maternal role has encompassed giving, caring, feeding, consoling, and loving. These qualities have been recognized and accepted, but whenever women have extended their role to become more active healers, rather than exclusive caregivers, they have been met with fear, suspicion, and mistrust.

The role of the caretaker, or mother surrogate, involves activity directed toward the well-being of another person, in whatever setting and in whatever way it needs to be fulfilled, e.g., by washing, holding, or listening. The role of healer has been more specifically directed toward tasks that are necessary to restore an individual to a functional status and generally occurs in specific health-care settings.

The mother surrogate (traditional feminine role) has evolved into the nursing role, while the healer (traditional masculine role) has become the physician role. Somewhere between has stood the midwife, always on uncertain territory because she has merged the active and passive characteristics and resisted the polarity created by the role restrictions of physician and nurse.

In order to understand women as health professionals, it is necessary to review briefly the evolution of their various roles.

Early history of women in health care

Women have always been healers as well as caretakers. They have been the pharmacists, nurses, abortionists, counselors, midwives, and "wise women," as well as the witches. There have also always been female physicians, although rarely were they permitted to perform in the same capacities and positions as men.

As early as 1500 B.C. women studied in the Egyptian medical school in Heliopolis. The Chinese record, in 1000 B.C., female physicians who functioned in positions that encompassed activities other than traditional midwife and herb-gathering roles. It appears that other medical roles also existed for women in the Greek and Roman civilizations.

Throughout history women have been special attendants—assisting with labor and delivery, advising women on the functions and disorders of their bodies, and tending the newborn. According to Sigerist, since childbirth was considered a physiological process it was not included as part of medicine. It is not clear when obstetrics and gynecology came to be considered part of medicine.

Soranas, a Roman, believed that women were divinely appointed to care for sick women and children. He defined criteria for those practicing —including literacy, anatomic understanding, a sense of patient responsibility, and ethical concerns, particularly about confidentiality. Although mention is repeatedly made of women in the practice of medicine, they appear to have practiced midwifery primarily.

Prior to A.D. 441, when the Council of Orange forbade their ordination, women apparently played a significant role in health care. They were called deaconesses and were ordained by the bishops with the consent of the congregation. Apparently they became the first parish workers and district nurses; little is known about their actual work (Shryock, 1959). They included such notable women as St. Monica, the mother of St. Augustine, and Fabiola, who founded a hospital at Astia in A.D. 398.

After the fall of the Roman Empire medicine diverged into two paths: Arabian medicine, which produced notable practitioners and established hospitals, and monastic medicine, which transmitted the heritage of Greek medicine through the hands and minds of those in convents and monasteries, which provided medical care and were staffed by male and female "nurses."

According to Corner, medical learning was established in the school at Salerno, which was founded in the ninth century and flourished in the tenth or eleventh century (Corner). At that time women apparently studied there. While little is known about most of those women, eleventh-century records reveal the existence of a woman doctor, Trotula, who wrote important texts on obstetrics and gynecology, and also headed a department of diseases of women. Her contributions were of major importance, since at that time all deliveries were performed by women, many of whom had no training. Trotula was not a doctor of medicine (M.D.). The degree itself was first awarded in 1180, but apparently only to men. A special diploma was offered to women in the thirteenth and fourteenth centuries. In 1430 Constanza Calenda became the first woman to obtain the degree.

Another medical woman of the Middle Ages was Hildegarde of Bingen (1098–1179), who was a scientific scholar and wrote two medical textbooks, *Liber Simplecis Medicinae* and *Liber Compositae Medicinae*. They were presumably written for the nurses in charge of the infirmaries of Benedictine monasteries. The books described a number of diseases, including their courses, symptoms, and treatment, as well as scientific data on the pulsation of blood and the regulation of vital activities by the nervous system. Hildegarde's writings also demonstrated an understanding of normal and abnormal psychology.

In the late medieval period wealthy women continued to be active in medicine, particularly in Italy where the universities were not closed to them. Those women who were qualified were permitted to practice in France, as well as in England and Germany. They generally had to practice in defined roles, including bleeding, administration of herbs and medicines, and reducing fractures, in addition to midwifery.

By the end of the fifteenth century medicine became established in various centers in Europe. The movement to exclude women from the formal practice of medicine gained momentum, and they were specifically limited to functioning as midwives. This movement coincided with the ideology of misogyny as encapsulated by Sprenger and Kraemer in *Malleus Maleficarum* (1486). Witch-hunting focused the restlessness of the population and capitalized on the "spiritual and mental" inferiority of women. Even when active witch-hunts subsided, their effects remained:

Women were effectively eliminated from roles other than the traditional caretaking one.

During the fifteenth and sixteenth centuries, when medicine and surgery were clearly differentiated, some of the male barber surgeons began to practice midwifery. Before the sixteenth century it was not possible for a male to be a widwife; in fact, it was a capital offense. The sixteenth to eighteenth centuries produced several outstanding female midwives, including Louyse Bourgeois (1563–1636), who in 1609 was the first midwife to publish a work on obstetrics. Nonetheless, with the invention of the obstetrical forceps in the seventeenth century by the Chamberlens, a family of male widwives and barber surgeons, obstetrics was pushed closer to the realm of the male practitioner. In 1634 Peter Chamberlen III attempted to establish a corporation of midwives in England with himself as governor—a move that was resented by female midwives. Increasingly, men began to participate and compete in this profession, particularly in serving the upper classes.

Women in health care: eighteenth century to the present

Women in early American medicine. In the United States the healing role of women was critical to the survival of the colonies. Ann Hutchinson (1571?–1643), the dissident religious leader, was a general practitioner and midwife. Since there were relatively few university-trained physicians, medicine was practiced by those who appeared to be particularly talented. An apprentice system began to evolve relatively early.

Eighteenth-century American medicine had no unified concept of medical care; there were a variety of views of practice and training, each offering a program that was generally an apprenticeship. In this setting, the role of women was extensive and complex, since the medical care of families was frequently the responsibility of the wife or of women. Although there were many female practitioners, they functioned primarily as midwives. Many went to Europe to train, as the first school for midwives in the United States was not started until 1762. The early training of midwives was based on the assumption that most obstetrical practice would remain in the hands of women. This, however, was not the outcome in the United States, although it was in many parts of Europe.

In 1765 Dr. John Morgan founded the first "regular" American medical school, which became part of the University of Pennsylvania. By excluding women, it began a tradition of barring them from formal medical training. Many women, however, did set up flourishing practices without diplomas and were trained in the homeopathic or eclectic traditions.

Women in nineteenth-century medicine. In 1847 Elizabeth Blackwell became the first woman to be admitted to a "regular" medical school in the United States. She was awarded a degree from the Geneva Medical School. The New York State Medical Association promptly censured the school, and when her sister, Emily Blackwell, applied a few years later she was rejected. Emily subsequently received her M.D. from Western Reserve.

In 1850 Harriet K. Hunt (1805–1875), who had established herself in an "irregular" practice in Boston in 1835, applied for admission to Harvard Medical School. She was admitted but was denied her seat when the all-male class threatened to leave if women and blacks were admitted. Not until almost one hundred years later, in 1946, did Harvard Medical School begin to admit women. By 1850 three all-female "irregular" medical colleges were founded—one in Boston (now Boston University), one in Philadelphia (now Medical College of Pennsylvania), and one in Cincinnati. The Boston Female Medical College was designed primarily to prevent male midwifery, which its founder, Dr. Samuel Gregory, felt trespassed on female delicacy.

In 1855 the National Eclectic Medical Association formally approved the education of women in medicine, and by 1870 it became the first medical society to accept them for membership. Traditional medical societies, however, continued to be closed to women. In his 1871 American Medical Association presidential address Dr. Alfred Stille criticized female physicians for being women who seek to rival men, who "aim toward a higher type than their own" (Ehrenreich and English, p. 26).

The road continued to be difficult even for those women who managed to obtain training. Not only did medical societies refuse them admission; hospitals denied them appointments. As a result, female physicians in the United States began to open their own hospitals and clinics. In 1857 Drs. Elizabeth and Emily Blackwell founded the New York Infirmary for Women, where they cared largely for indigent women, and by 1865 the Women's Medical College of the New York Infirmary was opened.

Women in Europe also had a difficult time. In 1862 the Royal College of Physicians in Edinburgh refused to grant medical diplomas to women. The attacks on female students from peers, however, prompted some public support from people who were outraged that these indelicate and ungentlemanly men would be seeing female patients.

Dr. James Barry (1797–1865), who became Inspector General of the British Army Medical Department in 1858, was discovered to be a woman after her death. It was not until 1870 that Elizabeth Garrett was entitled to use the M.D. in England. Sir William Jenner said in 1878 that he would rather follow his daughter's bier to the grave than see her become a medical student. In general, however, many of the women who were graduated from medical school were from middle-class or upper-class backgrounds. Often they had fathers or other family members in medicine; they entered the profession to join the family practice.

The role of women in medicine continued to be hotly debated. The productivity and life-style of female physicians were questioned then as they are now. In 1881 Rachel Bodley, Dean of the Women's Medical College of Pennsylvania, surveyed the 244 living graduates of the school and found that, despite the persistent mythology to the contrary, the overwhelming majority were in active practice, and those who had married reported that their profession had no adverse effect on their marriages, nor had marriage interfered with work.

Nineteenth-century midwifery.   There was considerable opposition to the practice of midwifery by women in the nineteenth century. In 1820 John Ware wrote his *Remarks on the Employment of Females as Practitioners of Midwifery*. In it he raised objections based on "the nature of their moral qualities." He continued:

Where the responsibility in scenes of distress and danger does not fall upon them when there is someone on whom they can lean, in whose skill and judgment they have entire confidence, they retain their collection and presence of mind; but where they become the principal agents, the feelings of sympathy are too powerful for the cool exercise of judgment.

Economic and class issues also appeared to be of major importance in this controversy. While midwives came primarily from working-class, rural, and poor backgrounds and charged less for their services, physicians came from upper-class families and received more money. Physicians feared economic competition from midwives.

Objections were also raised on grounds of the quality of health care. During the time when physicians were attempting to improve care they complained of the inferior quality of midwives —though not always with accuracy. In the 1840s Drs. Holmes and Semmelweiss reported on the spread of puerperal sepsis (childbirth infection); and Semmelweiss found that there was a lower incidence of it in women delivered by midwives. He deduced that, because medical students and physicians did not wash their hands when they moved from autopsy to delivery room, they spread disease. The warning of both doctors was ignored by most of the medical profession at that time, and controversy continued about the adequacy of midwives.

By the turn of the century about fifty percent of all babies were delivered by midwives, who, however, were still publicly attacked and held responsible for childbirth illness, namely, puerperal sepsis and neonatal ophthalmia (inflammation of the eyes generally related to maternal gonorrhea). It was felt that proper training would have taught them to prevent these illnesses. The pressure was intense, and many states began to pass laws forbidding midwifery. Many of those laws remain in effect today, despite the growing evidence of the important contributions of the midwife.

Evolution of nursing in the nineteenth century. Nursing continued to be primarily involved with the church until the mid-eighteenth century, when the London Infirmary appointed a lay "nurse." Records show long working hours and low pay. Nursing was seen as a low-status occupation. Dickens's *Martin Chuzzlewit*, 1844, focused attention on the quality of the nursing care given by pardoned criminals, aging prostitutes, and other women of "questionable" morality and interest who functioned as nurses.

Florence Nightingale (1820–1910), at the time of the Crimean War (1854–1857), responded to the need for nursing reform and proceeded to establish military and then civilian nursing. She founded a school for nurses in 1860 in London with a rigorous curriculum and specific guidelines for nursing as a profession. She met opposition from the medical profession, many of whose members felt that "nurses are in much the same position as housemaids and need little teaching beyond poultice-making and the enforcement of cleanliness and attention to the patient's wants" (Dolan, p. 230).

The first nursing schools recruited upper-class women who were "refugees from the enforced leisure of Victorian ladyhood" (Ehrenreich and English, p. 34). Despite their aristocratic image, nursing schools began to change and to attract women from working-class and lower-middle-class homes. The originators of nursing saw the nurse as the embodiment of Victorian femininity and nursing as a natural vocation for women, second only to motherhood. Nightingale viewed women as instinctive nurses, not physicians. In fact, she wrote of the few female physicians: "They have only tried to be men, and they have succeeded only in being third-rate men" (ibid., p. 36). Nursing, however, was established as an acceptable profession for women.

Women in twentieth-century medicine. By the beginning of the twentieth century, women began to seek entry into medical schools in increasing numbers; those who were not accepted in U.S. schools went to European schools. Flexner, in his 1910 Report, states:

Medical education is now, in the United States and Canada, open to women upon practically the same terms as men. If all institutions do not receive women, so many do, that no woman desiring an education in medicine is under any disability in finding a school to which she may gain admittance.

He went on to state: "Now that women are freely admitted to the medical profession, it is clear that they show a decreasing inclination to enter it."

Flexner's Report established medicine as an academic discipline with high standards for training and practice. It resulted in the closing of many medical schools: Unfortunately, they were often the only ones that would admit women.

The number of female physicians in the United States continued to be exceedingly low almost until the 1970s. The 1974–1975 enrollment of women in medical schools was twenty-two percent.

	1910	1920	1930	1940	1950	1960	1974
Women M.D.s (%)	6.0	5.0	4.0	4.6	6.1	6.8	8.7

Adapted from: United States Bureau of the Census, 1963, Vol. 1, Table 202, pp. 528–533; United States Department of Labor, 1954, p. 57; Association of American Medical Colleges, 1974, Chicago, Illinois.

Other countries report a greater percentage of female physicians. In 1965 the Soviet Union reported 65 percent female physicians, Poland 30 percent, the Philippines 25 percent, the German Federal Republic 20 percent, Italy 19 percent, United Kingdom and Denmark 16 percent, and Japan 9 percent. In that year 7 percent of U.S. physicians were women.

Medicine has been a paradoxical profession for women in the United States. The caretaking functions do not inherently contradict "traditional" views of women and women's roles, but the technological and instrumental aspects do. Even a revolutionary society like Cuba demonstrates the persistence of traditional roles. While thirty to forty percent of physicians are women, virtually all nurses and midwives are women.

An important aspect of a consideration of the roles of women in medicine involves a look at the choice of specialty as well as the specific positions held by women within their fields of expertise. Women in the United States have also characteristically entered pediatrics, internal medicine, psychiatry, and family practice. These areas continue to be the most popular for women, although they are entering other fields. There is more diversification in choice of fields for women in other countries, where, for example, obstetrics-gynecology has been more popular. Thus, despite its focus on women—a reason for the choice of obstetrics-gynecology for female physicians in other countries—U.S. female physicians have not been encouraged to pursue this specialty.

Within each specialty there are also some important differentiations in status and role. In the United States and other countries, academic and administrative appointments as well as other decision-making positions are almost exclusively held by men, whereas women tend to be involved in direct patient care (ninety percent of female physicians in the United States). The fact that women assume this role has been used, in the 1970s, as an argument for increasing their numbers in medical school, on the grounds that they could be counted on to meet the needs of the health-care system in delivering primary care.

This kind of role-stereotyping is pervasive and is seen in other fields as well. Francoise Giroud, State Secretary for the Condition of Women in France, stated at the International Conference on Women and Health (August 1975) that the positions women occupy in government in most countries generally involve hos..., prisoners, housing, and welfare. She ...children, that these are areas that do not threaten ... roles or status and furthermore are consid... less important, substantive, or critical in terms of national pride or prestige.

In countries where women have made significant progress in their influence on the health fields, the changes have occurred most often in times of war, physician shortages, or major cultural reorganization. In the Soviet Union midwives proved themselves to be effective as doctors in the Russo-Turkish War of 1870, thus beginning the influx of women into medical schools. After the 1917 revolution a trend in another direction reduced the prestige of medicine, and women were admitted in great numbers to medical school. The *feldscher* (semiprofessional health worker officially known as a physician's assistant) has become a female role in the Union of Soviet Socialist Republics. Thus, the person who performs more routine medical work is the woman. Furthermore, as medicine has resumed a more prestigious position, the number of female physicians has fallen from seventy-eight percent in 1959 to a point where today fifty-six percent of the medical students in the Soviet Union are women.

The rise of female health professionals in China has occurred along with the reorganization of the medical care system and of the society in general. Currently, thirty to forty percent of physicians are women. In 1950, 50,000 midwives were reeducated as local health workers, since the Chinese have emphasized hospital deliveries by fully trained obstetricians. In the countryside, "barefoot doctors" (peasants who have had basic medical training and provide medical care without leaving productive work) meet the needs of fellow workers. Women primarily fill this role.

Contemporary issues for women as health professionals

Family considerations and role development. In the United States a special aspect of the problem of medical training and practice is its rigidity and inflexibility. These factors make the simultaneous attainment of other life goals exceedingly difficult. In addition, the kind of sex role definitions existing within families has demanded the full attention of one parent partner (usually the mother) to the family, allowing for the exclusion of the other (usually the father).

This coincidcine. Thus career and family con- ..th the expectations and demands ofcially around childbearing and child-
flicts, are a significant problem for women.
..ince the time of medical training is also the
optimal physiological time for childbearing, conflicts that seem unresolvable may be posed for
the women.

In the United States part-time work, maternity
or paternity leave, or reduction in extra work are
often regarded as compromising to career aspirations. These attitudes are not found universally. Other countries, notably Sweden, have
made changes in the training system, which
have resulted in increased time off for men and
women during this period. They do not feel, as
many American physicians do, that this compromises training, nor do men appear to feel that
family issues are the sole responsibility of
women. Another approach, in the Union of
Soviet Socialist Republics and other countries,
has been to arrange for female students to have
adequate maternity leave and flexible schedules
—a policy that extends to all women in the work
force and thus is not a special privilege for some
women. In China, work expectations include
active participation in childrearing as well as
the involvement of extended families and day-
care centers. Thus a dual commitment, career
and family, is not a deviant but an expected
position.

Family and career conflicts tend to lead
women to choose less demanding and more flexible pursuits. They often choose to work at salaried jobs rather than in private practice or in
competitive academic positions. Fields like social
work, nursing, and paramedical specialties present a bridge between medical technology and
humanistic caretaking concerns. However,
women often choose them for pragmatic reasons
rather than because of true interest or talent.
Thus these professions tend to be almost totally
dominated by women and may foster male–female work separation and stereotyping.

Dilemmas and directions. Women in the
health professions are among the large number
of women who now work outside the home. In
1970 in the United States fifty percent of women
with young children worked. Women have continued to enter the work force in increasing
numbers. Most often they remain in low-status
jobs with limited goals, partly because of the
limits of training opportunities and flexible work
situations, and partly because of their own self-
image and the difficulty they have seeing themselves in active, instrumental roles outside of the
home.

It is useful to look at the complexity of some
of the dilemmas encountered by health professionals in order to assess the nature and extent
of the problems and to formulate appropriate
plans. The dependency of others upon the caretakers and healers makes their position unique;
the responsibilities are comparable to those of
parenthood. For the parent who is also a health
professional, the demands are doubled. Couples
have attempted many solutions, including the
use of live-in help, day-care centers, and help
from their families. Each solution presents obvious limits—in time, finances, and the quality of
help obtained. The traditional solution—the
wife's assumption of responsibility for household
and children—is not a real option in a society
in which both parents have serious commitments to careers in addition to their families.
Since societal structures are slow to change to
accommodate shifting values and norms,
mothers have often adapted, with guilt and conflict, frequently jeopardizing their careers.

These human problems force us to look at the
system that has evolved and to consider the human cost of either preventing talented people
from reaching their goals or not responding to
their needs when they do begin to take steps
toward autonomous choices. There are few available models and no simple solutions. Currently
each situation tends to be viewed as a separate
and unique problem—an attitude that avoids the
ethical and moral dilemmas arising from decisions made on the basis of stereotyping and
fixed expectations.

Changing roles and responsibilities. It is clear
that the current health system is hierarchical in
a way that may not be productive of best results;
it also demands superhuman performance that
may foster the omnipotence of those at the top
of the hierarchy and erodes the family roles of
those striving to achieve success within it. The
current structure of roles in health care results
in limited expectations and performance for
those lower in the hierarchy. As a result, the
wide range of talents and abilities of many providers is not utilized. A 1973 Michigan court decision considering malpractice liability for nurses
stated:

A nurse, although obviously skilled and well trained,
is not in the same category as a physician who is
required to exercise his independent judgment on
matters which may mean the difference between
life and death. Her primary function is to observe

and record the symptoms and reactions of patients. A nurse is not permitted to exercise judgment in diagnosing or treating any symptoms which develop. Her duty is to report them to the physician. Any treatment or medication must be prescribed by a licensed physician. A nurse by the very nature of her occupation is prohibited from exercising an independent judgment [*Kambas* v. *St. Joseph's Mercy Hospital*].

This statement clearly illustrates a view of reduced function for the nurse, which is contrary to some current directions in health care. The nurse practitioner is expected to perform autonomously, to make judgments about appropriate consultation, and to integrate the caretaking and healing roles at the level of direct patient care. Thus, while the court decision is regressive, it illustrates the current ambiguity about the nurse's roles and responsibilities.

The blurring of roles and overlapping of areas of function in a number of fields have caused considerable confusion. What are the similarities and differences among the functions of a psychologist, psychiatrist, psychiatric social worker, and psychiatric nurse? Among those of a primary care physician, a physician's assistant, and a nurse practitioner? In these situations, similar functions may be performed by people who have somewhat different training and/or skills. It is often difficult to differentiate what are appropriate functions and responsibilities.

Economic factors, rather than expertise or experience, can become the determinants of choice. If payment of fees by outside agencies is only for the services of specifically designated professionals, then the consumer/patient is forced to choose from those designated categories. On the other hand, if there is no funding, then a less skilled practitioner may be chosen when the particular condition might have required the services of another, more skilled person. Conflicts are currently found—particularly in the areas of psychotherapy, sexual therapy, routine physical exams, obstetrical, and minor medical and surgical procedures—where professionals of varied backgrounds and training may provide similar services.

In many of these areas women have functioned as the less highly trained professionals and paraprofessionals. Since skills are not as easily identifiable as are training and credentials, and since the accountability of certain professions is increasingly important, the woman may find herself again in the position of the nineteenth-century midwife—namely, as one who has the potential and expertise but not the credentials. She may thus find herself displaced and superseded unless training and recognition validate her skills. Since women have always been important providers of care, future planning calls for ways of utilizing this resource creatively and widely in the healing professions.

CAROL C. NADELSON AND
MALKAH T. NOTMAN

[*For further discussion of topics mentioned in this article, see the entries:* MEDICAL ETHICS, HISTORY OF, *section on* NEAR AND MIDDLE EAST AND AFRICA, *article on* ANCIENT NEAR EAST; NURSING; *and* MEDICINE, SOCIOLOGY OF. *Directly related is the other article in this entry,* WOMEN AS PATIENTS AND EXPERIMENTAL SUBJECTS. *For further information on women as health professionals, see the entry* MEDICAL ETHICS, HISTORY OF, *section on* EUROPE AND THE AMERICAS. *See also:* MEDICAL SOCIAL WORK.]

BIBLIOGRAPHY

ALEXANDER, FRANZ G., and SELESNICK, SHELDON T. *The History of Psychiatry: An Evaluation of Psychiatric Thought and Practice from Prehistoric Times to the Present.* New York: Harper & Row, 1966.

Association of American Medical Colleges. "Issue: Should More Women Be Encouraged to Enter the Medical Profession?" *Issues, Policies, Programs.* Washington: 1974, p. VII–4.

BOWERS, JOHN Z. "Special Problems of Women Medical Students." *Journal of Medical Education* 43 (1968): 532–537.

BROWN, JANET W. "International Conference on Women in Health." *Science* 189 (1975): 784.

CALDER, JEAN MCKINLAY. *The Story of Nursing.* 4th rev. ed. Methuen's Outlines. London: Methuen, 1963.

CORNER, GEORGE W. "The Rise of Medicine at Salerno in the Twelfth Century." *Lectures on the History of Medicine: A Series of Lectures at the Mayo Foundation and the Universities of Minnesota, Wisconsin, Iowa, Northwestern, and the Des Moines Academy of Medicine, 1926–1932.* Philadelphia: W. B. Saunders Co., 1937, pp. 371–399.

CUTTER, IRVING S., and VIETS, HENRY R. *A Short History of Midwifery.* Philadelphia: W. B. Saunders Co., 1964. Reprint of Cutter's chapter on the history of obstetrics in *Obstetrics and Gynecology.* Edited by Arthur A. Curtis. Philadelphia: W. B. Saunders Co., 1933.

DOLAN, JOSEPHINE. *Goodnow's History of Nursing.* 11th ed. Philadelphia: W. B. Saunders Co., 1963. First edition by Minnie Goodnow, 1916.

EHRENREICH, BARBARA, and ENGLISH, DEIDRE. *Witches, Midwives, and Nurses: A History of Women Healers.* 2d ed. Glass Mountain Pamphlet, no. 1. Old Westbury, N.Y.: Feminist Press, 1973.

FIELD, MARK G. *Soviet Socialized Medicine: An Introduction.* New York: Free Press, 1967.

FLEXNER, ABRAHAM. *Medical Education in the United States and Canada: A Report to the Carnegie Foundation for the Advancement of Teaching.* Bulletin of the

Carnegie Foundation for the Advancement of Teaching, no. 4 (1910). Reprint. Washington: Science & Health Publications, 1960. New York: Arno Press, 1972.

GUTHRIE, DOUGLAS. *A History of Medicine.* Introduction by Samuel C. Harvey. Philadelphia: J. B. Lippincott Co., 1946.

HENLEY, ARTHUR. "Current Scene: New Roles for Women Physicians." *Physicians World* 3, no. 4 (1975), pp. 53–56.

HUME, RUTH FOX. *Great Women of Medicine.* New York: Random House, 1964.

INGLIS, BRIAN. *A History of Medicine.* Cleveland: World Publishing Co., 1965.

JACOBSON, BEVERLY, and JACOBSON, WENDY. "Only Eight Percent: A Look at Women in Medicine." *Civil Rights Digest* 7, no. 4 (1975), pp. 20–27.

Kambas v. St. Joseph's Mercy Hospital. 205 N.W. 2d 431. 389 Mich. 249 (1973).

KAPLAN, HAROLD I. "Women Physicians: The More Effective Recruitment and Utilization of Their Talents and Resistance to It—The Final Conclusion of a Seven Year Study." *New Physician* 20, no. 1 (1971), pp. 10–19.

LOPATE, CAROL. *Women in Medicine.* Baltimore: Josiah Macy, Jr., Foundation, Johns Hopkins Press, 1968.

MARKS, GEOFFREY, and BEATTY, WILLIAM K. *Women in White.* New York: C. Scribner's Sons, 1972.

MEAD, KATE CAMPBELL HURD. *A History of Women in Medicine: From the Earliest Times to the Beginning of the Nineteenth Century.* Haddam, Conn.: Haddam Press, 1938.

NADELSON, CAROL M. "Adjustment: New Approaches to Women's Mental Health." *The American Woman: Who Will She Be?* Edited by Mary Louise McBee and Kathryn A. Blake. Beverly Hills, Calif.: Glencoe Press, 1974, pp. 21–36.

———, and NOTMAN, MALKA [Malkah T.]. "Success or Failure: Women as Medical School Applicants." *Journal of the American Medical Women's Association* 29 (1974): 167–172.

———, and NOTMAN, MALKAH T. "The Woman Physician." *Journal of Medical Education* 47 (1972): 176–183.

NOTMAN, MALKAH T., and NADELSON, CAROL. "Medicine: A Career Conflict for Women." *American Journal of Psychiatry* 130 (1973): 1123–1127.

PIRADOVA, M. D. "USSR—Women Health Workers." *Women and Health* 1, no. 3 (1976), pp. 24–29.

RENSHAW, JOSEPHINE E., and PENNELL, MARYLAND Y. "Distribution of Women Physicians, 1969." *Journal of the American Medical Women's Association* 26 (1971): 187–195.

SCHULMAN, SAM. "Basic Functional Roles in Nursing: Mother Surrogate and Healer." *Patients, Physicians and Illness: A Sourcebook in Behavioral Science and Health.* Edited by E. Gartly Jaco. New York: Free Press, 1958, chap. 54, pp. 528–537.

SHRYOCK, RICHARD H. *The History of Nursing: An Interpretation of the Social and Medical Factors Involved.* Philadelphia: W. B. Saunders Co., 1959.

———. "Women in American Medicine." *Journal of the American Medical Women's Association* 5 (1950): 371–379.

SIDEL, VICTOR W., and SIDEL, RUTH. *Serve the People: Observations on Medicine in the People's Republic of China.* The Macy Foundation Series on Medicine and Public Health in China. New York: Josiah Macy, Jr., Foundation, 1973.

SPURLOCK, JEANNE. "Sexism in Medicine and Psychiatry." *Psychiatric Annals* 6, no. 1 (1976), pp. 7–9.

United States, Bureau of the Census. *U.S. Census of Population, 1960: United States Summary—Detailed Characteristics.* Final Report PC(1)-1D. Washington: Government Printing Office, 1963, vol. 1, table 202, p. 528.

———, Department of Labor, Women's Bureau. *Changes in Women's Occupations, 1940–1950.* Women's Bureau Bulletin, no. 253. Washington: Government Printing Office, 1954, p. 57.

WARE, JOHN. *Remarks on the Employment of Females as Practitioners in Midwifery: By a Physician.* Boston: Cummings & Hilliard, 1820. *American Imprints,* no. 4171.

Women's Work Project of the Union for Radical Political Economics. "USA—Women Health Workers." *Women and Health* 1, no. 3 (1976), pp. 14–23.

XYY AND XXY GENOTYPES

See GENETIC ASPECTS OF HUMAN BEHAVIOR, *articles on* MALES WITH SEX CHROMOSOME ABNORMALITIES (XYY AND XXY GENOTYPES) *and* PHILOSOPHICAL AND ETHICAL ISSUES.

ZYGOTE BANKING or ZYGOTES

See REPRODUCTIVE TECHNOLOGIES, *articles on* SPERM AND ZYGOTE BANKING, ETHICAL ISSUES, *and* LEGAL ASPECTS.

APPENDIX

Codes and Statements Related to Medical Ethics

Contents

INTRODUCTION

    CODES OF THE HEALTH-CARE PROFESSIONS *by Ronald S. Gass*   1725

SECTION I. GENERAL CODES FOR THE PRACTICE OF MEDICINE

    OATH OF HIPPOCRATES [SIXTH CENTURY B.C.–FIRST CENTURY A.D.?]   1731

    OATH OF INITIATION (CARAKA SAMHITA) [FIRST CENTURY A.D.?]   1732

    OATH OF ASAPH [THIRD CENTURY–SEVENTH CENTURY A.D.?]   1733

    ADVICE TO A PHYSICIAN, ADVICE OF HALY ABBAS
    (AHWAZI) [TENTH CENTURY A.D.]   1734

    FIVE COMMANDMENTS AND TEN REQUIREMENTS [1617]   1735

    A PHYSICIAN'S ETHICAL DUTIES FROM *KHOLASAH AL HEKMAH* [1770]   1736

    DAILY PRAYER OF A PHYSICIAN ("PRAYER OF MOSES MAIMONIDES")
    [1793?]   1737

    CODE OF ETHICS, AMERICAN MEDICAL ASSOCIATION [1847]   1738

    VENEZUELAN CODE OF MEDICAL ETHICS, NATIONAL ACADEMY OF
    MEDICINE [1918]   1746

    DECLARATION OF GENEVA, WORLD MEDICAL ASSOCIATION [1948]   1749

    INTERNATIONAL CODE OF MEDICAL ETHICS, WORLD MEDICAL
    ASSOCIATION [1949]   1749

    PRINCIPLES OF MEDICAL ETHICS [1957], WITH REPORTS AND
    STATEMENTS, AMERICAN MEDICAL ASSOCIATION   1750

    OATH OF SOVIET PHYSICIANS [1971]   1754

    ETHICAL AND RELIGIOUS DIRECTIVES FOR CATHOLIC HEALTH
    FACILITIES, UNITED STATES CATHOLIC CONFERENCE [1971]   1755

    MEDICAL ETHICS: STATEMENTS OF POLICY DEFINITIONS AND
    RULES, BRITISH MEDICAL ASSOCIATION [1974]   1758

SECTION II. DIRECTIVES FOR HUMAN EXPERIMENTATION

    NUREMBERG CODE [1946]   1764

    RESPONSIBILITY IN INVESTIGATIONS ON HUMAN SUBJECTS,
    MEDICAL RESEARCH COUNCIL, GREAT BRITAIN [1963]   1765

    EXPERIMENTAL RESEARCH ON HUMAN BEINGS, BRITISH MEDICAL
    ASSOCIATION [1963]   1769

    DECLARATION OF HELSINKI, WORLD MEDICAL ASSOCIATION
    [1964 AND 1975]   1769

    ETHICAL GUIDELINES FOR CLINICAL INVESTIGATION, AMERICAN
    MEDICAL ASSOCIATION [1966]   1773

    U.S. GUIDELINES ON HUMAN EXPERIMENTATION (INSTITUTIONAL
    GUIDE TO DHEW POLICY ON PROTECTION OF HUMAN SUBJECTS)
    [1971]   1774

SECTION III. PATIENTS' BILLS OF RIGHTS

    A PATIENT'S BILL OF RIGHTS, AMERICAN HOSPITAL ASSOCIATION
    [1973]   1782

    PATIENTS' RIGHTS: REGULATIONS FOR SKILLED NURSING
    FACILITIES, U.S. DEPARTMENT OF HEALTH, EDUCATION
    AND WELFARE [1974]   1783

DECLARATION OF GENERAL AND SPECIAL RIGHTS OF THE MENTALLY
RETARDED, INTERNATIONAL LEAGUE OF SOCIETIES FOR THE
MENTALLY HANDICAPPED [1968]   1785

PEDIATRIC BILL OF RIGHTS, NATIONAL ASSOCIATION OF
CHILDREN'S HOSPITALS AND RELATED INSTITUTIONS [1975]   1786

SECTION IV. CODES OF SPECIALTY HEALTH-CARE ASSOCIATIONS

INTERNATIONAL COUNCIL OF NURSES, CODE FOR NURSES [1973]   1788

AMERICAN NURSES' ASSOCIATION, CODE FOR NURSES [1976]   1789

AMERICAN CHIROPRACTIC ASSOCIATION, CODE OF ETHICS [1973]   1799

AMERICAN DENTAL ASSOCIATION, PRINCIPLES OF ETHICS [1974]   1802

AMERICAN OSTEOPATHIC ASSOCIATION, CODE OF ETHICS [1965]   1804

AMERICAN PHARMACEUTICAL ASSOCIATION, CODE OF ETHICS [1969]   1806

AMERICAN PSYCHIATRIC ASSOCIATION, PRINCIPLES OF
MEDICAL ETHICS WITH ANNOTATIONS ESPECIALLY APPLICABLE
TO PSYCHIATRY [1973]   1807

AMERICAN PSYCHOLOGICAL ASSOCIATION, ETHICAL STANDARDS
OF PSYCHOLOGISTS [1972]   1811

INTRODUCTION

Codes of the Health-Care Professions

The following article, which serves as an introduction to most of the contemporary professional codes in this Appendix as well as many other codes not included here, is based on a survey of health-care organizations in the United States and some other countries.

The survey was conducted under the auspices of Georgetown University's Kennedy Institute and the Encyclopedia of Bioethics *project during the spring of 1974. Letters were sent to approximately 525 organizations representing a broad cross section of the health-care professions. Each organization was requested to express its ethical concerns by forwarding (1) official codes, statements, guidelines, policies, etc. which might reflect its interest in ethical issues; (2) editorials, articles, conference proceedings, or individual commentary written by members under the auspices of the organization; and (3) a brief, informal statement outlining its ethical activities or concerns. The question of what constituted an "ethical" issue was left to the individual organization to define. The Kennedy Institute is grateful to the responding organizations for making possible a unique collection of materials upon which much of the following article and this Appendix is based.*

Portions of the following article were revised in April 1977 to reflect changes in the codes of several health-care organizations.

For a more detailed historical and ethical analysis of the pivotal codes of medical ethics, see the Encyclopedia *entry* CODES OF MEDICAL ETHICS, *articles on* HISTORY *and* ETHICAL ANALYSIS.

Ethical policy for the health-care professions is fashioned by two principal forces. One is a formal and relatively public political process which generates codes of ethics, policy statements, oaths, pledges, creeds, vows, and bylaws. The other is an informal and less palpable process which fosters the development of influential oral traditions that may supplement, or even supplant, the ethical views expressed in codes or statements. While oral traditions undoubtedly play a significant role in the translation of codes of ethics into every-day practice, the extent of their influence is difficult to assess. Thus, this article will focus on the health-care professions' formal responses to ethical issues as made manifest by their written codes and policy statements. It should serve as an introduction and guide to the distinctive ethical concerns and omissions of these professions.

Contrary to what one might expect, namely, a strong emphasis on the resolution of important bioethical issues, we find that the ethical issues usually addressed by health-care professions fall mainly into two categories. The first is characterized by broad moral imperatives reminiscent of the Ten Commandments and the Golden Rule, and the second by detailed statements regarding the commercial aspects of professional practice.

Common Features of Codes

The broad ethical concerns of the major health-care professions—medicine, dentistry, nursing, pharmacy, and psychology—are generally predictable. For example, a typical code exhorts practitioners to preserve human life, to be good citizens, to prevent the exploitation of patients, to promote the highest-quality health care available, to perform their duties with objectivity and accuracy, to strive for professional excellence through continuing education, to avoid discriminatory practices, to promote the interest and ideals of the profession, to expose unethical or incompetent colleagues, to encourage public health through health-care education, to render service in times of public emergencies, to promote harmonious relations with other health-care professions, and to protect the welfare, dignity, and confidentiality of patients. Most of these imperatives are vague and of limited value, since they do not go beyond the fundamental humanitarian concerns we would expect of every member of society.

In contrast, the specific though mundane ethical guidelines address advertising, billing procedures, self-aggrandizement, conflicts of interest, professional courtesy, public and media relations, employment and supervision of auxiliary personnel, use of secret remedies and exclusive methods, as well as the location and physical appearance of the office practice.

Frequently, the more elaborate codes of ethics are accompanied by complex peer review mechanisms designed to enforce the code and discipline violators through censure, suspension, or, for particularly heinous conduct, expulsion. While disciplinary actions may prove detrimental to a practitioner's professional reputation, they seldom affect the right to practice. For those professions subject to state licensure, the judicial actions of health-care organizations rarely trigger official investigations, and when they do license revocation is the exception rather than the rule. Control over the unlicensed health-care professions (e.g., in the United States, medical technologists, dieticians, occupational therapists, physical therapists, and social workers) is even less formal.

A few codes specify distinct grounds for disciplinary action, including conviction of a felony or a crime involving moral turpitude, suspension or termination of licensure, self-aggrandizement, improper financial dealings, incompetence, solicitation of patients, unprofessional conduct, violation of the state or local society's bylaws, and even failure to pay dues. While professional organizations rarely report violations of their codes of ethics in forums readily accessible to the public, the limited evidence available suggests that a majority of complaints relate to business practices, especially restrictions on advertising, and not to transgressions of broad ethical principles. The American Physical Therapy Association reported in 1973 that its Judicial Committee adjudicated grievances falling into three general categories: telephone listing violations, improperly printed communications, and miscellaneous infractions including misuse of the association insignia, product endorsements, and failure to give loyalty and support.

Relatively new health-care professions (e.g., physicians' assistants and medical technologists) and subspecialties (e.g., bariatric medicine, legal medicine, endodontics, and nurse midwifery) have sought alternative ways of addressing ethical issues, if they do so at all. Subspecialties tend to endorse, in toto or with slight modifications, the code of ethics that dominates their major health-care field, and only in a few instances are these codes supplemented by the subspecialty's own code and/or policy statements. The American College of Foot Surgeons simply endorses the code of the American Podiatry Association; the Society for Pediatric Radiology endorses the codes of the American College of Radiology (1969) and the American Medical Association; the American College of Apothecaries has adopted its own *Code of Professional Practice* (n.d.) as well as (in 1969) that of the American Pharmaceutical Association; and the interdisciplinary Association for Advancement of Behavior Therapy endorses the codes of the American Medical Association, the American Psychiatric Association, and the American Psychological Association. One rarity is the American College of Legal Medicine (1960), which has adopted the code of a health-care organization, the American Medical Association, as well as that of a non-health-care profession, the American Bar Association's *Code of Professional Responsibility and Code of Judicial Conduct* (adopted, 1969; revised, 1975).

Abortion

Despite the generalities and even banalities that characterize many of the codes, a few health-care professions have expressed their concern about important bioethical issues in their codes of ethics. A brief but nonetheless controversial reference to therapeutic abortion was included in an early draft of the World Medical Association's *International Code of Medical Ethics* adopted in 1949. It noted that this procedure should be performed only if the conscience of the physician and the national laws permit. This broad statement was subsequently deleted from the final version of the code, and the issue did not formally reemerge until the adoption in 1970 of a separate statement, the *Declaration of Oslo*, which elaborates rough guidelines for physicians as to when a pregnancy must be terminated as a therapeutic measure. The time between the deletion and adoption of a statement on therapeutic abortion may be indicative of the difficulties professional organizations encounter, particularly on the international level, when controversial issues must be resolved by convention. A brief reference to abortion appears in the American Medical Association's *Opinions and Reports of the Judicial Council* (1972), a detailed commentary on its *Principles of Medical Ethics* (1957). It states that physicians are not prohibited from performing abortions if they are done in accordance with good medical practice and do not violate the laws of the community. A statement on abortion from the American College of Nurse-Midwives, in contrast, is more narrowly drawn, noting that abortion should be considered an operative procedure to be performed by a qualified physician with hospital privileges.

In connection with health-care problems or procedures that may provoke personal moral conflicts in general, the eleven-point *Code for Nurses* (adopted, 1950; revised, 1976) of the American Nurses' Association firmly supports the nurse's right to refuse to participate in morally offensive activities but not to the detriment of the nursing client. Before a nurse may withdraw from a case, the code requires that the client be advised of alternative sources of information or health-care delivery.

Research and Experimentation

The ethics of human experimentation and the special responsibilities of the research nurse, acting as an investigator directly involved with the research or as a practitioner providing care for research subjects, is discussed in the American Nurses' Association's *Code for Nurses* (1976). The Association's interest in this issue is further underscored by its publication of *Human Rights Guidelines for Nurses in Clinical and Other Research: Statement of the ANA Commission on Nursing Research* (1975), which is devoted to such topics as the evolving scope of nurses' responsibilities in research settings, nursing activities and their relation to ethical issues, the patient's right to freedom from intrinsic risk or injury and to privacy and dignity, the definition of a research subject, mechanisms for assuring the protection of patients' rights through informed consent and through reviews of research protocols by the sponsoring institutions and agencies, and the nurse's personal responsibilities in this special area.

Many of the problems associated with psychological research are discussed in the American Psychological Association's *Ethical Standards of Psychologists* (adopted, 1963; revised, 1972), including voluntary and informed consent, the minimization of psychological stress, the use of deception techniques, responsibility for testing consequences, confidentiality, animal research, and the use of experimental drugs (e.g., hallucinogenic or psychedelic substances) on human subjects. These and other important research dilemmas are examined in a comprehensive guide prepared by the Association expressly for the research psychologist entitled *Ethical Principles in the Conduct of Research with Human Participants* (adopted, 1972).

The World Medical Association's *Declaration of Helsinki* (Recommendations Guiding Doctors in Biomedical Research Involving Human Subjects, adopted, 1964; revised, 1975) discusses informed consent and research design in the context of both therapeutic and nontherapeutic research. In its commentary on one of the *Principles of Medical Ethics*, the American Medical Association's *Opinions and Reports* (1972), addresses three significant research areas: experimentation involving new drugs or procedures, ethical guidelines for clinical investigation (1966), and guidelines for organ transplantation (1968). Prior to their incorporation into the *Opinions and Reports*, the latter two statements were published separately in the years indicated.

The only reference to research appearing in the American Dental Association's *Principles of Ethics* (1974) states that dentists must seek fully informed consent from patients used for research or teaching purposes; however, no procedures for ensuring adequate consent are specified.

Confidentiality

While most of the codes mention the protection of patient confidentiality, a few health-care organizations have explored the ethical dimensions of this issue in greater detail. The American Psychological Association's code (1972) imposes an affirmative duty on the psychologist to inform clients as to the limits of this obligation. Problems do arise, however, when clients are minors seeking treatment without parental consent or patients reveal during the course of therapy that they intend to harm someone else. It is unclear whether a psychologist has a duty to seek parental consent before treating a minor or to warn third parties when a client threatens violence. Another area of potential conflict between client and psychologist is access to treatment records and test results. At the time of this survey (1974), the Association favored the position that this information should be released only to persons qualified to interpret and to use them properly, essentially leaving access to such materials to the discretion of the individual psychologist and not to the client. The American Medical Association's *Principles* establishes a similar policy with regard to patient access to medical records.

Death and Dying

The ethical problems associated with death and dying have also received attention from some health-care professions. The American Nurses' Association's code (1976) includes a moving statement on nursing care and the treatment of the terminally ill or dying patient. The World

Medical Association's *Declaration of Sydney: A Statement on Death* (adopted, 1968), is devoted exclusively to the problem of the determination of death and the related issues of maintaining life by artificial means and organ transplantation. The *Report on the Physician and the Dying Patient* (1973), prepared by the Judicial Council of the American Medical Association, includes the following recommendations: discussion of the reciprocal rights and duties of physicians and terminally ill patients should be promoted by the various medical societies; no particular form should be used to express an individual's wishes regarding prospective terminal care, although patients have a right to express such wishes; and physicians should respect these decisions but should also feel free to challenge them if the situation warrants. Although the report strongly condemns "mercy killings" or the intentional termination of life, the decision to terminate extraordinary life-support measures is the prerogative of the patient and/or the immediate family when there is irrefutable evidence that biological death is imminent.

Patients' Rights

Recent interest in patients' rights has prompted a few professional organizations to devote special attention to this field. For example, the *Standards of Bariatric Practice* (1974) of the American Society of Bariatric Physicians, which is dedicated to the study and treatment of the overweight patient, states that patients have the right to request information about their treatment regimen except under unusual circumstances. The American Occupational Therapy Association issued a statement in 1973 regarding increased consumer involvement in the evaluation of occupational therapy services. The ethical agenda of the National Association of Social Workers is replete with such consumer rights issues as citizens' participation in the treatment decisions affecting them or their families, the right to the most complete knowledge possible about one's health, the ownership of medical records, the right to choose or reject treatment procedures, the rights of children and adolescents to treatment without parental consent (e.g., abortion, contraception, treatment for drug use), the confidentiality of health records and data banking, informed consent and human experimentation, the rights of the elderly to self-determination, and the rights of the individual versus the family and/or the community in cases of mental illness. It has also published statements regarding national health care and

the allocation of health resources. The International Chiropractors Association advocates the provision of health-care services at reasonable cost and annual license renewal requirements.

In contrast, some codes tend to limit consumer involvement in the delivery of health care. As mentioned above, those of the American Medical Association and the American Psychological Association reserve for the practitioner the right to limit or deny patient access to treatment records. The American Medical Technologists' *Code of Ethics* (n.d.) states that members should report their findings only to the attending physician. The *Code of Ethics* (adopted, 1970; revised, 1973) of the American Academy of Oral Pathology maintains that laboratory reports should not be issued directly to patients without the permission of the attending dentist or physician. Under the section entitled "Transfer of Orthodontic Patients" in the American Association of Orthodontics' *Principles of Ethics* (1972), practitioners are urged not to criticize another's faulty diagnosis or treatment in the presence of patients so as not to undermine their confidence in the course of treatment or in the profession. While "unjust criticism" provisions are typical of many codes, they may operate to prevent patients from learning that they have been victims of incompetent treatment despite the fact that they generally must bear the expense of whatever remedial care is required. The American Dental Association's *Principles* states that a dentist has an obligation to refrain from making disparaging remarks about the services of another without justification, and the section entitled "Justifiable Criticism and Expert Testimony" comments that the dentist has an obligation to report instances of incompetent treatment to the local dental society and may provide expert testimony in any legal or administrative proceeding that results. It is unclear whether such information is to be conveyed directly to the patient in question.

The *Code of Professional Practice* (n.d.) of the American College of Apothecaries urges pharmacists to balance their commitment to confidentiality against the best interests of the patient but forbids them to discuss the therapeutic value and/or effect of a prescription or the details of its composition—information the prescriber may have intentionally withheld—with the patient. Instead, the pharmacist is obliged to refer the patient directly to the prescribing physician. Similarly, the American Pharmaceutical Association's *Code of Ethics* (1969) states that pharmacists should respect patient confidentiality except in instances where the patient's best interest or the law demands otherwise. Many codes purport to protect "the best interests of the patient," but all too often this is an empty catch-phrase for efforts by the profession to retain discretionary power over the delivery of health care at the expense of patient autonomy.

An unusual twist on the patients' rights theme appears in the American Chiropractic Association's *Code of Ethics* (adopted, 1966; revised, 1973). In addition to discussing the duties of chiropractors to their patients, to each other, and to the public, the code includes sections on the obligations of patients to their chiropractors and the public to the chiropractic profession. For example, a chiropractor should not be dismissed for light reasons, patients must be completely candid about their illness and not deviate from the prescribed treatment regimen, and the public should give the profession its utmost consideration in light of the important benefits and services conferred by chiropractors. Furthermore, the public should be willing to assist in the endowment of nonprofit chiropractic institutions and to demand that chiropractic services become available to the inmates of all state institutions.

Policy Statements on Ethical Issues

Many professional organizations appear more comfortable dealing with provocative ethical issues in the form of policy statements prepared by committees commissioned expressly for that purpose. The relative flexibility and informality afforded by such forums is considered preferable to the rigid, political, and more public process often associated with the adoption or amendment of a code of ethics. Generally, policy statements need only be ratified by an executive committee rather than the entire membership. Many of the professions that have not developed codes of ethics address important ethical issues through this mechanism. For example, the American Federation for Clinical Research, the American Society for Pharmacology and Experimental Therapeutics, and the American Society for Experimental Pathology are all interested in the ethics of human experimentation, especially the problem of informed consent, the evaluation of the benefit–harm calculus in research, and the proper use of animals in experimentation; the American College of Legal Medicine has issued several statements on such medico-legal topics as the administration of blood with regard to legal theories of strict liability and implied warranty and alternative methods for resolving malpractice disputes; the American Academy of Pediatrics

has established a variety of committees to investigate teenage pregnancy and abortion, drug abuse in adolescents, physical abuse and maltreatment of children, foster and long-term care of physically and mentally handicapped children, and drug testing in children; the American Society of Hospital Pharmacists has published statements regarding the use of investigational drugs in hospitals, charging the principal investigator with the responsibility for securing proper consent and urging hospitals to foster research that adequately safeguards patients; the National Catholic Pharmacists Guild of the United States seeks to promote the Church's ethical positions on such matters as contraception, abortion, euthanasia, and the sale of pornographic and indecent literature in pharmacies; the American Association on Mental Deficiency has published statements on the rights of the mentally retarded and on such issues as sterilization, human rights review and protection boards, guardianship for mentally retarded persons, and guidelines for research; the Association for Advancement of Behavior Therapy has policy statements concerning behavior modification and the U.S. Department of Health, Education, and Welfare's guidelines for the protection of human subjects; and the American Association for Respiratory Therapy has examined the ethical problems associated with the use of heart–lung machines and resuscitation techniques.

A number of professions have been silent on ethical issues that one would expect to be of vital importance to them. For example, the North American Clinical Dermatologic Association and the Pacific Dermatologic Association attempt to enhance the dialogue between physicians specializing in dermatology and venereology but make no mention of the patient confidentiality issues associated with the treatment of sexually transmitted diseases—e.g., Do physicians have a duty to inform public health officials, as may be required by law, or the patient's other sexual contacts if revealed during the course of treatment? Neither the American Thoracic Society nor the American Society of Internal Medicine has discussed the ethical implications of organ transplantation or the allocation of scarce medical resources; the latter organization indicated that its activities were limited to the "social and economic" aspects of health care. The American Urological Association has not promulgated any statements regarding sterilization or its attendant ethical problems.

Commercial Aspects

Other professional organizations tend to concentrate on the comparatively trivial commercial aspects of health-care practice rather than specific ethical issues. The American Dental Association's *Principles* is largely intended to influence the image the individual dentist presents to the public and how it affects the quality of dental care provided. Matters pertaining to advertising receive the bulk of the Association's attention, as indicated by the number of advisory opinions issued by its Council on Judicial Procedures, Constitution and Bylaws. Two of the three points included in the Pan-American Association of Ophthalmology's code, which appears as a part of its *Bylaws* (1972), address the organization's property rights over materials presented at its meetings and restrictions on advertising to the lay public. The American Psychopathological Association indicated that its primary interest was psychiatric research, and it has not found it necessary to elaborate on the ethical dimensions of this field. The American College of Surgeons issued a series of ethical position statements regarding premature publicity stemming from organ transplantation operations or other new techniques, the dispensing of spectacles or contact lenses by ophthalmic surgeons, and human experimentation and the public disclosure of research results; yet those statements did not discuss the ethical implications of organ transplantation, human experimentation, informed consent, or the allocation of scarce medical resources. Similarly, one of the Society of Thoracic Surgeons' fundamental concerns is the undue self-aggrandizement that may arise from news articles announcing innovative medical techniques, particularly heart transplantations or other cardiovascular surgery. It has even established a Committee on Training, Standards and Medical Ethics to advise the membership on what is described as its most troublesome problem, press publicity and self-aggrandizement. All of the interpretive statements relating to the *Code of Ethics* (revised, 1965) of the American Osteopathic Association concern business practices such as telephone listings, office signs, stationery, and billing procedures for services rendered. The American Physical Therapy Association's *Guide for Professional Conduct* (1973) also emphasizes commercial matters and includes an entire appendix devoted to the proper format for telephone listings. Neither the American Academy of Neurological Surgery nor the Neurosurgical Society of America has formally addressed such ethical issues as psychosurgery or electrical stimulation of the brain. The allocation of scarce medical resources and the rights of the terminally ill have not been examined by the American Society of Extra-Corporeal Technology, an organization serving members of the health-care team involved with life-sustaining technologies such as renal dialysis and heart-lung machines. The American Veterinary Medical Association's *Principles of Veterinary Medical Ethics* (1973) makes no reference to the ethics of using animals in research.

Conclusion

The proliferation of codes of ethics and policy statements by the health-care professions is disappointing to anyone who expects thoughtful and provocative discussions of bioethical issues. The scope of most codes is predictably limited to either broad moral imperatives or principles governing the commercial aspects of health-care delivery. This split suggests that the professions' formal mechanisms for resolving ethical dilemmas are not well suited to the task of analyzing the specific bioethical problems encountered by practitioners. A few health-care organizations have assumed the lead in this area. They have begun to redefine the role codes of ethics and policy statements are to play for their professions by addressing distinctive policy issues without weakening them with generalities. As health-care technology grows increasingly sophisticated and the issues more complex, the professions will find it necessary to resolve them, or society will.

RONALD S. GASS

BIBLIOGRAPHY

The primary resource materials for this article were the codes of ethics and policy statements furnished by the various professional organizations. The most comprehensive listings of health-care organizations can be found in the following two sources.

"Health and Medical Organizations." *Encyclopedia of Associations.* 9th ed. 3 vols. Edited by Margaret Fisk. Detroit: Gale Research Co., 1975, vol. 1, section 8, pp. 683–780.

"Organizations of Medical Interest." *Journal of the American Medical Association.* Reference directory appears in the 3d issue of the month in February, April, June, August, October, and December.

OTHER SOURCES

BENNION, FRANCIS A. R. *Professional Ethics: The Consultant Professions and Their Code.* London: Charles Knight & Co., 1969.

CLAPP, JANE. *Professional Ethics and Insignia.* Metuchen, N.J.: Scarecrow Press, 1974.

DERBYSHIRE, ROBERT C. "Medical Ethics and Discipline." *Journal of the American Medical Association* 228 (1974): 59–62.

VEATCH, ROBERT M. "Generalization of Expertise." *Hastings Center Studies* 1, no. 2 (1973), pp. 29–40.

——. "Medical Ethics: Professional or Universal?" *Harvard Theological Review* 65 (1972): 531–559.

SECTION I

General Codes for the Practice of Medicine

OATH OF HIPPOCRATES
Sixth Century B.C.–First Century A.D.?

Assumed to have been written by Hippocrates, the Oath exemplifies only the Pythagorean school rather than Greek thought in general. The Oath of Hippocrates is one of the earliest and most important statements on medical ethics. Estimates of its actual date of origin vary from the sixth century B.C. to the first century A.D. Not only has the Oath provided the foundation for many succeeding medical oaths, e.g., the Declaration of Geneva, but it is still administered by many medical schools to graduating medical students either in its original form or in a slightly altered version.

I swear by Apollo Physician and Asclepius and Hygieia and Panaceia and all the gods and goddesses, making them my witnesses, that I will fulfil according to my ability and judgment this oath and this covenant:

To hold him who has taught me this art as equal to my parents and to live my life in partnership with him, and if he is in need of money to give him a share of mine, and to regard his offspring as equal to my brothers in male lineage and to teach them this art—if they desire to learn it—without fee and covenant; to give a share of precepts and oral instruction and all the other learning to my sons and to the sons of him who has instructed me and to pupils who have signed the covenant and have taken an oath according to the medical law, but to no one else.

I will apply dietetic measures for the benefit of the sick according to my ability and judgment; I will keep them from harm and injustice.

I will neither give a deadly drug to anybody if asked for it, nor will I make a suggestion to this effect. Similarly I will not give to a woman an abortive remedy. In purity and holiness I will guard my life and my art.

I will not use the knife, not even on sufferers from stone, but will withdraw in favor of such men as are engaged in this work.

Whatever houses I may visit, I will come for the benefit of the sick, remaining free of all intentional injustice, of all mischief and in particular of sexual relations with both female and male persons, be they free or slaves.

What I may see or hear in the course of the treatment or even outside of the treatment in regard to the life of men, which on no account one must spread abroad, I will keep to myself holding such things shameful to be spoken about.

If I fulfil this oath and do not violate it, may it be granted to me to enjoy life and art, being honored with fame among all men for all time to come; if I transgress it and swear falsely, may the opposite of all this be my lot.

[Ludwig Edelstein. "The Hippocratic Oath: Text, Translation and Interpretation." *Bulletin of the History of Medicine*, Supplement 1. Baltimore: Johns Hopkins Press, 1943, p. 3. Reprinted with the permission of The Johns Hopkins University Press.]

OATH OF INITIATION
(Caraka Saṃhitā)
First Century A.D.?

This ancient Indian oath for medical students appears in the Caraka Saṃhitā *(or, Charaka Saṃhitā), a medical text written around the first century A.D. by the Indian physician Caraka. Unlike the Hippocratic Oath, which exemplified only one school of Greek thought, the Oath of the* Caraka Saṃhitā *reflects concepts and beliefs found throughout ancient nonmedical Indian literature.*

1. The teacher then should instruct the disciple in the presence of the sacred fire, Brāhmanas [Brahmins] and physicians.

2. [saying] "Thou shalt lead the life of a celibate, grow thy hair and beard, speak only the truth, eat no meat, eat only pure articles of food, be free from envy and carry no arms.

3. There shall be nothing that thou should not do at my behest except hating the king, causing another's death, or committing an act of great unrighteousness or acts leading to calamity.

4. Thou shalt dedicate thyself to me and regard me as thy chief. Thou shalt be subject to me and conduct thyself for ever for my welfare and pleasure. Thou shalt serve and dwell with me like a son or a slave or a supplicant. Thou shalt behave and act without arrogance, with care and attention and with undistracted mind, humility, constant reflection and ungrudging obedience. Acting either at my behest or otherwise, thou shalt conduct thyself for the achievement of thy teacher's purposes alone, to the best of thy abilities.

5. If thou desirest success, wealth and fame as a physician and heaven after death, thou shalt pray for the welfare of all creatures beginning with the cows and Brāhmanas.

6. Day and night, however thou mayest be engaged, thou shalt endeavour for the relief of patients with all thy heart and soul. Thou shalt not desert or injure thy patient for the sake of thy life or thy living. Thou shalt not commit adultery even in thought. Even so, thou shalt not covet others' possessions. Thou shalt be modest in thy attire and appearance. Thou shouldst not be a drunkard or a sinful man nor shouldst thou associate with the abettors of crimes. Thou shouldst speak words that are gentle, pure and righteous, pleasing, worthy, true, wholesome, and moderate. Thy behaviour must be in consideration of time and place and heedful of past experience. Thou shalt act always with a view to the acquisition of knowledge and fullness of equipment.

7. No persons, who are hated by the king or who are haters of the king or who are hated by the public or who are haters of the public, shall receive treatment. Similarly, those who are extremely abnormal, wicked, and of miserable character and conduct, those who have not vindicated their honour, those who are on the point of death, and similarly women who are unattended by their husbands or guardians shall not receive treatment.

8. No offering of presents by a woman without the behest of her husband or guardian shall be accepted by thee. While entering the patient's house, thou shalt be accompanied by a man who is known to the patient and who has his permission to enter; and thou shalt be well-clad, bent of head, self-possessed, and conduct thyself only after repeated consideration. Thou shalt thus properly make thy entry. Having entered, thy speech, mind, intellect and senses shall be entirely devoted to no other thought than that of being helpful to the patient and of things concerning only him. The peculiar customs of the patient's household shall not be made public. Even knowing that the patient's span of life has come to its close, it shall not be mentioned by thee there, where if so done, it would cause shock to the patient or to others.

Though possessed of knowledge one should not boast very much of one's knowledge. Most people are offended by the boastfulness of even those who are otherwise good and authoritative.

9. There is no limit at all to the Science of Life, Medicine. So thou shouldst

apply thyself to it with diligence. This is how thou shouldst act. Also thou shouldst learn the skill of practice from another without carping. The entire world is the teacher to the intelligent and the foe to the unintelligent. Hence, knowing this well, thou shouldst listen and act according to the words of instruction of even an unfriendly person, when his words are worthy and of a kind as to bring to you fame, long life, strength and prosperity."

10. Thereafter the teacher should say this—"Thou shouldst conduct thyself properly with the gods, sacred fire, Brāhmanas, the guru, the aged, the scholars and the preceptors. If thou has conducted thyself well with them, the precious stones, the grains and the gods become well disposed towards thee. If thou shouldst conduct thyself otherwise, they become unfavorable to thee." To the teacher that has spoken thus, the disciple should say, "Amen."

[A. Menon and H. F. Haberman. "Oath of Initiation" (From the *Caraka Saṃhitā*). *Medical History* 14 (1970): 295–296. Reprinted with the permission of *Medical History*.]

OATH OF ASAPH
Third Century–Seventh Century A.D.?

The Oath of Asaph appears at the end of the Book of Asaph the Physician (Sefer Asaph ha-Rofe), *which is the oldest Hebrew medical text. It was written by Asaph Judaeus, also known as Asaph ben Berachyahu, a Hebrew physician from Syria or Mesopotamia, who lived sometime between the third and the seventh centuries A.D., probably in the sixth century. The Oath, which in part resembles the Oath of Hippocrates, was taken by medical students when they received their diplomas.*

And this is the oath adminstered by Asaph, the son of Berachyahu, and by Jochanan, the son of Zabda, to their disciples; and they adjured them in these words: Take heed that ye kill not any man with the sap of a root; and ye shall not dispense a potion to a woman with child by adultery to cause her to miscarry; and ye shall not lust after beautiful women to commit adultery with them; and ye shall not disclose secrets confided unto you; and ye shall take no bribes to cause injury and to kill; and ye shall not harden your hearts against the poor and the needy, but heal them; and ye shall not call good evil or evil good; and ye shall not walk in the way of sorcerers to cast spells, to enchant and to bewitch with intent to separate a man from the wife of his bosom or woman from the husband of her youth.

And ye shall not covet wealth or bribes to abet depraved sexual commerce.

And ye shall not make use of any manner of idol-worship to heal thereby, nor trust in the healing powers of any form of their worship. But rather must ye abhor and detest and hate all their worshippers and those that trust in them and cause others to trust in them, for all of them are but vanity and of no avail, for they are naught; and they are demons. Their own carcasses they cannot save; how, then, shall they save the living?

And now, put your trust in the Lord your God, the God of truth, the living God, for He doth kill and make alive, smite and heal. He doth teach man understanding and also to do good. He smiteth in righteousness and justice and healeth in mercy and lovingkindness. No crafty device can be concealed from Him, for naught is hidden from His sight.

He causeth healing plants to grow and doth implant in the hearts of sages skill to heal by His manifold mercies and to declare marvels to the multitude, that all that live may know that He made them, and that beside Him there is none to save. For the peoples trust in their idols to succour them from their afflictions, but they will not save them in their distress, for their hope and their trust are in the Dead. Therefore it is fitting that ye keep apart from them and hold aloof from all the abominations of their idols and cleave unto the name of the Lord God of all flesh. And every living creature is in His hand to kill and to make alive; and there is none to deliver from His hand.

Be ye mindful of Him at all times and seek Him in truth uprightness and rectitude that ye may prosper in all that ye do; then He will cause you to prosper and ye shall be praised by all men. And the peoples will leave their gods and their idols and will yearn to serve the Lord even as ye do, for they will perceive that they have put their trust in a thing of naught and that their labour is in vain; (otherwise) when they cry unto the Lord, He will not save them.

As for you, be strong and let not your hands slacken, for there is a reward for your labours. God is with you when ye are with Him. If ye will keep His covenant and walk in His statutes to cleave unto them, ye shall be as saints in the sight of all men, and they shall say: "Happy is the people that is in such a case; happy is that people whose God is the Lord."

And their disciples answered them and said: All that ye have instructed us and commanded us, that will we do, for it is a commandment of the Torah, and it behooves us to perform it with all our heart and all our soul and all our might: to do and to obey and to turn neither to the right nor to the left. And they blessed them in the name of the Highest God, the Lord of Heaven and earth.

And they admonished them yet again and said unto them: Behold, the Lord God and His saints and His Torah be witness unto you that ye shall fear Him, turning not aside from His commandments, but walking uprightly in His statutes. Incline not to covetousness and aid not the evildoers to shed innocent blood. Neither shall ye mix poisons for a man or a woman to slay his friend therewith; nor shall ye reveal which roots be poisonous or give them into the hand of any man, or be persuaded to do evil. Ye shall not cause the shedding of blood by any manner of medical treatment. Take heed that ye do not cause a malady to any man; and ye shall not cause any man injury by hastening to cut through flesh and blood with an iron instrument or by branding, but shall first observe twice and thrice and only then shall ye give your counsel.

Let not a spirit of haughtiness cause you to lift up your eyes and your hearts in pride. Wreak not the vengeance of hatred on a sick man; and alter not your prescriptions for them that do hate the Lord our God, but keep his ordinances and commandments and walk in all His ways that ye may find favour in His sight. Be ye pure and faithful and upright.

Thus did Asaph and Jochanan instruct and adjure their disciples.

[Translated by Dr. Suessman Muntner for *Medical Ethics: A Compendium of Jewish Moral, Ethical and Religious Principles in Medical Practice.* Edited by M. D. Tendler. 5th ed. New York: Committee on Religious Affairs, Federation of Jewish Philanthropies, 1975, pp. 7–9. Reprinted with the permission of the Federation.]

ADVICE TO A PHYSICIAN
Advice of Haly Abbas (Ahwazi)
Tenth Century A.D.

A leading Persian figure in medicine and medical ethics, Haly Abbas (Ahwazi), who died in 994 A.D., devoted the first chapter of his work Liber Regius (Kamel Al Sanaah al Tibbia) *to the ethics of medicine. An excerpt of his ethical admonition follows. The translation is by Rahmatollah Eshraghi.*

The first advice is to worship God and obey his commands; then be humble toward your teacher and endeavor to hold him in esteem, to serve and show gratitude to him, to hold him equally dear as you do your parents, and to share your possessions with him as with your parents.

Be kind to the children of your teachers and if one of them wants to study medicine you are to teach him without any remuneration.

You are to prohibit the unsuited and undeserving from studying medicine.

A physician is to prudently treat his patients with food and medicine out of good and spiritual motives, not for the sake of gain. He should never prescribe or use a harmful drug or abortifacient.

A physician should be chaste, pious, religious, well-spoken, and graceful, and must avoid any kind of sinfulness or impurity. He should not look upon women with lust and never go to their home except to visit a patient.

A physician should respect confidences and protect the patient's secrets. In protecting a patient's secrets, he must be more insistent than the patient himself. A physician should follow the Hippocratic counsels. He must be kind, compassionate, merciful and benevolent, and give himself unstintingly to the treatment of patients, especially the poor. He must never expect remuneration from the poor but rather provide them free medicine. If it is not impossible, he must visit them graciously whenever it is necessary, day or night, especially when they suffer from an acute disease, because the patient's condition changes very quickly with this kind of disease.

It is not proper for a physician to live luxuriously and become involved in pleasure-seeking. He must not drink alcohol because it injures the brain. He must study medical books constantly and never grow tired of research. He has to learn what he is studying and repeat and memorize what is necessary. He has to study in his youth because it is easier to memorize the subject at this age than in old age, which is the mother of oblivion.

A medical student should be constantly present in the hospital so as to study disease processes and complications under the learned professor and proficient physicians.

To be a learned and skillful physician, he has to follow this advice, develop an upright character and never hesitate to put this advice into practice so as to make his work effective, to win the patient's trust, and to receive the benefit of the patient's friendship and gratitude.

The Almighty God knows better than all...."

FIVE COMMANDMENTS AND TEN REQUIREMENTS
1617

The Five Commandments and Ten Requirements of physicians constitute the most comprehensive statement on medical ethics in China. They were written by Chen Shih-kung, an early seventeenth-century Chinese physician, and appear in his work An Orthodox Manual of Surgery. *The Five Commandments are reproduced below.*

1. Physicians should be ever ready to respond to any calls of patients, high or low, rich or poor. They should treat them equally and care not for financial reward. Thus their profession will become prosperous naturally day by day and conscience will remain intact.

2. Physicians may visit a lady, widow or nun only in the presence of an attendant but not alone. The secret diseases of female patients should be examined with a right attitude, and should not be revealed to anybody, not even to the physician's own wife.

3. Physicians should not ask patients to send pearl, amber or other valuable substances to their home for preparing medicament. If necessary, patients should be instructed how to mix the prescriptions themselves in order to avoid suspicion. It is also not proper to admire things which patients possess.

4. Physicians should not leave the office for excursion and drinking. Patients should be examined punctually and personally. Prescriptions should be made according to the medical formulary, otherwise a dispute may arise.

5. Prostitutes should be treated just like patients from a good family and gratuitous services should be given to the poor ones. Mocking should not be

indulged for this brings loss of dignity. After examination physicians should leave the house immediately. If the case improves, drugs may be sent but physicians should not visit them again for lewd reward.

[Translated by T'ao Lee. *Bulletin of the History of Medicine* 13 (1943): 271–272. Reprinted with the permission of The Johns Hopkins Press.]

A PHYSICIAN'S ETHICAL DUTIES
From *Kholasah Al Hekmah*
1770

During Persia's Islamic era, Mohamad Hosin Aghili of Shiraz wrote the work Kholasah Al Hekmah *in 1770* A.D. *The first chapter of that work contains a list of a physician's ethical duties. They have been translated and condensed by Rahmatollah Eshraghi.*

1. A physician must not be conceited; he should know that the actual healer is God.

2. He should praise his teachers and professor and return thanks to them for their kindnesses.

3. He should never slander another physician. The fault of others should occasion the recognition of his own fault, not be the occasion for pride and conceit.

4. He must speak to patients with civility and good humor and never get angry at the misbehavior and insults of patients.

5. He must protect the patients' secrets and not betray them, especially to those the patients do not want to know.

6. In case of the transmission of disease, the physician must not turn the second patient against the first.

7. He must be energetic in studying diseases and drugs and earnest in the diagnosis and treatment of a patient or disease.

8. He must never be tenacious in his opinion, and continue in his fault or mistake but, if it is possible, he is to consult with proficient physicians and ascertain the facts.

9. If someone mentions a useless or wrong idea, he must not turn it down definitely but say politely, "Maybe it is true in some cases but, in my opinion, in this case it is more probably such and such."

10. If a prior physician has a better knowledge of a patient or disease, he has to encourage the patient to return to the first physician.

11. If he is not successful in the treatment of a case or if he has found the patient did not have confidence in his work or that the patient would like to refer to another physician, it is better to offer an excuse and ask him to consult another physician.

12. He must not be prejudiced against any method of treatment and never continue any wrong practice.

13. In the treatment of disease, he must begin with simple medicine and not recommend any drug as long as the nature of the diease is resistant to it and it would not be effective.

14. If a patient has several diseases, first of all he has to cure the main disease which may be the cause of complications.

15. He should never recommend any kind of fatal, harmful or enfeebling drugs; he has to know that as a physician he has to do what is conducive to the patient's temperament, and temperament itself is an efficient corrector and protector of the body, not fatal or destructive.

16. He must not be proud of his class or his family and must not regard others with contempt.

17. He must not withhold medical knowledge; he should teach it to everyone in medicine without any discrimination between poor or rich, noble or slave.

18. He must not hold his students or his patients under his obligation.

19. He must be content, grateful, generous and magnanimous, and never be covetous, greedy, ravenous or jealous.

20. He must never covet another's property. If someone offers him a present while he himself is in need of it, he must not accept it.

21. He must never claim that he can cure an impoverished patient who has gone to many physicians, and should not jeopardize his own reputation.

22. He should never be gluttonous and become involved in pleasure-seeking, buffoonery, drinking, and other sins.

23. He must not look upon women with lust but must look at them as he looks at his daughter, sister, or mother.

DAILY PRAYER OF A PHYSICIAN
("Prayer of Moses Maimonides")
1793?

Although there is considerable debate about this prayer's true authorship, it was first attributed to Moses Maimonides, a twelfth-century Jewish physician in Egypt. Many now believe it was in fact authored by Marcus Herz, a German physician, pupil of Immanual Kant, and physician to Moses Mendelssohn. The prayer first appeared in print in 1793 as "Tägliches Gebet eines Arztes bevor er seine Kranken besucht—Aus der hebräischen Handschrift eines berühmten jüdischen Arztes in Egypten aus dem zwölften Jahrhundert" ("Daily prayer of a physician before he visits his patients—From the Hebrew manuscript of a renowned Jewish physician in Egypt from the twelfth century"). The "Prayer of Moses Maimonides" and the Oath of Hippocrates are probably the best known of the older statements on medical ethics.

Almighty God, Thou has created the human body with infinite wisdom. Ten thousand times ten thousand organs hast Thou combined in it that act unceasingly and harmoniously to preserve the whole in all its beauty—the body which is the envelope of the immortal soul. They are ever acting in perfect order, agreement and accord. Yet, when the frailty of matter or the unbridling of passions deranges this order or interrupts this accord, then forces clash and the body crumbles into the primal dust from which it came. Thou sendest to man diseases as beneficent messengers to foretell approaching danger and to urge him to avert it.

Thou has blest Thine earth, Thy rivers and Thy mountains with healing substances; they enable Thy creatures to alleviate their sufferings and to heal their illnesses. Thou hast endowed man with the wisdom to relieve the suffering of his brother, to recognize his disorders, to extract the healing substances, to discover their powers and to prepare and to apply them to suit every ill. In Thine Eternal Providence Thou hast chosen me to watch over the life and health of Thy creatures. I am now about to apply myself to the duties of my profession. Support me, Almighty God, in these great labors that they may benefit mankind, for without Thy help not even the least thing will succeed.

Inspire me with love for my art and for Thy creatures. Do not allow thirst for profit, ambition for renown and admiration, to interfere with my profession, for these are the enemies of truth and of love for mankind and they can lead astray in the great task of attending to the welfare of Thy creatures. Preserve the strength of my body and of my soul that they ever be ready to cheerfully help and support rich and poor, good and bad, enemy as well as friend. In the sufferer let me see only the human being. Illumine my mind that it recognize what presents itself and that it may comprehend what is absent or hidden. Let it not fail to see what is visible, but do not permit it to arrogate to itself the power to see what cannot be seen, for delicate and indefinite are the bounds of the great art of caring for the lives and health of Thy creatures. Let me never be absent-minded. May no strange thoughts divert my attention at the bedside of the sick, or disturb my mind in its silent labors, for great and sacred are the thoughtful deliberations required to preserve the lives and health of Thy creatures.

Grant that my patients have confidence in me and my art and follow my directions and my counsel. Remove from their midst all charlatans and the whole host of officious relatives and know-all nurses, cruel people who arrogantly frustrate the wisest purposes of our art and often lead Thy creatures to their death.

Should those who are wiser than I wish to improve and instruct me, let my soul gratefully follow their guidance; for vast is the extent of our art. Should conceited fools, however, censure me, then let love for my profession steel me against them, so that I remain steadfast without regard for age, for reputation, or for honor, because surrender would bring to Thy ceatures sickness and death.

Imbue my soul with gentleness and calmness when older colleagues, proud of their age, wish to displace me or to scorn me or disdainfully to teach me. May even this be of advantage to me, for they know many things of which I am ignorant, but let not their arrogance give me pain. For they are old and old age is not master of the passions. I also hope to attain old age upon this earth, before Thee, Almighty God!

Let me be contented in everything except in the great science of my profession. Never allow the thought to arise in me that I have attained to sufficient knowledge, but vouchsafe to me the strength, the leisure and the ambition ever to extend my knowledge. For art is great, but the mind of man is ever expanding.

Almighty God! Thou hast chosen me in Thy mercy to watch over the life and death of Thy creatures. I now apply myself to my profession. Support me in this great task so that it may benefit mankind, for without Thy help not even the least thing will succeed.

[Translated by Harry Friedenwald. *Bulletin of the Johns Hopkins Hospital* 28 (1917): 260–261.]

CODE OF ETHICS
American Medical Association
1847

The first code of ethics drawn up by the American Medical Association can be understood only in light of the work in medical ethics done by the Englishman Thomas Percival. Percival wrote the first comprehensive modern statement of medical ethics in response to a request on the part of the trustees of the Manchester Infirmary to draw up a "scheme of professional conduct relative to hospitals and other medical charities" which would resolve conflicts among infirmary physicians and prevent future conflicts. In 1794, after three years of writing and revising, Percival privately distributed a book titled Medical Ethics. *It was finally published in 1803, with the subtitle:* A Code of Institutes and Precepts, Adapted To The Professional Conduct of Physicians and Surgeons.

Percival's Medical Ethics *consists of four chapters entitled "Of Professional Conduct Relative to Hospitals or Other Medical Charities," "Of Professional Conduct in Private or General Practice," "Of the Conduct of Physicians Towards Apothecaries," and "Of Professional Duties in Certain Cases Which Require a Knowledge of Law."* Medical Ethics *served for many years as a model for the codes of ethics of medical societies in both England and the United States.*

When the American Medical Association was founded in 1847, its first tasks were to set up standards for medical education and to formulate a code of ethics. Because most of the existing American codes of medical ethics relied heavily upon Thomas Percival's work, the American Medical Association fol-

lowed suit, frequently preserving Percival's wording from his chapter on private practice. The Code of 1847, adopted by both the American Medical Association and the New York Academy of Medicine, is printed in its entirety below.

Chapter I. OF THE DUTIES OF PHYSICIANS TO THEIR PATIENTS, AND OF THE OBLIGATIONS OF PATIENTS TO THEIR PHYSICIANS

ART. I—*Duties of Physicians to their Patients*

1. A physician should not only be ever ready to obey the calls of the sick, but his mind ought also to be imbued with the greatness of his mission, and of the responsibility he habitually incurs in its discharge. Those obligations are the more deep and enduring, because there is no tribunal other than his own conscience, to adjudge penalties for carelessness or neglect. Physicians should, therefore, minister to the sick with due impressions of the importance of their office; reflecting that the ease, the health, and the lives of those committed to their charge, depend on their skill, attention and fidelity. They should study, also, in their deportment, so to unite *tenderness* with *firmness*, and *condescension* with *authority*, as to inspire the minds of their patients with gratitude, respect and confidence.

2. Every case committed to the charge of a physician should be treated with attention, steadiness and humanity. Reasonable indulgence should be granted to the mental imbecility and caprices of the sick. Secrecy and delicacy, when required by peculiar circumstances, should be strictly observed; and the familiar and confidential intercourse to which physicians are admitted in their professional visits, should be used with discretion, and with the most scrupulous regard to fidelity and honor. The obligation of secrecy extends beyond the period of professional services;—none of the privacies of personal and domestic life, no infirmity of disposition or flaw of character observed during professional attendance, should ever be divulged by him except when he is imperatively required to do so. The force and necessity of this obligation are indeed so great, that professional men have, under certain circumstances, been protected in their observance of secrecy by courts of justice.

3. Frequent visits to the sick are in general requisite, since they enable the physician to arrive at a more perfect knowledge of the disease,—to meet promptly every change which may occur, and also tend to preserve the confidence of the patient. But unnecessary visits are to be avoided, as they give useless anxiety to the patient, tend to diminish the authority of the physician, and render him liable to be suspected of interested motives.

4. A physician should not be forward to make gloomy prognostications, because they savor of empiricism, by magnifying the importance of his services in the treatment or cure of the disease. But he should not fail, on proper occasions, to give to the friends of the patient timely notice of danger, when it really occurs; and even to the patient himself, if absolutely necessary. This office, however, is so peculiarly alarming when executed by him, that it ought to be declined whenever it can be assigned to any other person of sufficient judgment and delicacy. For, the physician should be the minister of hope and comfort to the sick; that, by such cordials to the drooping spirit, he may smooth the bed of death, revive expiring life, and counteract the depressing influence of those maladies which often disturb the tranquillity of the most resigned, in their last moments. The life of a sick person can be shortened not only by the acts, but also by the words or the manner of a physician. It is, therefore, a sacred duty to guard himself carefully in this respect, and to avoid all things which have a tendency to discourage the patient and to depress his spirits.

5. A physician ought not to abandon a patient because the case is deemed incurable; for his attendance may continue to be highly useful to the patient, and comforting to the relatives around him, even to the last period of a fatal malady, by alleviating pain and other symptoms, and by soothing mental anguish. To decline attendance, under such circumstances, would be sacrificing

to fanciful delicacy and mistaken liberality, that moral duty, which is independent of, and far superior to all pecuniary consideration.

6. Consultations should be promoted in difficult or protracted cases, as they give rise to confidence, energy, and more enlarged views in practice.

7. The opportunity which a physician not unfrequently enjoys of promoting and strengthening the good resolutions of his patients, suffering under the consequences of vicious conduct, ought never to be neglected. His counsels, or even remonstrances, will give satisfaction, not offence, if they be proffered with politeness, and evince a genuine love of virtue, accompanied by a sincere interest in the welfare of the person to whom they are addressed.

ART. II—*Obligations of Patients to their Physicians*

1. The members of the medical profession, upon whom are enjoined the performance of so many important and arduous duties towards the community, and who are required to make so many sacrifices of comfort, ease, and health, for the welfare of those who avail themselves of their services, certainly have a right to expect and require, that their patients should entertain a just sense of the duties which they owe to their medical attendants.

2. The first duty of a patient is, to select as his medical adviser one who has received a regular professional education. In no trade or occupation do mankind rely on the skill of an untaught artist; and in medicine, confessedly the most difficult and intricate of the sciences, the world ought not to suppose that knowledge is intuitive.

3. Patients should prefer a physician whose habits of life are regular, and who is not devoted to company, pleasure, or to any pursuit incompatible with his professional obligations. A patient should also confide the care of himself and family, as much as possible, to one physician, for a medical man who has become acquainted with the peculiarities of constitution, habits, and predispositions, of those he attends, is more likely to be successful in his treatment than one who does not possess that knowledge.

A patient who has thus selected his physician, should always apply for advice in whatever may appear to him trivial cases, for the most fatal results often supervene on the slightest accidents. It is of still more importance that he should apply for assistance in the forming stage of violent diseases; it is to a neglect of this precept that medicine owes much of the uncertainty and imperfection with which it has been reproached.

4. Patients should faithfully and unreservedly communicate to their physician the supposed cause of their disease. This is the more important, as many diseases of a mental origin simulate those depending on external causes, and yet are only to be cured by ministering to the mind diseased. A patient should never be afraid of thus making his physician his friend and adviser; he should always bear in mind that a medical man is under the strongest obligations of secrecy. Even the female sex should never allow feelings of shame and delicacy to prevent their disclosing the seat, symptoms and causes of complaints peculiar to them. However commendable a modest reserve may be in the common occurrences of life, its strict observance in medicine is often attended with the most serious consequences, and a patient may sink under a painful and loathsome disease, which might have been readily prevented had timely intimation been given to the physician.

5. A patient should never weary his physician with a tedious detail of events or matters not appertaining to his disease. Even as relates to his actual symptoms, he will convey much more real information by giving clear answers to interrogatories, than by the most minute account of his own framing. Neither should he obtrude the details of his business nor the history of his family concerns.

6. The obedience of a patient to the prescriptions of his physician should be prompt and implicit. He should never permit his own crude opinions as to their fitness, to influence his attention to them. A failure in one particular may render an otherwise judicious treatment dangerous, and even fatal. This remark is equally applicable to diet, drink, and exercise. As patients become con-

valescent, they are very apt to suppose that the rules prescribed for them may be disregarded, and the consequence, but too often, is a relapse. Patients should never allow themselves to be persuaded to take any medicine whatever, that may be recommended to them by the self-constituted doctors and doctoresses, who are so frequently met with, and who pretend to possess infallible remedies for the cure of every disease. However simple some of their prescriptions may appear to be, it often happens that they are productive of much mischief, and in all cases they are injurious, by contravening the plan of treatment adopted by the physician.

7. A patient should, if possible, avoid even the *friendly visits of a physician* who is not attending him—and when he does receive them, he should never converse on the subject of his disease, as an observation may be made, without any intention of interference, which may destroy his confidence in the course he is pursuing, and induce him to neglect the directions prescribed to him. A patient should never send for a consulting physician without the express consent of his own medical attendant. It is of great importance that physicians should act in concert; for, although their modes of treatment may be attended with equal success when employed singly, yet conjointly they are very likely to be productive of disastrous results.

8. When a patient wishes to dismiss his physician, justice and common courtesy require that he should declare his reasons for so doing.

9. Patients should always, when practicable, send for their physician in the morning, before his usual hour of going out; for, by being early aware of the visits he has to pay during the day, the physician is able to apportion his time in such a manner as to prevent an interference of engagements. Patients should also avoid calling on their medical adviser unnecessarily during the hours devoted to meals or sleep. They should always be in readiness to receive the visits of their physician, as the detention of a few minutes is often of serious inconvenience to him.

10. A patient should, after his recovery, entertain a just and enduring sense of the value of the services rendered him by his physician; for these are of such a character, that no mere pecuniary acknowledgment can repay or cancel them.

Chapter II. OF THE DUTIES OF PHYSICIANS TO EACH OTHER AND TO THE PROFESSION AT LARGE

ART. I—*Duties for the support of professional character*

1. Every individual, on entering the profession, as he becomes thereby entitled to all its privileges and immunities, incurs an obligation to exert his best abilities to maintain its dignity and honor, to exalt its standing, and to extend the bounds of its usefulness. He should therefore observe strictly, such laws as are instituted for the government of its members;—should avoid all contumelious and sarcastic remarks relative to the faculty, as a body; and while, by unwearied diligence, he resorts to every honorable means of enriching the science, he should entertain a due respect for his seniors, who have, by their labors, brought it to the elevated condition in which he finds it.

2. There is no profession, from the members of which greater purity of character and a higher standard of moral excellence are required, than the medical; and to attain such eminence, is a duty every physician owes alike to his profession, and to his patients. It is due to the latter, as without it he cannot command their respect and confidence; and to both, because no scientific attainments can compensate for the want of correct moral principles. It is also incumbent upon the faculty to be temperate in all things, for the practice of physic requires the unremitting exercise of a clear and vigorous understanding; and, on emergencies for which no professional man should be unprepared, a steady hand, an acute eye, and an unclouded head, may be essential to the well-being, and even life, of a fellow creature.

3. It is derogatory to the dignity of the profession, to resort to public advertisements or private cards or handbills, inviting the attention of individuals

affected with particular diseases—publicly offering advice and medicine to the poor gratis, or promising radical cures; or to publish cases and operations in the daily prints, or suffer such publications to be made;—to invite laymen to be present at operations—to boast of cures and remedies—to adduce certificates of skill and success, or to perform any other similar acts. These are the ordinary practices of empirics, and are highly reprehensible in a regular physician.

4. Equally derogatory to professional character is it, for a physician to hold a patent for any surgical instrument, or medicine; or to dispense a secret *nostrum*, whether it be the composition or exclusive property of himself or of others. For, if such nostrum be of real efficacy, any concealment regarding it is inconsistent with beneficence and professional liberality; and, if mystery alone give it value and importance, such craft implies either disgraceful ignorance, or fraudulent avarice. It is also reprehensible for physicians to give certificates attesting the efficacy of patent or secret medicines, or in any way to promote the use of them.

Art. II—*Professional services of Physicians to each other*

1. All practitioners of medicine, their wives, and their children while under the paternal care, are entitled to the gratuitous services of any one or more of the faculty residing near them, whose assistance may be desired. A physician afflicted with disease is usually an incompetent judge of his own case; and the natural anxiety and solicitude which he experiences at the sickness of a wife, a child, or any one who by the ties of consanguinity is rendered peculiarly dear to him, tend to obscure his judgment, and produce timidity and irresolution in his practice. Under such circumstances, medical men are peculiarly dependent upon each other, and kind offices and professional aid should always be cheerfully and gratuitously afforded. Visits ought not, however, to be obtruded officiously; as such unasked civility may give rise to embarrassment, or interfere with that choice on which confidence depends. But, if a distant member of the faculty, whose circumstances are affluent, request attendance, and an honorarium be offered, it should not be declined; for no pecuniary obligation ought to be imposed, which the party receiving it would wish not to incur.

Art. III—*Of the duties of Physicians as respects vicarious offices*

1. The affairs of life, the pursuit of health, and the various accidents and contingencies to which a medical man is peculiarly exposed, sometimes require him temporarily to withdraw from his duties to his patients, and to request some of his professional brethren to officiate for him. Compliance with this request is an act of courtesy, which should always be performed with the utmost consideration for the interest and character of the family physician, and when exercised for a short period, all the pecuniary obligations for such service should be awarded to him. But if a member of the profession neglect his business in quest of pleasure and amusement, he cannot be considered as entitled to the advantages of the frequent and long-continued exercise of this fraternal courtesy, without awarding to the physician who officiates the fees arising from the discharge of his professional duties.

In obstetrical and important surgical cases, which give rise to unusual fatigue, anxiety and responsibility, it is just that the fees accruing therefrom should be awarded to the physician who officiates.

Art. IV—*Of the duties of Physicians in regard to consultations*

1. A regular medical education furnishes the only presumptive evidence of professional abilities and acquirements, and ought to be the only acknowledged right of an individual to the exercise and honors of his profession. Nevertheless, as in consultations, the good of the patient is the sole object in view, and this is often dependent on personal confidence, no intelligent regular practitioner, who has a license to practise from some medical board of known and acknowledged respectability, recognised by this association, and who is in good moral and professional standing in the place in which he resides, should be fastidiously excluded from fellowship, or his aid refused in consultation

when it is requested by the patient. But no one can be considered as a regular practitioner, or fit associate in consultation, whose practice is based on an exclusive dogma, to the rejection of the accumulated experience of the profession, and of the aids actually furnished by anatomy, physiology, pathology, and organic chemistry.

2. In consultations, no rivalship or jealousy should be indulged; candor, probity, and all due respect, should be exercised towards the physician having charge of the case.

3. In consultations, the attending physician should be the first to propose the necessary questions to the sick; after which the consulting physician should have the opportunity to make such farther inquiries of the patient as may be necessary to satisfy him of the true character of the case. Both physicians should then retire to a private place for deliberation; and the one first in attendance should communicate the directions agreed upon to the patient or his friends, as well as any opinions which it may be thought proper to express. But no statement or discussion of it should take place before the patient or his friends, except in the presence of all the faculty attending, and by their common consent; and no *opinions* or *prognostications* should be delivered, which are not the result of previous deliberation and concurrence.

4. In consultations, the physician in attendance should deliver his opinion first; and when there are several consulting, they should deliver their opinions in the order in which they have been called in. No decision, however, should restrain the attending physician from making such variations in the mode of treatment, as any subsequent unexpected change in the character of the case may demand. But such variation and the reasons for it ought to be carefully detailed at the next meeting in consultation. The same privilege belongs also to the consulting physician if he is sent for in an emergency, when the regular attendant is out of the way, and similar explanations must be made by him, at the next consultation.

5. The utmost punctuality should be observed in the visits of physicians when they are to hold consultation together, and this is generally practicable, for society has been considerate enough to allow the plea of a professional engagement to take precedence of all others, and to be an ample reason for the relinquishment of any present occupation. But as professional engagements may sometimes interfere, and delay one of the parties, the physician who first arrives should wait for his associate a reasonable period, after which the consultation should be considered as postponed to a new appointment. If it be the attending physician who is present, he will of course see the patient and prescribe; but if it be the consulting one, he should retire, except in case of emergency, or when he has been called from a considerable distance, in which latter case he may examine the patient, and give his opinion in *writing* and *under seal*, to be delivered to his associate.

6. In consultations, theoretical discussions should be avoided, as occasioning perplexity and loss of time. For there may be much diversity of opinion concerning speculative points, with perfect agreement in those modes of practice which are founded, not on hypothesis, but on experience and observation.

7. All discussions in consultation should be held as secret and confidential. Neither by words nor manner should any of the parties to a consultation assert or insinuate, that any part of the treatment pursued did not receive his assent. The responsibility must be equally divided between the medical attendants—they must equally share the credit of success as well as the blame of failure.

8. Should an irreconcilable diversity of opinion occur when several physicians are called upon to consult together, the opinion of the majority should be considered as decisive; but if the numbers be equal on each side, then the decision should rest with the attending physician. It may, moreover, sometimes happen, that two physicians cannot agree in their views of the nature of a case, and the treatment to be pursued. This is a circumstance much to be deplored, and should always be avoided, if possible, by mutual concessions, as far as they can be justified by a conscientious regard for the dictates of

judgment. But in the event of its occurrence, a third physician should, if practicable, be called to act as umpire; and if circumstances prevent the adoption of this course, it must be left to the patient to select the physician in whom he is most willing to confide. But as every physician relies upon the rectitude of his judgment, he should, when left in the minority, politely and consistently retire from any further deliberation in the consultation, or participation in the management of the case.

9. As circumstances sometimes occur to render a *special consultation* desirable, when the continued attendance of two physicians might be objectionable to the patient, the member of the faculty whose assistance is required in such cases, should sedulously guard against all future unsolicited attendance. As such consultations require an extraordinary portion both of time and attention, at least a double honorarium may be reasonably expected.

10. A physician who is called upon to consult, should observe the most honorable and scrupulous regard for the character and standing of the practitioner in attendance: the practice of the latter, if necessary, should be justified as far as it can be, consistently with a conscientious regard for truth, and no hint or insinuation should be thrown out, which could impair the confidence reposed in him, or affect his reputation. The consulting physician should also carefully refrain from any of those extraordinary attentions or assiduities, which are too often practised by the dishonest for the base purpose of gaining applause, or ingratiating themselves into the favor of families and individuals.

ART. V—*Duties of Physicians in cases of interference*

1. Medicine is a liberal profession, and those admitted into its ranks should found their expectations of practice upon the extent of their qualifications, not on intrigue or artifice.

2. A physician in his intercourse with a patient under the care of another practitioner, should observe the strictest caution and reserve. No meddling inquiries should be made; no disingenuous hints given relative to the nature and treatment of his disorder; nor any course of conduct pursued that may directly or indirectly tend to diminish the trust reposed in the physician employed.

3. The same circumspection and reserve should be observed, when, from motives of business or friendship, a physician is prompted to visit an individual who is under the direction of another practitioner. Indeed, such visits should be avoided, except under peculiar circumstances; and when they are made, no particular inquiries should be instituted relative to the nature of the disease, or the remedies employed, but the topics of conversation should be as foreign to the case as circumstances will admit.

4. A physician ought not to take charge of or prescribe for a patient who has recently been under the care of another member of the faculty in the same illness, except in cases of sudden emergency, or in consultation with the physician previously in attendance, or when the latter has relinquished the case or been regularly notified that his services are no longer desired. Under such circumstances, no unjust and illiberal insinuations should be thrown out in relation to the conduct or practice previously pursued, which should be justified as far as candor, and regard for truth and probity will permit; for it often happens, that patients become dissatisfied when they do not experience immediate relief, and, as many diseases are naturally protracted, the want of success, in the first stage of treatment, affords no evidence of a lack of professional knowledge and skill.

5. When a physician is called to an urgent case, because the family attendant is not at hand, he ought, unless his assistance in consultation be desired, to resign the care of the patient to the latter, immediately on his arrival.

6. It often happens, in cases of sudden illness, or of recent accidents and injuries, owing to the alarm of friends, that a number of physicians are simultaneously sent for. Under these circumstances, courtesy should assign the patient to the first who arrives, who should select from those present, any additional assistance that he may deem necessary. In all such cases, however,

the practitioner who officiates should request the family physician, if there be one, to be called, and, unless his further attendance be requested, should resign the case to the latter on his arrival.

7. When a physician is called to the patient of another practitioner, in consequence of the sickness or absence of the latter, he ought, on the return or recovery of the regular attendant, and with the consent of the patient, to surrender the case.

8. A physician, when visiting a sick person in the country, may be desired to see a neighboring patient who is under the regular direction of another physician, in consequence of some sudden change or aggravation of symptoms. The conduct to be pursued on such an occasion is to give advice adapted to present circumstances; to interfere no farther than is absolutely necessary with the general plan of treatment; to assume no future direction, unless it be expressly desired; and, in this last case, to request an immediate consultation with the practitioner previously employed.

9. A wealthy physician should not give advice *gratis* to the affluent; because his doing so is an injury to his professional brethren. The office of a physician can never be supported as an exclusively beneficent one; and it is defrauding, in some degree, the common funds for its support, when fees are dispensed with, which might justly be claimed.

10. When a physician who has been engaged to attend a case of midwifery is absent, and another is sent for, if delivery is accomplished during the attendance of the latter, he is entitled to the fee, but should resign the patient to the practitioner first engaged.

Art. VI—*Of differences between Physicians*

1. Diversity of opinion, and opposition of interest, may, in the medical, as in other professions, sometimes occasion controversy and even contention. Whenever such cases unfortunately occur, and cannot be immediately terminated, they should be referred to the arbitration of a sufficient number of physicians, or a *court-medical.*

As peculiar reserve must be maintained by physicians towards the public, in regard to professional matters, and as there exist numerous points in medical ethics and etiquette through which the feelings of medical men may be painfully assailed in their intercourse with each other, and which cannot be understood or appreciated by general society, neither the subject-matter of such differences nor the adjudication of the arbitrators should be made public, as publicity in a case of this nature may be personally injurious to the individuals concerned, and can hardly fail to bring discredit on the faculty.

Art. VII—*Of Pecuniary Acknowledgments*

1. Some general rules should be adopted by the faculty, in every town or district, relative to *pecuniary acknowledgments* from their patients; and it should be deemed a point of honour to adhere to these rules with as much uniformity as varying circumstances will admit.

Chapter III. OF THE DUTIES OF THE PROFESSION TO THE PUBLIC, AND OF THE OBLIGATIONS OF THE PUBLIC TO THE PROFESSION

Art. I—*Duties of the profession to the public*

1. As good citizens, it is the duty of physicians to be ever vigilant for the welfare of the community, and to bear their part in sustaining its institutions and burdens: they should also be ever ready to give counsel to the public in relation to matters especially appertaining to their profession, as on subjects of medical police, public hygiene, and legal medicine. It is their province to enlighten the public in regard to quarantine regulations,—the location, arrangement, and dietaries of hospitals, asylums, schools, prisons, and similar institutions,—in relation to the medical police of towns, as drainage, ventilation, &c.,—and in regard to measures for the prevention of epidemic and contagious diseases; and when pestilence prevails, it is their duty to face the danger, and to continue their labors for the alleviation of the suffering, even at the jeopardy of their own lives.

2. Medical men should also be always ready, when called on by the legally constituted authorities, to enlighten coroners' inquests and courts of justice, on subjects strictly medical,—such as involve questions relating to sanity, legitimacy, murder by poisons or other violent means, and in regard to the various other subjects embraced in the science of Medical Jurisprudence. But in these cases, and especially where they are required to make a post-mortem examination, it is just, in consequence of the time, labor and skill required, and the responsibility and risk they incur, that the public should award them a proper honorarium.

3. There is no profession, by the members of which, eleemosynary services are more liberally dispensed, than the medical; but justice requires that some limits should be placed to the performance of such good offices. Poverty, professional brotherhood, and certain public duties referred to in section 1 of this chapter, should always be recognised as presenting valid claims for gratuitous services; but neither institutions endowed by the public or by rich individuals, societies for mutual benefit, for the insurance of lives or for analogous purposes, nor any profession or occupation, can be admitted to possess such privilege. Nor can it be justly expected of physicians to furnish certificates of inability to serve on juries, to perform militia duty, or to testify to the state of health of persons wishing to insure their lives, obtain pensions, or the like, without a pecuniary acknowledgment. But to individuals in indigent circumstances, such professional services should always be cheerfully and freely accorded.

4. It is the duty of physicians, who are frequent witnesses of the enormities committed by quackery, and the injury to health and even destruction of life caused by the use of quack medicines, to enlighten the public on these subjects, to expose the injuries sustained by the unwary from the devices and pretensions of artful empirics and impostors. Physicians ought to use all the influence which they may possess, as professors in Colleges of Pharmacy, and by exercising their option in regard to the shops to which their prescriptions shall be sent, to discourage druggists and apothecaries from vending quack or secret medicines, or from being in any way engaged in their manufacture and sale.

Art. II—*Obligations of the public to Physicians*

1. The benefits accruing to the public directly and indirectly from the active and unwearied beneficence of the profession, are so numerous and important, that physicians are justly entitled to the utmost consideration and respect from the community. The public ought likewise to entertain a just appreciation of medical qualifications;—to make a proper discrimination between true science and the assumption of ignorance and empiricism,—to afford every encouragement and facility for the acquisition of medical education,—and no longer to allow the statute books to exhibit the anomaly of exacting knowledge from physicians, under liability to heavy penalties, and of making them obnoxious to punishment for resorting to the only means of obtaining it.

[*Code of Medical Ethics.* New York: H. Ludwig & Co., 1848.]

VENEZUELAN CODE OF MEDICAL ETHICS
National Academy of Medicine
1918

The Venezuelan Code, first promulgated by the National Academy of Medicine of Venezuela in 1918, was largely the work of Dr. Luis Razetti and for this reason is sometimes called the "Razetti Code." It served as a model for other codes of medical ethics in Latin America (Colombia, 1919; Peru, 1922). The Sixth Latin American Medical Congress, meeting in Havana in 1922, recommended that the Venezuelan Code (slightly revised in 1922) serve to unify medical ethical concerns in Latin America. The First Brazilian Medical

Congress, held in Rio de Janeiro in 1931, was similarly influenced by the Venezuelan Code.

The Venezuelan Code of 1918 includes many elements characteristic of the codes of its day, with heavy emphasis on the protection of the dignity of the profession, the maintenance of high standards of competence and training, duties toward patients (even regarding their health habits), the rendering of professional services to other doctors, obligations regarding substitute physicians and consultants, professional discipline, fees, etc.

There are several interesting features in the Venezuelan Code which deserve comparison with other codes:

1. The Code insists that there are "rules of medical deontology" which apply to the entire "medical guild"—physicians, surgeons, pharmacists, dentists, obstetricians, interns, and nurses.

2. It places emphasis on physicians' virtues and qualities of character—circumspection, honesty, honor, good faith, respect, etc.—which serve as a basis for those practices of etiquette that support the honorable practice of medicine.

3. The Code prohibits abortion and premature childbirth (morally and legally), except "for a therapeutic purpose in cases indicated by medical science"; but it permits embryotomy if the mother's life is in danger and no alternative medical skills are available.

4. In the excerpt below, there is an interesting and detailed set of instructions on "medical confidentiality." It combines a strong affirmation of the moral obligation of health professionals to observe confidentiality with many attenuations of that obligation in the interests of the public welfare.

Chapter IX. On Medical Confidentiality

<u>Article 68.</u>   Medical confidentiality is a duty inherent in the very nature of the medical profession; the public interest, the personal security of the ill, the honor of families, respect for the physician, and the dignity of the art require confidentiality. Doctors, surgeons, dentists, pharmacists, and midwives as well as interns and nurses are morally obligated to safeguard privacy of information in everything they see, hear, or discover in the practice of their profession or outside of their services and which should not be divulged.

<u>Article 69.</u>   Confidential information may be of two forms: that which is explicitly confidential—formal, documentary information confided by the client —and that which is implicitly confidential, which is private due to the nature of things, which nobody imposes, and which governs the relations of clients with medical professionals. Both forms are inviolable, except for legally specified cases.

<u>Article 70.</u>   Medical professionals are prohibited from revealing professionally privileged information except in those cases established by medical ethics. A revelation is an act which causes the disclosed fact to change from a private to a publicly known fact. It is not necessary to publish such a fact to make it a revealed one: it suffices to confide it to a single person.

<u>Article 71.</u>   Professionally confidential information belongs to the client. Professionals do not incur any responsibility if they reveal the private information received by them when they are authorized to do so by the patient in complete freedom and with a knowledge of the consequences by the person or persons who have confided in them, provided always that such revelation causes no harm to a third party.

<u>Article 72.</u>   A medical person incurs no responsibility when he reveals private information in the following cases:

1. When in his capacity as a medical expert he acts as a physician for an insurance company giving it information concerning the health of the applicant sent to him for examination; or when he is commissioned by a proper authority to identify the physical or mental health of a person; or when he has been designated to perform autopsies or give medico-legal expert knowledge of any kind, as in civil or criminal cases; or when he acts as a doctor

of public health or for the city; and in general when he performs the functions of a medical expert.

2. When the treating physician declares certain diseases infectious and contagious before a health authority; and when he issues death certificates.

In any of the cases included in (1), the medical professional may be exempt from the charge of ignoring the right of privacy of a person who is the object of his examination if said person is his client at the time or if the declaration has to do with previous conditions for which the same doctor was privately consulted.

Article 73. The physician shall preserve utmost secrecy if he happens to detect a venereal disease in a married woman. Not only should he refrain from informing her of the nature of the disease but he should be very careful not to let suspicion fall on the husband as responsible for the contagion. Consequently, he shall not issue any certification or make any disclosure even if the husband gives his consent.

Article 74. If a physician knows that one of his patients in a contagious period of a venereal disease plans to be married, he shall take pains to dissuade his patient from doing so, availing himself of all possible means. If the patient ignores his advice and insists on going ahead with his plan to marry, the physician is authorized without incurring responsibility not only to give the information the bride's family asks for, but also to prevent the marriage without the bridegroom's prior consultation or authorization.

Article 75. The doctor who knows that a healthy wet-nurse is nursing a syphilitic child should warn the child's parents that they are obligated to inform the nurse. If they refuse to do so, the doctor without naming the disease will impose on the nurse the necessity of immediately ceasing to nurse the child, and he should arrange to have her remain in the house for the time needed to make sure that she has not caught the disease. If the parents do not give their consent and insist that the wet-nurse continue to nurse the child, the doctor shall offer the necessary arguments, and if they nevertheless persist he shall inform the nurse of the risk she runs of contracting a contagious disease if she continues to nurse the child.

Article 76. The doctor can without failing in his duty denounce crimes of which he may have knowledge in the exercise of his profession, in accord with article 470 of the [Venezuelan] Penal Code.

Article 77. When it is a matter of making an accusation in court in order to avoid a legal violation the doctor is permitted to disclose private information.

Article 78. When a doctor is brought before a court as a witness to testify to certain facts known to him, he may refuse to disclose professionally private facts about which he is being interrogated, but which he considers privileged.

Article 79. When a doctor finds himself obliged to claim his fees legally, he should limit himself to stating the number of visits and consultations, specifying the days and nights, the number of operations he has performed, specifying the major and minor ones, the number of trips made outside the city to attend the patient, indicating the distance and time involved in travel in each visit, etc., but in no case should he reveal the nature of the operations performed, nor the details of the care that was given to the patient. The explanation of these circumstances, if necessary, shall be referred by the doctor to the medical experts so designated by the court.

Article 80. The doctor should not answer questions concerning the nature of his patient's disease; however, he is authorized not only to tell the prognosis of the case to those closest to the patient but also the diagnosis if on occasion he considers it necessary, in view of his professional responsibility or the best treatment of his patient....

["Código Venezolano de Moral Médica," in Luis Razetti, *Obras Completas: I. Deontología Médica.* Caracas: Ministerio de Sanidad y Asistencia Social, 1963, pp. 111–135. The excerpt translated here is found on pp. 124–127.]

DECLARATION OF GENEVA
World Medical Association
1948

Adopted by the General Assembly of the World Medical Association at Geneva in 1948 and amended by the 22d World Medical Assembly at Sydney in 1968, the Declaration of Geneva was one of the first and most important actions of the Association. It is a declaration of physicians' dedication to the humanitarian goals of medicine, a declaration that was especially important in view of the medical crimes which had just been committed in Nazi Germany. The Declaration of Geneva was intended to update the Oath of Hippocrates, which was no longer suited to modern conditions. Of interest is the fact that the World Medical Association considered this short Declaration to be a more significant statement of medical ethics than the succeeding International Code of Medical Ethics. The words in italics were added to the Declaration in 1968.

At the time of being admitted as a member of the medical profession:

I solemnly pledge myself to consecrate my life to the service of humanity;
I will give to my teachers the respect and gratitude which is their due;
I will practice my profession with conscience and dignity;
The health of my patient will be my first consideration;
I will respect the secrets which are confided in me, *even after the patient has died;*
I will maintain by all the means in my power, the honor and the noble traditions of the medical profession;
My colleagues will be my brothers;
I will not permit considerations of religion, nationality, race, party politics or social standing to intervene between my duty and my patient;
I will maintain the utmost respect for human life from the time of conception; even under threat, I will not use my medical knowledge contrary to the laws of humanity.

I make these promises solemnly, freely and upon my honor.

[*World Medical Journal* 3 (1956), Supplement, pp. 10–12. Reprinted with the permission of the *World Medical Journal.*]

INTERNATIONAL CODE OF MEDICAL ETHICS
World Medical Association
1949

Adopted by the Third General Assembly of the World Medical Association at London in October 1949, the International Code of Medical Ethics states the most general principles of ethical medical practice. It was modeled after the Declaration of Geneva and the codes of ethics of most modern countries. But unlike most national codes, the International Code omits reference to specific unethical practices as well as to judiciary procedures. The original draft included a statement on therapeutic abortion (in italics below), which, because of its controversial nature, was deleted from the adopted version of the International Code of Medical Ethics (World Medical Association Bulletin, vol. 1, no. 3, October 1949, pp. 109, 111).

Duties of Doctors in General

A doctor must always maintain the highest standards of professional conduct.

A doctor must practice his profession uninfluenced by motives of profit. The following practices are deemed unethical:

a. Any self advertisement except such as is expressly authorized by the national code of medical ethics.
b. Collaborate in any form of medical service in which the doctor does not have professional independence.
c. Receiving any money in connection with services rendered to a patient other than a proper professional fee, even with the knowledge of the patient.

Any act, or advice which could weaken physical or mental resistance of a human being may be used only in his interest.

A doctor is advised to use great caution in divulging discoveries or new techniques of treatment.

A doctor should certify or testify only to that which he has personally verified.

Duties of Doctors to the Sick

A doctor must always bear in mind the obligation of preserving human life *from conception. Therapeutic abortion may only be performed if the conscience of the doctors and the national laws permit.*

A doctor owes to his patient complete loyalty and all the resources of his science. Whenever an examination or treatment is beyond his capacity he should summon another doctor who has the necessary ability.

A doctor shall preserve absolute secrecy on all he knows about his patient because of the confidence entrusted in him.

A doctor must give emergency care as a humanitarian duty unless he is assured that others are willing and able to give such care.

Duties of Doctors to Each Other

A doctor ought to behave to his colleagues as he would have them behave to him.

A doctor must not entice patients from his colleagues.

A doctor must observe the principles of "The Declaration of Geneva" approved by The World Medical Association.

[Reprinted with the permission of the *World Medical Journal.*]

PRINCIPLES OF MEDICAL ETHICS (1957)
WITH REPORTS AND STATEMENTS
American Medical Association

Until 1957 the American Medical Association's Code of Ethics had been basically that adopted in 1847, although there were revisions in 1903, 1912, and 1947. A major change in the code's format occurred when the current Principles of Medical Ethics were adopted in 1957. These ten principles, which replace the forty-eight sections of the older code, are intended as expressions of the fundamental concepts and requirements of the earlier code, unencumbered by easily outdated practical codifications. From time to time the Association's principles are interpreted and applied to contemporary ethical and professional problems, usually in the form of Opinions and Reports of the Judicial Council. (The Opinions and Reports of the Judicial Council, *including the Principles of Medical Ethics, have been published several times; a revised edition was being prepared as this encyclopedia neared completion.) Printed below are the AMA's (1) Principles of Medical Ethics, followed by a selection from the AMA's statements and reports on (2) Guidelines for Organ Transplantation (1968), (3) Report on the Physician and the Dying Patient (1973), and (4) Report on Human Artificial Insemination (1974). Ethical Guidelines for Clinical Investigation (1966) are printed in Section II of this Appendix, where directives for human experimentation can be found.*

I. Principles of Medical Ethics (1957)

<u>Preamble.</u>   These principles are intended to aid physicians individually and collectively in maintaining a high level of ethical conduct. They are not laws but standards by which a physician may determine the propriety of his conduct in his relationship with patients, with colleagues, with members of allied professions, and with the public.

<u>Section 1.</u>   The principal objective of the medical profession is to render service to humanity with full respect for the dignity of man. Physicians should merit the confidence of patients entrusted to their care, rendering to each a full measure of service and devotion.

<u>Section 2.</u>   Physicians should strive continually to improve medical knowledge and skill, and should make available to their patients and colleagues the benefits of their professional attainments.

<u>Section 3.</u>   A physician should practice a method of healing founded on a scientific basis; and he should not voluntarily associate professionally with anyone who violates this principle.

<u>Section 4.</u>   The medical profession should safeguard the public and itself against physicians deficient in moral character or professional competence. Physicians should observe all laws, uphold the dignity and honor of the profession and accept its self-imposed disciplines. They should expose, without hesitation, illegal or unethical conduct of fellow members of the profession.

<u>Section 5.</u>   A physician may choose whom he will serve. In an emergency, however, he should render service to the best of his ability. Having undertaken the care of a patient, he may not neglect him; and unless he has been discharged he may discontinue his services only after giving adequate notice. He should not solicit patients.

<u>Section 6.</u>   A physician should not dispose of his services under terms or conditions which tend to interfere with or impair the free and complete exercise of his medical judgment and skill or tend to cause a deterioration of the quality of medical care.

<u>Section 7.</u>   In the practice of medicine a physician should limit the source of his professional income to medical services actually rendered by him, or under his supervision, to his patients. His fee should be commensurate with the services rendered and the patient's ability to pay. He should neither pay nor receive a commission for referral of patients. Drugs, remedies or appliances may be dispensed or supplied by the physician provided it is in the best interests of the patient.

<u>Section 8.</u>   A physician should seek consultation upon request; in doubtful or difficult cases; or whenever it appears that the quality of medical service may be enhanced thereby.

<u>Section 9.</u>   A physician may not reveal the confidences entrusted to him in the course of medical attendance, or the deficiencies he may observe in the character of patients, unless he is required to do so by law or unless it becomes necessary in order to protect the welfare of the individual or of the community.

<u>Section 10.</u>   The honored ideals of the medical professional imply that the responsibilities of the physician extend not only to the individual, but also to society where these responsibilities deserve his interest and participation in activities which have the purpose of improving both the health and the well-being of the individual and the community.

II. Guidelines for Organ Transplantation (1968)

1. In all professional relationships between a physician and his patient, the physician's primary concern must be the health of his patient. He owes the patient his primary allegiance. This concern and allegiance must be preserved in all medical procedures, including those which involve the transplantation of an organ from one person to another where both donor and recipient are patients. Care must, therefore, be taken to protect the rights of both the donor and the recipient, and no physician may assume a responsibility in organ transplantation unless the rights of both donor and recipient are equally protected.

2. A prospective organ transplant offers no justification for a relaxation of the usual standard of medical care. The physician should provide his patient, who may be a prospective organ donor, with that care usually given others being treated for a similar injury or disease.

3. When a vital, single organ is to be transplanted, the death of the donor shall have been determined by at least one physician other than the recipient's physician. Death shall be determined by the clinical judgment of the physician. In making this determination, the ethical physician will use all available, currently accepted scientific tests.

4. Full discussion of the proposed procedure with the donor and the recipient or their responsible relatives or representatives is mandatory. The physician should be objective in discussing the procedure, in disclosing known risks and possible hazards, and in advising of the alternative procedures available. The physician should not encourage expectations beyond those which the circumstances justify. The physician's interest in advancing scientific knowledge must always be secondary to his primary concern for the patient.

5. Transplant procedures of body organs should be undertaken (a) only by physicians who possess special medical knowledge and technical competence developed through special training, study, and laboratory experience and practice, and (b) in medical institutions with facilities adequate to protect the health and well-being of the parties to the procedure.

6. Transplantation of body organs should be undertaken only after careful evaluation of the availability and effectiveness of other possible therapy.

7. Medicine recognizes that organ transplants are newsworthy and that the public is entitled to be correctly informed about them. Normally, a scientific report of the procedures should first be made to the medical profession for review and evaluation. When dramatic aspects of medical advances prevent adherence to accepted procedures, objective, factual, and discreet public reports to the communications media may be made by a properly authorized physician, but should be followed as soon as possible by full scientific reports to the profession.

[Reprinted with the permission of the American Medical Association from *American Medical Association Proceedings of the House of Delegates*, A–68: 101–103.]

III. Report on the Physician and the Dying Patient (1973)

(In response to resolutions concerning "death with dignity," i.e., practices and policies regarding terminal medical care, and after wide consultation, the Judicial Council of the AMA made the following Recommendations, which were adopted by the AMA House of Delegates, December, 1973.)

1. The Council recommends that the several state, county and specialty medical societies encourage and promote discussions of the reciprocal rights and duties of physicians and patients-suffering-terminal-illness.

2. The Council recommends that the House not endorse any particular form to express an individual's wishes which relate prospectively to his final illness but recognize that individuals have the right to express such wishes.

Physicians may, and indeed should, be encouraged to discuss death and terminal illness with patients. Physicians may, and indeed should, respect expressions of patient's wishes regarding medical care during terminal illness but may, and indeed should, feel free to question those wishes with patient's competent legal representative or by appropriate judicial proceedings when the circumstances of a particular situation seem to require it.

3. The Council recommends that the House adopt the following statement to serve as a guideline for physicians:

The intentional termination of the life of one human being by another—mercy killing —is contrary to that for which the medical profession stands and is contrary to the policy of the American Medical Association.

The cessation of the employment of extraordinary means to prolong the life of the body when there is irrefutable evidence that biological death is imminent is the decision of the patient and/or his immediate family. The advice and judgment of the physician should be freely available to the patient and/or his immediate family.

[Reprinted with the permission of the American Medical Association from *American Medical Association Proceedings of the House of Delegates*, C–73: 137–140.]

IV. Report on Human Artificial Insemination (1974)

Human artificial insemination has been a part of the American physician's medical armamentarium for half a century or more. In that time an untold number of women have become pregnant and borne children as a result of the procedure. The procedure has been used to overcome natural impediments to conception.

It is to the credit of American physicians that complaints of ethical infractions have been absent in this delicate, sensitive human procedure. Nonetheless, in view of the concern of members of the House of Delegates of the American Medical Association and because of the recent experience of the British Medical Association, a statement of ethical principles relating to human artificial insemination is timely.

The ethical issues in the procedure of human artificial insemination are, of course, the same as in any other medical or surgical procedure. The nature of the procedure, however, requires emphasis of: (1) the importance of the *concern* the physician must have for his patient, her spouse, and the child which may result from the procedure; (2) the need for *consent* arrived at intellectually rather than emotionally; (3) the *competence* of the physician who assumes this unique responsibility; and (4) the need for preservation of *confidentiality* by the physician and his staff.

Concern.   Human artificial insemination is a medical procedure used to overcome frustration of a basic biological drive. It should be performed by a physician who is deeply imbued with appreciation of the emotional and psychological aspects of the procedure. The physician must be an advisor and counsellor to the woman and her husband. A warm, friendly but professional concern for the importance of this decision and its accomplishment should characterize the physician in this intimate relationship.

Consent.   Even as the physician shows concern for the woman and her desire for motherhood, he must ensure that emotions do not adversely affect those judgments which must be sound and reasoned. Because a family is involved, the patient's spouse must participate in discussions regarding the procedure and its purpose. An additional member of a family involves economics as well as parental responsibilities which should be jointly undertaken by wife and husband.

The procedure directly affects the husband as an individual, as a prospective parent and as spouse of the woman who undergoes the procedure. The consent of both the woman seeking the procedure and her husband must be secured. This consent must be voluntary and informed.

Competence.   Because human artificial insemination is a medical procedure, the medical profession should exert its influence and efforts to the fullest extent necessary to ensure that the procedure is performed only by individuals licensed to practice medicine or osteopathy. Physicians without special knowledge and competence in the field should refrain from engaging in the procedure. Referrals to fellow physicians engaged in this practice and who possess the requisite knowledge regarding the selection of proper donors is ethically mandatory.

Confidentiality. The utmost medical secrecy by the attending physician and his entire staff is essential in all aspects of the procedure. All medical records regarding the procedure must be securely protected from invasion.

In addition to the above guidelines, the Judicial Council feels obligated to comment on (a) genetic screening and (b) use of frozen semen in connection with this procedure.

Knowledge is developing daily in the field of genetics. Possession of current knowledge of genetics and application of this knowledge are expected of the physician who engages in the practice of human artificial insemination. In the past, physicians who performed this procedure attempted to ensure, insofar as possible, that the child conceived of an artificial insemination would possess physical characteristics consonant with those of the mother and her husband. Now the genetic background of the donor must also be known to the extent currently possible. Selecting and screening donors to control the transmission of infectious and genetic disease insofar as current knowledge permits is ethically required.

In using frozen semen, adequate physical, mental, and genetic examinations must have been made of the donor. The use of frozen human sperm is relatively new; it must still be recognized as experimental. There must be concern about the insemination and equal concern about the child resulting from the use of frozen, stored human sperm. The mandate *primum non nocere* is particularly applicable.

It must be remembered by the physician and explained by him to the prospective parents that any child conceived and born of an artificial insemination is possessed of and entitled to all the rights of a child conceived naturally.

[Reprinted with the permission of the American Medical Association from *American Medical Association Proceedings of the House of Delegates*, A–74: 126–127.]

OATH OF SOVIET PHYSICIANS
1971

On 26 March 1971, the Presidium of the Supreme Soviet approved the text of this Oath and ordered that all physicians and graduating medical students take and abide by it. The ruling went into effect 1 June 1971. Distinctive features of this Oath are: (1) the dedication to preventive medicine, and (2) the national requirement that all graduating medical students take this Oath and sign a copy of it.

Having received the high title of physician and beginning a career in the healing arts, I solemnly swear:

to dedicate all my knowledge and all my strength to the care and improvement of human health, to treatment and prevention of disease, and to work conscientiously wherever the interests of the society will require it;

to be always ready to administer medical aid, to treat the patient with care and interest, and to keep professional secrets;

to constantly improve my medical knowledge and diagnostic and therapeutic skill, and to further medical science and the practice of medicine by my own work;

to turn, if the interests of my patients will require it, to my professional colleagues for advice and consultation, and to never refuse myself to give advice or help;

to keep and to develop the beneficial traditions of medicine in my country, to conduct all my actions according to the principles of the Communistic morale, to always keep in mind the high calling of the Soviet physician, and

the high responsibility I have to my people and to the Soviet government.
I swear to be faithful to this Oath all my life long.

[Translated by Zenonas Danilevicius. *Journal of the American Medical Association* 217 (1971): 834. Copyright 1971, American Medical Association. Reprinted with permission.]

ETHICAL AND RELIGIOUS DIRECTIVES FOR CATHOLIC HEALTH FACILITIES
United States Catholic Conference
1971

While most religions avoid the use of codes of medical ethics, a notable exception is the Catholic Church, which has published codes of medical ethics in several parts of the world, principally though not exclusively for use in its hospitals. These codes are considered binding not only on individuals but also on institutions: The medical staff, patients, and employees, regardless of their religion, are frequently expected to abide by such a code.

In the United States, a set of Ethical and Religious Directives for Catholic Hospitals was published in 1949 and revised in 1954. The 1971 Directives, which are printed below, were approved as the national code by the National Conference of Catholic Bishops. Most distinctive are the directives on abortion, hysterectomy, sterilization, and artificial insemination. A concluding section on spiritual ministrations to the sick has been omitted.

I. General

1. The procedures listed in these Directives as permissible require the consent at least implied or reasonably presumed, of the patient or his guardians. This condition is to be understood in all cases.

2. No person may be obliged to take part in a medical or surgical procedure which he judges in conscience to be immoral; nor may a health facility or any of its staff be obliged to provide a medical or surgical procedure which violates their conscience or these Directives.

3. Every patient, regardless of the extent of his physical or psychic disability, has a right to be treated with a respect consonant with his dignity as a person.

4. Man has the right and the duty to protect the integrity of his body together with all of its bodily functions.

5. Any procedure potentially harmful to the patient is morally justified only insofar as it is designed to produce a proportionate good.

6. Ordinarily the proportionate good that justifies a medical or surgical procedure should be the total good of the patient himself.

7. Adequate consultation is recommended, not only when there is doubt concerning the morality of some procedure, but also with regard to all procedures involving serious consequences, even though such procedures are listed here as permissible. The health facility has the right to insist on such consultations.

8. Everyone has the right and the duty to prepare for the solemn moment of death. Unless it is clear, therefore, that a dying patient is already well-prepared for death as regards both spiritual and temporal affairs, it is the physician's duty to inform him of his critical condition or to have some other responsible person impart this information.

9. The obligation of professional secrecy must be carefully fulfilled not only as regards the information on the patient's charts and records but also as regards confidential matters learned in the exercise of professional duties. Moreover, the charts and records must be duly safeguarded against inspection by those who have no right to see them.

10. The directly intended termination of any patient's life, even at his own request, is always morally wrong.

11. From the moment of conception, life must be guarded with the greatest care. Any deliberate medical procedure, the *purpose* of which is to deprive a fetus or an embryo of its life, is immoral.

12. Abortion, that is, the directly intended termination of pregnancy before viability, is never permitted nor is the directly intended destruction of a viable fetus. Every procedure whose sole immediate effect is the termination of pregnancy before viability is an abortion, which, in its moral context, includes the interval between conception and implantation of the embryo.

13. Operations, treatments, and medications, which do not directly intend termination of pregnancy but which have as their purpose the cure of a proportionately serious pathological condition of the mother, are permitted when they cannot be safely postponed until the fetus is viable, even though they may or will result in the death of the fetus. If the fetus is not certainly dead, it should be baptized.

14. Regarding the treatment of hemorrhage during pregnancy and before the fetus is viable: Procedures that are designed to empty the uterus of a living fetus still effectively attached to the mother are not permitted; procedures designed to stop hemorrhage (as distinguished from those designed precisely to expel the living and attached fetus) are permitted insofar as necessary, even if fetal death is inevitably a side effect.

15. Caesarean section for the removal of a viable fetus is permitted, even with risk to the life of the mother, when necessary for successful delivery. It is likewise permitted, even with risk to the child, when necessary for the safety of the mother.

16. In extrauterine pregnancy the dangerously affected part of the mother (e.g., cervix, ovary, or fallopian tube) may be removed, even though fetal death is foreseen, provided that:

a. the affected part is presumed already to be so damaged and dangerously affected as to warrant its removal, and that
b. the operation is not just a separation of the embryo or fetus from its site within the part (which would be a direct abortion from a uterine appendage), and that
c. the operation cannot be postponed without notably increasing the danger to the mother.

17. Hysterectomy, in the presence of pregnancy and even before viability, is permitted when directed to the removal of a dangerous pathological condition of the uterus of such serious nature that the operation cannot be safely postponed until the fetus is viable.

II. Procedures Involving Reproductive Organs and Functions

18. Sterilization, whether permanent or temporary, for men or for women, may not be used as a means of contraception.

19. Similarly excluded is every action which, either in anticipation of the conjugal act, or in its accomplishment, or in the development of its natural consequences, proposes, whether as an end or as a means, to render procreation impossible.

20. Procedures that induce sterility, whether permanent or temporary, are permitted when: (a) they are immediately directed to the cure, diminution, or prevention of a serious pathological condition and are not directly contraceptive (that is, contraception is not the purpose); and (b) a simpler treatment is not reasonably available. Hence, for example, oophorectomy or irradiation of the ovaries may be allowed in treating carcinoma of the breast and metastasis therefrom; and orchidectomy is permitted in the treatment of carcinoma of the prostate.

21. Because the ultimate personal expression of conjugal love in the marital act is viewed as the only fitting context for the human sharing of the divine act of creation, donor insemination and insemination that is totally artificial are morally objectionable. However, help may be given to a normally performed conjugal act to attain its purpose. The use of the sex faculty outside the legitimate use by married partners is never permitted even for medical or other laudable purpose, e.g., masturbation as a means of obtaining seminal specimens.

22. Hysterectomy is permitted when it is sincerely judged to be a necessary means of removing some serious uterine pathological condition. In these cases, the pathological condition of each patient must be considered individually and care must be taken that a hysterectomy is not performed merely as a contraceptive measure, or as a routine procedure after any definite number of Cesarean sections.

23. For a proportionate reason, labor may be induced after the fetus is viable.

24. In all cases in which the presence of pregnancy would render some procedure illicit (e.g., curettage), the physician must make use of such pregnancy tests and consultation as may be needed in order to be reasonably certain that the patient is not pregnant. It is to be noted that curettage of the endometrium after rape to prevent implantation of a possible embryo is morally equivalent to abortion.

25. Radiation therapy of the mother's reproductive organs is permitted during pregnancy only when necessary to suppress a dangerous pathological condition.

III. Other Procedures

26. Therapeutic procedures which are likely to be dangerous are morally justifiable for proportionate reasons.

27. Experimentation on patients without due consent is morally objectionable, and even the moral right of the patient to consent is limited by his duties of stewardship.

28. Euthanasia ("mercy killing") in all its forms is forbidden. The failure to supply the ordinary means of preserving life is equivalent to euthanasia. However, neither the physician nor the patient is obliged to use extraordinary means.

29. It is not euthanasia to give a dying person sedatives and analgesics for the alleviation of pain, when such a measure is judged necessary, even though they may deprive the patient of the use of reason, or shorten his life.

30. The transplantation of organs from living donors is morally permissible when the anticipated benefit to the recipient is proportionate to the harm done to the donor, provided that the loss of such organ(s) does not deprive the donor of life itself nor of the functional integrity of his body.

31. Post-mortem examinations must not be begun until death is morally certain. Vital organs, that is, organs necessary to sustain life, may not be removed until death has taken place. The determination of the time of death must be made in accordance with responsible and commonly accepted scientific criteria. In accordance with current medical practice, to prevent any conflict of interest, the dying patient's doctor or doctors should ordinarily be distinct from the transplant team.

32. Ghost surgery, which implies the calculated deception of the patient as to the identity of the operating surgeon, is morally objectionable.

33. Unnecessary procedures, whether diagnostic or therapeutic, are morally objectionable. A procedure is unnecessary when no proportionate reason justifies it. *A fortiori*, any procedure that is contra-indicated by sound medical standards is unnecessary.

• • •

[Reprinted with the permission of the Department of Health Affairs, United States Catholic Conference.]

MEDICAL ETHICS
Statements of Policy Definitions and Rules
British Medical Association
1974

The British Medical Association (B.M.A.), which was founded in 1832, takes the view that one of its most important functions is to advise and assist its members on ethical problems. In 1974 it published a very helpful 58-page book-let titled Medical Ethics, *which incorporates resolutions, regulations, and codes drawn up earlier by the same organization and by other groups and public authorities.*

After presenting the text of a number of important internationally known codes and statements on medical ethics and human experimentation, this lengthy document offers many detailed rules and recommendations, principally pertaining to professional etiquette, on the following topics: confidentiality, the establishment of a practice, location of premises, advertising, rules for the physician–physician relationship regarding consultation, the acceptance of patients, examination of a patient by a third party, the duties of physicians in occupational medicine, the interprofessional relationships of physicians, the physician's involvement in commercial undertakings especially drug business, the resolution of disputes, and contacts with the general public. Some excerpts from this document are printed below. In these excerpts, A.R.M. stands for Annual Representative Meeting, and M.D.U. for Medical Defence Union.

Professional Confidence

• • •

1. The English text of the International Code of Medical Ethics, which stems from the Hippocratic Oath as revised by the W.M.A. in 1947, states "a doctor shall preserve absolute secrecy on all he knows about his patient because of the confidence entrusted in him". This forms the basis of the doctor/patient relationship. On the doctor's side an awareness of the patient's trust serves to invoke the observance of ethical standards and the need to act always in the best interests of the patient. The principles are set out in the following terms:

A. General

(i) It is a doctor's duty (except as below) strictly to observe the rule of professional secrecy by refraining from disclosing voluntarily to any third party, information which he has learned directly or indirectly in his professional relationship with the patient. The death of the patient does not absolve the doctor from the obligation to maintain secrecy.

(ii) There are some exceptions to this principle: if the doctor is in doubt before making any such exception in disclosing information he should seek advice from his defence organization, the B.M.A. or an experienced colleague. The exceptions to the general principle are: (a) the patient or his legal adviser gives valid consent; (b) the information is required by law; (c) the information regarding a patient's health is given in confidence to a relative or other appropriate person, in circumstances where the doctor believes it *undesirable on medical grounds* to seek the patient's consent; (d) rarely, the public interest may persuade the doctor that his duty to the community may override his duty to maintain his patient's confidence; (e) information may be disclosed for the purposes of any medical research project specifically approved for such exception by the B.M.A. including information for cancer registration.

(iii) If, in the doctor's opinion, disclosure of confidential information to a third party is in the best interests of the patient, it is the doctor's duty to make every reasonable effort to persuade the patient to allow the information to be so given. If the patient still refuses, then only very exceptionally will the doctor feel entitled to overrule that refusal. Again if in doubt, he should seek advice as above.

(iv) A doctor should be prepared to justify his action in disclosing confidential information.

B. Minors

(v) Section 8 of the Family Law Reform Act 1969 provides that the consent to treatment by a minor of 16 years shall be effective consent. A person having reached the age of consent to treatment is entitled to appropriate professional confidence.

(vi) When the patient is under 16 the doctor should act with the consent of the parent or legal guardian, but there may be occasions when his duty to the patient, a minor, conflicts with his obligation to the parent. In such cases the doctor, if in any doubt, should seek advice (as in A (ii) above).

C. Others

(vii) In the case of a person too ill to comprehend the situation, or incapable of giving valid consent to the disclosure of confidential information, consent should be sought where possible from the appropriate relative, guardian or legal adviser.

Courts of Law

2. The doctor's usual course when asked in a court of law for medical information concerning a patient in the absence of that patient's consent is to demur on the ground of professional secrecy. The court, however, may overrule this contention and direct the medical witness to supply the required information. The doctor must then decide whether or not to obey the court knowing that his refusal may lead to a fine or imprisonment or both.

3. Where a suspect refuses consent to a medical examination, the doctor, unless directed to the contrary by a court of law, should refuse to make any statement based on his observation of the suspect other than to advise the police whether or not the suspect appears to require immediate treatment or removal to hospital. This does not, of course, preclude the doctor from making a statement in court based on such observation in circumstances where the accused later gives his consent to disclosure.

4. Generally speaking, the State has no right to demand information from a doctor about his patient save when some notification is required by statute, as in the case of infectious disease. There is no legal compulsion upon him to provide information concerning criminal abortion or venereal diseases. When in doubt concerning matters that have legal implications a doctor would be wise to consult his defence organization.

5. The administration of the Welfare State has brought doctors into close contact with government departments, hospital boards and many other bodies composed partly or wholly of non-medical persons, with the result that requests are made by both medical and lay officials for clinical records or other information concerning patients. The Representative Body has passed the following resolutions relating to this problem:

A.R.M. Resolutions

(i) That this Meeting considers that wherever practicable the exchange of medical details concerning patients should take place only between doctors and deplores the increasing tendency to exchange confidential medical details with lay persons. (A.R.M. 1955.)

(ii) Medical records should be lent to the medical officers employed by government departments only when written consent has been given by or on behalf of the patient. (A.R.M. 1955.)

(iii) Wherever practicable, and particularly where disclosure of information may have an adverse psychological effect upon the patient, the practitioner who compiled the record or, if he is not available, one nominated by the hospital authority for the purpose, should be consulted on the wisdom of disclosing to the patient all of the confidential information contained therein, and should take the opportunity of reviewing the notes before they leave the hospital. (A.R.M. 1955.)

(iv) That this Meeting agrees with the principle that specialists and general practitioners should not comply with requests from lay officials of local authorities for reports, as such requests should be made through the Medical Officer of Health. (A.R.M. 1968.)

(v) That medical information should be absolutely confidential between doctor and patient and should only be divulged to para medical workers working in direct professional relationship with the doctor. (A.R.M. 1969.)

6. Other third parties who frequently seek information from a doctor are employers who request reports on the medical condition of absent or sick employees, insurance companies requiring particulars about the past history of proposers for life assurance or deceased policy holders and solicitors engaging in threatened or actual legal proceedings. In all such cases where medical information is sought the doctor should refuse to give any information in the absence of the consent of the patient. B.M.A. policy established by the A.R.M. in 1962 is that practitioners be strongly recommended not to issue "duration certificates". Any practitioner experiencing difficulty in implementing this recommendation is advised to consult the B.M.A.

· · ·

Medical Records—Computers

10. The above principles apply to the computerization of medical information about patients. The responsibility of a doctor for the safe custody of his confidential records is the same whether the records are conventional or kept in a computer.

11. A doctor whose records are kept in the conventional way can reasonably be expected to supervise the measures that are taken to safeguard them when they are kept, for example, in his own surgery. When they are kept in a hospital records department, the doctor is usually dependent upon the hospital records officer for an assurance that there are adequate arrangements to prevent improper access; the procedure adopted can be quite easily understood. In general, doctors in hospitals will take the confidentiality of hospital records departments on trust, but if they have doubt about it they are in a position to insist upon appropriate safeguards.

12. A doctor who is considering committing confidential medical information to a computer or another form of data recording machine, should bear in mind that in the end he is responsible for the results of his decision. It follows that before such information is recorded the doctor should have an assurance that disclosure will be possible only to the people and to the extent that he has decided, and that the technical resources of the system will be properly used to ensure this result. He need not necessarily understand the technicalities of the system but he should be satisfied (as far as is reasonably possible) that the person from whom he has the assurance of confidentiality is competent and trustworthy.

13. It is considered that there is need, which is becoming increasingly urgent, for statutory sanctions to protect the confidentiality of sophisticated methods of keeping records.

14. The British Medical Association's Planning Unit has prepared a Report on Computers in Medicine (1969), and the Council endorses whole-heartedly chapter 5 of this Report which discusses in detail ethical problems associated with this complex field. Copies of this Report are available on application to the Secretary, price 25p.

· · ·

The Doctor and His Colleagues

• • •

Sterilisation

Since the M.D.U. first advised on this subject after taking leading Counsel's opinion in 1961, it is now accepted that sterilisation of the male or female is not unlawful whether it is performed on therapeutic, eugenic or any other grounds, provided that there is full and valid consent by the patient.

Recent legislation in the field of human sterilisation is to be found in the N.H.S. Reorganization Act of 1973. Under the provisions of this Act:

"It shall be the duty of the Secretary of State to make arrangements, to such extent as he considers necessary to meet all reasonable requirements in England and Wales, for the giving of advice on contraception, the medical examination of persons seeking advice on contraception, the treatment of such persons and the supply of contraceptive substances and appliances; and it is hereby declared that the power conferred by Section 1(1) of the National Health Service Act 1952 to provide for the making and recovery of charges includes power to provide for the making and recovery of charges for the supply of any such substances or appliances."

The Minister of State, Department of Health and Social Security, was asked in the House of Lords in 1973 whether "it is a fact that either under English or under Scottish Law a woman must obtain her husband's permission for a sterilisation operation, but a man can have a vasectomy performed without the permission of his wife?". He replied that he had been advised that there was no statutory requirement either under English or Scottish Law that the consent of a spouse must be obtained to the sterilisation of the partner. However, the Association's Solicitor has advised that it is debatable whether at Common Law a man has a legal right to the opportunity of having children by his wife and whether, if deprived of that right without his agreement, he could claim damages against the surgeon. Accordingly, doctors would be wise to continue to obtain signatures of both spouses whenever possible until an actual court case arises which would set a precedent in either English or Scottish Law.

Undisclosed Sharing of Fees (Dichotomy)

A practice which on occasion has brought the profession into disrepute is that of dichotomy, i.e. the secret division by two or more doctors of fees on a basis of commission or other defined method. Any undisclosed division of professional fees, save in a medical partnership publicly known to exist, is highly improper. In certain circumstances it is also illegal.

Attendance upon Colleagues

Every effort should be made to maintain the traditional practice of the medical profession whereby attendance by one doctor upon another or upon his dependents is without direct charge.

• • •

The Doctor and Commercial Undertakings

A general ethical principle is that a doctor should not associate himself with commerce in such a way as to let it influence, or appear to influence, his attitude towards the treatment of his patients. Some of the particular directions in which the danger of unethical conduct may arise are mentioned below.

Pharmaceutical Products

It is undesirable for a doctor to have a special direct and personal financial interest in the sale of any pharmaceutical preparation he may have to recommend to a patient. If such be unavoidable for any good and sufficient reason, he should disclose his interest when ordering that preparation or article. This is not held to apply to the acquisition of shares in a public company marketing pharmaceutical products.

Testimonials written by doctors on the value of proprietary products have often been abused by the manufacturers. A doctor should refrain from writing a testimonial on a commercial product unless he receives a legally enforceable guarantee that his opinion will not be published without his consent.

Commercial Enterprises

The Central Ethical Committee disapproves of the direct association of a medical practitioner with any commercial enterprise engaged in the manufacture or sale of any substance which is claimed to be of value in the prevention or treatment of disease and which is recommended to the public in such a fashion as to be calculated to encourage the practice of self-diagnosis and of self-medication or is of undisclosed nature or composition.

The Central Ethical Committee takes a similar view of the association of a medical practitioner with any system or method of treatment which is not under medical control and which is advertised in the public press.

In neither of the above findings does the Central Ethical Committee pretend to interfere with the right of a medical practitioner to be associated (save as above) with any legitimate business enterprise.

In general, a doctor should not allow his professional status to enhance the business or, conversely, allow the business to enhance his professional status.

• • •

The Doctor and the General Public

Modern life brings the doctor into contact with the general public in numerous ways, both directly and indirectly, and raises for him problems of conduct unknown to his predecessors. The general public interest in medical knowledge, the dissemination of medical information through radio and television, and the press interview, all demand the exercise of the utmost caution by the doctor, whose professional standards condemn self-advertisement and publicity. In 1968 the Council drew up a report which was approved by the Representative Body to serve as a guide to the profession, and further amendments were made in 1974.

Report on Advertising and the Medical Profession
(Approved by the Representative Body in 1968 and 1974)

Attention is drawn to the statement of the General Medical Council on advertising, which appears in the pamphlet issued by the G.M.C. on "Professional Discipline". The Association is in agreement with this statement.

N.B.—Ultimate responsibility in all these matters rests with the individual concerned, but practitioners finding themselves in any difficulty in deciding upon their course of action or in doubt as to the safeguards necessary are advised to seek guidance from the Secretary of the Association.

Advertising

1. The word "advertising" in connection with the medical profession must be taken in its broadest sense, to include all those ways by which a person is made publicly known, either by himself or by others without objection on his part, in a manner which can fairly be regarded as for the purpose of obtaining patients or promoting his own professional advantage.

2. It is generally accepted by the profession that certain customs are so universally practised that it cannot be said that they are for the person's own advantage, as, for instance, a door plate with the simple announcement of the doctor's name and qualifications. Even this, however, may be abused by undue particularity or elaboration.

Avoidance of Publicity

3. Any publicity by or on behalf of or condoned by a doctor which has as its object the personal advertisement of the doctor is highly undesirable, unethical, and in contravention of paragraph (viii) of "Professional Discipline" issued by the General Medical Council, Part II.

4. Therefore no active steps should be taken by any medical practitioner to achieve publicity as a doctor otherwise than as provided below. A doctor should take all possible steps to avoid or prevent publicity where it can be shown to be unnecessary or to be to his advantage as a doctor.

Newspapers, Radio, Television

5. The public has a legitimate interest in the advances made in the science and art of medicine, and it is of advantage that medical information discreetly presented should reach the public through such media, both for the general instruction of the inquiring layman and for the particular purpose of "health education".

6. Great caution is necessary in public discussions on theories and treatment of disease owing to the misleading interpretation that may be put on these by an uninformed public to the subsequent embarrassment of the individual doctor and the patient. Sensational presentation should be avoided at all costs. The discussion of controversial medical matters, particularly in relation to treatment, is more appropriate to medical journals or professional societies.

7. Medical practitioners who possess the necessary knowledge and talent may properly participate in the presentation and discussion of medical or semimedical topics through such media.

The Representative Body, in 1974, resolved:

"That a clear distinction be made between discussions solely of general principles of medicine, where no objection would be made to the naming of the doctor involved, and those discussions which result in any particular reference by that named doctor to the way in which he approached clinical problems."

• • •

[*Medical Ethics*. London: British Medical Association, 1974, pp. 13–16, 17, 28–29, 34–35, 38–39. Reprinted with the permission of the British Medical Association.]

SECTION II

Directives for Human Experimentation

NUREMBERG CODE
1946

The Nuremberg Military Tribunal's decision in the case of the United States
v. Karl Brandt et al. *includes what is now called the Nuremberg Code, a ten-
point statement delimiting permissible medical experimentation on human
subjects. According to this statement, humane experimentation is justified only
if its results benefit society and it is carried out in accord with basic principles
that "satisfy moral, ethical, and legal concepts." To some extent, the Nuremberg Code has been superseded by the Declaration of Helsinki as a guide for
human experimentation.*

1. The voluntary consent of the human subject is absolutely essential.

This means that the person involved should have legal capacity to give consent; should be so situated as to be able to exercise free power of choice, without the intervention of any element of force, fraud, deceit, duress, over-reach-
ing, or other ulterior form of constraint or coercion; and should have sufficient
knowledge and comprehension of the elements of the subject matter involved
as to enable him to make an understanding and enlightened decision. This
latter element requires that before the acceptance of an affirmative decision
by the experimental subject there should be made known to him the nature,
duration, and purpose of the experiment; the method and means by which it is
to be conducted; all inconveniences and hazards reasonably to be expected;
and the effects upon his health or person which may possibly come from his
participation in the experiment.

The duty and responsibility for ascertaining the quality of the consent rests
upon each individual who initiates, directs or engages in the experiment. It is
a personal duty and responsibility which may not be delegated to another with
impunity.

2. The experiment should be such as to yield fruitful results for the good of
society, unprocurable by other methods or means of study, and not random
and unnecessary in nature.

3. The experiment should be so designed and based on the results of animal
experimentation and a knowledge of the natural history of the disease or other
problem under study that the anticipated results will justify the performance
of the experiment.

4. The experiment should be so conducted as to avoid all unnecessary physical and mental suffering and injury.

5. No experiment should be conducted where there is an *a priori* reason to
believe that death or disabling injury will occur; except, perhaps, in those experiments where the experimental physicians also serve as subjects.

6. The degree of risk to be taken should never exceed that determined by
the humanitarian importance of the problem to be solved by the experiment.

7. Proper preparations should be made and adequate facilities provided to
protect the experimental subject against even remote possibilities of injury,
disability, or death.

8. The experiment should be conducted only by scientifically qualified per-

sons. The highest degree of skill and care should be required through all stages of the experiment of those who conduct or engage in the experiment.

9. During the course of the experiment the human subject should be at liberty to bring the experiment to an end if he has reached the physical or mental state where continuation of the experiment seems to him to be impossible.

10. During the course of the experiment the scientist in charge must be prepared to terminate the experiment at any stage, if he has probable cause to believe, in the exercise of the good faith, superior skill and careful judgment required of him that a continuation of the experiment is likely to result in injury, disability, or death to the experimental subject.

["Permissible Medical Experiments." *Trials of War Criminals before the Nuernberg Military Tribunals under Control Council Law No. 10: Nuernberg October 1946– April 1949.* Washington: U.S. Government Printing Office (n.d.), vol. 2, pp. 181– 182.]

RESPONSIBILITY IN INVESTIGATIONS ON HUMAN SUBJECTS
Medical Research Council, Great Britain
1963

Ten years prior to the appearance of this document on 16 October 1953, the British Medical Research Council issued its Memorandum on Clinical Investigations (Memorandum MRC 53/649). *(See Irving Ladimer and Roger W. Newman, eds.* Clinical Investigation in Medicine. *Boston: Boston University Law–Medicine Research Institute, 1963, pp. 152–154.) The following, more extensive statement was published in 1963.*

During the last fifty years, medical knowledge has advanced more rapidly than at any other period in history. New understandings, new treatments, new diagnostic procedures and new methods of prevention have been, and are being, introduced at an ever-increasing rate; and if the benefits that are now becoming possible are to be gained, these developments must continue.

Undoubtedly the new era in medicine upon which we have now entered is largely due to the marriage of the methods of science with the traditional methods of medicine. Until the turn of the century, the advancement of clinical knowledge was in general confined to that which could be gained by observation, and means for the analysis in depth of the phenomena of health and disease were seldom available. Now, however, procedures that can safely, and conscientiously, be applied to both sick and healthy human beings are being devised in profusion, with the result that certainty and understanding in medicine are increasing apace.

Yet these innovations have brought their own problems to the clinical investigator. In the past, the introduction of new treatments or investigations was infrequent and only rarely did they go beyond a marginal variation on established practice. Today, far-ranging new procedures are commonplace and such are their potentialities that their employment is no negligible consideration. As a result, investigators are frequently faced with ethical and sometimes even legal problems of great difficulty. It is in the hope of giving some guidance in this difficult matter that the Medical Research Council issues this statement.

A distinction may legitimately be drawn between procedures undertaken as part of patient-care which are intended to contribute to the benefit of the individual patient, by treatment, prevention or assessment, and those procedures which are undertaken either on patients or on healthy subjects solely for the purpose of contributing to medical knowledge and are not themselves designed to benefit the particular individual on whom they are performed. The former fall within the ambit of patient-care and are governed by the ordinary rules of professional conduct in medicine; the latter fall within the ambit of investigations on volunteers.

Important considerations flow from this distinction.

Procedures Contributing to the Benefit of the Individual

In the case of procedures directly connected with the management of the condition in the particular individual, the relationship is essentially that between doctor and patient. Implicit in this relationship is the willingness on the part of the subject to be guided by the judgment of his medical attendant. Provided, therefore, that the medical attendant is satisfied that there are reasonable grounds for believing that a particular new procedure will contribute to the benefit of that particular patient, either by treatment, prevention or increased understanding of his case, he may assume the patient's consent to the same extent as he would were the procedure entirely established practice. It is axiomatic that no two patients are alike and that the medical attendant must be at liberty to vary his procedures according to his judgment of what is in his patients' best interests. The question of novelty is only relevant to the extent that in reaching a decision to use a novel procedure the doctor, being unable to fortify his judgment by previous experience, must exercise special care. That it is both considerate and prudent to obtain the patient's agreement before using a novel procedure is no more than a requirement of good medical practice.

The second important consideration that follows from this distinction is that it is clearly within the competence of a parent or guardian of a child to give permission for procedures intended to benefit that child when he is not old or intelligent enough to be able himself to give a valid consent.

A category of investigation that has occasionally raised questions in the minds of investigators is that in which a new preventive, such as a vaccine, is tried. Necessarily, preventives are given to people who are not, at the moment, suffering from the relevant illness. But the ethical and legal considerations are the same as those that govern the introduction of a new treatment. The intention is to benefit an individual by protecting him against a future hazard; and it is a matter of professional judgment whether the procedure in question offers a better chance of doing so than previously existing measures.

In general, therefore, the propriety of procedures intended to benefit the individual—whether these are directed to treatment, to prevention or to assessment—are determined by the same considerations as govern the care of patients. At the frontiers of knowledge, however, where not only are many procedures novel but their value in the particular instance may be debatable, it is wise, if any doubt exists, to obtain the opinion of experienced colleagues on the desirability of the projected procedure.

Control Subjects in Investigations of Treatment or Prevention

Over recent years, the development of treatment and prevention has been greatly advanced by the method of the controlled clinical trial. Instead of waiting, as in the past, on the slow accumulation of general experience to determine the relative advantages and disadvantages of any particular measure, it is now often possible to put the question to the test under conditions which will not only yield a speedy and more precise answer, but also limit the risk of untoward effects remaining undetected. Such trials are, however, only feasible when it is possible to compare suitable groups of patients and only permissible when there is a genuine doubt within the profession as to which of two treatments or preventive regimes is the better. In these circumstances it is justifiable to give to a proportion of the patients the novel procedure on the understanding that the remainder receive the procedure previously accepted as the best. In the case when no effective treatment has previously been devised then the situation should be fully explained to the participants and their true consent obtained.

Such controlled trials may raise ethical points which may be of some difficulty. In general, the patients participating in them should be told frankly that two different procedures are being assessed and their cooperation invited. Occasionally, however, to do so is contra-indicated. For example, to awaken patients with a possibly fatal illness to the existence of such doubts about effective treatment may not always be in their best interest; or suspicion may have arisen as to whether a particular treatment has any effect apart from suggestion and it may be necessary to introduce a placebo into part of the trial to determine this. Because of these and similar difficulties, it is the firm opinion of the Council that controlled clinical trials should always be planned and supervised by a group of investigators and never by an individual alone. It goes without question that any doctor taking part in such a colleetive controlled trial is under an obligation to withdraw a patient from the trial, and to institute any treatment he considers necessary, should this, in his personal opinion, be in the better interests of his patient.

Procedures Not of Direct Benefit to the Individual

The preceding considerations cover the majority of clinical investigations. There remains, however, a large and important field of investigations on human subjects which aims to provide normal values and their variations so that abnormal values can be recognized. This involves both ill persons and "healthy" persons, whether the latter are entirely healthy or patients suffering from a condition that has no relevance to the investigation. In regard to persons with a particular illness, such as metabolic defect, it may be necessary to know the range of abnormality compatible with the activities of normal life or the reaction of such persons to some change in circumstances such as an alteration in diet. Similarly it may be necessary to have a clear understanding of the range of a normal function and its reaction to changes in circumstances in entirely healthy persons. The common feature of this type of investigation is that it is of no direct benefit to the particular individual and that, in consequence, if he is to submit to it he must volunteer in the full sense of the word.

It should be clearly understood that the possibility or probability that a particular investigation will be of benefit to humanity or to posterity would afford no defence in the event of legal proceedings. The individual has rights that the law protects and nobody can infringe those rights for the public good. In investigations of this type it is, therefore, always necessary to ensure that the true consent of the subject is explicitly obtained.

By true consent is meant consent freely given with proper understanding of the nature and consequences of what is proposed. Assumed consent or consent obtained by undue influence is valueless and, in this latter respect, particular care is necessary when the volunteer stands in special relationship to the investigator as in the case of a patient to his doctor, or a student to his teacher.

The need for obtaining evidence of consent in this type of investigation has been generally recognized, but there are some misunderstandings as to what constitutes such evidence. In general, the investigator should obtain the consent himself in the presence of another person. Written consent unaccompanied by other evidence that an explanation has been given, understood and accepted is of little value.

The situation in respect of minors and mentally subnormal or mentally disordered persons is of particular difficulty. In the strict view of the law parents and guardians of minors cannot give consent on their behalf to any procedures which are of no particular benefit to them and which may carry some risk of harm. Whilst English law does not fix any arbitrary age in this context, it may safely be assumed that the Courts will not regard a child of 12 years or under (or fourteen years or under for boys in Scotland) as having the capacity to consent to any procedure which may involve him in an injury. Above this age the reality of any purported consent which may have been obtained is a question of fact and as with an adult the evidence would, if necessary, have to show that irrespective of age the person concerned fully understood the implications to himself of the procedures to which he was consenting.

In the case of those who are mentally subnormal or mentally disordered the reality of the consent given will fall to be judged by similar criteria to those which apply to the making of a will, contracting a marriage or otherwise taking decisions which have legal force as well as moral and social implications. When true consent in this sense cannot be obtained, procedures which are of no direct benefit and which might carry a risk of harm to the subject should not be undertaken.

Even when true consent has been given by a minor or a mentally subnormal or mentally disordered person, considerations of ethics and prudence still require that, if possible, the assent of parents or guardians or relatives, as the case may be, should be obtained.

Investigations that are of no direct benefit to the individual require, therefore, that his true consent to them shall be explicitly obtained. After adequate explanation, the consent of an adult of sound mind and understanding can be relied upon to be true consent. In the case of children and young persons the question whether purported consent was true consent would in each case depend upon facts such as the age, intelligence, situation and character of the subject and the nature of the investigation. When the subject is below the age of 12 years, information requiring the performance of any procedure involving his body would need to be obtained incidentally to and without altering the nature of a procedure intended for his individual benefit.

Professional Discipline

All who have been concerned with medical research are aware of the impossibility of formulating any detailed code of rules which will ensure that irreproachability of practice which alone will suffice where investigations on human beings are concerned. The law lays down a minimum code in matters of professional negligence and the doctrine of assault. But this is not enough. Owing to the special relationship of trust that exists between a patient and his doctor, most patients will consent to any proposal that is made. Further, the considerations involved in a novel procedure are nearly always so technical as to prevent their being adequately understood by one who is not himself an expert. It must, therefore, be frankly recognized that, for practical purposes, an inescapable moral responsibility rests with the doctor concerned for determining what investigations are, or are not, proposed to a particular patient or volunteer. Nevertheless, moral codes are formulated by man and if, in the everchanging circumstances of medical advance, their relevance is to be maintained, it is to the profession itself that we must look, and in particular to the heads of departments, the specialized Societies and the editors of medical and scientific journals.

In the opinion of the Council, the head of a department where investigations on human subjects take place has an inescapable responsibility for ensuring that practice by those under his direction is irreproachable.

In the same way the Council feel that, as a matter of policy, bodies like themselves that support medical research should do everything in their power to ensure that the practice of all workers whom they support shall be unexceptionable and known to be so.

So specialized has medical knowledge now become that the profession in general can rarely deal adequately with individual problems. In regard to any particular type of investigation, only a small group of experienced men who have specialized in this branch of knowledge are likely to be competent to pass an opinion on the justification for undertaking any particular procedure. But in every branch of medicine specialized scientific societies exist. It is upon these that the profession in general must mainly rely for the creation and maintenance of that body of precedents which shall guide individual investigators in case of doubt, and for the critical discussion of the communications presented to them on which the formation of the necessary climate of opinion depends.

Finally, it is the Council's opinion that any account of investigations on human subjects should make clear that the appropriate requirements have been fulfilled and, further, that no paper should be accepted for publication if there are any doubts that such is the case.

The progress of medical knowledge has depended, and will continue to depend, in no small measure upon the confidence which the public has in those who carry out investigations on human subjects, be these healthy or sick. Only insofar as it is known that such investigations are submitted to the highest ethical scrutiny and self-discipline will this confidence be maintained. Mistaken, or misunderstood, investigations could do incalculable harm to medical progress. It is our collective duty as a profession to see that this does not happen and so to continue to deserve the confidence that we now enjoy.

[Reprinted with the permission of the Medical Research Council.]

EXPERIMENTAL RESEARCH ON HUMAN BEINGS
British Medical Association
1963

1. New drugs or other therapy should not be prescribed unless prior investigation as to the possible effects upon the human body has been fully adequate.

2. Before a new drug is used in treatment, the clinician should ensure that the distributors of the drug are reputable and the claims made for the products include reference to independent evidence of its effects.

3. No new technique or investigation shall be undertaken on a patient unless it is strictly necessary for the treatment of the patient, or, alternatively, that following a full explanation the doctor has obtained the patient's free and valid consent to his actions, preferably in writing.

4. A doctor wholly engaged in clinical research must be at special pains to remember the responsibility to the individual patient when his experimental work is conducted through the medium of a consultant who has clinical responsibility for the patient.

5. The patient must never take second place to a research project nor should he be given any such impression. Before embarking upon any research the doctor should ask himself these questions:

a. Does the patient know what it is I propose to do?
b. Have I explained fully and honestly to him the risks I am asking him to run?
c. Am I satisfied that his consent has been freely given and is legally valid?
d. Is this procedure one which I would not hesitate to advise, or in which I would readily acquiesce, if it were to be undertaken upon my own wife or children?

[*British Medical Journal Supplement* 2 (1963): 57. Reprinted with the permission of the British Medical Association.]

DECLARATION OF HELSINKI
World Medical Association
1964 and 1975

The first document reproduced below, which offers recommendations for conducting experiments using human subjects, was adopted in 1962 and revised by the 18th World Medical Assembly at Helsinki, Finland, in 1964. The second document is the Declaration of Helsinki as revised by the 29th World Medical Assembly in Tokyo in 1975. Revisions in the second document are noted in italics.

1. The Helsinki Declaration of 1964

Introduction

It is the mission of the doctor to safeguard the health of the people. His knowledge and conscience are dedicated to the fulfillment of this mission.

The Declaration of Geneva of The World Medical Association binds the doctor with the words: "The health of my patient will be my first considera-tion" and the International Code of Medical Ethics which declares that "Any act or advice which could weaken physical or mental resistance of a human being may be used only in his interest."

Because it is essential that the results of laboratory experiments be applied to human beings to further scientific knowledge and to help suffering human-ity, the World Medical Association has prepared the following recommenda-tions as a guide to each doctor in clinical research. It must be stressed that the standards as drafted are only a guide to physicians all over the world. Doctors are not relieved from criminal, civil and ethical responsibilities under the laws of their own countries.

In the field of clinical research a fundamental distinction must be recog-nized between clinical research in which the aim is essentially therapeutic for a patient, and the clinical research, the essential object of which is purely scientific and without therapeutic value to the person subjected to the research.

I. Basic Principles

1. Clinical research must conform to the moral and scientific principles that justify medical research and should be based on laboratory and animal experi-ments or other scientifically established facts.

2. Clinical research should be conducted only by scientifically qualified per-sons and under the supervision of a qualified medical man.

3. Clinical research cannot legitimately be carried out unless the importance of the objective is in proportion to the inherent risk to the subject.

4. Every clinical research project should be preceded by careful assessment of inherent risks in comparison to foreseeable benefits to the subject or to others.

5. Special caution should be exercised by the doctor in performing clinical research in which the personality of the subject is liable to be altered by drugs or experimental procedure.

II. Clinical Research Combined with Professional Care

1. In the treatment of the sick person, the doctor must be free to use a new therapeutic measure, if in his judgment it offers hope of saving life, reestab-lishing health, or alleviating suffering.

If at all possible, consistent with patient psychology, the doctor should ob-tain the patient's freely given consent after the patient has been given a full explanation. In case of legal incapacity, consent should also be procured from the legal guardian; in case of physical incapacity the permission of the legal guardian replaces that of the patient.

2. The doctor can combine clinical research with professional care, the ob-jective being the acquisition of new medical knowledge, only to the extent that clinical research is justified by its therapeutic value for the patient.

III. Non-Therapeutic Clinical Research

1. In the purely scientific application of clinical research carried out on a human being, it is the duty of the doctor to remain the protector of the life and health of that person on whom clinical research is being carried out.

2. The nature, the purpose and the risk of clinical research must be ex-plained to the subject by the doctor.

3a. Clinical research on a human being cannot be undertaken without his free consent after he has been informed; if he is legally incompetent, the con-sent of the legal guardian should be procured.

3b. The subject of clinical research should be in such a mental, physical and legal state as to be able to exercise fully his power of choice.

3c. Consent should, as a rule, be obtained in writing. However, the responsibility for clinical research always remains with the research worker; it never falls on the subject even after consent is obtained.

4a. The investigator must respect the right of each individual to safeguard his personal integrity, especially if the subject is in a dependent relationship to the investigator.

4b. At any time during the course of clinical research the subject or his guardian should be free to withdraw permission for research to be continued.

The investigator or the investigating team should discontinue the research if in his or their judgment, it may, if continued, be harmful to the individual.

2. The Helsinki Declaration of 1975

Introduction

It is the mission of the medical doctor to safeguard the health of the people. His *or her* knowledge and conscience are dedicated to the fulfillment of this mission.

The Declaration of Geneva of The World Medical Association binds the doctor with the words "The health of my patient will be my first consideration," and the International Code of Medical Ethics declares that "Any act or advice which could weaken physical or mental resistance of a human being may be used only in his interest."

The purpose of biomedical research involving human subjects must be to improve diagnostic, therapeutic and prophylactic procedures and the understanding of the aetiology and pathogenesis of disease.

In current medical practice most diagnostic, therapeutic or prophylactic procedures involve hazards. This applies a fortiori to biomedical research.

Medical progress is based on research which ultimately must rest in part on experimentation involving human subjects.

In the field of *biomedical* research a fundamental distinction must be recognized between *medical* research in which the aim is essentially *diagnostic or* therapeutic for a patient, and *medical* research, the essential object of which is purely scientific and without *direct diagnostic or* therapeutic value to the person subjected to the research.

Special caution must be exercised in the conduct of research which may affect the environment, and the welfare of animals used for research must be respected.

Because it is essential that the results of laboratory experiments be applied to human beings to further scientific knowledge and to help suffering humanity, The World Medical Association has prepared the following recommendations as a guide to every doctor in *biomedical* research *involving human subjects. They should be kept under review in the future.* It must be stressed that the standards as drafted are only a guide to physicians all over the world. Doctors are not relieved from criminal, civil and ethical responsibilities under the laws of their own countries.

I. Basic Principles

1. *Biomedical* research *involving human subjects* must conform to *generally accepted* scientific principles and should be based on *adequately performed* laboratory and animal experimentation *and on a thorough knowledge of the scientific literature.*

2. *The design and performance of each experimental procedure involving human subjects should be clearly formulated in an experimental protocol which should be transmitted to a specially appointed independent committee for consideration, comment and guidance.*

3. *Biomedical* research *involving human subjects* should be conducted only by scientifically qualified persons and under the supervision of a *clinically*

competent medical *person. The responsibility for the human subject must always rest with a medically qualified person and never rest on the subject of the research, even though the subject has given his or her consent.*

4. *Biomedical* research involving human subjects cannot legitimately be carried out unless the importance of the objective is in proportion to the inherent risk to the subject.

5. Every *biomedical* research project *involving human subjects* should be preceded by careful assessment of *predictable* risks in comparison with foreseeable benefits to the subject or to others. *Concern for the interests of the subject must always prevail over the interests of science and society.*

6. *The right of the research subject to safeguard his or her integrity must always be respected. Every precaution should be taken to respect the privacy of the subject and to minimize the impact of the study on the subject's physical and mental integrity and on the personality of the subject.*

7. *Doctors should abstain from engaging in research projects involving human subjects unless they are satisfied that the hazards involved are believed to be predictable. Doctors should cease any investigation if the hazards are found to outweigh the potential benefits.*

8. *In publication of the results of his or her research, the doctor is obliged to preserve the accuracy of the results. Reports of experimentation not in accordance with the principles laid down in this Declaration should not be accepted for publication.*

9. *In any research on human beings, each potential subject must be adequately informed of the aims, methods, anticipated benefits and potential hazards of the study and the discomfort it may entail. He or she should be informed that he or she is at liberty to abstain from participation in the study and that he or she is free to withdraw his or her consent to participation at any time. The doctor should then obtain the subject's freely given informed consent, preferably in writing.*

10. *When obtaining informed consent for the research project the doctor should be particularly cautious if the subject is in a dependent relationship to him or her or may consent under duress. In that case the informed consent should be obtained by a doctor who is not engaged in the investigation and who is completely independent of this official relationship.*

11. *In the case of legal incompetence, informed consent should be obtained from the legal guardian in accordance with national legislation. Where physical or mental incapacity makes it impossible to obtain informed consent, or when the subject is a minor, permission from the responsible relative replaces that of the subject in accordance with national legislation.*

12. *The research protocol should always contain a statement of the ethical considerations involved and should indicate that the principles enunciated in the present Declaration are complied with.*

II. Medical Research Combined with Professional Care (Clinical Research)

1. In the treatment of the sick person, the doctor must be free to use a new *diagnostic or* therapeutic measure, if in his *or her* judgment it offers hope of saving life, reestablishing health or alleviating suffering.

2. *The potential benefits, hazards and discomfort of a new method should be weighed against the advantages of the best current diagnostic and therapeutic methods.*

3. *In any medical study, every patient—including those of a control group, if any—should be assured of the best proven diagnostic and therapeutic method.*

4. *The refusal of the patient to participate in a study must never interfere with the doctor–patient relationship.*

5. *If the doctor considers it essential not to obtain informed consent, the specific reasons for this proposal should be stated in the experimental protocol for transmission to the independent committee.* (I, 2).

6. The doctor can combine medical research with professional care, the objective being the acquisition of new medical knowledge, only to the extent

that medical research is justified by its *potential diagnostic or* therapeutic value for the patient.

III. Non-therapeutic Biomedical Research Involving Human Subjects (Non-clinical Biomedical Research)

1. In the purely scientific application of *medical* research carried out on a human being, it is the duty of the doctor to remain the protector of the life and health of that person on whom *biomedical* research is being carried out.

2. *The subjects should be volunteers—either healthy persons or patients for whom the experimental design is not related to the patient's illness.*

3. The investigator or the investigating team should discontinue the research if in his, *her or their* judgment it may, if continued, be harmful to the individual.

4. *In research on man, the interest of science and society should never take precedence over considerations related to the well-being of the subject.*

[Reprinted with the permission of *The World Medical Journal.*]

ETHICAL GUIDELINES FOR CLINICAL INVESTIGATION
American Medical Association
1966

At the 1966 Annual Convention of its House of Delegates, the American Medical Association endorsed the ethical principles set forth in the 1964 Declaration of Helsinki *of the World Medical Association. The 1966 Ethical Guidelines for Clinical Investigation, which are printed below, were intended to enlarge on the Nuremberg Code and the Declaration of Helsinki, as well as on the fundamental concepts found in the AMA* Principles of Medical Ethics. *In 1974, when asked to establish mechanisms and procedures to protect the rights of the institutionalized in clinical investigations, the AMA House of Delegates reaffirmed the 1966 guidelines; emphasized the ethical responsibility of each investigator; endorsed the principle that precautions must be taken to protect the rights of subjects whose ability to consent knowingly and voluntarily is impaired; and affirmed the goal of establishing uniformity of standards and procedures for medical experimentation throughout the world.*

1. A physician may participate in clinical investigation only to the extent that his activities are a part of a systematic program competently designed, under accepted standards of scientific research, to produce data which is scientifically valid and significant.

2. In conducting clinical investigation, the investigator should demonstrate the same concern and caution for the welfare, safety and comfort of the person involved as is required of a physician who is furnishing medical care to a patient independent of any clinical investigation.

3. In clinical investigation *primarily for treatment—*

A. The physician must recognize that the physician-patient relationship exists and that he is expected to exercise his professional judgment and skill in the best interest of the patient.

B. Voluntary consent must be obtained from the patient, or from his legally authorized representative if the patient lacks the capacity to consent, following: (a) disclosure that the physician intends to use an investigational drug or experimental procedure, (b) a reasonable explanation of the nature of the drug or procedure to be used, risks to be expected, and possible therapeutic benefits, (c) an offer to answer any inquiries concerning the drug or procedure, and (d) a disclosure of alternative drugs or procedures that may be available.

    i.   In exceptional circumstances and to the extent that disclosure of information concerning the nature of the drug or experimental procedure or risks would be expected to materially affect the health of the patient and would be detrimental to his best interests, such information may be withheld from the patient. In such circumstances such information shall be disclosed to a responsible relative or friend of the patient where possible.

    ii.   Ordinarily, consent should be in writing, except where the physician deems it necessary to rely upon consent in other than written form because of the physical or emotional state of the patient.

    iii.   Where emergency treatment is necessary and the patient is incapable of giving consent and no one is available who has authority to act on his behalf, consent is assumed.

4. In clinical investigation *primarily for the accumulation of scientific knowledge—*

A. Adequate safeguards must be provided for the welfare, safety and comfort of the subject.

B. Consent, in writing, should be obtained from the subject, or from his legally authorized representative if the subject lacks the capacity to consent, following: (a) a disclosure of the fact that an investigational drug or procedure is to be used, (b) a reasonable explanation of the nature of the procedure to be used and risks to be expected, and (c) an offer to answer any inquiries concerning the drug or procedure.

C. Minors or mentally incompetent persons may be used as subjects only if:

    i.   The nature of the investigation is such that mentally competent adults would not be suitable subjects.

    ii.   Consent, in writing, is given by a legally authorized representative of the subject under circumstances in which an informed and prudent adult would reasonably be expected to volunteer himself or his child as a subject.

D. No person may be used as a subject against his will.

[Reprinted with the permission of the American Medical Association from *American Medical Association Proceedings of the House of Delegates, C–66; 189–190 and A–74: 127–131.*]

U.S. GUIDELINES ON HUMAN EXPERIMENTATION
(Institutional Guide to DHEW Policy on Protection of Human Subjects)
1971

This institutional guide, also known as the "yellow book," contains the first set of federal guidelines for human experimentation applicable to all U.S. Department of Health, Education and Welfare (DHEW) programs. Prior to 1971 here had been a series of guideline statements issued by various agencies within DHEW.

The first federal guidelines for human experimentation were established in 1953 by the Clinical Center of the National Institutes of Health (NIH). However, these guidelines were not a formal statement of NIH policy, and they applied only to research programs conducted at the Clinical Center. In 1966 the Public Health Service (PHS) issued a formal policy statement for all PHS supported research involving human subjects. NIH revised this statement in 1969 when it set up guidelines for research projects involving human subjects funded by NIH in the document titled "Protection of the Individual as a Research Subject."

Finally, in 1971 DHEW established department-wide guidelines modeled after those of the PHS and NIH, and supplemented these general guidelines with a set of interpretive statements. The guidelines were published in a booklet titled Institutional Guide to DHEW Policy on Protection of Human Subjects. *Printed below are excerpts from these guidelines, which include both official policy (in boldface type) and interpretive statements (in lightface type).*

The guidelines contained in the 1971 Institutional Guide *were revised slightly and officially published (30 May 1974) as part of the Code of Federal Regulations (Title 45, Subtitle A, Part 46). However, the earlier document of 1971—which is still an important and basic document—is being printed here, because the 1974 revisions included only minor changes and because the interpretive statements were not included in the 1974 regulations.*

Several additional documents governing research with special populations, such as fetuses, minors, prisoners, the institutionalized, and the mentally retarded were in various stages of preparation when this Appendix was assembled (1976). Since it was anticipated that those regulations would probably be subject to development and revision for several years, they have not been reproduced here.

(For the texts of regulations published in 1973 and 1974, see United States Senate, Subcommittee on Health of the Committee on Labor and Public Welfare. Federal Regulation of Human Experimentation, *1975, 94th Congress, 1st Session. Washington, D.C.: U.S. Government Printing Office, May 1975, pp. 30–91.)*

Policy

Safeguarding the rights and welfare of human subjects involved in activities supported by grants or contracts from the Department of Health, Education, and Welfare is the responsibility of the institution which receives or is accountable to the DHEW for the funds awarded for the support of the activity.

In order to provide for the adequate discharge of this institutional responsibility, it is the policy of the Department that no grant or contract for an activity involving human subjects shall be made unless the application for such support has been reviewed and approved by an appropriate institutional committee.

This review shall determine that the rights and welfare of the subjects involved are adequately protected, that the risks to an individual are outweighed by the potential benefits to him or by the importance of the knowledge to be gained, and that informed consent is to be obtained by methods that are adequate and appropriate.

In addition the committee must establish a basis for continuing review of the activity in keeping with these determinations.

The institution must submit to the DHEW, for its review, approval, and official acceptance, an assurance of its compliance with this policy. The institution must also provide with each proposal involving human subjects a certification that it has been or will be reviewed in accordance with the institution's assurance.

No grant or contract involving human subjects at risk will be made to an individual unless he is affiliated with or sponsored by an institution which can and does assume responsibility for the protection of the subjects involved.

Since the welfare of subjects is a matter of concern to the Department of Health, Education, and Welfare as well as to the institution, no grant or contract involving human subjects shall be made unless the proposal for such support has been reviewed and approved by an appropriate professional committee within the responsible component of the Department. As a result of this review, the committee may recommend to the operating agency, and the operating agency may require, the imposition of specific grant or contract terms providing for the protection of human subjects, including requirements for informed consent.

Applicability

A. General

This policy applies to all grants and contracts which support activities in which subjects may be at risk.

B. Subject

This term describes any individual who may be at risk as a consequence of participation as a subject in research, development, demonstration, or other activities supported by DHEW funds.

This may include patients; outpatients; donors of organs, tissues, and services; informants; and normal volunteers, including students who are placed at risk during training in medical, psychological, sociological, educational, and other types of activities supported by DHEW.

Of particular concern are those subjects in groups with limited civil freedom. These include prisoners, residents or clients of institutions for the mentally ill and mentally retarded, and persons subject to military discipline.

The unborn and the dead should be considered subjects to the extent that they have rights which can be exercised by their next of kin or legally authorized representatives.

C. At Risk

An individual is considered to be "at risk" if he may be exposed to the possibility of harm—physical, psychological, sociological, or other—as a consequence of any activity which goes beyond the application of those established and accepted methods necessary to meet his needs. The determination of when an individual is at risk is a matter of the application of common sense and sound professional judgment to the circumstances of the activity in question. Responsibility for this determination resides at all levels of institutional and departmental review. Definitive determination will be made by the operating agency.

D. Types of Risks and Applicability of the Policy

1. Certain risks are inherent in life itself, at the time and in the places where life runs its course. This policy is not concerned with the ordinary risks of public or private living, or those risks associated with admission to a school or hospital. It is not concerned with the risks inherent in professional practice as long as these do not exceed the bounds of established and accepted procedures, including innovative practices applied in the interest of the individual patient, student or client.

Risk and the applicability of this policy are most obvious in medical and behavioral science research projects involving procedures that may induce a potentially harmful altered physical state or condition. Surgical and biopsy procedures; the removal of organs or tissues for study, reference, transplantation, or banking; the administration of drugs or radiation; the use of indwelling catheters or electrodes; the requirement of strenuous physical exertion; subjection to deceit, public embarrassment, and humiliation are all examples of procedures which require thorough scrutiny by both the Department of Health, Education, and Welfare and institutional committees. In general those projects which involve risk of physical or psychological injury require prior written consent.

2. There is a wide range of medical, social, and behavioral projects and activities in which no immediate physical risk to the subject is involved: e.g., those utilizing personality inventories, interviews, questionnaires, or the use of observation, photographs, taped records, or stored data. However, some of these procedures may involve varying degrees of discomfort, harassment, invasion of privacy, or may constitute a threat to the subject's dignity through the imposition of demeaning or dehumanizing conditions.

3. There are also medical and biomedical projects concerned solely with organs, tissues, body fluids, and other materials obtained in the course of the routine performance of medical services such as diagnosis, treatment and care, or at autopsy. The use of these materials obviously involves no element of physical risk to the subject. However, their use for many research, training, and service purposes may present psychological, sociological, or legal risks to the subject or his authorized representatives. In these instances, application of the

policy requires review to determine that the circumstances under which the materials were procured were appropriate and that adequate and appropriate consent was, or can be, obtained for the use of these materials for project purposes.

4. Similarly, some studies depend upon stored data or information which was often obtained for quite different purposes. Here, the reviews should also determine whether the use of these materials is within the scope of the original consent, or whether consent can be obtained.

E. Established and Accepted Methods

Some methods become established through rigorous standardization procedures prescribed as in the case of drugs or biologicals, by law or, as in the case of many educational tests, through the aegis of professional societies or non-profit agencies. Acceptance is a matter of professional response, and determination as to when a method passes from the experimental stage and becomes "established and accepted" is a matter of judgment.

In determining what constitutes an established and accepted method, consideration should be given to both national and local standards of practice. A management procedure may become temporarily established in the routine of a local institution but still fail to win acceptance at the national level. A psychological inventory may be accepted nationally, but still contain questions which are disturbing or offensive to a local population. Surgical procedures which are established and accepted in one part of the country may be considered experimental in another, not due to inherent deficiencies, but because of the lack of proper facilities and trained personnel. Diagnostic procedures which are routine in the United States may pose serious hazards to an undernourished, heavily infected, overseas population.

If doubt exists as to whether the procedures to be employed are established and accepted, the activity should be subject to review and approval by the institutional committee.

F. Necessity to Meet Needs

Even if considered established and accepted, the method may place the subject at risk if it is being employed for purposes other than to meet the needs of the subject. Determination by an attending professional that a particular treatment, test, regimen, or curriculum is appropriate for a particular subject to meet his needs limits the attendant risks to those inherent in the delivery of services, or in training.

On the other hand, arbitrary, random, or other assignment of subjects to differing treatment or study groups in the interests of a DHEW supported activity, rather than in the strict interests of the subject, introduces the possibility of exposing him to additional risk. Even comparisons of two or more established and accepted methods may potentially involve exposure of at least some of the subjects to additional risks. Any alteration of the choice, scope, or timing of an otherwise established and accepted method, primarily in the interests of a DHEW activity, also raises the issue of additional risk.

If doubt exists as to whether the procedures are intended solely to meet the needs of the subject, the activity should be subject to review and approval by the institutional committee.

Institutional Review

A. Initial Review of Projects

1. Review must be carried out by an appropriate institutional committee. The committee may be an existing one, such as a board of trustees, medical staff committee, utilization committee, or research committee, or it may be specially constituted for the purpose of this review. Institutions may utilize sub-

committees to represent major administrative or subordinate components in those instances where establishment of a single committee is impracticable or inadvisable. The institution may utilize staff, consultants, or both.

The committee must be composed of sufficient members with varying backgrounds to assure complete and adequate review of projects and activities commonly conducted by the institution. The committee's membership, maturity, experience, and expertise should be such as to justify respect for its advice and counsel. No member of an institutional committee shall be involved in either the initial or continuing review of an activity in which he has a professional responsibility, except to provide information requested by the committee. In addition to possessing the professional competence to review specific activities, the committee should be able to determine acceptability of the proposal in terms of institutional commitments and regulations, applicable law, standards of professional conduct and practice, and community attitudes. The committee may therefore need to include persons whose primary concerns lie in these areas rather than in the conduct of research, development, and service programs of the types supported by the DHEW.

If an institution is so small that it cannot appoint a suitable committee from its own staff, it should appoint members from outside the institution. . . .

2. The institution should adopt a statement of principles that will assist it in the discharge of its responsibilities for protecting the rights and welfare of subjects. This may be an appropriate existing code or declaration or one formulated by the institution itself. It is to be understood that no such principles supersede DHEW policy or applicable law.

3. Review begins with the identification of those projects or activities which involve subjects who may be at risk. In institutions with large grant and contract programs, administrative staff may be delegated the responsibility of separating those projects which do not involve human subjects in any degree; i.e., animal and nonhuman materials studies. However, determinations as to whether any project or activity involves human subjects at risk is a professional responsibility to be discharged through review by the committee, or by subcommittees.

If review determines that the procedures to be applied are to be limited to those considered by the committee to be established, accepted, and necessary to the needs of the subject, review need go no further; and the application should be certified as approved by the committee. Such projects involve human subjects, but these subjects are not considered to be at risk.

If review determines that the procedures to be applied will place the subject at risk, review should be expanded to include the issues of the protection of the subject's rights and welfare, of the relative weight of risks and benefits, and of the provision of adequate and appropriate consent procedures.

Where required by workload considerations or by geographic separation of operating units, subcommittees or mail review may be utilized to provide preliminary review of applications.

Final review of projects involving subjects at risk should be carried out by a quorum of the committee. Such review should determine, through review of reports by subcommittees, or through its own examination of applications or of protocols, or through interviews with those individuals who will have professional responsibility for the proposal project or activity, or through other acceptable procedures that the requirements of the institutional assurance and of DHEW policy have been met, specifically that:

a. The rights and welfare of the subjects are adequately protected.

Institutional committees should carefully examine applications, protocols, or descriptions of work to arrive at an independent determination of possible risks. The committee must be alert to the possibility that investigators, program directors, or contractors may, quite unintentionally, introduce unnecessary or unacceptable hazards, or fail to provide adequate safeguards. This possibility is particularly true if the project crosses disciplinary lines, involves new and untried procedures, or involves

established and accepted procedures which are new to the personnel applying them. Committees must also assure themselves that proper precautions will be taken to deal with emergencies that may develop even in the course of seemingly routine activities.

When appropriate, provision should be made for safeguarding information that could be traced to, or identified with, subjects. The committee may require the project or activity director to take steps to insure the confidentiality and security of data, particularly if it may not always remain under his direct control.

Safeguards include, initially, the careful design of questionnaires, inventories, interview schedules, and other data gathering instruments and procedures to limit the personal information to be acquired to that absolutely essential to the project or activity. Additional safeguards include the encoding or enciphering of names, addresses, serial numbers, and of data transferred to tapes, discs, and printouts. Secure, locked spaces and cabinets may be necessary for handling and storing documents and files. Codes and ciphers should always be kept in secure places, distinctly separate from encoded and enciphered data. The shipment, delivery, and transfer of all data, printouts, and files between offices and institutions may require careful controls. Computer to computer transmission of data may be restricted or forbidden.

Provision should also be made for the destruction of all edited, obsolete or depleted data on punched cards, tapes, discs, and other records. The committee may also determine a future date for destruction of all stored primary data pertaining to a project or activity.

Particularly relevant to the decision of the committees are those rights of the subject that are defined by law. The committee should familiarize itself through consultation with legal counsel with these statutes and common law precedents which may bear on its decisions. The provisions of this policy may not be construed in any manner or sense that would abrogate, supersede, or moderate more restrictive applicable law or precedential legal decisions.

Laws may define what constitutes consent and who may give consent, prescribe or proscribe the performance of certain medical and surgical procedures, protect confidential communications, define negligence, define invasion of privacy, require disclosure of records pursuant to legal process, and limit charitable and governmental immunity (see e.g., the University of Pittsburgh Law Manual).

b. The risks to an individual are outweighed by the potential benefits to him or by the importance of the knowledge to be gained.

The committee should carefully weigh the known or foreseeable risks to be encountered by subjects, the probable benefits that may accrue to them, and the probable benefits to humanity that may result from the subject's participation in the project or activity. If it seems probable that participation will confer substantial benefits on the subjects, the committee may be justified in permitting them to accept commensurate or lesser risks. If the potential benefits are insubstantial, or are outweighed by risks, the committee may be justified in permitting the subjects to accept these risks in the interests of humanity. The committee should consider the possibility that subjects, or those authorized to represent subjects, may be motivated to accept risks for unsuitable or inadequate reasons. In such instances the consent procedures adopted should incorporate adequate safeguards.

Compensation to volunteers should never be such as to constitute an undue inducement.

No subject can be expected to understand the issues of risks and benefits as fully as the committee. Its agreement that consent can reasonably be sought for subject participation in a project or activity is of paramount practical importance.

"The informed consent of the subject, while often a legal necessity is a goal toward which we must strive, but hardly ever achieve except in the simplest cases." (Henry K. Beecher, M.D.)

c. The informed consent of subjects will be obtained by methods that are adequate and appropriate.

Note: In the United States, adherence to the regulations of the Food and Drug Administration (21 CFR 130) governing consent in projects involving investigational new drugs (IND) is required by law.

Informed consent is the agreement obtained from a subject, or from his authorized representative, to the subject's participation in an activity.

The basic elements of informed consent are:

1. A fair explanation of the procedures to be followed, including an identification of those which are experimental;
2. A description of the attendant discomforts and risks;
3. A description of the benefits to be expected;
4. A disclosure of appropriate alternative procedures that would be advantageous for the subject;
5. An offer to answer any inquiries concerning the procedures;
6. An instruction that the subject is free to withdraw his consent and to discontinue participation in the project or activity at any time.

In addition, the agreement, written or oral, entered into by the subject, should include no exculpatory language through which the subject is made to waive, or to appear to waive, any of his legal rights, or to release the institution or its agents from liability for negligence.

[*The foregoing definition of informed consent might be compared with the definition given in the 1974 revision of this document (Federal Register, Vol. 39, No. 105, May 30, 1974, p. 18917):*

"Informed consent" means the knowing consent of an individual or his legally authorized representative, so situated as to be able to exercise free power of choice without undue inducement or any element of force, fraud, deceit, duress, or other form of constraint or coercion. The basic elements of information necessary to such consent include:

1. *A fair explanation of the procedures to be followed, and their purposes, including identification of any procedures which are experimental;*
2. *a description of any attendant discomforts and risks reasonably to be expected;*
3. *a description of any benefits reasonably to be expected;*
4. *a disclosure of any appropriate alternative procedures that might be advantageous for the subject;*
5. *an offer to answer any inquiries concerning the procedures; and*
6. *an instruction that the person is free to withdraw his consent and to discontinue participation in the project or activity at any time without prejudice to the subject.*]

Informed Consent Must be Documented

Consent should be obtained, whenever practicable, from the subjects themselves. When the subject group will include individuals who are not legally or physically capable of giving informed consent, because of age, mental incapacity, or inability to communicate, the review committee should consider the validity of consent by next of kin, legal guardians, or by other qualified third parties representative of the subjects' interests. In such instances, careful consideration should be given by the committee not only to whether these third parties can be presumed to have the necessary depth of interest and concern with the subjects' rights and welfare, but also to whether these third parties will be legally authorized to expose the subjects to the risks involved.

The review committee will determine if the consent required, whether to be secured before the fact, in writing or orally, or after the fact following debriefing, or whether implicit in voluntary participation in an adequately advertised activity, is appropriate in the light of the risks to the subject, and the circumstances of the project.

The review committee will also determine if the information to be given to the subject, or to qualified third parties, in writing or orally, is a fair explanation of the project or activity, of its possible benefits, and of its attendant hazards.

Where an activity involves therapy, diagnosis, or management, and a professional/patient relationship exists, it is necessary "to recognize that each patient's mental and emotional condition is important...and that in discussing the element of risk, a certain amount of discretion must be employed consistent with full disclosure of fact necessary to any informed consent."

Where an activity does not involve therapy, diagnosis, or management, and a professional/subject rather than a professional/patient relationship exists, "the subject is entitled to a full and frank disclosure of all the facts, probabilities, and opinions which a reasonable man might be expected to consider before giving his consent."

When debriefing procedures are considered as a necessary part of the plan, the committee should ascertain that these will be complete and prompt....

SECTION III

Patients' Bills of Rights

A PATIENT'S BILL OF RIGHTS
American Hospital Association
1973

On 6 February 1973 the American Hospital Association's House of Delegates approved A Patient's Bill of Rights. Other historically significant documents in the United States, which predated this Bill of Rights, were a document drafted by the National Welfare Rights Organization (1970) and the preamble to the Standards of the Joint Commission on Accreditation of Hospitals. The AHA Patient's Bill of Rights, printed in full below, has been influential in the development of similar documents in other parts of the world.

The American Hospital Association presents a Patient's Bill of Rights with the expectation that observance of these rights will contribute to more effective patient care and greater satisfaction for the patient, his physician and the hospital organization. Further, the Association presents these rights in the expectation that they will be supported by the hospital on behalf of its patients, as an integral part of the healing process. It is recognized that a personal relationship between the physician and the patient is essential for the provision of proper medical care. The traditional physician-patient relationship takes on a new dimension when care is rendered within an organizational structure. Legal precedent has established that the institution itself also has a responsibility to the patient. It is in recognition of these factors that these rights are affirmed.

1. The patient has the right to considerate and respectful care.

2. The patient has the right to obtain from his physician complete current information concerning his diagnosis, treatment, and prognosis in terms the patient can be reasonably expected to understand. When it is not medically advisable to give such information to the patient, the information should be made available to an appropriate person in his behalf. He has the right to know by name, the physician responsible for coordinating his care.

3. The patient has the right to receive from his physician information necessary to give informed consent prior to the start of any procedure and/or treatment. Except in emergencies, such information for informed consent, should include but not necessarily be limited to the specific procedure and/or treatment, the medically significant risks involved, and the probable duration of incapacitation. Where medically significant alternatives for care or treatment exist, or when the patient requests information concerning medical alternatives, the patient has the right to such information. The patient also has the right to know the name of the person responsible for the procedures and/or treatment.

4. The patient has the right to refuse treatment to the extent permitted by law, and to be informed of the medical consequences of his action.

5. The patient has the right to every consideration of his privacy concerning his own medical care program. Case discussion, consultation, examination, and treatment are confidential and should be conducted discreetly. Those not directly involved in his care must have the permission of the patient to be present.

6. The patient has the right to expect that all communications and records pertaining to his care should be treated as confidential.

7. The patient has the right to expect that within its capacity a hospital must make reasonable response to the request of a patient for services. The hospital must provide evaluation, service, and/or referral as indicated by the urgency of the case. When medically permissible a patient may be transferred to another facility only after he has received complete information and explanation concerning the needs for and alternatives to such a transfer. The institution to which the patient is to be transferred must first have accepted the patient for transfer.

8. The patient has the right to obtain information as to any relationship of his hospital to other health care and educational institutions insofar as his care is concerned. The patient has the right to obtain information as to the existence of any professional relationships among individuals, by name, who are treating him.

9. The patient has the right to be advised if the hospital proposes to engage in or perform human experimentation affecting his care or treatment. The patient has the right to refuse to participate in such research projects.

10. The patient has the right to expect reasonable continuity of care. He has the right to know in advance what appointment times and physicians are available and where. The patient has the right to expect that the hospital will provide a mechanism whereby he is informed by his physician or a delegate of the physician of the patient's continuing health care requirements following discharge.

11. The patient has the right to examine and receive an explanation of his bill regardless of source of payment.

12. The patient has the right to know what hospital rules and regulations apply to his conduct as a patient.

No catalogue of rights can guarantee for the patient the kind of treatment he has a right to expect. A hospital has many functions to perform, including the prevention and treatment of disease, the education of both health professionals and patients, and the conduct of clinical research. All these activities must be conducted with an overriding concern for the patient, and, above all, the recognition of his dignity as a human being. Success in achieving this recognition assures success in the defense of the rights of the patient.

[Reprinted with the permission of the American Hospital Association.]

PATIENTS' RIGHTS
Regulations for Skilled Nursing Facilities
U.S. Department of Health, Education and Welfare
1974

The following list of patients' rights forms part of the regulations approved for the Social Security Administration of the U.S. Department of Health, Education and Welfare, effective 2 December 1974, for skilled nursing facilities which participate in Medicare and Medicaid health insurance programs for the aged and disabled. These regulations are significant because they have the force of law in all fifty states of the United States.

These regulations were extended, with appropriate changes, to institutions for the mentally retarded or for persons with related conditions (intermediate care facilities), effective 23 June 1976. Because of objections raised against the 1974 regulations, the italicized phrases were omitted from the regulations for intermediate care facilities.

Patients' Rights.   The governing body of the facility establishes written policies regarding the rights and responsibilities of patients and, through the administrator, is responsible for development of, and adherence to, procedures implementing such policies. These policies and procedures are made available to patients, to any guardians, next of kin, sponsoring agency(ies), or representative payees..., and to the public. The staff of the facility is trained and involved in the implementation of these policies and procedures. These patients' rights policies and procedures ensure that, at least, each patient admitted to the facility:

(1) Is fully informed, as evidenced by the patient's written acknowledgment, prior to or at the time of admission and during stay, of these rights and of all rules and regulations governing patient conduct and responsibilities;

(2) Is fully informed, prior to or at the time of admission and during stay, of services available in the facility, and of related charges including any charges for services not covered [by] the Social Security Act, or not covered by the facility's basic per diem rate;

(3) Is fully informed, by a physician, of his medical condition unless medically contraindicated (as documented, by a physician, in his medical record), and is afforded the opportunity to participate in the planning of his medical treatment and to refuse to participate in experimental research;

(4) Is transferred or discharged only for medical reasons, or for his welfare or that of other patients, or for non-payment of his stay (except as prohibited by titles XVIII or XIX of the Social Security Act), and is given reasonable advance notice to ensure orderly transfer or discharge, and such actions are documented in his medical record;

(5) Is encouraged and assisted, throughout his period of stay, to exercise his rights as a patient and as a citizen, and to this end may voice grievances and recommend changes in policies and services to facility staff and/or to outside representatives of his choice, free from restraint, interference, coercion, discrimination, or reprisal;

(6) May manage his pesonal financial affairs, or is given at least a quarterly accounting of financial transactions made on his behalf should the facility accept his written delegation of this responsibility to the facility for any period of time in conformance with State law;

(7) Is free from mental and physical abuse, and free from chemical and (except in emergencies) physical restraints except as authorized in writing by a physician for a specified and limited period of time, or when necessary to protect the patient from injury to himself or to others;

(8) Is assured confidential treatment of his personal and medical records, and may approve or refuse their release to any individual outside the facility, except, in case of his transfer to another health care institution, or as required by law or third-party payment contract;

(9) Is treated with consideration, respect, and full recognition of his dignity and individuality, including privacy in treatment and in care for his personal needs;

(10) Is not required to perform services for the facility that are not included for therapeutic purposes in his plan of care;

(11) May associate and communicate privately with persons of his choice, and send and receive his personal mail unopened, *unless medically contraindicated (as documented by his physician in his medical record);*

(12) May meet with, and participate in activities of, social, religious, and community groups at his discretion, unless medically contraindicated (as documented by his physician in his medical record);

(13) May retain and use his personal clothing and possessions as space permits, unless to do so would infringe upon rights of other patients, *and unless medically contraindicated (as documented by his physician in his medical record);* and

(14) If married, is assured privacy for visits by his/her spouse; if both are inpatients in the facility, they are permitted to share a room, *unless medically contraindicated (as documented by the attending physician in the medical record).*

All rights and responsibilities specified in paragraphs...(1) through (4) of this section–as they pertain to (a) a patient adjudicated incompetent in accordance with State law, (b) a patient who is found, by his physician, to be medically incapable of understanding these rights, or (c) a patient who exhibits a communication barrier–devolve to such patient's guardian, next of kin, sponsoring agency(ies), or representative payee (except when the facility itself is representative payee) selected pursuant to section 205(j) of the Social Security Act and Subpart Q of Part 404 of this chapter.

[*Federal Register*, vol. 39, no. 193, part II (3 October 1974), pp. 35775–35776, and *Federal Register*, vol. 41, no. 61 (29 March 1976), pp. 12884–12885.]

DECLARATION OF GENERAL AND SPECIAL RIGHTS OF THE MENTALLY RETARDED
International League of Societies for the Mentally Handicapped
1968

The following Declaration was adopted by the International League of Societies for the Mentally Handicapped in 1968. The United Nations General Assembly revised and amended this Declaration and officially adopted it on 20 December 1971 under the title of Declaration on the Rights of Mentally Retarded Persons.

Article I.   The mentally retarded person has the same basic rights as other citizens of the same country and same age.

Article II.   The mentally retarded person has a right to proper medical care and physical restoration and to such education, training, habilitation and guidance as will enable him to develop his ability and potential to the fullest possible extent, no matter how severe his degree of disability. No mentally handicapped person should be deprived of such services by reason of the costs involved.

Article III.   The mentally retarded person has a right to economic security and to a decent standard of living. He has a right to productive work or to other meaningful occupation.

Article IV.   The mentally retarded person has a right to live with his own family or with fosterparents; to participate in all aspects of community life, and to be provided with appropriate leisure time activities. If care in an institution becomes necessary it should be in surroundings and under circumstances as close to normal living as possible.

Article V.   The mentally retarded person has a right to a qualified guardian when this is required to protect his personal wellbeing and interest. No person rendering direct services to the mentally retarded should also serve as his guardian.

Article VI.   The mentally retarded person has a right to protection from exploitation, abuse and degrading treatment. If accused, he has a right to a fair trial with full recognition being given to his degree of responsibility.

Article VII.   Some mentally retarded persons may be unable due to the severity of their handicap, to exercise for themselves all of their rights in a meaningful way. For others, modification of some or all of these rights is appropriate. The procedure used for modification or denial of rights must contain proper legal safeguards against every form of abuse, must be based on an evaluation of the social capability of the mentally retarded person by qualified experts and must be subject to periodic reviews and to the right of appeal to higher authorities.

[Reprinted with the permission of the International League of Societies for the Mentally Handicapped.]

PEDIATRIC BILL OF RIGHTS
National Association of Children's Hospitals and Related Institutions
1975

The Pediatric Bill of Rights was endorsed and recommended by the (U.S.) National Association of Children's Hospitals and Related Institutions on 25 February 1975. A somewhat different version had been approved and published in 1974. Proposed for use in health care institutions, the Bill has historic significance because it has served as a focal point for discussions of the health-care rights of children. Furthermore, children's rights to medical and health care, including those mentioned in this Bill, are increasingly being acknowledged in U.S. law, with some variation among the states.

This Bill draws on earlier statements: (1) the Children's Charter, from the 1930 White House Conference on Child Health and Protection; (2) the Declaration of the Rights of the Child, approved by the United Nations in 1959; and (3) The Rights of Children: Report of the Forum, from the 1970 White House Conference on Children.

The Pediatric Bill of Rights raises the question of how to provide for children's rights and needs in relationship to parental rights and responsibilities, the rights and autonomy of physicians, the rights of health-care institutions, and the rights of the state (e.g., in preventing the spread of disease). The basic issue seems to be whether, in articulating the rights and the autonomy of children together with the corresponding duties of others, the assumption should be that the child's interests are best protected by the physician; by parents, guardian, or legal custodian; or by the state. Even in giving its endorsement to the Bill, the National Association of Children's Hospitals and Related Institutions indicated that it did not intend to deemphasize or negate the rights and responsibilities of parents in connection with the medical care of their children, but intended only to indicate that the right of the child to receive appropriate medical care and treatment should be regarded as paramount in cases where parents' views might be in direct conflict with the child's desire or need for appropriate care or treatment.

Another document which gives more detailed attention to the responsibilities of parents vis-à-vis the consent of minors is "A Model Act Providing for Consent of Minors for Health Services," Pediatrics 51 (1973): 293–296, which was approved by the Council on Child Health of the American Academy of Pediatrics.

Article 1.   Every person, regardless of age, shall have the right of timely access to continuing and competent health care.

Article 2.   Every person, regardless of age, shall have the right to seek out and to receive information concerning medically accepted contraceptive devices and birth control services in doctor-patient confidentiality. Every person, regardless of age, shall have the right to receive medically prescribed contraceptive devices in doctor-patient confidentiality.

Article 3.   Every person, regardless of age, shall have the right to seek out and to receive information concerning venereal disease; and every person, regardless of age, shall have the right to consent to and to receive any medically accepted treatment necessary to combat venereal disease in doctor-patient confidentiality.

Article 4.   Every person, regardless of age, shall have the right to seek out and to accept in doctor-patient confidentiality, the diagnosis and the treatment of any medical condition related to pregnancy. Every person, regardless of age, shall have the right to adequate and objective counseling relating to pregnancy and abortion in doctor-patient confidentiality; and every person shall have the right to request and to receive medically accepted treatment which will result in abortion, in doctor-patient confidentiality.

Article 5.   Every person, regardless of age, shall have the right to seek out and to receive psychiatric care and counseling in doctor-patient confidentiality.

Article 6.   Every person, regardless of age, shall have the right to seek out and to receive medically accepted counseling and treatment for drug or alcohol dependency in doctor-patient confidentiality.

Article 7.   Every person, regardless of age, shall have the right of immediate medical care, when the life or health of such person is in imminent danger. The decision of imminent danger to the life or health of such person is a decision to be made solely by the attending physician; and the attending physician shall decide which treatment is medically indicated under the circumstances.

Article 8.   Any person, regardless of age, who is of sufficient intelligence to appreciate the nature and the consequences of the proposed medical care, and if such medical care is for his own benefit, may effectively consent to such medical care in doctor-patient confidentiality.

Article 9.   In every case, in which a child is being examined by, being treated by, or under the medical care of a qualified medical practitioner, and where, in the opinion of that qualified medical practitioner, the child is in need of immediate medical care and where the parent or legal guardian of such child refuses to consent to such needed immediate medical treatment, said medical practitioner shall notify the juvenile court or the district court with juvenile jurisdiction immediately. The juvenile court or the district court with juvenile jurisdiction shall immediately appoint a guardian ad litem, who shall represent the child's interests in all subsequent legal proceedings. The juvenile court or the district court with juvenile jurisdiction shall immediately set a date for hearing, not to exceed 96 hours from the receipt of the initial report. The court shall determine at the hearing, based upon medical and other relevant testimony and the best interests of the child, whether or not said medical treatment should so be ordered by the court.

Article 10.   Every person, regardless of age, shall have the right to considered and respectful care. During examinations, every attempt shall be made to insure the privacy of every patient, regardless of age; and every person, regardless of age, has the right to know observers are present, what role the observer may have in regard to the patient's treatment and shall have the right to request that observers remove themselves from the immediate examining area.

Article 11.   Every person, regardless of age, shall have the right to know which physician is responsible for his care. Every person, regardless of age, shall have the right to be informed concerning his diagnosis, his treatment and his prognosis in language that is readily understandable to him. Every person, regardless of age, shall have the right to ask pertinent questions concerning the diagnosis, the treatment, tests and surgery done, on a day-to-day basis in a hospital setting; and every person, regardless of age, shall have the right to immediate response to the best of the attending physician's knowledge and in language that the patient clearly understands.

[The text of the Pediatric Bill of Rights is found in Brian G. Fraser, "The Pediatric Bill of Rights," *South Texas Law Journal* 16 (1975): 245–307, and is reprinted here with the permission of the *South Texas Law Journal*.]

SECTION IV
Codes of Specialty Health-Care Associations

INTERNATIONAL COUNCIL OF NURSES
Code for Nurses
1973

The International Council of Nurses approved an international code of ethics in 1973, which includes several notable changes over its earlier 1965 code. (1) The 1973 code makes explicit the nurse's responsibility and accountability for nursing care. It deletes the statement found in the 1965 code, "The nurse is under an obligation to carry out the physician's orders intelligently and loyally," which tended to abrogate the nurse's judgment and personal responsibility. (2) The 1965 code stated that "the nurse believes in the ... preservation of human life," adding: "The fundamental responsibility of the nurse is threefold: to conserve life, to alleviate suffering and to promote health." In its place, the 1973 code points to a fourfold responsibility: "...to promote health, to prevent illness, to restore health and to alleviate suffering," adding that "respect for life, dignity and rights of man are inherent in nursing." (3) The traditional concept of the virtuous nurse was expressed in the 1965 code: "In personal conduct nurses should not knowingly disregard the accepted pattern of behavior of the community in which they live and work." In its place, the 1973 code incorporates a statement that places emphasis on the profession: "The nurse when acting in a professional capacity should at all times maintain standards of personal conduct that would reflect credit upon the profession." The text of the 1973 Code for Nurses follows.

The fundamental responsibility of the nurse is fourfold: to promote health, to prevent illness, to restore health and to alleviate suffering.

The need for nursing is universal. Inherent in nursing is respect for life, dignity and rights of man. It is unrestricted by considerations of nationality, race, creed, colour, age, sex, politics or social status.

Nurses render health services to the individual, the family and the community and coordinate their services with those of related groups.

Nurses and People

The nurse's primary responsibility is to those people who require nursing care.

The nurse, in providing care, respects the beliefs, values and customs of the individual.

The nurse holds in confidence personal information and uses judgment in sharing this information.

Nurses and Practice

The nurse carries personal responsibility for nursing practice and for maintaining competence by continual learning.

The nurse maintains the highest standards of nursing care possible within the reality of a specific situation.

The nurse uses judgment in relation to individual competence when accepting and delegating responsibilities.

The nurse when acting in a professional capacity should at all times maintain standards of personal conduct that would reflect credit upon the profession.

Nurses and Society

The nurse shares with other citizens the responsibility for initiating and supporting action to meet the health and social needs of the public.

Nurses and Co-Workers

The nurse sustains a cooperative relationship with co-workers in nursing and other fields.

The nurse takes appropriate action to safeguard the individual when his care is endangered by a co-worker or any other person.

Nurses and the Profession

The nurse plays the major role in determining and implementing desirable standards of nursing practice and nursing education.

The nurse is active in developing a core of professional knowledge.

The nurse, acting through the professional organization, participates in establishing and maintaining equitable social and economic working conditions in nursing.

[Reprinted with the permission of the International Council of Nurses.]

AMERICAN NURSES' ASSOCIATION
Code for Nurses
1976

The 1976 Code for Nurses is a revised version of the code adopted by the American Nurses' Association in 1950. The eleven-point code and the interspersed Interpretive Statements together provide a framework for ethical decision making which is noteworthy in several respects: (1) It identifies the values and beliefs which undergird the ethical standards; (2) it shows a remarkable breadth of social and professional concerns; (3) it manifests an awareness of the ethical implications of shifting professional roles and of the complexity of modern health care; and (4) it goes beyond prescriptive statements regarding personal and professional conduct by advocating a sense of accountability to the client. The ANA Code for Nurses with Interpretive Statements is printed below in its entirety because of its distinctiveness among codes of ethics.

Point 1

The nurse provides services with respect for human dignity and the uniqueness of the client unrestricted by considerations of social or economic status, personal attributes, or the nature of health problems.

1.1 Self-Determination of Clients

Whenever possible, clients should be fully involved in the planning and implementation of their own health care. Each client has the moral right to determine what will be done with his/her person; to be given the information necessary for making informed judgments; to be told the possible effects of care; and to accept, refuse, or terminate treatment. These same rights apply to minors and others not legally qualified and must be respected to the fullest degree permissible under the law. The law in these areas may differ from state to state; each nurse has an obligation to be knowledgeable about and to protect and support the moral and legal rights to all clients under state laws and applicable federal laws, such as the 1974 Privacy Act.

The nurse must also recognize those situations in which individual rights to self-determination in health care may temporarily be altered for the common good. The many variables involved make it imperative that each case be considered with full awareness of the need to provide for informed judgments while preserving the rights of clients.

1.2 Social and Economic Status of Clients

The need for nursing care is universal, cutting across all national, ethnic, religious, cultural, political, and economic differences, as does nursing's responses to this fundamental need. Nursing care should be determined solely by human need, irrespective of background, circumstances, or other indices of individual social and economic status.

1.3 Personal Attributes of Clients

Age, sex, race, color, personality, or other personal attributes, as well as individual differences in background, customs, attitudes, and beliefs, influence nursing practice only insofar as they represent factors the nurse must understand, consider, and respect in tailoring care to personal needs and in maintaining the individual's self-respect and dignity. Consideration of individual value systems and life-styles should be included in the planning of health care for each client.

1.4 The Nature of Health Problems

The nurse's respect for the worth and dignity of the individual human being applies irrespective of the nature of the health problem. It is reflected in the care given the person who is disabled as well as the normal; the patient with the long-term illness as well as the one with the acute illness, or the recovering patient as well as the one who is terminally ill or dying. It extends to all who require the services of the nurse for the promotion of health, the prevention of illness, the restoration of health, and the alleviation of suffering.

The nurse's concern for human dignity and the provision of quality nursing care is not limited by personal attitudes or beliefs. If personally opposed to the delivery of care in a particular case because of the nature of the health problem or the procedures to be used, the nurse is justified in refusing to participate. Such refusal should be made known in advance and in time for other appropriate arrangements to be made for the client's nursing care. If the nurse must knowingly enter such a case under emergency circumstances or enters unknowingly, the obligation to provide the best possible care is observed. The nurse withdraws from this type of situation only when assured that alternative sources of nursing care are available to the client. If a client requests information or counsel in an area that is legally sanctioned but contrary to the nurse's personal beliefs, the nurse may refuse to provide these services but must advise the client of sources where such service is available.

1.5 The Setting for Health Care

The nurse adheres to the principle of non-discriminatory, non-prejudicial care in every employment setting or situation and endeavors to promote its acceptance by others. The nurse's readiness to accord respect to clients and to render or obtain needed services should not be limited by the setting, whether nursing care is given in an acute care hospital, nursing home, drug or alcoholic treatment center, prison, patient's home, or other setting.

1.6 The Dying Person

As the concept of death and ways of dealing with it change, the basic human values remain. The ethical problems posed, however, and the decision-making responsibilities of the patient, family, and professional are increased.

The nurse seeks ways to protect these values while working with the client and others to arrive at the best decisions dictated by the circumstances, the client's rights and wishes, and the highest standards of care. The measures used to provide assistance should enable the client to live with as much comfort, dignity, and freedom from anxiety and pain as possible. The client's nursing care will determine to a great degree how this final human experience is lived and the peace and dignity with which death is approached.

Point 2

The nurse safeguards the client's right to privacy by judiciously protecting information of a confidential nature.

2.1 Disclosure to the Health Team

It is an accepted standard of nursing practice that data about the health status of clients be accessible, communicated, and recorded. Provision of quality health services requires that such data be available to all members of the health team. When knowledge gained in confidence is relevant or essential to others involved in planning or implementing the client's care, professional judgment is used in sharing it. Only information pertinent to a client's treatment and welfare is disclosed and only to those directly concerned with the client's care. The rights, well-being, and safety of the individual client should be the determining factors in arriving at this decision.

2.2 Disclosure for Quality Assurance Purposes

Patient information required to document the appropriateness, necessity, and quality of care that is required for peer review, third party payment, and other quality assurance mechanisms must be disclosed only under rigidly defined policies, mandates, or protocols. These written guidelines must assure that the confidentiality of client information is maintained.

2.3 Disclosure to Others Not Involved in the Client's Care

The right of privacy is an inalienable right of all persons, and the nurse has a clear obligation to safeguard any confidential information about the client acquired from any source. The nurse-client relationship is built on trust. This relationship could be destroyed and the clients' welfare and reputation jeopardized by injudicious disclosure of information provided in confidence. Since the concept of confidentiality has legal as well as ethical implications, an inappropriate breach of confidentiality may also expose the nurse to liability.

2.4 Disclosure in a Court of Law

Occasionally, the nurse may be obligated to give testimony in a court of law in relation to confidential information about a client. This should be done only under proper authorization or legal compulsion. Privilege in relation to the disclosure of such information is a legal right that only the patient or his representative may claim or waive. The statutes governing privilege and the exceptions to them vary from state to state, and the nurse may wish to consult legal counsel before testifying in court to be fully informed about professional rights and responsibilities.

2.5 Access to Records

If, in the course of providing care, there is need for access to the records of persons not under the nurse's care, as may be the case in relation to the records of the mother of a newborn, the person should be notified and permission first obtained whenever possible. Although records belong to the agency where collected, the individual maintains the right of control over the information provided by him, his family, and his environment. Similarly, professionals may exercise the right of control over information generated by them in the course of health care.

If the nurse wishes to use a client's treatment record for research or nonclinical purposes in which confidential information may be identified, the client's consent must first be obtained. Ethically, this insures the client's right to privacy; legally, it serves to protect the client against unlawful invasion of privacy and the nurse against liability for such action.

Point 3

The nurse acts to safeguard the client and the public when health care and safety are affected by incompetent, unethical, or illegal practice of any person.

3.1 Role of Advocate

The nurse's primary commitment is to the client's care and safety. Hence, in the role of client advocate, the nurse must be alert to and take appropriate action regarding any instances of incompetent, unethical, or illegal practice(s) by any member of the health care team or the health care system itself, or any action on the part of others that is prejudicial to the client's best interests. To function effectively in the role, the nurse should be fully aware of the state laws governing practice in the health care field and the employing institution's policies and procedures in relation to incompetent, unethical, or illegal practice.

3.2 Initial Action

When the nurse is aware of inappropriate or questionable conduct in the provision of health care, concern should be expressed to the person carrying out the questionable practice and attention called to the possible detrimental effect upon the client's welfare. When factors in the health care delivery system threaten the welfare of the client, similar action should be directed to the responsible administrative person. If indicated, the practice should then be reported to the appropriate authority within the institution, agency, or larger system. There should be an established mechanism for the reporting and handling of incompetent, unethical, or illegal practice within the employment setting so that such reporting can go through official channels and be done without fear of reprisal. The nurse should be knowledgeable about the mechanism and be prepared to utilize it if necessary. When questions are raised about the appropriateness of behaviors of individual practitioners or practices of health care systems, documentation of the observed behavior or practice must be provided in writing to the appropriate authorities. Local units of the professional association should be prepared to provide assistance and support in reporting procedures.

3.3 Follow-Up Action

When incompetent, unethical, or illegal practice on the part of anyone concerned with the client's care is not corrected within the employment setting and continues to jeopardize the client's care and safety, additional steps need to be taken. The problem should be reported to other appropriate authorities such as the practice committees of the appropriate professional organizations or the legally constituted bodies concerned with licensing of specific categories of health workers or professional practitioners. Some situations may warrant the concern and involvement of all these groups. Reporting should be both factual and objective.

3.4 Peer Review

In addition to the role of advocate, the nurse should participate in the planning, establishment, and implementation of other activities or procedures which serve to safeguard clients. Duly constituted peer review activities in employment agencies directed toward the improvement of practice are one example. This ongoing method of review is based on objective criteria, it includes a mechanism for making recommendations to administrators for correction of deficiencies, it facilitates the improvement of delivery services, and it promotes the health, welfare, and safety of clients.

Point 4

The nurse assumes responsibility and accountability for individual nursing judgments and actions.

4.1 Acceptance of Responsibility and Accountability

The recipients of professional nursing services are entitled to high quality nursing care. Individual professional licensure is the protective mechanism legislated by the public to ensure basic and minimum competencies of the professional nurse. Beyond that, society has accorded to the nursing profession the right to regulate its own practice. The regulation and control of nursing practice by nurses demands that individual professional practitioners of nursing bear primary responsibility for the nursing care clients receive and be individually accountable for their practice.

4.2 Responsibility

Responsibility refers to the scope of functions and duties associated with a particular role assumed by the nurse. As nursing assumes functions, these functions become part of the responsibilities or expectations of performance of nurses. Areas of responsibilities expected of nurses include: data collection and assessment of the health status of the client; determination of the nursing care plan directed toward designated goals; evaluation of the effectiveness of nursing care in achieving the goals of care; and subsequent reassessment and revision of the nursing care plan as defined in the ANA Standards of Nursing Practice. By assuming these responsibilities, the nurse is held accountable for them.

4.3 Accountability

Accountability refers to being answerable to someone for something one has done. It means providing an explanation to self, to the client, to the employing agency, and to the nursing profession. Over and above the obligations such accountability imposes on the individual nurse, there is also a liability dimension to accountability. The nurse may be called to account to be held legally responsible for judgments exercised and actions taken in the course of nursing practice. Neither physician's prescriptions nor the employing agency's policies relieve the nurse of ethical or legal accountability for actions taken and judgments made. Accountability, therefore, requires evaluation of the effectiveness of one's performance of nursing responsibilities.

4.4 Evaluation of Performance

Self-evaluation. The nurse engages in ongoing evaluation of individual clinical competence, decision-making abilities, and professional judgments. The nurse also engages in activities that will improve current practice. Self-evaluation carries with it the responsibility for the continuous improvement of one's nursing practice.

Evaluation by peers. Evaluation of one's performance by peers is a hallmark of professionalism, and it is primarily through this mechanism that the profession is held accountable to society. The nurse must be willing to have practice reviewed and evaluated by peers. Guidelines for evaluating the appropriateness, effectiveness, and efficiency of nursing practice are emerging in the form of revised and updated nurse practice acts, ANA's Standards of Nursing Practice, and other quality assurance mechanisms. Participation in the development of objective criteria for evaluation that provide valid and reliable data is the responsibility of each nurse.

Point 5

The nurse maintains competence in nursing.

5.1 Personal Responsibilities for Competence

Nursing is concerned with the welfare of human beings, and the nature of nursing is such that inadequate or incompetent practice may jeopardize the client. Therefore, it is the personal responsibility and must be the personal commitment of each individual nurse to maintain competence in practice throughout a professional career. This represents one way in which the nurse fulfills accountability to clients.

5.2 Measurement of Competence in Nursing Practice

Competence is a relative term, and an individual's competence in any field may be diminished or otherwise affected by the passage of time and the emergence of new knowledge. This means that for the client's optimum well-being and for the nurse's own professional development, nursing care should reflect and incorporate new techniques and knowledge in health care as these develop and especially as they relate to the nurse's particular field of practice.

Measures of competence are developing; they include peer review criteria, outcome criteria, and ANA's program for certification.

5.3 Continuing Education for Continuing Competence

Nursing knowledge, like that in the other health disciplines, is rendered rapidly obsolete by mounting technological advances and scientific discoveries, changing concepts and patterns in the provision of health services, and the increasing complexity of nursing responsibilities. The nurse, therefore, should be aware of the need for continuous updating and expansion of the body of knowledge on which practice is based and should keep knowledge and skills current. The nurse should assess personal learning needs, should be active in finding appropriate resources, and should be skilled in self-directed learning. Such continuing education is the key to maintenance of individual competence.

5.4 Intraprofessional Responsibility for Competence in Nursing Care

All nurses, be they practitioners, educators, administrators, or researchers, share responsibility for quality nursing care. Therefore all nurses need thorough knowledge of the current scope of professional nursing practice. Advances in theory and practice made by one professional must be disseminated to colleagues. Since individual competencies vary in relation to educational preparation, experience, client population and setting, when necessary, nurses should refer clients to and/or consult with other nurses with expertise and recognized competencies, e.g. certified nurses and clinical specialists.

Point 6

The nurse exercises informed judgment and uses individual competence and qualifications as criteria in seeking consultation, accepting responsibilities, and delegating nursing activities to others.

6.1 Changing Functions

Because of the increased complexity of health care, changing patterns in the delivery of health services, continuing shortages in skilled health manpower, and the development and acceptance of evolving nursing roles, nurses are being requested or expected to carry out functions that have formerly been performed by physicians. In turn, nurses are assigning some nursing functions to variously prepared ancillary personnel. In this gradual shift of functions, as the scope of practice of each profession changes, the nurse must exercise judgment in seeking consultation, accepting responsibilities, and assigning responsibilities to others to ensure that clients receive quality care at all time.

6.2 Joint Policy Statements

Nurse practice acts are usually expressed in broad and general language in order to provide the necessary freedom for interpretation of the law so that future developments, new knowledge, and changing roles will not necessitate constant revision of the law. The nurse must not engage in practice prohibited by law or delegate to others activities prohibited by practice acts of other health care personnel or by other laws. Recognition by nurses of the need for a more definitive delineation of roles and responsibilities, however, has resulted in collaborative efforts to develop joint policy statements. These statements may involve other health care providers or associations and usually specify the functions that are agreed upon as appropriate and proper for the nurse to perform. Such statements represent a body of expert judgment that can be used as authority where responsibilities are not definitively outlined by legal statute.

6.3 Seeking Consultation

The provision of health and illness care to clients is a complex process that requires a wide range of knowledge and skills. Interdisciplinary team effort with shared responsibility is the most effective approach to provision of total health services. Nurses, whether practicing in clearly defined or new and emerging roles, must be aware of their own individual competencies. When the needs of the client are beyond the qualifications and competencies of the nurse, consultation must be sought from qualified nurses or other appropriate sources.

Discretion must be exercised by the nurse before intervening in diagnostic or therapeutic matters that are not recognized by the nursing profession as established nursing practice. Such discretion should be based on education, experience, legal parameters, and professional guidelines and policies.

6.4 Accepting Responsibilities or Delegating Activities

The nurse should look to mutually agreed upon policy statements for guidance and direction; but even where such statements exist, personal competence should be carefully assessed before accepting responsibility or delegating activities. Decisions in this area call for knowledge of and adherence to joint policy statements and the laws regulating medical and nursing practice as well as for the exercise of informed nursing judgments.

6.5 Accepting Responsibility

If the nurse does not feel personally competent or adequately prepared to carry out a specific function, the nurse has the right and responsibility to refuse. In so doing, both the client and the nurse are protected. The reverse is also true. The nurse should not accept delegated responsibilities that do not utilize nursing skill or competencies or that prevent the provision of needed nursing care to clients. Inasmuch as the nurse is responsible for the client's total nursing care, the nurse must also assess individual competence in assigning selected components of that care to other nursing service personnel. The nurse should not delegate to any member of the nursing team a function for which that person is not prepared or qualified to perform.

Point 7

The nurse participates in activities that contribute to the ongoing development of the profession's body of knowledge.

7.1 The Nurse and Research

Every profession must engage in systematic inquiry to identify, verify, and continually enlarge the body of knowledge which forms the foundations for its practice. A unique body of verified knowledge provides both framework and direction for the profession in all of its activities and for the practitioner in the provision of nursing care. The accrual of knowledge promotes the advancement of practice and with it the well-being of the profession's clients. Ongoing research is thus indispensable to the full discharge of a profession's obligations to society. Each nurse has a role in this area of professional activity, whether involved as an investigator in the furthering of knowledge, as a participant in research, or as a user of research results.

7.2 General Guidelines for Participating in Research

Before participating in research the nurse has an obligation:

1. To ascertain that the study design has been approved by an appropriate body.
2. To obtain information about the intent and the nature of the research.
3. To determine whether the research is consistent with professional goals.

Research involving human subjects should be conducted only by scientifically qualified persons or under such supervision. The nurse who participates in research in any capacity should be fully informed about both nurse and client rights and responsibilities as set forth in the publication *Human Rights Guidelines for Nurses in Clinical and Other Research* prepared by the ANA Commission on Nursing Research.

7.3 The Protection of Human Rights in Research

The individual rights valued by society and by the nursing profession have been fully outlined and discussed in *Human Rights Guidelines for Nurses in Clinical and Other Research*; namely, the right to freedom from intrinsic risks of injury and the rights of privacy and dignity. Inherent in these rights is respect for each individual to exercise self-determination, to choose to participate, to have full information, to terminate participation without penalty.

It is the duty of both the investigator and the nurse participating in research to maintain vigilance in protecting the life, health, and privacy of human subjects from unanticipated as well as anticipated risks. The subjects' integrity, privacy, and rights must be especially safeguarded if they are unable to protect themselves because of incapacity or because they are in a dependent relationship to the investigator. The investigation should be discontinued if its continuance might be harmful to the subject.

7.4 The Practitioner's Rights and Responsibilities in Research

Practitioners of nursing providing care to clients who serve as human subjects for research have a special need to clearly understand in advance how the research can be expected to affect treatment and their own moral and legal responsibilities to clients. Here, as in other problematic situations, the practitioner has the right not to participate or to withdraw under the circumstances described in paragraph 1.4 of this document. More detailed guidance about the rights and responsibilities of nurses in relation to research activities may be found in *Human Rights Guidelines for Nurses in Clinical and Other Research*.

Point 8

The nurse participates in the profession's efforts to implement and improve standards of nursing.

8.1 Responsibility to the Public

Nursing has the responsibility to admit to the profession only those who have demonstrated a capacity for those competencies believed essential to the practice of nursing. Areas of concern for nursing competence should include adequate performance of nursing skills, academic achievement, humanitarian concern for others, acceptance of responsibility for individual actions, and the desire to improve nursing practice. Nurses involved in the evaluation of student attainment carry a primary responsibility for ensuring that the profession's obligation to the public relative to entry qualifications for practice are met.

The nursing profession exists to give assistance to those persons needing nursing care. Standards of nursing practice provide guidance for the delivery of quality nursing care and are a means for evaluating that care received by clients. The nurse has a responsibility to the public for personally implementing and maintaining optimal standards.

8.2 Responsibility to the Discipline

The professional practice of nursing is founded on an understanding and application of a body of knowledge reflected in its standards. As the profession's organization for nurses, ANA has adopted standards for nursing practice, nursing service, and nursing education. The nurse has the responsibility to monitor these standards in everyday practice and through voluntary participation in the profession's ongoing efforts to implement and improve standards at the national, state, and local levels.

8.3 Responsibility to Nursing Students

The future of nursing rests with new recruits to the profession. Nursing has a responsibility to maintain optimal standards of nursing practice and education in schools of nursing and/or wherever students engage in learning activity. This places a particular responsibility on all nurses whose services are concerned with the educational process.

Point 9

The nurse participates in the profession's efforts to establish and maintain conditions of employment conducive to high quality nursing care.

9.1 Responsibility for Conditions of Employment

The nurse must be concerned with conditions of economic and general welfare within the profession. These are important determinants in the recruitment and retention of well-qualified personnel and in assuring that each practitioner has the opportunity to function optimally.

The provision of high quality nursing care is the responsibility of both the individual nurse and the nursing profession. Professional autonomy and self-regulation in the control of conditions of practice are necessary to implement standards of practice as established by organized nursing.

9.2 Collective Action

Defining and controlling the quality of nursing care provided to the client is most effectively accomplished through collective action. Collective action may include assistance and representation from the professional association in negotiations with employers to achieve employment conditions in which the professional standards of practice can be implemented and which are commensurate with the qualifications, functions, and responsibilities of the nurse. The Economic and General Welfare program of the professional association is the appropriate channel through which the nurse can work constructively, ethically, and with professional dignity. This program, encompassing commitment to the principle of collective bargaining, promotes the right and responsibility of the individual nurse to participate in determining the terms and conditions of employment conducive to high quality nursing practice.

9.3 Individual Action

A nurse may enter into an agreement with individuals or organizations to provide health care, provided that the agreement is in accordance with the Standards of Nursing Practice of the American Nurses' Association and the nurse practice law of the state and provided that the agreement does not permit or compel practices which are in violation of this Code.

Point 10

The nurse participates in the profession's effort to protect the public from misinformation and misrepresentation and to maintain the integrity of nursing.

10.1 Advertising Services

A nurse may make factual statements that indicate availability of services through means that are in dignified form, such as:

A professional card identifying the nurse by name and title, giving address, telephone number, and other pertinent data.

Listing name, title, and brief biography in reputable directories and reputable professional publications. Such published data may include the following: Name, address, phone, field of practice or concentrates; date and place of birth; schools attended, with dates of graduation, degrees, and other scholastic distinctions; offices held; public or professional honors; teaching positions; publications; memberships and activities in professional societies; licenses; names and addresses of references.

A nurse shall not use any form of public or professional communication to make self-laudatory statements or claims that are false, fraudulent, misleading, deceptive, or unfair.

10.2 Use of Titles and Symbols

The right to use the title "Registered Nurse" is granted by state governments through licensure by examination for the protection of the public. Use of that title carries with it the responsibility to act in the public interest. The nurse may use the title "R.N." and symbols of academic degrees or other earned or honorary professional symbols of recognition in all ways that are legal and appropriate. The title and other symbols of the profession should not be used, however, for personal benefit by the nurse or by those who may seek to exploit them for other purposes.

10.3 Endorsement of Commercial Products or Services

The nurse does not give or imply endorsement to advertising, promotion, or sale of commercial products or services because this may be interpreted as reflecting the opinion or judgment of the profession as a whole. Since it is a nursing responsibility to engage in health teaching and to advise clients on matters relating to their health, it is not unethical for the nurse to utilize knowledge of specific services and/or products in advising individual clients. In the course of providing information or education to clients or other practitioners about commercial products or services, however, a variety of similar products or services should be offered or described so that the client or practitioner can make an informed choice.

10.4 Protecting the Client from Harmful Products

It is the responsibility of the nurse to advise clients against the use of dangerous products. This is seen as discharge of nursing functions when undertaken in the best interest of the client.

10.5 Reporting Infractions

Not only should the nurse personally adhere to the above principles, but alertness to any instances of their violation by others should be maintained. The nurse should report promptly, through appropriate channels, any advertisement or commercial which involves a nurse, implies involvement, or in any way suggests nursing endorsement of a commercial product, service, or enterprise. The nurse who knowingly becomes involved in such unethical activities negates professional responsibility for personal gain, and jeopardizes the public confidence and trust in the nursing profession that have been created by generations of nurses working together in the public interest.

Point 11

The nurse collaborates with members of the health professions and other citizens in promoting community and national efforts to meet the health needs of the public.

11.1 Quality Health Care as a Right

Quality health care is mandated as a right to all citizens. Availability and accessibility to quality health services for all citizens require collaborative planning by health providers and consumers at both the local and national level. Nursing care is an integral part of quality health care, and nurses have a responsibility to help ensure that citizens' rights to health care are met.

11.2 Responsibility to the Consumer of Health Care

The nurse is a member of the largest group of health providers, and therefore the philosophies and goals of the nursing profession should have a significant impact on the consumer of health care. An effective way of ensuring that nurses' views regarding health care and nursing service are properly represented is by involvement of nurses in poltical decision making.

11.3 Relationships with Other Disciplines

The complexity of the delivery of health care service demands an interdisciplinary approach to delivery of health services as well as strong support from allied health occupations. The nurse should actively seek to promote collaboration needed for ensuring the quality of health services to all persons.

11.4 Relationship with Medicine

The interdependent relationship of the nursing and medical professions requires collaboration around the need of the client. The evolving role of the nurse in the health delivery system requires joint practice as colleagues, deliberations in determining functional relationships, and differentiating areas of practice between the two professions.

11.5 Conflict of Interest

Nurses who provide public service and who have financial or other interests in health care facilities or services should avoid a conflict of interest by refraining from casting a vote on any deliberation affecting the public's health care needs in those areas.

[Reprinted with the permission of the American Nurses' Association.]

AMERICAN CHIROPRACTIC ASSOCIATION
Code of Ethics
1973

Adopted by the American Chiropractic Association in 1966 and revised in 1973, the Code of Ethics rests on two fundamental principles: (1) that the chiropractor should strive for the greatest good for the patient, and (2) that the chiropractor should be guided by the Golden Rule in his dealings with other chiropractors and with patients. The Code, portions of which are excerpted below, bears a strong resemblance to the American Medical Association Code of Medical Ethics of 1847 in the wording and ordering of its articles and subsections. In addition, the present American Chiropractic Association Code preserves the opinion expressed in the 1847 American Medical Association Code that "medical ethics, as a branch of general ethics, must rest on the basis of religion and morality."

A Statement of Purpose

We believe that the chiropractic profession of America should occupy that place in its own and the public esteem to which it is entitled and that the chiropractor should be a leader in his community—in character, in learning, in dignified bearing, and in courteous relations with his professional colleagues. We believe that these things can be accomplished only by organized efforts and do hereby resolve ourselves into an organized association dedicated and pledged to the following objectives:

1. To maintain the science and art of chiropractic as a separate and distinct health profession dedicated to the service of mankind.
2. To maintain unimpaired the chiropractic principle and practice based on the premise that the relationship between structure and function in the human body is a significant health factor.
3. To protect, promote, and promulgate the advancement of the philosophy, science and art of chiropractic and the professional welfare of members of this association in every legitimate and ethical way. This to the end that people in every locality shall have knowledge of the health benefits of chiropractic and the unhampered right and opportunity of obtaining the qualified service of doctors of chiropractic of unquestionable standing and ability.

Since they serve humanity in the specialized "science and art which utilizes the inherent recuperative powers of the body and the relationship between the musculoskeletal structures and functions of the body, particularly of the spinal column and the nervous system in the restoration and maintenance of health," doctors of chiropractic have a unique health service to offer not available from any other source.

Members are authorized to do all things necessary and proper and to exercise such power and authority as are consistent with the general purposes of the organization, in the best interests of the profession and the public health and welfare under the Code of Ethics and the Bylaws and the ACA Master Plan.

Code of Ethics

The scope of a Code of Chiropractic Ethics comprises duties and obligations of chiropractors and patients, the duties and obligations of chiropractors to each other, and the reciprocal obligations of chiropractors and the public.

Fundamental Principles

The transcendent principles upon which chiropractic ethics are based are these:

1. The ultimate end and object of the chiropractor's effort should be: "The greatest good for the patient."
2. The rules of conduct of chiropractor and patient, and of chiropractors toward each other, should be but facets of the Golden Rule: "Therefore all things whatsoever ye would that men should do to you, do ye even so to them."

It naturally follows that the various articles of this Code are but special applications of these great principles.

PART 1. RECIPROCAL DUTIES AND OBLIGATIONS OF CHIROPRACTORS AND THEIR PATIENTS

Article I. Duties of the Chiropractor to the Patient

Section 1. The chiropractic profession has for its objective the greatest service it can render humanity. Therefore, financial gain becomes a secondary consideration.

Section 2. The chiropractor should hold himself in constant readiness to respond to calls of the sick. He should bear in mind the great responsibility his vocation involves and should so conduct himself as to acquire the confidence and respect of his patients. The chiropractor is bound to keep secret whatever he may hear or observe respecting the private affairs of his patient and the family, while in the discharge of his professional duties. Should it be evident, however, that such secrecy would result in harm to others, it becomes his duty to protect the innocent party or parties. Occasions may arise, however, when he may be compelled by law to reveal some such confidences in the interests of the commonwealth.

Section 3.   The chiropractor should attend his patient as often as is necessary to insure continued favorable progress, but should avoid unnecessary visits lest he expose himself to being accused of mercenary motives.

Section 4.   A chiropractor should not express gloomy forebodings regarding a patient's condition nor magnify the gravity of the case. He should endeavor to be cheerful and hopeful in mind and manner, thus inspiring confidence and courage in the patient. However, it is the chiropractor's duty to acquaint some judicious friend or relative of the patient with the true facts, should the case prove to be of a serious nature.

Section 5.   While the chiropractor has the right to select his cases, once having accepted one he should not abandon it because it seems incurable or for any other reason, unless he gives the patient or the patient's friends or relatives sufficient notice of withdrawal to permit them to secure other attendance.

Section 6.   Since a patient has the right to dismiss a chiropractor for reasons satisfactory to himself, so likewise the chiropractor may decline to attend patients when self respect or dignity seem to him to require this step; as, for example, when a patient persistently refuses to follow directions.

Section 7.   In difficult or protracted cases consultations are advisable, and the chiropractor should be ready to act upon any desire the patient may express for a consultation, even though he may not himself feel the need for it. Nothing is so likely to retain the patient's confidence as sincerity in this respect.

Section 8.   The intimate relation into which the chiropractor is brought with his patient gives him the opportunity to exercise a powerful moral influence, which should always be used in the best possible manner. The chiropractor may sometimes be asked to assist in practices of questionable propriety. Among these may be mentioned the pretense of disease in order to avoid jury or military duty; the concealment of organic disease in order to secure favorable life insurance; or the procurement of abortion when not necessary to save the life of the mother. To all such propositions the chiropractor should present an inflexible opposition.

Article II.   Duties of Patients to Their Chiropractors

Section 1.   Since chiropractors are required by the nature of their profession to sacrifice comfort, ease, and even their health for the welfare of their patients, it forthwith becomes the duty of patients to understand this and to realize that they have certain obligations toward their chiropractors.

Section 2.   The patient should select a chiropractor in whose knowledge, skill, and integrity he can place confidence. A chiropractor once having been selected should not be dismissed for light reasons, because the chiropractor who is acquainted with the conditions, tendencies, and temperaments of a family, can more successfully handle their cases.

Section 3.   The patient should consult his chiropractor as early as possible after signs of illness. He should unreservedly state any factors he may have in mind that might contribute to his condition, with the realization that all such statements are of a confidential nature.

Section 4.   The patient should obey his chiropractor's directions as regards frequency of adjustments, diet, sanitation, and other hygienic measures that may be indicated in his case. Nor should he permit himself to deviate from the outlined course through any advice from outsiders without first consulting his chiropractor.

Section 5.   If the patient desires a consultation, he should make a frank statement to that effect. On the other hand, if he wishes to dismiss his chiropractor he should, in justice and common courtesy, state his reasons in a friendly manner. Such a course need not of necessity change the social relations of the parties.

PART 2. DUTIES OF CHIROPRACTORS TO THE PROFESSION AND TO EACH OTHER

Article I. Duties to the Profession

Section 1. Inasmuch as the chiropractor has of his own free will and accord chosen chiropractic as his vocation, he must be willing to assume certain obligations. Since he is about to profit from the scientific labor of his predecessors and associates, it becomes his duty to enrich the scientific lore, to elevate the position of the profession; and always to conduct himself as a gentleman of pure character and high moral standards.

Section 2. The honor and dignity of the chiropractic profession may best be upheld, its sphere of influence expanded, and its science advanced through the association of all chiropractors in state and national organizations. Hence it is the duty of each chiropractor to associate himself with such bodies.

• • •

[Reprinted with the permission of the American Chiropractic Association.]

AMERICAN DENTAL ASSOCIATION
Principles of Ethics
1974

Amended in 1974, the Principles consist of twenty-two sections supplemented by advisory opinions of the American Dental Association. The twenty-two sections appear below.

Section 1. Education Beyond the Usual Level. The right of a dentist to professional status rests in the knowledge, skill, and experience with which he serves his patients and society. Every dentist has the obligation of keeping his knowledge and skill freshened by continuing education through all of his professional life.

Section 2. Service to the Public. The dentist's primary duty of serving the public is discharged by giving the highest type of service of which he is capable and by avoiding any conduct which leads to a lowering of esteem of the profession of which he is a member.

In serving the public, a dentist may exercise reasonable discretion in selecting patients for his practice. However, a dentist may not refuse to accept a patient into his practice or deny dental service to a patient solely because of the patient's race, creed, color, or national origin.

Section 3. Government of a Profession. Every profession receives from society the right to regulate itself, to determine and judge its own members. Such regulation is achieved largely through the influence of the professional societies, and every dentist has the dual obligation of making himself a part of a professional society and of observing its rules of ethics.

Section 4. Leadership. The dentist has the obligation of providing freely of his skills, knowledge, and experience to society in those fields in which his qualifications entitle him to speak with professional competence. The dentist should be a leader in his community, including all efforts leading to the improvement of the dental health of the public.

Section 5. Emergency Service. The dentist has an obligation when consulted in an emergency by the patient of another dentist to attend to the conditions leading to the emergency and to refer the patient to his regular dentist who should be informed of the conditions found and treated.

Section 6. Use of Auxiliary Personnel. The dentist has an obligation to protect the health of his patient by not delegating to a person less qualified any service or operation which requires the professional competence of a dentist. The dentist has a further obligation of prescribing and supervising the work of all auxiliary personnel in the interests of rendering the best service to the patient.

Section 7. Consultation.   The dentist has the obligation of seeking consultation whenever the welfare of the patient will be safeguarded or advanced by having recourse to those who have special skills, knowledge, and experience. A consultant will hold the details of a consultation in confidence and will not undertake treatment without the consent of the attending practitioner.

Section 8. Justifiable Criticism and Expert Testimony.   The dentist has an obligation to report to the appropriate agency of his component or constituent dental society instances of gross and continual faulty treatment by another dentist. If there is evidence of faulty treatment, the welfare of the patient demands that corrective treatment be instituted. The dentist may provide expert testimony when that testimony is essential to a just and fair disposition of a judicial or administrative action. A dentist has the obligation to refrain from commenting disparagingly, without justification, about the services of another dentist.

Section 9. Rebates and Split Fees.   The dentist may not accept or tender "rebates" or "split fees."

Section 10. Secret Agents and Exclusive Methods.   The dentist has an obligation not to prescribe, dispense, or promote the use of drugs or other agents whose complete formulas are not available to the dental profession. He also has the obligation not to prescribe or dispense, except for limited investigative purposes, any therapeutic agent, the value of which is not supported by scientific evidence. The dentist has the further obligation of not holding out as exclusive, any agent, method, or technique.

Section 11. Patents and Copyrights.   The dentist has the obligation of making the fruits of his discoveries and labors available to all when they are useful in safeguarding or promoting the health of the public. Patents and copyrights may be secured by a dentist provided that they and the remuneration derived from them are not used to restrict research, practice, or the benefits of the patented or copyrighted material.

Section 12. Advertising.   Advertising reflects adversely on the dentist who employs it and lowers the public esteem of the dental profession. The dentist has the obligation of advancing his reputation for fidelity, judgment, and skill solely through his professional services to his patients and to society. The use of advertising in any form to solicit patients is inconsistent with this obligation.

Section 13. Cards, Letterheads, and Announcements.   A dentist may properly utilize professional cards, announcement cards, recall notices to patients of record, and letterheads when the style and text are consistent with the dignity of the profession and with the custom of other dentists in the community.

Announcement cards may be sent when there is a change in location or an alteration in the character of practice, but only to other dentists, to members of other health professions, and to patients of record.

Section 14. Office Door Lettering and Signs.   A dentist may properly utilize office door lettering and signs provided that their style and the text are consistent with the dignity of the profession and with the custom of other dentists in the community.

Section 15. Use of Professional Titles and Degrees.   A dentist may use the titles or degrees Doctor, Dentist, D.D.S., or D.M.D., in connection with his name on cards, letterheads, office door signs, and announcements. A dentist who also possesses a medical degree may use this degree in addition to his dental degree in connection with his name on cards, letterheads, office door signs, and announcements. A dentist who has been certified by a national certifying board for one of the specialties approved by the American Dental Association may use the title "Diplomate" in connection with his specialty on his cards, letterheads, and announcements if such usage is consistent with the custom of dentists of the community. A dentist may not use his title or degree in connection with the promotion of any commercial endeavor.

The use of eponyms in connection with drugs, agents, instruments, or appliances is generally to be discouraged.

Section 16. Health Education of the Public.   A dentist may properly participate in a program of health education of the public involving such media as the press, radio, television, and lecture, provided that such programs are in keeping with the dignity of the profession and the custom of the dental profession of the community.

Section 17. Contract Practice. A dentist may enter into an agreement with individuals and organizations to provide dental health care provided that the agreement does not permit or compel practices which are in violation of these *Principles of Ethics.*

Section 18. Announcement of Limitation of Practice. Only a dentist who limits his practice exclusively to one of the special areas approved by the American Dental Association for limited practice may include a statement of his limitation in announcements, cards, letterheads, and directory listings (consistent with the customs of dentists of the community) provided at the time of the announcement, he has met the existing educational requirements and standards set by the American Dental Association for members wishing to announce limitation of practice.

In accord with established ethical ruling that dentists should not claim or imply superiority, use of the phrases "Specialist in..." or "Specialist on..." in announcements, cards, letterheads, or directory listings, should be discouraged. The use of the phrase "Practice limited to..." is preferable.

A dentist, who uses his eligibility to announce himself as a specialist to make the public believe that specialty services rendered in his dental office are being rendered by ethically qualified specialists when such is not the case, is engaged in unethical conduct. The burden is on the specialist to avoid any inference that general practitioners who are associated with him are ethically qualified to announce themselves as specialists.

Section 19. Directories. A dentist may permit the listing of his name in a directory provided that all dentists in similar circumstances have access to a similar listing and provided that such listing is consistent in style and text with the custom of the dentists in the community.

Section 20. Name of Practice. The name under which a dentist conducts his practice may be a factor in the selection process of the patient. The use of a trade name or an assumed name could mislead laymen concerning the identity, responsibility and status of those practicing thereunder. Accordingly, a dentist shall practice only under his own name, the name of a dentist employing him who practices in the same office, a partnership name composed only of the name of one or more of the dentists practicing in a partnership in the same office or a corporate name composed only of the name of one or more of the dentists practicing as employees of the corporation in the same office.

Use of the name of a dentist no longer actively associated with the practice may be continued for a period not to exceed one year.

The use of dentists' names in directories is covered entirely by Section 19.

Section 21. Corporate Designations. Corporate designations may be used.

Section 22. Judicial Procedure. Problems involving questions of ethics should be solved at the local level within the broad boundaries established in these *Principles of Ethics* and within the interpretation of the code of ethics of the component society. If a satisfactory decision cannot be reached, the question should be referred, on appeal, to the constituent society and the Council on Judicial Procedures, Constitution and Bylaws of the American Dental Association, as provided in Chapter XI of the *Bylaws* of the American Dental Association.

AMERICAN OSTEOPATHIC ASSOCIATION
Code of Ethics
1965

In addition to the Code of Ethics, which was revised in 1965, the American Osteopathic Association has also issued a statement interpreting sections 19, 20, 21, and 22 of the Code.

Section 1.   The physician shall keep in confidence whatever he may learn about a patient in the discharge of professional duties. Information shall be divulged by the physician when required by law or when authorized by the patient.

Section 2.   The physician shall give a candid account of the patient's condition to the patient or to those responsible for the patient's care.

Section 3.   A physician-patient relationship must be founded on mutual trust, cooperation, and respect. The patient, therefore, must have complete freedom to choose his physician. The physician must have complete freedom to choose patients whom he will serve. In emergencies, a physician should make his services available.

Section 4.   The physician shall give due notice to the patient or to those responsible for the patient's care when he withdraws from a case so that another physician may be summoned.

Section 5.   A physician is never justified in abandoning a patient.

Section 6.   A physician shall practice in accordance with the body of systematized knowledge related to the healing arts and shall avoid professional association with individuals or organizations which do not practice or conduct organization affairs in accordance with such knowledge.

Section 7.   A physician should join and actively support the recognized local, state, and national bodies representing the osteopathic profession and should abide by the rules and regulations of such bodies.

Section 8.   A physician shall not solicit patients, commercialize or advertise his services, or associate professionally with, or aid in any manner, individuals or organizations which indulge in such practices.

Section 9.   A physician shall not be identified in any manner with testimonials for proprietary products or devices advertised or sold directly to the public.

Section 10.   A physician shall not hold forth or indicate possession of any degree recognized as the basis for licensure to practice the healing art unless he is actually licensed on the basis of that degree in the state in which he practices.

Section 11.   A physician shall not seek or acquire any healing arts degree from institutions not approved by the American Osteopathic Association or not approved by a body recognized for the purpose by the American Osteopathic Association.

Section 12.   A physician shall designate his osteopathic school of practice in all professional uses of his name. Indications of specialty practice, membership in professional societies, and related matters shall be governed by rules promulgated by the Board of Trustees of the American Osteopathic Association.

Section 13.   A physician shall obtain consultation whenever requested to do so by the patient. A physician should not hesitate to seek consultation whenever he himself believes it advisable.

Section 14.   In any dispute between or among physicians involving ethical or organizational matters, the matter in controversy should be referred to the arbitrating bodies of the profession.

Section 15.   In any dispute between or among physicians regarding the diagnosis and treatment of a patient, the attending physician has the responsibility for final decisions, consistent with any applicable osteopathic hospital rules or regulations.

Section 16.   A physician shall not comment, directly, or indirectly, on professional services rendered by other physicians except before duly constituted professional bodies of inquiry or in public proceedings judicial in nature.

Section 17.   Illegal, unethical, or incompetent conduct of physicians shall be revealed to the proper tribunals.

Section 18.   A physician shall not assume treatment of a patient under the care of another physician except in emergencies and only during the time that the attending physician is not available.

Section 19.   Any fee charged by a physician shall be reasonable and shall compensate the physician for services actually rendered.

Section 20.   Division of any professional fees not based on actual services rendered is a violation which will not be tolerated within the membership of this Association.

    Section 21. A physician shall not pay or receive compensation for referral of patients.

    Section 22. The physician shall cooperate fully in complying with all laws and regulations pertaining to practice of the healing arts and protection of the public health.

    Section 23. No code or set of rules can be framed which will particularize all ethical responsibilities of the physician in the various phases of his professional life. The enumeration of obligations in the Code of Ethics is not exhaustive and does not constitute a denial of the existence of other obligations, equally imperative, though not specifically mentioned.

AMERICAN PHARMACEUTICAL ASSOCIATION
Code of Ethics
1969

Adopted in 1969, the Code has nine sections with explanatory annotations. The nine sections appear below.

    Preamble. These principles of professional conduct for pharmacists are established to guide the pharmacist in his relationship with patients, fellow practitioners, other health professionals and the public.

    Section 1. A pharmacist should hold the health and safety of patients to be of first consideration; he should render to each patient the full measure of his ability as an essential health practitioner.

    Section 2. A pharmacist should never knowingly condone the dispensing, promoting or distributing of drugs or medical devices, or assist therein, which are not of good quality, which do not meet standards required by law or which lack therapeutic value for the patient.

    Section 3. A pharmacist should always strive to perfect and enlarge his professional knowledge. He should utilize and make available this knowledge as may be required in accordance with his best professional judgment.

    Section 4. A pharmacist has the duty to observe the law, to uphold the dignity and honor of the profession, and to accept its ethical principles. He should not engage in any activity that will bring discredit to the profession and should expose, without fear or favor, illegal or unethical conduct in the profession.

    Section 5. A pharmacist should seek at all times only fair and reasonable remuneration for his services. He should never agree to, or participate in transactions with practitioners of other health professions or any other person under which fees are divided or which may cause financial or other exploitation in connection with the rendering of his professional services.

    Section 6. A pharmacist should respect the confidential and personal nature of his professional records; except where the best interest of the patient requires or the law demands, he should not disclose such information to anyone without proper patient authorization.

    Section 7. A pharmacist should not agree to practice under terms or conditions which tend to interfere with or impair the proper exercise of his professional judgment and skill, which tend to cause a deterioration of the quality of his service or which require him to consent to unethical conduct.

    Section 8. A pharmacist should not solicit professional practice by means of advertising or by methods inconsistent with his opportunity to advance his professional reputation through service to patients and to society.

    Section 9. A pharmacist should associate with organizations having for their objective the betterment of the profession of pharmacy; he should contribute of his time and funds to carry on the work of these organizations.

AMERICAN PSYCHIATRIC ASSOCIATION
Principles of Medical Ethics with Annotations Especially
Applicable to Psychiatry
1973

The medical specialty of psychiatry accepts as its ethical code the Principles of Medical Ethics of the American Medical Association. In 1973 the American Psychiatric Association formulated a set of annotations which interpret the Principles in light of the special ethical problems encountered in psychiatric practice. The Principles and annotations appear below.

Section 1

The principal objective of the medical profession is to render service to humanity with full respect for the dignity of man. Physicians should merit the confidence of patients entrusted to their care, rendering to each a full measure of service and devotion.

The patient may place his trust in his psychiatrist knowing that the psychiatrist's ethics and professional responsibilities preclude him from gratifying his own needs by exploiting the patient. This becomes particularly important because of the essentially private, highly personal, and sometimes intensely emotional nature of the relationship established with the psychiatrist.

The requirement that the physician "conduct himself with propriety in his profession and in all the actions of his life" is especially important in the case of the psychiatrist because the patient tends to model his behavior after that of his therapist by identification. Further, the necessary intensity of the therapeutic relationship may tend to activate sexual and other needs and fantasies on the part of both patient and therapist, while weakening the objectivity necessary for control. Sexual activity with a patient is unethical.

The psychiatrist should diligently guard against exploiting information furnished by the patient and should not use the unique position of power afforded him by the psychotherapeutic situation to influence the patient in any way not directly relevant to the treatment goals.

Physicians generally agree that the doctor-patient relationship is such a vital factor in effective treatment of the patient that preservation of optimal conditions for development of a sound working relationship between a doctor and his patient should take precedence over all other considerations. Professional courtesy may lead to poor psychiatric care for physicians and their families beause of embarrassment over the lack of a complete give-and-take contract.

Section 2

Physicians should strive continually to improve medical knowledge and skill, and should make available to their patients and colleagues the benefits of their professional attainments.

Psychiatrists are responsible for their own continuing education and should be mindful of the fact that theirs must be a lifetime of learning.

Section 3

A physician should practice a method of healing founded on a scienitific basis and he should not voluntarily associate professionally with anyone who violates this principle.

Section 4

The medical profession should safeguard the public and itself against physicians deficient in moral character or professional competence. Physicians should observe all laws, uphold the dignity and honor of the profession and accept its self-imposed disciplines. They should expose, without hesitation, illegal or unethical conduct of fellow members of the profession.

It would seem self-evident that a psychiatrist who is a lawbreaker might be ethically unsuited to practice his profession. When such illegal activities bear directly upon his practice, this would obviously be the case. However, in other instances, illegal activities such as those concerning the right to protest social injustices might not bear on either the image of the psychiatrist or the ability of the specific psychiatrist to treat his patient ethically and well. While no committee or board could offer prior assurance that any illegal activity would not be considered unethical, it is conceivable that an individual could violate a law without being guilty of professionally unethical behavior. Physicians lose no right of citizenship on entry into the profession of medicine.

A psychiatrist who regularly practices outside his area of professional competence should be considered unethical. Determination of professional competence should be made by peer review boards or other appropriate bodies.

Special consideration should be given to those psychiatrists who, because of mental illness, jeopardize the welfare of their patients and their own reputations and practices. It is ethical, even encouraged, for another psychiatrist to intercede in such situations.

Section 5

A physician may choose whom he will serve. In an emergency, however, he should render service to the best of his ability. Having undertaken the care of a patient, he may not neglect him; and unless he has been discharged he may discontinue his services only after giving adequate notice. He should not solicit patients.

A psychiatrist should not be a party to any type of policy that excludes, segregates, or demeans the dignity of any patient because of ethnic origin, race, sex, creed, age, or socioeconomic status.

Section 6

A physician should not dispose of his services under terms or conditions which tend to interfere with or impair the free and complete exercise of his medical judgment and skill or tend to cause a deterioration of the quality of medical care.

Contract practice as applied to medicine means the practice of medicine under an agreement between a physician or a group of physicians, as principals or agents, and a corporation, organization, political subdivision, or individual whereby partial or full medical services are provided for a group or class of individuals on the basis of a fee schedule, for a salary, or for a fixed rate per capita.

Contract practice per se is not unethical. Contract practice is unethical if it permits features or conditions that are declared unethical in these Principles of Medical Ethics or if the contract or any of its provisions causes deterioration of the quality of the medical services rendered.

The ethical question is not the contract itself but whether or not the physician is free of unnecessary nonmedical interference. The ultimate issue is his freedom to offer good quality medical care.

In relationships between psychiatrists and practicing licensed psychologists, the physician should not delegate to the psychologist or, in fact, to any nonmedical person any matter requiring the exercise of professional medical judgment.

When the psychiatrist assumes a collaborative or supervisory role with another mental health worker, he must expend sufficient time to assure that proper care is given. It is contrary to the interests of the patient and to patient care if he allows himself to be used as a figurehead.

In the practice of his specialty, the psychiatrist consults, associates, collaborates, or integrates his work with that of many professionals, including psychologists, psychometricians, social workers, alcoholism counselors, marriage counselors, public health nurses, etc. Furthermore, the nature of modern psychiatric practice extends his contacts to such people as teachers, juvenile and adult probation officers, attorneys, welfare workers, agency volunteers, and neighborhood aides. In referring patients for treatment, counseling, or rehabilitation to any of these practitioners, the psychiatrist should ensure that the allied professional or paraprofessional with whom he is dealing is a recognized member of his own discipline and is competent to carry out the therapeutic task required. The psychiatrist should have the same attitude toward members of the medical profession to whom he refers patients. Whenever he has reason to doubt the training, skill, or ethical qualifications of the allied professional, the psychiatrist should not refer cases to him.

Also, he should neither lend the endorsement of the psychiatric specialty nor refer patients to persons, groups, or treatment programs with which he is not familiar, especially if their work is based only on dogma and authority and not on scientific validation and replication.

In accord with the requirements of law and accepted medical practice, it is ethical for a physician to submit his work to peer review and to the ultimate authority of the medical staff executive body and the hospital administration and its governing body.

Section 7

In the practice of medicine a physician should limit the source of his professional income to medical services actually rendered by him, or under his supervision, to his patients. His fee should be commensurate with the services rendered and the patient's ability to pay. He should neither pay nor receive a commission for referral of patients. Drugs, remedies or appliances may be dispensed or supplied by the physician provided it is in the best interests of the patient.

The psychiatrist may also receive income from administration, teaching, research, education, and consultation.

• • •

Psychiatric services, like all medical services, are dispensed in the context of a contractual arrangement between the patient and the treating physician. The provisions of the contractual arrangement, which are binding on the physician as well as on the patient, should be explicitly established.

It is ethical for the psychiatrist to make a charge for a missed appointment when this falls within the terms of the specific contractual agreement with the patient.

Section 8

A physician should seek consultation upon request; in doubtful or difficult cases; or whenever it appears that the quality of the medical service may be enhanced thereby.

The psychiatrist should agree to the request of a patient for consultation or to such a request from the family of an incompetent or minor patient. The psychiatrist may suggest possible consultants, but the patient or family should be given free choice of the consultant. If the psychiatrist disapproves of the professional qualifications of the consultant or if there is a difference of opinion that the primary therapist cannot resolve, he may, after suitable notice, withdraw from the case. If this disagreement occurs within an institution or agency framework, the differences should be resolved by the mediation or arbitration of higher professional authority within the institution or agency.

Section 9

A physician may not reveal the confidences entrusted to him in the course of medical attendance, or the deficiencies he may observe in the character of patients, unless he is required to do so by law or unless it becomes necessary in order to protect the welfare of the individual or of the community.

Psychiatric records, including even the identification of a person as a patient, must be protected with extreme care. Confidentiality is essential to psychiatric treatment. This is based in part on the special nature of psychiatric therapy as well as on the traditional ethical relationship between physician and patient. Growing concern regarding the civil rights of patients and the possible adverse effects of computerization, duplication equipment, and data banks makes the dissemination of confidential information an increasing hazard. Because of the sensitive and private nature of the information with which the psychiatrist deals, he must be circumspect in the information that he chooses to disclose to others about a patient. The welfare of the patient must be a continuing consideration.

A psychiatrist may release confidential information only with the authorization of the patient or under proper legal compulsion. The continuing duty of the psychiatrist to protect the patient includes fully apprising him of the connotations of waiving the privilege of privacy. This may become an issue when the patient is being investigated by a government agency, is applying for a position, or is involved in legal action. The same principles apply to the release of information concerning treatment to medical departments of government agencies, business organizations, labor unions, and insurance companies. Information gained in confidence about patients seen in student health services should not be released without the student's explicit permission.

Clinical and other materials used in teaching and writing must be adequately disguised in order to preserve the anonymity of the individuals involved.

The ethical responsibility of maintaining confidentiality holds equally for the consultations in which the patient may not have been present and in which the consultee was not a physician. In such instances, the physician consultant should alert the consultee to his duty of confidentiality.

Ethically the psychiatrist may disclose only that information which is immediately relevant to a given situation. He should avoid offering speculation as fact. Sensitive information such as an individual's sexual orientation or fantasy material is usually unnecessary.

Psychiatrists are often asked to examine individuals for security purposes, to determine suitability for various jobs, and to determine legal competence. The psychiatrist must fully describe the nature and purpose and lack of confidentiality of the examination to the examinee at the beginning of the examination.

Psychiatrists at times may find it necessary, in order to protect the patient or the community from imminent danger, to reveal confidential information disclosed by the patient.

Careful judgment must be exercised by the psychiatrist in order to include, when appropriate, the parents or guardian in the treatment of a minor. At the same time the psychiatrist must assure the minor proper confidentiality.

When the psychiatrist is ordered by the court to reveal the confidences entrusted to him by patients he may comply or he may ethically hold the right to dissent within the framework of the law. When the psychiatrist is in doubt, the right of the patient to confidentiality and, by extension, to unimpaired treatment, should be given priority. The psychiatrist should reserve the right to raise the question of adequate need for disclosure. In the event that the necessity for legal disclosure is demonstrated by the court, the psychiatrist may request the right to disclosure of only that information which is relevant to the legal question at hand.

Section 10

The honored ideals of the medical profession imply that the responsibilities of the physician extend not only to the individual, but also to society where these responsibilities deserve his interest and participation in activities which have the purpose of improving both the health and the well-being of the individual and the community.

Psychiatrists should foster the cooperation of those legitimately concerned with the medical, psychological, social, and legal aspects of mental health and illness. Psychiatrists are encouraged to serve society by advising and consulting with the executive, legislative, and judiciary branches of the government. A psychiatrist should clarify whether he speaks as an individual or as a representative of an organization. Furthermore, psychiatrists should avoid clouding their public statements with the authority of the profession (e.g., "Psychiatrists know that...").

Psychiatrists may interpret and share with the public their expertise in the various psychosocial issues that may affect mental health and illness. Psychiatrists should always be mindful of their separate roles as dedicated citizens and as experts in psychological medicine.

On occasion psychiatrists are asked for an opinion about an individual who is in the light of public attention, or who has disclosed information about himself through public media. It is unethical for a psychiatrist to offer a diagnosis unless he has conducted an examination and has been granted proper authorization for such a statement.

The psychiatrist should not permit his certification to be used for the involuntary commitment of any person except when this is clearly necessary for the patient's own protection or the protection of others from probable injury at the patient's hands.

AMERICAN PSYCHOLOGICAL ASSOCIATION
Ethical Standards of Psychologists
1972

The American Psychological Association (APA) adopted the Standards in 1963, amending them in 1965 and 1972. All nineteen principles of the Standards and selected annotations appear below.

The psychologist believes in the dignity and worth of the individual human being. He is committed to increasing man's understanding of himself and others. While pursuing this endeavor, he protects the welfare of any person who may seek his service or of any subject, human or animal, that may be the object of his study. He does not use his professional position or relationships, nor does he knowingly permit his own services to be used by others, for purposes inconsistent with these values. While demanding for himself freedom of inquiry and communication, he accepts the responsibility this freedom confers: for competence where he claims it, for objectivity in the report of his findings, and for consideration of the best interests of his colleagues and of society.

Principle 1. Responsibility. The psychologist, committed to increasing man's understanding of man, places high value on objectivity and integrity, and maintains the highest standards in the services he offers.

a. As a scientist, the psychologist believes that society will be best served when he investigates where his judgment indicates investigation is needed; he plans his research in such a way as to minimize the possibility that his findings will be misleading; and he publishes full reports of his work, never discarding without explanation data which may modify the interpretation of results.

b. As a teacher, the psychologist recognizes his primary obligation to help others acquire knowledge and skill, and to maintain high standards of scholarship.

c. As a practitioner, the psychologist knows that he bears a heavy social responsibility because his work may touch intimately the lives of others.

Principle 2. Competence. The maintenance of high standards of professional competence is a responsibility shared by all psychologists, in the interest of the public and of the profession as a whole.

• • •

Principle 3. Moral and Legal Standards. The psychologist in the practice of his profession shows sensible regard for the social codes and moral expectations of the community in which he works, recognizing that violations of accepted moral and legal standards on his part may involve his clients, students, or colleagues in damaging personal conflicts, and impugn his own name and the reputation of his profession.

Principle 4. Misrepresentation.   The psychologist avoids misrepresentation of his own professional qualifications, affiliations, and purposes, and those of the institutions and organizations with which he is associated.

• • •

Principle 5. Public Statements.   Modesty, scientific caution, and due regard for the limits of present knowledge characterize all statements of psychologists who supply information to the public, either directly or indirectly.

• • •

Principle 6. Confidentiality.   Safeguarding information about an individual that has been obtained by the psychologist in the course of his teaching, practice, or investigation is a primary obligation of the psychologist. Such information is not communicated to others unless certain important conditions are met.

a. Information received in confidence is revealed only after most careful deliberation and when there is clear and imminent danger to an individual or to society, and then only to appropriate professional workers or public authorities.

b. Information obtained in clinical or consulting relationships, or evaluative data concerning children, students, employees, and others are discussed only for professional purposes and only with persons clearly concerned with the case. Written and oral reports should present only data germane to the purposes of the evaluation, every effort should be made to avoid undue invasion of privacy.

c. Clinical and other materials are used in classroom teaching and writing only when the identity of the persons involved is adequately disguised.

d. The confidentiality of professional communications about individuals is maintained. Only when the originator and other persons involved give their express permission is a confidential professional communication shown to the individual concerned. The psychologist is responsible for informing the client of the limits of the confidentiality.

e. Only after explicit permission has been granted is the identity of research subjects published. When data have been published without permission for identification, the psychologist assumes responsibility for adequately disguising their sources.

f. The psychologist makes provisions for the maintenance of confidentiality in the preservation and ultimate disposition of confidential records.

Principle 7. Client Welfare.   The psychologist respects the integrity and protects the welfare of the person or group with whom he is working.

a. The psychologist in industry, education, and other situations in which conflicts of interest may arise among various parties, as between management and labor, or between the client and employer of the psychologist, defines for himself the nature and direction of his loyalties and responsibilities and keeps all parties concerned informed of these commitments.

b. When there is a conflict among professional workers, the psychologist is concerned primarily with the welfare of any client involved and only secondarily with the interest of his own professional group.

c. The psychologist attempts to terminate a clinical or consulting relationship when it is reasonably clear to the psychologist that the client is not benefiting from it.

d. The psychologist who asks that an individual reveal personal information in the course of interviewing, testing, or evaluation, or who allows such information to be divulged to him, does so only after making certain that the responsible person is fully aware of the purposes of the interview, testing, or evaluation and of the ways in which the information may be used.

e. In cases involving referral, the responsibility of the psychologist for the welfare of the client continues until this responsibility is assumed by the professional person to whom the client is referred or until the relationship with the psychologist making the referral has been terminated by mutual agreement. In situations where referral, consultation, or other changes in the conditions of the treatment are indicated and the client refuses referral, the psychologist carefully weighs the possible harm to the client, to himself, and to his profession that might ensue from continuing the relationship.

f. The psychologist who requires the taking of psychological tests for didactic, classification, or research purposes protects the examinees by insuring that the tests and test results are used in a professional manner.

g. When potentially disturbing subject matter is presented to students, it is discussed objectively, and efforts are made to handle constructively any difficulties that arise.

h. Care must be taken to insure an appropriate setting for clinical work to protect both client and psychologist from actual or imputed harm and the profession from censure.

i. In the use of accepted drugs for therapeutic purposes special care needs to be exercised by the psychologist to assure himself that the collaborating physician provides suitable safeguards for the client.

Principle 8. Client Relationship.   The psychologist informs his prospective client of the important aspects of the potential relationship that might affect the client's decision to enter the relationship.

a. Aspects of the relationship likely to affect the client's decision include the recording of an interview, the use of interview material for training purposes, and observation of an interview by other persons.

b. When the client is not competent to evaluate the situation (as in the case of a child), the person responsible for the client is informed of the circumstances which may influence the relationship.

c. The psychologist does not normally enter into a professional relationship with members of his own family, intimate friends, close associates, or others whose welfare might be jeopardized by such a dual relationship.

Principle 9. Impersonal Services.   Psychological services for the purpose of diagnosis, treatment, or personalized advice are provided only in the context of a professional relationship, and are not given by means of public lectures or demonstrations, newspaper or magazine articles, radio or television programs, mail, or similar media.

•   •   •

Principle 10. Announcement of Services.   A psychologist adheres to professional rather than commercial standards in making known his availability for professional services.

•   •   •

Principle 11. Interprofessional Relations.   A psychologist acts with integrity in regard to colleagues in psychology and in other professions.

•   •   •

Principle 12. Remuneration.   Financial arrangements in professional practice are in accord with professional standards that safeguard the best interest of the client and the profession.

•   •   •

Principle 13. Test Security.   Psychological tests and other assessment devices, the value of which depends in part on the naivete of the subject, are not reproduced or described in popular publications in ways that might invalidate the techniques. Access to such devices is limited to persons with professional interests who will safeguard their use.

•   •   •

Principle 14. Test Interpretation.   Test scores, like test materials, are released only to persons who are qualified to interpret and use them properly.

•   •   •

Principle 15. Test Publication.   Psychological tests are offered for commercial publication only to publishers who present their tests in a professional way and distribute them only to qualified users.

• • •

Principle 16. Research Precautions.   The psychologist assumes obligations for the welfare of his research subjects, both animal and human.

The decision to undertake research should rest upon a considered judgment by the individual psychologist about how best to contribute to psychological science and to human welfare. The responsible psychologist weighs alternative directions in which personal energies and resources might be invested. Having made the decision to conduct research, psychologists must carry out their investigations with respect for the people who participate and with concern for their dignity and welfare. The Principles that follow make explicit the investigator's ethical responsibilities toward participants over the course of research, from the initial decision to pursue a study to the steps necessary to protect the confidentiality of research data. These Principles should be interpreted in terms of the contexts provided in the complete document offered as a supplement to these Principles.

a. In planning a study the investigator has the personal responsibility to make a careful evaluation of its ethical acceptability, taking into account these Principles for research with human beings. To the extent that this appraisal, weighing scientific and humane values, suggests a deviation from any Principle, the investigator incurs an increasingly serious obligation to seek ethical advice and to observe more stringent safeguards to protect the rights of the human research participants.

b. Responsibility for the establishment and maintenance of acceptable ethical practice in research always remains with the individual investigator. The investigator is also responsible for the ethical treatment of research participants by collaborators, assistants, students, and employees, all of whom, however, incur parallel obligations.

c. Ethical practice requires the investigator to inform the participant of all features of the research that reasonably might be expected to influence willingness to participate, and to explain all other aspects of the research about which the participant inquires. Failure to make full disclosure gives added emphasis to the investigator's abiding responsibility to protect the welfare and dignity of the research participant.

d. Openness and honesty are essential characteristics of the relationship between investigator and research participant. When the methodological requirements of a study necessitate concealment or deception, the investigator is required to ensure the participant's understanding of the reasons for this action and to restore the quality of the relationship with the investigator.

e. Ethical research practice requires the investigator to respect the individual's freedom to decline to participate in research or to discontinue participation at any time. The obligation to protect this freedom requires special vigilance when the investigator is in a position of power over the participant. The decision to limit this freedom gives added emphasis to the investigator's abiding responsibility to protect the participant's dignity and welfare.

f. Ethically acceptable research begins with the establishment of a clear and fair agreement between the investigator and the research participant that clarifies the responsibilities of each. The investigator has the obligation to honor all promises and commitments included in that agreement.

g. The ethical investigator protects participants from physical and mental discomfort, harm and danger. If the risk of such consequence exists, the investigator is required to inform the participant of that fact, secure consent before proceeding, and take all possible measures to minimize distress. A research procedure may not be used if it is likely to cause serious and lasting harm to participants.

h. After the data are collected, ethical practice requires the investigator to provide the participant with a full clarification of the nature of the study and to remove any misconceptions that may have arisen. Where scientific or humane values justify delaying or withholding information, the investigator acquires a special responsibility to assure that there are no damaging consequences for the participant.

i. Where research procedures may result in undesirable consequences for the participant, the investigator has the responsibility to detect and remove or correct these consequences, including, where relevant, long-term aftereffects.

j. Information obtained about the research participants during the course of an investigation is confidential. When the possibility exists that others may obtain access to such information, ethical research practice requires that this possibility, together with the plans for protecting confidentiality, be explained to the participants as a part of the procedure for obtaining informed consent.

k. A psychologist using animals in research adheres to the provisions of the Rules Regarding Animals, drawn up by the Committee on Precautions and Standards in Animal Experimentation and adopted by the American Psychological Association.

l. Investigations of human subjects using experimental drugs (for example: hallucinogenic, psychotomimetic, psychedelic, or similar substances) should be conducted only in such settings as clinics, hospitals, or research facilities maintaining appropriate safeguards for the subjects.

Principle 17. Publication Credit.   Credit is assigned to those who have contributed to a publication, in proportion to their contribution, and only to these.

• • •

Principle 18. Responsibility toward Organization.   A psychologist respects the rights and reputation of the institute or organization with which he is associated.

• • •

Principle 19. Promotional Activities. The psychologist associated with the development or promotion of psychological devices, books, or other products offered for commercial sale is responsible for ensuring that such devices, books, or products are presented in a professional and factual way.

• • •

[Reprinted and edited from the *American Psychologist*, January 1963, and as amended by the APA Council of Representatives in September 1965 and December 1972. Copyrighted by the APA, January 1963. Reprinted with permission of the APA.]

Alphabetical List of Articles

A

ABORTION
    I. Medical Aspects   *André E. Hellegers*
    II. Jewish Perspectives   *David M. Feldman*
    III. Roman Catholic Perspectives
        John R. Connery
    IV. Protestant Perspectives   *James B. Nelson*
    V. Contemporary Debate in Philosophical and Religious Ethics   *Charles E. Curran*
    VI. Legal Aspects   *J. M. Finnis*

ACTING AND REFRAINING   *Harold F. Moore*

ADOLESCENTS   *Daniel Offer and Judith B. Offer*

ADVERTISING BY MEDICAL PROFESSIONALS
    Clark C. Havighurst

AGING AND THE AGED
    I. Theories of Aging and Anti-aging Techniques
        Leonard Hayflick
    II. Social Implications of Aging
        Bernice L. Neugarten
    III. Ethical Implications in Aging
        Drew Christiansen
    IV. Health Care and Research in the Aged
        Ernlé W. D. Young

ALCOHOL, USE OF   *Mark Keller*

ANIMAL EXPERIMENTATION
    I. Historical Aspects   *Richard D. French*
    II. Philosophical Perspectives   *Peter Singer*

B

BEHAVIOR CONTROL
    I. Ethical Analysis   *Robert Neville*
    II. Freedom and Behavior Control   *Joel Feinberg*

BEHAVIORAL THERAPIES
    Kenneth E. Lloyd and Margaret E. Lloyd

BEHAVIORISM
    I. History of Behavioral Psychology
        Juris G. Draguns
    II. Philosophical Analysis   *Alasdair MacIntyre*

BIOETHICS   *K. Danner Clouser*

BIOLOGY, PHILOSOPHY OF   *Irwin Savodnik*

BLOOD TRANSFUSION   *Michael J. Garland*

BUDDHISM   *Hajime Nakamura*

C

CADAVERS
    I. General Ethical Concerns   *Christian A. Hovde*
    II. Jewish Perspectives   *Walter S. Wurzburger*

CARE   *Stanley Hauerwas*

CHILDREN AND BIOMEDICINE   *Norman C. Fost*

CHRONIC CARE
    Anselm Strauss and Elihu M. Gerson

CIVIL DISOBEDIENCE IN HEALTH SERVICES
    Edward H. Madden and Peter H. Hare

CODES OF MEDICAL ETHICS
  I. History   *Donald Konold*
  II. Ethical Analysis   *Robert M. Veatch*

COMMUNICATION, BIOMEDICAL
  I. Media and Medicine
       Lois DeBakey and Selma DeBakey
  II. Scientific Publishing   *Lois DeBakey*

CONFIDENTIALITY   *William J. Winslade*

CONFUCIANISM   *Paul U. Unschuld*

CONTRACEPTION   *John T. Noonan, Jr.*

CRYONICS   *J. A. Panuska*

D

DEATH
  I. Anthropological Perspective   *David Landy*
  II. Eastern Thought   *Frank E. Reynolds*
  III. Western Philosophical Thought
      James Gutmann
  IV. Western Religious Thought
    1. DEATH IN BIBLICAL THOUGHT *Lloyd Bailey*
    2. POST-BIBLICAL JEWISH TRADITION
      Seymour Siegel
    3. POST-BIBLICAL CHRISTIAN THOUGHT
      Milton McC. Gatch
    4. ARS MORIENDI *Brian P. Copenhaver*
  V. Death in the Western World *Talcott Parsons*

DEATH AND DYING: EUTHANASIA AND
  SUSTAINING LIFE
  I. Historical Perspectives *Gerald J. Gruman*
  II. Ethical Views *Sissela Bok*
  III. Professional and Public Policies
    Robert M. Veatch

DEATH, ATTITUDES TOWARD *Richard A. Kalish*

DEATH, DEFINITION AND DETERMINATION OF
  I. Criteria for Death *Gaetano F. Molinari*
  II. Legal Aspects of Pronouncing Death
    Alexander Morgan Capron
  III. Philosophical and Theological Foundations
    Dallas M. High

DECISION MAKING, MEDICAL *Edmond A. Murphy*

DENTISTRY
  I. Ethical Issues in Dentistry
    Clifton O. Dummett
  II. Professional Codes in American Dentistry
    Chester R. Burns

DOUBLE EFFECT *William E. May*

DRUG INDUSTRY AND MEDICINE
    Harris L. Coulter

DRUG USE
  I. Drug Use, Abuse, and Dependence
    Robert Neville
  II. Drug Use for Pleasure and Transcendent
  Experience *Sidney Cohen*

DYNAMIC THERAPIES *Thomas H. Morawetz*

E

EASTERN ORTHODOX CHRISTIANITY
    Stanley S. Harakas

ELECTRICAL STIMULATION OF THE BRAIN
    Joel Meister

ELECTROCONVULSIVE THERAPY
    Richard M. Restak

EMBODIMENT *Richard M. Zaner*

ENVIRONMENT AND MAN
  I. Western Thought *Ian G. Barbour*
  II. Eastern Thought *Hajime Nakamura*

ENVIRONMENTAL ETHICS
  I. Environmental Health and Human Disease
    Samuel S. Epstein
  II. Questions of Social Justice
    Norman J. Faramelli and Charles W. Powers
  III. The Problem of Growth
    Drew Christiansen and C. P. Wolf

ETHICS
  I. The Task of Ethics *John Ladd*
  II. Rules and Principles *Wm. David Solomon*
  III. Deontological Theories *Kurt Baier*
  IV. Teleological Theories *Kurt Baier*
  V. Situation Ethics *Joseph Fletcher*
  VI. Utilitarianism *R. M. Hare*
  VII. Theological Ethics *Frederick S. Carney*
  VIII. Objectivism in Ethics *Bernard Gert*
  IX. Naturalism *Carl Wellman*
  X. Non-Descriptivism *R. M. Hare*

XI. Moral Reasoning   *Philippa Foot*
XII. Relativism   *Carl Wellman*

EUGENICS
   I. History   *Kenneth M. Ludmerer*
  II. Ethical Issues   *Marc Lappé*

EUGENICS AND RELIGIOUS LAW
   I. Jewish Religious Laws   *David M. Feldman*
  II. Christian Religious Laws *William W. Bassett*

EUPHENICS   *Lee Ehrman and James J. Nagle*

EVOLUTION   *Antony G. N. Flew*

F

FETAL–MATERNAL RELATIONSHIP
                 Maurice J. Mahoney

FETAL RESEARCH   *André E. Hellegers*

FOOD POLICY   *Peter J. Henriot*

FREE WILL AND DETERMINISM   *Edmund L. Erde*

FUTURE GENERATIONS, OBLIGATIONS TO
                 Martin P. Golding

G

GENE THERAPY
   I. Enzyme Replacement   *Elizabeth F. Neufeld*
  II. Gene Therapy via Transformation
                Richard O. Roblin
  III. Gene Therapy via Transduction
                Richard O. Roblin
  IV. Cell Fusion and Hybridization   *George Poste*
  V. Production of Four-Parent Individuals
                Beatrice Mintz
  VI. Ethical Issues   *Roger L. Shinn*

GENETIC ASPECTS OF HUMAN BEHAVIOR
   I. State of the Art   *Irving I. Gottesman*
  II. Males with Sex Chromosome Abnormalities
    (XYY and XXY Genotypes)   *Ernest B. Hook*
  III. Race Differences in Intelligence
                John C. Loehlin
  IV. Genetics and Mental Disorders
               Irving I. Gottesman
  V. Philosophical and Ethical Issues
                Arthur L. Caplan

GENETIC CONSTITUTION AND ENVIRONMENTAL
  CONDITIONING   *René Dubos*

GENETIC DIAGNOSIS AND COUNSELING
   I. Genetic Diagnosis   *Robert F. Murray, Jr.*
  II. Genetic Counseling *Robert F. Murray, Jr.*

GENETIC SCREENING   *Tabitha M. Powledge*

GENETICS AND THE LAW   *Margery W. Shaw*

H

HEALTH AND DISEASE
   I. History of the Concepts   *Guenter B. Risse*
  II. Religious Concepts   *Frank De Graeve*
  III. A Sociological and Action Perspective
                Talcott Parsons
  IV. Philosophical Perspectives
        H. Tristram Engelhardt, Jr.

HEALTH AS AN OBLIGATION   *Samuel Gorovitz*

HEALTH CARE
   I. Health-Care System
        Philip R. Lee and Carol Emmott
  II. Humanization and Dehumanization of Health
    Care   *Jan Howard*
  III. Right to Health-Care Services
                Albert R. Jonsen
  IV. Theories of Justice and Health Care
                Roy Branson

HEALTH INSURANCE   *Stefan A. Riesenfeld*

HEALTH, INTERNATIONAL
    James R. Missett and Carl E. Taylor

HEALTH POLICY
   I. Evolution of Health Policy
            Stephen P. Strickland
  II. Health Policy in International Perspective
             Odin W. Anderson

HEART TRANSPLANTATION   *Harmon L. Smith*

HINDUISM   *A. L. Basham*

HOMOSEXUALITY
   I. Clinical and Behavioral Aspects *D. L. Creson*
  II. Ethical Aspects
    George A. Kanoti and Anthony R. Kosnik

HOSPITALS   *Kenneth J. Williams*

HUMAN EXPERIMENTATION
    I. History   *Gert H. Brieger*
    II. Basic Issues   *Alexander Morgan Capron*
    III. Philosophical Aspects   *Charles Fried*
    IV. Social and Professional Control
                         Mark S. Frankel

HYPNOSIS   *A. G. Hammer*

I

INFANTS
    I. Medical Aspects and Ethical Dilemmas
        John Michael Hemphill and John M. Freeman
    II. Ethical Perspectives on the Care of Infants
              Warren T. Reich and David E. Ost
    III. Public Policy and Procedural Questions
              Warren T. Reich and David E. Ost
    IV. Infanticide: A Philosophical Perspective
                    Michael Tooley

INFORMED CONSENT IN HUMAN RESEARCH
    I. Social Aspects   *Bradford H. Gray*
    II. Ethical and Legal Aspects
         Karen Lebacqz and Robert J. Levine

INFORMED CONSENT IN MENTAL HEALTH
                  Robert A. Burt

INFORMED CONSENT IN THE THERAPEUTIC
RELATIONSHIP
    I. Clinical Aspects   *Eric J. Cassell*
    II. Legal and Ethical Aspects   *Jay Katz*

INSTITUTIONALIZATION   *David B. Wexler*

ISLAM   *J. C. Bürgel*

J

JUDAISM   *Immanuel Jakobovits*

JUSTICE   *Joel Feinberg*

K

KIDNEY DIALYSIS AND TRANSPLANTATION
    Renée C. Fox and Judith P. Swazey

L

LAW AND MORALITY   *Baruch A. Brody*

LIFE
    I. Value of Life   *Peter Singer*
    II. Quality of Life   *Warren T. Reich*

LIFE-SUPPORT SYSTEMS
    Albert R. Jonsen and George Lister

M

MAN, IMAGES OF   *Julian N. Hartt*

MASS HEALTH SCREENING
    James R. Missett and Carl E. Taylor

MEDICAL EDUCATION   *Edmund D. Pellegrino*

MEDICAL ETHICS EDUCATION   *Robert M. Veatch*

MEDICAL ETHICS, HISTORY OF
    I. Primitive Societies   *Lucile F. Newman*
    II. Near and Middle East and Africa
        1. ANCIENT NEAR EAST *Darrel W. Amundsen*
        2. PERSIA   *Rahmatollah Eshraghi*
        3. CONTEMPORARY ARAB WORLD
                         Samuel P. Asper
                and Fuad Sami Haddad
        4. CONTEMPORARY MUSLIM PERSPECTIVE
                Muhammad Abdul-Rauf
        5. CONTEMPORARY ISRAEL   *Seymour Siegel*
        6. SUB-SAHARAN AFRICA   *Frederick T. Sai*
    III. South and East Asia
        1. GENERAL HISTORICAL SURVEY
                         Paul U. Unschuld
        2. INDIA   *O. P. Jaggi*
        3. PREREPUBLICAN CHINA *Paul U. Unschuld*
        4. CONTEMPORARY CHINA
             John J. Kao and Frederick F. Kao
        5. JAPAN THROUGH THE NINETEENTH
           CENTURY   *Joseph M. Kitagawa*
        6. TRADITIONAL PROFESSIONAL ETHICS IN
           JAPANESE MEDICINE   *Taro Takemi*
        7. CONTEMPORARY JAPAN: MEDICAL ETHICS
           AND LEGAL MEDICINE *Rikuo Ninomiya*
    IV. Europe and the Americas
        A. ANCIENT AND MEDIEVAL PERIODS
           1. ANCIENT GREECE AND ROME
                    Darrel W. Amundsen
           2. MEDIEVAL EUROPE: FOURTH TO
             SIXTEENTH CENTURY
                    Darrel W. Amundsen

B. Modern Period: Seventeenth to Nineteenth Century
1. introduction to the modern period in europe and the americas
Laurence B. McCullough
2. western europe in the seventeenth century Albert R. Jonsen
3. britain and the united states in the eighteenth century
Laurence B. McCullough
4. north america: seventeenth to nineteenth century
Chester R. Burns
5. central europe in the nineteenth century Guenter B. Risse
6. france in the nineteenth century Dora B. Weiner
7. britain in the nineteenth century M. Jeanne Peterson
C. Contemporary Period: The Twentieth Century
1. introduction to the contemporary period in europe and the americas
Laurence B. McCullough
2. eastern europe in the twentieth century Benjamin B. Page
3. western europe in the twentieth century Clarence Blomquist
4. britain in the twentieth century Gordon Wolstenholme
5. north america in the twentieth century
Albert R. Jonsen, Andrew L. Jameton, and Abbyann Lynch
6. latin america in the twentieth century Augusto Léon C.

Medical Ethics in Literature
Joanne Trautmann

Medical Ethics Under National Socialism F. C. Redlich

Medical Malpractice
George H. Hauck and David W. Louisell

Medical Profession
I. Medical Professionalism Martin S. Pernick
II. Organized Medicine James G. Burrow

Medical Social Work Kathryn K. Himmelsbach

Medicine, Anthropology of
Dorothea C. Leighton

Medicine, Philosophy of
H. Tristram Engelhardt, Jr. and Edmund L. Erde

Medicine, Sociology of David Mechanic

Mental Health
I. Mental Health in Competition with Other Values Alan Gettner
II. Religion and Mental Health
William J. Richardson

Mental Health Services
I. Social Institutions of Mental Health
Eugene B. Brody
II. Evaluation of Mental Health Programs
David Franklyn Allen

Mental Health Therapies
William M. Sullivan

Mental Illness
I. Conceptions of Mental Illness Robert Baker
II. Diagnosis of Mental Illness Robert Michels
III. Labeling in Mental Illness: Legal Aspects
Nicholas N. Kittrie

Mentally Handicapped Robert E. Cooke

Mind–Body Problem Sydney Shoemaker

Miracle and Faith Healing
I. Conceptual and Historical Perspectives
Harold Y. Vanderpool
II. Theological Perspective Helmut Thielicke

N

Natural Law Eric D'Arcy

Nursing Teresa Stanley

O

Obligation and Supererogation
Thomas J. Bole, III and Millard Schumaker

Organ Donation
I. Ethical Issues Andrew L. Jameton
II. Legal Aspects Jesse Dukeminier

Organ Transplantation
I. Medical Perspective
Richard J. Howard and John S. Najarian
II. Sociocultural Aspects Renée C. Fox
III. Ethical Principles Richard A. McCormick

Orthodoxy in Medicine Martin Kaufman

P

PAIN AND SUFFERING
   I. Psychobiological Principles
                     Daniel N. Robinson
  II. Philosophical Perspectives *Jerome A. Shaffer*
 III. Religious Perspectives   *John W. Bowker*

PASTORAL MINISTRY   *David C. Duncombe*

PATERNALISM   *Tom L. Beauchamp*

PATIENTS' RIGHTS MOVEMENT *George J. Annas*

PERSON   *A. G. M. van Melsen*

PHARMACY   *David L. Cowen*

POPULATION ETHICS: ELEMENTS OF THE
   FIELD
   I. Definition of Population Ethics
                     Arthur J. Dyck
  II. The Population Problem in Demographic
     Perspective   *Michael S. Teitelbaum*
 III. History of Population Theories
                    William Petersen
  IV. History of Population Policies
                  Joseph J. Spengler
  V. Ethical Perspectives on Population
                    Peter G. Brown
  VI. Normative Aspects of Population Policy
                    Ralph B. Potter

POPULATION ETHICS: RELIGIOUS TRADITIONS
   I. Jewish Perspectives   *J. David Bleich*
  II. Eastern Orthodox Christian Perspectives
                    Stanley S. Harakas
 III. Roman Catholic Perspectives *J. Bryan Hehir*
  IV. Protestant Perspectives   *Wilson Yates*
  V. Islamic Perspectives   *Basim F. Musallam*
  VI. A Hindu Perspective   *K. L. Seshagiri Rao*

POPULATION POLICY PROPOSALS
   I. Contemporary International Issues
                    Donald P. Warwick
  II. Differential Growth Rate and Population
     Policies
      1. DEMOGRAPHIC PERSPECTIVES
                    William Petersen
      2. ETHICAL ANALYSIS *Richard K. Sherlock*
 III. Governmental Incentives *Robert M. Veatch*
  IV. Social Change Proposals *Donald P. Warwick*
  V. Compulsory Population Control Programs
                    Wilson Yates
  VI. Population Distribution
     Martin P. Golding and Michael D. Bayles
 VII. Genetic Implications of Population Control
                    Carl Jay Bajema

VIII. Population Education *Stephen Viederman*

POVERTY AND HEALTH
   I. Poverty and Health in the United States
     Carter L. Marshall and Carol Paul Marshall
  II. Poverty and Health in International
     Perspective   *John H. Bryant*

PRAGMATISM   *Irwin C. Lieb*

PRENATAL DIAGNOSIS
   I. Clinical Aspects   *Aubrey Milunsky*
  II. Ethical Issues   *John C. Fletcher*

PRISONERS
   I. Medical Care of Prisoners *Leonard A. Sagan*
  II. Prisoner Experimentation *Roy Branson*
 III. Torture and the Health Professional
                    Leonard A. Sagan

PRIVACY   *Kent Greenawalt*

PROTESTANTISM
   I. History of Protestant Medical Ethics
                    James T. Johnson
  II. Dominant Health Concerns in Protestantism
                    Harold Y. Vanderpool

PSYCHOPHARMACOLOGY
     Gerald L. Klerman and Judith E. Izen

PSYCHOSURGERY   *Robert Neville*

PUBLIC HEALTH   *Harold Fruchtbaum*

PURPOSE IN THE UNIVERSE *Patrick A. Heelan*

R

RACISM
   I. Racism and Medicine   *James H. Jones*
  II. Racism and Mental Health *Aaron D. Gresson*

RATIONING OF MEDICAL TREATMENT
     James F. Childress

REDUCTIONISM
   I. Philosophical Analysis   *Ned Block*
  II. Ethical Implications of Psychophysical
     Reductionism   *Ruth Macklin*

RELIGIOUS DIRECTIVES IN MEDICAL ETHICS
   I. Jewish Codes and Guidelines
     Isaac N. Trainin and Fred Rosner
  II. Roman Catholic Directives *Bernard Häring*
 III. Protestant Statements *Thomas Sieger Derr*

REPRODUCTIVE TECHNOLOGIES
   I. Sex Selection   *Gale Largey*
  II. Artificial Insemination   *Mark S. Frankel*
 III. Sperm and Zygote Banking   *Mark S. Frankel*
 IV. In Vitro Fertilization   *Luigi Mastroianni, Jr.*
  V. Asexual Human Reproduction
        Robert L. Sinsheimer
 VI. Ethical Issues   *Richard A. McCormick*
VII. Legal Aspects   *John A. Robertson*

RESEARCH, BEHAVIORAL   *Herbert C. Kelman*

RESEARCH, BIOMEDICAL   *Robert J. Levine*

RESEARCH POLICY, BIOMEDICAL
        Charles R. McCarthy

RIGHT TO REFUSE MEDICAL CARE
        Alexander Morgan Capron

RIGHTS
   I. Systematic Analysis   *Joel Feinberg*
  II. Rights in Bioethics   *Ruth Macklin*

RISK   *James F. Childress*

ROMAN CATHOLICISM   *Charles E. Curran*

S

SCIENCE: ETHICAL IMPLICATIONS
        Abraham Edel

SCIENCE, SOCIOLOGY OF   *Jonathan R. Cole*

SELF-REALIZATION THERAPIES   *Kurt W. Back*

SEX THERAPY AND SEX RESEARCH
   I. Scientific and Clinical Perspectives
     Sallie Schumacher and Charles W. Lloyd
  II. Ethical Perspectives   *Ruth Macklin*

SEXUAL BEHAVIOR   *Perry London*

SEXUAL DEVELOPMENT   *Marcia Cavell Aufhauser*

SEXUAL ETHICS   *Margaret A. Farley*

SEXUAL IDENTITY
   Robert C. Solomon and Judith Rose Sanders

SMOKING   *Leonard J. Weber*

SOCIAL MEDICINE   *George A. Silver*

SOCIALITY   *Michael Gordy*

STERILIZATION
   I. Medical Aspects   *Louis M. Hellman*
  II. Ethical Aspects   *Karen Lebacqz*
 III. Legal Aspects   *Jane M. Friedman*

SUICIDE   *David H. Smith and Seymour Perlin*

SURGERY   *Judith P. Swazey and Paul S. Russell*

T

TAOISM   *Norman J. Girardot*

TECHNOLOGY
   I. Philosophy of Technology   *Carl Mitcham and Jim Grote*
  II. Technology and the Law   *Laurence H. Tribe and Kenneth M. Casebeer*
 III. Technology Assessment   *LeRoy Walters*

THERAPEUTIC RELATIONSHIP
   I. History of the Relationship
        Pedro Laín Entralgo
  II. Sociohistorical Perspectives
        Samuel W. Bloom
 III. Contemporary Sociological Analysis
        David Mechanic
 IV. Contemporary Medical Perspective
        Eric J. Cassell

TRUTH-TELLING
   I. Attitudes   *Robert M. Veatch*
  II. Ethical Aspects   *Sissela Bok*

V

VIOLENCE AND THERAPY   *Robert Baker*

W

WARFARE
   I. Medicine and War   *E. A. Vastyan*
  II. Biomedical Science and War
        Victor W. Sidel and Mark Sidel

WOMEN AND BIOMEDICINE
   I. Women as Patients and Experimental
     Subjects   *Malkah T. Notman and Carol C. Nadelson*
  II. Women as Health Professionals
     Carol C. Nadelson and Malkah T. Notman

APPENDIX
Codes and Statements Related to Medical Ethics

INTRODUCTION
    Codes of the Health-Care Professions
        Ronald S. Gass

SECTION I. GENERAL CODES FOR THE
  PRACTICE OF MEDICINE
    Oath of Hippocrates
    Oath of Initiation (*Caraka Saṃhitā*)
    Oath of Asaph
    Advice to a Physician, Advice of Haly Abbas
      (Ahwazi)
    Five Commandments and Ten Requirements
    A Physician's Ethical Duties from *Kholasah Al*
      Hekmah
    Daily Prayer of a Physician ("Prayer of Moses
      Maimonides")
    Code of Ethics, American Medical Association
    Venezuelan Code of Medical Ethics
    Declaration of Geneva
    International Code of Medical Ethics
    Principles of Medical Ethics, with Reports and
      Statements, American Medical Association
    Oath of Soviet Physicians
    Ethical and Religious Directives for Catholic
      Health Facilities
    Medical Ethics: Statements of Policy Defini-
      tions and Rules, British Medical Association

SECTION II. DIRECTIVES FOR HUMAN
  EXPERIMENTATION
    Nuremberg Code
    Responsibility in Investigations on Human
      Subjects, Medical Research Council
    Experimental Research on Human Beings,
      British Medical Association
    Declaration of Helsinki
    Ethical Guidelines for Clinical Investigation,
      American Medical Association
    U.S. Guidelines on Human Experimentation

SECTION III. PATIENTS' BILLS OF RIGHTS
    A Patient's Bill of Rights
    Patients Rights: Regulations for Skilled Nurs-
      ing Facilities
    Declaration of General and Special Rights of
      the Mentally Retarded
    Pediatric Bill of Rights

SECTION IV. CODES OF SPECIALTY
  HEALTH-CARE ASSOCIATIONS
    International Council of Nurses
    American Nurses' Association
    American Chiropractic Association
    American Dental Association
    American Osteopathic Association
    American Pharmaceutical Association
    American Psychiatric Association
    American Psychological Association

Systematic Classification of Articles

The classified list of articles that follows was compiled by the editor in chief to provide readers with a topical classification of all articles in the encyclopedia. This systematic list, which appears in skeletal form in the Introduction to this encyclopedia, is intended to be helpful in developing courses, pursuing research, or simply browsing in a particular area of bioethics or of ethics generally.

The six categories listed below indicate several levels of articles—from those discussing the most concrete problems in bioethics to others dealing with the principles, concepts, and ethical methods involved in their analysis. Every article in this encyclopedia has been listed at least once, and many articles are listed in more than one category.

OUTLINE

I. Concrete Ethical and Legal Problems
   1. The Therapeutic Relationship
   2. Codes of Professional Ethics
   3. Health Care
   4. Sociopolitical Problems in Biomedicine
   5. Biomedical and Behavioral Research
   6. Mental Health and Behavioral Issues
   7. Sexuality, Contraception, Sterilization, and Abortion
   8. Genetics
   9. Reproductive Technologies
   10. Organ and Tissue Transplantation and Artificial Organs
   11. Death and Dying
   12. Population
   13. Environment
II. Basic Concepts and Principles
III. Ethical Theories
IV. Religious Traditions
V. Historical Perspectives
VI. Disciplines Bearing on Bioethics

I. CONCRETE ETHICAL AND LEGAL PROBLEMS

The following articles, arranged under thirteen topics, represent the scope of concrete ethical problems included in this encyclopedia. Legal articles that deal with these bioethical issues are included in this first section because of the close interaction between ethics and the law: The law is a public policy expression of a preferred ethical position, and in many instances the law supplies concepts and principles useful for analyzing ethical issues.

1. The Therapeutic Relationship

ADOLESCENTS
AGING AND THE AGED
    THEORIES OF AGING AND ANTI-AGING TECHNIQUES
    SOCIAL IMPLICATIONS OF AGING
    ETHICAL IMPLICATIONS IN AGING
    HEALTH CARE AND RESEARCH IN THE AGED
CHILDREN AND BIOMEDICINE
CHRONIC CARE
CONFIDENTIALITY
DECISION MAKING, MEDICAL
DENTISTRY
    ETHICAL ISSUES IN DENTISTRY
    PROFESSIONAL CODES IN AMERICAN DENTISTRY
FETAL–MATERNAL RELATIONSHIP
INFANTS
    MEDICAL ASPECTS AND ETHICAL DILEMMAS
    ETHICAL PERSPECTIVES ON THE CARE OF INFANTS
    PUBLIC POLICY AND PROCEDURAL QUESTIONS
    INFANTICIDE: A PHILOSOPHICAL PERSPECTIVE
INFORMED CONSENT IN MENTAL HEALTH
INFORMED CONSENT IN THE THERAPEUTIC RELATIONSHIP
    CLINICAL ASPECTS
    LEGAL AND ETHICAL ASPECTS
INSTITUTIONALIZATION
LIFE-SUPPORT SYSTEMS
MEDICAL EDUCATION
MEDICAL ETHICS EDUCATION
MEDICAL ETHICS IN LITERATURE
MEDICAL MALPRACTICE
MEDICAL PROFESSION
    MEDICAL PROFESSIONALISM
    ORGANIZED MEDICINE
MEDICAL SOCIAL WORK
MENTALLY HANDICAPPED
NURSING
ORTHODOXY IN MEDICINE
PASTORAL MINISTRY
PATIENTS' RIGHTS MOVEMENT
PHARMACY
POVERTY AND HEALTH
    POVERTY AND HEALTH IN THE UNITED STATES
    POVERTY AND HEALTH IN INTERNATIONAL PERSPECTIVE
PRISONERS
    MEDICAL CARE OF PRISONERS
PRIVACY
RIGHT TO REFUSE MEDICAL CARE
SURGERY

THERAPEUTIC RELATIONSHIP
  HISTORY OF THE RELATIONSHIP
  SOCIOHISTORICAL PERSPECTIVES
  CONTEMPORARY SOCIOLOGICAL ANALYSIS
  CONTEMPORARY MEDICAL PERSPECTIVE
TRUTH-TELLING
  ATTITUDES
  ETHICAL ASPECTS
VIOLENCE AND THERAPY
WOMEN AND BIOMEDICINE
  WOMEN AS PATIENTS AND EXPERIMENTAL SUBJECTS
  WOMEN AS HEALTH PROFESSIONALS
APPENDIX: CODES AND STATEMENTS RELATED TO MEDICAL ETHICS
  INTRODUCTION. CODES OF THE HEALTH-CARE PROFESSIONS
  SECTION I. GENERAL CODES FOR THE PRACTICE OF MEDICINE
  SECTION III. PATIENTS' BILLS OF RIGHTS
  SECTION IV. CODES OF SPECIALTY HEALTH-CARE ASSOCIATIONS

2. Codes of Professional Ethics

CODES OF MEDICAL ETHICS
  HISTORY
  ETHICAL ANALYSIS
DENTISTRY
  PROFESSIONAL CODES IN AMERICAN DENTISTRY
RELIGIOUS DIRECTIVES IN MEDICAL ETHICS
  JEWISH CODES AND GUIDELINES
  ROMAN CATHOLIC DIRECTIVES
  PROTESTANT STATEMENTS
APPENDIX: CODES AND STATEMENTS RELATED TO MEDICAL ETHICS
  INTRODUCTION. CODES OF THE HEALTH-CARE PROFESSIONS
  SECTION I. GENERAL CODES FOR THE PRACTICE OF MEDICINE
  SECTION II. DIRECTIVES FOR HUMAN EXPERIMENTATION
  SECTION III. PATIENTS' BILLS OF RIGHTS
  SECTION IV. CODES OF SPECIALTY HEALTH-CARE ASSOCIATIONS

3. Health Care

ADOLESCENTS
AGING AND THE AGED
  THEORIES OF AGING AND ANTI-AGING TECHNIQUES
  SOCIAL IMPLICATIONS OF AGING
  ETHICAL IMPLICATIONS IN AGING
  HEALTH CARE AND RESEARCH IN THE AGED
CHILDREN AND BIOMEDICINE
CHRONIC CARE
DRUG INDUSTRY AND MEDICINE
FETAL–MATERNAL RELATIONSHIP
HEALTH CARE
  HEALTH-CARE SYSTEM
  HUMANIZATION AND DEHUMANIZATION OF HEALTH CARE
  RIGHT TO HEALTH-CARE SERVICES
  THEORIES OF JUSTICE AND HEALTH CARE
HEALTH INSURANCE
HEALTH, INTERNATIONAL
HEALTH POLICY
  EVOLUTION OF HEALTH POLICY
  HEALTH POLICY IN INTERNATIONAL PERSPECTIVE
HOSPITALS

INFANTS
    MEDICAL ASPECTS AND ETHICAL DILEMMAS
    ETHICAL PERSPECTIVES ON THE CARE OF INFANTS
    PUBLIC POLICY AND PROCEDURAL QUESTIONS
    INFANTICIDE: A PHILOSOPHICAL PERSPECTIVE
INSTITUTIONALIZATION
LIFE-SUPPORT SYSTEMS
MASS HEALTH SCREENING
MENTALLY HANDICAPPED
PRISONERS
    MEDICAL CARE OF PRISONERS
PUBLIC HEALTH
RATIONING OF MEDICAL TREATMENT
SMOKING
SOCIAL MEDICINE
WOMAN AND BIOMEDICINE
    WOMEN AS PATIENTS AND EXPERIMENTAL SUBJECTS
    WOMEN AS HEALTH PROFESSIONALS

4. Sociopolitical Problems in Biomedicine

ADVERTISING BY MEDICAL PROFESSIONALS
AGING AND THE AGED
    THEORIES OF AGING AND ANTI-AGING TECHNIQUES
    SOCIAL IMPLICATIONS OF AGING
    ETHICAL IMPLICATIONS IN AGING
    HEALTH CARE AND RESEARCH IN THE AGED
CIVIL DISOBEDIENCE IN HEALTH SERVICES
COMMUNICATION, BIOMEDICAL
    MEDIA AND MEDICINE
DRUG INDUSTRY AND MEDICINE
ENVIRONMENT AND MAN
    WESTERN THOUGHT
    EASTERN THOUGHT
ENVIRONMENTAL ETHICS
    ENVIRONMENTAL HEALTH AND HUMAN DISEASE
    QUESTIONS OF SOCIAL JUSTICE
    THE PROBLEM OF GROWTH
GENETIC SCREENING
HEALTH, INTERNATIONAL
HEALTH POLICY
    EVOLUTION OF HEALTH POLICY
    HEALTH POLICY IN INTERNATIONAL PERSPECTIVE
INSTITUTIONALIZATION
MASS HEALTH SCREENING
MEDICAL EDUCATION
MEDICAL PROFESSION
    MEDICAL PROFESSIONALISM
    ORGANIZED MEDICINE
PRISONERS
    TORTURE AND THE HEALTH PROFESSIONAL
PUBLIC HEALTH
RACISM
    RACISM AND MEDICINE
    RACISM AND MENTAL HEALTH
SOCIAL MEDICINE
WARFARE
    MEDICINE AND WAR
    BIOMEDICAL SCIENCE AND WAR

5. Biomedical and Behavioral Research

ADOLESCENTS
AGING AND THE AGED
   HEALTH CARE AND RESEARCH IN THE AGED
ANIMAL EXPERIMENTATION
   HISTORICAL ASPECTS
   PHILOSOPHICAL PERSPECTIVES
CADAVERS
   GENERAL ETHICAL CONCERNS
   JEWISH PERSPECTIVES
CHILDREN AND BIOMEDICINE
COMMUNICATION, BIOMEDICAL
   SCIENTIFIC PUBLISHING
DRUG INDUSTRY AND MEDICINE
FETAL RESEARCH
HEALTH, INTERNATIONAL
HUMAN EXPERIMENTATION
   HISTORY
   BASIC ISSUES
   PHILOSOPHICAL ASPECTS
   SOCIAL AND PROFESSIONAL CONTROL
INFORMED CONSENT IN HUMAN RESEARCH
   SOCIAL ASPECTS
   ETHICAL AND LEGAL ASPECTS
MENTALLY HANDICAPPED
PRISONERS
   PRISONER EXPERIMENTATION
RESEARCH, BEHAVIORAL
RESEARCH, BIOMEDICAL
RESEARCH POLICY, BIOMEDICAL
WOMEN AND BIOMEDICINE
   WOMEN AS PATIENTS AND EXPERIMENTAL SUBJECTS
APPENDIX: CODES AND STATEMENTS RELATED TO MEDICAL ETHICS
   INTRODUCTION. CODES OF THE HEALTH-CARE PROFESSIONS
   SECTION II. DIRECTIVES FOR HUMAN EXPERIMENTATION

6. Mental Health and Behavioral Issues

ADOLESCENTS
ALCOHOL, USE OF
BEHAVIOR CONTROL
   ETHICAL ANALYSIS
   FREEDOM AND BEHAVIOR CONTROL
BEHAVIORAL THERAPIES
BEHAVIORISM
   HISTORY OF BEHAVIORAL PSYCHOLOGY
   PHILOSOPHICAL ANALYSIS
DRUG USE
   DRUG USE, ABUSE, AND DEPENDENCE
   DRUG USE FOR PLEASURE AND TRANSCENDENT EXPERIENCE
DYNAMIC THERAPIES
ELECTRICAL STIMULATION OF THE BRAIN
ELECTROCONVULSIVE THERAPY
GENETIC ASPECTS OF HUMAN BEHAVIOR
   STATE OF THE ART
   MALES WITH SEX CHROMOSOME ABNORMALITIES (XYY AND XXY
      GENOTYPES)
   RACE DIFFERENCES IN INTELLIGENCE
   GENETICS AND MENTAL DISORDERS
   PHILOSOPHICAL AND ETHICAL ISSUES

HOMOSEXUALITY
   CLINICAL AND BEHAVIORAL ASPECTS
   ETHICAL ASPECTS
HYPNOSIS
INFORMED CONSENT IN MENTAL HEALTH
INSTITUTIONALIZATION
MENTAL HEALTH
   MENTAL HEALTH IN COMPETITION WITH OTHER VALUES
   RELIGION AND MENTAL HEALTH
MENTAL HEALTH SERVICES
   SOCIAL INSTITUTIONS OF MENTAL HEALTH
   EVALUATION OF MENTAL HEALTH PROGRAMS
MENTAL HEALTH THERAPIES
MENTAL ILLNESS
   CONCEPTIONS OF MENTAL ILLNESS
   DIAGNOSIS OF MENTAL HEALTH
   LABELING IN MENTAL ILLNESS: LEGAL ASPECTS
MENTALLY HANDICAPPED
PSYCHOPHARMACOLOGY
PSYCHOSURGERY
RACISM
   RACISM AND MENTAL HEALTH
SELF-REALIZATION THERAPIES
SEX THERAPY AND SEX RESEARCH
   SCIENTIFIC AND CLINICAL PERSPECTIVES
   ETHICAL PERSPECTIVES
SEX BEHAVIOR
SEXUAL DEVELOPMENT
SEXUAL IDENTITY
VIOLENCE AND THERAPY

7. Sexuality, Contraception, Sterilization, and Abortion

ABORTION
   MEDICAL ASPECTS
   JEWISH PERSPECTIVES
   ROMAN CATHOLIC PERSPECTIVES
   PROTESTANT PERSPECTIVES
   CONTEMPORARY DEBATE IN PHILOSOPHICAL AND RELIGIOUS ETHICS
   LEGAL ASPECTS
ADOLESCENTS
CONTRACEPTION
HOMOSEXUALITY
   CLINICAL AND BEHAVIORAL ASPECTS
   ETHICAL ASPECTS
MENTALLY HANDICAPPED
POPULATION POLICY PROPOSALS
   DIFFERENTIAL GROWTH RATE AND POPULATION POLICIES
   GOVERNMENTAL INCENTIVES
   SOCIAL CHANGE PROPOSALS
   COMPULSORY POPULATION CONTROL PROGRAMS
   POPULATION EDUCATION
PRENATAL DIAGNOSIS
   CLINICAL ASPECTS
   ETHICAL ISSUES
REPRODUCTIVE TECHNOLOGIES
   SEX SELECTION
   ARTIFICIAL INSEMINATION
   SPERM AND ZYGOTE BANKING
   IN VITRO FERTILIZATION

ASEXUAL HUMAN REPRODUCTION
ETHICAL ISSUES
LEGAL ASPECTS
SEX THERAPY AND SEX RESEARCH
SCIENTIFIC AND CLINICAL PERSPECTIVES
ETHICAL PERSPECTIVES
SEXUAL BEHAVIOR
SEXUAL DEVELOPMENT
SEXUAL ETHICS
SEXUAL IDENTITY
STERILIZATION
MEDICAL ASPECTS
ETHICAL ASPECTS
LEGAL ASPECTS

8. Genetics

EUGENICS
HISTORY
ETHICAL ISSUES
EUGENICS AND RELIGIOUS LAW
JEWISH RELIGIOUS LAWS
CHRISTIAN RELIGIOUS LAWS
EUPHENICS
EVOLUTION
GENE THERAPY
ENZYME REPLACEMENT
GENE THERAPY VIA TRANSFORMATION
GENE THERAPY VIA TRANSDUCTION
CELL FUSION AND HYBRIDIZATION
PRODUCTION OF FOUR-PARENT INDIVIDUALS
ETHICAL ISSUES
GENETIC ASPECTS OF HUMAN BEHAVIOR
STATE OF THE ART
MALES WITH SEX CHROMOSOME ABNORMALITIES (XYY AND XXY
GENOTYPES)
RACE DIFFERENCES IN INTELLIGENCE
GENETICS AND MENTAL DISORDERS
PHILOSOPHICAL AND ETHICAL ISSUES
GENETIC CONSTITUTION AND ENVIRONMENTAL CONDITIONING
GENETIC DIAGNOSIS AND COUNSELING
GENETIC DIAGNOSIS
GENETIC COUNSELING
GENETIC SCREENING
GENETICS AND THE LAW
POPULATION POLICY PROPOSALS
GENETIC IMPLICATIONS OF POPULATION CONTROL
PRENATAL DIAGNOSIS
CLINICAL ASPECTS
ETHICAL ISSUES
STERILIZATION
ETHICAL ASPECTS
LEGAL ASPECTS

9. Reproductive Technologies

GENE THERAPY
CELL FUSION AND HYBRIDIZATION
REPRODUCTIVE TECHNOLOGIES
SEX SELECTION

ARTIFICIAL INSEMINATION
SPERM AND ZYGOTE BANKING
IN VITRO FERTILIZATION
ASEXUAL HUMAN REPRODUCTION
ETHICAL ISSUES
LEGAL ASPECTS

10. Organ and Tissue Transplantation and Artificial Organs

BLOOD TRANSFUSION
CRYONICS
HEALTH CARE
   THEORIES OF JUSTICE AND HEALTH CARE
KIDNEY DIALYSIS AND TRANSPLANTATION
LIFE-SUPPORT SYSTEMS
ORGAN DONATION
   ETHICAL ISSUES
   LEGAL ASPECTS
ORGAN TRANSPLANTATION
   MEDICAL PERSPECTIVE
   SOCIOCULTURAL ASPECTS
   ETHICAL PRINCIPLES
RATIONING OF MEDICAL TREATMENT

11. Death and Dying

CADAVERS
   GENERAL ETHICAL CONCERNS
   JEWISH PERSPECTIVES
CRYONICS
DEATH
   ANTHROPOLOGICAL PERSPECTIVE
   EASTERN THOUGHT
   WESTERN PHILOSOPHICAL THOUGHT
   WESTERN RELIGIOUS THOUGHT
   DEATH IN THE WESTERN WORLD
DEATH AND DYING: EUTHANASIA AND SUSTAINING LIFE
   HISTORICAL PERSPECTIVES
   ETHICAL VIEWS
   PROFESSIONAL AND PUBLIC POLICIES
DEATH, ATTITUDES TOWARD
DEATH, DEFINITION AND DETERMINATION OF
   CRITERIA FOR DEATH
   LEGAL ASPECTS OF PRONOUNCING DEATH
   PHILOSOPHICAL AND THEOLOGICAL FOUNDATIONS
INFANTS
   MEDICAL ASPECTS AND ETHICAL DILEMMAS
   ETHICAL PERSPECTIVES ON THE CARE OF INFANTS
   PUBLIC POLICY AND PROCEDURAL QUESTIONS
   INFANTICIDE: A PHILOSOPHICAL PERSPECTIVE
LIFE
   VALUE OF LIFE
   QUALITY OF LIFE
LIFE-SUPPORT SYSTEMS
ORGAN DONATION
   ETHICAL ISSUES
   LEGAL ASPECTS
RIGHT TO REFUSE MEDICAL CARE
SUICIDE

12. Population

FOOD POLICY
POPULATION ETHICS: ELEMENTS OF THE FIELD
    DEFINITION OF POPULATION ETHICS
    THE POPULATION PROBLEM IN DEMOGRAPHIC PERSPECTIVE
    HISTORY OF POPULATION THEORIES
    HISTORY OF POPULATION POLICIES
    ETHICAL PERSPECTIVES ON POPULATION
    NORMATIVE ASPECTS OF POPULATION POLICY
POPULATION ETHICS: RELIGIOUS TRADITIONS
    JEWISH PERSPECTIVES
    EASTERN ORTHODOX CHRISTIAN PERSPECTIVES
    ROMAN CATHOLIC PERSPECTIVES
    PROTESTANT PERSPECTIVES
    ISLAMIC PERSPECTIVES
    A HINDU PERSPECTIVE
POPULATION POLICY PROPOSALS
    CONTEMPORARY INTERNATIONAL ISSUES
    DIFFERENTIAL GROWTH RATE AND POPULATION POLICIES
        DEMOGRAPHIC PERSPECTIVES
        ETHICAL ANALYSIS
    GOVERNMENTAL INCENTIVES
    SOCIAL CHANGE PROPOSALS
    COMPULSORY POPULATION CONTROL PROGRAMS
    POPULATION DISTRIBUTION
    GENETIC IMPLICATIONS OF POPULATION CONTROL
    POPULATION EDUCATION

13. Environment

ENVIRONMENT AND MAN
    WESTERN THOUGHT
    EASTERN THOUGHT
ENVIRONMENTAL ETHICS
    ENVIRONMENTAL HEALTH AND HUMAN DISEASE
    QUESTIONS OF SOCIAL JUSTICE
    THE PROBLEM OF GROWTH
FOOD POLICY
GENETIC CONSTITUTION AND ENVIRONMENTAL CONDITIONING
PUBLIC HEALTH
SMOKING
SOCIAL MEDICINE

II. BASIC CONCEPTS AND PRINCIPLES

The following articles offer explanations of concepts that clarify debates in bioethics and principles that are used to support ethical viewpoints and policy preferences.

ACTING AND REFRAINING
BEHAVIOR CONTROL
    FREEDOM AND BEHAVIOR CONTROL
BEHAVIORISM
    HISTORY OF BEHAVIORAL PSYCHOLOGY
    PHILOSOPHICAL ANALYSIS
CARE
CONFIDENTIALITY

DEATH
    ANTHROPOLOGICAL PERSPECTIVE
    EASTERN THOUGHT
    WESTERN PHILOSOPHICAL THOUGHT
    WESTERN RELIGIOUS THOUGHT
    DEATH IN THE WESTERN WORLD
DOUBLE EFFECT
EMBODIMENT
ENVIRONMENT AND MAN
    WESTERN THOUGHT
    EASTERN THOUGHT
EVOLUTION
FREE WILL AND DETERMINISM
FUTURE GENERATIONS, OBLIGATIONS TO
HEALTH AND DISEASE
    HISTORY OF THE CONCEPTS
    RELIGIOUS CONCEPTS
    A SOCIOLOGICAL AND ACTION PERSPECTIVE
    PHILOSOPHICAL PERSPECTIVES
HEALTH AS AN OBLIGATION
JUSTICE
LAW AND MORALITY
LIFE
    VALUE OF LIFE
    QUALITY OF LIFE
MAN, IMAGES OF
MENTAL HEALTH
    MENTAL HEALTH IN COMPETITION WITH OTHER VALUES
    RELIGIOUS AND MENTAL HEALTH
MENTAL ILLNESS
    CONCEPTIONS OF MENTAL ILLNESS
    DIAGNOSIS OF MENTAL ILLNESS
    LABELING IN MENTAL ILLNESS: LEGAL ASPECTS
MIND–BODY PROBLEM
NATURAL LAW
OBLIGATION AND SUPEREROGATION
PAIN AND SUFFERING
    PSYCHOBIOLOGICAL PRINCIPLES
    PHILOSOPHICAL PERSPECTIVES
    RELIGIOUS PERSPECTIVES
PATERNALISM
PERSON
PRIVACY
PURPOSE IN THE UNIVERSE
REDUCTIONISM
    PHILOSOPHICAL ANALYSIS
    ETHICAL IMPLICATIONS OF PSYCHOPHYSICAL REDUCTIONISM
RIGHTS
    SYSTEMATIC ANALYSIS
    RIGHTS IN BIOETHICS
RISK
SCIENCE: ETHICAL IMPLICATIONS
SOCIALITY
TECHNOLOGY
    PHILOSOPHY OF TECHNOLOGY
    TECHNOLOGY AND THE LAW
    TECHNOLOGY ASSESSMENT
VIOLENCE AND THERAPY

III. ETHICAL THEORIES

Systematic methods of explaining moral knowledge, choices, and norms are explained in the following articles.

BIOETHICS
ETHICS
 THE TASK OF ETHICS
 RULES AND PRINCIPLES
 DEONTOLOGICAL THEORIES
 TELEOLOGICAL THEORIES
 SITUATION ETHICS
 UTILITARIANISM
 THEOLOGICAL ETHICS
 OBJECTIVISM IN ETHICS
 NATURALISM
 NON-DESCRIPTIVISM
 MORAL REASONING
 RELATIVISM
EVOLUTION
NATURAL LAW
PRAGMATISM

IV. RELIGIOUS TRADITIONS

Most of this encyclopedia's articles dealing with specific ethical problems and underlying concepts and principles are based on both moral philosophy and religious ethics. While the previous section (III) of this classification of articles dealt principally with theories of moral philosophy, the following articles deal with systems of thought and topics of interest to religious ethics.

BUDDHISM
CONFUCIANISM
DEATH
 EASTERN THOUGHT
 WESTERN RELIGIOUS THOUGHT
EASTERN ORTHODOX CHRISTIANITY
ETHICS
 THEOLOGICAL ETHICS
HEALTH AND DISEASE
 RELIGIOUS CONCEPTS
HINDUISM
ISLAM
JUDAISM
MENTAL HEALTH
 RELIGION AND MENTAL HEALTH
MIRACLE AND FAITH HEALING
 CONCEPTUAL AND HISTORICAL PERSPECTIVES
 THEOLOGICAL PERSPECTIVE
PAIN AND SUFFERING
 RELIGIOUS PERSPECTIVES
PASTORAL MINISTRY
POPULATION ETHICS: RELIGIOUS TRADITIONS
 JEWISH PERSPECTIVES
 EASTERN ORTHODOX CHRISTIAN PERSPECTIVES
 ROMAN CATHOLIC PERSPECTIVES

PROTESTANT PERSPECTIVES
ISLAMIC PERSPECTIVES
A HINDU PERSPECTIVE
PROTESTANTISM
HISTORY OF PROTESTANT MEDICAL ETHICS
DOMINANT HEALTH CONCERNS IN PROTESTANTISM
RELIGIOUS DIRECTIVES IN MEDICAL ETHICS
JEWISH CODES AND GUIDELINES
ROMAN CATHOLIC DIRECTIVES
PROTESTANT STATEMENTS
ROMAN CATHOLICISM
TAOISM

V. HISTORICAL PERSPECTIVES

The history of medical ethics is surveyed in one large entry containing twenty-nine separate articles. Other articles discuss the history of specific questions in bioethics. The articles on religious traditions listed in the previous section (IV) also constitute part of the history of bioethics.

EUGENICS
HISTORY
HUMAN EXPERIMENTATION
HISTORY
MEDICAL ETHICS, HISTORY OF
PRIMITIVE SOCIETIES
NEAR AND MIDDLE EAST AND AFRICA
ANCIENT NEAR EAST
PERSIA
CONTEMPORARY ARAB WORLD
CONTEMPORARY MUSLIM PERSPECTIVE
CONTEMPORARY ISRAEL
SUB-SAHARAN AFRICA
SOUTH AND EAST ASIA
GENERAL HISTORICAL SURVEY
INDIA
PREREPUBLICAN CHINA
CONTEMPORARY CHINA
JAPAN THROUGH THE NINETEENTH CENTURY
TRADITIONAL PROFESSIONAL ETHICS IN JAPANESE MEDICINE
CONTEMPORARY JAPAN: MEDICAL ETHICS AND LEGAL MEDICINE
EUROPE AND THE AMERICAS
ANCIENT AND MEDIEVAL PERIODS
ANCIENT GREECE AND ROME
MEDIEVAL EUROPE: FOURTH TO SIXTEENTH CENTURY
MODERN PERIOD: SEVENTEENTH TO NINETEENTH CENTURY
INTRODUCTION TO THE MODERN PERIOD IN EUROPE AND THE AMERICAS
WESTERN EUROPE IN THE SEVENTEENTH CENTURY
BRITAIN AND THE UNITED STATES IN THE EIGHTEENTH CENTURY
NORTH AMERICA: SEVENTEENTH TO NINETEENTH CENTURY
CENTRAL EUROPE IN THE NINETEENTH CENTURY
FRANCE IN THE NINETEENTH CENTURY
BRITAIN IN THE NINETEENTH CENTURY
CONTEMPORARY PERIOD: THE TWENTIETH CENTURY
INTRODUCTION TO THE CONTEMPORARY PERIOD IN EUROPE AND THE AMERICAS

EASTERN EUROPE IN THE TWENTIETH CENTURY
WESTERN EUROPE IN THE TWENTIETH CENTURY
BRITAIN IN THE TWENTIETH CENTURY
NORTH AMERICA IN THE TWENTIETH CENTURY
LATIN AMERICA IN THE TWENTIETH CENTURY
MEDICAL ETHICS UNDER NATIONAL SOCIALISM
MEDICAL PROFESSION
   MEDICAL PROFESSIONALISM
   ORGANIZED MEDICINE
SCIENCE: ETHICAL IMPLICATIONS
THERAPEUTIC RELATIONSHIP
   HISTORY OF THE RELATIONSHIP

VI. DISCIPLINES BEARING ON BIOETHICS

The contributions of several key disciplines to the interdisciplinary field of bioethics have been included in earlier sections of this systematic list of articles —the biological and medical sciences, moral philosophy, religious studies and theology, ethics, law, and the social sciences. The articles listed below offer an overview of additional disciplines, together with an explanation of their bearing on bioethics.

BIOLOGY, PHILOSOPHY OF
LAW AND MORALITY
MEDICAL ETHICS IN LITERATURE
MEDICINE, ANTHROPOLOGY OF
MEDICINE, PHILOSOPHY OF
MEDICINE, SOCIOLOGY OF
SCIENCE, SOCIOLOGY OF
TECHNOLOGY
   PHILOSOPHY OF TECHNOLOGY
   TECHNOLOGY ASSESSMENT

Additional Resources
in Bioethics

There are several important resources available to aid the reader in keeping abreast of the literature in bioethics. The bibliographical tools mentioned below provide excellent up-to-date control of English-language materials on bioethical topics and thereby supplement the bibliographies that follow each article in this encyclopedia. Educational services in the field of bioethics are also included below.

Because the field is growing so rapidly, resources are continually in flux. Some of the publications referred to are no longer in print, but they are included in this list because of their importance as resources in bioethics. The periodicals listed are considered essential to a good, general collection in bioethics. Publication information for each document or serial is given at the end of this section.

Bibliographies

The *Bibliography of Bioethics*, a unique series of annual volumes, is a comprehensive source of English-language materials that includes listings of journal articles, books, essays in books, legislation, audio-visual media, and court cases. The *Bibliography*, compiled at the Kennedy Institute of Ethics, Georgetown University, represents the first attempt to develop a standardized indexing terminology and to provide a comprehensive guide to materials in the field. Each volume contains a Subject Entry Section, a Title Index, and an Author Index. With publication of Volume 4 in the fall of 1978, the *Bibliography* has cited more than 5,500 documents issued from 1973 to 1977. Future volumes will contain approximately 1,500 citations each.

BIOETHICSLINE, one of the computerized literature retrieval services of the National Library of Medicine (NLM), provides on-line access to all the citations that appear in the *Bibliography of Bioethics*. BIOETHICSLINE is available in most U.S. medical libraries and in a growing number of university and special libraries that participate in the on-line NLM network; it is updated every four months.

The Center for Bioethics Library at the Kennedy Institute of Ethics, Georgetown University, distributes *New Titles in Bioethics*, a monthly listing of its current acquisitions. This is a classified compilation of acquired books, reports, hearings, special issues of journals, and audio-visuals. The Bioethics Library staff monitors bibliographical services, indexes, and automated data bases and seeks to obtain a copy of every new document published in the field. This tool is especially helpful to those who wish to order or recommend for purchase the latest monographs related to bioethics.

The *Bibliography of Society, Ethics and the Life Sciences* has been distributed each year since 1973 to subscribers of the *Hastings Center Report*. The *Bibliography* is a partially-annotated, highly selective source list and contains references to introductory works on the issues; background writings on technological developments; and articles by philosophers, theologians, legal scholars, scientists, etc. It is revised and updated annually; selected references from previous years are retained in subsequent editions.

A regular feature of the *Hastings Center Report* is titled "In the Literature"; this is an excellent source for learning about new books and articles in the field.

Bioethics Digest, published from May 1976 to May 1978, offered lengthy abstracts of selected documents in bioethics and occasionally included feature articles on subjects relevant to bioethics.

Periodicals

Bioethics has been fertile ground for the growth of new periodicals dedicated solely to value questions in biology and medicine. Perhaps the most widely circulated journal is the *Hastings Center Report*, a bimonthly report devoted entirely to discussions of bioethics. It is an essential source for keeping up-to-date with developments in the field. Publication began in 1971; from 1973 to 1974 there was a sister publication, the *Hastings Center Studies*.

Another significant journal in bioethics, the *Linacre Quarterly*, is published by the (U.S.) National Federation of Catholic Physicians' Guilds and began publication in 1936. Its 1977 circulation was approximately 9,000.

Other, newer periodicals and their initial dates of publication are: *Ethics in Science and Medicine* (formerly *Science, Medicine, and Man*), 1973; *Journal of Medical Ethics*, 1976; *The Journal of Medicine and Philosophy*, (sponsored by the Society for Health and Human Values, Philadelphia, Pa.), 1976; and *Man and Medicine*, 1975. These publications offer timely essays, book reviews, and announcements of conferences, workshops, teaching programs, and fellowships. Several newsletters, too numerous to list here, are channels of information for special-interest groups.

Due to the interdisciplinary nature of the field, readers may wish to consult the literature of several other disciplines for contemporary writings in bioethics. Some of the most prestigious British and American journals are: *British Medical Journal, Journal of the American Medical Association, The Lancet,* and *New England Journal of Medicine* for articles on medical ethics; *Nature, New Scientist, Perspectives in Biology and Medicine* and *Science* for contributions on science and ethics; *Ethics, Philosophy & Public Affairs,* and *Journal of Religious Ethics* for bioethical articles of special interest to the ethicist; and *American Journal of Law and Medicine* for essays dealing with legal aspects of bioethics. Readers interested in additional English-language periodicals may wish to refer to *Canadian Medical Association Journal, Nursing Mirror, Nursing Times,* and *South African Medical Journal;* and two publications that deal with health care from an international perspective: *International Digest of Health Legislation* and *World Medical Journal.*

Numerous journals in other languages have also published articles on bioethics. Among them are *Anime e corpi, Arzt und Christ, ASSIA, Cahiers*

Laënnec, Metamed: An International Journal for Metatheory and Methodology of Medicine, Res Medicae, Saint-Luc médical/Sint-Lucas tijdschrift, and *Zeitschrift für evangelische Ethik.*

Educational programs and services

Several key resources offer helpful information on academic programs in bioethics and related fields. The *EVIST Resource Directory: A Directory of Programs and Courses in the Field of Ethics and Values in Science and Technology* was published in 1978 by the American Association for the Advancement of Science. The Society for Health and Human Values publishes a series of reports listing and describing educational programs. In addition, the Institute of Society, Ethics and the Life Sciences offers assistance in designing courses and in obtaining materials for educational programs in bioethics. Reprints of many significant articles may be obtained through its Reading Packet series. Topics covered are: (1) Survey of Ethics and the Life Sciences, (2) Death and Dying, (3) Experimentation and Informed Consent, (4) Social Science Experimentation, (5) Client-Professional Relationship, (6) Genetics, (7) Behavior Control, (8) Health and Allocation of Scarce Resources, and (9) Introduction to Bioethics. The latter packet contains popularized news accounts of bioethical issues and is oriented particularly towards high school students.

The following are addresses for the documents, journals, and services discussed in this section.

American Journal of Law and Medicine
MIT Press
28 Carleton St.
Cambridge, Massachusetts 02142

Anime e corpi
Via Della Canonica
Varese, Italy

Arzt und Christ
Otto Müller Verlag
5021 Salzburg/Freilassing
Postfach 167
Austria

ASSIA: Original Articles, Abstracts and Reports on Matters of Halacha and Medicine
The Falk Schlesinger Institute for Medical Halachic Research
Shaare Zedek Hospital
Jerusalem
Israel

Bibliography of Bioethics
Gale Research Company
Book Tower
Detroit, Michigan 48226

Bibliography of Society, Ethics and the Life Sciences
The Institute of Society, Ethics and the Life Sciences
360 Broadway
Hastings-on-Hudson, NY 10706

Bioethics Digest
Information Planning Associates, Inc.
P. O. Box 1523
Rockville, Maryland 20850

BIOETHICSLINE
Office of Inquiries and Publications Management
National Library of Medicine
8600 Rockville Pike
Bethesda, Maryland 20014

British Medical Journal
Tavistock Square
London WC1H 9JR
England

Cahiers Laënnec
10 Rue Cassette
Paris, France

Canadian Medical Association Journal
Box 8650
Ottawa K1G 0G8
Canada

Ethics
University of Chicago Press
5801 Ellis Avenue
Chicago, Illinois 60637

Ethics in Science and Medicine
Maxwell House, Fairview Park
Elmsford, New York 10523

EVIST Resource Directory
Office of Science Education
American Association for the Advancement of Science
1776 Massachusetts Avenue, N.W.
Washington, D.C. 20036

Hastings Center Report
360 Broadway
Hastings-on-Hudson, New York 10706

International Digest of Health Legislation
World Health Organization
20 Avenue Appia
CH-1211 Geneva 27
Switzerland

Journal of Medical Ethics
B.M.A. House
London WC1H 9JR
England

Journal of Medicine and Philosophy
University of Chicago Press
5801 Ellis Avenue
Chicago, Illinois 60637

Journal of Religious Ethics
Department of Religious Studies
University of Tennessee
Knoxville, Tennessee 37916

Journal of the American Medical Association
535 North Dearborn St.
Chicago, Illinois 60610

Lancet
c/o Little, Brown and Co.
34 Beacon St.
Boston, Massachusetts 02106

Linacre Quarterly
850 Elm Grove Road
Elm Grove, Wisconsin 53122

Man and Medicine
Columbia University College of Physicians and Surgeons
630 West 168th Street
New York, New York 10032

Metamed: An International Journal for Metatheory and Methodology of Medicine
Burg-Verlag
Postfach 1247
D-4542 Tecklenburg
West Germany

Nature
Macmillan Journals Ltd.
Brunel Road
Basingstoke, Hants. RG21 2XS
England

New England Journal of Medicine
10 Shattuck St.
Boston, Massachusetts 02115

New Scientist
King's Reach Tower
Stamford Street
London SE1 9LS
England

New Titles in Bioethics
Center for Bioethics Library
Kennedy Institute of Ethics
Georgetown University
Washington, D.C. 20057

Nursing Mirror
IPC Business Press Ltd.
33-40 Bowling Green Lane
London EC1R ONE
England

Nursing Times
Macmillan Journals Ltd.
4 Little Essex St.
London WC2R 3LF
England

Perspectives in Biology and Medicine
University of Chicago Press
5801 Ellis Ave.
Chicago, Illinois 60637

Philosophy and Public Affairs
Princeton University Press
Princeton, New Jersey 08540

Res Medicae
Fatebenefratelli
Via S. Vittore 12
20213 Milan
Italy

Saint-Luc médical/Sint-Lucas tijdschrift
Société Médicale Belge de Saint-Luc
Av. de l'Yser, 19
1040 Brussels
Belgium

Science
American Association for the Advancement of Science
1515 Massachusetts Avenue, N.W.
Washington, D.C. 20005

Society for Health and Human Values
723 Witherspoon Building
Philadelphia, Pennsylvania 19107

South African Medical Journal
Medical Association of South Africa
Box 643
Cape Town
South Africa

World Medical Journal
World Medical Association, Inc.
10 Columbus Circle
New York, New York 10019

Zeitschrift für evangelische Ethik
Guetersloher Verlagshaus Gerd Mohn
Koenigstr. 23
Postfach 2368
4830 Guetersloh
West Germany

ACKNOWLEDGEMENTS BY CONTRIBUTORS

The following contributors wish to extend their thanks for the special assistance they received in the preparation of their articles:

Sissela Bok to Paul Yock, who helped prepare the section devoted to direct and indirect killing in DEATH AND DYING: EUTHANASIA AND SUSTAINING LIFE, *article on* ETHICAL VIEWS.

Aubrey Milunsky to the U.S. Public Health Service Grants 1-PO1-HD-05515, 1-RO1-HD09281-01, 1-T32-GM07015-01, and the Amniocentesis Registry Contract Number NO1-HD-12451, for research support in preparing PRENATAL DIAGNOSIS, *article on* CLINICAL ASPECTS.

Warren T. Reich to the McMath Lecture Foundation of the Episcopal Diocese of Michigan and to the Metropolitan Detroit Theological Foundation, Inc., for support in preparing three articles: INFANTS, *the articles on* ETHICAL PERSPECTIVES ON THE CARE OF INFANTS *and* PUBLIC POLICY AND PROCEDURAL QUESTIONS, and LIFE, *article on* QUALITY OF LIFE; and to Carol Tauer for serving as research assistant in preparing the article on QUALITY OF LIFE.

Margery W. Shaw to the Medical Genetics Center (University of Texas) grant GM 19513, for research support in preparing GENETICS AND THE LAW.

Index

A

Abandonment of patients, 620, 1021
Abbing, P. J. Roscam, 984
Abelard, Peter, 1579
Abortifacients, 206–207, 1213, 1267
Abortion, 1–32, 552, 975
  in Africa, 900
  in ancient Egypt, 882
  in ancient Greece, 933
  in ancient Rome, 933
  anthropological perspective, 225–226
  Aquinas on, 18, 24, 943
  in Assyria–Babylonia, 882
  Augustine on, 943
  birth defects and, 2, 7–8, 30, 31, 896, 910, 998, 1109
    See also Prenatal diagnosis: followed by abortion
  in Canada, 29, 998–999
  in China, 915, 918, 919
  codes of ethics and, 167, 168, 169, 175–176, 1726–1727
  consequentialism and, 833–834, 837
  contemporary debate in philosophical and religious ethics, 17–25
    beginning of human life, 17–22
    survey of, 24–25
    values and rights of fetus, 22–24

cost-benefit analysis and, 834
deontological theory and, 414–416
direct, 11, 12–13, 318, 1531
Eastern Orthodox Christianity and, 350, 354
in Europe:
  Eastern, 979, 980
  medieval, 943–944, 946
  seventeenth century, 956
  Western, 983
felonious intercourse and, 28
fetal research and, 141–142, 491, 492, 493
foreign assistance funds for, 1279–1280
in France, 31, 1229
genetic diagnoses and, 555, 556–557
in Germany, 28, 31, 985
in Great Britain, 27–30, 990
Hinduism and, 662, 1271–1272
images of man and, 854
incest and, 28
in India, 909, 910, 1271–1272
indirect, 3, 11, 13, 23, 1531
interventionism and, 1222
Islam and, 787, 894, 1267
in Japan, 29, 928–929
Judaism and, 795, 797, 801, 896
  beginning of human life and, 8
  controversy in, 25
  Talmud and, 5–8, 25
  Torah and, 5–6, 9–10
in Latin America, 1006

legal aspects, 4, 1334–1335, 1649
  basic models, 26–32
  common law, 27, 485
  Jewish law, 5–10, 25
  prenatal diagnosis and, 1334–1335
  Roman Catholic law, 10
  Supreme Court ruling, 16, 27, 30, 31, 169, 198, 573, 820, 998, 1335, 1358, 1465, 1513, 1514, 1615
legislation of morality and, 820
medical aspects, 1–5
  complications, 4–5
  definition, 2–3
  ethical considerations, 4
  medical context, 1–2
  procedures, 3–4
medical malpractice and, 1026–1027
medical police concept and, 958
medical social work and, 1043
mind–body problem and, 18, 1117–1118
natural law and, 1338, 1526
normative relativism and, 455
nursing and, 1142
parental consent and, 38, 41
paternalism and, 1198
in Persia, 882, 885
as population control measure, 2, 23, 176, 1228, 1229, 1233, 1234, 1299, 1301, 1302
potentiality and, 23, 747, 826

Abortion (*Continued*)
  prenatal diagnosis followed by, 467, 521, 522, 555, 556–557, 1334–1335
    arguments against, 1337–1339
    arguments for, 1339–1341
    legal aspects, 1334–1335
    moral aspects, 883–884, 1334, 1337–1343
    parent's fear of defect and, 837, 1342
    public policy and, 1344–1345
    quality of life and, 833–834
    for reasons of sex preference, 1342–1343
    risks in, 1335
    special problems in, 1343
    timing of, 1343
    viewed as infanticide, 1341–1342
  Protestantism and, 13–16
    beginning of human life and, 14–16, 1437
    church statements on, 1436–1437
    contemporary perspectives, 15–16, 24–25
    early perspectives, 13–14
    in eighteenth and nineteenth centuries, 14–15
    solution of conflict situations and, 24
  purpose in the universe and, 1404
  quality of life and, 833–834, 837
  rape and, 24, 28, 928, 929, 998
  reductionism and, 128, 1427
  on request, 15, 16
  responsibility for fetus and, 488
  rights and, 1513, 1514
  Roman Catholicism and, 9–13, 818, 1256, 1257, 1527, 1529
    beginning of human life and, 10–12, 19, 25, 1531
    contemporary perspectives, 25, 1533
    Directives on, 169, 175, 176, 1434, 1527
    early perspectives, 10-11
    intentionality and, 11
    in medieval Europe, 943–944, 946
    modern perspectives, 11–13, 1524
    natural law and, 1526
    principle of double effect, 3, 11, 16, 23–24, 25, 34, 318, 1529
    scriptural influence, 9–10
    solution of conflict situations and, 23–24
  selective, *See* Abortion: prenatal diagnosis followed by
  situation ethics and, 423
  in Soviet Union, 29
  spontaneous, 1450

  supererogation and, 1152
  in Sweden, 28, 31, 983
  Taoism and, 1636
  therapeutic, 3, 6, 12–13, 25, 167, 896, 943–944, 990, 1338
  tort liability and, 1335
  truth-telling and, 1198
  in United States, 27–32, 998, 1563
    See also Supreme Court rulings: on abortion
  See also Infanticide
Abortion Act of 1967 (Great Britain), 29, 990
Absolute duty, 405, 414–415
Absolute existence, 374–376
Absolute prohibition, 414
Absolute rights, 104–105
Absolutism, 415, 416, 421, 454
Abstracts, scientific, 183, 193–194
Accessory qualities, 834, 835
Access to behavior control technologies, 92
Access to data, 385–386
Access to medical school, 866–867
Access to reproductive technologies, 1464–1466
Achaemenid dynasty, 885
ACPE, *See* Association for Clinical Pastoral Education
Acquiremental theory, 435
Acting and refraining, 32–38
  killing and letting die, 35–38, 318, 728–729, 747
  principle of double effect, *See* Double effect, principle of
  See also Euthanasia; Omission and commission
Action:
  in pragmatism, 1327–1331
  purpose and, 1399–1400
Actional center, human body as, 362–363
Action theory, 592–593
Act-utilitarianism, 411, 416, 421–424, 426-428
  bioethical issues and, 423–424
  coalescence with rule-utilitarianism, 426–428
  compulsory rules and, 420, 422
  defined, 421, 426
  duty and, 422-423
  guidance for individual deliberation and, 420
  love and, 422, 1370
  moral decision-making and, 405, 411, 422
  treatment of defective infants and, 731–732
Acupuncture, 912, 922, 923
Adab aṭ-ṭabīb, 789
Addiction to drugs, *See* Drug addiction
Addison, Joseph, 77

Ad hoc Committee on Ethical Standards in Psychological Research, 1479
Adler, Alfred, 1067, 1084, 1085, 1088
Adman, L. C., 654
Administrator, hospital, 678, 679, 681–682
Adolescents, 55
  medical care of, 38–43, 151–152
    age and psychological maturity, relationship between, 39
    confidentiality and, 41–42
    informed consent and, 42, 43
    judgement by physician on maturity, 40–41
    maturity as measure of self-determination, 39–40
    psychiatric treatment and, 38, 41
    research programs and, 42–43
    sexual development of, 1572–1574
Adrenalin, 842
Adrenal steroids, 1494
Adrenogenital syndrome, 474
Adult education, 873
Adultery:
  in ancient Greece, 1577
  in ancient Rome, 1577
  Aquinas on, 1580
  artificial insemination and, 1457, 1465
  Eastern Orthodox Christianity and, 353, 354
  Judaism and, 1576
  Luther on, 1581
Advaita Vedānta, 661
Advancement of Learning (Bacon), 261
Adventism, *See* Seventh-Day Adventism
"Adventure of the Speckled Band, The" (Conan Doyle), 1009
Advertising:
  of cigarettes, 1605
  codes of ethics and, 44, 167, 168, 179
  in medical journals, 193, 322–323
  of medical products, 47, 180, 187, 193, 322–323, 1211–1213, 1385
  by medical professionals, 44–47
    for abortions, 30
    in ancient Greece, 933
    in Arab nations, 889
    in dentistry, 312
    Hinduism and, 664
    impact on institutional providers, 46
    justifications for restrictions on, 45–46
    legal issues in, 46–47
    restrictions in United States, 44–46

of self-realization groups, 1548
subliminal, 97
Advocacy role, 1043–1044
Advocates, patients' rights, 1205
AEC, *See* Atomic Energy Commission
Aelred (Ethelred) of Rievaulx, 60
Aeschylus, 236
Aesclepiades, 1655
Affective psychosis, *See* manic–depressive disorders
AFPD, *See* American Federation of Physicians and Dentists
Africa:
    abortion in, 900
    contraception in, 208, 211, 899–900
    emigration from, 1304
    family planning in, 899
    grain production in, 495
    health care in, 898–899
    infanticide in, 226, 742
    medical ethics in, 897–900
    medical ethics education in, 872
    missionary activity in, 1367
    per capita expenditures on education, health, and defense in, 1323, 1324
    population control in, 899
    population education in, 1311
    population–physician ratio in, 1323–1324
    population policy in, 1297
    standards for medical practice in, 898
    taboo illness in, 1122
    traditional vs. scientific methods in, 897–898
    urban growth in, 1220
    See also specific countries
Africa Regional Conference on Abortion, 900
After-life:
    in biblical thought, 243–246
    Christianity and, 250–252, 256–257
    in Eastern thought, 231, 232
    in Western thought, 236, 241
Agapic love, 422, 431–432
Agassi, Joseph, 1639
Aged, *See* Aging and the aged
Age distribution, 54
Age-irrelevant society, 56
Ageism, 267
Agency:
    decision making by, *See* Decision making; Proxy consent
    determinism and, 506
Agency for International Development (AID), 1234, 1276, 1280, 1292
Agent-neutral theory, 418–419
Agent-relative theory, 418–419
Age structure, 1219, 1221, 1234
Agglutination, 1441
Aggression:
    "black," 1411
    genetics and, 544, 545, 1077
    population regulation with, 1307–1308
    psychosurgery and, 1387, 1389, 1391
Aging and the aged, 48–64
    anti-aging techniques, 50–53, 464
        ethical implications of, 62–64
        humanism and, 63–64
        improved nutrition as, 62
        metabolic-rate reduction as, 52, 63
        moral and anthropological effects of, 63
        prosthetic devices and, 62
        sleep-reduction as, 51–52
        social impact of, 63
        undernutrition as, 51
        use of, 62–63
    in Arab nations, 890–891
    chronic illness and, 156
    death and, *See* Death
    in Eastern Europe, 980
    Eastern Orthodox Christianity and, 351
    ethical implications in, 58–64
        analysis of problems, 61–62
        anti-aging techniques and, 62–64
        values and longevity, historical perspective of, 58–61
    in France, 971
    genetic causes of, 522
    health care and, 57, 65–68
        ethical considerations in, 61–62, 67–68
        medical and hospital services, 65–66
        mental health care, 67
        nursing homes, *See* Nursing homes
    rights and, 1512
    social implications of, 54–58
        changing relations between age groups, 54–55
        old-old persons, 54–55, 57–58
        population growth, 54, 57–58
        young-old persons, 54–57
    social medicine and, 1600
    theories of, 48–50
Agramont, Jacme d', 949, 950
Agrarian Justice (Paine), 624

Agudath Israel of America, 1430
AHA, *See* American Hospital Association
Ahiṃsā, 661, 907
Ahwazi, *See* Haly Abbas
AID, *See* Agency for International Development
AID, *See* Artificial insemination: by donor
AIH, *See* Artificial insemination: by husband
Aiken, Henry David, 1340
Air pollution, 380, 383, 387
Aitken-Swan, Jean, 1678
Akhavaynī, 887
Akinari, Ueda, 925
Alameda, Luis de, 923
Albertini, 1659
Albert the Great, 1523, 1580
Alcoholics Anonymous, 74, 333
Alcoholism, 71–74, 328, 1104, 1397
    as disease, 71–72
    genetic predisposition and, 539, 545, 1077
    institutionalization and, 1077
    libertarian view of, 330
    moral issue of, 72
    problems of response to alcoholics, 72–73
    rehabilitation programs and, 331–332
    research on, 73–74
Alcohol use, 69–74, 327, 334–335, 1384, 1386
    by adolescents, 38
    alcoholism, *See* Alcoholism
    in contemporary Arab world, 891
    drinking, 69–70, 71
    drunkenness, 70–71, 73, 853, 1021
    effects of, 335
    fetal development and, 487
    in Great Britain, 990
    Islam and, 70, 787
    Jehovah's Witnesses and, 1377
    Mormonism and, 1376
    permissive attitudes toward, 327
    for pleasure, 327, 335
    Seventh-Day Adventism and, 1376
Alexander, Leo, 1018
Alexander, Samuel, 443
Alexander the Great, 238
Alexandrian physicians, 685–686
Alexandrian school, 6
Alfidi, Ralph, 1681
Alienation:
    public health and, 1397
    technology and, 1640–1641
'Alī ibn 'Abbās al-Madjūsī (Haly Abbas), 786, 887
Advice to a Physician, 1734–1735

Allen, A. A., 1122
Allen, Norman, 293
Allison, Van Kleek, 159
Allocation of food, *See* Food policy
Allocation of scarce resources, *See* Scarce resources, allocation of
Allografts, *See* Heart transplantation
Allowing to die, *See* Acting and refraining; Death; Euthanasia; Right to refuse medical care
Alphonsianum Institute, Italy, 985
Altruism:
  blood donation and, 134
  dynamic therapies and, 340
  food policy and, 497
  genetic influence on, 132
  interpersonal conflicts and, 308
AMA, *See* American Medical Association
Ambisexuality, 668
Ambrose, St., 938
Ambulatory medical care, 1671
American Academy of Family Physicians, 1041
American Academy of Neurological Surgery, 1730
American Academy of Oral Pathology, Code of Ethics, 1728
American Academy of Pediatrics, 1729
  Model Act of 1973, 39, 40
American Anthropological Association:
  Principles of Professional Responsibility, 1479
  Statement of Human Rights, 454
American Association for Respiratory Therapy, 1729
American Association of Medical Colleges, 1032
American Association of Orthodontics, Principles of Ethics, 1728
American Association of Physicians and Surgeons, 1041
American Bar Association, 300, 1103, 1347
  Code of Professional Responsibility and Code of Judicial Conduct, 1726
American Board of Ophthalmology, 1039
American Cancer Society, 649
American Chiropractic Association, Code of Ethics, 1729
  text of, 1799–1802
American Civil Liberties Union, National Prison Project, 1351
American College of Apothecaries, Code of Professional Practice, 1726, 1728
American College of Foot Surgeons, 1726
American College of Legal Medicine, 1726, 1729

American College of Nurse-Midwives, 1726
American College of Obstetricians and Gynecologists, 4
  Nurses' Association of, 1142
American College of Physicians, 1039, 1202
American College of Radiology, 1726
American College of Surgeons, 1038–1039, 1202, 1730
American Correctional Association, 1350, 1352
American Correctional Health Services Association, 1348
American Dental Association, 1039
  Principles of Ethics, 313, 314-315
  text of, 1802–1804
American Federation for Clinical Research, 1729
American Federation of Physicians and Dentists (AFPD), 1040
American Health Care Association, 1141
American Heart Association, 649
American Hospital Association (AHA), 73, 169, 198, 639, 645, 648, 998, 1039, 1041, 1043
  A Patient's Bill of Rights, 169, 172, 176, 177, 198, 998, 1141, 1197, 1203, 1363, 1430, 1515, 1683
    text of, 1783–1785
  Right of the Patient to Refuse Treatment, 1515
American Indians, 1285, 1304, 1307
  See also American Plains Indians; names of specific tribes
American Institute of Homeopathy, 1174
American Journal of Nursing, 1138
American Law Institute, 28, 998, 1107, 1112
  Model Penal Code (1962), 673
American Medical Association (AMA), 161, 408, 624, 1033, 1038–1039, 1141, 1202, 1347, 1711, 1726
  on advertising by medical professionals, 44–47
  centrality of, 1041
  Code of Ethics of, 166–167, 172, 321, 770, 965–967, 995, 996, 1174, 1175, 1683
    text of, 1738–1746
  on confidentiality, 178
  Council on Drugs, 323
  Council on Medical Education, 1032
  on delegation of surgery, 1628
  Ethical Guidelines for Clinical Investigation, 1773
  on euthanasia, 176, 279, 735
  founding of, 952, 1030, 1037
  global work of, 1039

growth of, 1038–1039
  guidelines for treatment of terminal illness, 168
  Health Care in Correctional Institutions Project, 1348
  health insurance and, 639–640, 648, 649, 994, 1039–1040, 1041
  on human experimentation, 42, 656, 758, 1352, 1773–1774
  medical education and, 993, 1031, 1037–1038
  Opinions and Reports of the Judicial Council, 1726
  Opinions of the Judicial Council of, 770
  on organ transplantation, 168, 656
  political role of, 1041
  Principles of Medical Ethics of, 44, 173, 175, 179, 197, 575, 770, 1683, 1727
    text of, 1750–1754
  Report on the Physician and the Dying Patient (Judicial Council), 1728
  Statement on Heart Transplantation, 656
  on treatment of alcoholics, 73
  unionization and, 1040, 1041
American Medical Colleges, 645
American Medical Technologists, Code of Ethics, 1728
American Methodist Board of Christian Social Concern, 1437
American Nurses' Association (ANA), 172, 175–176, 177, 648, 995, 1039, 1141
  Code for Nurses, 1138–1139, 1142, 1143, 1727
    text of, 1789–1799
  human rights guidelines, 1143
  Human Rights Guidelines for Nurses in Clinical and Other Research: Statement of the ANA Commission on Nursing Research, 1727
American Occupational Therapy Association, 1728
American Osteopathic Association, 177–178, 1730
  Code of Ethics, 1730
    text of, 1804–1806
American Pharmaceutical Association, 1211, 1212, 1726
  Code of Ethics, 1728–1729
    text of, 1806
American Philosophical Association, Committee on Medicine and Philosophy, 1000
American Physical Therapy Association, 1726
  Guide for Professional Conduct, 1730
American Plains Indians, 879
American Podiatry Association, 1726

American Protestant Hospital Association (APHA), 1367

American Psychiatric Association, 670, 1565, 1726
  Nomenclature Committee, 1096
  Principles of Medical Ethics with Annotations Especially Applicable to Psychiatry, 1807–1811

American Psychological Association, 172, 1479, 1726
  Ethical Principles in the Conduct of Research with Human Participants, 1727
  Ethical Standards of Psychologists, 1727
  text of, 1811–1815

American Psychopathological Association, 1730

American Public Health Association (APHA), 648, 1039, 1319, 1394

American Society for Experimental Pathology, 1729

American Society for Experimental Therapeutics, 1729

American Society for Pharmacology and Experimental Therapeutics, 1729

American Society of Bariatric Physicians, 1728

American Society of Extra-Corporeal Technology, 1730

American Society of Hospital Pharmacists, 1729

American Society of Internal Medicine, 1729

American Society of Newspaper Editors, 180

American Sociological Association, Code of Ethics, 1479

American Thoracic Society, 1729

American Urological Association, 1729

American Veterinary Medical Association, Principles of Veterinary Medical Ethics, 1730

Ames, William, 1365

Amniocentesis, 2, 8, 461, 467, 490, 556, 569, 577, 999, 1332–1333, 1336, 1441, 1644
  commitment to abort and, 1335
  followed by abortion, *See* Prenatal diagnosis: followed by abortion
  historical perspective, 1332
  procedure, 1333
  risks in, 1333, 1335, 1336–1337
  timing of, 1343

Amniotic fluid, 1332

examination of, *See* Amniocentesis

Amphetamines, 89, 335, 1381, 1383

Amulets, 587, 588, 589

ANA, *See* American Nurses' Association

Anabaptists, 1376

Anal intercourse, 1563, 1564

Analytical ethics, *See* Metaethics

Anatomy, 1484, 1639

Anatomy Acts of 1832 and 1871 (Great Britain), 141

Anatomy and Pathology Laws of 1953 (Israel), 896

Anatomy of Melancholy (Burton), 1008

Ancestor worship, 221

Ancestral medicine, 912

Androgenic hormones, 1590

Anectine, 780, 1355

Anencephaly, 732, 835

Anesthetics, 2, 76, 265, 312, 1707
  in animal experimentation, 76, 80
  discovery of, 1031
  used for pleasure, 336

Angiography, 1681

Anglican Church, 1122, 1261
  See also Protestantism

Animal experimentation, 75–83, 123, 689, 1486
  in ancient Greece, 75, 936
  in ancient Rome, 936
  behaviorism and, 107
  cryonics, 217
  eugenics in, 462
  fetal, 489–490
  gene therapy and, 514, 517, 519, 520, 523
  in Great Britain, 77, 78, 80, 81, 989
  historical aspects, 75–79
    current situation in, 78–79
    institutionalization of, 76–77
    opposition to, 77–78, 689
    origins of, 75–76
  Islam and, 893
  legislation of morality and, 820
  organ transplantation, 654–655, 1160, 1168
  pain and, 76, 79, 80, 82, 1179–1180
  Pavlovian conditioning and, 101
  philosophical perspectives, 79–83
    case against, 81–82
    case for, 81
    legislation, 80–81
    moral status of animals, 82–83, 729, 745, 822, 827–828
    nature and extent of experiments, 80
  suffering and, 79–83, 1180

Animals:
  diseases of, 602
  experimentation on, *See* Animal experimentation
  love of, 377

Animal Welfare Act of 1970, 81

Animate organism, human body as, 363, 364

Animation of fetus, 10–12, 18

Anime e corpi, 985

Annales d'hygiène publique et de médecine legale, 972

Anomie, 95, 223, 622, 1619

Anorectics, 335

Anscombe, Elizabeth, 1135

Anselm, St., 251

Anthony of Cordova, 11

Anthony of Egypt, 60

Anthropocentrism, 397–398

Anthropology:
  of death, 221–228, 1048
    cannibalism, 225
    feticide, infanticide, and death of children, 225–226
    homicide, 223–224
    implications for bioethics, 228
    natural death and desire for immortality, 221–223
    senilicide and death of the aged, 226–228
    suicide, 223–225
    war, 225
  defined, 1045
  of homosexuality, 669
  influence on ethics, 1536
  of medicine, 1045–1049
    ascribed cause of illness, 1046–1047
    catalog of recognized diseases, 1046
    death, 1048
    defined, 1046
    ethical considerations, 1048–1049
    usual treatment of illness, 1047–1048
  theological, of Eastern Orthodox Christianity, 347–348

Anti-aging techniques, 50–53, 464
  ethical implications of, 62–64
  humanism and, 63–64
  improved nutrition as, 62
  metabolic-rate reduction as, 52, 63
  moral and anthropological effects of, 63
  prosthetic devices and, 62
  sleep-reduction as, 51–52
  social impact of, 63
  undernutrition as, 51
  use of, 62–63

Antianxiety drugs, 1381–1383
Antibiotics, 2, 169, 271, 1173
impact on diagnoses, 324
overprescription of, 323
Antidepressant drugs, 1380–1381
Antimodernism, 267
Antipaternalism, 1196, 1197, 1198, 1200
Antipsychiatry, 1092, 1094–1096, 1101
Antipsychotic drugs, 1379–1380
Antitrust laws, 47
Antivivisection movement, 77–79, 81–82, 685, 689, 690, 974
Antley, Mary Ann, 1339
Antonelli, Giuseppi, 871, 1525
Antoninus, St. (Archbishop of Florence), 10, 943, 1530
APHA, *See* American Protestant Hospital Association
APHA, *See* American Public Health Association
Apnea, 293, 294
Apocalypticism, 250
Apology (Plato), 237
Apology for Astrology (Servetus), 1366
Apothecaries:
in colonial America, 1030
in eighteenth century England, 1036
in medieval Europe, 942, 946, 947–948
in nineteenth-century Great Britain, 974
See also Pharmacy
Apothecaries Act of 1815 (Great Britain), 1037
Apothecaries Society, 1036
Appeal, behavioral, 88–89
Appeal to authority, 97, 402–403
Application of President of Georgetown College (1964), 1501, 1502, 1054
Applied ethics, 1216–1217
Aptowitzer, Viktor, 6
Aquapendente, Fabricius ab, 489
Aquinas, St. Thomas, 472, 1065, 1170, 1400
on abortion, 18, 24, 943
on animation of fetus, 18
on consanguineous marriages, 471
on contraception, 209, 1226
on death, 239
on double effect principle, 24, 33, 34
"Fifth Way" of, 480
on killing in self-defense, 274, 317, 319
on marriage, 1226, 1580
on natural law, 818, 1132, 1133, 1134, 1136, 1524, 1526
on physician's fees, 942
on resurrection, 252

on rights of animals, 81
sexual ethics of, 1580
on suicide, 275, 823, 943, 1620, 1621, 1623
on supererogation, 1148, 1149
on truth and lying, 1685, 1686
on virtue theory, 436
Arab nations:
medical ethics in, 888–891
Muslim perspective, 892–895
per capita expenditures on education, health, and defense in, 1323, 1324
population education in, 1311
See also specific nations
Arantius, 489
Arapaho Indians, 226
Arbitrariness, 809
Arbitrary inequality, 803
Arbitration, 1025
Archetypes, 1067
Archimedes, 1699
Aretaeus, 935
Argentina, Permanent Committee on Medical Education, 1006
Argentine Congress of Medical Ethics (1958), 1006
Arginosuccinicaciduria, 474
Argumentation, method of, 403
Arguments to design, 480
Ariès, Philippe, 151, 241, 242, 251, 252
Aristophanes, 236
Aristotle, 14, 59, 239, 403, 418, 435, 442, 489, 590, 685, 882, 1602
on animation of fetus 9–12
antiequalitarian position of, 804
on contraception, 205, 206
on death, 236, 237, 238
on friendship, 1577
on infanticide, 742, 826
influence on Islam of, 785
on justice, 1237
on liability, 545
on man's dominion over nature, 367
on mental health, 1061
moral reasoning of, 451, 452, 453
on moral rules, 409
on moral vs. legal status, 813
on natural law, 442, 1131
on population, 1225, 1233
prescriptivist elements in philosophy of, 448–449
sexual ethics of, 1578
on suicide, 1620–1621, 1623
on therapeutic relationship, 1655
on truth and lying, 1685
Arm's-length aspects of therapy, 341–342
Arnobius, 938
Arnold, John, 1352
Arrowsmith (Lewis), 1012–1013
Ars moriendi, or The Art of Dying, 253–255

Artha, 661
Arthashastra, 1235
Arthritis Commission, 1496
Artificial heart, 631, 634–635, 636, 659–660, 843, 845, 848, 1155, 1519, 1651–1652
Artificial insemination, 169, 557, 1444–1445
in Arab nations, 890
consent agreement for, 1445
by donor (AID), 467, 1444, 1445, 1454–1460, 1462, 1465–1469, 1531, 1533
donor selection, 1445
in Eastern Europe, 979
Eastern Orthodox Christianity and, 354–355
ethical issues, 1454-1460
eugenic use of, 1445
by husband (AIH), 1444, 1454, 1458, 1531, 1533
Judaism and, 797, 800, 1457, 1458
legal aspects, 1445, 1464–1469
legitimacy of child and, 1445, 1468
marriage and, 1444–1445, 1456–1459, 1468–1469
motive for, 1454
normative relativism and, 455
parenthood and, 1444, 1445, 1456–1459
procedure in, 1444
Protestantism and, 1437, 1457–1458
Roman Catholicism and, 1433, 1456–1457, 1458, 1531, 1533
situation ethics and, 423
ultimate factors in decision-making, 1459–1460
Artificial kidney, *See* Kidney dialysis
Artificial respiration, 840
Artificial support, *See* Life-supporting systems
Art of Ministering to the Sick, The (Cabot and Dick), 1367
Art of War, The (Sun Tzu), 1695
'*Arukh ha-Shulḥan,* 1251
Aruzi, Nizami, 887
Aryans, 270, 885
Arzt und Christ, 985, 1522
Asceticism, 1187
Ascribed cause of illness, 1046–1047
Asexual human reproduction, *See* Cloning
Ashby, Lord, 989
Asher ben Yehiel, 1418, 1429
Asia:
contraception in, 211–212
grain production in, 495
per capita expenditures on education, health, and defense in, 1323, 1324
population–physician ratio in, 1323, 1324

poverty in, 1321
urban growth in, 1220
See also specific countries
Asia Minor, 207
Aśoka, King of Magadha, 665
Asphyxia, 1108
Aspilcueta, Martin, *See* Navarrus
Assault, 1021
Assessing Biomedical Technologies: An Inquiry into the Nature of the Process (Committee on the Life Sciences and Social Policy), 1652–1653
Assia, 896
Assises de la Cour des Bourgeois, 946
Association for Advancement of Behavior Therapy, 1726, 1729
Association for Clinical Pastoral Education (ACPE), 1192
Association for the Advancement of Medicine by Research (Great Britain), 78
Association for Voluntary Sterilization, 1612
Association of American Medical Colleges, 1039, 1041
Association of American Medical Schools, 648
Assyria:
exorcism in, 1121
medical ethics, history of, 880–883
taboo illness in, 1121
Astrology, 1366
Astronomy, 1375
Astrophysics, 1403
Athenian Mercury, 181
Ātman, 661
Atmospheric testing, 1702
Atomic Energy Act, 577
Atomic Energy Commission (AEC), 383, 1350
Attachment, maternal–fetal, 485–486
Attorneys, *See* Lawyers
Attribution:
in help-seeking behavior, 1669
in medical reporting, 182–183
Aubert, Jean-Marie, 1136
Audiovisual sex therapy, 1554
Augustine, St., 238, 239, 434, 1232, 1371, 1400, 1523
on abortion, 943
on contraception, 207–208, 209
sexual ethics of, 1579, 1581
on the soul, 250–251, 436–437, 1524
on suicide, 275, 943
on truth and lying, 1685
Augustus, Emperor, 1226, 1233
Aune, Bruce, 35, 318

Austin, John, 819
Austin, John L., 505
Australia:
abortion laws in, 28
infanticide in, 742
Medibank system of, 641, 642
medical ethics education in, 872
net immigration in, 1221
urban growth in, 1220
Austria:
animal experimentation in, 78
brain death studies in, 296
eugenic societies in, 458
health insurance in, 637
health-related expenditures in, 650
population policy in, 1235
sterilization in, 1616
Authority:
appeal to, 97, 402–403
behavior control and, 87
of educators, 90–91
of nurses, 1140–1141, 1142
technical vs. moral, 1669
Authorship, 189–190, 192–193
Autoerotic activity, *See* Masturbation
Autoexperimentation, 688–689, 1487
Autonomy, 149
of the aged, 61
behavior control and, 94–95, 98
of children, 154
determinism and, 503–506
dynamic therapies and, 340, 343, 344
eugenic policy and, 466
human experimentation and, 700, 701, 703, 706
humanization and dehumanization of care and, 620, 621
informed consent and, 755, 759, 767
in physicians' decision-making, 279
private decisions and, 1358–1362
regulation of health care by government and, 612
rights and, 625–626, 823, 1500
treatment decisions and, 1693
See also Self-determination
Autopsy, 139–140, 583
Islam and, 891, 893
Judaism and, 144, 246, 798, 801–802, 894–895, 896, 1026
Roman Catholicism and, 140
Autosomal dominant traits, 556, 557
Average, normality as, 40
Average utilitarianism, 428, 508–509
Averroës, 239, 893, 1065, 1400
Aversive therapies, 97, 99, 101, 104, 109, 780, 1073

Avesta, 885
Avicenna (Ibn Sīnā), 208, 209, 239, 786, 887, 893, 1065, 1267
Avis au peuple sur sa santé (Tissot), 971
Avoiding harm, principle of, 694–695, 734–735, 754, 760, 775, 1124, 1355
Ayer, A. J., 448, 453, 542
Āyurveda, 663, 666, 906–907
Azathioprine, 1162

B

Babeuf Conspiracy, 624
Babylonia, medical ethics in, 880–883
Babylonian Talmud, 205
Bachrach, Yair, 7
Bacon, Francis, 62, 240, 261, 262, 367, 1375, 1659
Bacon, Roger, 261, 262, 1523
Bad behavior, 90
Baghdadi, Al-, 888
Bahamas, animal experimentation in, 78
Bahrain, health care in, 890
Baier, Kurt, 421, 439
Bailey, Derrick S., 1583
Baird, William, 160
Balikci, Asen, 224, 226, 227
Ballerini, 12
Baltazar, E. R., 1610
Balter, Mitchell B., 1383
Bandt, Karl, 1016
Bandura, Albert, 1086
Bangladesh:
population policies in, 1224
poverty in, 1321
Baptists, 70
Barber, Bernard, 1472, 1544
Barber surgeons, 1714
Barbiturates, 328, 1355, 1381–1382
Bard, John, 1030
Bard, Samuel, 959–960, 961, 964, 1030
Bardwick, Judith, 669
Barefoot doctors, 919, 1717
Bariatric medicine, 1726
Barnard, Christiaan N., 186, 296, 655, 657, 659, 1162
Barr, M. L., 1332
Barry, James, 1715
Barth, Karl, 15, 212, 434, 674, 1368–1372, 1583, 1610
Basho, 234
Basil, St., 349, 350, 938, 939
Bastardy, 469

Bateson, William, 541

Bates v. State Bar of Arizona (1977), 47

Battery, law of, 755, 759, 771, 772–773, 1021

Battie, William, 1091–1092

Baumrind, Diana, 760

Baylor University Hospital, 639

Beach, Wooster, 1173

Beals, Walter B., 1018

Bearers of rights, 1512–1513

Beatty, R. A., 1455

Beauchamp, Tom, 631, 636

Beaumont, William, 686, 687

Bechterev, Vladimir M., 107

Becker, Ernest, 289

Bede, 472

Beecher, Henry, 997

Beers, Clifford, 1080

Beginning of life, *See* Life, beginning of

Behavioral genetics, *See* Genetic aspects of human behavior

Behavioral modification, *See* Behavior control; Behavioral therapies; Behaviorism; Mental illness therapies

Behavioral observation, 1471–1472

Behavior research, 1470–1480
 consent in, 1472–1474
 deception in, 1472–1474, 1477
 protection and accountability in, 1479–1480
 risks in:
  entailed by research processes, 1474–1478
  entailed by research products, 1478–1479
 types of, 1470–1472
 See also Behavior control; Human experimentation

Behavioral therapies, 101–106
 alcoholism and, 72, 73–74
 classification of, 1086
 the institutionalized and, 104–105, 780–781
 practice of, 101–106, 1086
  conditioning, 101, 107, 109, 1086
  controversial issues related to, 102–104
  ethical issues related to, 105–106
  historical review of, 102
 sex therapy with, 1553
 See also Behavior control; Behaviorism; Mental illness therapies

Behavior control, 85–100, 125, 551, 1641
 ethical analysis of, 85–92
  controlled and free behavior, 87–89, 505–506
  dimensions, 86–87
  innovations, 85–86

right of access, 92
 role-systems, 87, 89–92
 freedom and, 87–89, 93–100
  effects of behavior control on freedom, 96–98
  free action, 93–94
  free person, 94–95
  free will, 95–96, 100, 502–503
  value of freedom, 98–100
 images of man and, 856
 in mental hospitals, 1073
 mental retardation and, 1112
 paternalism and, 1198–1199
 prisoners and, 999, 1199, 1347, 1348
 specific therapies in, *See* Mental health therapies
 television and, 86, 87
 See also Behavioral therapies; Behaviorism

Behaviorism, 107–114
 history of, 107–109
  antecedents, 107
  comprehensive learning theories, 108
  origins, 107
  recent developments, 108
  social impact, 108–109
 mind–body problem and, 1115–1116, 1421, 1425–1426
 philosophical analysis of, 110–114
  accounting for human actions, 112–113, 502–503
  inner states or events, 111–112
  overt behavior, 110–111
  Skinner, theory of, 108, 109, 113–114, 1068, 1425–1426
 religion and mental health and, 1067–1068
 See also Behavior control; Behavioral therapies; Free will; Mental health therapies; Reductionism

Beigelböck, W., 1018

Being and Nothingness (Sartre), 1594

Being and Time (Heidegger), 304

Belgium:
 abortion laws in, 27–32
 contraception in, 211, 213
 population growth in, 1286
 population policy in, 1235

Beliefs:
 in pragmatism, 1327–1331
 religious:
  privacy and, 1360, 1361
  sexuality and, 1560–1561
 See also Values

Benedict, Ruth, 456

Benedict, St., 371

Benedictine Order, 371

Benedict the Levite, 472

Beneficial experimentation, 693–694
 See also Therapeutic experimentation

Beneficial research, *See* Therapeutic research

Benefit paternalism, 1197

Bennet, Hughes, 1661

Bennett, Jonathan, 36

Bentham, Jeremy, 82, 173, 264, 413, 424, 428, 450, 451, 1292, 1401
 on acting and refraining, 35
 on contraception, 210
 on distributive justice, 543, 805
 on law and morality, 819
 on obligation to future generations, 508
 pleasure-pain calculus of, 1653
 on private ethics, 419–420
 on truth and lying, 1686

Benzoquinolines, 1379

Bérard, Joseph, 1661

Berger, Peter L., 1603

Bergson, Henri, 127, 129, 241, 362, 363, 1641

Berkeley, George, 421, 448

Berlin, Isaiah, 95, 97, 1062

Berlin, Naphtali, 1251

Berman, E. F., 654

Bernard, Claude, 76, 584, 689–690, 692

Bernard, Jean, 985

Berne, Eric, 1087

Bernheim, 711, 1661

Berreman, Gerald D., 878

Bert, Paul, 689

Bertalanffy, Ludwig von, 128, 130

Bertram, E. G., 1332

Besant, Annie, 210

Bestiality, 353, 1561, 1564, 1592

Bestowed rights, 124

Bethe, Hans, 1700

Bethune, Norman, 920

Beyond Freedom and Dignity (Skinner), 98–99

Bhagavadgītā, 1270

Bible:
 on abortion, 5–6, 9–10, 14, 15
 on contraception, 205–207
 on death, 239, 243–246
 on duty to preserve life and health, 793
 on feeding the hungry, 497
 on health and disease, 582, 588
 on homosexuality, 672
 Jewish medical ethics and, 792, 793
 on man's dominion over nature, 366–367, 397, 826
 on man's stewardship over nature, 371
 on miracle and faith healing, 1121, 1122–1123, 1126–1127, 1128
 on population control, 1250
 on suicide, 1622

Bibliography of Bioethics, 1000

Bibliography of the Philosophy of Technology, 1639

Bibring, Grete L., 485
Bichat, Marie François Xavier, 265, 266, 600, 972, 1482
Bieber, Irving, 668, 1592
Bieganski, W., 1051
Bierce, Ambrose, 988
Big Bang theories, 1403
Bills of rights, 1515
   of American Hospital Association, *See* Patient's Bill of Rights, A model, 1204–1205
Binding, Karl, 282, 983
Bini, L., 359
Biochemistry, 1484
Bioengineering, 1639
Bioethics, 115–127
   as natural response to new dilemmas, 115–116
   public policy and, 126–127
   science and, 118–119, 125–126, 1545–1546
   viewed as traditional ethics, 120–125
      medical ethics case, 116–120
Bioethics: Bridge to the Future (Potter), 118
Bioethics movement, 994, 996–1001
Biological aging theories, 48–50
Biological clocks, tampering with, 52–53
Biological criterion for beginning of human life, 17–20, 1338
Biological-functional model of human nature, 1088
Biological sex, 1589–1590
Biological weapons, 1308, 1700, 1701–1703
Biologists, 1000
Biology:
   bioethics and, 125
   philosophy of, 127–132
      defined, 127
      ethics and, 130–132
      holism, 130
      mechanism, 129, 130, 367–368, 619, 1419
      reductionism, *See* Reductionism
      vitalism, 129–130
Biomedical communication, *See* Communication, biomedical
Biomedical research, 1481–1491
   conflicts between medical practice and, 1486–1488
   domain of medicine, 1481–1484
   images of man and, 856
   law and, 1493–1494, 1644–1648
   publication of, *See* Communication, biomedical
   public policy and, 1492–1497
      ethical and policy dimensions, 1496–1497

history of development in United States, 1488–1489, 1493–1496
   value implications, 1492–1493
   in relation to medicine, 1484–1486
   socialization of, 1488–1490
   specific ethical issues in, *See* Animal experimentation; Human experimentation
Biostatistics, 2
Birth:
   beginning of human life viewed as, 8, 12, 18, 730–731, 1340–1341, 1469
   Jewish definition of, 795
Birth attendants, 897, 898
Birth control, *See* Contraception; Family planning; Population ethics; Population policy proposals; Sexual abstinence
Birth defects:
   abortion and, 2, 7–8, 30, 31, 896, 910, 998, 1109
      See also Prenatal diagnosis: followed by abortion
   alcohol consumption in pregnancy and, 487
   in Arab nations, 890
   clinical aspects of, 717–724
      agency in decision making, 723–724
      conflicting interests, 722–723
      conflicting principles and, 722
      management of untreated infants, 721–722
      therapy in newborns, 718–721
   drug caused, 80, 183, 324, 381, 487, 1349
   environmentally induced, 381, 1335
   ethical perspectives on, 724–735
      consequentialist theories, 731–732, 834–837
      deontological theories, 726–729, 833, 838
      equality theory of justice, 837
      ethic of care, 733–734
      extraordinary means principle, 727–729, 838
      medical criteria, 724–726
      personhood theories, 726–727, 729–732, 834–836
      principle of avoiding harm, 734–735
      slippery slope argument, 821, 836–837
      wrongful life theory, 835–836, 837
      See also Infanticide
   euphenics and, 474–478
   Hinduism and, 664

prenatal diagnosis of, *See* Prenatal diagnosis
public policy and procedural questions, 735–740
   on decision making, 737–739
   on euthanasia and sustaining life, 735–737
   on macroallocation, 739–740
   reproductive technologies and, 1450, 1461–1462, 1467
   socioeconomic factors and, 465
   See also Genetic counseling; Genetic screening; Infanticide
Birth Defects Institute (New York State), 571
Birthmarks, 719
Birth rate, *See* Fertility rate
Bisexuality, 668, 669
Bismarck, Otto von, 647, 1662
Black Death, *See* Plague
Black Elk, 879
Black Elk Speaks (Neilhardt), 879
Black magic, 586
Blacks, discrimination against, *See* Race differences in intelligence; Racism
Blackstone, William, 27
Blackwell, Barry, 1383
Blackwell, Elizabeth, 1715
Blake, Judith, 1296
Blake, William, 369
Blane, Sir Gilbert, 1051
Blastocyst reimplantation, 1441
Blind experiment, 695, 1488
Blindness, 719
Blomquist, Clarence, 985
Blood, oxygen transport by, 842
Blood banking, 1156
Blood donation, 987, 1153, 1154
Bloodletting, 1173, 1406, 1488
Blood pressure:
   in mass health screening, 857
   pronouncement of death and, 292–293, 294, 298
Blood sampling, 857
Blood transfusion, 2, 271, 842
   Eastern Orthodox Christianity and, 350
   ethical problems, 133–134
   exchange transfusion, 842
   Islam and, 893
   Jehovah's Witnesses and, 133, 271, 1361, 1377, 1426, 1512, 1514
   paternalistic principle and, 1195
   procedure, 133
Blood typing, 1160
Blue Cross Association, 639
Blue Cross Plans, 639, 640
Blue Shield Plans, 640
Blumgart, Herrman L., 191

VOLUME INDICATOR

Blumhardt, Johann Christoph, 1125
BMA, *See* British Medical Association
Board of Medical Specialties, 1041
Böckle, Franz, 985
Bodily enactments, 364
Bodin, Jean, 819, 1226, 1235
Bodley, Rachel, 1715
Body temperature, pronouncement of death and, 292
Boerhaave, Hermann, 1659
Boethius, Anicius, 1206, 1400
Bogomil of Bulgaria, 208
Bohannan, Paul, 223
Bohemia, contraception in, 211
Bohn, Johannes, 955, 956
Boil-openers, 909
Bok, Sissela, 22, 735
Bone, Hugh, 1494
Bone–Magnuson Act (P.L. 75–244), 1494
Bone marrow transplantation, 475
Bone-setters, 909
Bonhoeffer, Dietrich, 15, 421, 1583, 1610
Bonner v. Moran (1941), 153
Boorde, Andrew, 1091, 1092
Boorse, Christopher, 601, 602
Borderline situations, 1369
Berdyaev, 1585
Borelli, Giovanni, 954
Boros, Ladislaus, 302
Borough, The (Crabbe), 1008
Boston Medical Police, 965
Boston University Symposium on the Identity and Dignity of Man, 1001
Botero, Giovanni, 210, 1235
Boudewyns, Michiel, 1525
Boulding, Kenneth, 213
Boundary-breaker (image of man), 855–856
Bourgeois, Louyse, 1714
Bourke, M. P., 871
Bower manuscripts, 136–137
Boyle, Robert, 954
Boyle's Law, 1543
Boylston, Zabdiel, 686–687
Bradlagh, Charles, 210
Brāhmanas, 232
Brahmanism:
  alcohol use and, 70
  death and, 231, 232
Brain:
  electrical stimulation of, *See* Electrical stimulation of the brain (ESB)
  pain and, 1178
  surgery of, *See* Psychosurgery
Brain death, 18–19, 20, 259, 266, 292–298, 998
  cerebral circulation and, 294, 295, 296, 300

clinical experience and, 293–294
collaborative study of, 294–295
Eastern Orthodox Christianity and, 351–352
individual–biological criterion and, 18–19
irreversible coma, 292, 293, 294, 846
irreversible destruction of entire brain, 293, 295
legal aspects of, 298, 299
mind–body problem and, 304, 1118
organ transplantation and, 141, 296, 298, 303, 656, 1155
philosophical perspectives, 303–304
prolonged nonfunctional state, 293, 296, 300
relational criterion and, 20
Scandinavian criteria and, 294
termination of life-support systems and, 846, 847
terminology of, 292
Brain function:
  beginning of human life and, 18–19, 21
  personhood and, 746
  treatment of defective infants and, 725
Branch, C. H., 1678
Brandeis, Louis D., 704
Brandt, R. B., 21, 421, 1620
Branscomb, Herman, 286, 290
Braun, Wernher von, 1700
Brave New World (Huxley), 97, 100, 1385
Brazil:
  animal experimentation in, 81
  contraception in, 211
  health expenditures in, 1322
  health status by level of per capita income and, 1321
Brazilian Medical Congress (1931), 1005
Breach of express contract, 1021
Breast cancer, 1708–1709
Breggin, Peter, 1391
Bretonneau, Pierre F., 583
Bridgman, P. W., 111
Brihad-Aranyaka Upanishad, 205
Britain, *See* Great Britain
British Advisory Group, 707
British Association for the Advancement of Science, 989
British Broadcasting Company, 186, 187–188, 988
British East India Company, 908
British Medical Association (BMA), 44, 184, 192, 656, 973, 988
  code of ethics of, 173, 174, 175
  Statement on Experimental Research on Human Beings, 1769

Statements of Policy Definitions and Rules, 1758–1763
British Medical Journal, 192
Broad, C. D., 413, 414, 416
Brookings Foundation, 1033
Broussais, François J. V., 583–584, 603, 1053
Broverman, Donald M., 1709
Broverman, Inge K., 1709
Brown, J. B., 658
Brown, John, 583, 1051
Brown, Martin, 1703
Brown, Peter G., 1475
Browne, S. G., 872
Brunner, 1583
Bucer, Martin, 1259
Büchner, Georg, 1009
Buck v. Bell (1927), 574, 1108, 1397, 1614, 1617
Buddha, 134–135, 137
Buddhadāsa, King of Ceylon, 136
Buddhism, 134–137, 201–203, 901, 903, 904, 907, 911, 922, 1064
  alcohol use and, 70
  death and, 233–234
  environment and man and, 374–379
  "Four Noble Truths" of, 134–135
  genetic policy and, 463
  health care and, 135–136
  infanticide and, 742
  medical ethics, history of, 915, 923–924
  medical science in literature of, 136–137
  mental health and, 1065–1066
  mutilation and, 137
  pain and, 1182, 1183, 1187–1188
  suffering and, 137, 138, 1187–1188
  suicide and, 137, 1621–1623
  theological ethics and, 429
  value of animal life and, 827–828
Bulgaria, abortion laws in, 29
Bulletin of the Atomic Scientists, 1700
Bullough, Vern L., 670
Bumke, Oswald, 1016
Bunge, Mario, 1639
Burchard of Worms, 208, 940
Burger, Warren E., 777
Burial, 142, 144, 247, 798, 891
Burr, Robert, 1350
Burt, Robert, 736
Burton, Robert, 1008
Burundi:
  health status by level of per capita income and, 1321
  population policy in, 1283
Burzuya, 886
Butler, Joseph, 421, 542
Butyrophenones, 1379
By-line, of scientific article, 192

C

Cabot, Richard C., 1043, 1367, 1368
Cadavers, 139–145
  autopsy, 139–140, 583
    Islam and, 891, 893
    Judaism and, 144, 246, 798,
      801–802, 894–895, 896, 1026
    Roman Catholicism and, 140
  burial, 142, 144, 247, 798, 891
  cremation, 142–143, 144, 246
  donation of organs from:
    ethical perspective, 140–141,
      1154–1155, 1163, 1165, 1169,
      1172
    legal aspects, 1157–1158
    medical perspective, 1161
    salvaging organs, 1158–1159
    sociocultural aspects, 1167
  embalming, 141, 142
  fetal, research on, 141–142, 491,
    492
  Hinduism and, 663, 665
  Judaism and, 142, 144–145, 246,
    247, 248, 798, 801–802, 894–
    895, 896, 1026, 1427
  significance of the body, 139
  See also Cryonics
Caesar, Julius, 1136
Caesarea, 1657
Caesarean section, 2, 3, 1531
Caesarius of Arles, 208
Caffeine, 326, 327, 328, 334–336
Cahiers Laënnec, 985, 1522
Cajetan, Thomas de Vio, 34, 317
Calcium EDTA, 842
Calenda, Constanza, 1714
California, University of, Medical
  Center at San Francisco, 875,
  1001
California Natural Death Act of
  1976, 998
California Physicians' Service, 639
Callahan, Daniel, 21, 22, 477, 510,
  1000, 1340, 1341
"Calling," doctrine of, 1366, 1435
Calomel, 1173
Calvin, John, 239, 1066, 1232, 1365,
  1373
  on abortion, 14
  on after-life, 252
  on contraception, 209
  on ensoulment, 14
  on marriage, 209, 1259, 1581
  on miracles, 1375
  on sickness, 1366
  virtue theory of, 235
Calvinism, 432, 1133–1134, 1366,
  1400

Camara, Dom Helder, 1402
Cambodia:
  Buddhist health care in, 136
  forced migration in, 1305
  free medical service in, 665
Cameralism, 1235
Cameroun, population of, 899
Campanella, Tommaso, 1233
Campbell, A. G. M., 160, 736, 737
Campbell, Donald T., 1473
Camus, Albert, 1013
Canada:
  abortion laws in, 29, 998–999
  amniocentesis studies in, 1337
  bioethics movement in, 994, 996–
    1001
  codes of ethics in, 966–967
  contraception in, 213
  education in:
    medical, 993
    medical ethics, 1001
  eugenics in, 999
  grain production in, 495, 1223
  health care in, 618, 654, 993–994,
    998
  health care financing in, 611, 612
  health insurance in, 992, 994
  hospitals in, 992
  human experimentation in, 705,
    706–707, 994, 997, 998
  medical ethics, history of:
    seventeenth to nineteenth centu-
      ry, 964–967
    twentieth century, 992–1001
  medical licensure in, 964
  medical schools in, 964, 993
  net immigration in, 1221
  nursing schools in, 1004
  organ transplantation in, 997
  peer review in, 705
  Roman Catholic Directives in,
    1432, 1433
  specialists in, 993
  sterilization in, 999
Canada Council, 998
Canadian Catholic Conference, 996
Canadian Human Tissue Gift Acts,
  997
Canadian Medical Association
  (CMA), Code of Ethics, 966,
  995, 996
*Canadian Medical Association Jour-
  nal*, 1001
Canadian Nurses' Association, 995
Cancer, 169, 271, 1483
  breast, 1708–1709
  deaths from, 50, 51
  environmentally induced, 380–
    381, 382, 384, 1599, 1600
  gene therapy and, 519

  mass health screening and, 859
  prescription practices and, 323
  research on, 1494, 1496
  truth-telling and, 42, 1678–1681
  uterine, 33, 34
Cancer Institute, 1496
Cancer Ward (Solzhenitsyn), 1013
Candide (Voltaire), 240
Cangliamilla, F. E., 1525, 1660
Cannibalism, 139, 225
Cannula-shunt apparatus, 811
Canon of Medicine (Avicenna), 208,
  209, 786, 887, 1267
Canterbury Tales (Chaucer), 209
Canterbury v. Spence (1972), 773,
  774
Cantillon, Richard, 1226
Capacity, problem of, 597
Capellmann, Carl, 871, 1525
Capital (Marx), 480
Capitation, 1057
Capron, Alexander M., 705, 755, 756
Caraka, 664–665
Caraka Saṃhitā, 163, 172, 176, 177,
  663, 664–665, 870, 906–907
  text of, 1732–1733
Cardiac transplantation. *See* Heart
  transplantation
Cardiorespiratory death, 259, 292–
  294, 298–300
Cardiovascular disease, 50, 51, 62
  See also Heart disease
Cardozo, Benjamin, 755, 1154, 1198,
  1512
Care, concept of:
  value implications of, 145–149
  See also Health care; Medical care
Carnap, Rudolph, 448
Carnegie Foundation, 1033
Caro, Joseph, 248
Carpenter, William, 1140, 1143, 1661
Carrel, Alexis, 654, 1160
Carrier screening, 568–569
Carritt, E. F., 415, 421
Carroll, James, 687
Carroll House, Johns Hopkins Hospi-
  tal, 1000
Carr-Saunders, Alexander M., 1228
Carrying capacity, 394
Carson, Rachel, 181, 370, 393
Cartesian dualism, 18, 112, 240, 361–
  362, 367, 370, 501, 502, 603–
  604, 1050, 1052, 1115, 1117–
  1119, 1206, 1426, 1427
Cartwright, Samuel A., 1405–1406
Cases of Conscience (Ames), 1365
Case Western Reserve University,
  875
Casework therapy, 1087
Cassiodorus, 939

Casti Connubii (Pius XI), 13, 212, 213, 1170, 1255, 1256, 1527, 1582
Castiglioni, Arturo, 792
Castration:
    Judaism and, 469, 796
    in National Socialist Germany, 1016, 1018
    Roman Catholicism and, 1526
    of sexual offenders, 1348
Castro, Rodericus à, 954–955, 956
Casuistry, 1365
Cataracts, inherited, 474
Catastrophic Health Insurance Plan Act of 1974, 640
Catel, Werner, 983
Catharism, 208–209
Catherine of Siena, 209
Catholic Hospital Association, 281, 996, 1432
Catholic Medical Quarterly, 1522
Catholic Theological Society of America, 1434
Cattell, Raymond B., 1308
Causal explanation, 129, 1399–1400
Causal theory of mind, *See* Functionalism
Cause, scientific conception of, 503
Cavendish, Henry, 1543
Celibacy, 1578, 1581
Cell fusion and hybridization, 517–518, 523
Celsus, 685–686, 690, 935
Center for Bioethics, Kennedy Institute of Ethics, Georgetown University, 1000, 1001, 1193
Center for Interdisciplinary Research, University of Bielefeld, 985–986
Center for the Study of Democratic Institutions, 1638
Central African Republic, population of, 899
Central America:
    population growth in, 1228
    taboo illness in, 1122
    See also specific countries
Central Europe:
    medical ethics in nineteenth century, 968–970
    temporary migrants in, 1221
Centralized choice, 1647, 1648
Centrifugation, 1441, 1449
Cephalic reflexes, pronouncement of death and, 293, 294
Cerebral circulation, pronouncement of death and, 294, 295, 296, 300
Cerebral death, *See* Brain death
Cerletti, U., 359
Ceylon, *See* Sri Lanka
Chadwick, Sir Edwin, 627, 1394, 1662
Chamberlain–Kahn Act of 1918, 1493

Chamberlen, Peter, III, 1714
Chamousset, 958, 959
Chang Chieh-pin, 203
Chang Kao, 915
Chan-Kuo (Warring States period), 376
Chaplains, 1191–1192, 1367
Character armor, 1085
Charaka Saṃhitā, See Caraka Saṃhitā
Charcot, Jean-Martin, 1124, 1661
Charisma, 878
Charity:
    Christian, 939–942, 958, 1149
    food policy and, 499
Charity care, 651–652
Charlatans, 954, 957, 1395
Charleton, 489
Chateauneuf, L. F. Benoiston de, 972
Chaucer, Geoffrey, 209
Chauliac, Guy de, 941, 949
Chemical weapons, 1699–1700, 1702
Chemistry, reduction of mental phenomena to, *See* Reductionism
Chemotherapy, *See* Psychopharmacology
Ch'en Shih-kung, 165, 177, 916
Cherubino de Siena, 209
Cheselden, William, 1660
Chesler, Phyllis, 1710
Chest X-rays, 857–858, 862
Chiavacci, 19
Ch'ien-chin fang (Sun Ssu-miao), 913–914, 1636
Child abuse, 151, 152
Child guidance movement, 1080
Childlessness, motivation for, 1706–1707
Child-rearing, 63, 104–106, 121–122
Children:
    anthropological perspective on death of, 225–226
    definitional problems, 150
    experimentation on, 152–155, 759, 819, 820, 1497, 1648
    health care and, 151–152
    historical aspects, 151
    hyperkinetic, 1199, 1383–1384, 1388
    legitimacy of, artificial insemination and, 1445, 1468
    organ donation and, 1154, 1157
    proxy consent and, 153–155, 491, 577, 759
    rights of, 1512
    right to refuse medical care and, 1198, 1505
    sex research and, 1554
    sexual development in, 1570–1572
    socialization of, 1590
    See also Adolescents; Infants
Chile:
    health status by level of per capita income in, 1321
    Protomedicato in, 1005

China:
    abortion in, 915, 918
    acupuncture in, 912
    ancestral medicine in, 912
    Buddhism in, *See* Buddhism
    child abuse in, 151
    codes of ethics in, 165, 905–906, 918–919
    Confucianism in, *See* Confucianism
    contraception in, 210
    death, conceptions of, 230–231
    demonic medicine in, 912
    disposal of cadavers in, 142
    environment and man, conceptions of, 374–379
    forced migration in, 1305
    health and disease, conception of, 581
    heart transplantation in, 655
    infanticide in, 210, 226, 742
    magico–religious medicine in, 1655
    medical ethics, history of, 902–906, 911–921
        contemporary, 917–921; *See also* People's Republic of China
        prerepublican, 903–906, 911–916
    missionary activity in, 1367
    population policy in, 1234–1235, 1296
    suicide in, 1622
    Taoism in, *See* Taoism
    Western physicians in, 918
    women health professionals in, 1713, 1717
    See also People's Republic of China
China Medical Association, 918–919
Chiropractors, 1175, 1317
Chi-tsang, 375
Chloramphenicol, 721
Chloroprothixene, 1379
Chlorpromazine, 999, 1354, 1379
Cholera experiments, 688
Cholinesterase deficiency, 474
Chomsky, Noam, 113–114, 503, 1423
Choron, Jacques, 236, 239
Chou, Shelley N., 293
Chou dynasty, 230
Christian Church Fathers, 6
Christianity, 1064
    abortion and, 825
    agapic love in, 431
    authoritarian elements in ethics of, 402
    cryonics and, 218
    death and, 239
        biblical thought, 245–246
        post-biblical thought, 249–253, 256–257
    deontological theory in, 413–414
    disposal of cadavers and, 142
    doctrine of rewards and punishments in, 436
    eugenics and, 471–472

euthanasia and, 274–275
exorcism and, 1121
as healing faith, 1122–1123
health and disease, conception of, 582, 588
homosexuality and, 672
infanticide and, 743
influence on North American medical ethics, 963
informed consent and, 755
life as divine gift in, 525
love, concept of, 1657
man's dominion over nature and, 397–398
medieval medical ethics and, 938–950
mental health and, 1065, 1068–1070
Oath of Hippocrates and, 164
pain and, 1186–1187
penal understanding of disease and, 1122
purpose in the universe and, 1400, 1401–1403
sexual ethics and, 1578–1583, 1592–1593
status of the aged and, 58, 59–60
suffering and, 1186–1187
theological ethics and, 429
therapeutic relationship and, 1656–1660
value of life and, 825–826
virtue theory of theological ethics and, 435
visitation of the sick and, 1191
See also Eastern Orthodox Christianity; Protestantism; Roman Catholicism
Christian Science, 1174, 1175, 1361, 1377
alcohol use and, 70
faith healing in, 1123, 1124, 1126, 1365, 1377
pain and, 1183
Chromosomal abnormalities, 531–533, 543, 568, 571, 1333
Chromosomal sex, 1590
Chromosome screening, 568
Chronic illness, 156–158, 595, 615
care for, 157–158
in France, 971
iatrogenic disease and, 323
incidence of, 156
normalization as ethical problem, 158
poverty and, 1056, 1317
properties of, 157
Chuang-tzu, 374, 375, 903, 1631, 1633
Chuang-tzu, 1631, 1634
Chu Hsi, 202–203

Church, Frank, 1142
Church Dogmatics (Barth), 1369
Churches' Council of Healing, 1125
Church of Christ, Scientist, 589
See also Christian Science
Ciba Foundation (Great Britain), 988
Cicchetti, Charles, 394
Cicero, 1233
on aging, 59
on man's dominion over nature, 367
on moral vs. legal status, 818
on natural law, 442, 443, 1131, 1132
on truth-telling, 934
Cigarette smoking, *See* Smoking
Citation of references, 193
Citrullinemia, 474
City of God, The (Augustine), 251
City of the Sun (Campanella), 1233
Civic harms, population policy and, 1243
Civil commitment, 763–765, 779, 1072–1073, 1103–1105
Civil disobedience, 159–161
dissent in medicine, 161
in health services, 159–161
meaning of, 159
Civil liberties, 1238–1239
Civil rights, 625, 626, 1072, 1105, 1106, 1111–1112, 1201, 1408, 1409
Civil Service Commission, 1565
Claims:
generic concept of, 1508–1509
rights in bioethics as, 1511–1513
Classical conditioning, 101, 107, 109
Classical psychoanalysis, 1084
Clean Air Act, 577
Cleft lip and palate, 719
Clement of Alexandria, 207, 943, 1524
Clement III, Pope, 944
Clement VI, Pope, 140
Clergy, *See* Pastoral ministry
Clergy-psychotherapist, 1191
Client-centered therapy, 1085–1086
Client characterization, 561
Clinical education, 868–869
Clinical research, *See* Biomedical research; Human experimentation
Clinical Research, 1001
Clinician:
pastor distinguished from, 1069
researcher distinguished from, 43
Clinic population, mass health screening of, 862
Clinics:
clergy roles in, 1190
in Eastern Europe, 978

response of, to alcoholics, 73
See also Hospitals
Clock-tampering, 52–53
Cloning, 518, 549, 855, 999, 1027, 1450–1453, 1644
ethical issues, 1453, 1462–1463
legal aspects, 1464–1465
nuclear transplantation and, 518, 1452
social issues, 1453
Club of Rome, 370
Cluff, Leighton, 323
CMA, *See* Canadian Medical Association
CMHC, *See* Community Mental Health Centers
Cnidian School, 581
Coal workers' pneumoconiosis, 380
Coan School, 581
Cobb, John B., Jr., 389
Cobbe, Frances P., 77
Cobbs v. Grant (1972), 1679
Cocaine, 335
Code de la Famille, 1235
Code International de Déontologie Pharmaceutique, 1211
Code of Canon Law, 1523
Code of Ethics or Canons of Journalism, 180
Code of Hammurabi, 647, 792, 882, 884–885, 888, 1020, 1232
Code of Justinian, 672
Code of Medical Ethics for Catholic Hospitals, 1432
Code of Theodosius, 672
Code of Thuringia, 282
Code of Wuerttemberg, 282
Codes, rights established in, 1515
Codes of journalistic ethics, 180–181
Codes of medical ethics, 61, 120, 162–170, 172–179
advertising by medical professionals and, 44
in Canada, 966–967
Caraka Saṃhitā, 163, 172, 176, 177, 663, 664–665, 906–907
in China, 165, 905–906, 918–919
confidentiality and, 168, 169, 174–175, 177, 197–198
Declaration of Indian Code of Medical Ethics, 908
for dentistry, 313–315, 1727, 1728
text of, 1802–1804
ethical analysis of, 172–179
central ethic, 172–174
ethical languages, 172
ethics of professional relations, 178–179
specific ethical injunctions, 174–178
historical development of, 952–953

Codes of medical ethics (*Continued*)
  human experimentation and, 168, 703, 1479
  institutional responsibility and, 681
  Islamic, 893
  in Latin America, 1005–1006
  in Lebanon, 889
  medical prayers, 162–163
  oaths for physicians, 163–165
    See also Oath of Hippocrates
  from outside the profession, 169
  texts of, 1741–1763
  truth-telling and, 176–177, 1682–1683
  in United States, 959, 965–967, 995
    See also American Medical Association: Code of Ethics of
  See also Religious directives in medical ethics
Codes of nursing ethics:
  of American Nurses' Association, 1138–1139, 1142, 1143, 1727
    text of, 1789–1799
  of International Council of Nurses, 1139
    text of, 1788–1789
Codes of pharmaceutical ethics, 1211–1212, 1726, 1728–1729
    text of, 1806
Codes of specialty health-care associations, 1725–1729
    text of, 1788–1815
Codes of the health-care professions
  abortion and, 1726–1727
  commercial aspects of, 1730
  common features of, 1725–1726
  confidentiality and, 1727
  death and dying and, 1728
  human experimentation and, 1727
  patients' rights and, 1728–1729
  policy statements on ethical issues of, 1729
  research and, 1727
  See also Codes of medical ethics; Codes of nursing ethics; Codes of pharmaceutical ethics; Codes of specialty health-care associations
Code theory of pain, 1178
Codification in the sciences, 1545
Codronchi, Giovanni, 954
Coercion:
  behavior control and, 94, 96–97, 99, 104
  human experimentation and, 1198, 1472
  informed consent and, 757, 758, 763–766, 782
  legislation of morality and, 819, 820–821
  mass health screening and, 862
  organ donation and, 1157
  population policy and, 1217, 1237,

1245–1246, 1262, 1275, 1277–1278, 1293, 1302
    See also Compulsory population control programs; Paternalism
Cognition:
  development of, 1570–1574
  informed consent and, 768
  menstruation and, 1707–1708
  personhood and, 746
Cognitive behaviorists, 108
Cognitivism, 448
Coitus interruptus:
  in France, 1229
  Islam and, 787, 1264–1266, 1268
  Judaism and, 205, 206, 796
  in primitive cultures, 1228
  rationalism and, 210
Coke, Sir Edward, 27
Colbert, Jean Baptiste, 1235
Colleges of Physicians and Surgeons (Canada), 993, 995
Collusion, codes of ethics and, 167
Colombia:
  code of ethics in, 1005
  distribution of physicians in, 1324
  health expenditures in, 1322
  health status by level of per capita income in, 1321
  population growth in, 1230
Coma, irreversible, 292, 293, 294, 846
Commentary on Genesis (Calvin), 1581
Commerce, U.S. Department of, 386
Commission and omission, *See* Acting and refraining; Double effect, principle of; Euthanasia; Omission and commission; Sustaining life; Truthtelling
Commission on Ethical and Religious Directives for Catholic Hospitals, 1434
Commission on Hereditary Disorders, 571, 574
Commission on the Teaching of Bioethics, 873, 875
Commitment, *See* Mental institutionalization
Committee for Medical Research, 1494
Committee of 100, 649
Committee of Physicians for the Improvement of Medical Care, 1039
Committees, review, 190–191, 280, 738–739, 752, 753, 755, 759, 760, 1145, 1198, 1490, 1495
Commoner, Barry, 372, 398, 525, 1703
Common law:
  abortion and, 27, 485
  death, definition and determination of, 297

euthanasia and, 282
  informed consent and, 771, 1157
Communication:
  between dying patient and caretakers, 290
  biomedical, *See* Communication, biomedical
  as criterion for humanhood, 835
Communication, biomedical, 180–194
  international, 643
  media and medicine, 180–188
    corrections, 187
    ethical problems, 183–187
    historical basis of journalistic ethics, 180–182
    human experimentation and, 190, 191, 708–709
    regulations, 187–188
    responsible journalism, 182–183
  scientific publishing, 188–194, 1001, 1542
    advertising, 193
    authorship and the by-line, 192–193
    of behavioral research, 1477, 1478–1479
    biocommunication ethics, 189
    citation of references, 193
    confidentiality, 181, 185, 189, 191–192, 1477
    editorial criteria for ethical research, 190–191, 1490
    establishment of priority, 189
    growth of specialties and, 1544
    human experimentation control and, 704–705, 1489, 1490
    multiple publication, 191
    patterns of information exchange, 1544
    peer reviews of manuscripts, 183, 189–190
    pre-meeting abstracts and oral presentation, 183, 193–194
    retraction and refutation, 192
    reward systems and, 1543
    in Western Europe, 985
Communication model of sexuality, 1593–1594
Communism (community), 1542
Community cancer, 380–381
Community development, 1322, 1324–1326
Community health centers, 67
  See also Social medicine
Community Mental Health Act of 1975, 1080
Community Mental Health Centers (CMHC), 1074–1076
Community Mental Health Centers Act of 1963, 1080
Community planning and organization, medical, 1043

Community practice standard, 1022–1023

Compassion, 147, 1661
  in Christian thought, 941
  informed consent and, 776

Compatibilism, 502, 504, 1425

Compendium Theologiae Moralis (Gury), 317

Compensation boards, 1024

Compensation for professional negligence, 1026

Compensation of experimental subjects, 708

Compensation of physicians, 611, 612, 617
  in Africa, 899
  in ancient Greece, 932
  in ancient Near East, 882
  in ancient Rome, 932
  capitation, 1057
  in China, 914
  in Europe:
    medieval, 941–942, 946, 947
    seventeenth-century, 954
  fee-for-service, 612, 617, 1056–1057
  productivity and, 1056–1057
  regulation of, 613, 882
  salary, 1057

Competency:
  informed consent and, 758–759
  mental, 781, 1105, 1106
  of physicians, 866
  refusal of medical care and, 1504–1506

Competition, physicians and, 45–46, 1543–1544

Complexity-consciousness, universal law of, 1402

Compulsion, freedom and, 94

Compulsory genetic screening, 574–575

Compulsory health insurance, 637–639, 652

Compulsory population control programs, 1299–1303
  ethical issues, 1301–1303
  genetic implications of, 1309–1310
  methods of control, 1300–1301
  population policy orientations, 1299–1300

Compulsory reporting of contagious diseases, 1396

Compulsory sterilization, 213, 574, 1706
  Draconian/coercive interventionism and, 1222
  ethical aspects, 1611–1612
  Hinduism and, 1272
  in India, 1301

in Japan, 928
legal aspects, 459, 1614–1616
of mentally unfit, 31, 459–460, 1108–1109, 1111, 1395, 1397, 1614–1616
in National Socialist Germany, 1016, 1018
paternalism and, 1199
population control with, 1222, 1301
in United States, 459–460, 1108–1109

Computers, confidentiality and, 197

Comroe, Julius H., Jr., 1489

Comstock law of 1873, 210

Comte, Auguste, 241, 265, 1402

Conception, beginning of human life viewed as, 14, 19, 22, 25, 1531

Concept of Mind, The (Ryle), 112

Concubinage, 1576

Conditioning, 101, 107, 109, 1086

"Condition of the Working Class in England, The" (Engels), 1394

Condoms, 210, 800, 1299

Condorcet, Marie Jean de, 240, 264, 265, 1226

Conferences:
  in United States, 1000
  in Western Europe, 985–986

Conferred rights criterion for beginning of human life, 17, 21–22, 23

Confidentiality, 194–199, 1357–1360, 1362
  American Medical Association on, 178
  in ancient Greece, 932
  biomedical communication and, 181, 185, 189, 191–192, 1477
  codes of medical ethics and, 168, 169, 174–175, 177, 197–198, 1727
  conceptual analysis of, 194–196
    essential elements, 194
    scope, 195–196
    value, 196
  dynamic therapies and, 198, 199, 343
  in Eastern Europe, 978
  genetic counseling and, 564, 575
  genetic screening and, 570–571
  Judaism and, 799
  limitations on, 199
  in medical care of adolescents, 41–42
  medical malpractice and, 1021
  medical police concept and, 958
  medical social work and, 1044
  Oath of Hippocrates and, 163–164, 932, 1359
  pastoral counselors and, 1191

in patients' bills of rights, 1203, 1204
  pharmacy and, 1212
  practice conception of, 412
  privacy and, 195–196, 1357–1360, 1362
  protection of, 196–199
    bills of rights, 198
    legal, 197, 198–199
    restriction of information, 196–197
    virtue of those entrusted, 197–198
  right to, 1511–1512
  Roman Catholicism and, 1530
  sex chromosome abnormalities and, 531–532
  sex therapy and research and, 1559

Confinement to mental institutions, *See* mental institutionalization

Conflict:
  abortion and, 23–24
  of interest, 404
  in medical decision-making, 309, 310–311
  of moral demands problems, 404–405
  of rights, 1512, 1513, 1515–1516

Conflict model of therapeutic relationship, 1666

Conformity to nature, 374, 376

Confucianism, 200–204, 901, 904, 911, 922
  conformity to nature and, 374, 376
  death and, 200, 230, 231
  heart transplantation and, 655
  medical ethics, history of, 903, 904, 912–916
  Taoism and, 1631–1633

Confucius, 202–203, 231, 374

Congenital defects, *See* Birth defects

Congressional Commission on Obscenity and Pornography, 1564

Congress of International Organizations of Medical Sciences, 985

Congress on Recent Progress in Biology and Medicine: Its Social and Ethical Implications, 985

Consanguinity, 467, 468, 470–472

Consciousness, 112, 118
  definition of death and, 299, 303–304
  technology and, 1639
  See also Mind–body problem; Personhood

Consensus hominum, appeal to, 403
Consent:
  informed, *See* Informed consent
  Judaism and, 799
  medical information and, 1362
  to organ donation, 1155, 1157, 1158
  parental, *See* Parental consent
  proxy, *See* Proxy consent
  rape and, 1709
  scientific publishing and, 191
Consent forms, 753, 756, 761, 1043
Consequentialism, 174, 415, 416, 418, 421, 423, 424–425
  abortion following prenatal diagnosis and, 833–834
  infanticide and, 747
  principle of double effect and, 318, 319
  treatment of defective infants and, 731–732, 834–837
  See also Utilitarianism
Conservation, 371–372
Conservative justice, 804
Console, A. Dale, 323, 324
Conspiracy of silence, 1021
Constantine, Emperor, 1226, 1657
Constantinople, 207
Constitution on the Church (Second Vatican Council), 1533
Constitution of the United States
  Eighth Amendment, 780, 783, 1072
  First Amendment, 47, 86, 780, 1159, 1466, 1512, 1514
  Fourteenth Amendment, 30, 574, 1072
  Seventh Amendment, 1025
Constitution on the Church in the Modern World, The (Second Vatican Council), 1432–1433
Constraints, freedom from, 93–95
Consultations:
  in ancient Greece, 935
  in ancient Rome, 935
  in Central Europe, 969
  codes of medical ethics and, 166, 167, 168
  in Great Britain, 961, 973
  in medieval Europe, 940
Consulting room, 1661-1662
Consumer movement, 1201
Contemplation, neonaturalist vs. technological humanist view of, 64
Contraception, 204–214, 1229, 1245, 1299
  in Africa, 208, 211, 899–900
  in ancient Greece, 205, 206
  in ancient Rome, 205, 206
  in Arab nations, 890
  Augustine on, 207–208, 209
  Catharism and, 208–209
  in China, 210, 919

civil disobedience and, 159–161
cultural impact of, 1282–1283
early methods of, 204–205
Eastern Orthodox Christianity and, 212, 353–354
in Great Britain, 990, 1261
Hinduism and, 205, 1271
in India, 211–212, 909
interventionism and, 1222
Islam and, 208, 787, 894, 1264–1268
Judaism and, 205–206, 212, 795, 796–797, 800, 1576
in Latin America, 1283
Manicheanism and, 207
medieval ethical thought on, 208–209
for the mentally retarded, 1111
modern developments in, 210–213
parental consent and, 38, 41
pharmacy and, 1213
potentiality and, 747, 748
Protestantism and, 209–210, 212, 1260–1261, 1436
recent issues in, 213–214
research on, 1711
Roman Catholicism and:
  Aquinas on, 209, 1226
  Augustine on, 207–208
  Directives on, 1433
  disagreement on, 212–213, 1532, 1533, 1582
  moral principles and, 1529
  natural law and, 1526
  in penitentials, 1524
  population policy and, 1254–1258
  principle of double effect and, 1213
  sterilization, 11, 169, 1256, 1257, 1433, 1526, 1529, 1533, 1609–1610, 1612
sexual freedom and, 1563
sterilization:
  in Arab nations, 890
  in Canada, 999
  compulsory, *See* Compulsory sterilization
  Eastern Orthodox Christianity and, 355
  ethical aspects of, 1609–1611
  government incentives and, 1291
  Hinduism and, 1272, 1609, 1610–1611
  hysterectomy, 1608, 1705–1706
  informed consent and, 1606, 1608–1609, 1616
  Judaism and, 795, 796, 800, 1610
  legal aspects, 1616–1617
  nursing and, 1142
  preconditions for, 1617
  Protestantism and, 1436, 1609–1612

Roman Catholicism and, 11, 169, 1256, 1257, 1526, 1529, 1533, 1609–1610, 1612
tubal, 1607–1608
in United States, 999, 1616–1617
vasectomy, 1606, 1607
Supreme Court ruling on, 211, 462, 573, 818, 821, 1358, 1615
women, impact on, 1706
Contraceptives:
  distribution of, 1282
  implants, 1301
  testing of, 1281–1282
Contractarian method, 805
Contract theory, *See* Social-contract theory
Controlled behavior, *See* Behavior control
Controlled studies, 699
Convulsive therapy, *See* Electroconvulsive therapy (ECT)
Conyers, John, Jr., 388
Cook, Joyce M., 757
Cooley, Denton A., 659, 997
Cooper, Alan J., 1554
Core conception of tissue, 1095
Cornaro, Luigi, 262
Cornea transplantation, 141, 799, 928, 1153
Corner, George W., 1714
Corporate ethics of medical schools, *See* Medical schools: obligations of
Corpus Hippocraticum, *See* Hippocratic Corpus
Corrections, medical reporting and, 187
Correns, Karl, 541
Cortical death, *See* Brain death
Corvisart de Marets, Jean, 972
Cosmetic surgery, Judaism and, 800
Cosmetic toxicity tests, in animal experimentation, 80
Cosmic decline, doctrine of, 662
Cosmic guilt, 562
Cosmological myths, 1400
Cost-benefit analysis, 1520–1521
  abortion and, 834
  advantages of, 1520
  criticisms of, 1520
  defined, 1520
  environment and, 381–383
  euthanasia and, 835
  heart transplantation and, 657–658, 1162
  life-support systems and, 847
  in mass health screening, 860–861
  self-realization therapies and, 1549
  treatment of defective infants and, 725
  utility of health care and, 631
  value of human life and, 824–825

values and, 1520–1521
Council of Biology Editors, 704
Council of Constance, 254
Council of Elvira, 10
Council of Europe, 983
Council of Medical Ethics (Japan), 929
Council of Orange, 1713
Council of Trent, 252, 1582
Council on Environmental Quality, 577
Counseling, genetic, *See* Genetic counseling
Counseling in Medical Genetics (Reed), 559
Counselors:
   pastoral, 1191, 1368
   women as, 1713
Counterinsurgency activities, 1478
Counterpulsation, 842
Countertransference, 341
"Country Doctor, A" (Kafka), 1011
County hospitals, 67
Cour de Cassation, 1020
Courtesy, 179, 1203
Courts, *See* Law; Supreme Court of the United States
Covenant, 755, 756
Crabbe, George, 1008
Crammond, W. A., 1167
Craniofacial anomalies, 719
Craniotomy, 12–13
Cranston, Maurice, 1507
Crawford, Johnson T., 1018
Cremation, 142–143, 144, 246
Crigler–Najjar syndrome, 474
Criminal Abortion Act of 1861 (Great Britain), 990
Criminal behavior:
   behavior control and, 99–100
   drug use and, 330–331
   genetics and, 544-545
   males with sex chromosome abnormalities and, 531
   nonconsensual mental health care and, 765–766
   psychiatric inquiry into, 1073
   sex offenders, 1554, 1559
Criminal commitment, 765–766, 779
Criminal responsibility of the retarded, 1112
Critical medical decisions, 308
Critique of Judgment (Kant), 258
Crito (Plato), 237
Croizier, Ralph C., 919
Crosby, Edwin L., 1044
Cross-linking theory of aging, 49
"Crossover" design, 696
Crow, James F., 1340
Crude birthrate, 1219
Crude death rate, 1219

Crude rate of net migration, 1219
Cruelty to Animals Act of 1876 (Great Britain), 77, 81
Cryobiology, 216
Cryonics, 210, 216–219
   defined, 216
   in Enlightenment medicine, 264
   freezing, 216, 217–218
   hibernation, 63, 217
   hypothermia, 216, 217
   moral issues in, 217–219
   sperm banking and, 1446–1448
      ethical issues, 1446–1447, 1459
      eugenic applications, 1447–1448
      legal aspects, 1447, 1465–1469
      procedure, 1446
Cuba:
   contraception in, 211
   family planning in, 1282
   health status by level of per capita income in, 1321
   public health in, 1398
   women health practitioners in, 1717
Cude v. State (1964), 151
Culdoscopy, 1607
Cullen, William, 583, 600
Cults of the dead, 221
Cultural attitudes:
   blood transfusion and, 133
   homosexuality and, 671–672
   infanticide and, 742–743
Cultural development, beginning of human life viewed as, 20, 21
Cultural impact of contraception, 1282–1283
Cultural implications of drug use, 330
Cultural justification for peak experiences, 337–338
Cultural privacy, 1477
Cultural relativism, 454–455, 1090, 1133
Cultural rights, 624–625
Cultural settings, privacy in, 1358–1360
Cultural variations in sexual behavior, 1560–1561, 1583
Culver, Charles M., 1196
Cunningham, Bert J., 1170
Cur Deus Homo? (Anselm), 251
Curing vs. caring, 148
Curran, Charles E., 19, 675, 1136, 1610
Curreri, Anthony R., 1678
Custom, ethics distinguished from, 401
Cynics, 238
Cyprian, 939
Cyrenaics, 238

Cyrus the Great, 885
Cystic fibrosis, 475, 476, 522, 563, 720
Cystinosis, 475
Czechoslovakia, organ donation in, 1158

D

"D & C" (dilation and curettage), 3, 4
Daily Prayer of a Physician (Maimonides), 162–163
   text of, 1737–1738
Damages, in malpractice suits, 1021–1022, 1025
Damascus, University of, 889
Dangerousness, mental illness and, 1103
Daniel M'Naghten's Case (1843), 1106, 1112
Dante, 239, 251
D'Arcy, Eric, 1136
Darling decision (1965), 678
Darshan, 878
Dar-ul-Fanun, 887
Darwin, Charles, 127, 369–370, 373, 457, 479–482, 529, 1134, 1307, 1536, 1543
   See also Evolution, Darwin's theory of
Darwish, Ziad, 889
Daube, David, 1172
Davenport, Charles B., 458
Davidson, Donald, 1422
Davis, Nathan Smith, 1031
Deaconesses, 1713
Deafness, 719
De anatomicis administrationibus (Galen), 76
De Anima (Aristotle), 237
Death, 221–295
   of the aged, 54, 57
      anthropological perspective, 226–228
      biblical thought, 243
   animal experimentation and, 79, 80, 82
   anthropological perspective, 221–228, 1048
      cannibalism, 225
      feticide, infanticide, and death of children, 225–226
      homicide, 223–224
      implications for bioethics, 228
      natural death and desire for immortality, 221–223

VOLUME INDICATOR

Vol. 1: pp. 1-484   Vol. 2: pp. 485-900   Vol. 3: pp. 901-1404   Vol. 4: pp. 1405-1816

Death
  anthropological perspective *(Cont.)*
    senilicide and death of the aged,
      226–228
    suicide, 223–225
    war, 225
  attitudes toward, 286–290
    of nurses, 1144–1145
    of persons facing their own im-
      minent death, 287–288
    of persons not facing their own
      imminent death, 288–289
    of professionals, 289–290
  codes of ethics and, 1727–1728
  definition and determination of,
    141, 292–307
    belief in human soul and, 302,
      351
    brain death, *See* Brain death
    cardiorespiratory death, 259,
      292–294, 298–300
    Christian, 253
    Declaration of Sidney and, 168
    Eastern Orthodox Christian,
      351
    Judaic, 801
    legal aspects of, 296–301
    philosophical perspective, *See*
      Philosophy: death, definition
      of
    reductionism and, 1427
    Roman Catholic, 1532
    in Soviet Union, 979
  with dignity, 253
    See also Acting and refraining;
      Euthanasia; Right to refuse
      medical care
  Eastern thought, 229–235
    Buddhist, 233–234
    Sinitic, 200, 230–231
    Vedic-Hindu, 231–233
  humanism and, 63–64
  of infants:
    maternal grief and, 486
    See also Infant care; Infanti-
      cide
  medical social work and, 1044
  population policy and, 1243
  truth-telling and, *See* Truth-telling
  Western thought, 235–260
    ancient Greek, 236–237
    Ars Moriendi, 253–255
    biblical, 239, 243–246
    conceptualization of human in-
      dividual, 255–256, 259
    early modern, 239–240
    Freudian, 255, 259–260
    Hellenistic, 237–239
    Kantian, 240, 241, 257–258
    medieval, 239, 251–255, 261
    modern, 240–241
    post-biblical Christian, 249–253,
      256–257
    post-biblical Jewish, 246–249

    recent and contemporary, 241–
      242
    scientific orientations, 257, 258,
      259
    See also Cadavers; Euthanasia
Death and Western Thought
  (Choron), 236
Death of Ivan Ilych, The (Tolstoy),
  1687
Death rate, *See* Mortality rate
De augmentis scientarum (Bacon),
  76
DeBakey, M. E., 659
Debray, Jean-Robert, 985
Debreyne, Pierre J. C., 1525
Debriefing of subjects, 1473, 1474,
  1475, 1480
Decarceration, movement toward,
  779, 1110, 1165, 1379–1380
Deceit, *See* Deception
Decent minimum of health care,
  633–634
Deception:
  in behavioral research, 1472–
    1474, 1477
  debates among philosophers
    about, 1684–1685
  in human experimentation, 760
  in hypnosis, 712–713
  intentional, 712–713, 1683–1684
  medical malpractice and, 1021
  misleading omission, 1685
  in sex research, 1558
  unintentional, 1683–1684
*De Christiana ac tuta medendi
  ratione* (Codronchi), 954
Decision making, medical, 307–311
  decisive medical decisions, 308
  euthanasia and sustaining life
    and, 278–285, 735–740
    consequentialist criteria, 836
    by hospital committee, 280,
      738–739
    for infants, 737–739, 836
    by patients, lay persons, and
      public bodies, 280–285
    by physicians, 278–280, 738
  formal theory in, 309–310
  general characteristics of, 307–
    309
  in genetic counseling, 561, 562,
    564
  humanization and dehumaniza-
    tion of care and, 620, 621
  infant care and:
    ethical perspectives, 726–735
    medical criteria, 724–726
  informed consent and, 755, 764,
    765, 844
    by patients, 771, 774–775
    by physicians, 771, 775–777
  interpersonal decisions, 308, 311
  intrapersonal decisions, 308, 310–
    311

  life-support systems and, 843–847
    continuation of care, 845–846
    initiation of care, 844–845
    termination of care, 846–847
    weaning from system, 845
  in medical ethics education, 873–
    874
  probability and, 768
  pronouncement of death, *See*
    Brain death; Death, defini-
    tion and determination of
  public involvement in, 386
  technological assessment and,
    1652–1653
  See also Diagnosis
Declaration Concerning Medicine
  and Human Rights (Japan),
  929
Declaration of General and Special
  Rights of the Mentally Retarded, 172, 1515, 1516, 1785
Declaration of Geneva, 164–165,
  172, 173, 174, 175, 177, 920,
  989, 1598, 1602, 1683
  text of, 1749
Declaration of Helsinki, 68, 153,
  172, 455, 656, 770, 928, 985,
  1486, 1487, 1727
  text of, 1769–1773
Declaration of Independence
  (1776), 624, 1512
Declaration of Oslo, 169, 1726
Declaration of Sydney, 168, 1728
Declaration of the Indian Code of
  Medical Ethics, 908
Declaration of the Rights of Man
  and of Citizens (1789), 624,
  1512
Declaration of Tokyo, 1347–1348,
  1356
*Declaration on Certain Questions
  Concerning Sexual Ethics*
  (1975), 675
Declarations, rights established in,
  1515
Decretals (Gregory IX), 943, 944,
  945, 1524
Decretum (Gratian), 1524
De distinctione mentis a corpore
  (Boerhaave), 1659
Defamation, 1021
Default, moral, 436
Default of obligation, theory of, 927
Defective infants, *See* Birth defects
Defense, U.S. Department of, 696,
  1702
Defense mechanisms, 502, 503
Defensive medicine, 1026
Defilement, sense of, 1585
Degradation, *See* Dehumanization
Dehala, Maneckji N., 885
Dehumanization:
  in behavioral research, 1476
  causes of, 621–622

connotations of, 619–620
images of man and, 856
in Nazi concentration camps, 1019
overprotection as, 757
technology and, 998, 1645
See also Depersonalization
Deinstitutionalization, 779, 1110, 1165, 1379–1380
De Institutione Reipublicae (Patrizzi), 1234
Deism, 210
Delafield, Francis, 967
Delgado, José, 91–92
dell'Olio, Anselma, 1611
Dellums, Ronald V., 388
DeMause, Lloyd, 151
Democritus, 236, 238
Demographic transition, 1228–1229
Demonic medicine, 587, 877, 878–879, 903, 904, 905, 912, 923, 1065, 1121–1122, 1128–1129, 1523
Denial of death, 287, 288, 289
Denis the Carthusian, 1580
Denmark:
    abortion laws in, 28, 31
    animal experimentation in, 78, 81
    organ salvaging in, 1158
    sterilization in, 1616, 1617
    women physicians in, 1717
Dental schools, 313
Dentistry, 312–315
    code of ethics in, 313–315
        text of, 1802–1804
    dentist–patient relationship, 313
    education, 312–313
    ethical issues in, 312–313
    social issues in ethics of, 313–314
Denturism, 312
De officio medici duplici, clinici nimirum ac forensis, hoc est: Qua ratione ille se gerere debeat penes infirmos pariter (Bohn), 955
Deontological theories, 174, 405, 413–417, 463, 835
    abortion and, 414–416
    contract theory, *See* Social contract theory
    Hebrew–Christian, 413–414
    Kantian, *See* Kant, Immanuel
    obligation and supererogation in, 1147, 1148–1149
    Oxford Intuitionist, 415–416
    quality of life and, 726–729, 833, 835, 838
    teleological theories and, 413, 417
De ortu infantium (Raynadus), 1545

Dependence:
    of the aged, 60, 61
    of children, 1571, 1572
    on drugs, *See* Drug dependence
    of fetus, 486–487
    of patient:
        on physician, 1705
        on therapist, 341–342, 343, 1557–1558
Depersonalization, 616–620, 1140, 1641
    See also Dehumanization
Depo-Provera, 1282
Depressant drugs, 336
Depression:
    antidepressant drugs and, 1380–1381
    electroconvulsive therapy (ECT) and, 359, 360
    manic, *See* Manic depressive disorders
    women and, 1709–1710
Depthelectrodes, 357
De relationibus medicorum (Fideli), 955
Dermatologists, 1680, 1681
Descartes, René, 79, 240, 361–363, 367, 370, 501, 1050, 1066, 1091, 1115, 1183, 1401, 1659
    See also Cartesian dualism
Descent of Man, The (Darwin), 127, 369, 479
Descriptive relativism, 454–455, 457
    See also Cultural relativism
Descriptivist theories, 447–448
    See also Descriptive relativism; Intuitionism; Naturalism
De Senectute (Cicero), 59
Design of experiments, 695–696
Dessauer, Friedrich, 1638
Dessoir, Max, 970
Detached concern, 596
Detail men, 322
Determinism, 501–506, 1207
    bioethics and, 505–506
    biological sciences and, 502
    defined, 501
    genetic, 545–546
    "hard," 503
    images of man and, 853
    physical sciences and, 501–502
    realm of freedom and, 503–504
    reductionism and, 1419, 1425–1426
    "soft," 502, 504, 545
Deterrence principle, 1022
Detoxification programs, 332
Deutsche Aerztevereinsbund, 970
Developing countries:
    contraceptive testing and distribu-

tion in, 1281–1282
economic growth in, 1322–1323
health care in, 1321–1326
health expenditures in, 1321
health status by level of per capita income in, 1321
per capita public expenditures on education, health, and defense in, 1323, 1324
population aid to, 1276–1281
population education in, 1311, 1315
population of, 1220, 1223
population–physician ratio in, 1323–1324
sex preferences in, 1443
urbanization of, 1306
Developmentalists, 1274
Devereux, George, 225, 226
Deviance:
    labeling of, 1100–1101
    homosexuality and, 670
    illness and, 596
    research on, 1478
Devlin, Lord, 820
Dewey, John, 241, 443, 1329–1330, 1539
Dharma, 661, 664, 1269, 1270, 1272
Diabetes, 80, 474, 496, 593, 859
Diabetes Commission, 1496
Diagnosis, 615, 1481, 1482, 1670
    development of practice of, 1656, 1658, 1661
    of homosexuality, 668
    of mental illness, 1098–1102
        labeling of deviance, 1100–1101
        mental illness vs. normality and physical illness, 1099–1100
        sick role and, 1099
        types of data use in, 1101
    prenatal, *See* Prenatal diagnosis
    screening distinguished from, 858
Dialectical method, 403
Dialogues (Gregory I), 251
Dialogues concerning Natural Religion (Hume), 480
Dialysis, *See* Kidney dialysis
Diamat, 1403
Diaphragm, 211, 800, 1299, 1563
Diazepoxide derivatives, 1381–1382
Dickens, Charles, 1080, 1716
Dicks, Russell L., 1367, 1368
Didache, 6, 10
Diderot, Denis, 240, 479, 1401
Diethylstibestrol (DES), 1706
Differential population growth rate, 1285–1290
    demographic perspectives, 1285–1288
    ethical analysis, 1288–1290

Differential psychology, 528, 529
Dight Institute, University of Minnesota, 559
Digitalis, 842
Dignity:
  of the aged, 61
  death with, 253
    See also Acting and refraining; Euthanasia; Right to refuse medical care
  electrical stimulation of the brain (ESB) and, 357–358
  prenatal diagnosis and, 1338
  right to refuse medical care and, 1500
  suicide and, 1624
  value of, 98–99
Dinkard, 883
Dionysiatou, Gabriel, *See* Gabriel Dionysiatou
Dioscorides, 205, 785
Direct abortion, 11, 12–13, 318, 1531
Direct intention, 425
Directives:
  for human experimentation, 1764–1781
  legal, 1645–1646
  religious, *See* Religious directives in medical ethics
Direct killing, 272–274
Disadvantaged populations:
  as research subjects, 1478–1479
  See also Minority groups; Poverty
Disagreement, ethical, 405
Disclosure, *See* Confidentiality; Informed consent; Privacy; Truth-telling
"Discourse of the Damned Art of Witchcraft, A" (Perkins), 1367
Discourse on the Duties of a Physician (Bard), 959–960
Discourses (Epictetus), 238
Discrimination, 802, 803
  on basis of personhood, 731
  in dental school admissions, 313
  inherent worth concept and, 620
  in mental hospital admissions, 1076
  racial, 398, 1289, 1306, 1319
  reverse, 867
  women and, 1707
Disease:
  aging and, 50, 51
  alcoholism as, 71–72
  anthropology of medicine and:
    ascribed cause of illness, 1046–1047
    catalog of recognized diseases, 1046
    usual treatment of illness, 1047–1048
  Christian attitudes toward, 938–939
  chronic, *See* Chronic illness

environmentally induced, 379–387
  birth defects, 381, 1335
  burden-of-proof and, 383
  cancer, 380–381, 382, 384, 1599, 1600
  chemical products and processes, 382
  chronic respiratory disease, 380
  cost-benefit analysis and, 381–383
  generation and interpretation of data base, 383–385
  mutations, 381
  nuclear energy and, 382–383
  psychobehavioral defects, 381
  public interest movement and, 385–386
  social medicine and, 1599
germ theory of, 1396, 1408, 1485
history of concept, 579–585
  ancient, 581–582
  medieval, 582
  modern, 582–584, 1481–1483
iatrogenic, 323
philosophical perspectives, 599–605
  discovered vs. invented concepts, 601–603
  ethical force of nosologies, 604–605
  illness and well-being, disease and health, 599–601
  mental vs. somatic disease, 603–604
religious concepts, 585–589
  divine healers, 587
  forms of healing, 586–587
  Hinduism, 663–664, 902–903
  human healers, 587
  instruments of healing, 587–588
  monotheistic biblical tradition, 587–589
  Protestantism, 1374–1377
  Roman Catholicism, 1522
society and, 1394–1396
sociological and action perspective, 590–598
  definition of health, 591–593
  health as interaction medium, 597–598
  illness and life expectancy, 593
  social distribution, 1056
  social role of sickness, 593–597
Disease models, 600–601, 602
Disinherited, The (Lucian), 933, 936
Disinterestedness, 1542
Disputatio de ministrando baptismo (Florentinius), 1525
Disraeli, Benjamin, 649
Dissection, *See* Vivisection
Dissent in medicine, 161
Dissertatio theologico-medica (Hoffman), 1660
Distributionism, 1222

Distributive justice, *See* Justice
Divination, 922, 924
Divine Comedy (Dante), 251
Divine energies, 348
Divine power, healing by, 587, 1122–1123
  See also Miracle and faith healing
Divorce, 1563, 1567, 1576, 1577, 1581
Dix, Dorothea Lynde, 1080, 1093
DNA, recombinant, 1490, 1493, 1497, 1641, 1645, 1646
  See also Gene therapy
Dobzhansky, Theodosius, 524, 528–529, 542, 1402
Doctor directories, 1201
Doctor-induced disease, 323
Doctor–patient relationship, *See* Therapeutic relationship
Doctors, *See* Physicians
Doctor's Dilemma, The (Shaw), 918, 1011–1012
Doctor Thorne (Trollope), 1009
Dodson, Ruth, 878
Doe v. Bolton (1973), 16, 30, 169
Doe v. Charleston Area Medical Center (1975), 1617
Dōgen, Master, 376, 377
Dogmatism, ethical, 402
Dogs, experiments on, 80
Dominican Order, 209, 254
Dominion over nature, 372, 379
  animal experimentation and, 81
  Bible on, 366–367, 397, 826
  Christianity and, 397–398
  Eastern Orthodox Christianity and, 1253
  growth of science and technology and, 367–368
  Judaism and, 397–398
  Protestantism and, 1260
  in United States, 368
Doms, Herbert, 213
Donabedian, Avedis, 1081
Donaldson v. O'Connor (1975), 1072, 1105, 1514
Donation cards, 1155, 1157–1158
Donation of blood, 987, 1153, 1154
Donation of organs, *See* Organ donation
Donation of ova, 1447, 1450, 1462, 1468–1469
Donation of sperm, 467, 1444, 1445, 1447, 1454–1460, 1462, 1465–1469, 1531, 1533
Donceel, Joseph, 18
"Do no harm" principle, 694–695, 734–735, 754, 760, 775, 1124, 1355
Donor–recipient relationship, 813
Doṣa, 663
Double-blind technique, 1488
Double effect, principle of, 33–35, 316–319
  abortion and, 3, 11, 16, 23–24, 25, 34, 318, 1529

contemporary debates on, 318–319
contraception and, 1213
description of, 316, 1529
historical development of, 316–318
rejection of, 1533
See also Acting and refraining; Omission and commission
Double Helix, The (Watson), 181
Douglas, William O., 198, 1615
Douglass, William, 686-687
Dowling, Harry, 323
Down's syndrome, 531, 569, 571, 718, 728, 732, 738, 834, 835, 836, 1108, 1111, 1144
Dow v. Kaiser Foundation (1970), 772
Draconian/coercive intervention, 1222
Draft Act for the Hospitalization of the Mentally Ill of 1952, 1103
Dreams, interpretation of, 85
Driesch, Hans, 129, 130, 241
Drinking, *See* Alcohol use
Dripps, Robert D., 1489
Droit à la mort, Le (Heuse), 985
Drug Act of 1976 (Germany), 708
Drug dependence, 328, 1104
   dispensing of drugs and, 891, 1213–1214
   institutionalization and, 1077
   public health and, 1397
Drug industry, medical profession and, 320–325, 383–384
   advertising and marketing, 322–323
   drug trials, *See* Drug trials
   Food and Drug Administration and, 324
   informed consent and, 321
   overprescription of drugs and, 323–324, 1382
   pharmacological education, 320–321
   See also Pharmacy
Drugless Practitioners Act of 1925 (Canada), 995
Drug-resistant disease, 323
Drugs:
   addiction to, *See* Drug dependence
   advertising of, 47, 193, 322–323, 1385
   in behavior control, *See* Psychopharmacology
   depressant, 336
   euthanasia and, 273, 274
   immunosuppressive, 323, 812, 814, 1160, 1161, 1162
   pharmaceutical, 1211–1214
   psychoactive (psychotropic), *See* Psychopharmacology

stimulant, 335–336
Drug trials, 1628
   blind procedures in, 695, 1488
   duration of, 321–322
   informed consent in, 321, 756, 1488
   insurance for, 708
   labeling and, 322
   prisoners used in, 1349–1350, 1353
   reporting and, 322, 383–384
   risks in, 756
Drug use, 326–338
   as abuse, 328–333
      criminality and, 330–331
      dependence and, *See* Drug dependence
      Eastern Orthodox Christianity and, 351
      rehabilitation and, 331–333
   behavior control through, *See* Psychopharmacology
   coma and, 293, 294
   moral attitudes toward, 326–328
   for pleasure, 327, 328, 329, 334–338
      acceptable euphoriants, 334–335, 1384, 1385
      cultural justification, 337–338
      depressants, 336
      stimulants, 335–336
      value issues, 334, 1384–1385
   privacy and, 1361–1362
   Roman Catholicism and, 1531
   for transcendent experience, 327, 336–337
   See also Drug industry, medical profession and
Drunkenness, 70–71, 73, 853, 1021
Duae Viae, 10
Dualism, *See* Cartesian dualism
Dubos, René, 371–372, 1061, 1062, 1320, 1485–1486
Due care, 1020, 1022–1023, 1519–1520
Duff, R. A., 34
Duff, Raymond S., 160, 736, 737
Dugard, Samuel, 471
Dukeminier, Jesse, Jr., 1416
Dunant, Henri, 972, 1696
Dunton, John, 181
Durham v. United States (1954), 1106–1107, 1112
Durkheim, Emile, 95, 222, 223, 265, 266, 1502, 1619
Durrenmatt, Friedrich, 1009
Durustpat (master of health), 885
Duty:
   absolute, 405, 414–415
   benevolence and, 959–960
   prima facie, 174, 405, 415, 438

public vs. private, 1503
to relieve suffering, 960
rights and:
   in bioethics, 1513
   generic concept of, 1509–1510
situation ethics and, 422–423
to the state, 957–958
in theological ethics, 429, 433-435
See also Deontological theories; Obligation
Dworkin, Gerald, 1196, 1197, 1518
Dyck, Arthur J., 1338
Dying, *See* Death
Dynamic therapies, 85, 86, 87, 89–90, 97, 338–344, 505, 506, 596, 603, 1094
   basic values, 339–341, 1085
   classification of, 1084–1085
   confidentiality and, 198, 199, 343
   for criminal conduct, 765–766
   defined, 338–339
   determinism and, 502
   development of, 1085, 1661, 1662
   genetic counseling and, 562, 563
   goals of, 1084
   hypnosis in, 713, 714
   informed consent and, 340
   medical profession's acceptance of, 1482
   philosophy of mind and, 1053
   reductionism and, 1427
   responsibilities of patient, 342
   responsibilities of therapist, 341–344
   sex therapy with, 1552–1553, 1584
   social role of, 344
Dyscrasiac conception of tissue, 1095
Dysthanasia, 979–980

E

Early Han dynasty, 376
Easson, E. C., 1678
Eastern Europe:
   medical ethics in, 975, 977–981
   medical ethics education in, 872
   population policy in, 1235
   urban growth in, 1220
   See also specific countries
Eastern Orthodox Christianity, 347–355
   abortion and, 350, 354
   aging and, 351
   artificial insemination and, 354–355
   basic doctrine of, 347

Eastern Orthdox Christianity (*Cont.*)
  contraception and, 212, 353–354
  death, definition of, 351
  divine power, healing by, 1123
  doctrinal teachings of, 347–349
  drug dependence and, 351
  eugenics and, 471
  euthanasia and, 352
  genetic counseling and screening and, 355
  healing techniques and, 588–589
  health care and, 349
  human experimentation and, 349–350
  justice and, 1253–1254
  life-support systems and, 351–352
  man's dominion over nature and, 1253
  marriage and, 1252–1253
  mental health and, 351
  organ transplantation and, 350–351
  philanthropy, doctrine of, 1253
  population ethics and, 354, 1251–1254
  protection of life and, 349–352
  rights of patients and, 349
  sexuality and, 352–353
  transmission of life and, 352–355
Eastern thought, *See* Buddhism; Confucianism; Hinduism; Taoism
East Germany, *See* Germany
Eastman, Nicholson J., 1606
Eccles, Sir John C., 191, 303, 501, 502
Eckhart, Meister, 336
Eclecticism, 1173, 1174
École Polytechnique, 887
Ecological harms, population policy and, 1243
Ecological limits, population policy and, 1245, 1248
Ecological resiliency, 394
Ecology, *See* Environmental ethics; Environment and man
Ecology movement, 369–371
Economic effects of drug use, 329–330
Economic growth, 1322–1323
  environment and, 392–398
    criticism of traditional ethos and its ethics, 397–398
    debate among economists, 393–394
    global survival and, 395–397
    nature of the problem, 393
    obligation to future generations and, 397
    types of limits, 394–395
  population policy and, 1217, 1222, 1223, 1227–1228, 1230, 1234, 1235, 1237, 1243–1245, 1274
  public health and, 1397–1398

Economic rights, 624–627
ECT, *See* Electroconvulsive therapy
Ecuador:
  health expenditures in, 1322
  health status by level of per capita income in, 1321
Eddy, Mary Baker, 589, 1123, 1174, 1377
Edelstein, Ludwig, 173–174, 176, 930, 933, 935
Edict of Milan, 1657
Editorial criteria for ethical research, 190–191
Editorial revision, 193
Education:
  behavior control and, 86, 90–92
  dental, 312–313
  in genetic counseling process, 561
  health, 613, 615, 1396
  health status and, 1318–1319
  medical, 863–869
    in Africa, 898, 899
    American Medical Association and, 993, 1031, 1037–1038
    in Canada, 964, 993
    in China, 918
    in France, 972
    human experimentation control and, 703
    institutional ethics, 869
    ministers in, 1192–1193
    North American, 967
    obligations to faculty, students, and patients, 867–869
    obligations to society in general, 865–867
    philosophy and ethos of, 863–864
    social medicine in, 1601–1602
    sources and nature of obligations, 864–865
    in United States, 993, 1031, 1032–1033
  medical ethics, 870–875
    in Arab nations, 889
    in Canada, 1001
    concepts and goals of, 873–875
    contemporary, 871–873
    in Eastern Europe, 980–981
    in Germany, 984–985
    in Great Britain, 872, 988
    history of, 871
    in Latin America, 1006–1007
    in People's Republic of China, 872, 919–920
    in United States, 871, 872–873, 1001
    in Western Europe, 984–985
  nursing, 1138, 1139–1140
  per capita public expenditures on, 1323, 1324
  pharmacological, 320–321
  population, 1311–1316
    defined, 1311–1312

    goals of, 1312–1313
    population policy and, 1315–1316
    values in planning and implementation, 1313–1315
  sex, 1282–1283, 1566
Edwards, Jonathan, 436, 1066
Edwards, R. G., 1456, 1460–1461
Edwin Smith Papyrus, 580, 581, 881
EEG, *See* Electroencephalogram
Efficacy:
  genetic therapy and, 515
  good will and, 504
  heart transplantation and, 656–657
  of life-support systems, 845, 847
  of sex therapy, 1554
Egalitarianism, 635, 636, 1238
Eger, Akiva, 212
Egoism, ethical, 418, 419
Egoistic suicide, 1619
Ego therapies, 1084–1085
Egypt:
  health status by level of per capita income and, 1321
  population growth in, 1228, 1230
Egypt, ancient:
  abortion in, 882
  authoritarian elements in ethics of, 402
  contraception in, 204–205
  divine healing in, 1123
  entombment practices in, 142
  euthanasia in, 881–882
  healers in, 587
  health and disease, conception of, 580–581
  magico-religious medicine in, 1655
  medical ethics, history of, 880–883
  regulation of medical profession in, 882
  suicide in, 881–882
  women physicians in, 1713
Ehrlich, Paul R., 213, 370
Eichmann, Adolf, 1061
Einstein, Albert, 257, 482, 1403
Eisenstadt v. Baird (1972), 211, 462, 1615
EKG, *See* Electrocardiogram
Ekken, Kaibara, 924
Elamite civilization, 884–885
Elder, Robert E., Jr., 1283
Elderly, *See* Aging and the aged
Electrical stimulation of the brain (ESB), 85, 91, 97, 98, 356–358, 551
  ethical issues, 357–358
  reductionism and, 1427
  state of the art, 357
Electric shock:
  in animal experimentation, 80
  in human experimentation, 1474–1475, 1476

Electrocardiogram, 490, 862
Electroconvulsive therapy (ECT), 86, 87, 91, 359–361, 1087, 1381
  bioethical problems associated with, 359–360
  informed consent and, 360, 765
  in mental hospitals, 360, 1073
  nature and effect of treatment, 359
  prisoners and, 1347
Electroencephalogram (EEG), 293, 294, 296
Electrophoresis, 1441
Elements of Medical Logic (Blane), 1051
Elgood, Cyril L., 885
Eliminative materialism, 1116
Eliot, George, 265, 1009–1010
Elitism, ethical, 418, 419
Elizabeth I, Queen of England, 1366
Elkinton, J. R., 1001
Ellis, Albert, 1085
Ellis, Havelock, 1552, 1562, 1585
Elliston, Frederick, 1585
Ellul, Jacques, 212, 1538, 1583, 1638, 1639, 1640
Emmanuel Movement, 1367
Embalming, 141, 142, 144
Embodiment, 361–365
Embourgeoisement, 1227
Embryo:
  definitional problems, 150
  production of four-parent individuals, 519
  transfer, 1437, 1449, 1450–1451
    ethical issues, 1450–1451, 1460
    legal aspects, 1464, 1465, 1468
    motive for, 1450, 1454–1455
Emergency treatment:
  of the aged, 65, 66
  decision to initiate life support and, 844
  poverty and, 1318
  right to, 1204
Emergentism, 130, 131
Emery v. Emery (1955), 151
Emigration, 1219
Emotion, control over, 86
Emotional state, informed consent and, 768
Emotive meaning, 448
Emotivism, 438, 440, 448
Empathy, 42, 620, 621, 1574
Empedocles, 236
Emphatic reiteration, 97
Emphysema, 1596
Empiricism, 252, 1655
  See also Natural law; Science
Enchiridion Medicum (Hufeland), 969

Encounter groups, 1085, 1087, 1547, 1548, 1550
Encyclopaedia Judaica, 792
Endodontics, 1726
End-state values, 1275
Enemy of the People, An (Ibsen), 1010–1011, 1012
Energy crisis, 1642
Engelhardt, H. Tristam, Jr., 20, 730
Engels, Friedrich, 480, 1394, 1402, 1585
Enger, Erik, 985
England:
  abortion in, 14, 27–28
  child abuse and, 151
  contraception in, 210, 211, 213
  differential population growth in, 1286
  embourgeoisement in, 1227
  eugenic societies in, 458
  Industrial Revolution in, 1393
  medical malpractice in, 1020
  new towns in, 1306
  organ donation in, 1155
  organized medicine, development of, 1035–1036
  passive euthanasia in, 151
  peer review system in, 1495
  population policy in, 1235
  self-realization therapies in, 1549
  surgeons in, 615
  women health practitioners in, 1714
  See also Great Britain; United Kingdom
Enlightenment, 236, 240, 264, 395, 959, 962, 965, 976, 1401–1402
Ensoulment:
  Aquinas on, 18
  Aristotle on, 9–12
  contemporary perspective, 18
  Islam and, 1267
  Protestantism and, 14–16
  Roman Catholicism and, 10–12, 1524
  See also Personhood; Soul
Entelechy, 129, 237
Entitlement to health care, 631–633
Entombment, 142
Entralgo, P. Laín, *See* Laín Entralgo, P.
Environmental conditioning, *See* Genetic constitution and environmental conditioning
Environmental ethics, 379–398
  economic growth, 392–398
    criticism of traditional ethos and its ethics, 397–398

    debate among economists, 393–394
    global survival and, 395–397
    nature of the problem, 393
    obligation to future generations and, 397
    types of limits, 394–395
  environmental health and human disease, 379–387
    birth defects, 381
    burden-of-proof and, 383
    cancer, 380-381, 382, 384, 1599, 1600
    chemical products and processes, 382
    chronic respiratory disease, 380
    cost-benefit analysis and, 381–383
    generation and interpretation of data base, 383–385
    mutations, 381
    nuclear energy and, 382–383
    psychobehavioral defects, 381
    public interest movement and, 385–386
    social medicine and, 1599
  justice and, 388–392
    need for adequate theory of, 390–391
    public policy and, 390, 391
    rights, duties, and concern for, 389–390
    rights of human beings vs. rights of the environment, 389, 390
Environmental movement, 393
Environmental Protection Agency (EPA), 384, 386, 577, 1521
Environmental sanitation, 614
Environment and man, 366–379
  Eastern thought, 374–379
    action and change as reality, 376
    conformity to nature, 374
    contemporary implications, 378–379
    exploitation of nature, 378
    harmony with nature, 378
    love of animals, 377
    love of natural beauty, 376–377
    nature as the absolute, 374–376
    relationship between heaven and man, 376
    sentience of surroundings, 377–378
  heredity and, 459, 460, 577
  images of man and, 853, 855, 856
  law and, 1646–1647
  mental disorders and, 539

Environment and man *(Continued)*
  race differences in IQ and, 534, 535
  Western thought:
    continuing issues, 372–373
    dominion over nature, 366–368, 372, 397–398
    participation in nature, 368–373
    stewardship of nature, 371–372, 373
Enzyme replacement, 513–514
EPA, *See* Environmental Protection Agency
Epictetus, 238, 1065, 1578
Epicureanism:
  death and, 236, 237, 238
  freedom from constraint and, 93–94
  nature and, 369
  suicide and, 1620, 1623
Epicurus, 238
Epidemias, 1656
Epidemics, 890, 1394–1395
Epidemiology, 2
Epilepsy, 157, 1104
  in ancient Greece, 582
  electrical stimulation of the brain (ESB) and, 357
  electroconvulsive therapy (ECT) and, 359
  institutionalization and, 1077
Epilepsy Commission, 1496
Episcopal Church, 1365
  See also Protestantism
Epistemology, 20
Epistle of Barnabas, 10
Eppinger, H., 1018
Equal access to health services, 635–636, 653–654
Equalitarianism in practitioner–patient relations, 620, 621
Equality in distribution of resources, 613
  See also Scarce resources, allocation of
Equality of opportunity, 537
Equality theory of justice, 837
Equilibrium society, 394, 396
Equus (Shaffer), 1013
Era of Moral Treatment, 1080
Erasistratus, 75, 685, 935
Erhard, Johann B., 952, 953, 969
Erikson, Erik, 1068, 1084, 1570, 1573
Error theories of aging 48–49
Ervin, Frank, 1389
Ervin Act, 1103
Esalen, 1547
ESB, *See* Electrical stimulation of the brain
Eschatology, 251, 252–253
Eschbach, Alphons, 1525
Eskimo tribes, 223, 224, 226
Esmein, Adhémar, 471
Essay on the Principle of Population,

An (Malthus), 210, 479, 1226, 1227, 1234
Essenes, 206
Estate of Marriage, The (Luther), 1581
Eternal life, 245, 256, 257, 258
  See also Immortality
Ethical and Religious Directives for Catholic Health Facilities, 996, 1430–1434, 1530
  on abortion, 169, 172, 175, 176, 1434, 1527
  in Canada, 1432
  text of, 1755–1757
  in United States, 1432–1434
Ethical Basis of Medical Care, The (Sperry), 871
Ethical Committee of the World Psychiatric Association, 985
Ethical Culture, 1402
Ethical dogmatism, 402
Ethical drugs, 1214
Ethical egoism, 418, 419
Ethical elitism, 418, 419
Ethical legalism, 422
Ethical naturalism, *See* Natural law
Ethical nihilism, 454
Ethical parochialism, 418, 419
Ethical Principles in the Conduct of Research with Human Participants (American Psychological Association), 1727
Ethical relativism, *See* Relativism
Ethical skepticism, 402
Ethical universalism, 418
Ethics, 400–457
  biology and, 130–132
  codes of, *See* Codes of ethics
  defined, 877
  deontological theories, 174, 405, 413–417, 463, 835
    contract theories, *See* Social contract theory
    Hebrew–Christian, 413–414
    Kantian, *See* Kant, Immanuel
    obligation and supererogation in, 1147, 1148–1149
    Oxford Intuitionist, 415–416
    quality of life and, 726–729, 833, 835, 838
    teleological theories and, 413, 417
  environmental, *See* Environmental ethics
  evolutionary, 131–132, 1402–1403
    See also Evolution, Darwin's theory of; Natural law
  moral reasoning, 406, 449–453
    criteria of morality and, 450
    defined, 450
    mental health program evaluation and, 1082
    as practical reasoning, 451–453
  naturalism, 406, 439, 442–447, 458, 542, 1402, 1584

bioethics and, 444–446
    diversities in, 441–443
    images of man and, 852
    market, 1222
    Marxian, 443, 1222
    naturalistic fallacy and, 131–132, 443–444, 542
    personhood and, 1206–1207
    purpose in the universe and, 1400–1404
    See also Evolution, Darwin's theory of; Science
  natural law, 442–443, 446, 607, 608, 817–819, 1131–1137
    abortion and, 1338, 1526
    bioethics and, 446
    contemporary revival of, 1135–1137
    defined, 817–818
    diversities in, 818, 1131–1133
    illustrative examples of, 1131–1132
    naturalistic fallacy and, 1134–1135
    personhood and, 1206–1207
    principal objections to, 818–819, 1133–1135
    purpose in the universe and, 1400–1404
    Roman Catholicism and, 818, 1134–1135, 1136, 1524, 1526, 1532
    theological ethics and, 436
  non-descriptivism, 406, 443, 447–449
  objectivism in, 405, 438–441
    as guide to conduct, 438–439
    images of man and, 855–856
    rationality and desire, 440–441
    rationality and impartiality, 439–440
    See also Intuitionism
  relativism, 264, 438, 440, 448, 454–457, 1536
    cultural, 454–455, 1090, 1133
    descriptive, 454–455, 457
    distinguished from nihilism, 454
    images of man and, 856
    metaethical, 456, 457
    normative, 455–456, 457
    See also Situation ethics
  rules and principles, 406–412
    in classical ethical theory, 409–410
    general features of, 408–409
    in intuitionism, 415–416
    legal status and, 817–819
    moral justification and, 410–412
    in natural law, 446
    in theological ethics, 433–435
    See also Codes of ethics; Deontological theories; Teleological theories; Utilitarianism

science and, 1535–1540
  formulation of moral problems, 1540
  historical instances of influence of science on ethics, 1535–1536
  impact of technology, 1538, 1540
  moral problems aided by science, 1538–1539
  moral responsibility of science and technology, 1540
  theoretical conflicts between, 118–119, 125–126, 444–446, 1536–1538
  theoretical shifts in moral philosophy, 1539
  See also Natural law; Pragmatism
situation, 405, 421–424, 1135
  bioethical issues and, 423–424
  central thesis of, 456
  codes of ethics and, 177–178
  duty and, 422–423
  images of man and, 856
  love and, 422, 434
  moral decision-making and, 405, 411, 422, 423, 434
  theological advocates of, 421–422
  See also Act-utilitarianism; Relativism
task of, 400–406
  distinctive nature of, 401–402
  methods of, 402–403
  subject matter of, 403–406
  terminology of, 400–401
teleological theories, 417–421, 1134, 1399–1400
  criticisms of, 420–421
  defined, 417
  deontological theories and, 413, 417
  main problematic issues in, 417–420
  natural law theory and, 1134
  obligation and supererogation in, 1147–1148
  vitalism and, 129–130
  See also Utilitarianism
theological, 429–437, 732
  meaning of, 429–430
  method of authority and, 402–403
  obligation theory, 430, 433–435
  theistic orientation, 430–433
  value theory, 430, 436–437
  virtue theory, 430, 435–436
traditional, bioethics viewed as, 120–125
medical ethics case, 116–120

Ethics and Language (Stevenson), 453
Ethiopia:
  health expenditures in, 1322
  health status by level of per capita income in, 1321
Ethnic groups, counts of, 1285–1286
Ettinger, Robert C. W., 216, 218
Eudemos (Aristotle), 237
Eudemus, 932
Eugenic Protection Law of 1948 (Japan), 29, 211, 928, 929
Eugenics, 357–472, 538–539, 550, 834, 1277, 1308, 1309–1310, 1395
  in Canada, 999
  Christianity and, 471–472
  defined, 457
  in Eastern Europe, 979
  ethical issues, 462–467
    defining "desirable" and "undesirable" genes, 465
    defining genetic status quo, 464–465
    justice, 466–467
    minimal ethical considerations, 463
    objectives and means in practice, 462
    problems in changing genetic status quo, 465
    validating eugenic policy, 463–464
    value questions in genetic intervention, 462–463
  history of, 457–461, 550, 559, 1223
    background and origins, 457–458
    birth of movement, 458–459
    decline and rebirth of movement, 460–461
    impact of movement, 459–460
  in Japan, 458, 928–929
  Judaism and, 468–470, 792
  in National Socialist Germany, 460, 462, 541, 1015, 1016
  negative, 458, 460, 511–512, 550, 563, 1199, 1448, 1455
  obligations to future generations and, 463, 510–512
  paternalism and, 1199
  positive, 458–459, 460, 511, 1199, 1448, 1455–1456
  Protestantism and, 471
  purpose in the universe and, 1404
  Roman Catholicism and, 471, 472
  sperm and zygote banking and, 1447–1448
  See also Compulsory sterilization; Euphenics; Gene therapy; Genetic aspects of human be-

havior; Genetic constitution and environmental conditioning; Genetic diagnoses and counseling; Genetic screening
Eugenics Education Society, 559
Eugenics Society Record Office, 559
Euphenics, 474–478, 550–551
  defined, 474
  distribution of medical care and, 476
  genetic conservation and, 477–478
  genetic deterioration and, 475–476
  medical strategies used in, 474–475
  partially treatable genetic defects and, 476–477
  See also Eugenics; Gene therapy; Genetic aspects of human behavior; Genetic constitution and environmental conditioning; Genetic diagnoses and counseling; Genetic screening
Euphoria, *See* Drug use: for pleasure
Euripides, 236
Europe:
  medical ethics, history of:
    ancient, 930–937
    eighteenth century, 952, 957, 960–962
    medieval, 938–950
    nineteenth century, 952, 968–974
    seventeenth century, 952, 954–956
    twentieth century, 975–991
  medical ethics education in, 871
  per capita public expenditures on education, health, and defense in, 1324
  population education in, 1311
  population growth in, 1220–1221, 1223
  population policy in, 1235
  urban growth in, 1220
  See also Central Europe; Eastern Europe; Medieval Europe; Western Europe; specific countries
European Association of Editors of Biological Periodicals, 704
European Convention on Human Rights, 1499
European Science Foundation, 983
Eusebius, 939
Euthanasia, 32, 261–285
  American Medical Association on, 168, 279, 735
  in ancient Egypt, 881–882
  in ancient Greece, 261, 934–935

Euthanasia (*Continued*)
  in ancient Rome, 261, 934–935
  in Assyria–Babylonia, 881
  birth defects and, 151, 152, 160, 1109
    clinical aspects, 721–722, 724–726
    deontological theories, 726–729, 833, 838
    equality theory of justice, 837
    ethic of care, 733–734
    extraordinary means principle, 727–729, 838
    personhood theories, 726–727, 729–732, 834–836
    principle of avoiding harm, 734–735
    public policies, 735–739
    slippery-slope argument, 821, 836–837
    wrongful life theory, 835–836, 837
    See also Infanticide
  codes of medical ethics and, 167, 168, 171, 176
  in Eastern Europe, 979–980
  Eastern Orthodox Christianity and, 352
  in Germany, 969
    National Socialist, 267, 282–283, 426–427, 794, 846, 983, 1016–1017, 1696
  in Great Britain, 282, 283, 990–991
  historical perspectives, 261–267
    in Enlightenment, 264
    mercantilism, 262–264
    neopositivism, 265, 266–267
    positivist mortalism, 265–266
    Renaissance humanism, 262
  indirect, 34, 423
  Islam and, 894–895
  in Japan, 922, 928–929
  Judaism and, 793, 794, 795, 797–798, 801
  legislation of morality and, 819, 820, 821
  meanings of, 261–262
  medical malpractice and, 1026–1027
  medical social work and, 1043
  in medieval Europe, 942–943
  mind–body problem and, 1117, 1118
  naturalism and, 445
  natural law and, 446
  non-descriptivism and, 449
  normative relativism and, 455
  omission and commission, 269–277, 1502
    direct and indirect acts, 272–274
    ordinary and extraordinary means, 168, 176, 262, 270–271, 727–728

stopping vs. not starting a procedure, 271–272
voluntary and involuntary dying, 274–277
    See also Acting and refraining; Double effect, principle of
  paternalism and, 1197, 1199
  in Persia, 881
  potentiality and, 732, 835
  Protestantism and, 1369–1372, 1437
  public policy on, 278–285, 735–740
    decision-making by hospital committee, 280, 738–739
    decision-making by patients, lay persons, and public bodies, 280–285
    decision-making by physicians, 278–280, 738
    decision-making for infants, 737–739
    legal policies, 735–737
  purpose in the universe and, 1403, 1404
  quality of life and, 834–836
  reductionism and, 128
  respect for freedom and, 823
  right to die and, 37, 275–276
  Roman Catholicism and, 818, 942–943, 1531, 1533
  sanctity of life ethics and, 837–838
  situation ethics and, 423, 456
  teleological theory and, 416
  United States legislation and, 282–285, 735–736, 998
  utilitarianism and, 420, 835
  voluntary, 274–277, 280–285, 286–287, 290
    See also Right to refuse medical care; Suicide
  in Western Europe, 983–984
Euthanasia Bill of 1936 (Great Britain), 990
Euthanasia Educational Council, 280, 281
Euthanasia Society of America, 280, 282
Evaluation:
  in genetic counseling process, 561
  of mental health programs, 1080–1082
Evangelical United Brethren, 1596
Evangelische Ethik, 985
Evans, Frederick J., 711
Evdokimov, Paul, 1252
Evil:
  ethics of, *See* Normative ethics
  pain as, 82, 1182, 1183, 1189
  rightful causing of, *See* Double effect, principle of
  sex as, *See* Sexual ethics
Evolution, Darwin's theory of, 479–483

essentials of, 479–480
  eugenics and, 457–458, 483
  influence on ethics, 1536
  Lamarckian theory and, 482–483
  progress and, 481–482
  religion and, 480
  Social Darwinism, 458, 460, 480–481, 529, 1080, 1536
  See also Natural selection
Evolutionary ethics, 131–132, 1402–1403
  See also Evolution, Darwin's theory of; Natural law
Ewing, A. C., 421
Exchange transfusion, 842, 843
Excommunication, abortion and, 11, 12
Existentialism, 1085, 1539
  death and, 241, 242, 304–305
  man's participation in nature and, 370
  moral rules and, 411
Exorcism, 924, 1121–1122, 1128, 1376, 1523
Experimental manipulation, 1470–1471, 1477
Experimental psychology, 112
Experimentation, *See* Animal experimentation; Behavioral research; Biomedical research; Human experimentation
Experiments and Research with Humans: Values in Conflict (conference, 1975), 1000
Expert role, 1209–1210, 1669, 1673–1674
Expert witness, therapist as, 343–344
Explicitness in medical decisions, 307
Exploitation:
  of fellow man, 619–620, 645, 802, 803
  of nature, 368, 378
Exploiter (image of man), 855, 856
Extensive paternalism, 1196
External control, 108
Extortion, 97
Extracorporeal membrane oxygenator, 841–842, 844
Extramarital sex, 1581, 1583
Extraordinary means:
  codes of medical ethics and, 168, 176
  medical vs. moral use of term, 846–847
  quality of life and, 727–729, 838
  Renaissance humanism and, 262
  Roman Catholicism and, 176, 270, 271, 272, 727, 728, 1531–1532
  treatment of defective infants and, 727–729, 838
Eysenck, Hans J., 1086

F

Fabiola, 1713
FACA, *See* Federal Advisory Committee Act of 1972
Facial deformity, 719
Fairness, 1586
Faith healing, *See* Miracle and faith healing
Falk–Schlesinger Institute for Medical Halachic Research, 896
Falsehood, 1684, 1685–1686
False imprisonment, 1021
Family:
    genetic disease and, 475–476, 722, 728
    Hinduism and, 662
    relations of the aged with, 55–56, 60–61
    sexual revolution and, 1567
    women health professionals and, 1717–1718
Family medicine specialists, 613, 1661
Family Oracle of Health, The, 687
Family planners, 1274–1275
Family planning, 211, 213, 563, 1245–1246, 1249, 1289, 1296
    abortion and, 2, 23, 176
    in Africa, 899
    in Arab nations, 890
    concept of, 1299
    in Cuba, 1282
    education, 1315
    foreign assistance and, 1276–1281
    in India, 909–910, 1283
    policymaker acceptance of, 1300
    Protestantism and, 1436
    rights and, 1283
    in Taiwan, 1230
    See also Contraception; Population ethics; Population policy proposals
Family Planning International Assistance (FPIA), 1280
Family Planning Services and Population Research Act of 1970, 211
Family policy, 1229
Family therapy, 1087
Fang-shih, 1632
FAO, *See* United Nations Food and Agriculture Organization
Faraday, Michael, 1699
Farberow, Norman L,, 1619, 1710
Farmers' Daughters, The (Williams), 1013
Farrell, B. A., 112
Fascism, *See* National Socialism

Faulhaber, Cardinal, 1017
Fault, concept of, 1022
FDA, *See* Food and Drug Administration
Fear:
    of death, 289, 290
    informed consent and, 768, 769
    of pain, 1180
Federal Advisory Committee Act of 1972 (FACA), 386
Federal advisory committees, 386, 1497
Federal Bureau of Prisons, 1350, 1353
Federal Council of Churches of the United States, Committee on Marriage and Home, 1261
Federal Energy Corporation, 1646
Federal Insecticide Act, 577
Federal Reports Act, 1497
Federal Republic of Germany, *See* Germany
Federal Rule of Civil Procedure 56, 1024
Federal subsystem, 617
Federal Trade Commission, 45, 47
Federation of American Scientists, 1700
Federation of Jewish Philanthropies of New York, Committee on Religious Affairs of, 1429
Feedback techniques, 1547
Fee-for-service, 612, 617, 1056–1057
Fee-splitting, 167, 168, 1211
Feinberg, Joel, 507–508, 625, 627, 629, 1196–1197, 1352
Feinstein, Alvan R., 308, 756, 1051
Feldscher, 1717
Felix, Minucius, 943
Felonious intercourse, 28
Feminine role, 1713
Feminist Women's Health Center, 160
Fendall, N. R. E., 898
Ferdowsi, Abulghasem, 884
Fertility control, *See* Abortion; Birth control; Contraception; Family planning; Population ethics; Sterilization
Fertility control agents, 1300–1301
Fertility rate, 1217, 1274
    debates about factors affecting, 1221–1223
    demographic transition and, 1228
    of developing nations, 1220
    efforts to reduce, 1229–1230, 1234, 1235, 1245–1246, 1249
        See also Contraception; Family planning
    embourgeoisement and, 1227
    in India, 1271, 1321

    patterns in, 1219–1220
    per capita income and, 1321
    of the poor, 1317
    of primitive man, 1228
    sex selection and, 1439, 1443
    See also Population growth
Fertilization:
    beginning of life viewed as, 1460
    in vitro, *See* In vitro fertilization
Fetal biopsies, 577
Fetal blood samples, 577
Fetal development, 486–487
Feticide, *See* Abortion
Fetishism, 1592
Fetoscopy, 577, 1336, 1343
Fetus:
    care of, in Judaic law, 470
    definitional problems, 150
    –maternal relationship, 20, 485–488
        fetal well-being, 486–487
        interests and responsibilities, 487–488
        maternal psychology, 485–486
    research on, 489–493
        in animals, 489–490
        in cadavers, 141–142, 491, 492
        in Eastern Europe, 979
        ethical positions on, 491–492
        historical background of, 489
        informed consent and, 490–491, 492
        methods of, 489–490
        moral status of fetus and, 491
        regulation of, 492–493, 1497
        situation ethics and, 423
    rights of, 1337–1338, 1512, 1513
    screening for defects in, *See* genetic screening
    status of, 826
        contemporary debate about, 22–25
        fetal research and, 491
        Islam and, 894
        Judaism and, 5–10, 25, 795
        legal, *See* Law: abortion and
        medical perspective on, 1
        Protestantism and, 14–16, 24–25
        Roman Catholicism and, 10–12, 23–24
        See also Life: beginning of; Personhood
Feuerbach, Ludwig, 241, 1066, 1126
Fichte, Johann, 241
Fideli, 955
Fidelity, 149
Field experiments, 1471, 1476
Fienus, Thomas (De Feynes), 11–12
Fieser, Louis, 1700

Financing:
  health care, 610–612, 617, 627–628
  See also Health insurance
  research, 1488–1490, 1496
Findlay, John, 502
Finnis, John M., 1132, 1136
"First come, first treated," 1415–1418
First Continental Survey on Important Ethical Themes in Latin America, 1005
First-party insurance coverage, 1025
First-person quality-of-life criteria, 836
Fish catch, global, 495
Fisher, Bernard, 776
Fitts, William T., Jr., 1679, 1681
Five Commandments (Chen Shih-kung), 1735
"Fixation of Belief, The" (Peirce), 402
Fixity of cost, diagnoses and, 309–311
Fletcher, John, 485, 562, 1341, 1342
Fletcher, Joseph F., 825, 871, 996, 1193, 1368, 1416
  on abortion, 20, 1340, 1342
  on allocation of scarce resources, 1416
  on artificial insemination, 1457
  on cloning, 1462–1463
  conflict with Ramsey, 177, 1370
  on double effect principle, 318
  on euthanasia, 272, 731, 835, 1370, 1371
  on health-care delivery, 631
  on in vitro fertilization, 1460
  on love, 434, 1136
  on personhood, 731, 835, 1109, 1340, 1370–1371
  on sterilization, 1609, 1611
  on truth and lying, 1687
Flexner, Abraham, 1032–1033, 1716
Flexner Report, 993, 1032–1033, 1484, 1716
Fliedner, Theodor M., 985
Florentinius, P., 1525
Fluoridation, compulsory, 151
Flying Doctor, The (Molière), 1008
Fodor, Jerry A., 1421
Fogarty, John, 1495
Foligno, Gentile da, 950
Folk practitioners, 877–879, 1317
Followup, in genetic counseling process, 561
Food, Drug, and Cosmetic Act of 1965, 324, 997
Food additives, 1397
Food aid, 496–499, 1277
Food and Drug Administration (FDA), 152, 192, 193, 322, 324, 384, 577, 706, 707, 1384, 1518, 1521, 1711
"Food for Peace" program, 496, 497
Food policy, 493–500
  Eastern Orthodox Christianity

and, 1253–1254
  ethical frameworks, 497–499
  perspectives and policies, 496
  population growth and, 495, 496, 1222
  world food situation, 494–496, 1223
Food production, 494–496, 1223, 1326, 1398
Foot, Philippa, 318, 1135
Forced feeding, 1347–1348
Ford, Donald H., 1083
Ford, John, 72, 1582, 1609
Forecaster (image of man), 856–857
Foreign Assistance Act of 1971, 211
Foreign assistance programs, 1276–1281, 1297
Foresight, intention distinguished from, 35, 318
Forest Service, 371
Formalist Theory, 174
Former Han dynasty, 200
Forrester, Jay W., 395, 398
Forward-looking teleological theories, 418
Fost, Norman, 737, 738
Fourier, Charles, 1585
Four-parent individuals, production of, 519–520
Fourth Lateran Council (1215), 209, 940, 943, 945, 1523
Fox, George, 1123
Fox, Renée C., 272, 595, 596, 1169, 1665–1666
Fox, Sir Theodore, 1601
FPIA, *See* Family Planning International Assistance
Fracastoro, Girolamo, 582, 600
France:
  abortion in, 31, 1229
  animal experimentation in, 77, 80, 81
  brain death studies in, 296
  contraception in, 210, 211, 213
  definition of death in, 300
  differential population growth in, 1286
  eugenic societies in, 458
  health care in, 611, 652
  health insurance in, 638
  health-related expenditures in, 650
  Marxism in, 1402
  medical ethics, history of:
    eighteenth century, 958–959
    nineteenth century, 953, 971–972
  medical malpractice in, 1020
  organ donation in, 1155, 1158
  organ salvaging in, 1158
  population growth in, 1289
  population policies in, 1226, 1235, 1291
  public health in, 971–972
  scientific publications in, 985
  women health practitioners, 1714

Francis, St., 369, 371
Francoeur, R., 1456
Frank, Johann Peter, 627, 952, 953, 956, 957–958, 969, 1393, 1659
Frankel, Fred H., 713
Frankena, William K., 417, 422
Frankl, Victor, 1017, 1085, 1088
Franklin, Benjamin, 264, 1401
Fraud, 1021
Frazer, James G., 222
Frederick II, Holy Roman Emperor, 140, 946, 947, 1035
Free action, 93–94
Free association, 97, 342
Free behavior, *See* Freedom
Free choice, *See* Free will
Freedman, Benjamin, 1200
Freedom:
  the aged and, 60
  anti-aging techniques and, 64
  behavior control and, 87–89, 93–100
    effects of behavior control on freedom, 96–98
    free action, 93–94
    free person, 94–95
    free will, 95–96, 100, 502–503
    value of freedom, 98–100
  from bodily assault, right of, 1512
  of conscience, 1289
  electrical stimulation of the brain (ESB) and, 357–358
  genetic counseling and, 564–565
  migration and, 1275, 1304–1305
  personhood and, 1207, 1209
  population policy and, 1238–1239, 1245–1246, 1249, 1262
    compulsory control and, 1302
    governmental incentives and, 1293
    social change proposals and, 1296
  of the press, 180, 185
  rationality and, 1149
  reproductive, 1275
  of research, 83
  right to life and, 823
  selective abortion and, 1340
  situation ethics and, 423
  sociality and, 1604
Freedom of Information Act of 1967, 386, 1489, 1497
Freehof, Soloman B., 1457
Freeman, John M., 737
Freeman, Milton M. R., 226
Freeman, Walter, 1387
Free person, 94–95
Free will, 100, 105, 500–506
  behavior control and, 95–96, 100, 502–503
  bioethics and, 500–501, 505–506
  biological sciences and, 502
  environmental conditioning and, 552–553
  genetic determinism and, 545, 546
  images of man and, 853

informed consent and, 764, 765
philosophy of biology and, 130
physical sciences and, 501–502
psychology and, 502–503
realm of freedom, 503–504
reductionism and, 1425
"soft" determinism and, 502, 504
See also Determinism; Self-determination
Freezing of human bodies, 216, 217–218
See also Cryonics
Freidson, Eliot, 1666
Freigabe der Vernichtung lebensunwerten Lebens, Die (Binding and Hoche), 282, 983
French Edict of 1666, 1235
Freud, Anna, 775
Freud, Sigmund:
on death, 255, 259–260, 1536
on mental health, 1064
on morality, 1536
on psychosexual development, 1553, 1562, 1569–1572
on religion and mental health, 1066–1067, 1068
sexuality, theory of, 1584, 1585, 1587, 1593
on sexual object choice, 1591
on suicide, 1619
Freund, Paul, 807, 808, 1416
Fried, Charles, 148, 149, 196, 633–634, 1517, 1519
Friesen, Stanley R., 1678
Fritsch, Ahasverius, 955
Fromm, Erich, 1068, 1084, 1088
Fructose intolerances, 474
Fuchs, Fritz, 1336
Fuchs, Josef, 213, 1136, 1582
Fuchs, Victor, 1063
Fulgentius, St., 7
Fuller, J. L., 541
Fuller, Lon, 1135
Full ownership, 1154
Functionalism, 603, 1116–1117, 1119, 1421, 1422
Functional research on fetuses, 489–490
Fundamentalist Protestantism, 1365
Fürstenspiegel, 785
Fusion of human cells, 517–518
Future contribution factor, 809, 810, 1416, 1418
Future generations, obligations to, 507–512
concept of, 507–508
environment and, 397
ethical basis of:
Golding on, 510
justice and, 509
love and, 509–510
Passmore on, 509–510

Rawls on, 509, 510
social ideal and, 510
utilitarianism and, 508–509
eugenics and, 463, 510–512
images of man and, 856–857
legislation of morality and, 820
population policy and, 1223–1224, 1246
purpose in the universe and, 1403–1404
rights and, 1512–1513
risk and, 1519
sterilization and, 1611
Future of an Illusion, The (Freud), 1066–1067
Fyodorov, Nicholas, 266

G

Gabon, population of, 899
Gabriel Dionysiatou, 1252
Galactosemia, 474, 476, 574
Galen, 14, 76, 79, 582, 785, 786, 789, 931, 932, 934, 936, 937, 1091, 1375, 1656
Galen, Count Christoph von, 1017
Galenic system of therapy, 785, 786
Galenism, 1173
Galileo, 1699
Gall, Franz Joseph, 502
Galton, Sir Francis, 457, 462, 483, 529, 1233, 1307
Gamma globulin, 474, 551, 1494
Gandhi, Mohandas, 1271, 1272
GAO, *See* General Accounting Office
Gaon, R. Ahai, 1251, 1428
Gardner, Pierce, 323
Garland, Michael J., 734
Garnett, A. C., 421
Garrett, Elizabeth, 1715
Gas exchange in the lungs, 841–842
Gassendi, Pierre, 1115
Gassner, Johann Joseph, 1123
Gaston, Jerry, 1544
Gate-control theory of pain, 1178
Gateless Gate, See Wu-Men-Kuan
Gaucher's disease, 551
"Gaudium et Spes," 1255
Gaylin, Willard, 1000
Gay rights, 670, 673, 1565
Gebhart, K., 1018
Gehenio, P. N., 216
Gender identity, 669, 1552, 1554, 1571–1572, 1589, 1590–1591, 1594
Gene frequencies, 465, 475
Gene mutation, 48–49, 381, 465, 467,

476, 511, 523–524, 577
Gene pool, 475
General Accounting Office (GAO), 322
General Electric Company, 1292
General Medical Council (Great Britain), 44, 987, 988
General population, mass health screening of, 861–862
General practitioners, 613, 617
Generic prescribing, 1213
Gene therapy, 513–527
cell fusion and hybridization, 517–518, 523
enzyme replacement, 513–514
ethical issues, 521–527
advantages to individuals and to the species, 524–525
genetic liability, 521–522
human manipulation, 525–526
risk and consent, 522–524
social context of decision, 526
production of four-parent individuals, 519–520
via transduction, 516, 523
via transformation, 514–515, 523
See also Eugenics; Euphenics; Genetic aspects of human behavior; Genetic constitution and environmental conditioning; Genetic diagnosis and counseling; Genetic screening
Genetic aspects of human behavior, 527–547
genetics and mental disorders, 538–541
males with sex chromosome abnormalities, 531–533, 543
philosophical and ethical issues, 541–547
distributive justice, 543–544
history, 541–543
methodological issues, 547
research, 547
retributive justice, 544–547
race differences in intelligence, 533–538
elements of the question, 533–535
ethical implications, 535–537
state of the art, 528–530
field of behavioral genetics, 528–529
genetic aspect, 529–530
historical development of behavioral genetics, 529
See also Eugenics; Euphenics; Gene therapy; Genetic constitution and environmental conditioning; Genetic diagnosis and counseling; Genetic screening

Genetic conservation, 477–478
Genetic constitution and environmental conditioning, 548–554
  behavior control and, 551
  determinants of individuality, 548–549
  individual vs. statistical morality, 553–554
  influence of environmental conditioning, 550–551
  manipulations of the genetic endowment, 549–550
  person vs. social group, 552–553
  social factors in environmental control, 551–552
  See also Eugenics; Euphenics; Gene therapy; Genetic aspects of human behavior; Genetic diagnosis and counseling; Genetic screening
Genetic control, 169
Genetic counselors, 524
Genetic deterioration, 464, 475
Genetic determinism, 544
Genetic diagnosis and counseling, 467, 555–565, 837
  confidentiality and, 564, 575
  defined, 559–560
  in Eastern Europe, 979
  Eastern Orthodox Christianity and, 355
  freedom and, 564–565
  genetic diagnosis, 555–558
  in Germany, 985
  historical aspects of, 559
  law and:
    confidentiality, 575
    informed consent, 576–577
    licensing, 575
    privacy, 573–574
  medical social work and, 1043
  outcome of, 563–564
  process of, 560–561
  psychological and social considerations, 562–563
  qualifications for, 561–562
  reasons for seeking, 560
  truth-telling and, 558, 565
  in United States, 999
  See also Eugenics; Euphenics; Gene therapy; Genetic aspects of human behavior; Genetic constitution and environmental conditioning; Genetic screening
Genetic engineering, 526, 549
  biological reductionism and, 128
  images of man and, 854, 855
  personhood and, 1209, 1210
  See also Eugenics; Euphenics; Gene therapy; Genetic constitution and environmental conditioning; Genetic diagnosis and counseling; Reproductive technologies
Geneticists, bioethics and, 1000

Genetic liability, 521–522
Genetic load, 464, 467, 524
Genetics:
  aging theories based on, 48–50
  beginning of human life and, 19
  law and, 573–577, 1644–1646, 1648
    confidentiality, 575
    environmental hazards, 577
    genetic counseling, 575, 576–577
    genetic screening, 574–576
    informed consent, 576–577
    prenatal torts, 575–576
    procreation and privacy, 573–574
  population control and, 1307–1310
    evolution by selection, 1307
    selection generated by compulsory population control, 1309–1310
    selection generated by population growth, 1307–1308
    selection generated by voluntary population control, 1308–1309
Genetic science, 458, 459
Genetic screening, 532, 567–572, 1450
  allocation of scarce resources and, 571–572
  carrier screening, 568–569
  chromosome screening, 568
  confidentiality and, 570–571
  defined, 567
  Eastern Orthodox Christianity and, 355
  informed consent and, 570
  Judaism and, 470
  laws, 574–576
  newborn metabolic screening, 567–568
  paternalism and, 1198
  with prenatal diagnoses, *See* Prenatal diagnosis
  public policy and, 1343–1345
  susceptibility screening, 570
  truth-telling and, 571, 1198
  See also Eugenics; Euphenics; Gene therapy; Genetic aspects of human behavior; Genetic constitution and environmental conditioning; Genetic diagnosis and counseling
Geneva, Declaration of, *See* Declaration of Geneva
Geneva Conventions:
  (1864), 1696, 1697
  (1949), 1697, 1698
Genocide, 1641
  in National Socialist Germany, 267, 283, 1017, 1307
  population regulation with, 1277, 1307–1308

population replacement policy due to, 1289
Genotype, 530, 1453
Gentlemanly class, ethic of, 178–179, 963–964, 1029–1030, 1031
Geographic distribution of physicians, 865
George Brown College, Toronto, 1001
Georgetown University, 875, 1000, 1001, 1193
Georgia Medical College, 875
German Catechism (Luther), 209
German Democratic Republic, *See* Germany
Germany:
  abortion in, 28, 31, 985
  animal experimentation in, 77, 80, 81
  brain death studies in, 296
  contraception in, 209–210, 211, 213
  eugenic societies in, 458
  euthanasia in, 969
  genetic counseling in, 985
  health care in, 615, 652
  health insurance in, 611, 627, 637, 638, 641–642, 970
  health-related expenditures in, 650
  medical ethics, history of, 957–958, 969–970
  medical ethics education in, 984–985
  medical police concept and, 957–958, 969
  National Socialism in, 818, 979, 1538, 1700
    eugenics, 460, 462, 541, 1015, 1016
    "euthanasia," 267, 282–283, 426–427, 794, 846, 983, 1016–1017, 1696
    general state of medicine, 1015–1016
    genocide, 267, 283, 1017, 1307
    human experimentation, 619, 690, 697, 700, 1015, 1017–1018, 1512, 1696
    Nuremberg trials, 190, 1016, 1018–1019, 1135
    plea of "superior orders" and, 1696
    population policy, 1230
    prison camps, 1355
  physicians in, 615, 616, 714, 1717
  population policy in, 1235
  scientific publications in, 985
  women health practitioners in, 1714, 1717
Germ conception of tissue, 1095
Germ theory of disease, 1396, 1408, 1485
Gerontology, *See* Aging and the aged
Gerson, Jean, 254
Gert, Bernard, 405, 1196
Gestalt Therapy, 1085, 1087

Ghana:
  compensation of physicians in, 899
  distribution of physicians in, 1324
  population incentives in, 1293
Ghana, University of, Medical School, 898
Ghazzālī, al-, 431, 1266
Ghoos, J., 317
Ghostwriting, 192–193
Gibbs, Jack P., 1076
Gibbs, Willard, 1664
Gift, The (Mauss), 812
Gilder, George, 673
Ginzburg, Ralph, 1562
Girtanner, 489
Gisu society, 223, 224
Glaser, Barney G., 288
Glass, Bentley, 462, 1455
Glaucoma, mass health screening and, 859
Gleitman v. Cosgrove (1967), 576
Global survival, 395–397
Gluber, 1661
Glucosuria, 862
Gnosticism, 1064
  man's dominion over nature and, 367
  sexual ethics and, 206–209, 1578, 1579
Goal-directed action, 1399
Goal ethics, *See* Teleological theories
Goal-intended action, 1399
Goddard, James, 322
Godwin, William, 1226
Goering, Hermann, 1017
Goethe, Johann von, 240–241, 369, 1126
Goffman, Erving, 86, 1351, 1517
Goiter, 474
Goldberg, M., 654
Goldfarb v. Virginia State Bar (1975), 47
Golding, Martin P., 477, 507, 508, 510
Goldman, Emma, 159
Goldstein, Joseph, 758
Goodness, 1061
Good samaritan laws, 820
Good will, 504
Goren, Shlomo, 896
Gorer, Geoffrey, 242
Gorgias (Plato), 237, 1577
Gormley, William J., 712
Gosney, E. S., 1611
Goulet, Denis, 1279
Gout, 474
Gove, Walter R., 1709
Government:
  code of ethics, 167, 170
  financing of health care by, 611–612

incentives:
  population control and, 1290–1295, 1302
  technological choice and, 1646–1647, 1648
information systems, 197, 198–199
role in health, *See* Health policy
social programs, 1296
See also Health policy; Law; Public policy
Graham, Sylvester, 1376
Grain production, 494–496, 1223
Grant, George, 1640
Grant, Madison, 459
Grasset, Joseph, 1005
Gratian, 10, 472, 943, 1524
Gratitude, 174
Graunt, John, 1226
Great Britain:
  abortion in, 27–30, 990
  alcohol use in, 990
  animal experimentation in, 77, 78, 80, 81, 989
  blood donation in, 987
  consultation in, 961, 973
  contraception in, 990, 1261
  euthanasia in, 282, 283, 990–991
  fetal research in, 141, 492, 493
  General Medical Council in, 987, 988
  genetic screening in, 567, 571
  health care in:
    financing, 611, 612, 627
    policy, 652–653, 654
    regulation, 612
  homosexuality in, 990
  human experimentation in, 961, 974, 989–990
  legalization of narcotics in, 331, 332
  medical ethics, history of:
    eighteenth century, 957, 960–962
    nineteenth century, 952–953, 973–974
    twentieth century, 987–991
  medical ethics education in, 872, 988
  medical etiquette in, 987–988
  medical schools of, 988, 989
  organ donation in, 1158
  parental consent in, 151
  peer review committees in, 705
  pharmacy in, 1211, 1212
  public health in, 1392, 1393
  social conscience, development of, 987–988
  social ethics in, 991
  truth-telling in, 1678
  vivisection in, 974

women physicians in, 1715
See also England; United Kingdom
Greatness of Cities (Botero), 210
Greatrakes, Valentine, 1374
Greece, ancient, 930–937
  abortion in, 933
  advertising in, 933
  animal experimentation in, 75, 936
  authoritarian elements in ethics of, 402
  confidentiality in, 932
  consultations in, 935
  contraception in, 205, 206
  death, philosophy on, 236–238
  dissemination of medical knowledge in, 937
  divine healing in, 1123
  divorce in, 1577
  euthanasia in, 261, 934–935
  fees in, 932
  giving or withholding treatment in, 933–934
  health and disease, conception of, 581–582
  homosexuality in, 671, 1577
  human experimentation in, 684–686, 935–936
  ideal physician, concept of, 930–931
  infanticide in, 226, 742, 826
  influence on Islamic medicine, 785–787
  influence on organized medicine, 1035
  man's participation in nature and, 369
  marriage in, 1225, 1577
  medical ethics, history of, 885–886, 930–937
  medical etiquette in, 931–932
  medical malpractice in, 882, 936
  mental illness in, 1065
  population polices in, 1225
  public physicians in, 936
  scientific treatment, development in, 1655–1657
  sexual conduct in, 932–933, 1577–1578
  social responsibility of physicians in, 936–937
  status of the aged in, 58, 59
  suicide in, 934
  surgery in, 933, 934
  treatment of relatives by physicians in, 933
  truth-telling in, 934
  vivisection in, 935–936
  See also Hippocratic Corpus; Hippocratic medicine; Oath of Hippocrates

Greece, forced emigration and, 1304
Greek Orthodox Church, *See* Eastern
 Orthodox Christianity
Green, R. M., 22
Green, Ronald, 634–635
Green Revolution, 495, 496
Greenspoon, Shirley, 1679, 1680
Gregory, James, 961–962
Gregory, John, 871, 952, 953, 960–
 962, 973, 1030
Gregory, Samuel, 1715
Gregory of Nazianzus, 938
Gregory of Nyssa, 250
Gregory I (the Great), Pope, 251, 472
Gregory IX, Pope, 11, 943, 944, 945,
 1524
Grene, Marjorie, 502
*Grenzsituationen des Lebens: Beitrag
 zum Problem der begrenzten
 Euthanasie* (Catel), 983
Grief, 562–563, 734, 789
Griesbach, Eberhard, 421
Griffith, Belver, 1544
Griscom, John H., 1394
Grisez, Germain G., 18, 19, 316–319,
 1136
Griswold v. Connecticut (1965), 211,
 462, 573, 818, 821, 1358, 1615
Grotius, Hugo, 624, 625, 818
Grotjahn, Alfred, 1598, 1662
*Groundwork of the Metaphysics of
 Morals* (Kant), 504
Group differences, research on, 1471
Group for the Advancement of Psy-
 chiatry, 1068
Group health insurance, 638
Group practice, 614
Group practice prepayment pro-
 grams, 612
Group therapies, 1087–1088
 self-realization, *See* Self-realiza-
  tion therapies
 sex therapy, 1559
Group work, medical, 1043
Growth momentum, 1219
Growth therapies, 1087
*Grundlinien einer Philosophie der
 Technik* (Kapp), 1639
Grunwald, Max, 470
Guardianship:
 of incompetents, 1105–1106,
  1110–1111, 1505
 of medical knowledge, 867
Guardini, Romano, 1402
Guatemala:
 health status by level of per capita
  income in, 1321
 Protomedicato in, 1005
Guérin, Jules, 1598
Guide de la mort (Heuse), 985
Guidelines, professional, 703
Guild of Pastoral Psychology, 1125
Guilds, 947, 1035
Guillotin, Joseph-Ignace, 971
Guilt, cosmic, 562

Gunavarman, 376
Gury, Jean Pierre, 213, 317
Gustafson, James M., 24, 463, 1341
Gut feelings, appeal to, *See* Intuition-
 ism
Guthrie, C. C., 654, 1160
Guthrie, Edwin Ray, 108
Guttentag, Otto E., 1710
Gynecologists, *See* Obstetrician–gyn-
 ecologists

H

Habit, 108
Hadith Ash Sharif, 889
Haeckel, Ernst, 266
Haemmerli, Urs Peter, 279, 984
Hägerström, Axel, 448
Hahnemann, Samuel, 1030, 1173
Haiti, distribution of physicians in,
 1324
Halakhah, 1250
Hale, Matthew, 27, 1235
Hales, Stephen, 77
Haley, Jay, 1084
Halfway technologies, 1489, 1899
Haller, Albrecht, 955
Hallucinogens, 335, 336–337
Haloperidol, 1354, 1379
*Halushka v. University of Saskatche-
 wan* (1965), 997
Haly Abbas (Ahwazi), (ʿAlī ibn ʿAb-
 bās al-Madjūsī), 786, 887
 Advice to a Physician, 1734–1735
Hamburger, Jean, 985, 1171–1172
Hamilton, Alexander, 368
Hamilton, Bernice, 1137
Hamilton, Michael, 1459
Hamilton, William, 1456
Hammurabi, Code of, *See* Code of
 Hammurabi
Hampson, Joan G., 1590
Hampson, John L., 1590
Handicapped persons, *See* Birth de-
 fects; Chronic care; Mentally
 handicapped; Mental retarda-
 tion
Han dynasty, 200, 230, 376
Hanson, Norwood R., 503
Harakiri, 1619, 1622
Hardin, Garrett, 21, 370, 497, 1309
Hardware behavioral technologies,
 87
Hardy, J. D., 655
Hardy, James, 1162
Hare, R. M., 23, 411, 453, 1585
Häring, Bernard, 18, 24, 213, 985,
 1582, 1609, 1610
Harlow, Harry F., 1560
Harmony:
 Islamic concept of, 786
 with nature, 378

Harm paternalism, 1197
Harm principle, 1195, 1197, 1198
Harms, anticipated, population pol-
 icy and, 1242–1243, 1248
Harrington, Michael, 1317
Harrison Act, 330
Hart, H. L. A., 1132, 1135, 1196
Hartland, Edwin S., 221
Hartley, David, 1091–1092
Hartshorne, Charles, 302, 303
Hart v. Brown (1972), 153, 1154
Harvard Committee on Irreversible
 Coma, 293, 296, 302
Harvard Medical School, 1037, 1715
 Ad Hoc Committee to Examine the
  Definition of Brain Death,
  846
Harvard Program on Technology and
 Society, 1641
Harvard University, 875, 998
 Kennedy Interfaculty Program in
  Medical Ethics at, 1001
Harvey, John F., 674
Harvey, William, 1, 76, 77, 489, 583,
 692, 954, 1375
Hashish, 1384
Hastings Center Report, 1000
Hatcher, Sherry L. M., 39
Hathaway v. Worcester City Hospital
 (1973), 1617
Hauerwas, Stanley, 365, 733–734
Havighurst, Clark C., 631, 636
Hawi (Razi), 1267
Hawkins, Henry, 27
Hawthorne, Nathaniel, 1009
Hayes-Bautista, David, 619
Hays, Isaac, 966
Headlines, of medical news story,
 187
Healers, 881, 1065, 1317
 in Africa, 897
 in ancient Near East, 877–883
 divine, 587, 1122–1123
 in East Asia, 905
 folk practitioners, 877–879, 1317
 in India, 909
 ministers as, 1048, 1191
 primitive, 877–879
 Taoist, 1633, 1635–1636
 women as, 1713
 See also Physicians
Health:
 environmental, *See* Environmental ethics
 history of concept, 579–585
  ancient, 581–582
  medieval, 582
  modern, 582–584, 1481–1483
 international, 643–646
  continuing problems in, 645–
   646
  defined, 643
  motivation for work in, 643–644
  responsibilities in, 644–645
  understanding the problem, 643

mental, *See* Mental health

normality as, 39–40

as an obligation, 606–609

philosophical perspectives, 599–605

discovered vs. invented concepts, 601–603

ethical force of nosologies, 604–605

illness and well-being, disease and health, 599–601

mental vs. somatic disease, 603–604

policy, *See* Health policy

public, *See* Public health

religious concepts, 585–589

disease, 586

divine healers, 587

forms of healing, 586–587

Hinduism, 663–664, 902–903

human healers, 587

instruments of healing, 587–588

monotheistic biblical tradition, 587–589

Protestantism, 1373–1378

right to, 123, 627, 953, 971

sexual behavior and, 1567–1568

shifting orientation toward, 1483–1484

sociological and action perspective, 590–598

definition of health, 591–593

health as interaction medium, 597–598

illness and life expectancy, 593

social distribution, 1056

social role of sickness, 593–597

Health, Education, and Welfare (HEW), U.S. Department of, 141, 153, 190, 493, 649, 696, 706, 997, 1039, 1103, 1350, 1352, 1353, 1495, 1497, 1596, 1702, 1729

Final Report of the Task Force on Homosexuality, 673

Final Report of the Task Force on Prescription Drugs, 320

Institutional Guide to DHEW Policy on Protection of Human Subjects, 1774–1781

regulations for skilled nursing facilities, 1783–1785

Health and Social Security, British Department of, 707

Health and Welfare, Canadian Department of, 706, 707

Health care, 585, 976

in Africa, 898–899

for the aged, 57, 65–68

ethical considerations in, 61–62, 67–68

medical and hospital services, 65–66

mental health care, 67

nursing homes, *See* Nursing homes

in Arab nations, 889–890

of blacks, 1407, 1409

Buddhism and, 135–136

in Canada, 618, 654, 993–994, 998

of children, 151–152

chronic illness, 156–158, 595, 615

care for, 157–158

in France, 971

iatrogenic disease and, 323

incidence of, 156

normalization as ethical problem, 158

poverty and, 1056, 1317

properties of, 157

Confucianism and, 200

in developing countries, 1321–1326

in Eastern Europe, 978

Eastern Orthodox Christianity and, 349

health care system, 584, 610–618

the aged and, 65–66

delivery of services, 613–615

financing of, 610–612, 617, 627–628; *See also* Health insurance

organization of services, 616–617

policy choices of, 617–618

regulation of, 612–613

resources of, 615–616, 1323–1324

in hospitals, *See* Hospitals; Nursing

humanization and dehumanization of, 619–622, 1140

causes of dehumanization, 621–622

connotations of, 619–620

ingredients of humanized care, 620–621

in India, 909

Islamic, 893

justice and, 610, 630–636, 650, 1319, 1325–1326

decent minimum of health care, 633–634

entitlement to health care, 631–633

equal access to equal levels of health, 635–636

maximum level of health care, 634–635

utility of health care, 631

medical care distinguished from, 643, 1319–1320

oral, *See* Dentistry

in People's Republic of China, 920

poverty and, 616, 617, 1316–1326

accessibility of services, 1318

availability of services, 1318

ethical considerations, 1319–1320

international perspective, 1321–1326

relationship of, 1317–1319

in United States, 1316–1320

religious curing, role of, 1124

right to health care services, 610–611, 613, 623–629, 647, 1513

entitlement position, 631–633

human rights, 626–627

of institutionalized patients, 779–780, 1072, 1077, 1105

rights in general, 624–626

right to health, 627

right to medical care, 627–629, 1604–1605

of women, 1705–1710

Health Care and Changing Values (conference, 1973), 1000

Health-care professions, codes of the, *See Codes of the Health-Care Professions*

Health Disciplines Act of 1974 (Canada), 995

Health education, 613, 615, 1396

Health information, access to, 62

Health insurance, 637–642

the aged and, 65

American Medical Association and, 639–640, 648, 649, 994, 1039–1040, 1041

in Canada, 992, 994

compulsory, 637–639, 652

in Germany, 611, 627, 638, 641–642, 970

group, 638

national, 56, 611, 612, 622, 637–638, 641–642, 648, 649, 680, 994, 1039, 1205, 1318, 1397–1398

poverty and, 1317, 1318

private, 637–642, 652

purpose of, 637

in United States, 611–612, 618, 638–641, 648, 649, 994

outside United States, 611, 641–642

Health Insurance Act of 1974 (Australia), 642

Health Insurance Association of America, 648

Health Insurance Plan of Greater New York, 640

Health labor force, 615–616

Health Maintenance Organization Act of 1973 (PL 93–222), 46, 640

Health Maintenance Organizations (HMOs), 46, 612

Health policy, 646–654
  evolution of, 647–650
    history in United States, 647–649
    history of concept, 647
    responsive and responsible policy, 649–650
  international, 651–654
    equalizing access to health services, 653–654
    ethical issues and public policy, 651–652
    Great Britain, 652–653, 654
    types of health services, 651
    U.S.S.R., 653, 654

Health Policy Advisory Center (Health-PAC), 161

Health Research Group, 649

Health screening, *See* Genetic screening; Mass health screening

Health Systems Agency of Northern Virginia v. Virginia State Board of Medicine (1976), 47

Healy, Edwin F., 996, 1530

Hearing defects, mass health screening and, 859

Heartbeat, pronouncement of death and, 259, 292, 296, 298

Heart disease, 496, 570, 720, 842, 860, 1483, 1596

Heart support systems:
  artificial heart, 634–635, 636, 659–660, 843, 845, 848, 1155, 1519, 1651–1652
  counterpulsation, 842, 843
  drugs, 842
  external massage, 842
  pacemakers, 296, 842, 843

Heart transplantation, 141, 296, 654–660
  allocation of resources and, 808
  brain death and, 141, 296, 298, 303, 656
  Confucianism and, 655
  cost of, 1165
  Eastern Orthodox Christianity and, 350–351
  efficacy of, 656–657
  histocompatibility and, 657–659
  historical development of, 654–655, 1162
  in India, 655, 909
  intercultural aspects of, 655
  in Japan, 928
  Judaism and, 800
  law and, 656
  medical regulation of, 655–656
  medical reporting and, 183, 186, 190, 656, 659, 708–709

procurement and, 656
psychological aspects of, 658
risk-benefit and, 657–658, 1162
sociocultural aspects, 1166–1167
in United States, 997

Heatstroke, experiments in, 80

Hebrew–Christian ethics, *See* Bible; Christianity; Judaism

Hedonism, 264
  psychotropic, 1385

Hedonistic egoism, 418

Hegel, Georg, 241, 419, 1149, 1151, 1402, 1603

Heidegger, Martin, 236, 237, 242, 304–305, 1638, 1639

Heilbroner, Robert, 1642

Heisenberg, Werner, 502, 1403

Held, Virginia, 1239, 1240

Hellegers, André, 1000

Hellenistic period, *See* Greece, ancient

Helmholz, Hermann von, 584, 1661

Helmont, Jan Baptista van, 582, 583

Help-seeking behavior, 1055–1056, 1669–1671

Helsinki, Declaration of, *See* Declaration of Helsinki

Hemodialysis, *See* Kidney dialysis; Kidney transplantation

Hemoglobin, 842

Hemophilia, 465–466, 469, 474, 475, 476, 1343, 1439

Henderson, Lawrence J., 1664–1665, 1686

Henotheism, 430

Henry VIII, King of England, 987, 1036

Hepatitis experiment, 700, 997

Heraclitus, 189, 236

Herbal cauterization, 912

Herberg, Will, 248

Herder, Johann G. von, 240, 1402

Hereditary Genius (Galton), 529

Hereditary Health Law of 1933 (Germany), 460

Hereditary principle, 469

Heredity, *See* Genetics

Herodotus, 59, 205, 236, 581

"Heroic" medicine, 1173–1174

Heroin maintenance, 332

Herophilus, 75, 685, 935

Hertz, Robert, 222

Herz, Marcus, 162

Heschel, Abraham, 248

Hesian period, 923

Hesiod, 236

Heterologous artificial insemination, *See* Artificial insemination: by donor (AID)

Heterozygote detection, 555–558

Hettlinger, Richard F., 674

Heuse, Georges, 985

HEW, *See* Health, Education, and Welfare (HEW), U.S. Department of

Heydecker, J. J., 1018

Hibernation, 52, 63, 217

High school medical ethics courses, 873

High technology, 1485

Hildegarde of Bingen, 1714

Hilgard, Ernest R., 712, 713

Hilgard, Josephine R., 713

Hill, Lister, 1495, 1496

Hill, Sir Austin Bradford, 695

Hill–Burton Hospital Act of 1946, 648, 992

Hiltner, Seward, 1368

Himmler, Heinrich, 1017, 1018, 1019

Hinduism, 661–666, 901
  abortion and, 662, 1271–1272
  Ayurveda medicine and, 663, 666, 906–907
  Caraka Saṃhitā, 163, 172, 176, 177, 663, 664–665, 870, 906–907
    text of, 1732
  contraception and, 205, 1271
  cosmic decline, doctrine of, 662
  death and, 231–233
  family and, 662
  gods and demons, battle between, 661–662
  health and disease, ethics of, 663–664, 902–903
  heart transplantation and, 655
  individual conduct and, 662–663
  karma, doctrine of, 431, 436, 586, 661–664, 903, 1183, 1188
  marriage and, 1270, 1271
  medical ethics of, 664–665
    history of, 902–903, 904, 906–910
  medical system of, 663
  mental health and, 665–666
  pain and, 1182, 1183, 1187–1188
  population ethics and, 1269–1272
  principles of ethics of, 1269–1270
  quality of life and, 1270
  sanctity of life and, 832
  sexual abstinence and, 1271
  social norms in, 662
  social service medicine and, 665
  soul in, 661, 903
  sterilization and, 1272, 1609, 1610–1611
  suffering and, 664, 1187–1188
  suicide and, 1621
  theological ethics and, 429
  transmigration, doctrine of, 661
  value of animal life and, 827
  See also India

Hippocrates, 489, 685, 785, 786, 886, 888, 889, 930, 937, 1065, 1091, 1095, 1486, 1656
  See also Hippocratic Corpus; Hippocratic medicine; Oath of Hippocrates

Hippocratic Corpus, 581, 930–937, 1095, 1486, 1656

on advertising, 933
on confidentiality, 932
on consultations, 935
on euthanasia, 934
on fees, 932
on general etiquette, 931–932
on giving or withholding treatment, 933–934
on ideal physician, 930–931
influence on organized medicine, 1035
on sexual conduct, 932
on theorizing, 1050
on truth-telling, 934
See also Oath of Hippocrates
Hippocratic medicine, 775
influence on medieval Europe, 940–941
scientific treatment, development of, 1655, 1657
violence and, 1689–1690
vis medicatrix naturae, 590
See also Hippocratic Corpus; Oath of Hippocrates
Hippocratic Oath, *See* Oath of Hippocrates
Hirata Atsutane, 925
Hirsch, Fred, 394
Hirschhorn, Kurt, 1340, 1342–1343, 1455
Hirth, A., 1018
Histocompatibility, 570, 657-659, 1153, 1160
Historical-entitlement view of justice, 632
Historical method of organization, 874
History of Animals (Aristotle), 206
History of the Persian Wars (Herodotus), 59, 236
Hitler, Adolf, 283, 460, 481, 1015, 1016, 1017, 1019, 1183
Hobbes, Thomas, 416, 501-502, 542, 819, 1115, 1292, 1509, 1535
Hocart, Arthur, 221
Hoche, Alfred, 983
Hoebel, Edward A., 227
Hoess, Rudolf, 1017
Hoffman, Friedrich, 871, 956, 1659
Holbach, Paul d', 240, 501, 502
Holism, 130
Holland, *See* Netherlands
Hollenbach, David, 1255
Hollender, Marc H., 1665
Holman, 658
Holmes, Oliver Wendell, Jr., 1108, 1614
Holmes, Oliver Wendell, Sr., 325, 1405, 1686, 1716
Holy man, 878, 879
Holy Office, 12

Hölzloher, A., 1017
Home health care, 66, 67
Homeopathy, 1173, 1174, 1377
Homeostasis, 584
Homer, 139, 236
Homicide, anthropological perspective of, 223–224
Hominization, *See* Life, beginning of
Homocentrism, 389
Homocystinuria, 574
Homologous artificial insemination, *See* Artificial insemination: by husband (AIH)
Homosexual act, 671
Homosexual condition, 671
Homosexuality, 667–675, 853, 1557, 1561, 1566, 1589, 1590-1592, 1593
in ancient Greece, 671, 1577
in ancient Rome, 1577
clinical and behavioral aspects, 109, 667–670
changing homosexual behavior, 670
normal and abnormal, 669–670
nature and causes of, 668–669
problems in definition and diagnosis, 667–668
contemporary attitudes toward, 1563
cultural variation in, 1583
Eastern Orthodox Christianity and, 353
ethical aspects, 671–675
cultural and religious attitudes, 671–672
ethical positions, 673–675
problems in definition, 671
society and homosexuality, 672–673
in Great Britain, 990
hormonal levels and, 1591
Judaism and, 672, 1576–1577
parent–child relationship and, 1591–1592
pedophilic, 1387
Protestantism and, 1581, 1583
public attitudes toward, 1565
Victorianism and, 1561
Honesty, in dynamic therapy, 342
Hong Kong, abortion laws in, 29
Honolka, Bert, 1016
Hooke, Robert, 1543
Hooker, Worthington, 966, 1031
Hopi Indians, 227, 1046
Horace, 371
Horney, Karen, 1084, 1088
Horrobin, David F., 1051
Hospital chaplains, 1191–1192
Hospital committees, 280, 738–739, 752, 753, 755, 759, 760, 1145

See also Institutional Review Boards (IRBs)
Hospital Construction and Survey Act of 1946, 1202
Hospitalization, *See* Mental institutionalization
Hospitals, 677–683, 1048, 1661
administration–board relationships, 681–682
the aged in, 65–66
alcoholics in, 73
Buddhist, 201
Byzantine, 1657
in Canada, 992
Christian, origin and development of, 939–940
chronic care in, 157
clergy-directed, 1190, 1365, 1367, 1428, 1430–1434, 1523
confidentiality of medical records and, 197
in contemporary society, 677–683
governance and management of, 678, 679, 681
historical perspective of, 677–678
human experimentation in, 685
in India, 907–908, 909
institutional responsibility and, 680–681
Islamic, 788
Jewish, 1190, 1428, 1430
lack of social concern in, 1056
mass health screening in, 862
medical education in, *See* Medical education
mental, *See* Mental hospitals
North American, rise of, 967–968
patients' rights and, 169, 682, 994, 1201–1205
consumer demands, 1202
history of, 1202
institutional scope of, 1203–1204
international scope of, 1203
Judaism and, 1430–1431
medical malpractice litigation, reaction to, 1203
model bill of rights, 1204–1205
patients' rights advocate, 1205
Roman Catholicism and, 1530
See also Patient's Bill of Rights, A (American Hospital Association)
in Persia, 885
the poor in, 1317, 1318
primary care in, 614, 616
privacy in, 1363
problems facing, 679–680
purpose of, 680
quality control in, 682–683
regulation of, 613, 680

VOLUME INDICATOR

Hospitals (*Continued*)
    Roman Catholic, 1431–1434, 1523
    secondary care in, 614
    segregation in, 1408
    sterilization and, 1616–1617
    therapeutic relationship in, 1671
    in United States, 967–968, 992, 993, 994
Hospital trustees, 679, 681, 682
Hostiensis, 943
Howard, 1660
Howard v. Lecher (1965), 576
Hsien, 1632, 1635–1636
Hsü Ch'un-fu, 203
Hsü-tzu, 374
Hsü Yen-tso, 916
Huang-ti nei-ching (Yellow Emperor's Inner Classic), 903, 905, 1632, 1634, 1635, 1636
Hua Shan Hospital (Shanghai), 872
Hua Tu, 871
Hua-yen sect, 375
Hufeland, Christoph W., 969
Hugh of St. Victor, 1523
Huizinga, Johan, 254
Hull, Clark L., 108, 111, 112, 114, 711
Human actions, accounting for, 112–113
Humanae Vitae (Paul VI), 25, 213, 1136, 1256, 1257, 1433, 1527, 1533, 1582
Human Betterment Foundation, 1612
Human dignity, *See* Dignity
Human experimentation, 683–709, 975
    on adolescents, 42–43
    on the aged, 68
    on alcoholics, 73–74
    American Medical Association on, 42, 656, 758, 1352, 1773–1774
    in ancient Greece, 684–686, 935–936
    in ancient Near East, 882–883
    in ancient Rome, 935–936
    autoexperimentation, 688–689, 1487
    basic issues in, 692–697
        conceptual clarifications, 692–694
        design of experiments, 695–696
        ethical, 694–695
        experimentation as social practice, 692
        requisites for conduct, 696–697
    behavioral, *See* Behavioral research
    on blacks, 1409
    in Canada, 705, 706–707, 994, 997, 998
    on children, 152–153, 759, 819, 820, 1497, 1648
    codes of ethics and, 168, 703, 1479, 1727
    coercion and, 1198, 1472

competition for scientific rewards and, 1544
    in contemporary Arab world, 891
    contraceptive testing, 1281
    drug trials, 1628
        blind procedures in, 695, 1488
        duration of, 321–322
        informed consent and, 321, 756, 1488
        insurance for, 708
        labeling and, 322
        prisoners used in, 1349–1350, 1353
        reporting and, 322, 383–384
        risks in, 756
    in Eastern Europe, 979
    Eastern Orthodox Christianity and, 349–350
    electrical stimulation of the brain (ESB) as, 357
    Flexner Report and, 1033
    foundations and goals of, *See* Biomedical research
    gene therapy, 523–524
    genetic screening, 570
    in Great Britain, 961, 974, 989–990
    history of, 684–690
        autoexperimentation, 688–689
        Claude Bernard and, 689–690
        criticisms of, 689
        deliberate experimentation involving second parties, 685–688
        experimentation incidental to medical treatment, 684–685
        natural experiments, 684
    images of man and, 854
    informed consent in, 410, 697, 751–761
        adolescents and, 42–43
        the aged and, 68
        alcoholics and, 73
        in behavioral research, 1472–1474
        children and, 152–155, 759
        conditions and exceptions, 757–760
        drug trials and, 321, 756, 1488
        in Eastern Europe, 979
        electrical stimulation of the brain (ESB) and, 357
        ethical aspects of, 754–761
        fetal research and, 490–491, 492
        functions of, 755–756
        gene therapy and, 523
        genetic screening and, 570
        grounding of, 754–755
        international aspects of, 645
        interpretation of concept, 756–757
        law and, 755
        legislation of morality and, 819
        mass health screening and, 860, 862

        moral justification and, 410
        Nuremberg Code and, 1512
        operational meaning and, 751–752
        origin of concern, 751
        philosophical basis of, 754–755
        prisoners and, 757, 758, 1350–1351
        quality of, 752–753
        religious basis of, 755
        self-realization therapies and, 1549
        sex research and, 1558–1559
        social aspects of, 751–753
        as social control problem, 753
        therapeutic relationship as barrier to, 753
        value conflicts and, 1544
        women and, 1710
    in vitro fertilization as, 1449–1450, 1461
    Islam and, 893
    in Japan, 928
    Judaism and, 796, 799
    kidney dialysis and transplantation as, 812
    law and, 706, 707, 1648
    legislation of morality and, 819, 820
    medical malpractice and, 1022
    medical reporting of, 190, 191, 704–705, 708–709, 1489, 1490
    medical social work and, 1044
    on the mentally retarded, 1112–1113, 1497
    in National Socialist Germany, 619, 690, 697, 700, 1015, 1017–1018, 1512, 1696
    on newborn, 721
    Nuremberg Code and, 153, 172, 656, 697, 754, 757–760, 1018–1019, 1113, 1486, 1487, 1512
        text of, 1764–1765
    nursing and, 1143
    organ transplantation as, 1164–1165
    in pain, 1179
    paternalism and, 1195, 1198, 1351–1352
    in patients' bills of rights, 1203, 1204
    in People's Republic of China, 920
    philosophical aspects of, 699–702
        duties of physicians, 700
        fairness, 701–702
        obligation to participate, 700–702
        problem of definition, 699–700
    policy statements on, 1729
    on prisoners, 1198, 1349–1353, 1478, 1497, 1559, 1648
        informed consent, 757, 758, 1350–1351
        policies, 1352–1353

practices, 1349–1350
principles, 1350–1352
sex research, 1559
privacy and, 1362
public policy and, 1352–1353,
1495
regulation of, 656, 1479, 1497
rights of patients in, 1515
risks in, 689, 693, 694–695, 697,
1198
Roman Catholicism and, 1532
situation ethics and, 423–424
social and professional control of,
702–709
professional control, 703–706
public and quasi-public controls,
706–709
in surgery, 1628–1629
on terminally ill, 1648
texts of directives for, 1764–1781
in United States, 975, 994, 997–998
value conflicts and, 1544, 1665–
1666
vivisection, 76, 139–140, 144, 685–
686, 689–690, 798
on women, 1710–1711
See also Fetus: research on
Humanhood, *See* Life, beginning of;
Personhood
Humani Generis (Pius XII), 1527
Humanism, 1402
anti-aging techniques and, 63–64
euthanasia and, 262
sustaining life and, 262
Humanistic medical education, 864
Humanization:
of health care, 619–621, 623
See also Life: beginning of; Per-
sonhood
Human Life, *See* Life
Human nature:
models of, 1088
theories of, *See* Determinism; En-
vironment and man; Free
will; Images of man; Mental
health therapies; Mind–body
problems; Natural law; Per-
sonhood
Human nature and Conduct
(Dewey), 1330
Human rights, 626–627
Human Rights Guidelines for
Nurses in Clinical and Other
Research: Statement of the
ANA Commission on Nursing
Research, 1727
See also Rights
Human self-determinism, 546
See also Self-determination
Human Sexual Inadequacy (Masters
and Johnson), 1566

Human Tissue Act of 1961 (Great
Britain), 141, 300, 492
Hume, David, 240, 448, 480, 501,
952, 957, 962, 1066, 1235,
1535
on cause, 503
on distributive justice, 803
on marriage, 1584
on moral rules, 409
naturalistic fallacy and, 131, 444,
1134
on reasoning, 95, 451, 452
on relativism, 264
on suicide, 276–277, 1620, 1623
on sympathy, 960
Hume, Dr. David, 1160
Hume, Edward H., 1367
Humility, 1049
Humoral theory of disease, 581–582
Humphrey, Laud, 1472
Humphrey Clinker (Smollett), 1008
Hungary:
abortion laws in, 29
medical ethics education in, 872
Hunger, *See* Food policy
Hung Liang-chi, 210, 1233
Hunt, Harriet K., 1715
Hunt, Morton, 1563–1564, 1565,
1568, 1583
Hunter, John, 688, 1660
Huntington's chorea, 466, 511, 529,
555, 558
Huntington's Chorea Commission,
1496
Huron Indians, 225
Husserl, Edmund, 363
Hutcheson, Francis, 957, 959
Hutchinson, Ann, 1714
Huxley, Aldous, 100, 1384, 1385,
1386, 1566
Huxley, Sir Julian, 127, 131, 481,
482, 511, 542, 1402, 1537
Huxley, Thomas H., 190, 480, 1536,
1537
Huygens, Christian, 1050
H-Y antigen, 1440
Hybridization of human cells, 517–
518
Hybrid vigor, 475
Hygiene:
Seventh-Day Adventism and, 1376
See also Public health
Hylomorphism, 18
Hyperammonemia, 474
Hyperbilirubinemia, 474
Hypercholesterolemia, 556
Hyperkinetic learning disorders,
1199, 1383–1384, 1388
Hypertension, 496, 570, 857
Hypnosedatives, 336
Hypnosis, 85, 710–714

defined, 710
historical origins of misunderstandings about, 710–711
law and, 713–714
professional practitioners, concerns of, 712–713
social anxiety about hypnotic powers, 711–712
unanticipated consequences of,
714
Hypospadias, 719
Hypothermia, 216, 217
Hysterectomy, 1531, 1608, 1705–1706
Hysteroscopy, 1607, 1608
Hysterotomy, 3, 4, 318

I

Iatrogenic disease, 323
Ibn Abi Usaybia, 888–889
Ibn Ezra, Abraham, 239, 791
Ibn Hazm, 1265, 1266
Ibn Khaldun, 1264
Ibn Qayyim al-Jawziyya, 1266
Ibn Radwan, 888
Ibn Sīnā, *See* Avicenna
Ibn Taymīhah, 1264
Ibn Tibbons, 791
Ibsen, Henrik, 1010–1011
Ideal observer theories, 439, 449
Ideals, 504
Identity thesis, 303–304, 1116–1117,
1420–1421
Ideological reduction, 1420–1421,
1427
Ido, concept of, 924
Iglesias, F., 655
Ill-education, behavior control and,
90–91
Illich, Ivan, 1053
Illness, 599–601
biological vs. theological view of,
1127–1128
chronic, *See* Chronic illness
phenomenon of, 1672–1673
See also Anthropology of medicine; Disease
Images of man, 620, 851–857
pilgrim vs. stranger, 854
provincial vs. boundary maker,
855–856
singular creature vs. odd specimen, 851–852
sinner vs. victim, 852–853
soul-self vs. plastic man, 853–854
steward vs. exploiter, 855
struggle among, 856–857
worker vs. player, 854–855

Imaginary Invalid, The (Molière), 1008
Imago dei, 1368
Imitation, 109
Immanuel ben Solomon of Rome, 791
Immanuel Movement, 1125
Immigration, 1219, 1221, 1233, 1235
    restriction of, 460, 1304–1305
Immigration Restriction Act of 1924, 460
Immoral people, 90
Immortality:
    anthropological perspective of, 221–223
    Aristotle on, 237
    in biblical thought, 244, 245
    Calvinism and, 252
    Christianity and, 256
    in Eastern thought, 230
    Epicureanism and, 238
    in Hellenistic thought, 238, 250
    humanism and, 64
    Judaism and, 246–247, 248
    Kant on, 257
Immune system, biological decrement theory and, 48
Immunization, 151, 593, 594, 614, 1484, 1485
Immunology, 77
Immunosuppressive drugs, 323, 812, 814, 1160, 1161, 1162
Impartial rationality, 439–440, 449
Imperative theory of law, 819
Implantation, *See* Artificial heart
Incantations, 587–588, 923
Incarceration, *See* Mental institutionalization; Prisoners
Incentives:
    fee-for-service, 1056–1057
    population control, 1290–1295, 1302
    technological choice, 1646–1647, 1648
Incest:
    abortion and, 28
    Eastern Orthodox Christianity and, 353
    Judaism and, 468–472
Income, health and, *See* Poverty; health care and
Incompetency, 781, 1105, 1106
    informed consent and, 758–759
    to stand trial, 1106
Indeterminacy, principle of, 1425
India:
    abortion in, 909, 910, 1271–1272
    amulet investiture in, 588
    Buddhism in, *See* Buddhism
    contraception in, 211–212, 909
    current trends in, 909–910
    darshan, concept of, 878
    death, conceptions of, 231–233
    divine healers in, 587
    environment and man, conceptions of, 374–378
    European medicine in, 908
    family planning in, 909–910, 1283
    future outlook for, 910
    health and disease, conception of, 581
    health care in, 909
    health expenditures in, 1322
    health status by level of per capita income in, 1321
    heart transplantation and, 655, 909
    Hinduism in, *See* Hinduism
    hospitals in, 907–908, 909
    infanticide in, 226
    magico–religious medicine in, 1655
    Maria aborigines of, 224
    missionary activity in, 1367
    1956 code of conduct of, 908–909
    oaths for physicians in, 163, 164, 177, 664–665
    population of, 1271
        education of, 1311
        growth in, 1228, 1230, 1269
    population policy in, 1224, 1235, 1289
    poverty in, 1321
    sex preferences in, 1442
    sterilization in, 910, 1283, 1291, 1301, 1397
    suicide in, 1621–1622
    Tantrism in, 205, 907
    Yūnāni (Unani), medicine in, 789, 907–908
Indian Oath of Initiation, 172
Indirect abortion, 3, 11, 13, 23
Indirect euthanasia, 34, 423
Indirect killing, 272–274
Individual–biological criterion for beginning of human life, 17–20, 1338
Individual ethics, 121–122
Individualism, 64, 1260, 1535
Individuality:
    beginning of human life and, 19
    determinants of, 548–549
Individual morality, 553–554
Indonesia:
    contraception in, 211, 213
    health status by level of per capita income in, 1321
    poverty in, 1321
Industrial Accident Insurance Act of 1884 (Germany), 970
Industrialization, 1393–1394, 1641–1642
Infant care:
    clinical aspects, 717–724
        agency in decision-making, 723–724
        conflicting interests, 722–723
        conflicting principles and, 722
        management of untreated infants, 721–722
    therapy in newborns, 718–721
    ethical perspectives on, 724–735
        consequentialist theories, 731–732, 834–837
        deontological theories, 726–729, 833, 838
        equality theory of justice, 837
        ethic of care, 733–734
        extraordinary means principle, 727–729, 838
        medical perspective, 724–726
        personhood theories, 726–727, 729–732, 834–836
        principle of avoiding harm, 734–735
        slippery slope argument in, 821, 836–837
        wrongful life theory, 835–836, 837
    in France, 971
    public health and, 1396
    public policy and procedural questions, 735–740
        on decision making, 737–739
        on euthanasia and sustaining life, 736–737
        on macroallocation, 739–740
    See also Infanticide
Infanticide, 151, 276, 552, 826
    abortion following prenatal diagnosis viewed as, 1341–1342
    in Africa, 226, 742
    in ancient Greece, 226, 742, 826
    anthropological perspective, 226
    Buddhism and, 742
    in China, 210, 226, 742
    Hinduism and, 662
    in India, 226
    medical police concept and, 958
    normative relativism and, 455
    philosophical perspective of, 742–750
        destruction of latent persons issue, 744, 748
        destruction of potential persons issue, 744, 746–748
        equated to morality of abortion, 747, 1341–1342
        historical considerations, 742–743
        infants as persons issue, 729–731, 743–746, 826
        principle of avoiding harm, 734–735
        undesirable consequences issue, 744, 748–750
    as population control measure, 1228
    Taoism and, 1636
    tolerance of, 151
    See also Abortion; Euthanasia
Infantile autism, 539
Infant mortality rate, 1321, 1396
Informational privacy, 1357–1360, 1362–1363

Information-containing molecules, aging theories based on, 48–50

Information control, 86, 89

Informed consent, 46, 178, 1518
artificial insemination and, 1445
behavior control and, 90, 97–98, 104, 125
coercion and, 757, 758, 763–766, 782
doctrine of, 1498–1499
euthanasia and, 275, 276
free will and determinism and, 505
in human experimentation, 410, 697, 751–761
on adolescents, 42–43
on the aged, 68
on alcoholics, 73
in behavioral research, 1472–1474
on children, 152–155, 759
conditions and exceptions, 757–760
drug trials and, 321, 756, 1488
in Eastern Europe, 979
electrical stimulation of the brain (ESB) and, 357
ethical aspects of, 754–761
fetal research and, 490–491, 492
functions of, 755–756
gene therapy and, 523
genetic screening and, 570
grounding of, 754–755
international aspects of, 645
interpretation of concept, 756–757
law and, 755
legislation of morality and, 819
mass health screening and, 860, 862
moral justification and, 410
Nuremberg Code and, 1512
operational meaning and, 751–752
origin of concern, 751
philosophical basis of, 754–755
on prisoners, 757, 758, 1350–1351
quality of, 752–753
religious basis of, 755
self-realization therapies and, 1549
sex research and, 1558–1559
social aspects of, 751–753
as social control problem, 753
therapeutic relationship as barrier to, 753
value conflicts and, 1544
on women, 1710
hypnosis and, 713

medical malpractice and, 1023–1024
medical social work and, 1043–1044
in mental health, 762–766
drug therapy and, 765
dynamic therapies and, 340
electroconvulsive therapy (ECT) and, 360, 765
vs. informed consent in physical health care, 763
justification for nonconsensual health care, 763–765
law and, 781–782, 1105
legislation of morality and, 820
mental retardation and, 1112
nonconsensual care in criminal justice system, 765–766
psychosurgery and, 765, 1389
nurses and, 1142–1143
organ transplantation and, 1157
paternalism and, 1197, 1199–1200
in patients' bills of rights, 1203, 1204
prenatal diagnosis and, 1335
reproductive technologies and, 1445, 1447, 1466
self-determination and, 755, 761, 771–777
sterilization and, 1606, 1608–1609, 1616
in therapeutic relationship, 767–778, 1558–1559, 1693
adolescents and, 42–43
ambiguous nature of, 768–769
clinical aspects, 767–769
decision making by patients, 771, 774–775
decision making by physicians, 771, 775–777
decision to initiate life-support systems and, 844
dentistry and, 312
genetic counseling and, 576–577
infant care and, 737, 738
vs. informed consent in mental health, 763
in Japan, 927
law and, 769–774
nature of, 767–768
obstacles to, 768
the poor and, 1056
purpose of, 767
self-realization therapies and, 1549
sex therapy and, 1558–1559
surgery and, 1627–1628
Ingelfinger, F. J., 183, 190
Inherent worth concept, 620
Ink-therapy, 789

Inmates of Boy's Training School vs. Affleck (1972), 104
"In need of care and treatment," 1103
Inner-city poor, health care for, 616
Inner states or events, 111–112
Innocent III, Pope, 10, 11, 254, 472, 945
Innocent XI, Pope, 11, 12
In personam rights, 1509, 1510
Inquiry, doctrine of, 1327, 1328
Inquisition, 209, 1187
In re *Estate of Brooks* (1965), 1504, 1505
In re *Gault* (1967), 151
In re *Joseph Lee Moore* (1976), 574, 1614
In re *Lynch* (1972), 783
In rem rights, 1509–1510
In re *Quinlan* (1976), 1505
In re *Richardson* (1973), 153
In re *Yetter* (1973), 1505
Insanity, *See* Mental illness
Insanity defense, 1106–1107
Insemination, artificial, *See* Artificial insemination.
Instinctive help, 1655
Instinct therapy, 1085
Institute for Child Health and Human Development, 1495
Institute for Environmental Health Sciences, 1495
Institute for General Medical Sciences, 1495
Institute of Religion, Texas Medical Center, 1000
Institute of Society, Ethics and the Life Sciences (Hastings Center), 1000, 1193, 1278, 1280
Institute on Aging, 1495
Institutes of the Christian Religion (Calvin), 1366, 1581
Institutional change, 1222
Institutional ethics, 869
Institutionalization:
of the aged, 66–67
See also Nursing
of animal experimentation, 76–77
mental, *See* Mental institutionalization
Institutionally centered legal intervention, 1647, 1648–1649
Institutional practices, ethics distinguished from, 401
Institutional review boards (IRBs), 190–191, 1198, 1490, 1495
Institutional review committees, 1479, 1490
Institutional therapy, 1087
Institutiones theologiae moralis, 1525

Insurance:
  health, *See* Health insurance
  medical malpractice, 1025
  no-fault, 1022, 1024-1025
Integrationist gerontologists, 60
Integrist understanding of homosexuality, 673, 674
Integrity, physicians', 866
Intelligence:
  fertility and, 1307, 1308–1309
  genetics and, 526, 544
  as indicator of personhood, 835, 1371
  race differences in, 533–538
Intelligence quotient, 1109
Intelligence tests, 1470
Intensive care, *See* life-support systems
Intent:
  abortion and, 11
  foresight and, 35, 318
  of good or evil, *See* Double effect, principle of
  to injure, 1519
  utilitarianism and, 425
Internal Revenue Service, 1159
International Association for Cross-Cultural Psychology, 1479
International Chiropractors Association, 1728
International Code of Medical Ethics, 44, 167–168, 172–175, 989, 1726
  text of, 1749–1750
International Conference on Abortion (1967), 1000
International Congresses of Medical Ethics, 985
International Council of Nurses, Code for Nurses, 1139
  text of, 1788–1789
International Covenant on Economic, Social, and Cultural Rights (1966), 623, 624
International health, 643–646
  continuing problems in, 645–646
  defined, 643
  motivations for work in, 643–644
  policy, 651–654
    equalizing access to health services, 653–654
    ethical issues and public policy, 651–652
    Great Britain, 652–653, 654
    types of health services, 651
    in U.S.S.R., 653, 654
  poverty and, 1321–1326
  responsibilities in, 644–645
  understanding the problem, 643
International League of Societies for the Mentally Handicapped, 1515
  Declaration on the Rights of Mentally Retarded Persons, 1785
International Medical Association for

the Study of the Conditions of Life and Health, 985
International migration, 1220–1221, 1304–1305
International Planned Parenthood Federation, 1277
International Red Cross, 134, 1696
International Society for Technology Assessment, 1650
International Symposium on the Medical Care of Prisoners (1972), 1348
Internists, 613
  truth-telling and, 1680
  women as, 1717
Interpersonal decisions, 308, 311
Interpersonal (ego) therapies, 1084–1085
Interpersonal life of the aged, 60–61
Interventionism, 1222–1223
Interviews, 1471
Intrapersonal decisions, 308, 310–311
Intrauterine devices (IUDs), 3, 213, 800, 1229, 1299
Intravenous feeding, 842
Intrinsicalism, 413–416
Intrinsically evil acts, 1132
Introduction à l'étude de la médecine expérimentale (Bernard), 76, 689
Intrusions on privacy, 185, 1021, 1356–1358
Intuitionism, 403, 415–416, 439, 443, 444, 447–448, 542
Invasion of privacy, *See* Privacy
Invectivae (Petrarch), 1658
In vitro fertilization, 999, 1446, 1448–1451
  ethical issues, 1454–1456, 1460–1462
  experimental and therapeutic purpose of, 1449–1451
  experimental nature of, 1449–1450, 1461
  legal aspects, 1464–1469
  motive for, 1454–1455
  status of fetus, 1469
  technical procedures in, 1448–1449
  technological assessment of, 1652–1653
Involuntary commitment, *See* Mental institutionalization
Involuntary dying, 274
Involuntary participation in experiments, 697
Involuntary sterilization, 1612, 1706
Iowa Security Medical Facility, 780
Iran, *See* Persia
Ireland, contraception in, 211, 213
Irenaeus of Lyons, 250
Iron lung, 841
Iroquois Indians, 225

Irreducible structure of life, 305–306
Irreversible coma, 292, 293, 294, 846
  See also Brain death
Isaac of Fez (Alfasi), 1428, 1429
Iscanus, Bartholomew, 940
Ishmael, Rabbi, 6
Isidore of Seville, 472
Islam, 785–789, 1064
  abortion and, 787, 894, 1267
  alcohol use and, 70, 787
  ancient Greek medicine and, 785–787, 789
  autopsy and, 891, 893
  blood transfusions and, 893
  charms and amulets in, 588
  contraception and, 208, 787, 894, 1264–1268
  defined, 785
  doctrine of rewards and punishments, 436
  ensoulment and, 1267
  environment and, 786
  euthanasia and, 894–895
  fasting and, 787
  harmony, concept of, 786
  health care and, 893
  jurisprudence of, 1264–1268
  Koran and, 208, 431, 432, 785, 786, 787, 889, 1065, 1186
  life-support systems and, 894–895
  medical care systems and methods, 788
  medical ethics, contemporary perspective, 892–895
  mental health care and, 894
  mutilation and, 788
  Oath of Hippocrates and, 164
  organ transplantation and, 893, 1171
  pain and, 1186
  Persian influences on, 785, 786
  pilgrimage and, 787
  population ethics and, 1264–1268
  prayer and, 787
  sexuality and, 787
  suffering and, 1186
  Sufism and, 786
  suicide and, 1622
  surgery and, 788
  sustaining life and, 894–895
  symmetry, concept of, 785–786, 789
  theological ethics and, 429, 435
  waning and resurgence of traditional values in medicine, 789
Isolation:
  chronic disease and, 157
  dehumanization and, 620
Israel, 1289
  medical ethics in, 895–896
  net immigration in, 1221
  new towns in, 1306
  World Health Organization and, 644

Issues method of organization, 874
Italy, 207
    contraception in, 208, 209, 211, 213
    eugenic societies in, 458
    health care financing in, 611
    organ salvaging in, 1158
    population policy in, 1235
    scientific publications in, 985
    sterilization in, 1616
    women health practitioners in, 1714, 1717
I-tsing, 137
Itzama, 587
IUDs, *See* Intrauterine devices
Ivory coast, compensation of physicians in, 899

J

Jackson, Drummond, 192
Jackson v. Indiana (1972), 783, 1106
Jacobs, Patricia, 568
Jacobson, Lenore, 1475
Jacobson v. Massachusetts (1905), 1396, 1501
Jainism:
    pain and suffering and, 1187–1188
    suicide and, 1621
    value of life and, 827, 828
    vivisection and, 907
Jakobovits, Immanuel, 871, 996, 1457, 1458
Jamaica:
    distribution of physicians in, 1324
    health expenditures in, 1322
    health status by level of per capita income in, 1321
    population policy in, 1297
James, William, 241, 337, 501, 503, 1329–1330
Janet, Pierre, 711, 1543
Jansenism, 1582
Janssens, Louis, 212, 318–319
Japan:
    abortion in, 29, 928–929
    animal experimentation in, 80, 81
    Buddhism in, *See* Buddhism
    Confucianism in, *See* Confucianism
    consent in, 927–928
    contraception in, 211, 213
    Council of Medical Ethics of, 929
    default of obligation, theory of, 927
    environment and man, conception of, 374, 376-378

eugenics in, 458, 928–929
euthanasia in, 922, 928–929
health insurance in, 638
health status by level of per capita income in, 1321
human experimentation in, 928
ido, concept of, 924
life-support systems in, 929
medical ethics, history of, 922–929
    contemporary, 926–929
    through the nineteenth century, 922–926
medical malpractice in, 926, 927
mental illness in, 929
mental institutionalization in, 1388
obligation of attention in, 927
organ transplantation in, 928
population policy in, 1235
Shintoism in, *See* Shintoism
sterilization in, 928
suicide in, 1622
women physicians in, 1717
Japan Bar Association:
    Committee for Protection of Human Rights, 928
    Declaration Concerning Medicine and Human Rights, 929
Japanese Society of Psychiatry, 928
Japanese Society of Transplantation, 928
Jaramillo, Don Pedrito, 878
Jayavarman VII, King of Cambodia, 136
JCAH, *See* Joint Commission on Accreditation of Hospitals
Jefferson, Thomas, 264, 368, 529, 647, 823, 1401
Jefferys, Margot, 1708
Jeffreys, M. D. W., 223
Jehovah's Witnesses, 1365, 1373, 1377
    alcohol use and, 1377
    blood transfusions and, 133, 271, 1026, 1361, 1377, 1426, 1512, 1514
    heart transplantation and, 655
Jencks, Christopher, 537
Jenner, Edward, 647, 592, 1393, 1484, 1655
Jenner, Sir William, 1715
Jensen, Arthur, 483
Jerome, 6, 938, 940, 943, 1524
Jesus, 206, 239, 245, 371, 497, 588, 963, 1121, 1122, 1123, 1126, 1127, 1128, 1135, 1149, 1187, 1376, 1431
Jewish Chronic Disease Hospital, Brooklyn, New York, 754, 997
Jewish Encyclopedia, 792

Jewish Medical Ethics (Jakobovits), 871, 996
Jewish Patients' Bill of Rights, The, 1430–1431
Jinsai Itō, 376
Job Corps, 1080
Joe Egg (Nichols), 1009
John Chrysostom, St., 354, 1252, 1579
John F. Kennedy Memorial Hospital v. Heston (1971), 1502
John of Arderne, 941
John of Burgundy, 949–950
John of Damascus, 1579
John of Naples, 10, 11, 943
John of Salisbury, 1658
John of St. Thomas, 317
John XXII, Pope, 1524
John XXIII, Pope, 13, 212, 1255, 1256
Johns Hopkins Hospital, 1000, 1144
Johns Hopkins School of Medicine, 559, 1032
Johnson, J., 1554
Johnson, Lyndon B., 185, 649, 1496
Johnson, Samuel, 77
Johnson, Virginia E., 1552, 1553, 1566
Joint Commission on Accreditation of Hospitals (JCAH), 678, 1081, 1202
    Accreditation Council for Long Term Care Facilities, 1141
Joint Commission on Mental Health and Illness, 1080
Jonas, Hans, 68, 756, 1166, 1639, 1642
Jonsen, Albert R., 66, 67–68, 734
Jordan, health care in, 890
Joseph P. Kennedy, Jr., Foundation, 1000
Josephus, 6, 206
Journal des Scavans, 189
Journalistic ethics, *See* Communication, biomedical
Journal of Medical Ethics, 988
Journal of Medicine and Philosophy, 1000
Journal of the American Medical Association, 1001, 1696, 1698
Journals, biomedical, *See* Scientific publishing
Judah the Patriarch, 1428
Judah the Pious, 470
Judaism, 429, 432, 791–802, 1064
    abortion and, 795, 797, 801, 896
    beginning of human life and, 8
    controversy in, 25
    Talmud on, 5–8, 25
    Torah on, 5–6, 9–10
    artificial insemination and, 797, 800, 1457, 1458

Judaism *(Continued)*
　autopsies and, 144, 246, 798, 801–
　　802, 894–895, 896, 1026
　beginning of life and, 8, 800–801
　birth, definition of, 795
　cadavers, treatment of, 142, 144–
　　145, 246, 247, 248, 798, 801–
　　802, 894–895, 896, 1026, 1427
　charms in, 588
　confidentiality and, 99
　consent and, 799
　contraception and, 205–206, 212,
　　795, 796–797, 800, 1576
　cosmetic surgery and, 800
　death and, 243–249
　　biblical thought on, 243–246
　　definition of, 801
　　philosophy on, 239
　　post-biblical tradition, 246–249
　demonology and, 1121
　deontological theory in, 413–414
　duty to preserve life and health
　　and, 793–794
　eugenics and, 468-470, 792
　euthanasia and, 793, 794, 795,
　　797–798, 801
　generation of life and, 795–797
　genetic policy and, 463
　genetic screening and, 470
　health services and, 1430–1431
　homosexuality and, 672, 1576–
　　1577
　human experimentation and, 795,
　　799
　immortality and, 246–247, 248
　incest and, 468–472
　informed consent and, 755
　life as divine gift in, 525
　life support and, 793, 801
　limits of life and, 795
　man's dominion over nature and,
　　397–398
　marriage and, 795, 1561, 1576
　masturbation and, 1576–1577
　medical ethics of:
　　authoritarian elements in, 402
　　codes of law, 1428–1430
　　guidelines, 1429–1430
　　historical antecedents, 791–792
　　recent sources and development,
　medical ethics education and, 871
　mental health and, 1065, 1068–
　　1070
　Oath of Asaph, 164, 174, 175, 176,
　　792
　organ transplantation and, 144–
　　145, 795, 798, 799–800, 1169,
　　1171
　pain and, 793–794, 1186
　patients' rights and, 1430–1431
　physician's duties, rights, and lia-
　　bilities and, 799, 1430
　population ethics and, 1250–1251
　procreation and, 795–796, 1561,
　　1576

purpose in the universe and, 1400
sanctity of life and, 8, 794–795,
　1429
sexuality and, 796–797, 1561,
　1576–1577
sponsorship of health facilities,
　1190, 1428, 1430
status of the aged and, 59
sterilization and, 795, 796, 800,
　1610
suffering and, 1186
suicide and, 247, 1622
surgery and, 799–800
Talmud and, 791, 792, 793, 1232,
　1250, 1251, 1428, 1430, 1440
　on abortion, 5–8, 25
　on artificial insemination, 797
　on contraception, 796
　definition of death of, 801
　on duty to preserve life and
　　health, 793
　on eugenics, 469–470, 792
　on procreation, 1250–1251
　on sanctity of life, 794, 795
　on taboo illness, 1122
　on treatment of cadavers, 798
theological ethics and, 429
Torah and, 793, 1428, 1429
　on abortion, 5–6, 9–10
　on autopsy, 896
treatment of defective infants and,
　727
truth-telling and, 798, 801
United States medical ethics and,
　996
value of life and, 25, 825–826
visitation of the sick and, 798–
　799, 1192
Judgment, 308–309
Judgmental injustice, 802–803
Jundishapur medical ethics, 886–
　887
Jundishapur Medical School, 886
Jung, Carl, 1067, 1084, 1085
Jünger, Ernst, 1640
Jurjānī, Ismā 'īl ibn Hasan al-, 887
Justice, 802–810
　concept of, 802–805
　cryonics and, 217
　in dental care, 312
　deontological theory and, 174
　Eastern Orthodox Christianity
　　and, 1253–1254
　environmental ethics and, 372,
　　388–392
　　need for adequate theory of,
　　　390–391
　　public policy and, 390, 391
　　rights, duties, and concern for,
　　　389–390
　　rights of human beings vs.
　　　rights of the environment,
　　　389, 390
　equality theory of, 837
　eugenic policy and, 466–467

food policy and, 499
genetic aspects of human be-
　havior and, 543–547
health care and, 610, 630–636,
　650, 1319, 1325–1326
　decent minimum of health care,
　　633–634
　entitlement to health care, 631–
　　633
　equal access to equal level of
　　health, 635–636
　maximum level of health care,
　　634–635
　utility of health care, 631
international, 1275
international health and, 644–
　645
meritarian, 1238
merit theory of, 837
obligations to future generations
　and, 509
organ donation and, 1155–1156
population policies and, 1237–
　1238, 1244–1245, 1262, 1289
　compulsory control and, 1303
　governmental incentives and,
　　1293–1295
　social change proposals and,
　　1296–1297
prisoner experimentation and,
　1352
retributive, 544–546
Roman Catholicism and, 1255–
　1256
scarce resources, allocation of,
　390, 806–810, 1414–1418
　artificial heart, 1652
　behavior control and, 89–90
　Eastern Orthodox Christianity
　　and, 349
　enzyme replacement and, 514
　genetic screening and, 571–572
　images of man and, 855
　kidney dialysis and, 808–809,
　　815, 1414, 1415, 1416, 1418
　obligation to future generations
　　and, 1519
　organ transplantation and, 807–
　　808, 815, 1163–1164, 1414,
　　1415
　paternalism and, 1518–1519
　population problem and, 1224
　practice conception of, 412
　quality of life and, 832
　randomization of, 809–810,
　　1416, 1417
　rights and, 1510–1511, 1513
　risk-taking and, 1518–1519
　rules for final selection, 809–
　　810, 1416–1418
　rules of exclusion, 809, 1415–
　　1416
　social justice and, 390
　social worth criteria, 809–810,
　　1415–1418

treatment of defective infants and, 739–740

triage and, *See* Triage

in United States, 1418

utilitarianism and, 419, 421, 809, 810, 1416–1417

science and, 1539

sexual ethics and, 1585–1587

social contract theory and, 1604–1605

social utility and, 805–806

utilitarianism and, 419, 421, 631, 636, 805–806, 809, 810, 1416–1417

Justice, U.S. Department of, 322

"Justice in the World" (Synod of Bishops), 1256

Justifiable abortion, 14, 15, 16, 23–24

Justification, *See* Moral justification

Justinian, Code of, 672

Just savings principle, 509

Jūṭhā, 663

K

Kafka, Franz, 1011

Kahn, Herman, 526

Kaibara Ekiken (Ekken), 924, 925

Kaimowitz v. Michigan Department of Mental Health (1973), 104, 758, 781, 1388

Kaira, Simon, 1428

Kaiser Foundation, 640

Kaiser-Permanente program, 858

Kalish, Richard A., 288

Kali yuga, 662

Kallman, F. J., 668

Kallman, Franz, 562

Kaltreider, N. B., 1706

Kāma, 661, 1270

Kambas v. St. Joseph's Mercy Hospital (1973), 1718–1719

Kansas, University of, 875

Kant, Immanuel, 95, 174, 404, 755, 1044, 1292, 1402, 1586

autonomy theory of, 625

on death, 240, 241, 257–258

on determinism, 501, 503–504

on duties to oneself, 607, 608

on human experimentation, 701, 755

on immortality, 240, 241

main theses of, 414

on marriage, 1584

on moral obligation, 414, 1147, 1148–1149, 1151

on moral reasoning, 450, 451

on moral rules, 409, 414, 504

prescriptivist elements in philosophy of, 448–449

principle of right of, 1519

on rights of animals, 81

on suicide, 277, 1621

on supererogation, 1151

on truth and lying, 1685–1686

Kantrowitz, A., 655

Kaplan, Abraham, 1640

Kapp, Ernst, 1639

Karaites, 6

Karma, doctrine of, 431, 436, 586, 661–664, 903, 1183, 1188

Karman, Harvey, 160

Karo, Joseph, 793, 1429

Karolinska Institute (Stockholm), 872, 984

Karp, Haskell, 659

Kasperak, Michael, 658

Kass, Leon R., 601, 602, 1503, 1337, 1338, 1456

Kastenbaum, Robert, 287

Katz, Jay, 705, 755, 1711

Kautzky, Rudolf, 985

Keane, A. H., 1045

Kefauver–Harris Drug Amendments of 1962, 324

Kelly, Gerald, 871, 996, 1582, 1609

Kelly, William D., 1678

Kelman, Herbert C., 1474

Kennedy, John F., 1074

Kennedy, Edward M., 1496

Kennedy Institute of Ethics, Center for Bioethics, Georgetown University, 1000, 1001, 1193

Kennedy Interfaculty Program in Medical Ethics, 1001

Kenny, Joan P., 1529

Kenya:

compensation of physicians in, 899

contraceptive distribution in, 1282

Kerr–Mills legislation of 1960, 1039

Keynes, John Maynard, 394

Khat, 336

Kidney dialysis, 553, 811–815, 842–845, 1155, 1156

allocation of scarce resources and, 808–809, 815, 1414, 1415, 1416, 1418

development of, 1160

ethical issues of, 811–812

experimental-therapy dilemma and, 812

history of, 811

in home, 813, 814

principle of, 842–843

quality of life and, 811, 813, 814, 1162

selection criteria, 1161

survival and, 1161–1162

termination of, 272, 845

in United States, 812, 996, 1418

Kidney donation:

from cadavers, 1154–1155, 1161, 1163, 1165, 1166, 1167

children and, 1154, 1157

from living donors, 1153–1154, 1161, 1163, 1167

risks in, 1161

sociocultural aspects, 1166, 1167

Kidney Foundation, 141

Kidney transplantation, 141, 153, 660, 811–815, 842–845

allocation of scarce resources and, 807–808, 815, 1163–1164, 1414–1415

cost of, 1165

development of, 1160

donation for, *See* Kidney donation; Organ donation

in Eastern Europe, 979

Eastern Orthodox Christianity and, 350

ethical issues of, 811–812

as euphenic measure, 475

experiment–therapy dilemma and, 812

gift-exchange aspects of, 812–813

history of, 811

immunosuppressive drugs and, 1162

in India, 909

in Japan, 928

Judaism and, 800

normative relativism and, 456

quality of life and, 811, 813–814, 1162

selection criteria, 1161

sociocultural aspects, 1166

success of, 1161–1162

Kierkegaard, Søren, 241, 1076

Killing:

direct, 272–274

distinction between letting die and, 35–38, 318, 728–729, 747, 1369

See also Abortion; Double effect, principle of; Euthanasia; Infanticide; Omission and commission

Kim, Jaegwon, 1420

Kindness, 340

King, Gregory, 1226

Kinsey, Alfred C., 668, 1552, 1562–1565, 1568, 1583, 1589

Kinyoun, Joseph J., 1493

Klaw, Spencer, 1703

Klerman, Gerald L., 327

Klett Verlag (Stuttgart), 985

Knauer, Peter, 318–319
Knecht v. Gillman (1973), 104, 105, 780, 1073
Knights Hospitallers of St. John of Jerusalem, 1695–1696
Knowledge:
    of own death, 287
    technology as, 1639
Knowlton, Charles, 210
Knox–Keene Health Care Service Act of 1975 (California), 46
Koch, Karl, 1017
Koch, Robert, 583, 594, 1032, 1396, 1485
Ko Ch'ien-sun, 915
Ko Hung, 1633, 1635–1636
Kolb, Lawrence C., 1692
Kōmyō, Empress of Japan, 136
Koran (Qu'ran), 208, 431, 432, 785, 786, 787, 889, 892, 1065, 1186, 1265, 1267
Korea:
    health expenditures in, 1322
    population education in, 1311
Koreamoku, 587
Kraemer, 1714
Krafft-Ebing, Richard von, 1552, 1562, 1585, 1593
Krebiozen, 183
Kremer, J. P., 1017
Kreuzelschreiber, Die (Honolka), 1016
Krieger, Knut, 1700
Kropotkin, Prince Pëtr, 1536
Ktenology, 1018
Kübler-Ross, Elisabeth, 287, 998
Kuhn, Thomas S., 1401, 1545
!Kung Bushmen, 1228
Kung Hsin, 915
Kung T'ing-hsien, 915–916
Kuwait:
    alcohol prohibited in, 891
    health care in, 890
    net immigration in, 1221

L

Labeling:
    of drugs, 322
    in mental illness, *See* Labeling in mental illness
    philosophical, 400–401
    sexual, 1590
Labeling in mental illness, 1071, 1073, 1078, 1098–1107, 1108
    diagnosis and, 1100–1101
    legal aspects of, 1102–1107
        confinement to mental institutions, 1102–1105
        guardianship, 1105–1106
        incompetence to stand trial, 1106

        insanity defense, 1106–1107
        psychosurgery and, 1389
Labor, Department of, Children's Bureau, 1396
Ladimer, Irving, 1000
Lady Chatterley's Lover (Lawrence), 1562
Laënnec, René, 972
Lai Fu-yang, 203
Laín Entralgo, Pedro, 984
Laing, R. D., 1085, 1088, 1096, 1101
Lakatos, Imre, 1545
Lake, Catherine, 1199
Lamarck, Chevalier de, 482, 483
Lambeth Conference (1930), 1261, 1582
Lambeth Conference (1958), 1436
La Mettrie, Julien Offray de, 1115
Lancet, The, 191, 1173, 1174, 1356
Lancini, 1659
Landau, Ezekiel, 798
Land-use regulation, 1305–1306
Lanfranc, 1658
Lanthanic diseases, 601
Lao-tzu, 374, 375, 914, 1631, 1633, 1636
Lao-tzu (Tao-te Ching), 1631, 1634
Laparoscopy, 1446, 1448, 1460, 1466, 1607–1608
Laparotomy, 1448
Laplace, Pierre de, 501, 502
Lappé, Marc, 1703
Largus, Scribonius, 936
Lasagna, Louis, 323
Lasker, Mary B., 1495
Lasswell, Harold, 1640
Latent consequences of social change, 1297–1298
Latent learning, 108
Latent personhood, 744, 748
Latin America:
    abortion in, 1006
    contraception in, 1283
    drug use in, 1383
    health status by level of per capita income in, 1321–1322
    Marxism, in, 1403
    medical ethics in, 1005–1007
    per capita public expenditures on education, health, and defense in, 1324
    population aid to, 1276
    population education in, 1311
    urban growth in, 1220
    See also specific countries
Latin American Medical Congress (1922), 1005
Latter-Day Saints, 70, 337, 1376–1377, 1596
Laughlin, Harry, 460
Laurent, E., 471
Lausier v. Pescinski (1975), 153
Laval University, 1001
Law:
    abortion and, 4, 1649
        basic models, 26–32

        common law, 27, 485
        Jewish law, 5–10, 25
        prenatal diagnosis and, 1334–1335
        Roman Catholic law, 10
        Supreme Court rulings, 16, 27, 30, 31, 169, 198, 573, 820, 998, 1335, 1358, 1465, 1513, 1514, 1615
    advertising by medical professionals and, 46–47
    animal experimentation and, 80–81
    artificial insemination and, 1445, 1464–1469
    behavioral therapies and, 104–105
    biomedical research and, 1493–1494, 1644–1648
    brain death and, 298, 299
    codes of medical ethics and, 167
    confidentiality and, 197, 198–199, 575
    criminal responsibility of the retarded and, 1112
    drug use and, 330–331
    dynamic therapies and, 343–344
    in Eastern Orthodox Christianity, 348
    ethics distinguished from, 401
    euthanasia and, 281–285, 735–737
    freedom of the press and, 185
    genetics and, 573–577, 1644–1646, 1648
        confidentiality, 575
        environment hazards, 577
        genetic counseling, 575, 576–577
        genetic screening, 574–576
        informed consent, 576–577
        prenatal torts, 575–576
        procreation and privacy, 573–574
    heart transplantation and, 656
    homosexuality and, 673
    hospitals and, 678
    human experimentation and, 706, 707, 1648
    hypnosis and, 713–714
    informed consent:
        genetics and, 576–577
        in human experimentation, 755
        medical malpractice and, 1023–1024
        in mental health, 763–766, 781–783, 1105
        in therapeutic relationship, 769–774
    Japanese, 927–928, 929
    Latin American, 1005–1006
    mass health screening and, 861–862
    medical malpractice and, 1020–1027
        alternatives to litigation, 1024–1026
        future, 1026–1027

historical background, 1020
informed consent and, 1023–1024
nature and purpose of law, 1020–1022
reasons for suits, 1024
standards of due care and, 1020, 1022–1023
medieval medicine and:
canon law, 942–945
secular law, 945–947
mental illness and:
civil commitment, 763–765, 779, 1072–1073, 1103–1105
guardianship, 1105–1106
incompetence to stand trial, 1106
insanity defense, 1106–1107
mental institutionalization and, 779–784
durational limits, 782–784
informed consent, 757, 758, 763–766, 779, 781–782
right to refuse treatment, 779–781
right to treatment, 779–780
morality and, 817–821
moral status and legal status, 817–819
use of legal system to enforce morality, 819–821
natural, *See* Natural law
organ donation and, 1157–1159
cadaver donorship, 1157–1158
live donorship, 1154, 1157
salvaging organs, 1158–1159
paternalism and, 1195
pharmacy and, 1211, 1212, 1213
population policy and, 1296
prenatal diagnosis and, 1334–1335
pronouncement of death and, 296–301
public health and, 1394–1396
racism and, 1408, 1409
rape and, 1709
reproductive technologies and, 573–574, 1464–1469
access and state regulation, 1464–1466
donor or surrogate relationship with child, 1468–1469
effect on marital relationship, 1468
status of child, 1455, 1467–1468
status of fetus, 1469
rights, 625, 626, 1508–1509, 1514–1515
right to refuse medical care and, 1499, 1500, 1504, 1506
schizophrenia and, 540
sterilization and, 459–460, 1613–1617

compulsory, 459, 1614–1616
voluntary, 1616–1617
suicide and, 1625–1626
supply of physicians and, 866
technology and, 1644–1649
comparison of available legal approaches, 1647–1648
means and ends in, 1644–1645
taxonomy of legal technique, 1645–1647
Law for the Prevention of Congenitally Ill Progeny (Germany), 1016
Law of Care and Custody of Mental Patients (Japan), 929
Law of Mental Health (Japan), 929
Law of Mental Hospitals (Japan), 929
Laws (Plato), 932, 1225, 1360, 1578, 1624, 1656
Law schools, 873
Law to Protect Genetic Health of 1935 (Germany), 1016
Lawyers:
bioethics and, 1000
medical malpractice suits and, 1024
Lazar houses, 677
Lazarus, Richard, 1086
Lazear, Jesse W., 687, 688
League for Spiritual Discovery, 337
Leake, Chauncey, 995–996
Learning theory, 107–108, 110–114, 503
Lebacqz, Karen A., 1338
Lebanese Order of Physicians, 889
Lebanese Society of Neurology, Neurosurgery, and Psychiatry, 889
Lebanon:
codes of ethics in, 889
differential population growth in, 1286
family planning in, 890
organ transplantation in, 891
population policy in, 1283
Lecky, William E. H., 743, 797
Lectures on Ethics (Kant), 1584
Lectures on the Duties and Qualifications of a Physician (John Gregory), 871, 960
Lederberg, Joshua, 20, 474, 1456, 1703
Leeb, J., 1018
Leffingwell, Albert, 689
Left ventricular assist device (LVAD), 659–660
Legalism, ethical, 422
Legal medicine, 1726
Legal moralism, 1195
Legal positivism, 818–819, 1134, 1135
Legal rights, 625, 626

in bioethics, 1511–1515
generic concept of, 1508–1509
Legislation, *See* Law
Lehman, Harvey Christian, 53
Lehmann, Paul, 421
Leibniz, Gottfried W. von, 240, 1402
Leibnizian optimism, 240
Léjeune, Jérôme, 985, 1332, 1337, 1338
Le Maistre, Martin, 212, 1580–1581
Lennard, Henry L., 1382
Leo I (the Great), Pope, 207
Leonardo da Vinci, 827, 1699
Leopold, Aldo, 370, 398
Lesbianism, *See* Homosexuality
Lesch-Nyhan syndrome, 474
Lessing, Doris, 1013
Lessius, Leonard, 34
Letting die:
distinction between killing and, 35–38, 318, 728–729, 747, 1369
See also Euthanasia
Leucotomies, *See* Lobotomies
Levels of health care, 613–614
Leventhal, Howard, 619
Levin, Amy, 1563, 1564
Levin, Robert, 1563, 1564
Lévi-Strauss, Claude, 878, 879
Levy, Howard B., 159, 160, 1697–1698, 1702
Lewis, C. I., 1330
Lewis, C. S., 372
Lewis, Denslow, 1552
Lewis, Sinclair, 1012–1013
Lexical ordering of health care, 634
Lexikon für Theologie und Kirche, 1433
Lex talionis, 9
Liaison Committee on Continuing Medical Education, 1041
Liber Compositae Medicinae (Hildegarde of Bingen), 1714
Liber Regius (Haly Abbas), 786, 887
Liber Simplecis Medicinae (Hildegarde of Bingen), 1714
Liberty, 1195, 1196
eugenic aims and, 466–467
population policy and, 1238–1239, 1242, 1245–1246
suicide and, 1624
See also Freedom
Liberty, Equality, and Fraternity (Stephen), 820
Liberty-limiting principles, 1194–1195
Libri Poenitentiales, 1524
Licensing:
in Canada, 964
codes of ethics and, 1726
of genetic counselors, 575
in Great Britain, 973

Licensing (*Continued*)
  to have children, 1301, 1310
  of hospitals, 1202
  human experimentation and, 704
  in medieval Europe, 946–947
  of sex therapists, 1557
  in United States, 964–965, 1030, 1032, 1037, 1174
  of users of technology, 1646
Lidz, Victor M., 1169
Lieber, Francis, 1696
Lieber Code, 1696
Liechtenstein, animal experimentation in, 78
Liefcort, 183
Life:
  beginning of, 17–22
    Aquinas on, 13
    Aristotle on, 9–12
    birth viewed as, 8, 12, 18, 730–731, 1340–1341, 1469
    conception viewed as, 14, 19, 22, 25, 1531
    conferred rights and, 17, 21–22, 23
    individual-biological criterion, 17–20, 1338
    in vitro fertilization and, 1460, 1469
    Judaism and, 8, 800–801
    multiple criterion, 17, 21, 1341
    Protestantism and, 14–16, 24–25, 1437
    relational criterion, 17, 20–21, 22–23, 1341
    Roman Catholicism and, 10–12, 19, 25, 1531
    See also Ensoulment; Personhood
  prolongation of, *See* Anti-aging techniques; Life-support systems; Sustaining life
  quality of, *See* Quality of life
  right to, 123, 726–731, 823, 1337, 1340, 1513, 1528
  sanctity of, *See* Sanctity of life
  value of, 22–25, 822–828, 1217
    animal life, 822, 826, 827–828
    anthropological perspective, 1048, 1049
    Buddhism and, 827–828
    capacity for consciousness and, 828
    Christianity and, 825–826
    cost-benefit approach, 824–825
    human being vs. person, 823, 825
    human life vs. nonhuman life, 825–826
    Judaism and, 25, 825–826
    population problem and, 1217
    possible persons, 827
    potential persons, 826
    Protestantism and, 16

  quality-of-life ethic and, 830–833
  Roman Catholicism and, 23–24
  sanctity of life, *See* Sanctity of life
  utilitarianism and, 823–824, 827, 828
  See also Fetus: status of
Lifeboat ethics, 497, 498, 499
Life expectancy:
  anti-aging techniques and, 50–53
  average, 54
  decline in infectious disease and, 615
  in developing vs. developed nations, 1220
  disease and, 593
  as factor in allocation of scarce resources, 810, 1416
  increase in, 54, 57, 259, 593
  of kidney donors, 1161
  per capita income and, 1321
  public health and, 1397
"Life extension" societies, 216
Life goals, 1060–1061
Life of Reason (Santayana), 237
Life-support systems, 62, 272, 296, 298, 300, 303, 593, 840–848
  in ancient Greece and Rome, 933–934
  blood transfusions, 2, 271, 842
    Eastern Orthodox Christianity and, 350
    ethical problems, 133–134
    exchange transfusion, 842
    Islam and, 893
    Jehovah's Witnesses and, 1026, 1361, 1377, 1426, 1512, 1514
    paternalistic principle and, 1195
    procedure, 133
  Eastern Orthodox Christianity and, 350–352
  extracorporeal membrane oxygenator, 841–842, 844
  function of, 840–843
  heart:
    artificial, 634–635, 636, 659–660, 843, 845, 848, 1155, 1519, 1651–1652
    counterpulsation, 842, 843
    drugs, 842
    external massage, 842
    pacemakers and, 296, 842, 843
    in United States, 997
  images of man and, 855
  iron lungs, 841
  Islam and, 893–895
  in Japan, 929
  Judaism and, 793, 801
  kidney dialysis, 553, 811–815, 842–845, 1155, 1156
    allocation of scarce resources and, 808–809, 815, 1414, 1415, 1416, 1418

  development of, 1160
  ethical issues of, 811–812
  experiment–therapy dilemma and, 812
  history of, 811
  in home, 813, 814
  principle of, 842–843
  quality of life and, 811, 813, 814, 1162
  selection criteria, 1161
  survival and, 1161–1162
  termination of, 272, 845
  in United States, 812, 996, 1418
  medical practice questions, 843–847
    continuation of care, 845–846
    limitation of care, 844–845
    termination of care, 846–847; *See also* Euthanasia
    weaning from system, 845
  medical social work and, 1043
  negative pressure ventilators, 841, 844
  nursing and, 1144
  nutrients, supply of, 842
  oxygen, supply of, 841–842
  parenteral nutrition, 842
  paternalistic principle and, 1195
  philosophical issues, 847–848
  policy questions, 847
  Protestantism and, 1371–1372, 1437
  refusal of, *See* Right to refuse medical care
  Roman Catholicism and, 1531–1532
  surgery and, 1629
  wastes, removal of, 842–843
Liguori, St. Alphonsus, 34, 1065, 1525, 1582
Li Han-chang, 204
Likelihood-of-success factor, 809, 1415, 1416
Limited paternalism, 1196
Limits of Growth, The (Meadows), 393–395
Linacre Quarterly, 996, 1522
Lind, James, 686, 1488
Lindesmith, Alfred R., 330
Linguistic analysis, 1532
Linnaeus (Carl von Linné), 583
Literature, medical ethics in, 1008–1014
Lithium, 1381
Lithotomy, 933
Littlefield, John W., 1337
Liver transplantation, 656, 808, 1162
Living wills, 271, 280–281, 1505
Lloyd, Charles W., 1554
Lobotomies, 98, 99, 999, 1073, 1180, 1182, 1348, 1387, 1526
Locke, John, 264, 403, 416, 625, 953, 971, 1292, 1375, 1401, 1482
  on divine ownership of life, 608

on freedom, 1238
on man's dominion over nature, 368
on mind–body problem, 1091, 1118
on right to integrity of body and freedom from bodily pain, 627
on right to life, liberty, and property, 263, 442, 624, 823
LoDagaa society, 223–224, 226, 227
Loeb, Jacques, 129
Logic, 1328, 1330
Logical analysis, 1051–1052
Logical behaviorism, 1115–1116
Logical Positivists, 448
Logic of Medicine, The (Murphy), 1051
Logika Medycyny (Bieganski), 1051
Lokasaṁgraha, 1270–1271
Lombard, Peter, 1579
London, Perry, 85, 86
London Barber-Surgeons Company, 1035
London Medical Group, 988
Longevity:
    gene therapy and, 522
    Hinduism and, 663–664
    thought and, 230, 231, 233
    values associated with, 58–61
    See also Anti-aging techniques; Life expectancy; Life-support systems; Sustaining life
Lorber, John, 725
Lorenz, Konrad, 541, 542
Lottery system, 809, 810, 867, 1301, 1353, 1416, 1417
Lourdes, healings at, 1123, 1125, 1126, 1127
Love:
    act-utilitarianism and, 422, 1370
    agapic, 422, 431–432
    of animals, 377
    Augustine on, 1579
    Christian concept of, 1657
    ethics and, 1135
    marital, 1582
    of natural beauty, 376–377
    natural law theory and, 1132, 1135
    obligation to future generations and, 509–510
    parental, 1458, 1459
    of self, 1621
    sexual, 1259, 1260, 1457, 1561, 1578, 1579, 1592
    situation ethics and, 422, 434
    theological ethics and, 437
    Victorian, 1561
Love's the Best Doctor (Molière), 1008

Lower, R. R., 655
Loyalties:
    mental health evaluation and, 1082
    population policies and, 1217, 1218
Loyola, St. Ignatius of, 1069
LSD, 332, 335, 337, 338, 1384, 1385
Lu Chih, 914
Lucian, 931, 933, 936
Lucidity of patient, 149
Luckmann, Thomas, 1603
Lucretius, 238, 369, 479
Ludwig, Carl, 584
Lugo, John de, 1170, 1531
Lu Hsün, 917
Lumpectomy, 1708
Lundberg, S., 1699
Lungs:
    cancer of, 381
    gas exchange in, 841–842
    oxygen delivery to, 841
    transplantation of, 1162–1163
Lunyü ("Analects"), 202
Luria, Solomon, 212
Luther, Martin, 282, 1066, 1232, 1372, 1373
    on abortion, 14
    on after-life, 252
    on calling, 1366
    on contraception, 209
    on ensoulment, 14
    on marriage, 209, 1259, 1581, 1587
    on sickness, 1374
    virtue theory of, 435
Lutheranism, 1133–1134
Luyet, Basile Joseph, 216
LVAD, *See* Left ventricular assist device
Lycurgus, King of Sparta, 8
Lying, *See* Deception
Lyman, Samuel, 647
Lysenko, T. D., 482
Lysenkoism, 979
Lysosomal enzyme deficiency diseases, 514
Lysosome, 513–514

M

Maastricht Medical School, Netherlands, 984
Macaulay, Lord, 908
MacDonald, Ramsay, 480–481
Machiavelli, Niccolò, 532, 1235
Ma Chih, 1633
MacIntyre, A. C., 503

Mackey v. Procunier (1973), 780, 1073
MacKinney, Loren C., 941
MacMurray, John, 1585
Macroallocational policies, *See* Scarce resources, allocation of
Macrocultural environment, redesign of, 1296
Madison, James, 647
Madness:
    cultural relativism and, 1090
    historical conceptions of, 1090–1091
    medical models of, 1090–1094, 1096, 1097
    metaphysical foundations of, 1091–1092
    Pinelian model of, 1092–1094, 1096, 1097
    See also Mental illness
Magendie, François, 76, 77, 584
Magic, 1065, 1126, 1127, 1281, 1523
    in Indian medicine, 909
    in Japanese medicine, 922, 923
    in primitive medicine, 878–879
    Roman Catholicism and, 1523
    See also Miracle and faith healing
Magical correspondence, 912
Magical expert, 881
Magicians, 881, 1632
Magico–religious treatment, 1655
    See also Miracle and faith healing
Magnuson, Warren G., 1494
Mahābhārata, 378
Mahāyāna Buddhism, 376
Mai, Franz A., 969
Mailer, Norman, 1594
Maimonides, Moses, 162, 239, 247, 787–788, 791, 1065, 1121, 1186, 1400, 1430
    on abortion, 6, 7
    on intercourse during pregnancy, 470
    Mishneh Torah, 1428, 1429
    "Prayer of," 162–163, 1598, 1602
    text, 1733–1738
    on sanctity of life, 794
    Yad Hachazak (Yad Ha-Hazakah), 248, 793
Mainstreaming, 1110
Mainstream medical care, 616
Majoussi, Al-, 888
Makura no Sōshi (Pillow Books), 377
Maladaptation conception of tissue, 1095
Malaria, 1047
Malawi:
    health expenditures in, 1322
    health status by level of per capita income in, 1321

Malaysia, population policy in, 1283, 1297

Maldistribution of health resources, 1323–1324

Mali, contraception in, 899

Malingering, 595

Malinin, Theodore I., 217

Malleus Maleficarum (Sprenger and Kraemer), 1714

Malnutrition, 1322, 1325, 1599
See also Food policy

Malpighi, Marcello, 954

Malpractice, *See* Medical malpractice

Malthus, Thomas, 210, 211, 394, 479, 496, 1226–1228, 1231, 1234, 1235

Malthusianism, 1217, 1222, 1226–1228, 1243

Malthusianism: The Crime of Genocide (Gabriel Dionysiatou), 1252

Man, images of, *See* Images of man

Man and environment, *See* Environment and man

Man and Nature (Marsh), 369, 393

Mandatory Prepaid Health Care Law of 1974, 640

Mangan, Joseph T., 317

Mani, 207

Manic–depressive disorders, 539–540, 1381
electroconvulsive therapy (ECT) and, 359
genetic predisposition and, 1077
universality of, 1077

Manicheanism, 207–208, 209, 239, 1064, 1579
contraception and, 207
man's dominion over nature and, 367
pain and suffering and, 1184

Manipulative behavior control, 96–98

Mankind at the Turning Point (Mesarovič and Pestel), 394

Man–machine symbiosis, 848

Mann, F. C. 654

Mannus v. State (1966), 151

Mansure, Al, 886

Manu, Code of, 1232

Manufacturing Chemists Association (MCA), 384

Maoism, 1402

Mao Tse-tung, 212, 378, 919, 920

Marcel, Gabriel, 242, 363

Marcus, E., 654

Marcus, Ioannes, 12

Marcus Aurelius, 238, 239, 932

Marcuse, Herbert, 1062, 1063, 1642

Margolis, A. G., 1706

Margolis, Joseph, 601, 602, 1585

Maria aborigines of India, 224

Marijuana, 328, 332, 336, 891, 1384, 1385

Marine Hospital Service, 627, 1493

Maritain, Jacques, 241

Marital counseling, 157

Mark, Vernon, 1389, 1691–1692

Marketable baby license system, 1301–1310

Marketing of drugs, 322–323

Market in organs, 1159

Market naturalism, 1222

Marmor, Judd, 668

Marriage:
in ancient Greece, 1225, 1577
in ancient Rome, 1225–1226, 1577
Aquinas on, 1226, 1580
Augustine on, 1579
Christianity and, 1561
Eastern Orthodox Christianity and, 1252–1253
eugenics and, 469–472
Gnosticism and, 1578
Hinduism and, 1270, 1271
Islam and, 787
Judaism and, 795, 1561, 1576
Malthus on, 1227, 1234
mental illness and, 1710
of mentally retarded, 1111
postponement of, 1227, 1228, 1229, 1271
Protestantism and, 1259, 1261, 1581, 1582
reproductive technologies and, 1444–1445, 1456–1459, 1468–1469
Roman Catholicism and, 208, 209, 1256, 1524, 1527, 1529, 1531, 1582
Victorian ideal of, 1561
See also, Sex therapy

Marriage and Concupiscence (Augustine), 1579

Marsh, George P., 369, 393

Martin Chuzzlewit (Dickens), 1716

Martyrdom of Man (Reade), 266

Marx, Karl, 419, 480, 1402
on environmental preservation, 372
on marriage, 1585
on morality, 1536
on private interest, 1603
on religion, 331, 1066
on technology, 1640–1641

Marx, Karl F. H., 969

Marx, Leo, 371

Marxian naturalism, 443, 1222

Marxism:
contraception and, 213–214
man and medicine and, 977
paternalism and, 1360
purpose in the universe and, 1402
as theology, 429
therapeutic relationship and, 1663, 1666–1667
view of human society, 1603, 1604, 1605

Maryland School of Medicine, University of, 1352

Masden v. Harrison (1957), 1154

Maslow, Abraham, 1068, 1085, 1088

Masona, Bishop of Merida, 939

Massachusetts General Hospital, 191, 280

Massachusetts Medical Society, 1037
Code of Ethics, 45

Massage, 922

Mass health screening, 857–862
abnormal test results, 861
cost-benefit calculations, 860–861
criteria for, 858–859
defined, 857–858
diagnosis distinguished from, 858
effectiveness of, 859
evaluation of, 859–860
of general population, 861–862
genetic, *See* Genetic screening
history of, 858, 1396
of hospital patients, 862
purposes of, 858
of school children, 862

Mass media, *See* Media

Mastectomy, 1708–1709

Masters, William H., 1552, 1553, 1566

Masturbation:
by animals, 1557
contemporary attitudes toward, 1557, 1563, 1564
cultural variations in attitudes toward, 1561, 1583
de-moralization of, 1568
Eastern Orthodox Christianity and, 353
incidence in United States, 1584
Judaism and, 1576–1577
in models of sexuality, 1592, 1593, 1594
semen obtained by:
for in vitro fertilization, 1449
Roman Catholicism and, 1433, 1530–1531, 1533
as therapeutic technique, 1556
Victorianism and, 1561

Mater et Magistra (John XXIII), 1255, 1256

Materialism, 370, 1115–1119, 1419–1423
See also Natural law; Reductionism

Maternal age, chromosomal abnormalities and, 1333

Maternal–fetal relationship, *See* Fetus: –maternal relationship

Maternal life, abortion and
Japanese perspective, 928–929
Judaism and, 6–9
legal aspects, 29, 31
medical perspective, 2
Protestantism and, 14, 16, 1437
Roman Catholicism and, 10, 11, 12, 16, 23, 1527

Maternity leave, 1718

Mate-selection, eugenics and, 469–472

Mate swapping, 1563, 1564
Mathé, Georges, 985
Mather, Cotton, 686–687, 963
Maturity, psychological, 39–41
Maupertuis, Pierre, 479
Mauriceau, 489
Mauss, Marcel, 256, 812, 813, 1168
Maximin level of health care, 634–635
Maximin rule, 806
Maximum awards, in malpractice suits, 1025–1026
May, Rollo, 1085
Mayeroff, Hans, 146
Mayr, Ernst, 591
McCormick, Richard A., 154, 319, 732, 759, 835, 1113
McFadden, Charles J., 871, 996, 1685
McGill University, 1001
McGreevey, William P., 1295
McIntosh, Jim, 1678
McKinley, Sonya M., 1708
McLuhan, Marshall, 1639
McNeill, John, 673, 675
Meadows, Donella H., 393–395
Mean time to failure concept, 50
Mechanic, David, 1666
Mechanical determinism, 501–502
Mechanical explanation, 129
Mechanism, 102–103, 129, 130, 367–368, 619, 1419
Mechanistic Conception of Life, The (Loeb), 129
Mechnikov, Ilya, 265
Medawar, Sir Peter, 184, 655, 658, 1455–1456, 1460, 1461
Media:
 display of sexual permissiveness and, 1561, 1562, 1564
 medicine and, 180–188
  corrections, 187
  ethical problems, 183–187
  historical basis of journalistic ethics, 180–182
  human experimentation and, 190, 191, 708–709
  regulations, 187–188
  responsible journalism, 182–183
  See also Scientific publishing
 television, *See* Television
Mediation, principle of, 1523
Medibank, 641, 642
Medicaid, 66, 611–612, 649, 680, 1201–1202, 1318
Medical acceptability, 1415
Medical Act of 1858 (Great Britain), 973, 988, 1037
Medical aidmen, 1697
Medical care, 145–149
 of adolescents, 38–43, 151–152
  age and psychological maturity,

 relationship between, 39
  confidentiality and, 41–42
  informed consent and, 42, 43
  judgment by physician on maturity, 40–41
  maturity as measure of self-determination, 39–40
  psychiatric treatment and, 38, 41
  research programs and, 42–43
 distribution of, 476
 health care distinguished from, 643, 1319–1320
 of infants, *See* Infant care
 Islamic, 788
 ministers and, 1190
 moral ambiguity of, 146
 organization of, 1056–1057
 as personal care, 146–147
 poverty and, 1317–1320, 1322, 1325
 primacy of patient's interest and, 147–148
 primary, 629, 613–617, 1668
 of prisoners, 1346–1348
  behavior control and, 999, 1199, 1347, 1348, 1390
  improvements in, 1348
  involuntary treatment, 1347–1348
  lack of, 1347
  mental health care, 1348
  standards of, 1347
 privacy and, 1363
 rationing of, *See* Scarce resources, allocation of
 respect and, 147, 148–149
 right to, 627–629, 1604–1605
 right to refuse, *See* Right to refuse medical care
 social distribution of, 1056
 sociality and, 1604–1605
 social medicine and, 1599–1600
 truth-telling and, 149
 See also Therapeutic relationship
Medical Care Act of 1966 (Canada), 994
Medical columns, 182
Medical Council of Canada, 967
Medical Council of India, 908–909
Medical Devices Act, 1497
Medical Economics, 322
Medical education, 863–869
 in Africa, 898, 899
 American Medical Association and, 993, 1031, 1037–1038
 in Canada, 993
 in China, 918
 in France, 972
 human experimentation control and, 703

 institutional ethics and, 869
 medical ethics teaching, *See* Medical ethics: education
 ministers in, 1192–1193
 North American, 967
 obligations to faculty, students, and patients, 867–869
 obligation to society in general, 865–867
 philosophy and ethos of, 863–864
 social medicine in, 1601–1602
 sources and nature of obligations, 864–865
 in United States, 993, 1031, 1032–1033
Medical Essays (Holmes), 1686
Medical ethics:
 codes of, *See* Codes of medical ethics
 education, 870–875
  in Arab nations, 889
  in Canada, 1001
  concepts and goals of, 873–875
  contemporary, 871–873
  in Eastern Europe, 980–981
  in Germany, 984–985
  in Great Britain, 872, 988
  history of, 871
  in Latin America, 1006–1007
  in People's Republic of China, 872, 919–920
  in United States, 871, 872–873, 1001
  in Western Europe, 984–985
 history of, *See* Medical ethics, history of
 in literature, 1008–1014
 National Socialism and, 1015–1019
  eugenics, 460, 462, 541, 1015, 1016
  "euthanasia," 267, 282–283, 426–427, 794, 846, 983, 1016–1017, 1696
  general state of medicine, 1015–1016
  genocide, 267, 283, 1017, 1307
  human experimentation, 619, 690, 697, 700, 1015, 1017–1018, 1512, 1696
  Nuremberg trials, 90, 1016, 1018–1019, 1135
 religious directives in, *See* Religious directives in medical ethics
 viewed as traditional ethics, 116–120
Medical Ethics (Committee on Religious Affairs of the Federation of Jewish Philanthropies of New York), 1429

Medical Ethics (Häring), 985
Medical Ethics (Percival), 166, 172, 770, 871, 952, 956, 965, 968, 973, 996, 1038
Medical ethics, history of, 876–1007
  Africa, sub-Saharan, 897–900
  Arab world, contemporary, 888–891
    Muslim perspective, 892–895
  Assyria–Babylonia, 880–883
  China, 902–906, 911–921
    contemporary, 917–921
    prerepublican, 903–906, 911–916
  Eastern world, general survey of, 901–906
  Egypt, ancient, 880–883
  Europe:
    ancient, 930–937
    Central, 968–970
    Eastern, 975, 977–981
    eighteenth-century, 952, 957, 960–962
    medieval, 938–950
    nineteenth-century, 952, 968–974
    seventeenth-century, 952, 954–956
    twentieth-century, 975–991
    Western, 954–956, 982–986
  France:
    eighteenth-century, 958–959
    nineteenth-century, 953, 971–972
  Great Britain:
    eighteenth-century, 957, 960–962
    nineteenth-century, 952–953, 973–974
    twentieth-century, 987–991
  Greece, ancient, 885–886
  India, 902–910
  Israel, contemporary, 895–896
  Japan, 922–929
    contemporary, 926–929
    through the nineteenth century, 922–926
  Latin America, contemporary, 1005–1007
  North America:
    seventeenth to nineteenth century, 963–968
    twentieth-century, 992–1001
  Persia (Iran), 880–887
  primitive societies, 877–879
  Rome, ancient, 930–937
  United States:
    contemporary, 992–1001
    modern, 952–953, 959–960, 963–968
Medical Ethics: A Compendium of Jewish Moral, Ethical and Religious Principles in Medical Practice (Tendler), 996
Medical Ethics for Nurses (McFadden), 871

Medical etiquette:
  in ancient Greece, 931–932
  in Great Britain, 987–988
  rules of, 408
  See also Codes of ethics
Medical exposés, 186
Medical Hypothesis, 1051
Medical journals, *See* Communication, biomedical
Medical League of Socialized Medicine (United States), 1039
Medical malpractice, 752, 755, 873, 1020–1027
  alternatives to litigation, 1024–1026
  in ancient Egypt, 882, 936
  in ancient Greece and Rome, 936
  anthropological perspective, 1048–1049
  in Arab nations, 889
  desire for patient autonomy and, 1674
  in England, 1020
  euthanasia and, 1026–1027
  in France, 1020
  future, 1026–1027
  historical background, 1020
  hospitals and, 1202, 1203
  impersonality of therapeutic relationship and, 1669
  informed consent and, 1023–1024
  in Japan, 926, 927
  in medieval Europe, 946, 947
  nature and purpose of law, 1020–1022
  reasons for suits, 1024
  standards of due care and, 1020, 1022–1023
  in United States, 998, 1020
Medical missions, 1365, 1367
Medical model, 610
  of mental illness, 1090–1094, 1096, 1097
  of therapy, 604
Medical Nemesis (Illich), 1053
Medical police, 952, 957–959, 969
Medical prayers, 162–163
Medical profession:
  advertising by, 44–47
    for abortions, 30
    in ancient Greece, 933
    in Arab nations, 889
    dentistry, 312
    Hinduism and, 664
    impact on institutional providers, 46
    justifications for restrictions on, 45–46
    legal issues in, 46–47
    restrictions in United States, 44–45
  in Africa, 898
  the aged, attitudes toward, 65
  alcoholics, attitudes toward, 72–73

death, attitudes toward, 289–290
dissent against, 161
drug industry and, *See* Drug industry: medical profession and
legal abortion and, 27, 28–29
medical professionalism, 1028–1033
  attributes of professions, 1028
  change and, 1029
  in colonial America, 1029–1030
  functions of, 1028–1029
  in nineteenth-century America, 1030–1031
  in twentieth-century America, 1031–1033
organized medicine, 1034–1041
  American Medical Association and, 1037–1041
  ancient legacy, 1035
  in colonial America, 1036–1037
  early post-Revolutionary trends, 1037
  era of retreat, 1037
  evolution in England, 1035–1036
  global medicine and, 1039
  in medieval Europe, 1035
  peer review and, *See* Peer review
  principal focus of, 1481–1482
  racism and, *See* Racism
  See also Health care; Medicine
Medical records, 197, 1359, 1362–1363
Medical Register (Great Britain), 973
Medical reporting, *See* Communication, biomedical
Medical Research Council (Great Britain), 153, 191, 705, 989, 998, 1000
  statement on responsibility in investigations on human subjects, 1765–1769
Medical schools:
  in Africa, 898
  biomedical research in, 1484
  blacks in, 1408, 1409
  in Canada, 964, 993, 1001
  chaplains in, 1191–1192
  in colonial America, 964
  in Great Britain, 988, 989
  human experimentation control and, 703
  medical ethics education in, 870–875
    in Arab nations, 889
    in Canada, 1001
    concepts and goals of, 873–875
    contemporary, 871–873
    in Eastern Europe, 980–981
    in Great Britain, 988
    history of, 871
    in Latin America, 1006–1007
    in People's Republic of China, 872, 919–920

in United States, 871, 872–873, 1001
in Western Europe, 984–985
Oath of Hippocrates and, 164
obligations of, 863–869
  to faculty, students, and patients, 867–869
  institutional ethics and, 869
  philosophy and ethos of medical education and, 863–864
  to society in general, 865–867
  sources and nature of, 864–865
in Republican China, 918
research in, 697
in United States, 967, 993, 1000, 1001, 1031, 1032–1033, 1037, 1714–1715
women in, 1715, 1716
Medical social work, 1042–1044
Medical societies, 167, 1037
Medical Society of New Jersey, 959
Medical Society of the State of New York, 279
Medical technologists, 1726
Medical Termination of Pregnancy Bill of 1971 (India), 910
Medical testimony, 1103, 1104, 1106
Medical treatment, *See* Health care
Medical University of Pécs (Hungary), 872
Medicare, 56, 66, 67, 611, 638–639, 641, 649, 680, 815, 994, 1040, 1201–1202, 1318
Medicina pastoralis (Antonelli), 871
Medicine:
  anthropology of, 1045–1049
    ascribed cause of illness, 1046–1047
    catalog of recognized diseases, 1046
    death, 1048
    defined, 1046
    ethical considerations, 1048–1049
    usual treatment of illness, 1047–1048
  bioethics and, 125
  biomedical research in relation to, 1484–1486
  as calling, 1366
  dissent in, 161
  domain of, 1481–1484, 1668
  media and, *See* Media: medicine and
  organized, *See* Organized medicine
  orthodoxy in, 1173–1175
  philosophy of, 1049–1054
    philosophy about medicine, 1049–1050, 1052–1053
    philosophy for medicine, 1049–1050–1051

philosophy in medicine, 1049, 1051–1052
philosophy of medicine, proper, 1049, 1050, 1053
primitive, 877–879
Protestant contribution to, 1375–1376
racism and, 1405–1409
  experimentation and, 1409
  health care and, 1407, 1409
  history of, 1405–1409
religion, relationship to, 1374
social, *See* Social medicine
sociology of, 1054–1058
  ethical dilemmas, 1058
  help-seeking and, 1055–1056
  organization of medical care, 1056–1057
  role of physician, 1055
  role of sociologist, 1054–1055
  scope of, 1054
  social distributions of health, illness, and medical care, 1056
  sociology of health occupations, 1057–1058
truth-telling and, 1686–1687
war and, 1695–1699
  conflicting obligations, 1695–1696
  Geneva conference, 1697–1698
  new organizations and codes, 1696
  plea of "superior orders," 1696–1697
  policies in Vietnam, 1697–1698, 1700
Medicine men, 587, 893, 1065
Medico–Chirurgical Society of Baltimore, 965
Medico–Moral Committees, 1432
Medico–Moral Guide, 996, 1432, 1433
Medico–Moral Problems (Kelly), 871
Medicus politicus, 957
Medicus Politicus (Hoffman), 871
Medicus–Politicus: sive de officiis medico–politicis tractatus (Castro), 954–955
Medieval Europe:
  contraception in, 208, 209
  death, conceptions of, 239, 251–255, 261
  disease, conceptions of, 582
  guilds in, 1035
  medical ethics, history of, 938–950
    apothecary regulation, 947–948
    canon law and moral/theological opinions, 942–945
    charity, 939–942

    disease and medicine, early attitudes, 938–939
    early hospitals, 939–940
    Hippocratic ideals, influence of, 940–941
    ideal physicians, 940
    obligations of physicians to community, 948
    plague, 948–950
    professional organizations, 947
    secular law, 945–947
  status of the aged in, 58, 59–60
  therapeutic relationship in, 1657–1658
  women health practitioners in, 1714
Meditations (Marcus Aurelius), 239
Medizinische Logik (Oesterlen), 1051
Medvedev, Zhores A., 48–49
Meir, Rabbi, 247
Melanchthon, Philip, 14, 1366
Melanesia, infanticide in, 742
Melbourne, University of, 872
Melden, Abraham I., 504
Meliorism, 262, 265, 267
Melsen, A. G. M. van, 984
Melville, Herman, 1009
Mémoires sur les hôpitaux de Paris (Tenon), 958
Memorial to the Managers of the Royal Infirmary (James Gregory), 961
Menace of the unfit, 458
Menahem ben Solomon Me'iri, 1251
Mencius, 200, 374
Mendel, Gregor, 480, 529, 541
Mendel's law, 458
Mendelssohn, Moses, 248
Mengele, Joseph, 1018
Meningitis, 1108
Meningomyelocele, *See* Spina bifida
Menninger, Karl, 1619, 1693
Mennonites, 1596
Menopause, 1708
Mensinger, Wilhelm, 211
Menstruation, 1707–1708
Mental age, 1109
Mental deficiency, *See* Mental illness; Mental retardation
Mental health:
  of the aged, 67
  Buddhism and, 1065–1066
  Christianity and, 1065, 1068–1070
  in competition with other values, 1059–1063
    life goals, 1060–1061
    meaning of mental health, 1059–1060
    moral worth of persons, 1061
    social policies, 1061–1063

Mental health (*Continued*)
Eastern Orthodox Christianity
and, 351
Hinduism and, 665–666
informed consent in, 762–766
drug therapy and, 765
dynamic therapies and, 340
electroconvulsive therapy
(ECT) and, 360, 765
vs. informed consent in physical health care, 763
justification for nonconsensual
health care, 763–765
law and, 781–782, 1105
legislation of morality and, 820
mental retardation and, 1112
nonconsensual care in criminal
justice system, 765–766
psychosurgery and, 765, 1389
racism and, 1410–1413
availability and efficacy of services, 1412
context of problem, 1410
new therapeutic approaches,
1413
parochialism and, 1410–1412
scope of problem, 1410
religion and, 1064–1070
clarification of terms, 1064
history of, 1064–1068
Judeo-Christianity case, 1068–
1070
services, *See* Mental health services
therapies, *See* Mental health therapies
of women, 1709–1710
Mental health services, 1071–1082
mental health programs, 1079–
1082
evaluation of, 1080–1082
history of, 1079–1080
social institutions of mental
health, 1071–1078
community centers, 67, 1074–
1076
mental institutionalization, *See*
Mental institutionalization
social role of psychiatrist, 1071–
1074
Mental health therapies:
aversive, 97, 99, 101, 104, 109,
780, 1073
dynamic therapies, 85, 86, 87,
89–90, 97, 338–334, 505, 506,
596, 603, 1094
basic values, 339–341, 1085
classification of, 1084–1085
confidentiality and, 198, 199,
343
for criminal conduct, 765–766
defined, 338–339
determinism and, 502
development of, 1085, 1661,
1662

genetic counseling and, 562,
563
goals of, 1084
hypnosis in, 713, 714
medical profession's acceptance
of, 1482
philosophy of mind and, 1053
reductionism and, 1427
responsibilities of patient, 342
responsibilities of therapist,
341–344
sex therapy with, 1552–1553,
1584
social role of, 344
electrical stimulation of the brain
(ESB) and, 85, 91, 97, 98,
356–358, 551
ethical issues, 357–358
reductionism and, 1427
state of the art, 357
electroconvulsive therapy (ECT),
86, 87, 91, 359–361, 1087,
1381
bioethical problems associated
with, 359–360
informed consent and, 360, 765
in mental hospitals, 360, 1073
nature and effect of treatment,
359
prisoners and, 1347
hypnosis and, 85, 710–714
defined, 710
historical origins of misunderstandings about, 710–711
professional practitioners, concerns of, 712–713
social anxiety about hypnotic
powers, 711–712
practice of, *See* Behavioral therapies: practice of
psychopharmacology, 85, 86, 89,
91, 97, 98, 326, 327, 328,
331, 358, 505, 506, 551, 765,
1087, 1378–1386, 1485
access to, 1385
antianxiety drugs, 1381–1383
antidepressant drugs, 1380–
1381
antipsychotic drugs, 1379–1380
defined, 1378
dispensing of drugs, 1214
experimental research and, 77
hyperkinetic learning disorders
and, 1383–1384
paternalism and, 1199
recreational use of, 1384–1386
reductionism and, 1427
psychosurgery, 85, 87, 91, 99, 505,
506, 765, 781, 999, 1387–
1391, 1397, 1644
defined, 1387
development of, 1387
human nature and, 1391
informed consent and, 765, 1389
lobotomy, 98, 99, 999, 1073,

1180, 1182, 1348, 1387, 1526
paternalism and, 1199
prisoners and, 999, 1347, 1348,
1390
public policy and, 1391
reductionism and, 1427
as social control, 1389–1390
social definition of therapeutic
goals, 1389
social setting of, 1388–1389
as therapy, 1388
self-realization therapies, 1547–
1551
assignment of responsibility in,
1548
basic ambiguities in, 1548
benefits in, 1549
defined, 1547
ethics of change and, 1548–1549
range of techniques, 1547–1548
risks in, 1549
social control and, 1549–1550
social implications of, 1550
sex therapy, *See* Sex therapy
values in, 1083–1088
classification of therapy systems, 1083–1086
definition and approach, 1083
general problem of, 1088–1089
three models of human nature,
1088
See also Behavior control; Behaviorism
Mental hospitalization, *See* Mental
institutionalization
Mental hospitals:
the aged in, 67
alcoholics, response to, 73
assumption of value of, 1077
behavior control in, 86, 91, 1073
Community Mental Health Centers
(CHMC), 1074–1076
discrimination in admissions to,
1076
electroconvulsive therapy (ECT)
in, 360, 1073
home care vs., 1075
in Japan, 929
lobotomies in, 1073
pastoral teaching programs in,
1192
as total institutions, 1076
in United States, 1079–1080
See also Mental institutionalization
Mental illness, 1095–1096, 1098–
1107
assumption of, in institutionalization, 1076–1077
behavior therapies and, 103–104
civil commitment laws and, 763–
765, 779, 1072–1073, 1103–
1105
conceptions of, 1090–1097
antipsychiatry, 1092, 1094–
1096

contemporary non-Pinelian models, 1093–1094
medical models, 1090–1094, 1096, 1097
medical vs. sociological, 1090
metaphysical foundations of mental illness, 1091–1092
Pinelian model, 1092–1094, 1096, 1097
somaiatric models, 1094
somatic models, 1091, 1094, 1096, 1097
diagnosis of, 1098–1102
labeling of deviance, 1100–1101
mental illness vs. normality and physical illness, 1099–1100
sick role and, 1099
types of data used in, 1101
dynamic therapies and, *See* Dynamic therapies
electroconvulsive therapy (ECT) and, 359
genetics and, 544
in Japan, 929
Judaism and, 1065
legal aspects of labeling in, 1102–1107
confinement to mental institutions, 1102–1105
guardianship, 1105–1106
incompetence to stand trial, 1106
insanity defense, 1106–1107
privacy and, 1362
See also Mentally handicapped; Mental institutionalization; Mental retardation
Mental institutionalization, 779–784
assumption of mental illness and, 1076–1077
assumption of value of hospitals and, 1077
behavioral therapies and, 104–105, 780–781
conflict of rights and, 1512
depersonalization and, 1140
duration of, 782–784, 1104–1105
informed consent and, 757, 758, 763–766, 779, 781–782
in Japan, 1388
justification for, 763–765, 1103
labeling and, 1103–1104
legal status of involuntary patients, 1105
of mentally retarded, 1110
movement toward decarceration, 779, 1105, 1379–1380
paternalism and, 1195, 1199
Pinelian revolution and, 1092–1093

privacy and, 1363
procedure for, 1104
right to refuse treatment, 779–781, 1072–1073, 1203, 1503–1504
right to treatment, 779–780, 1072, 1077, 1105, 1203, 1514–1515
social role of psychiatrists and, 1071–1074
social selection for, 1076
for sociopolitical reasons, 1071–1072, 1078
as torture, 1355
Mentally handicapped, 1108–1113
defined, 1108
general rights of, 1109–1112
labeling of, 1108
See also Birth defects; Mental retardation
Mental model of disease, 603–604
Mental model of madness, 1091
Mental pain, 1181
Mental retardation, 81, 82, 529, 1108–1113
amniocentesis and, 569
behavior control and, 1112
civil rights and, 1111–1112
classification of, 1108
compulsory sterilization and, 31, 459–460, 1108–1109, 1111, 1395, 1397
contraception and, 1111
criminal responsibility and, 1112
deinstitutionalization and normalization of, 1110
environmental factors in, 1108
eugenics and, 467
experimentation and, 1112–1113, 1497
genetics and, 538–539, 1108–1109
guardianship and, 1110–1111
informed consent and, 1112
institutionalization and, 1110
intelligence quotient and, 1109
mainstreaming of, 1110
marriage and, 1111
mental age and, 1109
personhood and, 1109
progressive conditions associated with, 718–719
reproduction and, 1111
right to survival and, 1109–1110
screening for, *See* Genetic screening; Prenatal diagnosis
static conditions associated with, 718
See also Birth defects; Mental illness
Mercantilism, 262–263, 1226, 1235
Merciful overdose, 273, 274
Mercy killing, *See* Euthanasia

Meritarian justice, 1238
Merit theory of justice, 837
Merleau-Ponty, Maurice, 363, 364, 1585
Merton, Robert K., 703, 1541, 1542, 1543, 1545
Mesarović, Mihajlo, 394
Mesmer, Franz Anton, 710–711, 1123, 1660
Mesmerism, 1123, 1376, 1377
Mesopotamia, 207, 580
Mesthene, Emmanuel G., 1642
Metabolic death, 259
Metabolic rate reduction, as anti-aging technique, 52, 63
Metabolic screening, 567–568
Metachromatic leukodystrophy (MLD), 718–719
Metaethical relativism, 456, 457
Metaethics, 1217
normative ethics distinguished from, 403–404, 1132–1133
See also Moral reasoning; Naturalism; Nondescriptivism; Objectivism in ethics
Metalogicus (John of Salisbury), 1658
Metaphysical model of sexuality, 1593
Metaphysics of Morals (Kant), 1685
Methadone maintenance, 332
Methodist Church, 70, 1374
Methylmalonic acidemia, 1333
Methylphenidate, 1381, 1383
Metropolitan Hospital (Baghdad), 886
Mexico, 1005
Meyer, 1080
Michigan, University of, 559
Micro–macrocosm analogy, 581
Microsocial environment, restructuring of, 1296
Middle class medical care, 616
Middlemarch (Eliot), 1009–1010, 1012
Midwifery, 897, 898, 971, 1047, 1713–1717, 1726
Mielke, F., 1018
Migration, 1217, 1219, 1245, 1274, 1315
illegal, 1221
internal, 1305–1306
international, 1220–1221, 1304–1305
interplanetary, 1304
of physicians, 645–646
rural to urban, 1220, 1224, 1233
Miklishanski, Y. K., 5
Milgram, Stanley, 1474–1475, 1476
Milieu therapy, 1087, 1379

Military:
  behavior control in, 91
  expenditures, 1323, 1324
Mill, John Stuart, 173, 424, 428, 432, 448, 543, 1051, 1292, 1585
  on equivalence of love and utilitarianism, 422
  on happiness, 542, 828
  on justice, 805, 806
  on law and morality, 819
  on liberty, 1195–1196, 1238, 1518
  on moral rules, 409
  on paternalism, 1103
  on population, 1234
  on "stationary state" economy, 394
Miller, David, 635
Miller, Jean Baker, 1704
Millon, Theodore, 1083
Milunsky, Aubrey, 1337, 1339, 1340
Mind and the World-Order (Lewis), 1330
Mind–body problem, 1091, 1114–1119
  abortion and, 18, 1117–1118
  behaviorism and, 1115–1116, 1421, 1425–1426
  brain death and, 304, 1118
  Cartesian dualism and, 18, 112, 240, 361–362, 367, 370, 501, 502, 603–604, 1050, 1052, 1115, 1117–1119, 1426, 1427
  causal theory of mind and, 1117
  embodiment and, 361–365
  euthanasia and, 1117–1118
  functionalism and, 1116–1117, 1119, 1421, 1422
  identity thesis and, 303–304, 1116–1117, 1420–1421
  materialism and, 1115–1119
  physicalism and, 1422
  process philosophy and, 370
  Protestantism and, 1375
  psychosurgery and, 1391
  Roman Catholicism and, 1532
  See also Personhood; Soul
Mindless phenomenon, human body as, 362–363
Ministers, See Pastoral ministry
Minnesota, University of, 559
Minnesota Multiphasic Personality Inventory (MMPI), 1411–1412
Minority groups:
  behavioral research and, 1477, 1479
  medical school admissions and, 866–867
  population policy and, 1289
  zoning and, 1306
  See also Discrimination; Racism
Minors:
  consent of, for health services, 39
  sterilization of, 1616

See also Children; Infant care
Miracle and faith healing, 589, 924, 1048, 1120–1129, 1191
  conceptual and historical perspectives, 1120–1124
    definitions, 1120
    exorcism, 924, 1121–1122, 1128, 1376, 1523
    faith healing, 1123
    forgiveness of sickness-producing sins, 1122
    healing by divine power, 587, 1122–1123
    significance of cures, 1123–1124
  theological perspective, 1125–1129
    debate about interpretation, 1125–1126
    extreme case of possession, 1128–1129
    faith and the object of faith, 1126–1127
    Protestantism, 1121–1123, 1124, 1365, 1374–1377
    role of medicine, 1127
    Roman Catholicism, 1121, 1523
    understanding of illness, 1127–1128
    word and miracle, 1127
Miracles, defined, 1120
Mishan, Ezra J., 394
Mishima, Yukio, 1622
Mishnah (Mishna), 7, 8, 469, 1428
Mishneh Torah (Maimonides), 1428, 1429
Misinformation in television broadcasting, 187
Misleading omission, 1685
Misquotations in medical reporting, 186–187
Mitscherlich, A., 1018
MMPI, See Minnesota Multiphasic Personality Inventory
Modeling, 109
Modern Medicine and Jewish Law (Rosner), 871, 996
Mohammedanism, See Islam
Mohandas, A., 293
Mohave Indians, 224
Moksha, 661, 1188
Molecular cross-linking theory of aging, 49
Molière, 1008, 1009, 1012
Molina, Louis, 317
Mondeville, Henri de, 941–942
Monetary population incentives, 1290–1291, 1293
Money, John, 1552, 1589–1590, 1591
Mongolia, population policy in, 1291
Mongolism, See Down's syndrome
Monica, St., 1713
Monistic teleological theories, 417–418

Monitoring, variety in, 490
Moniz, Egas, 1387
Monkeys, experiments on, 80, 82
Monoamine oxidase (MAO) inhibitors, 1381
Monopoly, 1326
Monopsony, 1326
Montaigne, Michel de, 240
Montanus, 1659
Montesquieu, Baron de La Brède et de, 1132
Montgomery v. Board of Retirement of the Kern County Employees' Retirement Association (1973), 1501
Montreal, University of, 1001
Montyon, Baron de (A. J.-B. Huget), 958
Mood changes, 169
Moods, control over, 86
Moore, George E., 173, 403, 417, 419, 420, 424, 426, 438, 448
  on naturalistic fallacy, 131, 443–444, 542, 1134, 1135
Moore, Thomas Verner, 1138
Moral agency, 81, 1574
Moral blackmail, 1153
Moral community, 510
Moral default, 436
Morales v. Thurman (1973), 104
Morality, See Ethics
Morality of Organic Transplantation, The (Cunningham), 1170
Moral justification, 410–412, 432
Morally normative statements, 831
Moral notions, 431–437
Moral obligation, See Obligation
Moral reasoning, 406, 449–453
  criteria of morality and, 450
  defined, 450
  mental health program evaluation and, 1082
  as practical reasoning, 451–453
Moral rights, 625
  in bioethics, 1511–1514
  generic concept of, 1507–1509
Moral rules, See Rules and principles
Morals, defined, 877
Morals and Medicine (Fletcher), 996, 1368, 1370, 1687
Morals in Medicine (O'Donnell), 871
Moral therapists, 1092
Moral worth of persons, 1061
Moratoria, clinical, 703–704
More, Sir Thomas, 262–263, 943, 1234
Morgagni, Giovanni, 600, 1659
Morgan, John, 964, 1714
Morgentaler, Henry, 999
Morison, Robert S., 302–303, 524, 1340
Mormonism, See Latter-Day Saints
Morris, Herbert, 506

Morris, Norval, 782–783
Morris, R. T., 313
Mortalism, 265–266, 267
Mortality rate, 1217, 1245, 1274
  of blacks, 1406–1407, 1408
  debates about factors affecting, 1221–1222
  decline in, 54
  demographic transition and, 1228
  in developing countries, 1220, 1282
  for iatrogenic disease, 323
  in India, 1271
  of infants, 1321, 1396
  patterns in, 1219–1220
  per capita income and, 1321
  of primitive man, 1228
  sex differences in, 55
Mosaics, cellular, 519–520
Moses and Monotheism (Freud), 1067
Moses ben Nachman, 1428
Mothers, surrogate, 557, 1450, 1454, 1462, 1467, 1468–1469, 1713
Mothner, Ira, 1704
Motivation:
  in dynamic theories, 1084
  electrical stimulation of the brain and, 357
  for international health work, 643–644
Motivational research, 92
Motive-utilitarianism, 427
Mo-tzu, 374, 1234
Mowrer, O. H., 1087
Moxibustion, 912, 922, 923
Muhammad, 431, 432, 434, 785, 786–787, 1186
Muir, John, 369, 371, 372
Muller, Charlotte, 1382
Muller, Hermann J., 462, 511, 527, 1455
Mullins, Nicholas, 1544
Multiphasic screening, 858
Multiple criterion for beginning of human life, 17, 21, 1341
Multiple publication, 191
Multiple Sclerosis Commission, 1496
Mumford, Lewis, 1639, 1640
Mummification, 142
Municipal physicians, 948
Munk, William, 265
Murngin society, 222, 227
Muromachi period, 923
Murphy, Edmond A., 1051
Murray, Gilbert, 238
Muscular dystrophy, 555, 557, 720, 1343
Muslims, *See* Islam
Musonius Rufus, 206, 1578

Mutability, 236
Mutagen, 577
Mutations, 48–49, 381, 465, 467, 476, 511, 523–524, 577
Mutilation:
  Buddhism and, 137
  Islam and, 788
  Judaism and, 144
  mastectomy and, 1709
  Roman Catholicism and, 818, 1170–1171, 1528–1529, 1609–1610
Mutual criticism of research and publications, 192
Mutuality, 966
Myelomeningocele, *See* Spina bifida
Myotonic dystrophy, 555
Mystery of Death, The (Boros), 302
Mystery of Love, The (Evdokimov), 1252
Mystical experience, drug use and, 336–337
Mystic–hasidic movement, 248
Mysticism, 1064
  See also Taoism
Myth, 1400, 1401, 1403

N

Nachmanides, 791
Nader, Ralph, 649
Nagel, Ernest, 1399
Nagel, Thomas, 632
Napalm, 1700
Napoleon III, Emperor, 972
Napoleonic Code, 992
Narcotics, 336, 1213–1214
  See also Opiates
Narveson, Jan, 508
NAS, *See* National Academy of Sciences
Natanson v. Kline (1960), 770, 771, 772
National Academy of Medicine of Venezuela, 1007
  Venezuelan Code of Medical Ethics, 1746–1748
National Academy of Sciences (NAS), 184, 386
  Board of Medicine, 703
  Institute of Medicine, 1000
  National Research Council, 1494
National Advisory Health Council, 1493
National Association of Science Writers, 181

National Association of Social Workers, 1728
National Board of Health, 1394
National Cancer Act of 1971, 1496
National Cancer Institute (NCI), 380, 382, 1494
National Catholic Pharmacists Guild, 1729
National centers, 614
National Commission for the Protection of Human Subjects of Biomedical and Behavioral Research, 142, 153, 492, 493, 707–708, 975, 997, 1000, 1198, 1350, 1352, 1353, 1487–1488, 1495, 1497
National Conference of Catholic Bishops, 169
National Cooley's Anemia Control Act of 1972, 1496
National Council for International Health, 1039, 1276
National Council of Churches, 1437
National Dental Association, 315
National development, 1322–1324, 1326
National Eclectic Medical Association, 1715
National Endowment for the Humanities, 1001
National Environmental Policy Act of 1970, 391
National Environmental Protection, 1497
National Federation of Catholic Physicians' Guilds, 996
National Hamdard Foundation, 789
National health insurance, 56, 611, 612, 622, 637–638, 641–642, 648, 649, 680, 994, 1039, 1205, 1318, 1397–1398
National Health Insurance (NHI), 1205
National Health Service (Great Britain), 29–30, 987, 990, 991, 1601
National Health Service Act of 1946 (Great Britain), 638
National Heart, Blood Vessel, Lung and Blood Act of 1972, 1496
National Heart and Lung Institute, 997
National Institute of Environmental Health Sciences, 577
National Institute of Occupational Safety and Health, 577
National Institute of Health (NIH), 1494
National Institute of Mental Health, 1494

National Institutes of Health (NIH), 524, 577, 649, 706, 707, 1074, 1489, 1494, 1496, 1646
  Artificial Heart Assessment Panel of the National Heart and Lung Institute, 1651–1652
  Cancer Institute, 1496
  Clinical Center, 1352, 1495
  Code for Self-experimentation, 1487
National Insurance Act of 1911 (Great Britain), 638
Nationalism, 1229
National League for Nursing (NLN), 1138, 1141
National Medical Association, 1031, 1039, 1041, 1408
National Medical Association of China, 918
National Physicians Council, 1040
National Prison Project, 1351
National Research Council, Committee on the Life Sciences and Social Policy, 1652–1653
National Science Foundation, 1489, 1494
National Sex Forum, 1554
National Sickle Cell Anemia Control Act of 1972, 1496
National Socialism, 818, 979, 1538, 1700
  eugenics and, 460, 462, 541, 1015, 1016
  "euthanasia," 267, 282–283, 426–427, 794, 846, 983, 1016–1017, 1696
  general state of medicine, 1015–1016
  genocide, 267, 283, 1017, 1307
  human experimentation, 619, 690, 697, 700, 1015, 1017–1018, 1512, 1696
  Nuremberg trials, 190, 1016, 1018–1019, 1135
  plea of "superior orders" and, 1696
  population policy in, 1230
  prison camps, 1355
National Society for Medical Research, 78
National Training Laboratory, 1547
National Welfare Rights Organization (NWRO), 1202
Native American Church of North America, 337
Natural beauty, love of, 376–377
Natural Death Act of 1976, 1506, 1514
Natural ends, 442, 1132, 1133
Natural experiments, 684
Natural increase, rate of, 1219
Naturalism, 406, 439, 442–447, 458, 542, 1402, 1584
  bioethics and, 444–446
  diversities in, 442–443
  images of man and, 852

market, 1222
Marxian, 443, 1222
naturalistic fallacy and, 131–132, 443–444, 542
personhood and, 1206–1207
purpose in the universe and, 1400–1404
  See also Evolution, Darwin's theory of; Science
Naturalistic fallacy, 131–132, 443–444, 542, 1134, 1135
Naturalistic observation, 1471
Naturalistic optimism, 1222
Natural law, 442–443, 446, 607, 608, 817–819, 1131–1137
  abortion and, 1338, 1526
  bioethics and, 446
  contemporary revival of, 1135–1137
  defined, 817–818
  diversities in, 818, 1132–1133
  illustrative examples of, 1131–1132
  naturalistic fallacy and, 1134, 1135
  personhood and, 1206–1207
  principal objections to, 818–819, 1133–1135
  purpose in the universe and, 1400–1404
  Roman Catholicism and, 818, 1134–1135, 1136, 1524, 1526, 1532
  theological ethics and, 436
Naturally purposive tendencies, 1134
Natural processes, intervention in, 130–131
Natural rights, 625
Natural selection, 479–480, 524, 1307
  generated by compulsory population control, 1309–1310
  generated by continued population growth, 1307–1308
  generated by voluntary population control, 1308–1309
Natural Theology: or Evidences of the Existence and Attributes of the Deity Collected from the Appearances of Nature (Paley), 480
Nature, *See* Environment and man; Environmental ethics; Naturalism; Natural law
Nature of Women 93, The, 205
Navaho Indians, 590, 877, 878, 1045, 1046, 1285
Navarro, Vicente, 1666
Navarrus (Martin Aspilcueta), 942–945
Nazism, *See* National Socialism
NCI, *See* National Cancer Institute
Necromancy, 922, 924
Necropsy, 1482

Needham, Joseph, 482, 1632, 1634, 1635
Needling, 912
Needs, 626–627
Neel, James V., 1340
Neely, Matthew M., 1493
Negative eugenics, 458, 460, 511–512, 550, 563, 1199, 1448, 1455
Negative pressure ventilators, 841, 844
Negative rights, 625, 1509, 1510
Negative utilitarianism, 428
Negligence, 755, 772, 773, 774, 1020, 1021, 1022, 1024, 1467
  See also Medical malpractice
Negotiations for informed consent, 755–756
Nehru, Jawaharlal, 1229
Neighborhood Health Centers, 617, 1319
Neilsen v. Regents of University of California (1973), 153
Neo-American Church, 337
Neo-Confucianism, 923–924
Neocortical function, as criterion for personhood, 835
Neo-Marxism, 1663, 1666–1667
Neonatal care, *See* Infant care
Neonaturalism, 63–64
Neo-Platonism, 239, 251, 367
Neopositivism, 265, 266–267
Neo-Pythagoreanism, 206, 239
Neo-Thomism, 252
Nerve gas testing, 1702
Nestorius, 886
Netherlands:
  animal experimentation in, 81
  contraception in, 213
  differential population growth in, 1286
  health care financing in, 611
  health-related expenditures in, 650
  influence on Japanese medicine, 924
  medical care, wartime history of, 1697, 1698
  medical ethics education in, 872
  medical schools in, 984
Net migration, rate of, 1219
Neuburger, Max, 792
Neumann, Salomon, 969
Neurohumoral theory of pain, 1178
Neurokinins, 1178, 1179
Neurological Society of America, 1730
Neurophysiological theories of pain, 1178
Neurotic condition, 339
Neville, Robert, 1691–1692
New Atlantis (Bacon), 367
Newborn infants:
  brain damage and, 2
  genetic screening of, 567–568

See also Infant care
New Deal, 648
New Dimensions in Legal and Ethical Concepts for Human Research, 1000
New England Journal of Medicine, The, 190, 191, 1001
New eugenics, *See* Genetic engineering
New group therapy, 1087–1088
New Jersey–Pennsylvania Income Maintenance Experiment, 1471
New Perspective on the Health of Canadians, A, 1601
Newspapers:
    advertising in, 180
    media reporting in, *See* Media
New Testament, 10, 1578, 1622
    on contraception, 206–207
    on death, 245–246
    disease, conception of, 588
    on miracle and faith healing, 1121, 1122–1123, 1126–1127, 1128
    on status of fetus, 15
    on supererogation, 1149–1150
    See also Bible
Newton, Sir Isaac, 240, 263, 367, 480, 501, 1543
New towns, 1306
New York Academy of Medicine, 1030
New York Infirmary for Women, 1715
New York State Medical Society, 965, 967
New York State Medical Society House of Delegates, 176
New Zealand:
    abortion laws in, 28
    accident and injury compensation in, 1026
    health insurance in, 638, 641, 642
    infanticide in, 742
    urban growth in, 1220
NHI, *See* National Health Insurance
Nicephorus, 589
Nichiren sect, 378
Nichols, Peter, 1009
Nichomachean Ethics (Aristotle), 59, 545, 785, 1237, 1577, 1685
Nicon, Patrinacos, 1253
Nicotine, *See* Smoking
Niebuhr, H. Richard, 1371
Niebuhr, Reinhold, 212, 248, 1583
Niedermeyer, Albert, 1525
Nielsen, Kai, 421
Nietzsche, Friedrich, 237, 241, 266, 418, 1066, 1584
Nigeria:
    census of, 1285–1286
    compensation of physicians in, 899
Nightingale, Florence, 995, 1696, 1716
NIH, *See* National Institute of Health; National Institutes of Health
Nihilism, ethical, 454
1984 (Orwell), 196, 267, 1385
Ninshō, 136, 923
Nirvana, 1188
Nixon, Richard M., 1496
NLN, *See* National League for Nursing
Noachide Code, 1251
Nobel, Alfred, 1699, 1700
"No-fault" concept, 1022, 1024–1025
Nolte, Ernst, 267
Nominalism, 1400
Nonbeneficial experimentation, 693–694, 695
Non-cognitivism, 448
Nonconsequentialist teleological theories, 418
Non-descriptivism, 406, 443, 447–449
Nonlogical characteristics, diagnoses and, 309–311
Nonmedical models of therapy, 604
Nonquantifiable teleological theories, 418
Nonsexual human reproduction, *See* Cloning
Nonsomatic models of disease, 603–604
Nontechnology of medicine, 1485
Nontheistic religions, 1064
Nontherapeutic abortions, 3
Nontherapeutic experimentation:
    on the aged, 68
    on children, 153–155
    on fetuses, 490, 492
    on the mentally retarded, 1113
    obligation to participate in, 700–702
    therapeutic experimentation distinguished from, 693–694, 699–700
Noonan, John T., 19, 1254
Norinaga, Motoori, 925
Normality:
    diagnoses of behavioral dysfunction and, 357
    perspectives of, 39–40
    vs. perversion, 1592–1595
    vs. physical and mental illness, 1099–1100
Normalization:
    chronic disease and, 158
    of the mentally retarded, 1110
Normative ethics, 1217
    metaethics distinguished from, 403–404, 1132–1133
    questions of, 403, 404–405
    See also Deontological theories; Rules and principles; Situation ethics; Teleological theories; Utilitarianism
Normative relativism, 455–456, 457
    See also Situation ethics
North America:
    history of medical ethics in:
        seventeenth to nineteenth century, 963–968
        twentieth century, 992–1001
    per capita public expenditures on education, health, and defense in, 1324
    population education in, 1311
    urban growth in, 1220
    See also Canada; United States
North American Clinical Dermatologic Association, 1729
Northern Ireland, differential population growth in, 1286
Norway:
    animal experimentation in, 78
    differential population growth in, 1286
    health insurance in, 637
    organ salvaging in, 1158
    Penal Code of 1902, 282
Noshisran, Khosrow, 886
Nosologia Methodica Sistens Morborum Classes Juxta Sydenhami Mentem et Botanicorum Ordinem (Sauvage de la Croix), 1051
Nosologies, ethical force of, 604–605
Nostrums, 994
Nott, Josiah Clark, 1405–1406
Nottingham Medical School (England), 872
Nouvelle Héloïse, La (Rousseau), 1584
Nozick, Robert, 632–633, 1604
Nuclear energy, 382–383, 389, 1224
Nuclear transplantation, 518, 1452
Nuclear weapons, 1641, 1699, 1700, 1702
Nuremberg Code, 153, 172, 656, 697, 754, 757–760, 1018–1019, 1113, 1486, 1487, 1512
    text of, 1764–1765
Nuremberg trials, 190, 983, 997, 1016, 1018, 1696
Nurse midwifery, 1726

Nurse practitioners, 616, 622, 1719
Nursing, 1138–1145
    abortion and, 1142
    blacks in, 1409
    codes of ethics, *See* Codes of nursing ethics
    constrained definition of roles in, 1058, 1718–1719
    defective children and, 723, 724, 738
    early history of, 1713
    education, 1138, 1139–1140
    ethics committees and, 1145
    general conflicts in, 1141–1142
    human experimentation and, 1143
    informed consent and, 1142–1143
    institutional bureaucracy and, 1140
    life-support systems and, 1144
    in nineteenth century, 1716
    physician–nurse relationship, 1140–1141
    responsibilities of profession, 1141
    right to know and, 1143
    Roman Catholicism and, 1529
    scope of, 1140
    suicide and, 1143
    terminal illness and, 1144
    truth-telling and, 1143–1144, 1680
Nursing Ethics for Hospital and Private Use (Robb), 1138
Nursing homes, 57, 66–67
    clergy-directed, 1190
    mistreatment in, 1600
    privacy in, 1363
    rights of patients in, 1203
Nutrients, supply of, 842
Nutrition:
    anti-aging and, 51, 62
    parenteral, 842
    See also Food policy
NWRO, *See* National Welfare Rights Organization
Nymman, 489

O

Oates, Joyce Carol, 1013, 1014
Oath of Asaf (Asaph Harofé), 164, 174, 175, 176, 792
Oath of Hippocrates, 86, 197, 206, 553, 647, 664, 684–685, 694, 770, 907, 982, 989, 1093, 1175, 1597–1598, 1602, 1656
    on abortion, 175, 933
    on confidentiality, 163–164, 174, 932, 963, 1359
    date of, 930
    on dissemination of medical knowledge, 937
    on euthanasia, 176, 934–935
    Islam and, 788–789

on justice, 177
    language used in, 172
    on medical teachers, 870
    on physician's primary obligation, 173–174, 1689, 1702
    on professional relations, 178
    text of, 1731
Oath of Initiation, *See Caraka Saṃhitā*
Oath of Soviet Physicians, 981
    text of, 1754–1755
Oaths for physicians, 163–165
Obedience research, 1471, 1474–1475, 1476
Object constancy, 1571
Objectification:
    of nature, *See* Mechanism
    of technology, 1639, 1640
Objective teleological theory, 418
Objectivism in ethics, 405, 438–441
    as guide to conduct, 438–439
    images of man and, 855–856
    rationality and desire, 440–441
    rationality and impartiality, 439–440
    See also Intuitionism
Objectivity, journalistic, 181
Object of Morality, The (Warnock), 1686
Obligation:
    of attention, 927
    to community, in medieval Europe, 948
    comparability of, 1180
    conflicting, between medicine and war, 1695–1696
    default of, theory of, 927
    to future generations, *See* Future generations, obligation to
    health as, 606–609
    of medical schools, 863–869
        to faculty, students, and patients, 867–869
        institutional ethics and, 869
        philosophy and ethos of medical education and, 863–864
        to society in general, 865–867
        sources and nature of, 864–865
    organ donation and, 1153, 1154
    to participate in experimentation, 700–702
    of practitioner, to science and medicine, 694, 700
    to prevent suicide, 1624–1626
    to prohibit suicide, 1620–1623
        to oneself, 1620–1621
        to other people, 1620
        religious, 1621–1623
    supererogation and, 1147–1152, 1166
        bioethics and, 1151–1152
        distinction between, 1147
        philosophical discussion of, 1150–1151
        theological discussion of, 1149–1150

theoretical basis for distinction, 1147–1149
    See also Duty
Obligation theories, *See* Ethics
Oblique intention, 425
Observation, 693
Observational studies, 699
"Observations on the Duties of a Physician and the Methods of Improving Medicine" (Rush), 960
Obstetrical forceps, 1714
Obstetrician–gynecologists, 614
    reproductive decisions and, 1705
    truth-telling and, 1680
    women as, 1717
Occupational counseling and retraining, 157
Occupational health, 381–382, 384–385, 1396
Occupational Safety and Health Administration, 577
O'Connor v. Donaldson (1975), 780, 783, 1203
Odd specimen (image of man), 852, 853
O'Donnell, Thomas J., 871, 1529
Oedipus at Colonus (Sophocles), 59
Oedipus complex, 1572
Oesterlen, F. R., 1051
Offense principle, 1195
Offer, Daniel, 1059
Office of Economic Opportunity, 1080
Office of Nursing Home Affairs, 67
    1975 Facility Improvement Survey, 66
"Of Polygamy and Divorces" (Hume), 1584
Ogburn, William F., 1641
Ogden, C. K., 448
Oken, Donald, 1679
Old age, *See* Aging and the aged
Old-old persons, 54–55, 57–58
Old Testament, 1592
    on contraception, 205–206
    on death, 243–245
    disease, conception of, 582
    on eugenics, 468–469
    on homosexuality, 672
    on miracle and faith healing, 1172
Oligospermia, 1444, 1454
Omen lore, 923
Omission and commission, 269–277, 807, 1502
    direct and indirect acts, 272–274
    ordinary and extraordinary means, 168, 176, 262, 270–271, 727–728
    potentiality and, 748
    stopping vs. not starting a procedure, 271–272
    truth-telling and, 1684
    voluntary and involuntary dying, 274–277
    See also Acting and refraining; Double effect, principle of

Omphalocele, 719
Onanism, 1250, 1251
Oncologists, 1680
On Liberty (Mill), 819, 1195, 1196, 1518
On Suicide (Hume), 1623
On the Good of Marriage (Augustine), 1579
On the Immortality of the Soul (Augustine), 251
On the Precautions That the Physician Must Observe (Arnold of Villanova), 871
On the Sacred Disease (Hippocrates), 1091
Ontological concept:
　of death, 304–305
　of disease, 579–583, 602–603
Ontological reduction, 1420–1421, 1427
Open awareness of dying persons, 287, 290
Open options, freedom as, 94–95, 98
Operant conditioning, 101, 109, 113
Operationalism, 111
Opiates, 328, 330–332
Opinion polling, 1470, 1475–1476
Opler, Marvin K., 674
Oppenheim, Paul, 1419–1420
Oppenheimer, J. Robert, 1700
Optimificity, 415–416, 420, 421
Optimum, population, 1227–1228, 1234
Oral period of sexual development, 1570–1572
Ordinary means:
　codes of medical ethics and, 176
　quality of life and, 727–729, 838
　Roman Catholicism and, 270, 271, 727, 728, 1531–1532
　treatment of defective infants and, 727–729
Orem, Dorothea E., 1140
Organ donation, 1152–1159
　in Arab nations, 891
　cadaver donorship:
　　ethical perspective, 140–141, 1154–1155, 1163, 1164, 1169, 1172
　　legal aspects, 1157–1158
　　medical perspective, 1161
　　salvaging organs, 1158–1159
　　sociocultural aspects, 1167
　compulsion and, 807–808
　in Eastern Europe, 929
　in France, 1155, 1158
　gift-exchange aspects, 812–813, 1168–1169
　in Great Britain, 1158
　live donorship:
　　ethical perspective, 1153–1154, 1163, 1170–1172

　　legal aspects, 1154, 1157
　　medical perspective, 1153, 1161
　　risks, 1161
　　sociocultural aspects, 1166–1167
　public policy and, 1155–1156
　sociological perspective, 1058, 1166–1169
　in United States, 997, 1155, 1157–1158
Organic growth, 394
Organized medicine, 1034–1041
　American Medical Association and, 1037–1041
　ancient legacy, 1035
　in colonial America, 1036–1037
　early post-Revolutionary trends, 1037
　era of retreat, 1037
　evolution in England, 1035–1036
　global medicine and, 1039
　in medieval Europe, 1035
Organized skepticism, 1542
Organs:
　cryopreservation of, 217, 218
　salvaging of, 1158–1159
　See also Organ donation; Organ transplantation
Organ transplantation:
　allocation of resources of, 807–808, 1163–1164, 1414, 1415
　American Medical Association on, 168
　in Arab nations, 891
　blood typing and, 1160
　brain death and, 141, 296, 298, 303, 656, 1155
　from cadavers, *See* Organ donation: cadaver donorship
　in Canada, 997
　choice of recipients, 1163–1164
　comparative value of, 1165
　corneas, 141, 799, 928, 1153
　defined, 1160
　determination of death and, 1161
　development of, 1160
　experimental aspects of, 1164–1165
　heart, 141, 296, 654–660
　　allocation of resources and, 808
　　brain death and, 141, 296, 298, 303, 656
　　Confucianism and, 655
　　cost of, 1165
　　Eastern Orthodox Christianity and, 350–351
　　efficacy of, 656–657
　　histocompatibility and, 657–659
　　historical development of, 654–655, 1162
　　in India, 655, 909
　　intercultural aspects of, 655
　　in Japan, 928

　　Judaism and, 800
　　law and, 656
　　medical regulation of, 655–656
　　medical reporting and, 183, 186, 190, 656, 659, 708–709
　　procurement and, 656
　　psychological aspects of, 658
　　risk-benefit and, 657–658, 1162
　　sociocultural aspects, 1166–1167
　　in United States, 997
　immunosuppressive drugs used in, 323, 812, 814, 1160, 1161, 1162
　infection and, 1161
　informed consent and, 1157
　Islam and, 893, 1171
　in Japan, 928
　Judaism and, 144–145, 795, 798, 799–800, 1169, 1171
　kidney, 141, 153, 660, 811–815, 842–845
　　allocation of scarce resources and, 807–808, 815, 1163–1164, 1414–1415
　　cost of, 1165
　　development of, 1160
　　donation for, *See* Kidney donation; Organ donation
　　in Eastern Europe, 929
　　Eastern Orthodox Christianity and, 750
　　ethical issues of, 811–812
　　as euphenic measure, 475
　　experiment–therapy dilemma and, 812
　　gift-exchange aspects of, 812–813
　　history of, 811
　　immunosuppressive drugs and, 1162
　　in India, 909
　　in Japan, 928
　　Judaism and, 800
　　normative relativism and, 456
　　quality of life and, 811, 813–814, 1162
　　selection criteria, 1161
　　sociocultural aspects, 1166
　　success of, 1161–1162
　limits on, 1171–1172
　liver, 656, 808, 1162
　lung, 1162–1163
　medical malpractice and, 1027
　medical perspective, 1160–1165
　naturalism and, 445
　natural law and, 446
　normative relativism and, 455
　pancreas, 1163
　philosophical perspectives, 1169–1172
　Protestantism and, 1171

Organ transplantation *(Continued)*
  public attitude toward, 140–141
  rejection of, 1160, 1161, 1162, 1168
  Roman Catholicism and, 1170–1171, 1172, 1531
  selection criteria and, 1161
  sociocultural aspects of, 1166–1169
  technological advances and, 1540
  theological perspectives, 1169–1172
  tissue typing and, 1160
  totality, principle of, 1170–1171
Origen, 239, 938, 940
Origin and Development of the Moral Ideas (Westermarck), 826
Origin of Species by Means of Natural Selection, The (Darwin), 369, 479, 481, 529
Orne, Martin T., 711
Ortega y Gasset, José, 1585, 1640
Orthodox Confucianists, 202, 203, 204
Orthodoxy in medicine, 1173–1175
Orwell, George, 196, 267, 1384, 1385
Osborn, Frederick, 1308
Osler, Sir William, 266, 1032
Oslo, Declaration of, 169, 1726
Osteopaths, 1174, 1175
Other America, The (Harrington), 1317
Other-control, 89, 92
Otherness phenomenon, human body as, 364
Otto, Rudolph, 1064, 1067
Outka, Gene, 635, 636
Ova:
  banking, 1446–1448, 1459
  donation of, 355, 1447, 1450, 1462, 1468–1469
Overprescription, 323–324, 654, 1382
Overt behavior, 110–111
Over-the-counter sales, 1214
Overzealousness of scientists, 184–185
Owens, Robert Dale, 210
Oxford Intuitionism, 415–416
Oxygen, supply of, 841–842
Oxygenators, 841–842, 844

P

Pacemakers, 296, 842, 843
Pacem in Terris (John XXIII), 1256
Pacific Dermatologic Association, 1729
Pacific School of Religion (Berkeley), 875, 1001
Paddock, Paul, 497
Paddock, William, 497

Padgett, E. C., 658
Page, Irving, 184
Pahlavi literature, 883
Pain, 602, 1177–1189
  animal experimentation and, 76, 79, 80, 82, 1179–1180
  drug use and, 328
  hypnosis and, 710, 714
  philosophical perspectives, 1181–1184
    meaning of, 1182–1184
    moral status of, 1182
    nature of, 1181–1182
  positivism and, 265
  psychobiological principles, 1177–1181, 1422
    clinical perspectives, 1179
    contextual determinants, 1180
    neurophysiological theories, 1178
    psychological and behavioral dimensions, 1179–1180
    relevance for bioethics, 1180–1181
    traditional perspective, 1177
  purpose in the universe and, 1403, 1404
  religious perspectives, 1185–1189
    Buddhism, 1182, 1183, 1187–1188
    Christianity, 1186–1187
    Christian Science, 1183
    Hinduism, 1182, 1183, 1187–1188
    Islam, 1186
    Jainism, 1187–1188
    Judaism, 793, 794, 1186
    Roman Catholicism and, 1531
  suffering, relationship to, 1180–1182
  suicide and, 1624
  treatment of defective infants and, 728, 729, 730
Paine, Thomas, 624, 1401
Pakistan:
  population growth in, 1230
  population policy in, 1291
  poverty in, 1321
Paley, William, 480
Palmer, D. D., 1175
Palm Springs General Hospital v. Martinez (1971), 1504
Palude, Peter de, 209
Panama, 1005
Pan–American Association of Ophthalmology, 1730
Pancreas transplantation, 1163
Panormitanus, 943
Papakostas, Seraphim G., 1252
Papyrus Ebers, 881
Paracelsus, 582, 583, 602, 1066, 1375, 1659
Paraprofessionals, 561–562, 1191, 1436, 1719
Paré, Ambrosio, 1655, 1660

Parens patriae, doctrine of, 151, 1103, 1105
Parental consent:
  experimentation in children and, 152–154
  medical care of adolescents and, 38–41, 151
  organ donation and, 1157
Parent–child relationship:
  behavior control in, 86, 87
  homosexuality and, 1591–1592
  See also Fetus: –maternal relationship; Paternal consent; Parenthood; Parents
Parent-Duchatelet, A. J. B., 972
Parenteral nutrition, 842
Parenthood:
  reproductive technologies and, 1444, 1445, 1456–1459, 1468
  Roman Catholicism and, 1530
Parents:
  defective children and:
    attitudes of, 723
    emotional impact on, 1339
    fear of defect, 837, 1342
    responsibility of, 733, 734, 1340
    role in decision making, 724, 737–738
  women health professionals as, 1717–1718
Pareto, Vilfredo, 1664
Parfit, Derek, 827
Paris Medical School, 583
Parker, Peter, 918, 1367
Parkinsonism, 1439
Park v. Chessin (1976), 576
Parliamentary Assembly of the Council of Europe, 1203
Parliament of Great Britain, 27–28
Parmenides, 236
Parochialism:
  ethical, 418, 419
  mental health and, 1410–1412
Parole:
  experimentation and, 758
  informed consent and, 782
Parsons, Talcott, 265, 604, 1071, 1169
  on illness, 1090, 1099
  on sick role, 1099, 1483, 1665, 1666, 1675–1676
  on therapeutic relationship, 1665, 1666, 1675–1676
Participant observation, 1471–1472, 1477
Participation in experimentation, 697 700–702
Participation in nature, 368–373
Pascal, Blaise, 362, 365
Passive euthanasia, *See* Acting and refraining; Omission and commission
Passmore, John A., 398, 508, 509–510
Pasteur, Louis, 583, 594, 690, 692, 972, 1032

Pastor:
clinician differentiated from, 1069
See also Pastoral ministry
Pastoral Constitution on the Church in the Modern World (Second Vatican Council), 25, 1530
Pastoral counseling, 1191, 1368
Pastoral-Médicin (Capellmann), 871
Pastoral ministry, 1189–1194
health planners, 1190–1191
medical education, 1192–1193
medical ethicists, 1193
medical school chaplains, 1191–1192
paramedical roles, 1191
physicians, 1190, 1523, 1658
providers of health care, 1190–1191, 1365, 1367–1368, 1428, 1430
providers of spiritual care, 1191–1192, 1368
role of, in medicine, 1193–1194
visitation of the sick, 1191–1192, 1366
Pastoral supervisors, 1191–1192
Past services rendered factor, 809, 810, 1416
Patent medicines, 994
Paternalism, 173, 604, 738, 774, 1194–1200, 1360, 1674, 1675
antipaternalism and, 1196, 1197, 1198, 1200
behavior control and, 1198–1199
biological control and, 1199
eugenics and, 1199
euthanasia and, 1197, 1199
extensive, 1196
genetic screening and, 1198
history in ethical theory, 1195–1196
human experimentation and, 1195, 1198, 1351–1352
informed consent and, 1197, 1199–1200
limited, 1196
meaning of, 1194–1195
mental institutionalization and, 1195, 1199
nature of, 1196, 1360
patient refusal of therapy and, 1197–1198
right to refuse medical care and, 1197–1198, 1500, 1518
risk and, 1517–1519
in therapeutic relationship, 1704
truth-telling and, 1198
types of, 1196–1197, 1360
women patients and, 1704
See also Compulsory population control programs
Paternalistic power, 779, 780, 781

Paternalistic principle, 1194–1200
Paternity leave, 1718
Paterson, Ralston, 1678
Pathfinder Fund, 1280
Pathologies, patients perceived as, 619
Pathology, 1484
Pathology theory of black personality, 1411, 1412, 1413
Patient as Person, The (Ramsey), 996, 1368, 1371
Patient benefit, principle of, 1689–1690
See also Codes of medical ethics: ethical analysis
Patient representative, 1205
Patient's Bill of Rights, A (American Hospital Association), 169, 172, 176, 177, 198, 998, 1141, 1197, 1203, 1363, 1430, 1515, 1683
text of, 1782–1783
Patients' bills of rights, 1515–1516
Jewish, 1430–1431
model, 1204–1205
pediatric, 172
texts of, 1782–1787
See also Patient's Bill of Rights, A
Patients' rights advocate, 1205
Patients' rights movement, 169, 682, 994, 1201–1205
codes of ethics and, 1728–1729
consumer demands, 1202
history of, 1202
institutional scope of, 1203–1204
international scope of, 1203
Judaism and, 1430–1431
medical malpractice litigation and, 1203
model bill of rights, 1204–1205
patients' rights advocate, 1205
Roman Catholicism and, 1530
See also Patients' bill of rights; Rights
Patristic Age, 1523–1524
Patrizzi, Francesco, 1234
Paul, Julius, 1612
Paul, St., 207, 209, 245, 371, 588, 1131, 1132, 1186, 1232
Paul VI, Pope, 13, 25, 161, 213, 1136, 1244, 1255–1258, 1527, 1582
Paulsen, Friedrich, 970
Paulson, Stanley, 1135
Pavlov, I. P., 107
Pavlovian conditioning, 107
Peace Corps, 1080
Pediatric Bill of Rights, 172
text of, 1786–1787
Pediatricians, 613
Pedophilic homosexuality, 1387
Peel Commission, 1113

Peer reviews:
codes of ethics and, 1726
in dentistry, 312
human experimentation and, 705–706
legislation establishing, 1040
of manuscripts, 183, 189–190
of nurses, 1139–1140
of research proposals, 1489–1490, 1495, 1497
Peirce, Charles S. S., 241, 402, 1327–1330
Peking Union Medical College, 918
Pelagius, 208
Pellegrino, Edmund D., 680
Peloponnesian War, 238
Peloponnesian War (Thucydides), 237
Penicillin, 1494
Penitentials, 1579
Pennsylvania, University of, 1715
Pennsylvania State Medical School at Hershey, 1001
Pennsylvania State University, 875
Pension systems, 55, 56
Pentecostal churches, 1121
People's Republic of China, 375
abortion in, 919
birth control in, 919
environmental record of, 372
health care in, 552, 614, 920
health care financing in, 627
human experimentation in, 920
medical ethics, history of, 919–921
medical ethics education in, 872, 919–920
medical practice, political ideology and, 920
national conferences in, 919
public health in, 1938
sex preferences in, 1442
social medicine, 1601
World Health Organization and, 644
See also China
People v. Sorenson (1968), 1468
Peptic ulcer, 1596
Perceptual organism, human body as, 363–364
Percival, Thomas, 165–166, 172, 173, 178, 770, 871, 952, 956, 957, 960, 965, 968, 969, 973, 996, 1038, 1661
Peregrine Pickle (Smollett), 1008
Periodic health exams, 859
Perlmutter, Johanna, 1708
Perls, Fritz, 1087
Persia, 207, 785–786
medical ethics, history of, 880–887
Person, *See* Personhood

Personal communication euthanasia policies, 280–281
Personal health services, 651–652
Personality theory, 1084
Personal perfectionism, 418
Person-centeredness, 1368
Personhood, 505, 1206–1210
  compulsory population control and, 1303
  consequentialism and, 834–836
  determination of, 746
  dualistic view of, 18, 112, 240, 361–362, 367, 370, 501, 502, 1206, 1207
  dynamic process of, 1208–1209
  freedom and, 1207, 1209
  heart transplantation and, 1166–1167
  humanhood vs. accessory qualities, 834–835, 836
  human life vs. nonhuman life, 825–826
  human vs. person, 729–731, 823, 825
  images of man and, 854
  latent, 744, 748
  materialistic view of, 1207
  mental retardation and, 1109
  natural order and, 1206–1207
  norms and, 1208–1209
  potentiality of:
    abortion and, 23, 747, 826
    beginning of life and, 18–20
    euthanasia and, 732, 835
    infanticide and, 744, 746–748
    value of potential persons, 826
  Protestant moralists and, 1369–1372
  reductionism and, 1426–1427
  responsibility and, 1207
  science, role of, 1209–1210
  social order and, 1207
  treatment of defective infants and, 726–727, 729–732, 735–737, 743–746, 834–836
  See also Embodiment; Life: beginning of; Mind–body problem; Soul
Person-neutral teleological theories, 418, 419
Person-relative teleological theories, 418
Perspectives in Biology and Medicine, 1001
Peru, 1005
Perversion:
  concept of, 1570
  vs. normalcy, 1592–1595
Pestel, Edward, 394
Petrarch, 1658
Petty, William, 1226
Phaedo (Plato), 237, 785, 823, 1597, 1622, 1624
Phantom limb, 1179
Pharisaic doctrine, 246

Pharmaceutical industry, *See* Drug industry, medical profession and
Pharmaceutical Manufacturers Association, 1350
Pharmaceutical rebates, 167
Pharmaceutical Society of Great Britain, 1211, 1212
Pharmacology, 1484
Pharmacy, 1211–1214
  bioethical issues in, 1212–1914
  changing role of, 1212
  codes of ethics in, 1211–212, 1728–1729
    text of, 1806
  medical profession, relations with, 1211, 1212
  policy statements on ethical issues, 1729
  professional etiquette in, 1211
  professional role of, 1211
  Roman Catholic norms of conduct in, 1213
  women in, 1713
  See also Psychopharmacology
Phenomenology, 1532
Phenomenology of Spirit (Hegel), 1603
Phenothiazines, 1379, 1381
Phenotype, 530
Phenylketonuria (PKU), 151, 474, 475, 476, 527, 539, 551, 567–568, 574, 1108, 1334
Philanthropy, doctrine of, 1253
Philebus (Plato), 1577
Philippines:
  medical ethics education in, 872
  population education in, 1311
  women physicians in, 1717
Philo, 6, 206
Philosophical Transactions, 189
Philosophie der Technik (Dessauer), 1638
Philosophy:
  abortion and, 17, 25, 999
  animal experimentation and, 79–83
    case against, 81–82
    case for, 81
    legislation, 80–81
    moral status of animals, 82–83, 729, 745, 822, 827–828
    nature and extent of experiments, 80
  behaviorism and, 110–114
    accounting for human actions, 112–113, 502–503
    inner states or events, 111–112
    overt behavior, 110–111
    Skinner, theory of, 108, 109, 113–114, 1068, 1425–1426
  of biology, 127–132
    defined, 127
    ethics and, 130–132
    holism, 130

    mechanism, 129, 130, 367–368, 619, 1419
    reductionism, *See* Reductionism
    vitalism, 129–130
  death, attitudes toward, 235–242
    ancient Greek, 236–237
    early modern, 239–240
    Hellenistic, 237–239
    Kantian, 140, 241, 257–258
    medieval, 239
    modern, 240–241
    recent and contemporary, 241–242
  death, definition of, 301–307, 1052
    belief in human soul and, 302
    brain oriented, 302–303
    irreducible structure of life and, 305–306
    logical approach, 305
    ontological approach, 304–305
    process view and, 302–303
  environment and man and, 370
  genetic aspects of human behavior and, 541–547
    distributive justice, 543–544
    history, 541–543
    methodological issues, 547
    research, 547
    retributive justice, 544–547
  health and disease and, 599–605
    discovered vs. invented concepts, 601–603
    ethical force of nosologies, 604–605
    illness and well-being, disease and health, 599–601
    mental vs. somatic disease, 603–604
  human experimentation and, 699–702
    duties of physicians, 700
    fairness, 701–702
    obligation to participate, 700–702
    problems of definition, 699–700
  infanticide and, 742–750
    destruction of latent persons issue, 744, 748
    destruction of potential persons issue, 744, 746–748
    equation to morality of abortion, 747, 1341–1342
    historical considerations, 742–743
    infants as persons issue, 729–731, 743–746, 826
    principle of avoiding harm, 734–735
    undesirable consequences issue, 744, 748–750
  informed consent and, 754–755
  life-support systems and, 847–848
  medical education and, 863–864
  of medicine, 1049–1054
    philosophy about medicine,

1049–1050, 1052–1053
philosophy for medicine, 1049, 1050–1051
philosophy in medicine, 1049, 1051–1052
philosophy of medicine, proper, 1049, 1050, 1053
North American bioethics and, 999–1000
organ transplantation and, 1169–1172
pain and, 1181–1184
meaning of, 1182–1184
moral status of, 1182
nature of, 1181–1182
pragmatism, 308, 1327–1331, 1426–1427, 1539
bioethics and, 1331
contemporary pragmatists, 1330–1331
defined, 1327
Dewey and, 1329–1330, 1539
James and, 1329–1330
Peirce and, 1327–1330
reductionism, 1419–1423
behaviorism, 1115–1116, 1421
Fodor–Putnam argument against, 1421–1422
functionalism, 1116–1117, 1119, 1421, 1422
identity thesis, 303–304, 1116–1117, 1420–1421
reducibility and methodology, 1423
weaker versions, 1422–1423
sexual ethics and, 1584–1585
sociality and, 1603–1605
supererogation and, 1150–1151
of technology, 1638–1642
defined, 1638
development of, 1638–1639
ethical issues, 1640–1642
metaphysical analyses, 1639–1640
See also Ethics; names of philosophers; specific philosophies
Philosophy and Technology: An Annual Compilation of Research, 1639
Philosophy of Right (Hegel), 1149
Phlebotomy, 945–946
PHMO, *See* Professional Health Maintenance Organizations
Physical dependence, 328
Physical examination, 859, 1482
Physicalism, *See* Reductionism
Physical pain, 1181
Physical suffering, 1182
Physician and Patient (Hooker), 966
Physician assistants, 616, 622, 1717
Physician in Spite of Himself, The

(Molière), 1008
Physician–nurse relationship, 1140–1141
Physician–patient relationship, *See* Therapeutic relationship
Physicians:
in Africa, 898–899
alcoholics, response to, 72
in Arab nations, 889–890
blacks as, 1408, 1409
compensation of, *See* Compensation of physicians
conflicts between researchers and, 1486–1488
consultations, *See* Consultations
death, attitudes toward, 290
decision making by, *See* Decision making, medical
defective infants and:
attitudes toward, 723
ethical views of, 724–726
responsibility of, 733
role in decision making, 723–724, 738
distribution of, 865, 1323–1324
as genetic counselors, 561, 562
group practice, 617
Hindu, 664–665
in hospitals, role of, 677–679
human experimentation, role in, 694, 700
ideals of:
in ancient Greece, 930–931
in ancient Near East, 883
early Christian, 940
integrity of, 866
international migration of, 645–646
licensing of, 1395
medical reporting by, 182
ministers as, 1190, 1523, 1658
municipal, 948
obligation of, to science of medicine, 674, 700
peer review of, *See* Peer review
Plato on role of, 1093
political action by, 1599, 1600, 1601
prenatal tort actions and, 576
professional role of, 594–597
as providers of primary care, 613–614, 615
religious obligations of, 944
social role of, *See* Social medicine; Sociology: of medicine; Therapeutic relationship
specialists, 613, 614, 615, 993, 1029, 1668–1669
strikes by, 161
supply of, 865–866
Taoist, 1633–1637

truth-telling, attitudes toward, 1679–1680
See also Truth-telling
in U.S.S.R., 653
weapons development and, 1701–1702
women as, 1713, 1715–1717
See also Codes of medical ethics; Healers; Health care; Medical care; Medical profession
Physician's assistants, 1726
Physician's Ethical Duties, A (from Kholasah Al Hekmah), 1736–1737
Physicians Forum, 1041
Physicians National Housestaff Association, 1040
Physicists, The (Dürrenmatt), 1009
Physicochemical explanation, 129
Physics, reduction of biology to, *See* Reductionism
Physiological concept of disease, 580–584
Physiology, 1484, 1639
Piaget, Jean, 363, 1088, 1570, 1573
Pickering, 310
Pierce v. Swan Point Cemetery (1872), 139
Pietism, 1372
Pike, James, 421
Pikuach Nefesh, 1169, 1171
Pilgrim (image of man), 854
Pilgrimages, 587, 588, 589, 787
Pillow Books, 377
Pinchot, Gifford, 371
Pindar, 587, 588
Pinel, Philippe, 583, 600, 971, 1053, 1079–1080, 1091–1094
Pinelian psychiatry, 1093
Pinelian revolution, 1092–1093
Pinel model of mental illness, 1092–1094, 1096, 1097
Pinocytosis, 514
Pisistratus, 205
Pitocin, 3, 4
Pittenger, Norman, 673, 675
Pituitary dwarfism, 474
Pituri leaves, 336
Pius II, Pope, 942
Pius V, Pope, 945
Pius IX, Pope, 11
Pius XI, Pope, 13, 212, 1170, 1255, 1256, 1527
Pius XII, Pope, 13, 34, 212, 270, 271, 272, 1170, 1255, 1256, 1267, 1456, 1458, 1527, 1528, 1530–1531, 1532, 1582
PKU, *See* Phenylketonuria
Place, Francis, 210
Placental glucocerebrosidase, 551
Plague, 948–950, 958, 972

Plague, The (Camus), 1013
Planned Parenthood movement, 211
Plastic man (image of man), 853–854
Plath, Sylvia, 1013–1014
Plato, 59, 95, 206, 250, 339, 364, 367, 785, 823, 932, 1050, 1062, 1065, 1593
   antiequalitarian position of, 804
   on death, 236, 237, 238
   on friendship, 1577
   on images of man, 852
   on infanticide, 742, 826
   influence on Islamic bioethics, 785
   on just state, 541–542
   on lying, 1685
   medical ethics teaching and, 870
   on mental health, 1060, 1061
   on moral reasoning, 450, 451, 452
   on moral rules, 409
   on paternalism, 1360
   on physician's role, 1093
   on population, 1225, 1233
   prescriptivist elements in philosophy of, 448
   sexual ethics of, 1577–1578
   on suicide, 1622, 1624
   on therapeutic relationship, 1656
Platt, 310
Platt, Gerald, 595, 596
Player (image of man), 854–855
Pleasure:
   drug use for, 327, 328, 329, 334–338
      acceptable euphoriants, 334–335, 1384, 1385
      cultural justification, 337–338
      depressants, 336
      stimulants, 335–336
      value issues, 334, 1384–1385
   self-realization therapies and, 1547, 1548
   sexual, *See* Sexual behavior
Pliny the Elder, 205, 932–933, 935
Pliny the Younger, 934
Pluralism, 1433, 1434
Pluralistic teleological theories, 418
Plutarch, 827, 935
Pneumoconioses, 380, 383
Poland:
   animal experimentation in, 78
   Penal Code of 1903, 282
   women physicians in, 1717
Polanyi, Michael, 305–306, 1400, 1401
Police power, 779, 780, 781, 1103, 1305
Policy statements on ethical issues, 1729
Political ethics, 398
Political limits to economic growth, 394
Political rights, 625, 626

Politics (Aristotle), 742, 1602
Politics of Experience, The (Laing), 1096
Politics of psychiatry, 1095–1096
Pollution, 372, 1397, 1642
   See also Environmental ethics
Polya, George, 309
Polycystic kidney disease, 475, 720
Polymorphism, 550
Polynesia, infanticide in, 742
Pomeroy operation, 1607
Pope, Alexander, 77, 81, 240
Popenoe, Paul, 1611
Popper, Karl, 1545
Population aid, 1276–1281
Population Council, 211
Population Debate, The (conference 1974), 1229
Population distribution, 1217, 1233, 1315
   internal, 1305–1306
   international migration, 1220–1221, 1304–1305
   interplanetary migration, 1304
   as population policy, 1304–1306
Population education, 1311–1316
   defined, 1311–1312
   goals of, 1312–1313
   population policy and, 1315–1316
   values in planning and implementation, 1313–1315
Population ethics, 1215–1272
   defined, 1216–1218
   ethical perspectives on population, 1237–1241
      freedom, 1238–1239
      general welfare, 1239–1241
      justice, 1237–1238
   history of population policies, 1232–1236
      control, 1233–1234
      distribution, 1233
      populationism, 1234–1235
      quality, 1233
   history of population theories, 1225–1231
      ancient, 1225–1226
      demographic transition, 1228–1229
      efforts to reduce fertility, 1229–1230
      Malthus and, 1226–1227
      medieval, 1226
      population optima, 1227–1228
      totalitarian theories, 1230
   normative aspects of population policy, 1241–1249
      anticipated harms, 1242–1243
      functions performed by normative elements, 1241–1242
      general formulation of population problem, 1244–1245
      recurring questions in debates, 1244

      recurring tensions among alternative solutions, 1245–1249
      risks of public debate, 1242
   population problem in demographic perspective, 1218–1225
      elements of, 1219
      ethical issues, 1223–1224
      factors affecting fertility and mortality, 1221–1223
      impact of population processes, 1221
      patterns in births and deaths, 1219–1221
   purpose in the universe and, 1403, 1404
   religious traditions, 1218, 1250–1272
      Eastern Orthodox Christianity, 354, 1251–1254
      Hinduism, 1269–1272
      Islam, 1264–1268
      Judaism, 1250–1251
      Protestantism, 1259–1262
      Roman Catholicism, 1226, 1254–1258
   See also Population policy proposals
Population genetics, *See* Eugenics
Population growth, 211, 1233
   the aged and, 54, 57–58
   blacks and, 1406
   in developing nations, 1220
   differential rate of, 1285–1290
      demographic perspectives, 1285–1288
      ethical analysis, 1288–1290
   encouragement of, 1226, 1233, 1234–1235, 1307–1308
   food policy and, 495, 496, 1222
   impact of anti-aging policy on, 63
   in India, 1228, 1230, 1269
   negative, 1308
   public health and, 1397
   rate of, 1219–1220
   urban, 1220, 1224, 1233, 1234, 1306
   zero, 1229, 1308
   See also Fertility rate; Mortality rate; Population ethics; Population policy proposals
Populationism, 1234–1235
Population optimum, 1227–1228, 1234
Population policy proposals, 1273–1316
   compulsory population control programs, 1299–1303
      ethical issues, 1301–1303
      genetic implications of, 1309–1310
      methods of control, 1300–1301
      population policy orientations, 1299–1300

contemporary international issues, 1274–1284
  contraceptive testing and distribution, 1281–1282
  foreign assistance, 1276–1281
  indirect consequences, 1282–1284
  schools of thought, 1274–1276
differential growth rate, 1285–1290
  demographic perspectives, 1285–1288
  ethical analysis, 1288–1290
genetic implications of, 1307–1310
  evolution by selection, 1307
  selection generated by compulsory population control, 1309–1310
  selection generated by population growth, 1307–1308
  selection generated by voluntary population control, 1308–1309
governmental incentives, 1283, 1290–1295, 1302
  ethical dimensions of, 1292–1295
  types of, 1290–1292
population distribution, 1304–1306
  international migration, 1304–1305
  interplanetary migration, 1304
  national migration, 1305–1306
population education, 1311–1316
  defined, 1311–1312
  goals of, 1312–1313
  population policy and educational policy, 1315–1316
  values in planning and implementation, 1313–1315
social change, 1295–1300
  acceptance of, by policymakers, 1300
  ethical issues, 1296–1298
  measures, 1295–1296, 1299
Populorum Progressio (Paul VI), 1255, 1257, 1258
Pornography, 1562, 1565
Porphyria, 556
Portugal:
  health care financing in, 611
  organ donation in, 1158
  physician–population ratio in, 615
  World Health Organization and, 644
Positive eugenics, 458–459, 460, 511, 1199, 1448, 1455–1456
Positive morality, ethics distin-

guished from, 401
Positive rights:
  in bioethics, 1513–1516
  generic concept of, 1507, 1509–1510
Positivism, 265–266, 453, 818–819, 863, 1134, 1135, 1402, 1537
Posner, Meir, 212
Possession, demonical, 1121–1122, 1128–1129
Posterity, duties to, 397
Post-hypnotic suggestion, 97
Postmortem examination, *See* Autopsy
Postprandial blood sugar, 862
Potentiality:
  abortion and, 23, 747, 826
  beginning of human life and, 18–20
  euthanasia and, 732, 835
  infanticide and, 744, 746–748
  value of potential persons, 826
Pott, Percivall, 1660
Potter, Charles, 282
Potter, Ralph B., 1217
Potter, Van Rensselaer, 118–119
Pound, Ezra, 1078
Poverty, 1316–1327, 1410
  chronic disease and, 1056
  in France, 958–959, 971
  in Germany, 969
  health care and, 616, 617, 1316–1326
    accessibility of services, 1318
    availability of services, 1318
    ethical considerations, 1319–1320
    international perspective, 1321–1326
    relationship of, 1317–1319
    in United States, 1316–1320
  Malthus on, 1227
  meaning of, 1316–1317
  in medieval Europe, 941, 947, 948
  population policies and, 1243
  social medicine and, 1599
Poverty assistance programs, 498
Power and Society (Lasswell and Kaplan), 1640
Power of attorney, euthanasia and, 281
Practical effects, 1327
Practicality in medical decision-making, 309
Practice conception of rules, 412
Practitioner, The, 191
Pragmatism, 308, 1327–1331, 1426–1427, 1539
  bioethics and, 1331
  contemporary, 1330–1331

defined, 1327
Dewey and, 1329–1330, 1539
James and, 1329–1330
Peirce and, 1327–1330
Roman Catholicism and, 1532
Prayers, medical, 162–163
Prednisone, 1160, 1161
Pregnancy, *See* Abortion; Fetus: -maternal relationship
Premarital sex, 1563, 1564, 1581, 1583
Premature claims of scientists, 184–185
Premature publication of scientific information, 183–184
Premenstrual tension, 1707
Prenatal diagnosis, 2, 521, 522, 531, 569–570, 1332–1345
  amniocentesis, 2, 8, 461, 467, 490, 566, 569, 577, 999, 1332–1333, 1336, 1441, 1644
  commitment to abort and, 1335
  historical perspective, 1332
  procedure, 1333
  risks in, 1333, 1335, 1336–1337
  timing of, 1343
  current status of, 1333–1338
  errors in, 1335
  fetoscopy, 1343
  followed by abortion, 467, 521, 522, 555, 556–557, 1334–1335
    arguments against, 1337–1339
    arguments for, 1339–1341
    legal aspects, 1334–1335
    moral aspects, 883–884, 1334, 1337–1343
    parent's fear of defect and, 837, 1342
    public policy and, 1344–1345
    quality of life and, 833–834
    for reasons of sex preference, 1342–1343
    risks in, 1335
    special problems in, 1343
    timing of, 1343
    viewed as infanticide, 1341–1342
  in Germany, 985
  grief reactions and, 486
  informed consent and, 1335
  methodologies of, 1336
  prenatal torts and, 575–576
  sex determination with, 1332–1335, 1342–1343
Prenatal torts, 575–576
Prepayment health plan, 637, 639–641
Prepayment programs, 612
Preponderance theories, 1239

Prescription of drugs:
    overprescription, 323–324, 654, 1382
    pharmacists and, 1211–1214
Prescriptivism, 440, 448–449
President's Task Force on Aging (1970), 67
Preventive medicine, 77, 614, 616, 629, 1396, 1397–1398, 1483, 1484
    See also Mass health screening
Price, Derek J. de Solla, 192, 1545
Price–Anderson Act, 383
Prichard, H. A., 415, 542
Prieras, Sylvester, 1524
Priesthood of all believers, 1366
Priest of Sekhmet, 881
Priests, 881
    See also Pastoral ministry
Prima facie duties, 174, 405, 415, 438
Primal therapy, 1085
Primary care, 613–617, 629, 1668
Primary preventive screening, *See* Mass health screening
Primitive medicine, 877–879
Primitive religions, 429
Principia Ethica (Moore), 443
Principles, *See* Rules and principles
Principles of Medical Ethics (AMA), 44, 173, 175, 179, 197, 575, 770, 1683, 1727
    text of, 1750–1754
Prior, Arthur N., 444
Priority, author's, 189
Priority disputes, 1543–1544
Prisoners, 979, 1346–1356
    experimentation on, 1198, 1349–1353, 1478, 1497, 1559, 1648
        informed consent and, 757, 758, 1350–1351
        policies, 1352–1353
        practices, 1349–1350
        principles, 1350–1352
        sex research, 1559
    medical care of, 1346–1348
        behavior control and, 1190, 1347, 1348
        improvements in, 1348
        involuntary treatment, 1347–1348
        lack of, 1347
        mental health care, 1348
        psychosurgery and, 999, 1347, 1348, 1390
        standards of, 1347
    rights of, 1512
    torture of, 1354–1356
        ethical principles, 1355–1356
        medical personnel and, 1355
        methods of, 1354–1355
Privacy, 1356–1363
    autonomy and, 1358–1362
    bioethics and, 1361–1363
    concept of, 1356–1358

confidentiality and, 195–196, 1357–1360, 1362
cultural, 1477
in cultural settings, 1358–1360
drug use and, 1361–1362
genetic counseling and, 573
genetic intervention and, 462
in hospitals, 1363
human experimentation and, 1362
informational, 1357–1360, 1362–1363
intrusions on, 185, 1021, 1356–1358
legislation of morality and, 821
medical care and, 1363
private situations, 1356–1357, 1360
procreational, 573–574, 1358, 1465, 1466, 1582, 1615–1616
religious beliefs and, 1360, 1361
right of, 30, 31, 105, 1073, 1203, 1204, 1358, 1359
    abortion and, 1513, 1514
    confidentiality, 198
    informed consent and, 1472
    sex therapy and research and, 1559
    sterilization and, 1615–1616
    Supreme Court on, 573
right to die and, 1361
right to refuse medical care and, 1361, 1500
Privacy Act of 1974, 198, 1497
Private health insurance, 637–642, 652
Private space, violation of, 1478
Privileged communication, 198
Probabilism, 1433, 1527–1528
Probability:
    decision making and, 768
    diagnoses and, 309–311
Problem of Anxiety (Freud), 259
Process, technology of, 1639–1640
Process philosophy:
    death and, 299, 302–303
    man's participation in nature and, 370–371
Procreation, 1592–1594
    Aquinas on, 1580
    Augustine on, 1579
    Christianity and, 1561
    Gnosticism and, 1578
    Judaism and, 795–796, 1561, 1576
    Lombard on, 1579
    Manicheanism and, 207
    Protestantism and, 1259–1260, 1436, 1457, 1582
    right of, 1334, 1615
    Roman Catholicism and, 208, 209, 1529, 1530–1531, 1579–1580, 1582
    Stoicism and, 1578–1579
    Victorianism and, 1561
    See also Population ethics; Popula-

tion policy proposals; Reproductive technologies; Sexual behavior; Sexual ethics
Procreational privacy, 573–574, 1358, 1465, 1466, 1582, 1615–1616
Professional control of human experimentation, 703–706
Professional Health Maintenance Organizations (PHMOs), 1040
Professionalism, medical, 1028–1033
    attributes of professions, 1028
    change and, 1029
    in colonial America, 1029–1030
    functions of, 1028–1029
    in nineteenth-century America, 1030–1031
    in twentieth-century America, 1031–1033
Professionalization, 622
Professional relations, ethics of, 178–179
Professional role, 595
Professional Standards Review Organizations (PSROs), 612, 678, 994, 1040
Profit motive, 168
Programmed genetic events, aging theory based on, 49–50
Project Camelot, 1479
Projections, technology as, 1639
Project on Cultural Values and Population Policy, 1278
Prolongation of life, *See* Sustaining life
Pronatalism, 1226, 1233, 1234–1235, 1307–1308
Propaganda, 97
Proper Marriage, A (Lessing), 1013
Property rights, 1305
Prophet (image of man), 856–857
Proportionality, 783
Proportionate reason, 319
Proprietary remedies, 321, 1214
Prostaglandins, 3, 4
Prosthetic devices, *See* Life-support systems
Prostitution, 1557
    in ancient Greece, 1577
    contemporary attitudes toward, 1563
    cultural variation and, 1561
    Eastern Orthodox Christianity and, 353
    Victorianism and, 1561
Protagoras, 447
Protein deficiency, 494
Protein synthesis, biological aging theory and, 48
Protestant Hospital Association (United States), 996
Protestantism, 1364–1378
    abortion and, 13–16
        beginning of human life and, 14–16, 1437

church statement on, 1436–1437
contemporary perspective, 15–16, 24–25
early perspectives, 13–14
in eighteenth and nineteenth centuries, 14–15
solution of conflict situations and, 24
antivivisectionist movement and, 78
artificial insemination and, 1437, 1457–1458
church statement, 1435–1437
  authority of, 1435–1436
  on health-care delivery, 1436
  on medical practice and research, 1436–1437
contraception and, 209–210, 212, 1260–1261, 1436
cremation and, 142–143
death and, 251–253
divine power, healing by, 1123, 1125
ensoulment and, 14–16
eugenics and, 471
euthanasia and, 1369–1372, 1437
exorcism and, 1121–1122
health concerns in, 1373–1378, 1436
  Adventism, 1376–1377
  cause of disease, 1374
  Christian Science, *See* Christian Science
  emergence of modern medicine, 1375–1376
  Jehovah's Witnesses, *See* Jehovah's Witnesses
  Mormonism, 1376–1377
  present concerns, 1376
  role of medicine, 1374–1375
homosexuality and, 1581, 1583
individualism and, 1260
life-support systems and, 1371–1372, 1437
man's dominion over nature and, 1260
marriage and, 1259, 1261, 1581, 1582
medical ethics, history of, 1364–1372
  contemporary, 1368–1372
  medical missions, 1367–1368
  personalist theme, 1368
  Reformation doctrines, 1366–1367
medical ethics education and, 871
medical missions and, 1365, 1367
mental health and, 1066
miracle and faith healing and, 1121–1122, 1124, 1365, 1374–1377

nurture of children and, 1259–1260
organ transplantation and, 1171
population ethics and, 1259–1262
procreation and, 1259–1260, 1436, 1457, 1582
right to refuse medical care and, 1437
sexuality and, 1259–1260, 1436, 1457, 1581, 1582–1583
sponsorship of health-care facilities, 1190, 1365, 1367, 1375
status of the aged and, 60
sterilization and, 1436, 1609–1612
sustaining life and, 1369–1372
United States medical ethics and, 996
value of life and, 16
visitation of the sick and, 1366
Protestant Reformation, 209–210, 239, 257, 1066, 1133–1134, 1150, 1259, 1260, 1365, 1366–1367, 1401, 1435
Protomedicato, 1005
Protrepticos (Aristotle), 237
Proudhon, Pierre Joseph, 210
Provincial (image of man), 855–856
Proxmire, William, 1552
Proxy consent, 1473–1474
  for the aged, 68
  for children, 153–155, 491, 577, 759
  for fetuses, 491
  for the mentally retarded, 577, 1110, 1112, 1113, 1611
  psychosurgery and, 1389
Proxy decision-making, 737–739
Proxy quality-of-life criteria, 836
Prussia, population policy in, 1235
Psilocybin, 1384
PSROs, *See* Professional Standards Review Organizations
Psychedelics, 1384
Psychiatric hospitalization, *See* Mental institutionalization
Psychiatric hospitals, 616
Psychiatric neurosurgery, *See* Psychosurgery
Psychiatrists:
  social role of, 1071–1074
  truth-telling and, 1680, 1681
  women as, 1717
Psychiatry, 1094
  adolescents and, 38, 41
  in Africa, 898
  the aged and, 67
  misused for political purposes, 980
  Pinelian, 1093
  politics of, 1095–1096

religion and, 1066
suicide and, 1625
See also Behavioral therapies; Behavior control; Behaviorism; Dynamic therapies; Mental health; Mental illness; Mental institutionalization
Psychic dependence, 328
Psychoactive drugs, *See* Psychopharmacology
Psychoanalysis, *See* Dynamic therapies
Psychobehavioral defects, 381
Psychological relativism, 454, 455
Psychological warfare, 1698
Psychology:
  behavior control and, 92
  bioethics and, 125
  determinism and, 502–503
  differential, 528, 529
  experimental, 112
  influence on ethics, 1536, 1537
  of pain, 1179–1180
  reduction to physics, *See* Reductionism
  of sexual development, 1569–1574
    adolescence, 1572–1574
    earliest years, 1570–1571
    from four to six, 1572
    Freud on, 1562, 1569–1572
    moral agency, 1574
    from two to four, 1571–1572
  See also Behavior control; Behavioral therapies; Behaviorism
Psychomotor stimulants, 1381
Psychoneurosis, 539
Psychopathia Sexualis (Krafft-Ebing), 1562
Psychopathology:
  of body-experience, 364
  homosexuality and, 667
Psychopharmacology, 85, 86, 89, 91, 97, 98, 326, 327, 328, 331, 358, 505, 506, 551, 765, 1087, 1378–1386, 1485
  access to, 1385
  antianxiety drugs, 1381–1383
  antidepressant drugs, 1380–1381
  antipsychotic drugs, 1379–1380
  defined, 1378
  dispensing of drugs, 1214
  experimental research and, 77
  hyperkinetic learning disorders and, 1383–1384
  paternalism and, 1199
  recreational use of, 1384–1386
  reductionism and, 1427
  torture and, 1354–1355
Psychophysical dualism, *See* Cartesian dualism

Psychosomatic illness, 596
Psychosurgery, 85, 87, 91, 99, 505, 506, 765, 781, 999, 1387–1391, 1397, 1644
  defined, 1387
  development of, 1387
  human nature and, 1391
  informed consent and, 765, 1389
  lobotomy, 98, 99, 999, 1073, 1180, 1182, 1348, 1387, 1526
  paternalism and, 1199
  prisoners and, 999, 1347, 1348, 1390
  public policy and, 1391
  reductionism and, 1427
  as social control, 1389–1390
  social definition of therapeutic goals, 1389
  social setting of, 1388–1389
  as therapy, 1388
Psychotherapy, *See* Dynamic therapies
Psychotic patients, 359, 846, 1077
Psychotropic drugs, *See* Psychopharmacology
Psych resorts, 1547
Ptolemies of Egypt, 685
Public access to data, 385–386
Public commissions, human experimentation and, 707–708
Public control of human experimentation, 706–709
Public figures, publication of medical information about, 185, 190
Public health, 627, 1392–1398, 1483
  blacks and, 1407–1408
  defined, 1392–1393
  domain of, 1484
  in Europe:
    in eighteenth century, 1393
    medieval, 948
    in nineteenth century, 1393
    in seventeenth century, 956
  in France, 971–972
  health and change, 1397–1398
  industrialization and, 1393
  medical reporting and, 183
  sanitary reform, 1394, 1483–1484
  social reform and, 1396–1397
  society and disease, 1394–1396
  See also Social medicine; War: biomedical science and
Public Health Acts of 1848 and 1875 (Great Britain), 1394
Public health laws, 197
Public Health Service, 611, 770, 997, 1350, 1396, 1407, 1493, 1494
Public Health Service Act of 1944 (P.L. 78-410), 1494, 1495
Public health services, 651–654
Public interest movement, 385–386
Publicity, sexual, 1561, 1562, 1564
Publick Occurrences, 181
Public Law 89–97 of 1965, *See* Medicare

Public Law 480 of 1954, *See* "Food for Peace" program
Public physicians, 936
Public policy:
  bioethics and, 126–127
  biomedical research and, 1492–1497
    ethical and policy dimensions, 1496–1497
    history of development in United States, 1488–1489, 1493–1496
    human experimentation, 1352–1353, 1495
    value implications, 1492–1493
  environment and, 381–385, 390, 391
  eugenics and, 462–468
  euthanasia and sustaining life and, 278–285, 735–740
    decision making by hospital committee, 280, 738–739
    decision making by patients, lay persons, and public bodies, 280–285
    decision making by physicians, 278–280, 738
    decision making for infants, 737–739
    legal policies, 735–737
  fetal research in Great Britain and, 141
  food policy, 493–500
    ethical frameworks, 497–499
    perspectives and policies, 496
    world food situation, 494–496
  genetic aspects of human behavior and, 543–546
  genetic intervention and, 462–463
  genetic screening and, 1343–1345
  health policy, *See* Health policy
  heterozygote testing and, 556
  life-support systems and, 847
  mental health as goal in, 1061–1063
  organ donation and, 1155–1156
  population and, *See* Population ethics; Population policy proposals
  pornography and, 1562
  prenatal diagnosis followed by abortion and, 1344–1345
  pronouncement of death and, 296–301
  psychosurgery and, 1391
  scientific views of risk and, 1521
  smoking and, 1597
  treatment of defective and diseased infants and, 735–740
    agency in decision making, 737–739
    euthanasia and sustaining life, 735–737
    macroallocation, 739–740
Public safety, confidentiality and, 199

Puerperal sepis, 1716
Puerto Rico:
  children born out of wedlock in, 225
  sterilization in, 1397
Pufendorf, Samuel von, 625
Pugwash Conference on Science and World Affairs (1962), 1071
Pump oxygenator, 656
Punitive sterilization, 1612, 1706
Pure Food and Drug Act of 1906, 1396
Purgatory, doctrine of, 251–252
Puritans, 14, 60, 368, 1259, 1360, 1365, 1375
Purpose in the universe, 1399–1404
  action, concept of, 1399–1400
  ethical implications, 1403–1404
  images of man and, 851–852
  modern view, 1401–1403
  traditional conceptions, 128, 1400–1401
Puruṣartha, 1269
Putnam, Hilary, 1419–1420, 1421
Pyloric stenosis, 474, 475–476
Pythagoras, 236, 827
Pythagoreans, 521, 1065
  on death, 236, 237
  Oath of Hippocrates and, 163, 173, 174, 176, 684, 870, 930, 933, 935
  sexuality and, 1577

Q

Qābusnāme, 785
Qatar, health care in, 890
Quacks, 957, 970, 994, 1031, 1174, 1175, 1557
Quack's Charter, 1036
Quadragesimo Anno, 1255
Quaestiones medico-legales (Zacchia), 956, 1524, 1660
Quakers, 70, 1393, 1583, 1596
Quality of life, 51, 829–838
  the aged and, 57, 58
  chronic care and, 157
  continuation of life-support systems and, 846
  Hinduism and, 1270
  images of man and, 855
  Jewish law and, 8
  kidney dialysis and transplantation and, 811, 813–814, 1162
  as morally normative, 830–831
  pain and, 1180
  vs. qualities of life, 832–833
  vs. quantity of life, 832
  sanctity-of-life distinguished from, 831–833
  treatment of defective infants and:
    clinical aspects, 717–723

consequentialist theories, 731–732, 834–838
deontological theories, 726–729, 833, 838
equality theory of justice, 837
ethic of care, 733–734
extraordinary means principle, 727–729, 838
medical criteria, 724–726
personhood theories, 729–731, 834–836
principle of avoiding harm, 734–735
slippery slope argument, 821, 836–837
wrongful life theory, 835–836, 837
See also Life: value of
Quantifiable teleological theories, 418
Quarantine, 1395
Quasi-public control of human experimentation, 706–709
Quesnay, François, 1226
Questioning of respondents, 1471, 1477
Questionnaires, 1471
Question of the Procreation of Children, The (Papakostas), 1252
Quickening, 485–486
Quine, W. V. O., 1330
Quinlan, Karen Ann, 280, 284, 998
Quintilian, 933
Quinton, A. M., 482
Quotas, immigration, 1304–1305
Qur'an, *See* Koran

R

Rabbinical tradition, 791, 792
abortion and, 6–9
death and, 246–247
genetic policy and, 463
procreation and, 1250
Race differences in intelligence, 533–538
elements of the question, 533–535
ethical implications, 535–538
Racial discrimination, 398, 1289, 1306, 1319
Racism, 1405–1413
eugenics and, 460, 462
medicine and, 1405–1409
experimentation and, 1409
health care and, 1407, 1409
history of, 1405–1409
mental health and, 1410–1413
availability and efficacy of services, 1412
context of problem, 1410

new therapeutic approaches, 1413
parochialism and, 1410–1412
scope of problem, 1410
population policies and, 1277
Radioactive wastes, 383, 389
Radiostimulators, 357
Rahawi, Al-, 888
Rahner, Karl, 1457, 1459–1460
Rāmāyana, 378
Ramazzini, 1659
Ramsey, Paul, 996
on abortion, 15, 19, 24, 1337–1338
on allocation of medical resources, 1417–1418
on artificial insemination, 1457, 1458
on care, 146–148
conflict with Fletcher (Joseph), 177, 1370
on double effect principle, 319
on eugenics, 462
on euthanasia, 272, 727, 728, 1371–1372
on informed consent, 756, 759
on organ transplantation, 1169, 1171
on research on the mentally handicapped, 1113
on sexuality, 673
on therapeutic relationship, 1368, 1371, 1372
Randomized clinical trial (RCT), 695–696, 699, 1164–1165, 1488, 1628
Random selection, 809–810, 816, 817, 1301, 1353, 1416, 1417
Rangel, Charles B., 388
Rank, Otto, 1084
Ransdell, Joseph, 1493
Rapaport, David, 1084
Rape, 1592, 1709
abortion and, 24, 28, 928, 929, 998
RAPID (genetic register system), 571
"Rappaccini's Daughter" (Hawthorne), 1009
Rascher, S., 1017, 1018
Rashdall, Hastings, 421
Rashi, 5, 7
Raspail, F.-V., 971
Rate of natural increase, 1219
Rate of population growth, 1219
Ratio iuris exigit (John XXII), 1524
Rational-contractor theory, 449
Rationalism, 210
Rationality:
desire and, 440–441
determinism and, 1426
freedom and, 1149
human rights and, 81
impartiality and, 439–440, 449
reductionism and, 1427

technology and, 1640
Rational persuasion, 96, 97
Rationing of medical treatment, *See* Scarce resources, allocation of; Triage
Ratnoff, Marian F., 193
Ratnoff, Oscar D., 193
Rau, Wolfgang Thomas, 957
Rauwolfia derivatives, 1379
Ravdin, I. S., 1679, 1681
Rawls, John, 177
contract theory of, 416–417, 449, 1604
difference principle of, 635
on justice, 67, 404, 406, 450, 543, 632, 634, 804–805, 806, 1325
on material wants vs. civil liberties, 1239
on obligation to future generations, 509, 510
Raymond, Henry J., 180
Raynaudus, Theophilus, 1525
Razetti, Luis, 1005
Razetti Code, 1005
Rāzi, al-, *See* Rhazes (al-Rāzi)
Rea, M. Priscilla, 1679, 1680
Reade, Winwood, 266
Reality-testing, 341
Receptor theory of pain, 1178
Reciprocity, 878
Recombinant DNA, 1490, 1493, 1497, 1641, 1645, 1646
Recreationalism, 673, 674
Recreational understanding of homosexuality, 673, 674–675
Recreational use of drugs, 1384–1385
Red Cross, 972
Redman, John, 964
Reductionism, 128–129, 130, 502, 546, 547, 863, 1419–1427
ethical implications, 1424–1427
as denial of Cartesian dualism, 1426
determinism and, 1425–1426
motivations for reductionist view, 1425
pragmatic consequences, 1426–1427
philosophical analysis, 1419–1423
behaviorism, 1115–1116, 1421
Fodor–Putnam argument against, 1421–1422
functionalism, 1116–1117, 1119, 1421, 1422
identity thesis, 303–304, 1116–1117, 1420–1421
reducibility and methodology, 1423
weaker versions, 1422–1423
Roman Catholicism and, 1532
Redundant message theory of aging, 48–49

Reed, J. D., 1166
Reed, S. C., 559
Reed, Walter, 687–688
Reemtsma, K., 655
References, citation of, 193
Reflexivity of human body, 363
Refraining, distinction between acting and, *See* Acting and refraining
Refusal of treatment, *See* Right to refuse medical care
Refutation of published information, 192
Regan, Augustine, 1170
Regino of Prüm, 11
Regional centers, 614
Regional planning, 1306
Regulatory agencies, 385, 386, 706–707
Rehabilitative ideal, 765, 766
Reinforcement:
  in behavioral therapies, 101, 102, 104–105
  in behaviorism, 113, 114
Rejection of transplanted organs, 656, 658, 811, 813, 814, 1160, 1161, 1167, 1168
Relational criterion for beginning of human life, 17, 20–21, 22–23, 25, 1341
Relational theory, 436
Relational understanding of homosexuality, 673, 674–675
Relativism, 264, 438, 440, 448, 454–457, 1536
  cultural, 454–455, 1090, 1133
  descriptive, 454–455, 457
  distinguished from nihilism, 454
  images of man and, 856
  metaethical, 456, 457
  normative, 455–456, 457
  See also Situation ethics
Relf v. Weinberger (1974), 1615–1616, 1617, 1706
Relics, 589
Religiomagical practices, 1065
Religion:
  anthropologies of, 1185
  Darwinism and, 480
  environment and, 398
  health and disease, concepts of, 585–589
    divine healers, 587
    forms of healing, 585–589
    Hinduism, 663–664, 902–903
    human healers, 587
    instruments of healing, 587–588
    monotheistic biblical tradition, 587–589
    Protestantism, 1373–1378
    Roman Catholicism, 1522
  medicine, relationship to, 1374
  mental health and, 1064–1070
    clarification of terms, 1064

history of, 1064–1068
Judeo–Christianity case, 1068–1070
pain and suffering and, 1185–1189
  Buddhism, 1182, 1183, 1187–1188
  Christianity, 1186–1187
  Christian Science, 1183
  Hinduism, 1182, 1183, 1187–1188
  Islam, 1186
  Jainism, 1187–1188
  Judaism, 793, 794, 1186
psychiatry and, 1066
science, conflict with, 1401–1403
See also names of specific religions
Religion and Health (Hiltner), 1368
Religious beliefs:
  privacy and, 1360, 1361
  sexuality and, 1560–1561
Religious directives in medical ethics, 1428–1437
  Jewish codes of law and guidelines, 1428–1431
    authority of, 1429–1430
    codes of law, 1428–1429
    guidelines, 1429
    health service, 1430–1431
  Protestant statements, 1435–1437
    authority of, 1435–1436
    on health-care delivery, 1436
    on medical practice and research, 1436–1437
  Roman Catholic, 996, 1430–1434, 1530
    on abortion, 169, 172, 175, 176, 1434, 1527
    in Canada, 1432
    text of, 1755–1757
    in United States, 1432–1434
Religious dissenters, 1289–1290
Religious experience, drug use and, 327, 336–337
Religious healing, *See* Miracle and faith healing
Religious obligations of physicians, 944
Remark on the Employment of Females as Practitioners of Midwifery (Ware), 1715
Renaissance, 58, 59, 77, 236, 239, 261, 262, 582
Renal dialysis, *See* Kidney dialysis
Renal Transplantation Registry, 812
Reparation, deontological theory and, 174
"Report: On the Rights of the Sick and Dying" (Council of Europe), 983
Reporting stage of drug trial, 322
Report of the Commission on the Teaching of Bioethics in the United States, 1138
Report . . . on an Inquiry into the Sanitary Condition of the

Labouring Population of Great Britain (Chadwick), 1394
Report on the Physician and the Dying Patient (AMA), 1728
Reproductive freedom, 1275
Reproductive technologies, 573, 1439–1443
  artificial insemination, 169, 557, 1444–1445
    in Arab nations, 890
    consent agreement for, 1445
    by donor (AID), 467, 1444, 1445, 1454–1460, 1462, 1465–1469, 1531, 1533
    donor selection, 1445
    in Eastern Europe, 979
    Eastern Orthodox Christianity and, 354–355
    ethical issues, 1454–1460
    eugenic use of, 1445
    by husband (AIH), 1444, 1454, 1458, 1531, 1533
    Judaism and, 797, 800, 1457, 1458
    legal aspects, 1445, 1464–1469
    legitimacy of child and, 1445, 1468
    marriage and, 1444–1445, 1456–1459, 1468–1469
    motive for, 1454
    normative relativism and, 455
    parenthood and, 1444, 1445, 1456–1459
    procedure in, 1444
    Protestantism and, 1437, 1457–1458
    Roman Catholicism and, 1433, 1456–1457, 1458, 1531, 1533
    situation ethics and, 423
    ultimate factors in decision making, 1459–1460
  cloning, 518, 549, 855, 999, 1027, 1450–1453, 1644
    ethical issues, 1453, 1462–1463
    legal aspects, 1464–1465
    nuclear transplantation and, 518, 1452
    social issues, 1453
  ethical issues, 1454–1463
    artificial insemination, 1456–1460
    cloning, 1453, 1462–1463
    interventions for personal purposes, 1456
    interventions for positive eugenics, 1455–1456
    in vitro fertilization, 1454–1456, 1460–1462
    motive for intervening, 1454–1455
  in vitro fertilization, 999, 1446, 1448–1451
    ethical issues, 1454–1456, 1460–1462

experimental and therapeutic purpose of, 1449–1451
experimental nature of, 1449–1450, 1461
legal aspects of, 1464–1469
motive for, 1454–1455
status of fetus, 1469
technical procedures, 1448–1449
technological assessment of, 1652–1653
legal aspects, 573–574, 1464–1469
access and state regulation, 1464–1466
donor or surrogate relationship with child, 1468–1469
effect on marital relationship, 1468
status of child, 1455, 1467–1468
status of fetus, 1469
sex selection, 1439–1443, 1644
gene therapy and, 520, 522
justification of, 1439
legal aspects, 1465
postconception methods, 1332–1335, 1342–1343, 1441
preconception methods, 1440–1441
research and development, 1440
social impact of, 1441–1443
sperm banking and, 1448
sperm and zygote banking, 1446–1448
ethical issues, 1446–1447, 1459
eugenic applications, 1447–1448
legal aspects, 1447, 1465–1469
procedure, 1446
Republic (Plato), 206, 237, 452, 541, 870, 1050, 1062, 1360, 1577, 1578, 1603, 1656
Rescher, Nicholas, 809, 810, 1416, 1417
Research, behavioral, 1470–1480
consent in, 1472–1474
deception in, 1472–1474, 1477
protection and accountability in, 1479–1480
risk:
entailed by research processes, 1474–1478
entailed by research products, 1478–1479
types of, 1470–1472
See also, Behavior control; Human experimentation
Research, biomedical, 1481–1491
conflicts between medical practice and, 1486–1488
domain of medicine, 1481–1484

images of man and, 856
law and, 1493–1494, 1644–1648
publication of, *See* Communication, biomedical
public policy and, 1492–1497
ethical and policy dimensions, 1496–1497
history of development in United States, 1488–1489, 1493–1496
value implications, 1492–1493
in relation to medicine, 1484–1486
socialization of, 1488–1490
specific ethical issues in, *See* Animal experimentation; Human experimentation
Research, sex, *See* Sex research
Research Defense Society (Great Britain), 78
Researcher:
distinguished from clinician, 43
–subject relationship, 752–753
Research Involving Prisoners, 1198
Resident physicians:
delegation of surgery to, 1628
training of, 868
Resignation, technological humanism and, 64
Res Medicae, 985
Resources:
distribution of, *See* Justice
health-care, 615–616
population policy and, 1244–1245, 1248
population problem and, 1217, 1222, 1237
Respect:
fundamental principle of, 1586
infanticide and, 748–749
informed consent and, 755–757
legislation of morality and, 821
for life, *See* Sanctity of life
for patients, 147, 148–149
Respirators, 270, 272, 296
Respiratory disease, environmentally induced, 380
Respiratory rate, pronouncement of death and, 259, 292–293, 298
Respiratory system failure, 841
Responsibility:
behavior control and, 87
in dynamic therapies:
of patient, 342
of therapist, 341–344
in Eastern Orthodox Christianity, 348
of hospitals, 677–683
institutional, 680–681
international, 644–645
medical vs. nonmedical models of therapy and, 604

mental illness and, 764, 1099
of mother for fetus, 487–488
of nurses, 1140–1141, 1142
personhood and, 1207
philosophical positions on, 545–546
of science and technology, 1540
in self-realization therapies, 1548
sick role and, 595, 604
in social medicine, 1600–1601
treatment of defective children and, 733–734
in weapons development:
of physician, 1701–1702
of scientist, 1699–1701
Responsible journalism, 182–183
Restraint, technological humanism and, 64
Resurrection:
in biblical thought, 243, 244, 245
Christianity and, 250, 251–252, 256, 257
Judaism and, 246, 247, 248
Resuscitation, 844
Retinoblastoma, 465–466, 474, 511
Retirement:
early, 55, 56
graduated, 61
impact of anti-aging policy on, 63
Retirement Income Security Act (PL 93–406), 641
Retraction of published information, 192
Retributive justice, 544–546
Retributive lid, 783
Retributive punishment, 102–108
Reuleaux, Franz, 1639
Reuther, Rosemary, 1610
Reverse discrimination, 867
Review committees, 190–191, 280, 738–739, 752, 753, 755, 759, 760, 1145, 1198, 1490, 1495
Reviewers, scientific, 183, 189–190
Revocability, medical decisions and, 307–308
Rewards and punishments, doctrine of, 436
Reward system of science, 1542–1543
Reward therapy, 781
Reymond, Emil DuBois, 584
Reynolds, David K., 288
Reza Shah, 887
Ṛgveda, 1270
Rhazes (al-Rāzi), 582, 789, 887, 893, 1065, 1267
Rh incompatibility, 474, 1332, 1333
Rhodesia:
population policy in, 1277
World Health Organization and, 644

Rhys, Jean, 1013
Rhythm method, 1256, 1267, 1533, 1582
Richards, D. A. J., 448, 449
Richter, Hermann E. F., 970
Ricoeuer, Paul, 1585
Rieff, Philip, 1061, 1567
Right and The Good, The (Ross), 1686
Right not to be born, 1340
Right of freedom from bodily assault, 1512
Right of free movement, 1304–1305
Right of parents to procreate, 1334, 1615
Right of privacy, 30, 31, 105, 1073, 1203, 1204, 1358, 1359
  abortion and 1513, 1514
  confidentiality and, 198
  informed consent and, 1472
  sex therapy and research and, 1559
  sterilization and, 1615–1616
  Supreme Court on, 573
Right of self-determination, 16, 22, 23, 27, 350, 998, 1154, 1512, 1513, 1611
Right of use or stewardship, 1528
Rights:
  absolute, 104–105
  of adolescents, *See* Adolescents: medical care of
  of the aged, 1512
  of animals, 81
  behavior control and, 87
  bestowed, 124
  in bioethics, 1511–1516
    as claims, 1511–1513
    conflicts of, 1512–1513, 1515–1516
    with correlative duties, 1513
    established in declarations, codes, and bills, 1515–1516
    legal, 1514–1515
    limits in satisfying, 1513–1514
    moral, 1511–1514
    positive, 1513–1516
  of children, 1512
  civil, 625, 626, 1072, 1105, 1106, 1111–1112, 1201, 1408, 1409
  concept of, 624–626
  cultural, 624–625
  Eastern Orthodox Christianity and, 349
  economic, 624–627
  family planning and, 1283
  of fetus, 1335, 1337–1338, 1340, 1341, 1512, 1513
  of future generations, *See* Future generations, obligations to
  genetic aspects of human behavior and, 546–547
  of human beings vs. rights of the environment, 389, 390

  of the institutionalized, 779–780, 1072, 1077, 1105
  of the mentally retarded, 1512
  in naturalism, 442, 443, 446
  of natural systems, 389, 390
  population policy and, 1262, 1276
  of prisoners, 1512
  property, 1305
  risk and, 1519
  Roman Catholicism and, 1530
  social conferral of, 17, 21–22
  systematic analysis of, 1507–1511
    as claims, 1508–1509
    with correlative duties, 1509–1510
    without correlative duties, 1510–1511
    legal, 1508–1509
    moral, 1507–1509
    negative, 1509, 1510
    positive, 1507, 1509–1510
  See also Confidentiality; Informed consent; Patients' rights movement; Privacy; specific rights; Truth-telling
Rights of Man (Paine), 624
Right to be free from hunger and malnutrition, 494, 499, 1510
Right to be gay, 670
Right to be left alone, 1514
Right to confidentiality, 1511–1512
Right to control one's own body, *See* Right of self-determination
Right to die, 37, 275–276, 1156, 1361, 1512, 1514
Right to health, 123, 627, 953, 971
Right to health-care services, 610–611, 613, 623–629, 647, 1513
  entitlement position, 631–633
  human rights, 626–627
  of institutionalized patients, 779–780, 1072, 1077, 1105
  rights in general, 624–626
  right to health, 627
  right to medical care, 627–629, 1604–1605
Right to know, 185, 1143
  See also Confidentiality; Informed consent; Truth-telling
Right to life, 133, 726–731, 823, 1337, 1340, 1513, 1528
Right to medical care, 627–629, 1604–1605
Right to refuse medical care, 275–276, 278, 281, 284–285, 845, 1498–1506, 1514
  balancing of public and private duties, 1503
  children and, 1198, 1505
  competency and, 1504–1505
  conflicting claims or interests, 1499–1503
    benefit to society, 1500–1502
    individual interests, 1500

    minimization of costs, 1501
    paternalism, 1500
    protection of others, 1501
    safeguarding of public feelings, 1501–1502
    sanctity of life and, 1502–1503, 1504
  importance of, 1499
  incompetency and, 1505–1506
  of institutionalized patients, 779–781, 1072–1073, 1203, 1503–1504
  legislation of morality and, 819
  paternalism and, 1197–1198, 1500, 1518
  in patients' bills of rights, 1203, 1204
  in practice, 1503–1504
  privacy and, 1361, 1500
  Protestantism and, 1437
  See also Euthanasia
Right to suicide, 1512, 1514
Riis, Povl, 985
Risk, 1516–1521
  of amniocentesis, 1333, 1335, 1336–1337
  cost-benefit analysis, 1520–1521
    abortion and, 834
    advantages of, 1520
    criticisms of, 1520
    defined, 1520
    environment and, 381–383
    euthanasia and, 835
    heart transplantation and, 657–658, 1162
    life-support systems and, 847
    in mass health screening, 860–861
    self-realization therapies and, 1549
    treatment of defective infants and, 725
    utility of health care and, 631
    value of human life and, 824–825
    values and, 1520–1521
  defined, 1516–1517
  disclosure of, *See* Informed consent
  in drug trials, 756
  gene therapy and, 522–524
  genetic, 562, 564
  health insurance and, 641
  human experimentation and, 689, 693, 694–695, 697, 1198, 1474–1479
  imposition of, 1519–1520
  involuntary, 1517
  organ donation and, 1161
  paternalism and, 1517–1519
  in reproductive technologies, 1461, 1466, 1467
  risk-taking conduct, 1517
    voluntary, 1517, 1518

in withdrawal of life-support systems, 85
Risk budget, 1517, 1518
Risk pool, 1519
"Risky-shift" phenomenon, 562
Ritchie, D. G., 81
Ritualism, 589
Robb, Isabel Hampton, 995, 1138
Robbins, John, 1277
Roberts, Oral, 1122
Robertson, John A., 736, 737, 738
Robins, Eli, 669
Robinson, J. A. T., 421
Robitscher, Jonas, 1611
Rochefoucauld-Liancourt, François Alexandre, Duc de la, 971
Rock, John, 212
Rockefeller, John D., III, 211, 480
Rockefeller Foundation, 1033, 1407
Roderick Random (Smollett), 1008
Roederer, 489
Roentgen, Wilhelm, 1489
Roe v. Wade (1973), 16, 27, 30, 31, 169, 198, 573, 820, 998, 1335, 1358, 1465, 1513, 1514, 1615
Roger II, King of Sicily, 946, 1035
Rogers, Carl, 1085, 1087, 1088, 1547
Rogers, Everett M., 1296
Rogers, Paul, 1496
Roman Catholicism, 1522–1533
  abortion and, 9–13, 818, 1256, 1257, 1527, 1529
    beginning of human of life and, 10–12, 19, 25, 1531
    contemporary perspectives, 25, 1533
    Directives on, 169, 175, 176, 1434, 1527
    early perspectives, 10–11
    intentionality and, 11
    in medieval Europe, 943–944, 946
    modern perspective, 11–13, 1524
    natural law and, 1526
    principle of double effect, 3, 11, 16, 23–24, 25, 34, 318, 1529
    scriptural influence, 9–10
    solution of conflict situations and, 23–24
  in Africa, 899
  antivivisectionist movement and, 78
  artificial insemination and, 1433, 1456–1457, 1458, 1531, 1533
  the arts and, 1523
  authoritative church teaching, 1431–1434, 1526–1527, 1532–1533

development of, 1527
Directives in Canada, 1432
Directives in United States, 1432–1434
dissent and, 1532
nature of, 1431–1432, 1527
autopsy and, 140
beginning of life and, 10–12, 19, 25, 1531, 1533
birth and, 1531
canon law, 942–945, 1523, 1524, 1527
care for health and, 1531
castration and, 1526
charity and, 939–942, 958
codes of medical ethics and, 169, 175, 176
confidentiality and, 1530
conscience, role of, 1527–1528
contraception and:
  Aquinas on, 209, 1226
  Augustine on, 207–208
  Directives on, 1433
  disagreement on, 212–213, 1532, 1533, 1582
  moral principles and, 1529
  natural law and, 1526
  in penitentials, 1524
  population policy and, 1254–1258
  principle of double effect and, 1213
  sterilization, 11, 169, 1256, 1257, 1433, 1526, 1529, 1533, 1609–1610, 1612
cooperation and, 1529–1530
cremation and, 142–143
current trends in, 1532–1533
death:
  definition of, 1532
  philosophy on, 250–253, 256
disease and, 938–939, 1522
double effect, principle of, 33–35
  abortion and, 3, 11, 16, 23–24, 25, 34, 318, 1529
  contemporary debates on, 318–319
  contraception and, 1213
  description of, 316, 1529
  historical development of, 316–318
  rejection of, 1533
  See also Acting and refraining; Omission and commission
drug use and, 1531
ensoulment and, 10–12, 1524
Ethical and Religious Directives for Catholic Health Facilities, 996, 1430–1434, 1530
on abortion, 169, 172, 175, 176,

1434, 1527
in Canada, 1432
text of, 1755–1757
in United States, 1432–1434
eugenics and, 471, 472
euthanasia and, 817, 942–943, 1531, 1533
exorcism and, 1121, 1523
healing and, 588–589, 1522–1523
  by divine power, 1123, 1125
homosexuality and, 673, 675
human experimentation and, 1532
human reason and, 1523
hypnosis and, 712
ideal physician, concept of, 940
in India, 909
justice and, 1255–1256
life-support systems and, 1531–1532
lobotomy and, 1526
marriage and, 208, 209, 1256, 1524, 1527, 1529, 1531, 1582
masturbation and, 1433, 1530–1531, 1533
mediation, principle of, 1523
medical ethics, history of: contemporary, 1525–1526
  medieval, 938–945, 1524
  modern, 1524–1525
  Patristic Age, 1523–1524
medical ethics education and, 871
mental health and, 1065–1066
mind–body problem and, 1532
mutilation and, 818, 1170–1171, 1528–1529, 1609–1610
natural law and, 818, 1134–1135, 1136, 1524, 1526, 1532
obligations of physicians and, 1530
ordinary and extraordinary means and, 176, 270, 271, 272, 727, 728, 1531–1532
organ donation and, 1154
organ transplantation and, 1170–1171, 1172, 1531
pain and, 1531
parenthood and, 1530
pastoral medicine, 1525
  clerics as physicians, 1523, 1658
health-care institutions, 939–940, 1190, 1431–1434, 1523
  medical schools, 1192
  teaching programs, 1192
patients' rights and, 1530
pharmacy and, 1213
philosophical thought, trends in, 1532
population ethics and, 1226, 1254–1258

Roman Catholicism (*Continued*)
  procreation and, 208, 209, 1529, 1530–1531, 1579–1580, 1582
  right to life and, 1528
  sacrament of anointing, 1522–1523
  sanctity of life and, 823
  scandal and, 1529–1530
  sexual abstinence and, 1234
  sexuality and, 1529, 1530–1531, 1579–1582
  sins of physicians, in medieval European thought, 942–945
  sponsorship of health facilities, 939–940, 1431–1434, 1523
  status of the aged and, 59–60
  stewardship, principle of, 1528, 1531
  suicide and, 275, 1531, 1623
  supererogation and, 1150
  surgery and, 1531
  theological thought, trends in, 1532
  totality, principle of, 1170–1171, 1528–1529, 1531, 1609–1610
  truth-telling and, 1530
Romano, V., 878
Romanticism:
  death and, 236, 241
  man's participation in nature and, 369
  technology and, 1640, 1641
Romberg, Ernst, 603
Rome, ancient:
  abortion in, 933
  animal experimentation in, 936
  confidentiality in, 932
  consultations in, 935
  contraception in, 205, 206
  dissemination of medical knowledge in, 937
  divine healing in, 1123
  divorce in, 1577
  euthanasia in, 261, 934–935
  fees in, 932
  giving or withholding treatment in, 933–934
  homosexuality in, 1577
  human experimentation in, 935–936
  infanticide in, 226, 742, 826
  marriage in, 1225–1226, 1577
  medical ethics, history of, 930–937
  medical malpractice in, 936
  population policies in, 1225–1226
  public physicians in, 936
  status of the aged in, 59
  suicide in, 934
  surgery in, 933
  truth-telling in, 934
  vivisection in, 935–936
Roosevelt, Franklin D., 1494
Roosevelt, Theodore, 371, 647–648
Rose, G., 1018
Rosebury, Theodor, 1700, 1701

Rose Case of 1703, 1036
Rosen, Joseph, 1251
Rosenberg, Alfred, 1019
Rosenfield v. United States (1957), 310
Rosenhan, David L., 1477
Rosensweig, Franz, 248
Rosenthal, Robert, 1475
Rosner, Fred, 871, 996, 1171
Ross, David, 542
Ross, Eleanor R. Rieff, 1081
Ross, William D., 174, 405, 415, 1686
Rotter, Julian B., 1086
Rouse v. Cameron (1966), 1514
Rousseau, Jean-Jacques, 416, 542, 953, 1226, 1292, 1401
  on coercion, 96
  ethical naturalism of, 442, 444
  "general will" theory of, 264
  on justice theories, 543
  on marriage, 1584
Rowland, 711
"Royal Book" [*Liber Regins*] ('Alī ibn 'Abbās al-Madjūsī) (Haly Abbas), 786, 887
Royal College of Physicians and Surgeons (Canada), 993
Royal College of Physicians of Edinburgh, 1715
Royal College of Physicians of London, 973, 989, 1030, 1036
Royal College of Surgeons of England, 973, 1036
Royal Commission on Capital Punishment, 283
Royal Society of Medicine, 988
Rubella, 576, 1108
Rüdin, E., 539, 1016
Ruff, Wilfried, 18
Rufus, 785
Rule by experts, 1062
Rule of St. Benedict, 939
Rules and principles, 406–412
  in classical ethical theory, 409–410
  general features of, 408–409
  in intuitionism, 415–416
  legal status and, 817–819
  moral justification and, 410–412
  in naturalism, 446
  in theological ethics, 433–435
  See also Codes of Ethics; Deontological theories; Teleological theories; Utilitarianism
Rule-utilitarianism, 406, 416, 422, 426–428
  coalescence with act-utilitarianism, 426–428
  compulsory rules and, 420
  defined, 421, 426
  guidance for individual deliberation and, 420
  health-care delivery and, 631
Rumania, abortion laws in, 29
Rural medical care, 617

Rural-to-urban population migration, 1220, 1223, 1224, 1305
Rush, Benjamin, 960, 961, 965, 1030, 1031, 1079–1080
Russell, Bertrand, 1585
Russell, E. S., 128
Russell, J. C., 1234
Russia:
  animal experimentation in, 80
  Penal Code of 1903, 282
  See also Union of Soviet Socialist Republics
Rwanda:
  health expenditures in, 1322
  population policy in, 1283
Ryle, Gilbert, 111–112, 114, 362, 504
Ryōkan, Master, 375

S

Sabshin, Melvin, 1059
Sackett, Walter, 283, 284
Sacra embryologia (Cangliamila), 1525, 1660
Sacramentals, 589
Sacra philosophia (Valles), 1660
Sacred Congregation for the Doctrine of the Faith, 25
Sacredness of human life, *See* Sanctity of life
Saghir, Mardel, 669
Saigyo, 234
Saint-Just, Louis de, 1226
Saint-Luc Medicale, 985, 1522
Sale of organs, 1159
Sales, Francis de, 1065
Salesmanship, 97
Salgo v. Stanford University (1957), 770, 772
Saline injections, as abortion procedure, 3, 4
Salmanticenses, 317
Salmond, John W., 1510
Salpingectomy, 3
Salvaging organs, 1158–1159
Salvation Army, 1596
Salvationism, 418
Samp, Robert J., 1678
Sample survey, 1471
Saṃsārā, 661, 1188
Sanchez, Thomas, 34, 212, 317, 471, 472
Sanctity of life, 823
  euthanasia and, 837–838
  Hinduism and, 832
  images of man and, 855
  Judaism and, 8, 794–795, 1429
  purpose in the universe and, 1403, 1404
  right to refuse medical care and, 1502–1503, 1504

quality-of-life distinguished from, 831–833
Roman Catholicism and, 823
Sand, René, 1598
Sanders, David, 1416
Sang, J. H., 464
Sanger, Margaret H., 159–160, 211, 998
Sanitary condition of the laboring class, 1393
Sanitary reforms, 1394, 1483–1484
Sanitation, *See* Public health
Santa Teresa, Domingo de, 317
Santayana, George, 237
Santorio, Santorio, 688
Sartre, Jean-Paul, 239, 242, 363, 411, 1585, 1594
Sassanian period, 883, 886
Saudi Arabia:
    alcohol use in, 891
    family planning in, 890
    health care in, 890
Sauvages de la Croix, François Boissier de, 600, 1051
SBA, *See* Small Business Administration
Scandinavia:
    eugenic societies in, 458
    fetal research in, 490
    health care financing in, 611
    health policy in, 652
    self-realization therapies in, 1549
    See also names of countries
Scarce resources, allocation of, 390, 806–810, 1414–1418
    artificial heart, 1652
    behavior control and, 89–90
    Eastern Orthodox Christianity and, 349
    enzyme replacement and, 514
    genetic screening and, 571–572
    images of man and, 855
    kidney dialysis and, 808–809, 815, 1414, 1415, 1416, 1418
    obligation to future generations and, 1519
    organ transplantation on, 807–808, 815, 1163–1164, 1414, 1415
    paternalism and, 1518–1519
    population problem and, 1224
    practice conception of, 412
    quality of life and, 832
    randomization of, 809–810, 1416, 1417
    rights and, 1510–1511, 1513
    risk-taking and, 1518–1519
    rules for final selection, 809–810, 1416–1418
    rules of exclusion, 809, 1415–1416
    social justice and, 390

social worth criteria, 809–810, 1415–1418
    treatment of defective infants and, 739–740
    triage and, *See* Triage
    in United States, 1418
    utilitarianism and, 419, 421, 809, 810, 1416–1417
Schambergen, Casper, 924
Scheel, Karl, 489
Scheff, Thomas J., 1666
Scheler, Max, 242
Schelling, Friedrich von, 241
Schiel, Jean Vincent, 884
Schizophrenia:
    chance of recovery and, 1073–1074
    electroconvulsive therapy (ECT) and, 359
    fertility and, 1075, 1076
    genetics and, 539, 540, 1077
    home care and, 1075
    public institutions and, 1076
    universality of, 1077
Schleiermacher, Friedrich, 241, 1582
Schlick, Moritz, 129, 542
Schloendorff v. Society of New York Hospital (1914), 1154, 1512
Schmidt, Gerhard, 1016
Schmidt, Heinrich, 970
Schneider, Richard, 688
Schneidman, Edwin S., 1710
Scholasticism, 209, 248, 1134
School of Salerno, 1658
Schopenhauer, Arthur, 239, 241, 1584
Schrödinger, Erwin, 1403
Schultze, Charles L., 1475
Schumacher, Sallie, 1554
Schumaker, Millard, 1150, 1151
Schutz, Alfred, 1603
Schweitzer, Albert, 827, 828, 832
Science:
    bioethics and, 118–119, 125–126, 1545–1546
    death and, 257, 258, 259
    determinism and, 501–502
    ethics and, 1535–1540
        formulation of moral problems, 1540
        historical instances of relationship between, 1535–1536
        impact of technology, 1538, 1540
        moral problems aided by science, 1538–1539
        moral responsibility of science and technology, 1540
        theoretical conflicts between, 118–119, 125–126, 444–446, 1536–1538

theoretical shifts in moral philosophy, 1539
        See also Natural law; Pragmatism
    man's dominion over nature and, 367–368
    personhood and, 1209–1210
    religion, conflict with, 1401–1403
    sociology of, 1541–1546
        bioethics and, 1545–1546
        communications among scientists, 1544
        ethos of science, 1542
        growth of scientific knowledge, 1544–1545
        growth patterns, 1542
        priority disputes, 1543–1544
        social stratification, 1542–1543
    technology as, 1639
    war and, 1699–1703
        continuing controversies, 1702–1703
        social responsibility of physician, 1701–1702
        social responsibility of scientist, 1699–1701
Science and Health with Key to the Scriptures (Eddy), 1377
Science writing, *See* Communication, biomedical
Scientific cosmology, 1402–1403
Scientific data, falsification of, 184
Scientific determinism, 545
Scientific knowledge, growth of, 1544–1545
Scientific limits to economic growth, 394
Scientific materialism, 257, 258
Scientific meetings, 183, 193–194
Scientific method, pragmatism and, 1328
Scientific publishing, 188–194, 1001, 1542
    advertising, 193
    authorship and the by-line, 192–193
    of behavioral research, 1477, 1478–1479
    biocommunication ethics, 189
    citation of references, 193
    confidentiality and, 181, 185, 189, 191–192, 1477
    editorial criteria for ethical research, 190–191, 1490
    establishment of priority, 189
    growth of specialties and, 1544
    human experimentation control and, 704–705, 1489, 1490
    multiple publication, 191
    patterns of information exchange, 1544

Science publishing (*Continued*)
  peer reviews of manuscripts, 183, 189–190
  pre-meeting abstracts and oral presentation, 183, 193–194
  retraction and refutation, 192
  reward systems and, 1543
  in Western Europe, 985
  See also Media: medicine and
Scientific rationalism, 398
Scott, J. P., 541
Screening, *See* Genetic screening; Mass health screening
Scriptures, *See* Bible
Searle, John R., 444
Sebring, Harold L., 1018
Secondary care, 614
Secondary screening, 858
Second Lateran Council, 209
Second Vatican Council, 12, 13, 25, 213, 1255, 1432, 1456, 1522, 1530, 1531, 1582
Secrecy, *See* Confidentiality
Sectarian practitioners, 167
Secular humanism, 429
Sedative hypnotics, 1381
Sedgwick, Peter, 1053
Sefer Asaf, 164
Segregation, 1408
Segregationist gerontologists, 60
Selective abortion, *See* Prenatal diagnosis: followed by abortion
Selectivity position on treatment of defective infants, 725
Self-awareness, 341, 672
Self-care, 614
Self-consciousness, as personhood criterion, 1369–1370, 1371
Self-control, 87, 89–91, 109
Self-determination, 504, 505
  Eastern Orthodox Christianity and, 347, 348
  informed consent and, 755, 761, 771–777
  maturity as measure of, 39–40
  paternalism and, 1198
  population policy and, 1245, 1246
  Protestantism and, 15, 16
  right of, 16, 22, 23, 27, 350, 998, 1154, 1512, 1513, 1611
  See also Autonomy; Free will; Right to refuse medical care
Self-development, 1209
Self-discovery, 339
Self-evidence, appeal to, *See* Intuitionism
Self-examination, 339
Self-experimentation, 688–689, 1487
Self-help clinics for women, 161
Self-image, 1474–1475
Self-knowledge, 339–340
Self-love, 1621
Self-observation, 109
Self-presentation, 1477

Self-realization therapies, 1547–1551
  assignment of responsibility in, 1548
  basic ambiguities in, 1548
  benefits in, 1549
  defined, 1547
  ethics of change and, 1548–1549
  range of techniques, 1547–1548
  risks in, 1549
  social control and, 1549–1550
  social implications of, 1550
Self-regarding actions, 607
Self-regarding obligations, 606–609
Self-regulation by media, 187–188
Self-revelation, 97
Semen, *See* Sperm
Semmelweiss, Ignaz, 1716
Senancour, Jean Baptiste Étienne de, 210
Seneca, Lucius Annaeus, 238, 239, 826, 931, 1065, 1578
Seneca, Marcus Annaeus (the Elder), 933
Senegal, compensation of physicians in, 899
Senghor, Léopold, 1402
Senilicide, 227–228
Senility, 1077
Sensationalism in medical reporting, 181, 185–186
Sensory deficits, mass health screening and, 861
Sensory fields, localization of, 363
Sentences (Lombard), 1579
Sentience of surroundings, 377–378
Septuagint, 9
Sermon on the Estate of Marriage, A (Luther), 1581
Servetus, 1366
Seventh Day Adventists, 70, 337, 1376–1377, 1596
Sex chromosome abnormalities, males with, 531–533, 543, 568, 571
Sex determination, *See* Sex selection
Sex education, 1282–1283, 1566
Sex hormones, 1590
Sexism, 1410, 1416
Sex-linked disease, 1333–1334, 1342, 1439, 1442, 1443
Sex predetermination, *See* Sex selection
Sex preferences, 1342–1343, 1442–1443
Sex ratio, 1442–1443, 1465
Sex research:
  ethical perspectives, 1554–1559
    confidentiality, 1559
    general moral considerations, 1556–1557
    informed consent, 1558–1559
    privacy, 1559
    therapist-patient intimacies, 1557–1558, 1566

  scientific and clinical perspectives, 1551, 1552
Sex selection, 1439–1443, 1644
  gene therapy and, 520, 522
  justification of, 1439
  legal aspects, 1465
  postconception methods, 1332–1335, 1342–1343, 1441
  preconception methods, 1440–1441
  research and development, 1440
  social impact of, 1441–1443
  sperm banking and, 1448
Sex therapy:
  ethical perspectives, 1554–1559
    confidentiality, 1559
    general moral considerations, 1556–1557
    informed consent, 1558–1559
    privacy, 1559
    therapist-patient intimacies, 1557–1558, 1566
  scientific and clinical perspectives, 1551–1554
    effectiveness of, 1554
    purpose of, 1552
    types of, 1552–1554
Sexual abstinence:
  cultural variation and, 1561
  Hinduism and, 1271
  Judaism and, 1251
  in primitive cultures, 1228
  Roman Catholicism and, 1234
Sexual Attitude Restructuring Process (SAR), 1554
Sexual behavior, 1560–1568
  contemporary problems:
    crime, 1567
    de-moralization of sex, 1567–1568
    in families, 1567
    limits of permissiveness, 1567
    sex therapy and, *See* Sex therapy
  contemporary sexual norms, 1563–1565
    changes in, 1563–1564
    display of permissiveness, 1564–1565
  homosexual, *See* Homosexuality
  of mentally retarded, 1111
  research on, *See* Sex research
  sexual revolution:
    background for, 1560–1561
    publicity and, 1561, 1562
    technology and, 1561–1563
  See also Sexual development; Sexual ethics
Sexual development, 1569–1574
  adolescence, 1572–1574
  earliest years, 1570–1571
  from four to six, 1572
  Freud on, 1562, 1569–1572
  moral agency, 1574
  from two to four, 1571–1572

Sexual differentiation studies, 1554
Sexual ethics, 1575–1587, 1592–1594
  in ancient Greece, 932–933, 1577–1578
  in ancient Rome, 1577
  Christianity and, 1578–1583, 1592–1593
  contemporary challenge to traditional norms, 1583–1587
  evolutionary analysis, 1585–1587
  factors contributing to, 1583–1585, 1593
  defined, 1589
  Eastern Orthodox Christianity and, 352–353
  Gnosticism and, 1578, 1579
  Islam and, 787
  Judaism and, 796–797, 1561, 1576–1577
  models of, 1592–1594
  Protestantism and, 1259–1260, 1436, 1457, 1581, 1582–1583
  Roman Catholicism and, 1529, 1530–1531, 1579–1582
  Stoicism and, 672, 1578–1579
  See also Sexual behavior; Sexual identity
Sexual health, 340–341
Sexual identity, 1589–1595
  biological sex, 1589–1590, 1594
  gender identity, 669, 1552, 1554, 1571–1572, 1589, 1590–1591, 1594
  problem of normalcy, 1594–1595
  sexual ethics, See Sexual ethics
  sexual orientation, 1589, 1591–1592, 1594
  See also Sex therapy
Sexuality, See Sexual behavior; Sexual ethics; Sexual identity
Sexual misconduct in literature, 1008
Sexual offenders, 1554, 1559
Sexual orientation, 1589, 1591–1592, 1594
Sexual promiscuity, 853
Sexual relations with patients, 989, 990, 1557–1558, 1566, 1704–1705
Sexual surrogates, 1566
Sexual surveys, 1552
Shaare Zedek Hospital (Jerusalem), 896
Shaffer, Peter, 1013
Shahmameh (The Book of Kings), 884
Shamans, 203, 587, 877, 878–879, 905, 1065, 1632
Sham operations, 1628
Shang, Lord of, 1235

Shang dynasty, 230
Shannon, James A., 1495
Shapiro, Samuel, 191
Shapur I, King of Persia, 886
Shapur II, King of Persia, 886
Shatin, Leo, 1416
Shattuck, Lemuel, 1394
Shaw, George Bernard, 689, 827, 918, 1011–1012
Sherlock, B. J., 313
Shetland, Margaret, 1140
Shiism, 786
Shingu Ryotei, 925–926
Shintoism, 376, 901, 922
Shneidman, Edwin S., 1619
Shockley, William, 213
Shock treatment, 359
Short gut syndrome, 719
Shōtoku, Prince of Japan, 136, 932
Shōzen, Kajiwara, 923
Shulhan Arukh (Karo), 248, 793, 794, 795, 798, 799, 1429
Shumway, N. E., 655, 657–658
Shurtleff, David B., 725
Sickle-cell disease, 157, 476, 511–512, 522, 550, 557, 563, 568, 569, 601, 720, 861
Sickness, See Disease; Illness
Sickness Insurance Act of 1883 (Germany), 647, 970
Sickness-producing sins, forgiveness of, 1122
Sick role, 594, 595–596, 604, 1091, 1093, 1094, 1099, 1483
Sick visitation, See Visitation of the sick
Siculus, Diodorus, 882
Sidgwick, Henry, 413, 420, 421, 438, 508, 804, 827, 1685, 1686
Siebold, P. F., 924
Sierra Club, 369
Sierra Leone, compensation of physicians in, 899
Sigerist, Henry E., 1481, 1663, 1713
Sigmoidoscopic examination, 862
Silent Spring (Carson), 181, 370, 393
Simmel, Georg, 242
Simmons, Leo Williams, 221
Simplicity in medical decision-making, 309
Simpson, G. G., 542
Simulation studies, 1471
Sin, sense of, 1585
Singapore, sterilization in, 1617
Singular creature (image of man), 851–852
Sinitsyn, H., 654
Sinner (image of man), 852–853

Situation ethics, 405, 421–424, 1135
  bioethical issues and, 423–424
  central thesis of, 456
  codes of ethics and, 177–178
  duty and, 422–423
  images of man and, 856
  love and, 422, 434
  moral decision-making and, 405, 411, 422, 423, 434
  theological advocates of, 421–422
  See also Act-utilitarianism; Relativism
Six Bookes of a Commonweale, The (Bodin), 1226
Sixtus V, Pope, 11, 795
Skepticism, ethical, 402
Skinner, B. F., 1062, 1068, 1086, 1088
  basic approach of, 108, 113–114
  on countercontrol by subjects, 109
  on freedom and dignity, 98–99, 100, 503, 1425–1426
  on reinforcement of the institutionalized, 105
Skinner box, 113
Skinner v. Oklahoma (1942), 1615
Skolimowski, Henryk, 1639
Slater v. Baker (1767), 689
Sleep-reduction, as anti-aging technique, 51–52
Slippery-slope arguments, 821, 836–837
Small, Henry, 1544
Small Business Administration (SBA), 386
Smallpox vaccination, 686–687, 1393, 1395
Smart, J. J. C., 421
Smith, Adam, 973, 1235, 1535
Smith, Audrey V., 217
Smith, Harmon L., 1368, 1458
Smoking, 326, 327, 328, 330, 334–335, 1384, 1385, 1518, 1596–1597
  Adventism and, 1376
  advertising and, 1605
  in Arab nations, 891
  fetal development and, 487
  health and, 70, 1597
  health of others and, 1597
  Jehovah's Witnesses and, 1377
  Mormonism and, 1376
  objections to, 1596–1597
  public health and, 1397, 1398
  tobacco industry and, 1597, 1601
Smollett, Tobias, 1008
Snake charmers, 909
Snezhnevsky, Andrei, 1078
Snow, John, 1484
Social casework, medical, 1043

VOLUME INDICATOR

Vol. 1: pp. 1-484   Vol. 2: pp. 485-900   Vol. 3: pp. 901-1404   Vol. 4: pp. 1405-1816

Social change population policy proposals, 1295–1300
  direct measures, 1295–1296
  ethical issues, 1296–1298
  indirect measures, 1295
  semidirect measures, 1295, 1296
Social context:
  of decision, 526
  of human research, 692
Social contract theory, 266, 416–417, 543, 1603–1605, 1668
  human experimentation and, 692
  implications for bioethics, 1604–1605
  obligation to future generations and, 509
Social control, 87, 89, 90, 91–92, 596–597
  of human experimentation, 702, 706–709
  medicine as, 1055
  psychiatrists as agents of, 1071–1074
  psychosurgery as, 1389–1390
  self-realization therapies and, 1549–1550
Social Darwinism, 458, 460, 480–481, 529, 1080, 1536
Social engineers, 482–483
Social ethics, 122
Social experiments, 1475, 1478
Social Gospel movement, 15
Social institutions of mental health, 1071–1078
  community centers, 67, 1074–1076
  mental institutionalization, *See* Mental institutionalization
  social role of psychiatrist, 1071–1074
Social insurance systems, 611–612, 618
Social-interactional model of human behavior, 1088
Sociality, 1603–1605
  implications for bioethics, 1604–1605
  neonaturalism and, 64
  philosophical thought on, 1603–1604
Socialization:
  of biomedical research, 1488–1490
  of children, 1590
Social medicine, 1597–1602
  as ethical model, 1598–1601
    environmental health, 1599
    medical care system, 1599–1600
    responsibility in, 1600–1601
  meaning of, 1598
  in medical education, 1601–1602
  origin of, 1598
  Taoism and, 1636
  See also Public Health
Social personhood theory, 730
Social policy, *See* Public policy

Social reform, 1396–1397
Social rights, 624–625, 626, 627
Social role:
  attitudes toward death and, 289
  of dynamic therapies, 344
  of psychiatrist, 1071–1074
  of sickness, 593–597
Social Security Act of 1935, 611, 638
Social vs. military expenditures, 1323, 1324
Social work:
  medical, 1042–1044
  truth-telling and, 1680
Social worth factors, 809–810, 1415–1418
Society:
  defective infants and, 723, 728
  disease and, 1394–1396
  homosexuality and, 672–673
  vs. the individual, 522, 1224, 1453
  medicine and, 976
  obligation of medical schools to, 865–867
  right to refuse medical care and, 1500–1502
  technology and, 1641–1642
  value of biomedical research to, 1497
Society for Health and Human Values, 1000, 1192
Society for Pediatric Radiology, 1726
Society for Social Responsibility in Science (Great Britain), 988, 1701
Society of Apothecaries of London, 973
Society of Jesus, 923
Society of Thoracic Surgeons, 1730
Socioeconomic factors in birth defects, 465
Socioeconomic institutions, modifications of, 1296
Sociological models of disease, 604
Sociology:
  bioethics and, 125
  health and disease and, 590–598
    definition of health, 591–593
    health as interaction medium, 597–598
    illness and life expectancy, 593
    social role of sickness, 593–597
  homosexuality and, 669
  of medicine, 1054–1058
    ethical dilemmas, 1058
    help-seeking and, 1055–1056
    organization of medical care, 1056–1057
    role of physician, 1055
    role of sociologist, 1054–1055
    scope of, 1054
    social distribution of health, illness, and medical care, 1056
    sociology of health occupations, 1057–1058

of mental illness, 1090
organ donation and, 1058, 1166–1169
of science, 1541–1546
  bioethics and, 1545–1546
  communications among scientists, 1544
  ethos of science, 1542
  growth of scientific knowledge, 1544–1545
  growth patterns, 1542
  priority disputes, 1543–1544
  social stratification, 1542–1543
of technology, 1639–1640
of therapeutic relationship, 1663–1671
  behavioral implications of organic systems, 1665–1666
  conflict model, 1666
  elaboration of relationship, 1671
  epidemiology of help-seeking, 1669–1671
  neo-Marxist, 1666–1667
  Parsonian model, 1665
  system model, 1664–1665
Socrates, 206, 339, 828, 870
  on death, 236, 237, 238
  prescriptivist elements in philosophy of, 448
Socratic method, 403
Sodium polystyrene sulfonate, 842
Sofer, Moses, 212
Solicitation of patients, 44–47
Solitude, 1357, 1360
Solomon ben Abraham Adret, 1251, 1428
Solovyev, 1585
Solzhenitsyn, Alexander, 1013, 1355
Somaiatric models of mental illness, 1094
Somatic models:
  of disease, 603–604
  of mental illness, 1091, 1094, 1096, 1097
Somatic Pinelianism, 1094
Somatic therapies, 1086–1087
  See also Electrical stimulation of the brain (ESB); Electroconvulsive therapy (ECT); Psychopharmacology; Psychosurgery
Some Medical Ethical Problems (Bourke), 871
Sommer, Barbara, 1707–1708
Son-preference, 1442–1443
Sons of Noah, Laws of, 6
Sophocles, 59, 236
Soranas, 1713
Soranus of Ephesus, 205, 933
Sorcerers, 877, 878, 879, 1065
Soul:
  ancient Greek philosophy on, 236, 237

Augustine on, 250–251, 436–437, 1524

Christian view of, 250–253

definition of death and, 302, 351

early modern philosophy on, 240

Eastern Orthodox Christian view of, 348

Hellenistic thought on, 238

in Hinduism, 661, 803

immortality of, *See* Immortality

Judaic view of, 246–247, 248

Kant on, 257

religious conceptions of disease and, 586

Roman Catholic view of, 256

value theory of theological ethics and, 436–437

See also Ensoulment; Mind-body problem

Soul-self (image of man), 853–854

South Africa:

blood transfusion, attitude towards, 133

population policy in, 1277, 1283

World Health Organization and, 644

South America:

eugenic societies in, 458

infanticide in, 742

See also names of countries

Southern Sung dynasty, 201

South Korea, contraception in, 211

South Sea Islands, infanticide in, 742

Souvenir de Solferino, Un (Dunant), 1696

Soviet Union, *See* Union of Soviet Socialist Republics

Soziale Pathologie (Grotjahn), 1598

Spain:

animal experimentation in, 81

contraception in, 211

differential population growth in, 1286

health care financing in, 611

medical ethics education in, 872, 984

population policy in, 1235

Protomedicato in, 1005

Spanish Edict of 1623, 1235

Spatiality of body, 362

Specialists, 167, 613, 614, 615, 1029, 1668–1669, 1717

Special obligations, 606–607

Species membership, 744

Species vs. individual, 524–525

Speciesism, 82, 826

Speck, Richard, 531

Spencer, Herbert, 479, 480, 529, 1402, 1536, 1537

Sperm:

banking, 1446–1448

ethical issues, 1446–1447, 1459, 1465

eugenic applications, 1447–1448

legal aspects, 1447, 1465–1469

procedure, 1446

donation of, 467, 1444, 1445, 1447, 1454–1460, 1462, 1465–1469, 1531, 1533

in vitro fertilization and, 999, 1446, 1448–1451

sex selection and, 1440–1441

Spermatogenesis, 1440

Sperry, R. W., 463

Sperry, Willard, 871

Spherocytosis, 474

Spilka, Bernard, 1679, 1680

Spina bifida, 474, 719–720, 725

Spinoza, Benedict de, 240, 362, 502, 1066

Split-brain operations, 1119

Spontaneous help, 1655

Sprenger, 1714

Śraddha, 662

Sri Lanka, 665

life expectancy in, 1229

population education in, 1311

Ssu-ma Ch'ien, 917

St. Martin, Alexis, 687

St. Thomas, University of (Philippines), 872

Stage theory of dying, 287

Stampfl, 1086

Standard of living:

population policy and, 1244–1245, 1247–1249

See also Quality of life

Standards of Bariatric Practice, 1728

Standards of Good Practice for Radio Broadcasters of the United States of America, 181

Stapf, A. J., 471

Star of Redemption (Rosensweig), 248

Starzl, Thomas E., 1162

State hospitals, 67

State of New York, University of, 1515

State University of New York at Stony Brook, 875

Static and sterile medical institutions, 620

Stationary state economy, 394, 396

Statistical analysis, 1488

Statistical morality, 553–554

Statistical theory, 695–696, 699

Steady-state economics, 394

Stearns, J. Brenton, 508–509

Stephen, James Fitzjames, 820

Stereotaxic surgery, 357

Stereotyped emotional responses, stimulation of, 97

Sterilization, 560, 1229, 1262

in Arab nations, 890

in Canada, 999

compulsory, 213, 574, 1706

Draconian/coercive interventionism and, 1222

ethical aspects, 1611–1612

Hinduism and, 1272

in India, 1301

in Japan, 928

legal aspects, 459, 1614–1616

of mentally unfit, 31, 459–460, 1108–1109, 1111, 1395, 1397, 1614–1616

in National Socialist Germany, 1016, 1018

paternalism and, 1199

population control with, 1222, 1301

in United States, 459–460, 1108–1109, 1395, 1397

Eastern Orthodox Christianity and, 355

government population incentives and, 1291

Hinduism and, 1272, 1609, 1610–1611

hysterectomy, 1608, 1705–1706

in India, 910, 1283, 1291, 1301, 1397

involuntary, 1612, 1706

Islam and, 788

Judaism and, 795, 796, 800, 1610

medical aspects of, 1606–1608

nursing and, 1142

Protestantism and, 1436

punitive, 1612, 1706

therapeutic, 355, 796, 1433, 1609

tubal, 1607–1608

vasectomy, 355, 1283, 1291, 1302, 1446, 1447, 1606, 1607

voluntary:

age-parity formulas and, 1610, 1611

Hinduism and, 1272, 1609, 1610–1611

informed consent and, 1606, 1608–1609, 1616

Judaism and, 1610

legal aspects, 1616–1617

motivation for childlessness and, 1706–1707

preconditions for, 1617

Protestantism and, 1609, 1610, 1611

Roman Catholicism and, 1530, 1609–1610

in United States, 1616–1617

Stevenson, Charles L., 448, 453
Steward (image of man), 855
Stewardship, 1154
  of nature, 371–372, 373
    Roman Catholicism and, 1528, 1531
Stewart v. Long Island College Hospital (1971), 574
Stieglitz, Johann, 969
Still, A. T., 1174
Stille, Alfred, 1715
Stimulant drugs, 335–336
Stoeckle, J. D., 777
Stoicism:
  contraception and, 206, 207, 208
  death and, 236–240
  freedom from constraint and, 93–94
  man's dominion over nature and, 367
  mental health and, 1065
  natural justice and, 818
  sexual ethics and, 672, 1578–1579
  status of the aged and, 59
  suicide and, 238–239, 1620, 1623
Stone, Christopher D., 123, 389
Stopping vs. not starting a procedure, 271–272
Storer, Norman, 1544
Stott, D. H., 486
Stranger (image of man), 854
Stratification system of science, 1542–1543
Strauss, Anselm L., 288
Strehler, Bernard L., 49
Strikes:
  physician, 161
  prisoner, 1347
Strip-mine land reclamation, 383
Stroke, 50, 51, 62, 1483
Strong paternalism, 1197, 1352
Structural functionalism, 1663, 1665, 1666, 1675-1676
Structural research on fetuses, 489
Struggles for existence, 479
Strunk v. Strunk (1969), 1154
Studies in the Psychology of Sex (Ellis), 1562
Study sections, 1489
Subject advocates, 705
Subjectivism, 438, 440, 447, 448
Subjectivity of human body, 363
Subliminal advertising, 97
Subspecialists, 614
Subspecialties, 1726
Substitution of drugs, 1211, 1213
Suburban medical care, 616
Suction curettage, 3, 4
Suddenly Last Summer (Williams), 1010
Suffering, 597
  abortion and, 2, 7, 8
  animal experimentation and, 79–83, 1180
  duty to relieve, 960

euthanasia and, *See* Euthanasia
  of fetus, 1339
  initiation of life-support systems and, 844
  pain, relationship to, 1180–1182
  of parents with defective children, 1339
  population policy and, 1243
  purpose in the universe and, 1403, 1404
  religious perspectives, 1185–1189
    Buddhism, 137, 138, 1187–1188
    Christianity, 1186–1187
    Hinduism, 664, 1187–1188
    Islam, 1185
    Jainism, 1187–1188
    Judaism, 1186
  risk of, *See* Informed consent
  treatment of defective infants and, 728, 733
Sufism, 431, 786
Suggestion, 97
Suicide, 276–277, 1618–1626
  in ancient Egypt, 881–882
  in ancient Greece and Rome, 934
  anomic, 95, 1619
  anthropological perspective, 223–225
  Aquinas on, 275, 823, 943, 1620, 1621, 1623
  Aristotle on, 1620–1621, 1623
  in Assyria–Babylonia, 881
  Augustine on, 275, 943
  barbiturates and, 1382
  Bible and, 1622
  Buddhism and, 137, 1621–1623
  in China, 1622
  Christianity and, 274, 275
  confidentiality and, 1511–1512
  "dialysis," 845
  electroconvulsive therapy (ECT) and, 359, 360
  as ethical question, 1620
  hedonism and, 264
  Hinduism and, 1621
  Hume on, 276–277
  incidence of, 1618–1619, 1625
  in India, 1621–1622
  Islam and, 1622
  Jainism and, 1621
  in Japan, 1622
  Judaism and, 247, 1622
  Kant on, 277, 1621
  law and, 1625–1626
  legislation of morality and, 819
  mercantilism and, 263
  moral character of persons who commit, 1623–1624
  nature of, 1618–1620
  nursing and, 1143
  obligations prohibiting, 1620–1623
    to oneself, 1620–1621
    to other people, 1620
    religious, 1621–1623

  obligation to prevent, 1624–1626
  pain and, 1624
  paternalistic principle and, 1195
  positivism and, 265
  premenstrual tension and, 1707
  privacy and, 1361
  psychiatry and, 1625
  vs. refusal of medical care, 1501–1503
  respect for freedom and, 823
  right to, 1512, 1514
  Roman Catholicism and, 275, 1531, 1623
  Stoicism and, 238–239, 1620, 1623
  in United States, 1618
Suicide prevention centers, 1625
Sulfanilamides, 1494
Sulfur injections, 1355
Sullivan, Harry Stack, 1084, 1088
Summa Contra Gentiles (Aquinas), 1580
Summae summarum (Antoninus), 1524
Summary conception, the, 411–412
Summary of Medicine (Descartes), 1050
Summa Theologiae (Aquinas), 317, 1149, 1226, 1524, 1580, 1685
Sumner, William Graham, 480
Sunnism, 786
Sun Ssu-miao, 165, 202, 203, 911, 913–914, 917, 925, 1633, 1636
Sun Tzu, 1695
Supererogation, 1147–1152, 1166
  bioethics and, 1151–1152
  distinction between obligation and, 1147
    theoretical basis for, 1147–1149
  philosophical discussion of, 1150–1151
  theological discussion of, 1149–1150
Super gregem (Pius VI), 944
"Superior orders," plea of, 1696–1697
Supernatural, 877–881, 1047–1048
  See also Miracle and faith healing
Superstition, 1523
Supply and demand, global availability of food and, 494–495, 497
Supreme Court rulings:
  abortion, 16, 27, 30, 31, 169, 198, 573, 820, 998, 1335, 1358, 1465, 1513, 1514, 1615
  advertising, 47, 1212
  contraception, 211, 462, 573, 818, 821, 1358, 1615
  mental institutionalization, 780, 783, 1203
  procreational privacy, 573–574, 1465
  reproductive acts, 462
  right to privacy, 573
  right to treatment, 780, 1072
  segregated education, 313

sterilization, 1614–1617, 1706
Surgery, 463, 614, 615, 1627–1630, 1690, 1693
abortion procedures, 3
in ancient Greece, 933, 934
in ancient Rome, 933
behavior control with, *See* Psychosurgery
clinical trials and, 1628–1629
ethical aspects of surgeon's role, 1627
as euphenic measure, 474–475
experimental research and, 77
informed consent and, 1627–1628
Islam and, 788
Judaism and, 799–800
Oath of Hippocrates and, 163, 164
prolongation and termination of treatment and, 1629
Roman Catholicism and, 1531
stereotaxic, 357
truth-telling, 1629, 1679, 1680
See also Organ transplantation
Surrogate consent mechanisms, 68
Surrogate mother, 557, 1450, 1454, 1462, 1467, 1468–1469, 1713
Surrogate partners in sex therapy, 1556–1557
Survival:
global, 395–397
heart transplantation and, 657–658
kidney dialysis vs. kidney transplantation, 1161–1162
mental retardation and, 1109–1110
in Western philosophical thought, 236, 240
See also Anti-aging techniques; Life-support systems; Risk; Sustaining life
Survivalists, 1275, 1277
Susceptibility screening, 570
Suspended animation, *See* Cryonics
Suśruta, 665
Suśruta Saṃhitā, 663, 907
Süssmich, Johann Peter, 1226
Sustaining institutions, 1668
Sustaining life:
of defective infants:
clinical aspects, 718–724
consequentialist theories, 731–732, 834–837
deontological theories, 726–729, 833, 838
equality theory of justice, 837
ethic of care, 733–734
extraordinary means principle, 727–729, 838
medical criteria, 724–726

personhood theories, 726–727, 729–732, 834–836
principle of avoiding harm, 734–735
slippery-slope argument, 821, 836–837
wrongful life theory, 835–836, 837
See also Infanticide
historical perspectives, 261–267
the Enlightenment, 264
mercantilism, 262–264
neopositivism, 265, 266–267
positivist moralism, 265–266
Renaissance humanism, 262
Islam and, 894–895
omission and commission, 269–277
direct and indirect acts, 272–274
ordinary and extraordinary means, 168, 176, 262, 270–271, 727–728
stopping vs. not starting a procedure, 271–272
voluntary and involuntary dying, 274–277
See also Acting and refraining; Double effect, principle of
organ donation and, 1155
Protestantism and, 1369–1372
public policy on, 278–285, 735–740
decision making by hospital committee, 280, 738–739
decision making by patients, lay persons, and public bodies, 280–285
decision making by physicians, 278–280, 738
decision making for infants, 737–739
legal policies, 735–737
Roman Catholicism and, 1531–1532
surgery and, 1629
See also Anti-aging techniques; Life-support systems; Organ transplantation
Swahili society, 742
Swanson, Terrance E., 1339
Swazey, Judith, 272
Swearingen, Victor C., 1018
Sweden:
abortion in, 28, 31, 983
animal experimentation in, 78
contraception in, 211
health care in:
expenditures, 654
financing, 611, 627
primary, 614

health insurance in, 641
health-related expenditures in, 650
medical ethics education in, 872
organ salvaging in, 1158
peer review system in, 1495
sterilization in, 1617
surgeons in, 615
Sweet, William, 1389
Swift, Jonathan, 1401
Swiss Academy of Medical Sciences, 279
Switzerland:
animal experimentation in, 78
contraception in, 211
differential population growth in, 1286–1287
physician discretion in, 279
Sydenham, Thomas, 583, 600, 602–603, 954, 1501, 1503
Sydney, Declaration of, 168
Sydney, Sir Philip, 263
Symmetry, concept of, 785, 786, 789
Sympathy, 960, 1152
Hume–Smith concept of, 1535–1536
Symposia:
in United States, 1000
in Western Europe, 985
Symposium (Plato), 237, 1577, 1593
Synanon, 333
Synergy, doctrine of, 1253
Synod of Bishops, 1255
Syphilis:
human experiments with, 688, 708, 754, 1320, 1409, 1472
mass health screening and, 859
Syria:
family planning in, 890
health care in, 890
Systematic correspondence, 912
System einer vollständingen medicinischen Polizey (Frank), 956, 957–958, 1393
System model of therapeutic relationship, 1664–1665
Systems dynamics school of thought, 398
Szasz, Thomas:
on abuse of the mentally ill, 505
antipaternalism of, 330, 1103, 1200
on mental illness as myth, 603, 604, 1077, 1094, 1095, 1096
on suicidal patients, 1624, 1625
on terminology of illness and health, 999, 1060, 1666
therapeutic relationship model of, 1665
on violence and therapy, 1690, 1691

T

Tabari, Al-, 888
Taboo illness, 1122
Tacitus, 238
T'ai-p'ing ching, 1636
T'ai-shang kan ying p'ing, 1636
Taittirīya Brāhmaṇa, 1270
Taiwan:
  contraception in, 211
  family planning in, 1230, 1292–1293
Talismans, 789
Talmud, 791, 792, 793, 1232, 1250, 1251, 1428, 1430, 1440
  on abortion, 5–8, 25
  on artificial insemination, 797
  on contraception, 796
  definition of death of, 801
  on duty to preserve life and health, 793
  on eugenics, 469–470, 792
  on procreation, 1250–1251
  on sanctity of human life, 794, 795
  on taboo illness, 1122
  on treatment of cadavers, 798
Tang dynasty, 904
Tantrism, 205, 907
Tanzania:
  health expenditures in, 1322
  health status by level of per capita income in, 1321
Tao Hung-ching, 1633
Taoism, 201, 202, 203, 901, 904, 911, 1064
  church, 1636–1637
  classical, 1633–1635
  Confucianism and, 1631–1633
  death and, 230, 231, 234, 235
  environment and man and, 369, 374, 1632, 1633
  esoteric, 1635–1636
  history of Chinese medicine and, 1632–1633
  infanticide and, 742, 1636
  Inner Classic, 903, 905, 1632, 1634, 1635, 1636
  medical ethics in, 903, 1631–1637
  universal principle of, 1631–1632
Tarasoff v. Regents of the University of California (1976), 199
Tarjan, George, 1111
Task Force on Consumer Health Education, 1141
Task Force on Genetics and Reproduction, Yale University, 1193
Tatian the Assyrian, 938–939, 1656
Tavistock Clinic, London, 1547
Taylor, Charles, 1135–1136
Taylor v. St. Vincent's Hospital (1976), 1617

Tay-Sachs disease, 470, 476, 522, 555, 556, 568–569, 718–819, 858, 861, 1334, 1344
Teaching chaplains, 1191–1192
Teal, Donn, 670
"Tearoom Trade" study, 754, 1558, 1559
Technicalization, 1640
Technique, technology as, 1640
Technological humanism, 64
Technological Society, The (Ellul), 1639, 1640
Technology, 1537, 1638–1654
  assessment of, 1650–1654
    appraisal of, 1653–1654
    biomedical fields and, 1651–1653
    concept of, 1650–1651
  environment and, 368, 372, 373, 375–376, 387, 1642
  food production and, 493–494, 496
  halfway, 1489, 1899
  high, 1485
  as knowledge, 1639
  law and, 1644–1649
    comparison of available legal approaches, 1647–1649
    means and ends in, 1644–1645
    taxonomy of legal technique, 1645–1647
  life-support, *See* Life-support systems
  as object, 1639, 1640
  philosophy of, 1638–1642
    defined, 1638
    development of, 1638–1639
    ethical issues, 1640–1642
    metaphysical analyses, 1639–1640
  as process, 1639–1640
  of sex, 1561–1562
  therapeutic relationship and, 1668–1669
  as volition, 1640
  of war, *See* War: biomedical science and
Technology and Culture, 1639
Technology Assessment, 1650
Teenagers, *See* Adolescents
Tehran, University of, 887
Teilhard de Chardin, Pierre, 128, 1402
Teleological theories, 417–421, 1134, 1399–1400
  criticisms of, 420–421
  defined, 417
  deontological theories and, 413, 417
  main problematic issues in, 417–420
  natural law theory and, 1134
  obligation and supererogation in, 1147–1148
  vitalism and, 129–130

See also Utilitarianism
Teleonymy, 591–593
Television:
  behavior control and, 86, 87
  interviews, physicians on, 45, 659
  medical reporting on, 182, 186, 187
Television Code of The National Association of Radio and Television Broadcasters, The, 181
Temkin, Owsei, 937
Temperance movement, 69–70
Temperate Life (Cornaro), 262
TEMPO, 1292
Tendai sect, 378
Tendler, M. D., 996
Tennessee, University of, 875, 1001
Tenon, Jacques, 958, 1660
Terminal illnesses, *See* Death; Euthanasia; Life-support systems
Tertiary care, 614
Tertullian, 6, 685, 938, 943, 1656
Test bias, 536
Testicular feminization, 565
Testosterone, 1591
Test-tube fertilization, *See* In vitro fertilization
Texas, University of, Medical Branch at Galveston, 875
Texas Medical Center, 1000
Textbooks, 1001
T4 program, 1016–1017
T-groups, 1547
Thackrah, Turner, 1662
Thailand:
  distribution of physicians in, 1324
  health expenditures in, 1322
  population education in, 1311
  population policy in, 1297
Thalassemia major, 522, 557
Thalidomide, 80, 183, 324, 381, 487, 1349
Theistic Hinduism, 661
Theistic orientation, 430–433, 1064
Theochemicals, 337
Theocritus, 371
Theodosius, Code of, 672
Theodulphus of Orléans, Bishop, 208
Theognis, 1233
Theological ethics, 429–437, 732
  meaning of, 429–430
  method of authority and, 402–403
  obligation theory, 430, 433–435
  theistic orientation, 430–433, 1064
  value theory, 430, 436–437
  virtue theory, 430, 435–436
Theological seminaries, 873
Theology:
  definition of death and, 301, 302
  miracle and faith healing and, 1125–1129
    debate about interpretation, 1125–1126
    extreme case of possession, 1128–1129

faith and the object of faith, 1126–1127
  Protestantism, 1121–1123, 1124, 1365, 1374–1377
  role of medicine, 1127
  Roman Catholicism, 1121, 1523
  understanding of illness, 1127–1128
  word and miracle, 1127
organ transplantation and, 1169–1172
supererogation and, 1149–1150
See also Ensoulment; names of religions; Soul; Theological ethics
Theory of Justice, A (Rawls), 450, 804
Therapeutic abortion, 3, 6, 12–13, 25, 167, 896, 943–944, 990, 1338
Therapeutic communities, 333
Therapeutic experimentation:
  the aged and, 68
  alcoholics and, 73–74
  fetuses and, 490, 492
  nontherapeutic experimentation distinguished from, 693–694, 699–700
Therapeutic innovation, 1487–1488
Therapeutic lag, 1411
Therapeutic privilege, 760, 774, 1687
Therapeutic relationship, 1654–1676
  in Arab nations, 889–890
  as barrier to consent, 753
  in Eastern Europe, 978
  history of, 1655–1662
    ancient scientific stage, 1655–1656
    Christianity and, 1656–1660
    empirico–magical stage, 1655
    medieval scientific stage, 1657–1658
    modern scientific stage, 1658–1662
  informed consent in, 767–768, 1558–1559, 1693
    adolescents and, 42–43
    ambiguous nature of, 768–769
    clinical aspects, 767–769
    decision making by patients, 771, 774–775
    decision making by physicians, 771, 775–777
    decision to initiate life-support systems and, 844
    dentistry and, 312
    genetic counseling and, 576–577
    infant care and, 737, 738
    vs. informed consent in mental health, 763

in Japan, 927
law and, 769–774
nature of, 767–768
obstacles to, 768
the poor and, 1056
purpose of, 767
self-determination and, 771–777
self-realization therapies and, 1549
sex therapy and, 1558–1559
surgery and, 1627–1628
in Japan, 926
medical perspective, contemporary, 1672–1676
  patient in, 1674
  phenomenon of illness, 1672–1673
  physician in, 1673–1674
  technico–social vs. technico–personal view, 1675
Muslim perspective, 892–893
sexualization of, 989, 990, 1557–1558, 1566, 1704–1705
social contract theory and, 1604
sociohistorical perspectives, 1663–1667
  behavioral implications of organic systems, 1665–1666
  conflict model, 1666
  neo-Marxist, 1666–1667
  Parsonian model, 1665
  system model, 1664–1665
sociological model, contemporary, 1668–1671
  elaboration of relationship, 1671
  epidemiology of help-seeking, 1669–1671
in Western Europe, 982-983
See also Confidentiality; Health care; Medical care; Medical malpractice; Truth-telling
Therapeutic research, *See* Therapeutic experimentation
Therapeutic role, 594–596
Therapeutic sterilization, 355, 796, 1433, 1609
Therapist–patient relationship, *See* Dynamic therapies
Therapy:
  behavioral, *See* Behavioral control; Behavioral therapies; Mental health therapies
  dynamic, *See* Dynamic therapies
  electroconvulsive, *See* Electroconvulsive therapy (ECT)
  experimentation vs., 693
  gene, *See* Gene therapy
  in newborns with birth defects, 718–721

of normals, 1547
psychosurgery as, 1388
sex, *See* Sex therapy
violence and, 1689–1693
  classical medicine and control of, 1689–1690
  conservatism and, 1690–1692
  liberalism and, 1692
  ultraliberalism and, 1692–1693
  ultratraditionalism and, 1690
Theravedic Buddhism, 463
Thermodynamics, Laws of, 394
Thielicke, Helmut, 421, 985, 1371, 1372, 1583
  on abortion, 15
  on artificial insemination, 1457, 1458
  on homosexuality, 674
  medical ethics of, 1369–1370
  on sterilization, 1610
Thinking, control over, 86
Thiothixene, 1379
Thioxanthene derivatives, 1379
Third parties:
  injuries to, 1021
  protection of, 1501
Third-party quality-of-life criteria, 836
Thomas, Lewis, 1485
Thomas Aquinas, St., *See* Aquinas, St. Thomas
Thompson, Judith J., 24
Thompson, Lewis R., 1493
Thompson, William (Lord Kelvin), 479
Thomson, Samuel, 1030
Thoreau, Henry David, 369, 372, 1309
Thorndike, Edward L., 107, 111
Thousand Golden Prescriptions, The (Sun Ssu-miao), 165
"Three Constantly Read Articles" (Mao Tse-tung), 920
Three Contributions to the Theory of Sex (Freud), 1593
Three Women (Plath), 1013
Thrita, 587
Thucydides, 236–237
Turingia, Code of, 282
Tic douloureux, 1179
T'ien-tai sect, 375
Tier systems, 781
Tifashi, al-, 1267–1268
Tillich, Paul, 421
Timaeus (Plato), 1050
Tissot, S. A., 971
Tissue:
  culture, 79, 82
  delivery of oxygen to, 842
  typing, 1160
Titmuss, Richard, 1168

Tiv society, 223
Tobacco, *See* Smoking
Tobacco industry, 1597, 1601
Togo, compensation of physicians in, 899
Token economics, 781
Tokyo, Declaration of, *See* Declaration of Tokyo
Tolman, Edward C., 108, 111
Tolstoy, Leo, 827, 1687
Tooley, Michael, 20, 36, 729, 825, 827
Too Many Asians (Robbins), 1277
Torah, 793, 1428, 1429
   on abortion, 5–6, 9–10
   on autopsy, 896
Toronto, University of, 1001
Torres, Camillo, 1402
Tort law, 1519
   malpractice branch of, *See* Medical malpractice
   prenatal, 575–576
Torture of prisoners, 1354–1356
   ethical principles, 1355–1356
   medical personnel and, 1355
   methods of, 1354–1355
Totalitarian theories of population, 1230
Totality, principle of, 1170–1171, 1528–1529, 1531, 1609–1610
Total utilitarianism, 428
Total utility, 508–509
Totem, 879
Totem and Taboo (Freud), 1066, 1067
Toulmin, Stephen, 1545
Toxic Substances Control Act, 577, 1497
Tractatus Logico–Philosophicus (Wittgenstein), 304
Traditions, 1265, 1266, 1267
Tragedy of the commons, 1309, 1310
Traité médico–philosophique sur l'aliénation mentale ou la manie (Pinel), 1092
Traits, 528, 529–530
Trance, *See* Hypnosis
Tranquilizers, 86, 91, 99, 327, 328, 336, 1381, 1385, 1386
Transactional analysis, 1087
Transactional systems, 40
Transcendental experience, 327, 336–337
Transcendentalists, 369
Transcendental Thomism, 1532
Transcultural psychiatry, 1410, 1413
Trans-Disciplinary Symposia on Philosophy and Medicine, 1000
Transduction, gene therapy via, 516, 523
Transference, 341, 1084
Transformation, gene therapy via, 514–515, 523

Transfusion, *See* Blood transfusion
Transmigration, doctrine of, 661
Transmitter theory of pain, 1178
Transsexualism, 1589
Transsexual operations, 1594
Transvestism, 1591
Treasury, U.S. Department of, 1493
Treatise of Man (Descartes), 1050
Treatise on Government (Locke), 263
Treatise on the various sins of princes, their ministers, of lawyers, accountants, physicians, merchants, etc. (Fritsch), 955
Treatment, *See* Health care; Medical care; Therapeutic relationship
Treatment refusal, *See* Right to refuse medical care
Triage, 1246–1247, 1249, 1417–1418
   food policy and, 497, 499
   initiation of life-support systems and, 845
   teleological theory and, 419
Tribe, Laurence, 1653
Tricyclic derivatives, 1380–1381
Trisomy 21, 531
Trobriand Islanders, 222
Trollope, Anthony, 1009
Trotula, 1714
Truman, Harry, 648
Trust:
   confidentiality and, 195, 196
   informed consent and, 767, 776
   neonaturalism and, 64
   in therapeutic relationship, 341, 1674
Trusteeship, hospital, 679, 681, 682,
Truth-telling, 149, 290, 1486, 1677–1687
   abortion and, 1198
   in ancient Greece and Rome, 934
   attitudes toward, 1677–1682
      ethical implications, 1680–1682
      of health-care professionals, 1679–1680
      of lay people, 1678–1679
   cancer patients and, 42, 1678–1681
   codes of medical ethics and, 176–177, 1682–1683
   deception, unintentional vs. intentional, 1683–1684
   deontological theory and, 174
   empathy and, 42
   ethical dilemmas in, 1682–1683
   in Europe, seventeenth century, 954–955, 956
   genetic counseling and, 565
   genetic diagnosis and, 558
   genetic screening and, 571, 1198
   in Great Britain, 1678
   Hinduism and, 665
   Judaism and, 798, 801
   medicine and, 1686–1687

nursing and, 1143–1144, 1680
paternalism and, 1198
philosophical debates about, 1684–1686
practice conception of, 412
psychiatrists and, 1680, 1681
religious curing and, 1124
Roman Catholicism and, 1530
sexual ethics and, 1586
situation ethics and, 422
in surgery, 1629, 1679, 1680
in United States, eighteenth century, 960
Tryon, R. C., 541
Tschermak, Armin, 541
Tsūan, Takenaka, 924
Tuang Fang, 918
Tubal sterilization, 1607–1608
Tuberculosis, 1394, 1396
   human experiments with, 688
   mass health screening and, 859, 861
Tucker v. Lower (1972), 298
Tudor, Jeannette F., 1709
Tuffier, Théodore, 658
Tuke, Daniel Hack, 1661
Tung Chung-shu, 376
Turgot, Anne Robert Jacques, 958, 959
Turkey, 645
   forced emigration and, 1304
   heart transplantation in, 655
   sterilization in, 1616
Turner, Victor W., 222
Turner's syndrome, 569
Tuskegee Syphilis Study, 708, 754, 1320, 1409
Twin studies, 539, 668, 1453
Two Sources of Morality and Religion, The (Bergson), 1641
Two-stage consent form, 753
Tylor, Edward B., 221
Typhoid, 861
Tyrosinemia, 574

U

Ultimate aim, in pragmatism, 1328–1329
Ultrasound studies, 490, 1332, 1333, 1336, 1387
Unani (Yūnānī) medicine, 789
   in India, 907–908
Uncertainty:
   kidney dialysis or transplantation and, 812, 814
   in medical decisions, 308
   truth-telling and, 777
Undernutrition, as anti-aging technique, 51

Understanding Media: The Extensions of Man (McLuhan), 1639
Uniform Anatomical Gift Acts, 140, 300, 997, 1155, 1157–1158, 1169, 1172
Uniform Code of Military Justice, 1697
Union of Concerned Scientists, 383
Union of Soviet Socialist Republics:
  abortion in, 29
  death, definition of, 979
  differential population growth in, 1286
  environmental record of, 372
  feldscher in, 1717
  forced migration in, 1305
  grain production in, 495
  health care in, 614
    expenditures, 654
    financing, 611, 627
    policy, 653, 654
  health insurance in, 611
  medical deontology in, 981
  medical ethics education in, 872, 875
  mental hospitalization in, 1078
  Oath of Soviet Physicians, 173, 175
    text of, 1754–1755
  physician-population ratio in, 615
  population policy in, 1230, 1286
  psychiatrist's responsibility in, 1071–1072
  torture in, 1355
  women health professionals in, 1717, 1718
  World Health Organization and, 644
Uniqueness, 549, 620–621
United Arab Emirates, health care in, 890
United Auto Workers, 649
United Company of Barbers and Surgeons, 1036
United Kingdom:
  abortion in, 28, 31, 990
  affective psychoses in, 540
  animal experimentation in, 80
  biomedical research in, 1492
  eugenics societies of, 529
  health care expenditures in, 612, 1322
  health insurance in, 638, 641
  organ donation in, 1158
  women physicians in, 1717
  See also England; Great Britain
United Ministries of Higher Education, 1000
United Nations, 644, 1234, 1539

Education, Scientific and Cultural Organization, 1311
Food and Agriculture Organization (FAO), 494, 495
"Standard Minimum Rules for the Treatment of Prisoners," 1347
Universal Declaration of Human Rights of, 455, 623, 624
World Food Conference (1974), 494, 496, 498
United Presbyterian Church, General Assembly of, 1376
United States:
  abortion in, 27–32, 998, 1563
    See also Supreme Court rulings: abortion
  advertising by medical professionals in, 44–47
  amniocentesis studies in, 1337
  animal experimentation in, 80, 81
  bioethics movement in, 994, 996–1001
  blood banking in, 1156
  blood transfusion, attitude towards, 133
  cancer deaths in, 380
  chemical weapons testing in, 1702
  child abuse statutes in, 151
  Christian burial rites in, 142
  codes of ethics in, 959, 965–967, 995
  commitment laws in, 999
  conferences in, 1000
  contraception in, 210–211, 213
  death, definition of, 300, 1161
  divorces in, 1567
  drug rehabilitation programs in, 331–333
  drug use in, 1382–1385
  dynamic therapies in, 999
  eugenics movement in, *See* Eugenics
  euthanasia legislation in, 282–285, 735–736, 998
  faith healers in, 1121–1122
  fetal research in, 141–142, 492–493
  genetic counseling in, 999
  grain production in, 494–495, 1223
  health care in, 993–994
    delivery of services, 613–614
    expenditures, 654
    financing, 611, 612, 617, 628, 994
    manpower resources, 615
    organization of services, 616–617
    policy, 647–649, 652
    primary, 613–614
    regulation of, 613

  health insurance in, 611–612, 618, 638–641, 648, 649, 994
  health status by level of per capita income in, 1321
  heart transplantation in, 997
  homosexuality in, 668
  hospitals in, 967–968, 992, 993, 994
  human experimentation in, 975, 994, 997–998
    public policy, 1488–1489, 1493–1497
  kidney dialysis in, 812, 996, 1418
  kidney transplantation in, 811
  land-use regulation in, 1305–1306
  medical education in, 993, 1031, 1032–1033
  medical ethics, history of
    contemporary, 992–1001
    modern, 952–953, 959–960, 963–968
  medical ethics education in, 871, 872–873, 1001
  medical licensure in, 964–965
  medical malpractice in, 998, 1020
  medical professionalism in, 1029–1033
    colonial, 1029–1030
    nineteenth-century, 1030–1031
    twentieth-century, 1031–1033
  medical schools in, 967, 993, 1000, 1001, 1031, 1032–1033, 1037, 1714–1715
  mental health programs in, 1079–1081
  mental institutionalization in, 1079–1080, 1105
  migration of physicians to, 645–646
  net immigration in, 1221
  nursing personnel in, 1139
  nursing schools in, 1001
  organ donation in, 957, 1155, 1157–1158
  organized medicine in, 1036–1041
    American Medical Association and, 1037–1041
    colonial, 1036–1037
    early post-Revolutionary trends, 1037
    era of retreat, 1037
  peer review in, 705
  per capita public expenditures on education, health, and defense, 1323, 1324
  philosophy of technology, development in, 1638–1639
  population aid from, 1276, 1279–1280
  population education in, 1311

VOLUME INDICATOR

Vol. 1: pp. 1-484   Vol. 2: pp. 485-900   Vol. 3: pp. 901-1404   Vol. 4: pp. 1405-1816

United States *(Continued)*
  poverty in, 1316–1320
  prisoner experimentation in, *See* Human experimentation
  psychosurgery in, 1387, 1388
  public health in, 1394–1397
  racism in, *See* Racism
  religious influences on medical ethics of, 996
  Roman Catholic Directives in, *See* Ethical and Religious Directives for Catholic Health Facilities
  self-realization therapies in, 1549
  sex preferences in, 1442, 1443
  specialists in, 993
  sterilization in, 459–460, 999, 1108–1109, 1397, 1614–1616
  suicide in, 1618
  symposia in, 1000
  unorthodox medical practices, history of, 1173–1175
  Vietnam War and, 1697–1698
  women physicians in, 1714–1717
United States Catholic Conference, Advisory Committee on Ethical and Religious Directives, 1434
United States congressional hearings and reports, 1000–1001
United States Marine Hospital Service, 1394, 1396
Universal Declaration of Human Rights of the United Nations 1948), 455, 623, 624
Universalism, 418, 1542
Universalizability, 449
Universalization of moral judgments, 427
Universe, purpose in, *See* Purpose in the universe
University medical centers, 614
Unterman, Isaar, 7, 8
Untermann, Yehuda, 896
Upanayana, 663
Upanisads (Upanishads), 232, 234, 1270, 1271, 1621
Upper class medical care, 616
Urban growth, 1220, 1224, 1233, 1234, 1306
Urban medical care, 616
Urmson, J. O., 1150, 1151
Uruguay:
  fetal research in, 490
  organ salvaging in, 1158
  Penal Code of 1933, 282
Useful life, 657
Uterus, cancer of, 33, 34
Utilitarianism, 404, 405, 406, 418, 419–421, 424–428, 463, 542, 834
  act-, 411, 416, 421–424, 426–428
    bioethical issues and, 423–424
    coalescence with rule-utilitari-

anism, 426–428
    compulsory rules and, 420, 422
    defined, 421, 426
    duty and, 422–423
    guidance for individual deliberation and, 420
    love and, 422, 1370
    moral decision-making and, 405, 411, 422
    treatment of defective infants and, 731–732
  act vs. consequences in, 424–425
  allocation of scarce resources and, 419, 421, 809, 810, 1416–1417
  animal experimentation and, 81, 82
  average, 428, 508–509
  compulsory population control and, 1301
  euthanasia and, 420, 835
  gene therapy and, 523–524
  health-care delivery and, 631
  Hippocratic ethic vs., 173
  human experimentation and, 697, 701, 705, 706–707, 1475
  informed consent and, 754–755
  justice and, 419, 421, 631, 636, 805–806, 809, 810, 1416–1417
  main problematic issues in, 418–420
  mental health program evaluation and, 1082
  metaethical vs. normative view of, 424
  motive, 427
  negative, 428
  non-descriptivism and, 447
  obligation to future generations and, 508–509
  paternalism and, 1195, 1196
  population policy and, 1289, 1292
  positive, 428
  prisoner experimentation and, 1350
  psychiatrist role and, 1073
  public health and, 1393
  rule-, 406, 416, 422, 426–428
    coalescence with act-utilitarianism, 426–428
    compulsory rules and, 420
    defined, 421, 426
    guidance for individual deliberation and, 420
    health-care delivery and, 631
  total, 428
  value of life and, 823–824, 827, 828
  See also Consequentialism
Utilitarianism (Mill), 542
Utility of health care, 631
Utopia (More), 263, 943, 1234
Utopian approach to normality, 40, 1059
Uziel, Ben Zion, 7, 896

V

Vaccines, *See* Immunization
Vāgbhata, 664
Vaidya, 664, 665
Valentine v. Chrestensen (1942), 47
Valles, 1660
Values:
  associated with longevity and aging, 58–61
  in cost-benefit analysis, 1520–1521
  defined, 877
  drug use for pleasure and, 334, 1384–1385
  in dynamic therapies, 339–341
  genetic intervention and, 462–463
  human experimentation and, 1544, 1665–1666
  law and technology and, 1645, 1647
  of medical education, 863–864
  mental health program evaluation and, 1082
  in mental health therapies, 1083–1088
    classification of therapy systems, 1083–1086
    definition and approach, 1083
    general problem of, 1088–1089
    three models of human nature, 1088
  in population education, 1313–1315
  in pragmatism, 1327–1331
  in scientific community, 1542
  of sex therapy and research, 1554–1555
  sexual development and, 1569
  technological assessment and, 1654
Value theories, *See* Ethics
Van der Marck, William H. M., 318–319
Van der Poel, Cornelius J., 318–319
Van Gennep, Arnold, 222
Varna, 662
Vasectomy, 355, 1283, 1291, 1302, 1446, 1447, 1606, 1607
Vasquez, Gabriel, 34
Vaux, Kenneth, 218, 1369
Vavilov, N. I., 483
Vayda, Andrew P., 225
VDRL exam, 857
Veatch, Robert, 327, 635–636, 760, 1384
Vedas, 231–232
Vedic-Hindu tradition, *See* Hinduism
Vegetative state, 847
Vendîdâd, 882
Venereal disease:
  adolescent, parental consent and, 39, 151, 152

public health reform and, 1396–1397
research program, 1493
See also Syphilis
Venezuela:
attitudes of physicians in, 1006
codes of ethics in, 1005
health expenditures in, 1322
health status by level of per capita income in, 1321
National Academy of Medicine of, 1007
Venezuelan Code of Medical Ethics, 1005
text of, 1746–1748
Ventilabrum medico-theologicum (Boudewyns), 1525
Ventilators, 841, 844
Vers la Médecine Sociale (Sand), 1598
Vesalius, Andreas, 76, 489, 1375
Vespasian, Emperor, 1123
Veterans Administration, 617
Viability, beginning of human life and, 18, 20, 21
Victim (image of man), 852–853
Victimless crimes, 819, 1196
Victorianism, 1561, 1582
Vienna Circle, 448
Vietnam, forced migration in, 1305
Vietnam War, 1697–1698, 1700, 1702
Villermé, L. R., 972, 1662
Violence, 1689–1693
classical medicine and control of, 1689–1690
conservatism and, 1690–1692
liberalism and, 1692
meaning of, 1689
psychosurgery and, 1387, 1389, 1391
ultraliberalism and, 1692–1693
ultratraditionalism and, 1690
Virchow, Rudolf, 969, 1053, 1319, 1320, 1598
Virgil, 371
Virginia State Board of Pharmacy v. Virginia Citizens' Consumer Council (1976), 47, 1212
Virtue theories, *See* Ethics
Visigothic law, 945–946
Vision of God, The (Augustine), 251
Vision of Paul, 251
Visitation of the sick, 798–799, 1191–1192, 1366, 1661
Vis medicatrix naturae, 590
Vista, 1080
Vital functions, support of, *See* Life-support systems
Vitalism, 129–130, 241
Vital signs, 294, 298, 299

Vitamin A deficiency, 494
Vives, Juan Luis, 1066
Vivisection, 76
in ancient Greece and Rome, 935–936
animal, 689
in Great Britain, 974
human, 76, 139–140, 144, 685–686, 689–690, 798
in India, 907, 908
Islam and, 893
Volition, technology as, 1640
Volkhart, Edmund H., 1666
Voltaire, 240, 1226, 1401
Voluntarism, 1222–1223, 1548
Voluntary action, 592
Voluntary euthanasia, 274–277, 280–285, 286–287, 290
See also Right to refuse medical care; Suicide
Voluntary Euthanasia Legislation Society, 282
Voluntary population control, 1308, 1310
Voluntary sterilization, *See* Sterilization: voluntary
von Hahn, H. P., 49
Voyage in the Dark (Rhys), 1013
Vries, Hugo de, 480
Vulgate of St. Jerome, 9

W

Waddington, C. H., 131, 542
Wagner-Jauregg, Julius von, 1016
Wagner National Health Bill of 1939, 1039
Wahlberg, Rachel Conrad, 22
Waismann, Friedrich, 111
Waitzkin, Howard, 777, 1666
Waldenberg, Zevi, 896
Wallace, Alfred, 1543
Walshe, Sir Francis, 303–304
Wang Huai-yin, 1633
Wang-pi, 374
Wang Ping, 1633, 1635
Wang Shi-to, 210
War, 1695–1703
anthropological perspective, 225
biomedical science and, 1699–1703
continuing controversies, 1702–1703
social responsibility of physician, 1701–1702
social responsibility of scientist,

1699–1701
medicine and, 1695–1699
conflicting obligations, 1695–1696
Geneva conference, 1697–1698
new organizations and codes, 1696
plea of "superior orders," 1696–1697
policies in Vietnam, 1697–1698, 1700
population regulation with, 1307–1308
technology and, 1641
Warburton Anatomy Act of 1832 (Great Britain), 798
Ward, Ingebord, 1591
Ware, John, 1715
Warmth, expression of, 620, 621
Warnock, Geoffrey J., 1686
Warren, Mary Anne, 825
Warwick, Donald P., 1472
Washington, University of, 559
Wasserstrom, Richard, 1585
Wastes, removal of, 842–843
Waterman, Barbara, 1666
Water Pollution Control Act, 577
Watson, James, 181
Watson, John B., 107, 108, 110–111
Watt, James, 1543
Watts, James W., 1387
Weak paternalism, 1197
Weapons development, *See* War
Weber, Max, 591, 1640
Weems v. United States (1910), 783
Weil, Andrew, 327
Weinberg, Alvin, 1642
Weisman, Avery D., 287
Weismann, August, 266, 458
Weiss, Carol H., 1081
Weitbrecht, H. J., 1016
Welch, William H., 1032
Welfare, population policy and, 1239–1240
Welfare principle, 1195
Well-being, 605
informed consent and, 774
population policy and, 1243
See also Health
Werdnig-Hoffman's disease, 720
Wernz, Franz X., 472
Wesley, John, 1123, 1374–1377
West, Cornel R., 757
West, D. J., 670
West, L. J., 326, 1384
West Bengal, compulsory sterilization in, 1301
Westermarck, Edward A., 471, 743, 826

Western Europe:
  biomedical research in, 1492
  differential population growth in, 1286
  drug use in, 1383
  medical ethics, history of:
    seventeenth-century, 954–956
    twentieth-century, 982–986
  medical ethics education in, 871–872
  population policy in, 1235
  urban growth in, 1220
West Germany, *See* Germany
Westminster Report (1956), 673
Wexler, David B., 104, 105
Weyer, Johann, 1066
WHDW principle, 581
White, Ellen G., 1376, 1377
White, Lynn, 367, 1251
White, R. J., 82
Whitehead, Alfred N., 241, 302, 370, 1402
White-Jacket (Melville), 1009
WHO, *See* World Health Organization
Widowhood, 55, 59
Wilberforce, Bishop, 480
Wilderness preservation, 369, 371, 1305
Wildlife preserves, 1647
Wilkür, 504
Will, *See* Autonomy; Free will
Willard, Frances, 70
Willful misconduct, 1021
William of Occam, 1659
William of Salicet, 941
Williams, Glanville, 21, 33, 34, 1611
Williams, Granville L., 318
Williams, Hyatt, 674
Williams, Tennessee, 1010
Williams, William Carlos, 1013
Williamson, W. E., 655
Willowbrook State School, New York, 694, 754, 997
Wilson, Edward O., 132, 483
Wilson's disease, 474
Windsor, Duchess of, 185
Winters v. Miller (1971), 1073
Wisconsin, University of, 559
Witchcraft, 909, 922, 1048, 1366–1367, 1713
Witch doctors, 909
Wittgenstein, Ludwig, 302, 304, 305, 504
WMA, *See* World Medical Association
Wohler, Friedrich, 129
Wolfenden Committee, 1195
Wolff, Christian, 1051
Wollstonecraft, Mary, 1584–1585
Wolpe, Joseph, 1086, 1088
Women, 1704–1719
  affective disorders among, 71
  in Arab nations, 889
  awareness of sexuality, 1584
  contemporary attitudes toward sex, 1563–1564
  discrimination against, 1707
  as experimental subjects, 1710–1711
  as health professionals, 1713–1719
    changing roles and responsibilities and, 1718–1719
    dilemmas in, 1718
    early history of, 1713–1714
    eighteenth century to the present, 1031, 1714–1717
    family considerations and, 1717–1718
    role development and, 1717–1718
    See also Nursing
  mastectomy and, 1708–1709
  menopause and, 1708
  menstruation and, 1707–1708
  mental health and, 1709–1710
  mortality rates for, 55
  rape and, 1592, 1709
    abortion and, 24, 28, 928, 929, 998
  reproductive decisions and, 1705–1707
    See also Abortion; Contraception; Reproductive technologies
  sexual revolution and, 1563
  suicide and, 1618, 1622
  in therapeutic relationship, 1704–1705
Women's liberation movement, 27, 29, 622, 994, 1058, 1201, 1422
Wonderland (Oates), 1013, 1014
Wood, Leonard, 688
Woodcock, Leonard, 388
Wootton, Barbara, 991, 1095–1096
Word and Object (Quine), 1330
Word association, 85
Wordsworth, William, 369
Worker (image of man), 854–855
Workmen's compensation, 1024
World Bank, 1234, 1326
World Congress on Biology and the Future of Man, 985
World Council of Churches, 212
  Christian Medical Commission, 1436
World Health Organization (WHO), 134, 592, 598, 605, 644, 1039, 1281, 1436, 1483, 1515, 1618
  definition of health of, 1062, 1483, 1515
  Expert Committee on Drug Dependence, 328
World Medical Association (WMA), 44, 68, 164, 167–168, 169, 656, 696, 928, 989, 1039
  Code of Ethics in Wartime, 1702
  Declaration of Geneva, 164–165, 172, 173, 174, 175, 177, 929, 989, 1598, 1602, 1683
    text of, 1749
  Declaration of Helsinki, 68, 153, 172, 455, 656, 770, 928, 985, 1486, 1487, 1727
    text of, 1769–1773
  Declaration of Sidney, 1728
  Declaration of Tokyo, 1347–1348, 1356
  International Code of Medical Ethics, 44, 167–168, 172–175, 989, 1726
    text of, 1749–1750
World Population Conference (1974), 1274, 1275, 1276, 1278, 1300, 1305
World Population Plan of Action (WPPA), 1275, 1276, 1280, 1305, 1306
Woyzeck (Büchner), 1009
WPPA, *See* World Population Plan of Action
Wrongful life actions, 576
Wrongful life theory, 835–836, 837
Wuerttemberg, Code of, 282
Wu-men Hui-k'ai, 377
Wu-men-kuan [Gateless Gate] (Wu-men Hui-k'ai), 377
Wunderlich, Carl, 603
Wurm, Theophil, 1017
Wu-wei, 1634
Wyatt v. Stickney (1972), 104, 779, 781, 999, 1073, 1514

X

X-linked infantile agammaglobulinemia, 477
X-linked recessive trait, 555–558
XXX genotypes, 1333
XXY genotypes, 1333
XYY genotypes, 531–533, 543, 568, 571

Y

Yad Hachazak (Yad Ha-Hazakah) (Maimonides), 248, 793
Yaka society, 587
Yang-chu, 374
Yang-sheng, 1632–1635
Yasunari, Kawabata, 1622
Yasunori, Tanba, 923

Yellow Emperor's Inner Classic, The (*Huang-ti nei-ching*), 903, 905, 1632, 1634, 1635, 1636
Yellow fever:
  epidemic, 1395
  experiment, 687–688
Yin–yang philosophy, 922
Yoga, 664, 1188, 1270
Young, 711
Young, Brigham, 1377
Young-old persons, 54–57
Yūnānī medicine, *See Unani* medicine
Yü Pien, 915

Z

Zacchia, Paolo, 12, 956, 1524–1525, 1660
Zachary, R. B., 725, 726
Zambia, abortion laws in, 29, 900
Zen Buddhism, 369, 375, 378, 923
Zend-Avesta, 883
Zepeda v. Zepeda (1963), 576, 1335
Zero population growth, 1229, 1308
Ziemssen, Hugo W. von, 970
Zimbardo, Philip G., 1476
Zohar, 247

Zola, Irving K., 1666
Zoning, population distribution and, 1305
Zoroaster, 885
Zoroastrianism, 207, 881, 883, 885, 886, 1064, 1184
Zuckerman, Harriet, 1545
Zuni Indians, 1046
Zusman, Jack, 1081
Zygote banking, 1446–1448
  ethical issues, 1446–1447, 1459
  eugenic applications, 1447–1448
  legal aspects, 1447, 1465–1469
  procedure, 1446

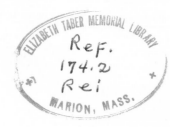